Watch over 50 surgical videos from the
second edition online at MediaCenter.thieme.com!

Simply visit MediaCenter.thieme.com and, when prompted during the
registration process, enter the code below to get started today.

W89Z-M55L-K4WG-4H64

	WINDOWS	MAC	TABLET
Recommended Browser(s)**	Recent browser versions on all major platforms and any mobile operating system that supports HTML5 video playback ** *all browsers should have JavaScript enabled*		
Flash Player Plug-in	Flash Player 9 or Higher* * *Mac users: ATI Rage 128 GPU does not support full-screen mode with hardware scaling*		Tablet PCs with Android OS support Flash 10.1
Recommended for optimal usage experience	Monitor resolutions: • Normal (4:3) 1024×768 or Higher • Widescreen (16:9) 1280×720 or Higher • Widescreen (16:10) 1440×900 or Higher DSL/Cable internet connection at a minimum speed of 384.0 Kbps or faster WiFi 802.11 b/g preferred.		7-inch and 10-inch tablets on maximum resolution. WiFi connection is required.

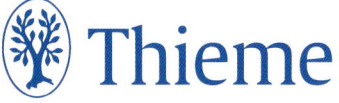

Phacoemulsification and Intraocular Lens Implantation

Mastering Techniques and Complications in Cataract Surgery

Second Edition

William J. Fishkind, MD, FACS
Clinical Professor
University of Utah
Salt Lake City, Utah
and
University of Arizona
Tucson, Arizona
and
Fishkind, Bakewell, Maltzman and Hunter
Eye Care and Surgery Center
Tucson, Arizona

With 643 illustrations

Thieme
New York • Stuttgart • Delhi • Rio de Janeiro

Executive Editor: William Lamsback
Managing Editor: Elizabeth Palumbo
Editorial Assistant: Haley Paskalides
Director, Editorial Services: Mary Jo Casey
International Production Director: Andreas Schabert
International Marketing Director: Fiona Henderson
International Sales Director: Louisa Turrell
Director of Sales, North America: Mike Roseman
Senior Vice President and Chief Operating Officer: Sarah Vanderbilt
President: Brian D. Scanlan
Production Editor: Barbara Chernow
Compositor: Carol Pierson, Chernow Editorial Services, Inc.

Library of Congress Cataloging-in-Publication Data

Names: Fishkind, William J., editor.
Title: Phacoemulsification and intraocular lens implantation :
   mastering techniques and complications in cataract surgery /
   [edited by] William J. Fishkind.
Other titles: Complications in phacoemulsification
Description: 2nd edition. | New York : Thieme, [2017] | Preceded by
   Complications in phacoemulsification : avoidance, recognition,
   and management / edited by William J. Fishkind. 2002. | Includes
   bibliographical references and index.
Identifiers: LCCN 2016040004 (print) | LCCN 2016040774 (ebook) |
   ISBN 9781626231290 | ISBN 9781626231306
Subjects: | MESH: Phacoemulsification—methods | Lens
   Implantation, Intraocular—methods
Classification: LCC RE451 (print) | LCC RE451 (ebook) | NLM WW
   260 | DDC 617.7/42059—dc23
LC record available at https://lccn.loc.gov/2016040004

Copyright © 2017 by Thieme Medical Publishers, Inc.
Thieme Publishers New York
333 Seventh Avenue, New York, NY 10001 USA
+1 800 782 3488, customerservice@thieme.com

Thieme Publishers Stuttgart
Rüdigerstrasse 14, 70469 Stuttgart, Germany
+49 [0]711 8931 421, customerservice@thieme.de

Thieme Publishers Delhi
A-12, Second Floor, Sector-2, Noida-201301
Uttar Pradesh, India
+91 120 45 566 00, customerservice@thieme.in

Thieme Publishers Rio de Janeiro, Thieme Publicações Ltda.
Edifício Rodolpho de Paoli, 25º andar
Av. Nilo Peçanha, 50 – Sala 2508
Rio de Janeiro 20020-906 Brasil
+55 21 3172 2297

Printed in India by Replika Press Ltd.

ISBN 978-1-62623-129-0

Also available as an e-book:
eISBN 978-1-62623-130-6

To our teachers, colleagues, and ophthalmic surgeons,
who collectively participate in the splendid mission
of restoring sight to our fellow human beings.

Contents

Video Contents

Foreword

When I was a new faculty member, I had the pleasure of spending time with an amazing resident, William Fishkind, who was already a fully trained internist and who, after practice in the Public Health Service, decided to start from scratch as an ophthalmology resident. I have known Bill as his teacher, his friend, his colleague, and ultimately as his student. Bill had a native curiosity that knew no bounds combined with an intense desire to learn. So many are afraid that a question may reveal a lack of knowledge and so hesitate to ask. Not Bill. I knew he would go far, and my expectations were greatly exceeded, as time has so well shown.

Bill is a natural teacher and has been an authority in the field of complex cataract and anterior segment surgery throughout his career. His work on the propagation of ultrasound during cataract surgery is a unique and important addition to the field. Such is also clearly the case with his first book on cataract surgery, which covered all aspects of surgery and related complications. I was honored to be asked to write a chapter for this book because I knew Bill would not accept anything but the best in this work, and the quality of the other authors made it an honor to be included.

Now we have the long-awaited second edition to this widely acclaimed book. Again, only luminaries (with the possible exception of yours truly) in the field have been asked to contribute, and Bill has made every effort to ensure that this new edition is encyclopedic in covering the general field of cataract surgery. Readers and students of all stripes in this field are in for a treat! I am proud to be asked to take part, proud of the final product, and fortunate to be able to call Bill a friend.

Randall J. Olson, MD

Foreword

Readers might wonder if we really need a second edition of Bill Fishkind's book. We definitely do, because cataract surgery is changing rapidly, and the rate of change is accelerating. At the beginning of my career, not so long ago, intracapsular cataract extraction (ICCE) was the universal technique, and a surgeon's hope was to get through the procedure without capsule rupture and vitreous loss. The incision was viewed solely as providing access to the cataract. Surgeons did not understand surgically induced astigmatism. Today there are multiple options for incision location, architecture, and construction techniques and devices. And today we almost never use the universal instrument of the past—scissors.

Except for grasping the cataract itself, ICCE entailed no intraocular maneuvers, and there was very little done to adequately address complications. Viscoelastics did not exist. Now we have multiple options and ever-evolving new substances, combinations, and properties, so our preferred viscoelastic depends on the immediate task.

There are numerous choices for capsular openings and multiple ways of achieving them. Hydrodissection and hydrodelineation, instrumentation, and techniques continue to evolve. The initial phaco machines required tuning for each case and utilized 100% power on, or off at zero power. The sophistication of the modern machines, with their myriad power modulations and fantastic fluidics with truly stable anterior chambers, were never even a dream when I began phaco surgery. Techniques for dissembling the nucleus and mobilizing the nucleus continue to evolve, making surgery easier for the surgeon and safer for the patient. Capsule rupture, vitreous loss, and endothelial cell loss, once common, have dramatically declined.

In early phaco surgery, most capsule ruptures occurred during cortical cleanup. New instrumentation and techniques and hand pieces have almost eliminated that.

Intraocular lens designs, materials, and optical properties have given us, and patients, options never previously conceived of, and they continue to improve, as do new available medications, used as eyedrops or intracameral infusions. Other devices such as capsular tension rings, capsular tension segments, and pupil expanders add to surgeon comfort and patient safety.

Early venturers into refractive lens exchange were viewed by most ophthalmologists as buccaneers. Currently, refractive results are considered a measure of the quality of the surgical procedure. Landing a man on the moon and outpatient cataract surgery under topical anesthesia with immediate visual rehabilitation would all have been viewed as equally impossible when I entered medical school.

So considering the scope, rate, and effects of the evolution of cataract surgery, we will always need updated surgical atlases and textbooks. No one entering an ophthalmology residency would ever anticipate that in the future they could be accused of selling day-old bread.

This second edition is adequately comprehensive, detailed and illustrated. It has the added advantage of adding fresh faces to well-recognized experts in the list of authors. Ophthalmologists involved in cataract surgery will appreciate this book for the new options that give surgeons more comfort and safety in performing cataract surgery and dealing with complications.

The reward as always will be pride, the respect of your peers, and the gratitude of your patients.

I. Howard Fine, MD

Preface to the Second Edition

In the first edition, my goal was to attempt a systematized presentation of ophthalmic surgical techniques. With the procedure documented, I then strove to clarify recognition of problems encountered and, finally, if avoidance was unattainable, management of the consequent complication.

I believe that textbook did a commendable job. However, some information is now out-of-date, and the issues themselves have become more intricate.

This new edition employs the equivalent systematized methodology. However, the scope of the book is significantly amplified. Now not only cataract surgery, with its up-to-date nuances, is presented, but lens implant surgery, with all its wide-ranging situations, is comprehensively included. Exhaustive, step-by-step descriptions, with explanatory figures, are designed to support surgeons with the assessment of the perceived challenge and then impart the essential strategies to prepare for, and undertake, the surgical procedure.

In addition, some decision making in contemporary ophthalmic surgery demands integration of "nonsurgical" data to predict complications such as lens implant construction, selection, function, dysphotopsia, and IOL instability both short and long term. Management of TASS, endophthalmitis, retinal complications, and well-known anatomical abnormalities requiring additional surgical planning are incorporated to provide thorough treatment of the subject.

To achieve these objectives I invited a distinguished group of surgeon authorities to contribute to this text. They were chosen for their expertise and proficiency in surgery, as well as their experience and understanding of surgical judgment and their proficiency in teaching and writing. They share an aspiration to improve the surgery we perform, and ultimately, the desire to help, through their contemporaries, enhance surgical outcomes. Other than this, they requested nothing in return. Further, analogous to a magnificent dessert at the conclusion of a meal, they have prepared exceptional videos to provide supplementary illustrations of the surgical procedures discussed in the text.

The purpose of this edition is as noble as it can be for educators. We are hopeful that our colleagues find something unique, valuable, or illuminating, conceivably a technical insight or a new approach to an old problem. If this book can strengthen our colleagues' capabilities to care for our patients, it will soar to be the success to which we authors aspire. Please read, scrutinize, study, and assimilate that material which you find valuable.

William J. Fishkind, MD, FACS

Acknowledgments

It takes three years and the work of many individuals to assemble a textbook of this merit.

The first round of thanks goes to the authors of the chapters in this book. There are 68 of them. They have given their time and knowledge. They unassumingly bore criticism and modified their work. They have endured deadlines. They have done all of this to drive higher the quality of the care we deliver to our patients.

I thank my family who provide the indispensable foundation on which I stand. Their inspiration makes available the personal fortitude to confront challenge, unscramble enigmas, and offer guidance to colleagues and patients. Wendy W. Fishkind, my wife and soul mate on this voyage entitled life, provides the reassuring companionship on which I have come to rely. My children, Jennifer and Bret, their spouses Andrew and Stephanie, and grandchildren, Tova and Ari, Bryn and Brayden, fill me with joy and ground me in recognizing what is important in life.

The next groups are my mentors. Teachers who stimulated me to achieve, provided me with fundamental knowledge, and persuaded me that I had the persistence to commit, and complete, any assignment, regardless of complexity. Stan Shulman, my swimming coach, who taught me that I had the fortitude to conquer physical challenges through stamina and determination. Lewis Love, my physics teacher, who taught me that any complex problem can be solved by breaking it up into its components, and then solving each component problem, one at a time. Jack Porter, my English teacher, who convinced me that I had the talent to write. The last individual of note is Warren Eickelberg, PHD, the Department Chairman at Adelphi University. He urged me to apply to medical school and personally sponsored me in attaining admission to Tufts University School of Medicine.

Then surgeons, champions, whom I respect and admire, have learned from and have relished their counsel: Randall Olson, MD, I. Howard Fine, MD, William Maloney, MD, Alan Crandall, MD, Manus Kraff, MD, C. Drew Sanders, MD, David Chang, MD. Then those colleagues with whom I have worked side by side. They individually imparted various instructive delicacies on a consistent basis: Roger Steinert, MD, Amar Agarwal, MD, Sam Market, MD, Bobby Osher, MD. My partners in my practice who every day support me: Brock K. Bakewell, MD, FACS, Jeff S. Maltzman, MD, FACS, Brian Hunter, MD, FACS, Rich Lewis, MD, Jeff Lewis, MD, Stewart Mecom, OD, and my office administrator, Beverly King.

I must recognize and thank the staff at Thieme Publishing who made available the infrastructure to complete this textbook. Haley Paskalides, editorial assistant, who daily wrote, called, persuaded, implored, and sometimes threatened me to get all the work done. Elizabeth Palumbo, managing editor, who never let me neglect the big picture. William Lamsback, executive editor, who kept everything on track. Owen Zurhellen, managing editor for Thieme, who continually had confidence that we would complete our project with a submission worthy of publication by Thieme and acquisition by our colleagues.

The last thank you goes to Tony Pazos, the medical illustrator who undertook the study of intricate ocular anatomy as well as surgical techniques, so that he could create fabulous and perceptive illustrations. These figures would add to our insight and the capability to undertake the surgical maneuver. He never lost patience with the chapter authors or me, and always created splendid illustrations.

Contributors

Amar Agarwal, MS, FRCS, FRCOphth
Professor
Chairman and Managing Director (CMD)
Dr. Agarwal's Eye Hospital Ltd.
Secretary General
Intraocular Implant and Refractive Society
Past President
International Society of Refractive Surgery/American
    Academy of Ophthalmology
Chenni, India

Iqbal Ike K. Ahmed, MD, FRCSC
Fellowship Director
Glaucoma and Anterior Segment Surgery (GAASS)
    Fellowship
Research Fellowship Director
Department of Ophthalmology and Vision Sciences
University of Toronto
Research Director
Kensington Eye Institute
University of Toronto
Chief
Division of Ophthalmology
Trillium Health Partners
Mississauga, Ontario
Medical Director
Prism Eye Institute
Mississauga and Brampton, Ontario
Co-Medical Director
TLC Mississauga
Mississauga, Ontario, Canada

Quentin B. Allen, MD
Florida Vision Institute
Stuart, Florida

Anika Amritanand, MD
Loma Linda University (Gimbel)
Loma Linda, California

Lisa Brothers Arbisser, MD
Adjunct Professor
Moran Eye Center
University of Utah
Salt Lake City, Utah

Paul N. Arnold, MD
Sneed Eye Associates
Ashland, Oregon

Steve A. Arshinoff, MD FRCSC
York Finch Eye Associates
Humber River Hospital
University of Toronto
Toronto, Ontario, Canada
McMaster University
Hamilton, Ontario, Canada

Ehud I. Assia, MD
Department of Ophthalmology
Meir Medical Center
Kfar Saba, Israel
Ein-Tal Eye Center
Tel Aviv, Israel
Sackler Faculty of Medicine
Tel Aviv University
Tel Aviv, Israel

Thomas D. Bailey, MD, FACS
Ophthalmologist
Loden Vision
Paris, Tennessee

Brock K. Bakewell, MD, FACS
Clinical Assistant Professor
Department of Ophthalmology
University of Utah
Fishkind, Bakewell, Maltzman Eye Care and Surgery Center
Tucson, Arizona

Graham D. Barrett, MD
Clinical Professor
Lions Eye Institute
Nedlands, Australia

John P. Berdahl, MD
Cataract Surgery, Corneal Surgery, and Glaucoma Surgery
Vance Thompson Vision
Sioux Falls, South Dakota

Thomas A. Berk, MD
Resident Physician
Department of Opthalmology
McGill University
Montreal, Quebec, Canada

Mark H. Blecher, MD
Codirector
Cataract Service
Wills Eye Hospital
Assistant Clinical Professor
Department of Ophthalmology
Thomas Jefferson University
Philadelphia, Pennsylvania

Hari Bodhireddy, MD
Visiting Instructor
Department of Ophthalmology and Visual Sciences
Moran Eye Center
University of Utah
Salt Lake City, Utah

Álvaro Fidalgo Broncano, MD
Resident in Ophthalmology
La Mancha-Centro Hospital
Ciudad Real, Spain

Charles M. Calvo, MD
Wills Eye Hospital Residency Program
Thomas Jefferson University
Philadelphia, Pennsylvania

David F. Chang, MD
Clinical Professor
Department of Ophthalmology
University of California–San Francisco
Los Altos, California

Kristin Ow Chapman, MD
Glaucoma Fellow
Department of Opthalmology and Visual
  Sciences
Moran Eye Center
University of Utah
Salt Lake City, Utah

Robert J. Cionni, MD
Medical Director
Eye Institute of Utah
Salt Lake City, Utah

Alan S. Crandall, MD
Moran Eye Center
University of Utah
Salt Lake City, Utah

James A. Davison, MD, FACS
Wolfe Eye Clinic
Marshalltown, Iowa

Uday Devgan, MD
Private Practice
Devgan Eye Surgery, Los Angeles and
  Beverly Hills
Chief of Ophthalmology
University of California at Los Angeles Medical
  Center
Clinical Professor of Ophthalmology
Jules Stein Eye Institute
University of California at Los Angeles
Los Angeles, California

Steven H. Dewey, MD
Colorado Springs Health Partners, PC
Colorado Springs, Colorado

David M. Dillman, MD
Founder
Dillman Eye Care Associates
Daville, Illinois

Mohammed Aabid Farukhi, MD
Ophthalmic Pathology and Research Fellow
Moran Eye Center
University of Utah
Salt Lake City, Utah

María José Domínguez Fernández, MD
Specialist in Ophthalmology
La Mancha-Centro Hospital
Ciudad Real, Spain

Jason M. Feurman, MD
Cornea and Refractive Surgery Fellow
Moran Eye Center
University of Utah
Salt Lake City, Utah

I. Howard Fine, MD
Professor of Ophthalmology
Casey Eye Institute
Oregon Health and Science University
Drs. Fine, Hoffman & Sims, LLC
Eugene, Oregon

William J. Fishkind, MD, FACS
Clinical Professor
University of Utah
Salt Lake City, Utah
and
University of Arizona
Tucson, Arizona
and
Fishkind, Bakewell, Maltzman and Hunter
Eye Care and Surgery Center
Tucson, Arizona

Harry W. Flynn, Jr., MD
Professor
Department of Ophthalmology
Bascom Palmer Eye Institute
University of Miami Health Center
Miami, Florida

Nicole R. Fram, MD
Clinical Instructor of Ophthalmology
David Geffen School of Medicine
Jules Stein Eye Institute
University of California at Los Angeles
Advanced Vision Care
Los Angeles, California

Howard V. Gimbel, MD, MPH, FRCSC
Gimbel Eye Centre
Calgary, Alberta, Canada

Fernando González del Valle, MD
Chief of Ophthalmology
Hospital General La Mancha Centro
Alcázar de San Juan, Spain

Harry B. Grabow, MD
Founder and Medical Director
Sarasota Cataract Institute
Sarasota, Florida

Anya Gushchin, MD
Visiting Instructor
Department of Ophthalmology
University of Utah
Salt Lake City, Utah

David R. Hardten, MD, FACS
Founding Partner
Minnesota Eye Consultants, PA
Minnetonka, Minnesota

Richard S. Hoffman, MD
Clinical Associate Professor of Ophthalmology
Casey Eye Institute
Oregon Health and Science University
Drs. Fine, Hoffman & Sims, LLC
Eugene, Oregon

Brian A. Hunter, MD, FACS
Cataract and Refractive Surgery
Comprehensive Ophthalmology
Fishkind, Bakewell, Maltzman, Hunter, & Associates Eye Care
    and Surgery Center
Clinical Assistant Professor
Department of Ophthalmology
University of Arizona
Tucson, Arizona

Mitchell A. Jackson, MD
Founder/CEO, Jacksoneye
Lake Villa, Illinois

**Leonard Joffe, MB, BCh (WITS), FCS (SA), FAAO, FRCS
    Edinburgh**
Retina Specialists of Southern Arizona
Tucson, Arizona

Paul S. Koch, MD
Founder and Medical Director
Koch Eye Associates
Warwick, Rhode Island

Manus C. Kraff, MD
Founder and President
Kraff Eye Institute
Chicago, Illinois

Brent A. Kramer
Fourth year medical student
Carver College of Medicine at the University
    of Iowa
Iowa City, Iowa

Stephen S. Lane, MD
Adjunct Clinical Professor
Ophthalmology
University of Minnesota
Medical Director
Associated Eye Care
Stillwater, Minnesota

Marc L. Leib, MD
Chief Medical Officer
Arizona Health Care Cost Containment Center
Phoenix, Arizona

James C. Loden, MD
Loden Vision Center
Goodlettsville, Tennessee

Francis S. Mah, MD
Director of Cornea and External Disease
Codirector of Refractive Surgery
Scripps Clinic
La Jolla, California

Jeff S. Maltzman, MD, FACS
Fishkind, Bakewell, Maltzman, & Hunter Eye Care
    and Surgery Center
Tucson, Arizona

Boris Malyugin, MD, PhD
Professor
Department of Ophthalmology
S. Fyodorov Eye Microsurgery Federal State Institution
Cataract and Implant Surgery Department
Moscow, Russian

Nick Mamalis, MD
Professor of Ophthalmology
Codirector, Intermountain Ocular Research Center
Director, Ocular Pathology
Moran Eye Center
University of Utah
Salt Lake City, Utah

Isabel Alonso Martínez, MD
Specialist in Ophthalmology
Hospital de Leganés
Madrid, Spain

Samuel Masket, MD
Founding Partner
Advanced Vision Care
Clinical Professor
David Geffen School of Medicine
University of California-Los Angeles
Los Angeles, California

Francisco Javier Lara Medina, PhD, MD
Specialist in Ophthalmology
La Mancha-Centro Hospital
Ciudad Real, Spain

Marc A. Michelson, MD
Associate Clinical Professor
University of Alabama at Birmingham
Callahan Eye Hospital
Birmingham, Alabama

Mark D. Mifflin, MD
Professor
Moran Eye Center
University of Utah
Salt Lake City, Utah

Esperanza López Mondéjar, MD
Specialist in Ophthalmology
La Mancha-Centro Hospital
Ciudad Real, Spain

Ramón Lorente Moore, PhD, MD
Head of Department
Specialist in Ophthalmology
Complexo Universitario de Ourense
Ourense, Spain

Louis D. "Skip" Nichamin, MD
Ophthalmic Surgeon and Consultant
Avon, Colorado

Gregory S.H. Ogawa, MD
Assistant Clinical Professor
University of New Mexico
Ophthalmologist
Eye Associates of New Mexico
Albuquerque, New Mexico

Randall J. Olson, MD
Professor, Chair, and CEO
Department of Ophthalmology and Visual Sciences
Moran Eye Center
University of Utah
Salt Lake City, Utah

Antonio Arias Palomero, MD
Specialist in Ophthalmology
La Mancha-Centro Hospital
Ciudad Real, Spain

Hreem N. Patel
Fellow
Moran Eye Center
University of Utah
Salt Lake City, Utah

Patricia Ann Ple-plakon, MD
Cornea and Refractive Surgery Fellow
Baylor College of Medicine
Houston, Texas

Marcelino Álvarez Portela, MD
Specialist in Ophthalmology
Complexo Universitario A Coruña
Coruña, Spain

Kenneth J. Rosenthal, MD, FACS
Surgeon Director
Rosenthal Eye Surgery
New York, New York

Jonathan B. Rubenstein, MD
Vice Chairman and Deutsch Family Professor
Department of Ophthalmology
Rush University Medical Center
Chicago, Illinois

Sanduk Ruit, MD
Cofounder
Himalayan Cataract Project
Waterbury, Vermont

Agustín Núñez Sánchez, MD
Specialist in Ophthalmology
La Mancha-Centro Hospital
Ciudad Real, Spain

Javier Celis Sánchez, MD
Head of Section
Specialist in Ophthalmology
La Mancha-Centro Hospital
Ciudad Real, Spain

Fani Segev, MD
Department of Ophthalmology
Meir Medical Center
Kfar Saba, Israel
Ein-Tal Eye Center
Tel Aviv, Israel
Sackler Faculty of Medicine
Tel Aviv University
Tel Aviv, Israel

Barry S. Seibel, MD
Clinical Assistant Professor of Ophthalmology
David Geffen School of Medicine
University of California at Los Angeles
Los Angeles, California

Annette Chang Sims, MD
Clinical Assistant Professor
Surgery
Western University of Health Sciences
Fine, Hoffman, and Sims Ophthalmologists
Eugene, Oregon

Harmanjit Singh, MD
Department of Ophthalmology and Vision Sciences
University of Toronto
Toronto, Canada

William E. Smiddy, MD
Professor
Department of Ophthalmology
Bascom Palmer Eye Institute
University of Miami Health System
Miami, Florida

Roger F. Steinert, MD
Irving H. Leopold Professor of Ophthalmology
Director, Gavin Herbert Eye Institute
Interim Dean, School of Medicine
University of California–Irvine
Irvine, California

Geoffrey Tabin, MD
Moran Eye Center
University of Utah
Salt Lake City, Utah
Himalayan Cataract Project
Waterbury, Vermont

Yokrat Ton, MD
Department of Ophthalmology
Meir Medical Center
Kfar Saba, Israel
Ein-Tal Eye Center
Tel Aviv, Israel
Sackler Faculty of Medicine
Tel Aviv University
Tel Aviv, Israel

Abhay R. Vasavada, MD, MS, FRCS (England)
Iladevi Cataract and IOL Research Centre
Raghudeep Eye Hospital
Ahmedabad, India

Vaishali Vasavada, MS
Raghudeep Eye Hospital
Memnagar, Ahmedabad, India

R. Bruce Wallace III, MD
Medical Director
Wallace Eye Associates
Alexandria, Louisiana

Charles H. Weber, MD
Adjunct Assistant Professor
Moran Eye Center
University of Utah
Eye Institute of Utah
Salt Lake City, Utah

Mitchell P. Weikert, MD
Associate Professor
Baylor College of Medicine
Houston, Texas

Arthur J. Weinstein, MD, FACP, MACR
Eye Associates of New Mexico
Albuquerque, New Mexico

Matthew J. Welch, MD
Clinical Assistant Professor
Loyola University Chicago
American Society of Retina Specialists
Associated Retina Consultants, Ltd.
Phoenix, Arizona

Liliana Werner, MD, PhD
Associate Professor; Codirector
Intermountain Ocular Research Center
Moran Eye Center
University of Utah
Salt Lake City, Utah

Ronald Yeoh, MD, FRCS FRCOphth, DO, FAMS
Consultant Eye Surgeon and Medical Director
Adjunct Assistant Professor
Duke–National University of Singapore Medical School
Eye and Retina Surgeons
Singapore National Eye Centre
Singapore

Section I Anesthesia

1 Complications of Ophthalmic Anesthesia

Kenneth J. Rosenthal

Complications of regional and topical anesthesia for ophthalmic surgery have become increasingly rare, which can be attributed to our improved understanding of anatomy and, consequently, the improved strategies for administering anesthetics, the development of safe and effective anesthetic substances, and the use of appropriate monitoring in the perioperative period. Nonetheless, although many anesthesia complications may be relatively innocuous, some may be sight- or even life-threatening. As such, the administration of anesthesia should be done with proper training and experience, and with care and respectful attention to detail.

Injectable Ophthalmic Anesthesia for Sedation and for General Anesthesia

General Considerations

Local anesthesia is the greatest single hazard in cataract surgery,[1-4] accounting for an incidence of adverse effects in as high as 3.5% of patients (orbital adverse effects in 2.6%, and systemic effects in 0.9%), according to a study by the Royal College of Ophthalmologists. A cataract surgeon in the United States has, on average, a 3% chance each year of being sued over cataract surgery,[5] and the majority of such cases relate to anesthesia complications, such as globe perforations, inadvertent intraocular injections and retinal detachment, and intraocular hemorrhage associated with these misadventures.[6]

The purpose of anesthesia is to convert an otherwise painful, anxiety-producing, and unpleasant experience into a tolerable, comfortable, and even pleasant and restful experience. In choosing the anesthesia, the least invasive and the safest method should always be employed. The extensiveness, duration, and complexity of surgery, factors that are often intertwined, should be evaluated in choosing the route, duration, and depth of anesthesia employed. Exposure to anesthesia in excess of that which is necessary adds unnecessary risk to the procedure, with no tangible benefit to the patient or the surgical team. Regional anesthesia is usually preferable to general anesthesia, producing safer, equally effective, and cost-efficient results. However, just as it is inappropriate for a surgeon to use the same technique for every surgical intervention, it is similarly incorrect to use the same anesthesia for each case. Although surgeons may subscribe to a particular practice of anesthesia for routine cases, it is important to assess each patient's needs and act appropriately for exceptional cases. Such exceptions may exist either because of the patient's medical conditions or personality, or because the surgical intervention may be more complex or is anticipated to be of longer duration than is routine.

Definition of Injectable Block

For the purposes of this discussion, I am using the term *injectable techniques* to refer to any anesthesia method involving the use of a sharp needle and an injectate, which includes peribulbar as well as retrobulbar techniques, unless otherwise disqualified. The procedures collectively are referred to as "regional orbital anesthetic block."[7] It has been suggested that a peribulbar block (also referred to as a periconal block), involving injection outside of the muscle cone, entails less risk of complication than a retrobulbar technique. However true this may be, complications have been observed with both techniques.[8]

Preoperative Assessment

Good planning is always part of the strategy to limit risk in anesthesia administration. Some authors believe that if the patient has preexisting systemic medical conditions, a history should be taken and a physical examination and laboratory testing should be performed. But there is considerable regional and international variation in these requirements; in fact, in some states, there are regulations that require a medical evaluation before major surgery, even on a perfectly healthy patient. However, no consistent standards have been established, and there is little evidence that such evaluations have a significant bearing on the safety of cataract surgery in general, and even less in healthy patients. A prospective multicenter clinical trial evaluating this issue in 19,557 elective cataract operations in the United States and Canada, conducted by the Study of Medical Testing for Cataract Surgery, randomized patients into either a No Routine Screening group or a Routine Screening group; in patients in the latter group, an electrocardiogram (ECG) was performed, and electrolytes/glucose and complete blood count (CBC) were assessed. Demographic, clinical, perioperative, and medical event data were collected for seven days postsurgery, and they demonstrated that "perioperative morbidity and mortality are not reduced by routine use of commonly ordered preoperative medical tests."[9] A study by Rosenfeld et al[10] similarly showed that the need for anesthesia intervention during cataract surgery was correlated neither with the presence of an abnormal preoperative ECG nor with the presence of diabetes, two tests almost always performed during a preoperative evaluation. Nonetheless, a history of systemic hypertension, pulmonary disease, renal disease, or cancer was associated with a statistically significant increase in the incidence of intervention, suggesting that at least a review of the patient's medical conditions may be prudent in the immediate preoperative assessment.

Some investigators have reported that the anesthesia team did not make use of reported results of preoperative tests and examinations, and that perioperative management was not influenced because of these investigations.[11] Findings from the National Survey of Local Anesthesia for Ocular Surgery in 1997 reveal further that in patients who had no preoperative tests, there was a very low rate of serious adverse events that would have been influenced by such tests.[12]

Because cataract surgery is most frequently performed on geriatric patients, a high incidence of systemic illnesses may coexist, such as diabetes, hypertension, coronary artery disease, obesity, chronic obstructive pulmonary disease, and arthritis. These conditions may pose special challenges to the surgical and anesthesia teams. To limit these risks, every effort should be made to ensure that the patient is in optimal condition for surgery. Nonetheless, in most instances cataract surgery can take place even in the presence of these conditions; there are almost no contraindications to surgery in patients whose medical condition has been optimized.

During the immediate preoperative consultation, the patient should provide a list of current medications so that any potential drug interactions can be anticipated, and to verify that the patient has taken the medications appropriately. It is useful to schedule surgery for diabetics during the early morning, so that their oral hypoglycemics or insulin dosage can be taken with food immediately after the surgery without interrupting their usual routine. Alternate strategies may make surgery safe during any time of the day; for example, diabetics can be scheduled during the early afternoon so that they can take their insulin and breakfast earlier in the day with enough time to fast prior to surgery. In any case, it is best to avoid conditions that place the patient at risk of hypoglycemia; elevated blood glucose levels can generally be managed postoperatively, if medically appropriate.

Considerations Regarding Anticoagulation

In general, it is advisable to continue patients on systemic anticoagulants during routine cataract surgery, particularly in cases of small-incision phacoemulsification. Discontinuation of anticoagulant therapy may bear a greater risk than that of significant intraoperative ocular bleeding, even with retrobulbar injection.[13] In these cases, however, it is of particular importance to use small needles and correct anatomic placement, and to avoid excessive manipulation during the injectable block. Studies to date, however, have not distinguished among the risks of discontinuing anticoagulation prior to cataract surgery vis-à-vis different medical indications. It is well known that stopping medications have different implications for risk depending on the condition for which the patient is being treated. For example, patients with mechanical heart valve replacement are at substantially higher risk for embolism or stroke than are patients with atrial fibrillation as the underlying reason for treatment; accordingly, mechanical heart valve replacement patients require higher routine levels of anticoagulation. These factors should be weighed carefully, in consultation with the patient's internist, in determining the systemic and ocular risks. In patients whose International Normalized Ratio (INR; a derivative of the prothrombin time) is above 2.0, consideration should be given to reducing anticoagulation therapy preoperatively. Depending on the complexity of the surgical intervention, discontinuation of anticoagulation therapy can be considered, although it is rarely necessary.

The Role of the Anesthesia Team in Systemic Sedation and General Anesthesia

In the United States, both Certified Registered Nurse Anesthetists (CRNAs) and anesthesiologists (MDs) have been trained to administer anesthesia, monitor and treat the patients' systemic condition, and provide sedation appropriate to the patient's need. Although there are regional variations in usage of anesthesia services both through the United States and internationally,[14] the role of this vital team member cannot be overlooked. In an era where cost containment has reached a high degree of consciousness, it is important to evaluate the necessity of each aspect of the care we provide. Rosenfeld et al[10] found that during cataract surgery, major anesthesia intervention (i.e., excluding verbal reassurance, hand holding, or physical restraint) was required in 28.6% of patients. Although intervention was required more often in patients with certain underlying diseases, almost a third of patients without predisposing factors required intervention of some type. This suggests that with current anesthesia methods it is impossible to predict preoperatively which patients will require intervention, thereby suggesting further that anesthesia monitoring is essential for avoiding perioperative complications, regardless of the patient's preoperative condition.

Intravenous Sedation and Monitoring

Considerable debate has persisted regarding the usefulness of intravenous (IV) sedation for cataract surgery, particularly with the use of topical anesthetic agents and minimally invasive surgical technique (for further discussion, see Chapter 2). It is important to understand what constitutes appropriate use of this mode of treatment. First, anesthesiologists must possess appropriate personality traits and communication skills that enable them to gain the patient's trust and confidence.[15] Second, they should inform the patient about the experience he or she is about to have. This discussion will help minimize anxiety and lower complications during the perioperative period.[16] Third, perioperative monitoring should generally consist of at least an ECG, pulse oximetry, and periodic blood pressure measurements.[13,17] The latter measurements should be kept to a minimum during critical surgical periods to avoid patient discomfort during surgery, which may cause undue anxiety or movement.

The goal of IV sedation should be to relieve anxiety while enabling the patient to remain stationary, calm, comfortable, and cooperative. The elderly generally require less pharmacological squelching of anxiety during surgery than do younger patients, both with regard to the absolute amount of the agent given and the level of consciousness attained; however, considerable variability exists in the amount of drug necessary to obtain the desired end point. It is usually desirable to produce anxiolysis without obtundation, because obtundation may result in a patient who is unpredictably still, then combative,[18-21] and may cause further depression of preexisting cardiac and respiratory instabilities.[22-26] Some newer sedatives, however, can achieve substantial levels of sedation without significant respiratory depression (see discussion in Chapter 2).

Excessive IV sedation should rarely be used to compensate for an incomplete regional anesthesia block. Rather, this should be managed by supplementation of the local anesthesia. However, occasionally it is necessary to provide a deeper level of sedation or systemic analgesia (e.g., narcotics) to supplement the regional anesthesia block, particularly in situations where the additional block is ineffective or cannot be administered because of ongoing surgical maneuvers.

Complications of Pharmacological Agents

Systemic toxicity of anesthetic agents is usually associated with inadvertent ectopic injection or overdose of a particular agent, allergic reactions, or vasovagal responses. Ectopic injection may be propagated by the intravascular route or through inadvertent direct central nervous system injection through the subdural route via penetration of the optic nerve sheath. These problems will each be discussed later in their respective sections. However, as a general measure, limitation of these problems can be accomplished by slow, patient injection of anesthetics[15] (no more than 2 cc/min) while monitoring the patient for any signs of systemic toxicity, and by gentle preinjection aspiration to ensure an extravascular location of the needle.

Although hyaluronidase is invaluable as a spreading agent, its use may result in allergic or frankly anaphylactic reactions.[27] As such, this proteolytic drug should be avoided in atopic individuals. A study by Prosser et al[28] suggests that hyaluronidase may not be necessary at least in peribulbar blocks.

Perforation and Penetration of the Globe

The administration of a regional orbital anesthetic block is a technique requiring specialized training and experience. In many institutions the block is given by the least experienced surgeon or by anesthesia personnel, often without adequate experience or training. This practice should be discouraged. A detailed study of the orbit, its nerves, its vasculature, and its soft tissue septa should be undertaken before administering injectable anesthesia. Regional orbital anesthesia requires an appreciation for the three dimensionality of the skill, and hands-on, one-to-one training is desirable.

This is the most common of the serious complications of injectable anesthesia and has been documented by numerous authors over the years.[29–32] Globe perforation and inadvertent intraocular injections also rank as two of the most common causes of litigation in cataract surgery.[6] Ocular penetration refers to the entry of a needle into the globe after which the needle is withdrawn. Ocular perforation suggests that the needle entered the eye and then exited through another part of the globe prior to having been withdrawn. Because the clinical pictures are similar, the terms are used interchangeably in this discussion.

The actual incidence of ocular penetration is difficult to determine, owing to the tremendous diversity of reports that have appeared in the literature. Reported incidences range from as few as one penetration in 16,224 consecutive cases,[33,34] to as many as 1 in 100 cases. Teichmann and Uthoff[35] reported an incidence of 0 in 21,000 cases using their technique. If the incidences reported in several available references are averaged, the occurrence rate is ~ 0.01%.

Because the risk of complication is directly related to the number of injections administered, every effort should be made to reduce the frequency with which multiple injections are given. Correct placement, use of hyaluronidase, and adequate volume of injectate will increase the likelihood of success of the "first take." Ocular compression devices such as the "superpinky" or the Honan's balloon[36–38] may likewise improve the distribution of anesthetic, although they must be used judiciously to avoid vascular compromise to the globe. A good end point for determination of adequate block should be the ablation of sensation to the area to be operated upon. Testing by lightly pinching the conjunctiva with a 0.12-mm Castroviejo forceps will give adequate indication of anesthesia. While providing a convenient measure as to the effectiveness of the block, it is not necessary to achieve akinesia or amaurosis in every case; insisting on achieving these end points has the effect of needing more frequent readministration of anesthesia injections than are necessary.

Perforation/Penetration: Anatomic Considerations

The incidence of ocular penetration is significantly higher in eyes that have axial lengths greater than 26 mm on ultrasonic biometry. This increased incidence is most likely due to the increased incidence of staphylomata or previous scleral buckle in this population. In fact, Duker et al[39] estimate the incidence at 1 in 140 cases in such eyes. The increased susceptibility of staphylomatous eyes is most likely due to the fact that, whereas non-staphylomatous eyes have predictable anterior-posterior shape and the location of the equator can be extrapolated, these proportions are distorted in eyes with staphylomata. In the latter, there is an elongated anterior-posterior dimension that is not entirely predictable,[40] in contrast even to nonpathologically myopic eyes[41] (**Fig. 1.1**). Because a misjudgment of even 1 or 2 mm can lead to globe penetration, it is incumbent upon the person administering the block to review the patient's chart and know the axial length of the eye prior to administering the injection.[42] The presence of a previously placed scleral buckle bears the additional risk that the retrobulbar needle may snag behind the buckle, causing a globe penetration.

As with staphylomatous eyes, small, tight orbits with deep-set eyes are also particularly at risk for injury,[43] owing primarily to the unexpectedly posterior position of the equator with respect to the lateral orbital rim, and the dearth of space between the orbital rim and the globe (**Fig. 1.2**).

Perforation/Penetration: Patient Movement

Patient cooperation is essential for any successful regional anesthesia. Nowhere is this more true than in orbital regional anesthesia. Critical structures within the orbit are in close proximity to one another, and any unanticipated movement may result in ocular perforation. As mentioned earlier, it is essential to obtain sedation appropriate to the patient's clinical status. This usually means administration of a light, anxiolytic dose of sedative without obtundation, in conjunction with a skillfully performed, "painless" anesthetic block as described, for example, by Hustead,[44] in which a subconjunctival injection of dilute anesthetic

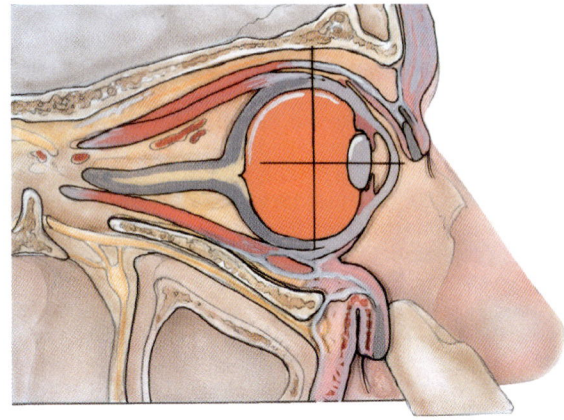

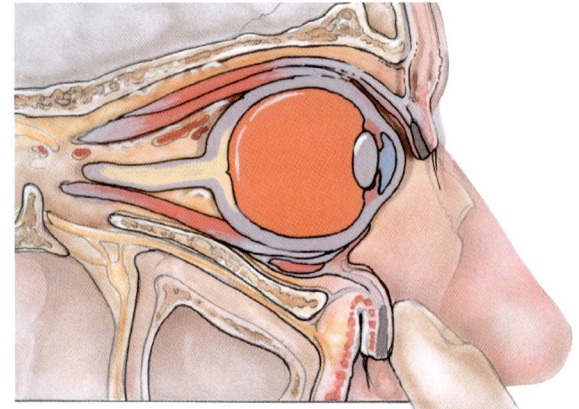

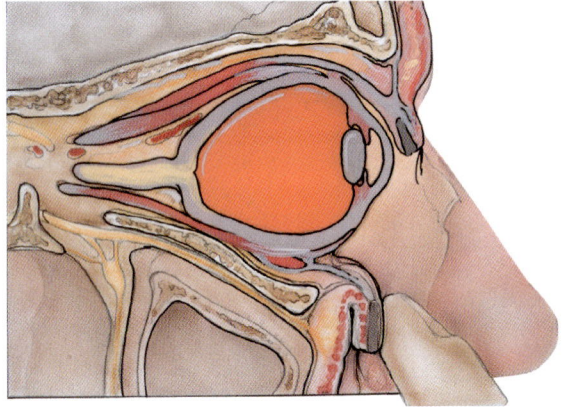

Fig. 1.1 **(a)** Normal eye: expected anterior-posterior dimension. The needle clears the equator. **(b)** Larger myopic eye with normal proportions but slight posterior displacement of the equator. **(c)** The staphylomatous eye has an abnormal anterior-posterior dimension that is unpredictable, making the risk of ocular perforation greater.

precedes the retrobulbar anesthetic injection. It is my opinion that sedation resulting in complete obtundation of patients can be quite hazardous because there is little predictability of such patients with regard to sudden, unexpected movement. Unpredictable movement can be elicited in patients with psychiatric or behavioral disorders, mental retardation, or neurologic movement disorders. And pain itself may cause the patient to move suddenly. Unwanted environmental stimuli such as loud noise, power failure, or uncomfortable or unstable patient positioning

may also lead to movement and should be avoided. Therefore, a quiet, comfortable room with proper head support and power backup should always be used during this critical step in cataract surgery.

Often, however, there are no known specific factors leading to perforation. In rare instances, well-trained, experienced practitioners working on quiet, cooperative patients will experience globe perforation. Therefore, the existence of a perforation is certainly not prima facie evidence of negligence or malpractice.[43]

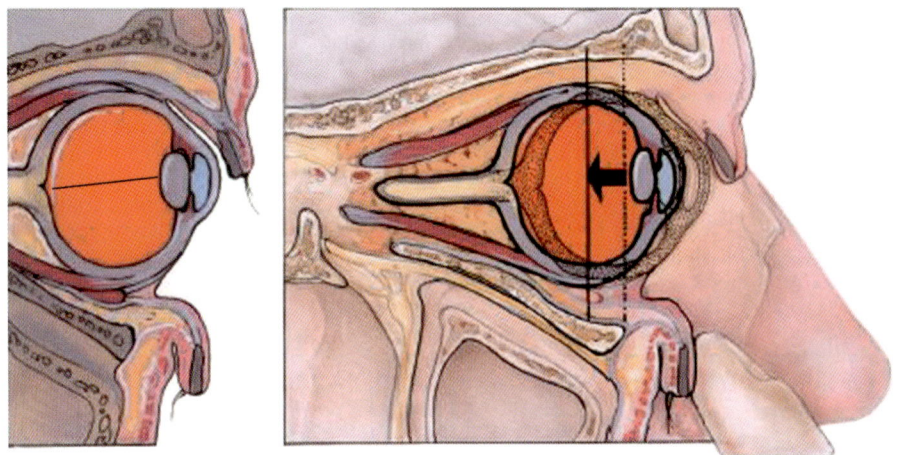

Fig. 1.2 **(a)** Normal set eye: the equator *(solid line)* is approximately at the level of the lateral orbital rim. **(b)** Deep-set eye: the equator *(solid line)* is retro-placed behind the lateral orbital rim *(dotted line)*, increasing the risk of ocular perforation.

Perforation/Penetration: Diagnosis

The occurrence of ocular penetration is often not apparent to the surgeon. Sometimes resistance to injection is appreciated at the time of injection, owing to the finite volume of the globe. Bullock et al[45] reported a case of inadvertent globe penetration in which such a large volume of fluid was injected into the vitreous cavity that it caused the eye to explode, extruding the ocular contents into the subconjunctival space. The investigators subsequently determined that 3,600 mm Hg pressure (from ~ 2 cc of injectate) was required to cause explosion in eye-bank eyes. However, in cases of complete perforation in which the needle enters and then exits from the posterior pole, injection may be without resistance. Indeed, the presence of a "perfect block" with total globe akinesia and anesthesia may result, owing to the posterior orbital location of the injection.

Conversely, globe hypotony may be observed if the needle penetration or perforation occurred without injection into the globe.

Severe pain may sometimes herald an ocular perforation, but this may vary according to the type of needle used (sharp versus dull), the type and amount of sedation used, and the pain tolerances of the patient.[43]

A popping sensation may be felt as the needle penetrates the globe. Because the practitioner sometimes feels this sensation during normal blocks when piercing a connective tissue septum, its significance may not be readily appreciated. This popping sensation can also be elicited from perforation of a blood vessel, the optic nerve sheath, or an extraocular muscle (EOM) as well.

A vitreous hemorrhage, retinal detachment, or retinal tear is seen in a majority of cases. The surgeon may be aware of a diminished red reflex in such patients. Frequently, the presence of these further complications, may not be appreciated until the postoperative office visits, even weeks later.

Perforation/Penetration: Prevention and Treatment

Treatment consists of early recognition of the problem, and, where appropriate, canceling the proposed surgery until the eye can be stabilized. In cases of intraocular injection, increased pressure elevation may cause closure of the central retinal artery. In such cases, consideration should be given to performing vitreous tap or even pars plana vitrectomy if needed, to lower the intraocular pressure. Mannitol may be used to create an osmotic deturgescence of the vitreous cavity. Vitreous hemorrhage or detachment requires treatment following the usual protocols.

This complication can be avoided by an awareness of the patient's axial length, preexamination of the orbit/globe relationship, and proper instruction to the patient regarding avoiding unnecessary movement. A history of prior difficulties with regional block in the companion eye should also be investigated, and etiologic factors delineated before proceeding with the second eye.

Numerous authors have described techniques that may reduce the likelihood of perforation. Current practice consists of a sharp needle technique with insertion either at the lateral canthus or slightly below the canthus, or, alternatively, at the medial canthus, preferably though the conjunctiva and not through the lid. The eye should be held open, remain in primary gaze, and be observed throughout the insertion and injection. The eye should not move during this maneuver, as this may indicate that the sclera has been engaged. The classic concept of looking "up and in" as popularized by Atkinson, should be avoided because it brings the optic nerve closer to the inferotemporal quadrant and places it on stretch, making it more susceptible to injury.

There is still some debate about the ideal needle for this task. Waller et al[46] recommend a dull needle, citing the theoretically greater force required to penetrate the sclera. This argument, however, fails when one considers that any needle sharp enough to penetrate the skin will probably have no trouble penetrating the sclera. Further, because eyes at high risk often have scleral ectasias, there would be sufficient thinning to allow even a dull needle to penetrate. I prefer a straight, sharp, 27-gauge needle no longer than 31 mm inserted as described above, with the bevel toward the globe, thus reducing the risk of damage to critical structures.

A medial orbital injection is also sometimes favored. In this technique the needle is placed at the caruncle, and injection is administered with the needle positioned with the bevel facing away from the globe so as to accommodate the sharply medio-posterior sloping of the medial orbital wall.

Retrobulbar Hemorrhage

Retrobulbar hemorrhage occurs in 0.44% to 3% of retrobulbar anesthetic cases.[47,48] Because of the extensive vascular plexus within the orbit, any vessel may be nicked and caused to bleed. This may be aggravated in patients taking anticoagulants, antiplatelet aggregation medications (e.g., aspirin), steroids, nonsteroidal anti-inflammatory drugs (NSAIDs),[13] or in the presence of poorly controlled hypertension or in cases of excessive manipulation of the needle.

Retrobulbar hemorrhages vary in severity. Although some are venous in origin and may spread slowly, arterial hemorrhages tend to be rapid and produce an aggressive orbital swelling, marked proptosis with immobility of the glove, and massive subconjunctival and eyelid blood staining. Serious vascular compromise to the globe may ensue.[49,50]

Retrobulbar Hemorrhage: Treatment and Prevention

Treatment of this condition depends entirely on its severity. If a tense orbit and globe are observed, prompt treatment is essential to avoid permanent visual loss. The central retinal artery should be immediately assessed, and if it is pulsatile or closed, immediate decompression of the anterior orbit must be performed. In these cases, lateral canthotomy should be performed, and if necessary a complete disinsertion of the lateral canthal tendon and incision of the lower fornix may provide further decompression. If surgery is canceled, the patient should be observed until the vision and circulation are stabilized, and periodic frequent measurement of visual acuity should be made for several hours postoperatively.

In milder cases, immediate compression of the globe with digital pressure, intravenous mannitol, and observation may be sufficient to limit the spread of blood. It is not unreasonable to proceed with surgery if the hemorrhage is sufficiently innocuous that ballottement of the globe is soft, there is no intraocular circulatory compromise, and visualization of the anterior segment is unimpeded.

This complication may be avoided in most cases by taking several precautions. First, gentle yet decisive insertion of the needle without tilting, jiggling, or continually stabbing with the needle will minimize the risk of piercing a vessel. Second, a small-diameter, disposable needle that does not exceed the desired orbital depth of penetration is preferable. A needle length of less than 31 mm will limit access to the most posterior vessels of the orbital apex,[51] which contains the largest vessels, and the small bore (27 gauge or less) will limit the amount of bleeding

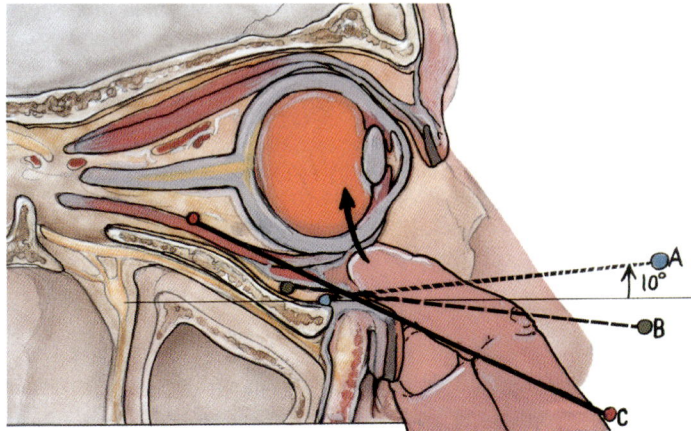

a

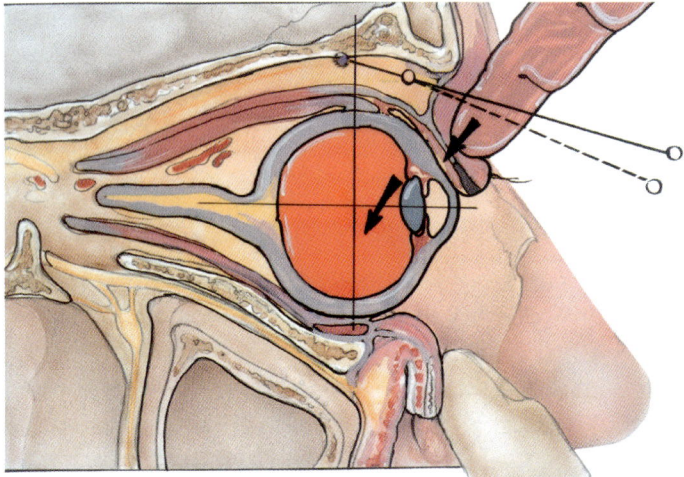

b

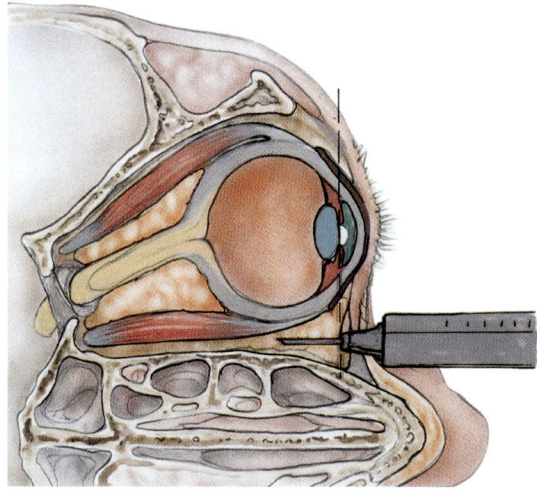

c

Fig. 1.3 (a) Inferotemporal block. The eye is held in primary gaze, and the injection is performed through the conjunctiva. The needle passes posteriorly at a 10-degree elevation from the coronal plane until the equator is reached. Then it is passed slightly medially and superiorly entering the cone. The globe is continually observed to detect movement, which may indicate an entering of the sclera. **(b)** Superotemporal pericone (peribulbar) block. The needle is directed through the lid 3 mm lateral to the lateral limbus and aimed toward the roof of the orbit. Slow injection and careful observation of the globe are performed. **(c)** Medial block. A 30-gauge, 20- to 25-mm, sharp disposable needle is placed just medial to the caruncle with the bevel pointed away from the globe. When the needle hub reaches the plane of the iris, the anesthetic is injected near the medial orbital wall. (Modified from Hamilton RC. Complications of ophthalmic regional anesthesia. Ophthalmol Clin North Am 1998;11:99–114.)

that may occur in the event that a vessel is pierced, because a smaller rent in the vessel will be created.

It is also possible that aggressive aspiration through the syringe to rule out an intravascular injection may cause traction on and subsequent rupture of a blood vessel. Although I prefer not to aspirate at all while administering a retrobulbar block, aspiration should be performed gently, if at all, prior to injection, withdrawing the needle slightly if intravascular position is suspected.

The anterior orbit is relative avascular in three sites: the inferotemporal quadrant (junction of the lateral one third and medial two thirds), the superotemporal quadrant in the sagittal plane of the lateral limbus, and directly nasally in the compartment nasal to the medial rectus. This avascular property makes these sites ideal for orbital injection.[52] The superotemporal quadrant is particularly suitable for pericone injection. The superonasal area is to be avoided because the end vessels of the ophthalmic artery and the trochlea of the superior oblique are located there (**Fig. 1.3**).

Subconjunctival Hemorrhage

Within the spectrum of orbital bleed, a less severe problem is that of subconjunctival bleed. These may occur with some frequency and, unfortunately, may be part of the criteria by which the patient evaluates the immediate postoperative success. Aside from their cosmetic appearance they are rarely of significance medically. If a patch is applied, the patient may be unaware of

the problem, but should be reassured as to the benign nature of the condition.

Extraocular Muscle Paresis

Transient and reversible akinesia is the hallmark of most injectable anesthesia. Many operators use this as the end point to determine the appropriateness of the block. The introduction of ropivacaine 1% as an agent for injection has been shown to have less motor neuron effect, with similar anesthetic effect,[53] with the result that there is a decrease in intra- and postoperative akinesia. In cases where peribulbar anesthesia is given, neither amaurosis nor akinesia will occur, obviating to some extent the need to patch the eye at the conclusion of the procedure.

In some cases the injection of local anesthetic has been shown to cause persistent or even permanent EOM paresis. It is important to realize that some postoperative diplopia may be due either to preexisting strabismus masked by the cataract, commonly from prolonged occlusion, or to preexisting ocular palsy.[54] Further, some postoperative diplopia is based on optical problems, for example anisometropia[55] or the decompensation of a previously compensated tropia, especially if there is decline in vision immediately following surgery. However, in many cases, the diplopia is likely due to injury related directly to the anesthetic injection.

Hamed[54] postulates that there is a direct mechanical injury due to injection directly into the belly of the EOM, or by laceration of the anterior ciliary arteries causing an intra-sheath hematoma, resulting in a compartment syndrome. Hypoperfusion, ischemia, inflammation, and permanent muscle fiber damage may then ensue. The inferior rectus muscle is most likely to be damaged.[56,57]

The role of direct chemical myotoxicity from the anesthetic agents has been studied but remains unclear. Animal studies using bupivacaine, lidocaine, and mepivacaine[58,59] found that when injected around but not into the EOMs, there was negligible effect, which was fully reversible in time. These findings are in contrast to the high degree of myotoxicity demonstrated in other skeletal muscles. However, when these drugs were injected directly into the EOMs, histological changes deemed to be severe enough to cause strabismus were observed.

In the 1990s, when Wydase (hyaluronidase, Wyeth) was unavailable, an increase in persistent postoperative diplopia was noted in patients undergoing cataract surgery with retrobulbar and peribulbar anesthesia.[55] One theory that may have explained this finding is that the absence of the hyaluronidase may have caused a pooling of anesthetic near the muscle for a prolonged period of time and that this may have in turn caused more toxicity than usual. With the current availability of hyaluronidase, these complications are rare.

Brainstem Anesthesia and Injection into the Optic Nerve

The optic nerve sheath is continuous with the dura of the brain. As such, injection beneath the sheath can result in injectate tracking back into the subarachnoid or subdural space. Symptoms of such "brainstem" anesthesia are protean and include respiratory arrest; cardiopulmonary arrest[60,61]; hypertension; tachycardia; dysarthria[62]; confusion; marked shivering; convulsions; loss of consciousness; hemi-, para-, or quadriplegia; and contralateral blockade of the optic nerve and the third, sixth, and twelfth cranial nerves.[63,64] Hamilton[65] has explained the occurrence of hypertension and tachycardia on the basis of a parasympathetic blockade after the anesthetic enters the cerebrospinal fluid. An alternate explanation suggests vagal blockade at the brainstem.[66]

Although the consequences of undetected brainstem anesthesia can be quite dire, immediate diagnosis and appropriate treatment and supportive measures usually result in an otherwise uneventful outcome. The onset is usually within 2 to 10 minutes of injection and resolves over several hours. It is therefore advisable that patients should not be draped for at least 15 minutes following retrobulbar injection so that in the event this complication occurs, it can be immediate recognized, and unobstructed access to the patient can be obtained.[61]

Treatment consists of ventilatory support with oxygen, intravenous fluid therapy, and use of systemic pharmacological agents such as vasopressors, vasodilators, or adrenergic blocking agents, and close monitoring of the vital signs.

Injection directly into the optic nerve causing severe visual loss or blindness has also been reported.[67]

Prevention of this problem may be accomplished in much the same way as prevention of other needle-related complications: proper placement of the needle, both with respect to orbital position and depth, avoidance of the "up-and-in" positioning of the eye, and awareness of the axial length.

Limitation of Ocular Blood Flow

Limitation of blood flow from retrobulbar hemorrhage has been discussed above. In addition, studies by Findl et al[68] have shown that peribulbar and retrobulbar anesthetics have a negative effect on the choroidal and retinal blood flow. This phenomenon may

not be clinically significant in every patient. However, for those with compromised circulation such as diabetics, hypertensives, and those in whom normal autoregulation of ocular blood flow is impaired, such as those with diabetic retinopathy or glaucoma, this phenomenon may take on increased significance, because even a small reduction in ocular perfusion in these patients may result in ischemia. These factors should be considered when evaluating a patient with underlying ocular or systemic disease for injectable anesthesia.

Ocular compression devices, which are used to enhance the spread of anesthetic and reduce intraocular pressure prior to surgery, have been implicated in the production of ischemia as well. Because blood flow to the retina is influenced by a balance between intraocular and extraocular arterial blood pressure, the application of external pressure from devices such as the Honan's balloon or "super-pinky" may cause an initial increase in intraocular pressure,[69–72] thus reducing blood flow in patients with arterial disease, diabetes, or glaucoma.[73–75]

The use of epinephrine in the injectate may similarly be implicated in production of ischemia,[76] and is probably both unnecessary and best avoided.

Oculocardiac Reflex

The oculocardiac reflex is commonly seen in conjunction with ocular surgery. Most commonly, it is seen under general anesthesia when the EOMs are stretched, but it also can be seen in conjunction with retrobulbar block. According to Hamilton,[52] the latter finding is attributable to the use of dull large-bore needles.

Because the afferent limb of this reflex is trigeminal, arising from within the orbit, and because the efferent limb is vagal, ablation of this reflex may be accomplished by administering retrobulbar lidocaine[77] (with a sharp small-bore needle) or by the aggressive administration of atropine[78] (2–3 mg in adults).

Facial Nerve Block

Although rarely used anymore as a separate injection during routine cataract surgery, seventh nerve blockade using the van Lint, O'Brien, or Nadbath techniques is sometimes required. Complications from this technique are reported most commonly with the Nadbath technique, in which injection in or near the stylomastoid foramen is accomplished. The complications include swallowing difficulty (spread to the glossopharyngeal nerve) and respiratory difficulty (vagus and spinal accessory blockade). Cases of permanent facial palsy are most commonly reported with the Nadbath approach as well.

Separate injection of the seventh nerve is best avoided, if possible. If an orbital injection is administered using hyaluronidase, a sufficiently high volume of anesthetic should be given and an ocular decompression device should be used to aid in the spread of the anesthetic; eyelid akinesia is accomplished by spreading anesthesia to the lids through the orbital septum, thus obviating the need for the painful percutaneous nerve block technique.[52] In cases where a separate injection is required as a supplement, avoiding hyaluronidase and limiting the injection to a superficial depth (no more than 12 mm) are recommended.[79,80]

Corneal Exposure

As the cornea may remain anesthetic for a period of time following surgery, it is prudent to take appropriate measures to protect it against inadvertent injury, particularly when lid akinesia exists concomitantly. An occlusive eye patch is most commonly employed for this purpose. However, with shorter duration anesthetics, appropriate patient counseling (frequent lubrication and blinking, avoidance of touching or rubbing the eye) may be sufficient until sensation returns. Advantages of using an occlusive dressing must be weighed against the potential hazards, such as contributing to the development of postoperative ptosis,[81] increased moisture and temperature enhancing the growth of pathogenic organisms,[82] and the patient's loss of peripheral vision and stereopsis, which may lead to accidental injury from a fall or bump.

Atonic Pupil

Postoperative atonic pupil is a rare but reported complication of cataract surgery. Suggestions that this may be related to damage to the ciliary ganglion or adjacent parasympathetic branches[83] have been countered by the observation that pilocarpine instilled in these eyes did not induce pupillary constriction, suggesting a direct iris sphincter malfunction as the etiology.[84] Although some patients are asymptomatic following this occurrence, patients who experience symptoms, such as photophobia, decreased vision, and glare, may require repair or implantation of an iris prosthetic device (see Chapter 32 for further discussion).

Summary

Complications related to regional orbital anesthesia occur infrequently, but their consequences can be substantial. Awareness of the potential for these problems, with meticulous attention to detail and the institution of prompt corrective measures, optimizes the outcomes in these cases. A summary of these conditions, their clinical presentations, and treatment is given in **Table 1.1**.

Topical and Intracameral Anesthesia

The continuing evolution of minimally invasive techniques for cataract surgery has been paralleled by a concomitant development of less invasive anesthesia techniques that have been used increasingly in recent decades.[85] The parallel improvement in both surgical and anesthetic technique is noteworthy for the relative paucity of complications.[86] Nonetheless, if these innovative procedures are to yield reproducible results with few complications, we must continue to evaluate the way in which we approach the patient and the surgical procedure.

What has usually been called "topical anesthesia" should more suitably be called "noninjection anesthesia" or "minimally invasive anesthesia," because it encompasses techniques such as parabulbar, sub-Tenon's, and pinpoint anesthesia, as well as intracameral techniques. Furthermore, the term *topical anesthesia* suggests the emphasis on the application of drugs to the ocular surface, or within the anterior chamber. In fact, the technique comprises a unique skill set that requires different interaction with the patient and balancing the topical anesthesia with systemic sedation or even general anesthesia. The adjunctive use of IV sedation varies greatly, particularly among geographic regions.[2] Perhaps, then, we ought to collectively call this array of ophthalmic anesthetic techniques "topically assisted anesthesia."

An understanding of this global approach is essential to the successful outcome of what we will call, for expedience's sake, "topical anesthesia" from this point on. In contradistinction to common usage, the word *anesthesia* in the context of intraocular surgery does not simply connote analgesia alone. It encompasses amaurosis, akinesia, sedation, and amnesia.[87] The absence of amaurosis and akinesia in patients receiving topical anesthetic with

IV sedation, and the absence of all four characteristics in patients receiving topical anesthetic alone, are the hallmarks of this multifaceted technique. Retention of vision during and immediately after surgical intervention is not merely window dressing. A parallel exists between the rapid return of visual function and the likelihood of return to activities enjoyed prior to the development of visual impairment.[88] Immediate vision, as an index of a successful outcome, is reassuring to surgeon and patient alike.

The introduction of femtosecond laser technology has created a two-step process for cataract surgery: The femtosecond laser procedure is generally performed without sedation, and requires absolute cooperation of the patient in lying still and fixating. Topical anesthetic drops alone are usually sufficient, although very anxious patients can be given mild sedation usually in the form of oral benzodiazepines (e.g., alprazolam, lorazepam, diazepam), although in some centers IV sedation is also available. Once the patient arrives in the surgical suite, IV sedation is generally administered for the cataract surgery itself.

Assessment of immediate postoperative vision can be useful in diagnosing increased intraocular pressure, retinal vascular compromise, and intraocular lens (IOL) power errors. Furthermore, several surgical techniques (for example, intraoperative wavefront aberrometry) are largely dependent on the patient's maintaining fixation, which can only be achieved with topical anesthetic techniques.

Preoperative Assessment and General Considerations

A patient undergoing topical anesthesia will have a different experience before, during, and after surgery than a patient having injection-based anesthesia. Therefore, in preparation for surgery, it is essential for a successful outcome that the patient receive careful and consistent counseling.

Patient Selection

The patient must be evaluated as to suitability for this type of anesthetic. Some authors have suggested that there is a correlation between the patient's preoperative responses to topical anesthetic drops or to preoperative testing using tonometry and ultra sound (such as the "drop then decide" method of Dinsmore[89] and the patient's suitability for topical anesthesia.[90] However, in my experience, usually patients who are candidates for injectable anesthesia are also candidates for topical anesthetics.[31] Nonetheless, patients who are demented, extremely anxious, or psychotic, or have certain movement disorders, as well as children, may not be candidates for any type of local anesthesia, and a general anesthetic with topical supplement should be considered for them (exceptions to this paradigm will be discussed later). Patients with hearing impairment or language barriers pose special challenges with topical anesthesia.[91] Preoperative counseling is essential, and a family member or friend can help in translation of information when language barriers exist. A predetermined series of signals should be developed between patient and operating room personnel to allow communications during surgery. These issues are discussed further below.

Finally, patients with movement disorders should not automatically be excluded from topical, or, for that matter, injection anesthetic procedures, because these movements are frequently ablated with sedation. Ophthalmic movement disorders (e.g., nystagmus) are frequently ablated with appropriate levels of IV sedation. Therefore, only if a tremor persists after induction of IV sedation should a general anesthetic be considered.

Table 1.1   Complications of Injectable Regional Ophthalmic Anesthesia: Clinical Presentation, Prevention, and Treatment

Complication	Signs and Symptoms	Prevention/Treatment
Perforation and penetration of the globe	Pain, "perfect block," hypotony, marked increase in intraocular pressure, vitreous hemorrhage, retinal detachment, loss of red reflex	Cancel cataract surgery, repair detachment, or hemorrhage as required; avoidance by correct placement and selection of needle
Retrobulbar hemorrhage	Increase in globe and orbit tension ("frozen orbit"), proptosis, conjunctival ballooning with hemorrhage, central retinal artery occlusion	Milder cases: observe, IV osmotic agents, digital pressure on orbit Severe cases: lateral canthotomy, cantholysis, disinsertion of lower fornix Avoidance by correct placement and selection of needle.
Subconjunctival hemorrhage	Ballooning and hemorrhage in anterior conjunctiva	Incise and drain only if interfering with surgeons view; otherwise no treatment
Extraocular muscle paresis	Diplopia with strabismus postoperatively (inferior rectus most likely to be involved with vertical paralytic strabismus)	Prevention by correct needle placement
Brainstem anesthesia	• Respiratory arrest • Cardiopulmonary arrest • Hypertension • Tachycardia • Dysarthria • Confusion • Marked shivering • Convulsions • Loss of consciousness • Hemi-, para-, or quadriplegia • Contralateral blockade of the optic nerve and the third, sixth, and twelfth cranial nerves	
Limitation of ocular blood flow	Loss of vision (difficult to diagnose with concomitant block), retinal artery occlusion	Prevention by avoiding use of epinephrine, judicious use of ocular compression devices, and use of minimal concentration and volume of anesthetics in susceptible individuals
Oculocardiac reflex	Bradycardia, dysrhythmia, nausea, hypertensives crisis, cardiac arrest	Prevention by limiting manipulation of extraocular muscles during general anesthesia, limiting volume of anesthetic during retrobulbar anesthesia Treatment: systemic atropine, local (intraconal) injection of lidocaine
Facial nerve damage	Dysphagia, respiratory distress, permanent facial paralysis	Avoidance of hyaluronidase and deep injection; block during orbital injection with appropriate technique (see text)
Corneal exposure	Open tonic lid, keratitis	Patch with lubricants, patient instruction (see text)
Atonic pupil	Presence of fixed dilated pupil postoperatively	Pilocarpine test (see text); treatment with masking contact lens, iris cerclage (pursestring suture) or insertion of iris prosthesis

Anesthetic for cataract surgery
ESCRS 2006-2013

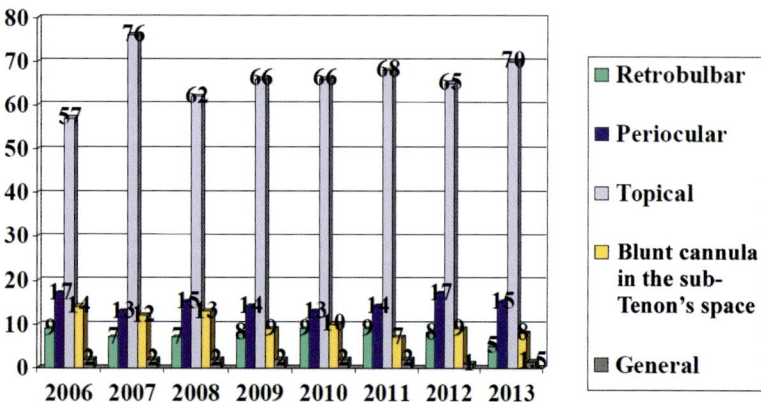

Fig. 1.4 Prevalence of anesthesia techniques. ASCRS, American Society of Cataract and Refractive Surgery; ESCRS, European Society of Cataract and Refractive Surgeons. (From Leaming DV. Practice style and preferences of ESCRS members: 2013 survey. Eurotimes, September 2014.)

ASCRS 2012: Retrobulbar = 7, Periocular = 12, Topical = 78, Blunt cannula = 3, General = 0

Preoperative Medications

Although practices vary considerably in pharmacological preparation for surgery, many surgeons prescribe a regimen of topical NSAIDs, antibiotics, and steroids for up to several days prior to surgery. Immediately prior to surgery, patients may be given a topical NSAID along with a dilation regimen in a single drop, combination drop, or gel formulation. In cases where deeper anesthesia is being considered, a surgical sponge may be soaked with combination of drugs and placed in the fornix (see Rosenthal Deep Topical, Fornix-Based, Nerve Block Anesthesia, below).

The NSAID has been shown to reduce patient discomfort and to aid in maintaining pupillary mydriasis during surgery, presumably by blocking the effect caused by prostaglandins secreted during the inflammatory cascade.

Methods of Noninjection Anesthesia

A brief description of the currently available noninjection and topical anesthesia techniques is useful in understanding the complications that may ensue.

Topical Drop

Knowledge of the topical anesthetic properties of cocaine date back to the 16th century. Pizarro, the Spanish conquistador, first became aware of these properties in the coca leaf. However, it was not until 1888 that the first human eye anesthesia technique was developed by Karl Koller (erroneously spelled "Carl" in some references). Deploying a technique that predates injectable anesthesia, he instilled cocaine onto the ocular surface, following the suggestion of his friend and colleague, Sigmund Freud.[92-96] Although an extremely effective anesthetic, cocaine had significant, sometimes severe, local and systemic toxicity, including severe keratitis and inflammation, hypertension, stroke, and death. Thus, despite the effectiveness and simplicity of topical anesthetics, they were supplanted by injectable anesthetics because of these problems. Additionally, injectable anesthetics provided deep anesthesia and akinesia at a time where comparatively invasive techniques of eye surgery required extensive anesthesia (**Fig. 1.4**).

In 1991, in concert with the development of increasingly noninvasive cataract surgery techniques, Fine et al[97] and Fichman[98] described the use of topical lidocaine as being sufficient and effective in cataract surgery. This technique has gained widespread popularity, especially in patients undergoing uncomplicated clear cornea surgery. In 2013, Leaming[99] surveyed the European Society of Cataract and Refractive Surgeons (ESCRS) membership via email. Among his findings was that 70% of respondents were using topical anesthesia for routine cataract surgery, and the use of retrobulbar anesthesia had decreased to nearly half of its 2006 level (5% down from 9%). By contrast, in 1993 only 4% of the American Society of Cataract and Refractive Surgery (ASCRS) respondents and in 1998 only 37% of respondents preferred topical anesthesia.

Intracameral Anesthesia

A natural evolution of the technique of application to the ocular surface was to instill anesthetic directly into the anterior segment, where abundant pain receptors exist. Fichman also later described, and Gills et al[100] popularized, the concept of instilling 1% lidocaine MPF (methylparaben free) intracameral anesthetics at the onset of the procedure. This alleviated a frequent complaint regarding topical instillation alone—that it may not always provide sufficient pain ablation, particularly with iris manipulation or in longer procedures. Gills and many others found that intracameral instillation alone or as a supplement to topical anesthetics produced an additional measure of anesthesia. Despite the fact that intracameral anesthesia is not, in its strictest sense, a "topical" technique, the approach to the patient using this method is similar to other topical methods and is therefore included in this discussion. Today intracameral anesthesia is often used in concert with topically applied 4% lidocaine for ocular surface anesthesia.

Shugarcaine

In 2006, Joel Shugar introduced an intracameral mixture of 1:1,000 preservative free epinephrine; balanced salt solution enriched with bicarbonate, dextrose, and glutathione, known as

BSS Plus; and 4% preservative free lidocaine in a buffered solution, which he named "Shugarcaine" (**Box 1.1**). This formulation had the advantage of being a nonstinging, physiologically balanced solution, due to being buffered to match the intraocular pH. Perhaps more significantly, it assists in pupillary dilation and increasing the iris sphincter tone in cases of intraoperative floppy iris syndrome (IFIS).[101-103]

Phenylephrine and Ketorolac Injection

Recently a proprietary solution of phenylephrine and ketorolac 1%/0.03% (Omidria; Omeros Corp., Seattle, WA) has been introduced. This mixture is instilled through the infusion line of the phaco machine, and has been reported to improve mydriasis as well as reduce postoperative pain. The ketorolac, an NSAID, inhibits cyclooxygenase enzymes (COX-1 and -2), which results in a decrease in tissue concentrations of prostaglandins, thus reducing pain. Some reports indicate it may be effective at reducing intraoperative pain as well.

Although this drug is costly, it is covered by some insurance carriers.

Rosenthal Deep Topical, Fornix-Based, Nerve Block Anesthesia

Because topical anesthesia alone could be inadequate for more complex or longer cases, I developed a method of anesthesia that combines the safety, comfort, ease of administration, and rapid onset of topical anesthesia with the deep, extensive, anatomic distribution of retrobulbar anesthesia.[104-107] In Rosenthal deep topical, nerve block anesthesia (RDTNBA), an absorbent cellulose sponge is soaked with an anesthetic mixture of 4% lidocaine MPF and 0.75% bupivacaine MPF in a 2:1 ratio. The sponge is then placed deep in the upper and lower fornices (**Fig. 1.5a**), and pressurized by the placement of a pressure device such as Honan's balloon. This encourages absorption of the anesthetic into both adjacent tissues and posteriorly, thus inducing a nerve block (**Fig. 1.5b**).

Because absorption occurs posteriorly into the peribulbar space (and possibly transconally into the retrobulbar space), the posterior ciliary nerves, which supply the anterior sclera, anterior conjunctiva, and limbus, as well as the iris and ciliary body, are anesthetized at their nerve roots.[108-110] The combination of the posterior placement, high concentration of anesthesia, prolonged exposure to the globe, and pressure produces a deep anesthetic effect comparable to injectable techniques. Lidocaine 4% was chosen for RDTNBA because of its low ocular toxicity and its ready commercial availability. In addition, because of its pharmacology, high potency, and ready absorption across mucous membranes[111] as an amide, it tends to bind to protein and is therefore extremely permeable across conjunctival membranes.

Placement of lidocaine 4% into the conjunctival fornix is similar in efficacy to similar placement of cocaine 4%, but with substantially less ocular toxicity. Its duration of action is adequate for most ocular surgical procedures. Selective supplementation with bupivacaine provides prolonged analgesia to control immediate postoperative discomfort. Experience over 7 years has proven this technique to be comparable to injectable methods[112] in the production of deep anesthesia for almost all anterior segment surgery.[113]

Sub-Tenon's or "Parabulbar" Anesthesia

To provide global ocular anesthesia along with akinesia, without needle injection, several techniques have evolved. They fall into

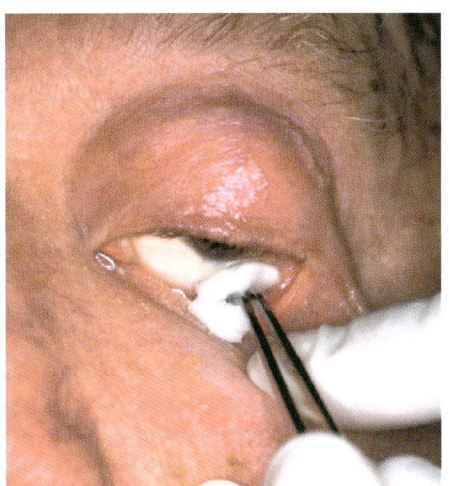
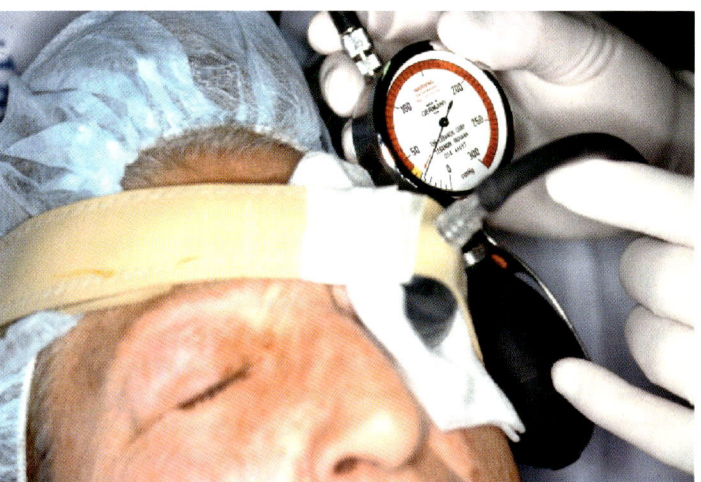

a　　　　　　　　　　　　　　　　　　　　　　　　　b

Fig. 1.5 **(a)** Rosenthal deep topical nerve block anesthesia. A cellulose sponge soaked with anesthetic is placed in the superior fornix. **(b)** Honan's balloon is applied to press anesthetic sponges against the globe.

the category of sub-Tenon's anesthesia and are administered by incising the anterior conjunctiva followed by a posteriorly directed anesthetic injection into the sub-Tenon's space through a blunt metal cannula.

Pinpoint Anesthesia (Fukasaku)

In pinpoint anesthesia, a long, curved, blunt-tipped cannula is inserted into the sub-Tenon's space and directed posteriorly until it reaches the area adjacent to the optic nerve.[114,115] Then the anesthetic agent of choice is injected. This technique provides akinesia as well as anesthesia.

Topical Gel Anesthesia

Topical Xylocaine 2% gel MPF[116–118] applied to the ocular surface prior to starting surgery has been shown to be an effective method of anesthesia for cataract surgery. It also has the added benefit of providing ocular surface lubrication. The gel can be applied for 5 to 30 minutes prior to surgery. No significant ocular surface toxicity has been observed with this method. Additionally the gel anesthetic has proven to be a useful adjunct to the RDTNBA method. The application of a small dollop of gel to the incision at the conclusion of the procedure is extremely effective in alleviating postoperative foreign-body sensation. This is presumably due to its combination of emollient and anesthetic properties.

Systemic Sedation: Balancing The Topical Anesthetic Technique

It is important to recognize that the sole effect of any regional anesthetic, whether administered by needle injection, topical application, or intracameral infusion, is to numb the eye. The role of systemic medication, on the other hand, is to control the behavior of the patient, thus creating an environment in which the patient can be both cooperative and comfortable.

Thus, a patient undergoing cataract surgery should receive the minimum amount of systemic medication required to produce anxiolysis, usually not to the point of creating obtundation with its attendant loss of patients' behavioral control. Not all patients require IV sedation, however, and a calm, comfortable patient can have successful surgery without sedation.[119] The anesthesiologist/anesthetist and the surgeon together should assess the patient's level of initial anxiety and titrate an initial dose of anxiolytic agent. During the surgery, the patient may experience additional anxiety related to feeling pressure or movement within the eye, or less commonly, discomfort or frank pain. Although the local anesthetic agents should be the primary agents of analgesia, it is necessary on occasion to provide a deeper level of sedation, coupled with system narcotics to alleviate pain as well.

The most common unpleasant distraction patients experience is the feeling of pressure within the eye, particularly when entering the eye on irrigation mode. The initial approach should be gentle reassurance of the patient that this is a normal experience and, further, to instruct the patient to identify the sensation as "pressure" rather than "pain." However, additional sedation can be administered to the patient who cannot tolerate this sensation.

Succinctly then, regional anesthetics control pain, and systemic agents regulate behavior. As with injectable methods of anesthesia, oversedation of a patient in an attempt to ablate pain is dangerous and inappropriate.[51] This may sometimes lead to a wildly uncooperative patient and ensuing potential surgical complications. As noted previously, patients who are candidates for injectable anesthesia are also candidates for topical anesthesia.

Conversely, patients who do not tolerate the topical anesthetic approach probably will not do well if converted to injectable block during surgery. Therefore, if the patient's cooperation cannot be secured with mild IV sedation, a light general anesthetic should be administered, while continuing to administer noninjectable regional anesthesia (intracameral or topical) to control pain. With this balanced technique, less general anesthesia can be given, with less risk to the patient and less likelihood of intra- and postoperative complications. The general anesthetic merely keeps the patient tranquil during surgery.

Agents Used in the Administration of Intravenous Sedation

Classically, IV sedation has consisted of a combination of IV narcotic with a hypnotic, typically an opioid, benzodiazepine, and/or propofol. This remains the most common combination anesthesia strategy. The administration of propofol has the added benefit of amnesia. However, any of these combinations, particularly when used in larger quantities for a patient who is uncooperative, excessively anxious, or experiencing pain, can result in cardiorespiratory depression; additionally, propofol requires a steady infusion of medication during the procedure. This is both an advantage and a disadvantage, in that it provides a rapid increase in sedation and rapid cessation in cases where this is required (e.g., uncooperative patient due to too much sedation), but it requires either a mechanical infusion device or constant monitoring by the anesthesiologist.

A newer addition to the sedative armamentarium is dexmedetomidine (Precedex; Hospira Worldwide, Lake Forest, IL). Precedex is a relatively selective α_2-adrenergic agonist widely used in intensive care settings for intubated and mechanically ventilated patients. Precedex is also effective in the surgical setting. It is capable of producing deep sedation without profound disorientation, or alternatively, quiet sedation of a patient without movement. Additionally, it is known to cause significantly less respiratory depression and hypotension at levels of sedation comparable to other agents. Accordingly deep sedation without respiratory support (e.g., intubation) is consistently possible. This drug can be used effectively in patients who suffer from dementia or moderate to severe systemic medical conditions who would be at greater risk for general anesthesia, with less concern about patients becoming combative or uncooperative, as they might when given typical sedative/hypnotics. It can also be used alone, without narcotic, in patients with narcotic sensitivities.

LoMonaco et al[120] studied the use of propofol versus dexmedetomidine in cataract surgery. They found that dexmedetomidine was superior both in terms of intraoperative blood pressure and heart rate stability, and that there was significantly less respiratory depression in the dexmedetomidine group. This underscores its advantage in patients with compromised cardiovascular states, or requiring greater sedation with less concern over cardiorespiratory instability.

Also, as an α-agonist it may be beneficial in counteracting some effects of α-antagonists, implicated in the development of IFIS, and may result in stabilization of the iris during cataract surgery. I am currently evaluating my recent discovery of this drug property in a prospective fellow-eye cohort study.

Significantly, in a survey of anesthetists, patients, and surgeons concerning the efficacy of each method of sedation, all respondents rated the quality of sedation higher for the dexmedetomidine. Probably the only downside to the use of this drug, then, is that it is significantly more costly than the alternatives. The care provider needs to assess the value proposition that this increased cost represents, over the quality of the surgical experience, patient comfort, and safety.

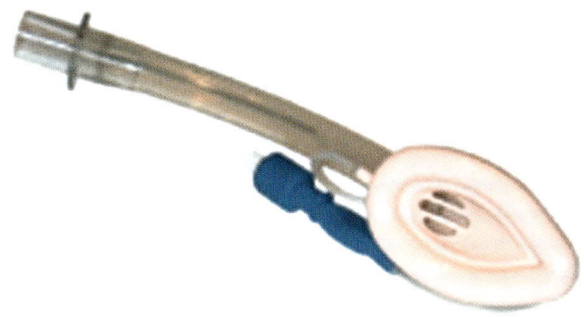

Fig. 1.6 The laryngeal mask airway.

For adult procedural sedation, it is recommended that a loading dose of 1 μg/kg over 10 minutes be given, followed by a maintenance infusion initiated at 0.6 μg/kg/h and titrated to achieve the desired clinical effect with doses ranging from 0.2 to 1 μg/kg/h.

Laryngeal Mask Anesthesia as an Adjunct to Topical Anesthesia

A useful adjunct to topical anesthesia requiring general anesthesia is the laryngeal mask airway (LMA) (**Fig. 1.6**). It was invented in 1981 by Archie Brain[90,121,122] at the London Hospital, Whitechapel, London. The aim was to form a direct connection with the patient's airway. In this way there would be assured greater security and convenience than with only the face mask. This device can be positioned rapidly and noninvasively without the use of a laryngoscope or traditional intubation technique. It does not generally interfere with the vocal cords, so that voice hoarseness does not occur, and it can be used in cases when the decision is made intraoperatively to convert to a general anesthetic.

Intraoperative Finesse: The Patient's Experience

The details of the patient's surgical history should be discussed during the preoperative evaluation in the office and repeated just prior to the patient's being brought to the operating room. Patients should also be reassured that, in the unlikely event that they are uncomfortable, they may tell the surgeon so that the problem can be promptly rectified.

It is important to counsel patients to expect to see bright lights, feel pressure (although not always), and feel the surgeon touching their eyelids. They should be aware that they will be expected to participate by looking in the direction that the surgeon requests.

With this information, and with appropriate intraoperative coaching in the form of calm reassurance, patients will be relaxed and cooperative. Many patients are aware of brilliant, prismatic lights during the surgery. They find these aesthetically pleasing. In fact, patients who are told to expect to see beautiful kaleidoscope-like lights find this an additional source of relaxation.

A remarkable amount of anxiety can be relieved just by telling patients that their experience, even if slightly unpleasant, is routine. It appears that patients' greatest fear is not discomfort but rather that these experiences are the unwarranted anticipation of a poor visual outcome.

The use of local/topical anesthesia in patients with a language barrier entails several requirements: (1) preoperative discussion with the patient using a translator (preferably a trusted friend or family member), (2) use of a translator during the sur-

gery, and (3) profound sedation (see discussion of Precedex, above). In all, a patient with a language barrier should not be deprived of a potentially safer procedure if possible.

The neophyte surgeon will find that the patients best suited for topical anesthesia are the elderly, as they tend to be more cooperative, more stoic, and less anxious, and they require less IV sedation.

The Operating Room Milieu: Making the Patient Comfortable

Patients undergoing topical anesthetic cataract surgery are generally more alert than their injectable anesthetic counterparts. The operating room team should avoid loud and boisterous talk or laughter. Instead, peaceful music should be played. Studies have shown that music played during cataract surgery actually lessens the requirement for IV sedation, and lowers heart rate and blood pressure.[123] Furthermore, surgeon performance is enhanced with music background selected by the surgeon.[124] The concept of "vocal local," that is, verbal reassurance and communication with the patient, is often key to ensuring a comfortable and cooperative patient experience.

Eye Movement

There is no ocular akinesia with topical anesthetic methods. Although the uninitiated may imagine a patient wildly looking about during surgery, in reality this is a very rare occurrence.[125] Most patients, when instructed to keep a steady fixation on the microscope light, or to gaze eccentrically, are able to follow instructions. The ability to cooperate is enhanced with mild IV sedation such as with propofol, or a balanced technique using midazolam and fentanyl.

For the experienced surgeon, the patient's voluntary eye movement becomes a natural and desirable feature of the procedure. Patient cooperation is excellent in most cases and obviates stretching the EOMs to produce the desired globe position. For example, the patient is encouraged to look directly into the microscope light during capsulorrhexis and phacoemulsification, and downward during incision and IOL insertion. The lack of EOM stretching may account for the rarity of surgically induced ptosis. In patients who have trouble self-positioning their eye, the surgeon must gently grasp and move the eye to the desired position (with the patient's cooperation). The patient is then requested to maintain that position. The eye is never forced into position, however; as in the unanesthetized EOM, the afferent limb of the oculocardiac reflex is intact, and stretching it may provoke bradycardia.

It is helpful to instruct the patient to keep the companion eye open during the procedure. Instillation of topical anesthetic in the companion eye prior to surgery is helpful in reducing the blink reflex and improves cooperation.

Virtual-Reality Fixation Device

To further aid in control of eye movement during anterior segment surgery, I have developed a virtual-reality fixation device (**Fig. 1.7**). This is a miniature computer monitor and visual simulation program that is presented to the companion eye during surgery. Static visual images can be used as fixation targets for patients who have retained ocular motility. The enhanced ability for patients to participate in surgery by controlling their eye movement facilitates the performance of surgical maneuvers and obviates the need for fixation instruments. Because a virtual image is projected out into space, the patient's sense of claustrophobia

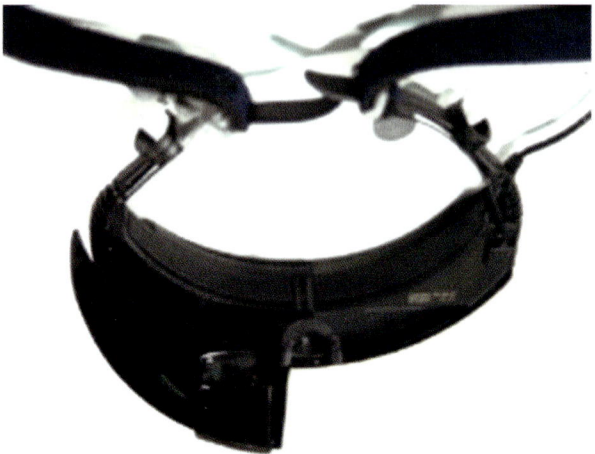

Fig. 1.7 The virtual-reality headset is placed in front of the unoperated eye. A small video monitor is mounted under the visor, causing a virtual image to be projected out into space in front of the patient.

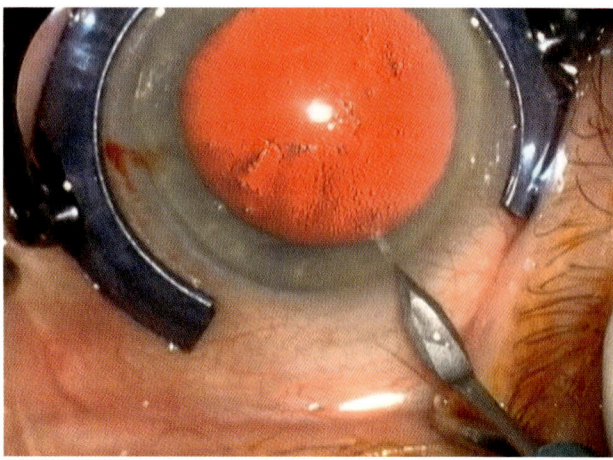

Fig. 1.8 A Fine-Thornton fixation ring stabilizes the globe with little uncomfortable external pressure and provides excellent countertraction for anterior chamber entry.

is diminished, thus enhancing the surgical experience. The requirement that the patient open the fellow eye also discourages squeezing against the eyelid speculum in the operated eye. Visual images such as scenes from nature can be delivered to encourage relaxation. The images can even be coordinated with auditory stimuli by an earpiece fitted in the ipsilateral ear. The ability to provide nonpharmacological relaxation by this means reduces the amount of IV sedation required compared with surgery without the device in the companion eye.[126] New technological developments, for example "Google Glass," may, if appropriately modified, provide further avenue for patient fixation and relaxation devices.

Complications Arising from Eye Movement

Inadvertent eye movement may be the result of inadequate anesthesia, but more often it is a manifestation of anxiety. Intravenous sedation as an appropriate adjunct is therefore essential. Unanticipated eye movement may create problems at any stage of the procedure. During creation of the incision, especially with super-sharp diamond knives, it is possible to extend the incision. A sudden movement during capsulorrhexis may cause it to tear into the equator. Posterior capsular rupture may occur during phacoemulsification, irrigation and aspiration (I/A), or IOL insertion.

One method to avoid unexpected eye movement is to gently stabilize the eye with a second instrument. This is accomplished by fixation of the globe with an atraumatic instrument; a Fine-Thornton fixation ring (**Fig. 1.8**), a cotton-tipped applicator, or an open 0.12-mm forceps placed 180 degrees from the incision can stabilize the globe. Once incisions are made, instruments placed in them can be used to "oarlock" the globe during phacoemulsification.

Alternatively, incision extension may be avoided by the use of diamond blades with unsharpened parallel sides (**Fig. 1.9**). The diamond blade enables a swift incision without tissue drag. Once inserted, the blunt parallel sides of the blade are within the incision, so that any lateral movement of the blade will fail to extend the incision.

Inadvertent movement during phaco, I/A, and IOL insertion can be similarly avoided by the use of two instruments, one through the phaco incision and the other through the paracen-

tesis incision. This will act to create an "oarlock," preventing voluntary ocular movement.

Posterior capsular rupture using topical anesthesia is rare. My experience is that the posterior capsule is torn less commonly than with retrobulbar anesthesia. The reason for this may lie in evolving improvement of surgical techniques, instrumentation, and perhaps the surgeon's heightened awareness of the patient's potential for movement.

Piovella et al[127] and Uusitalo et al[128] have collected data to demonstrate that complications secondary to eye movement occur more frequently during the early phase of the learning curve. However, with proper patient instruction and with the development over time of a "second sense" of anticipating patient eye movement, these potential problems can be reduced.

Eyelid Squeezing, Photophobia, and Phototoxicity

Any anesthesia technique that does not block the seventh cranial nerve creates the potential for squeezing. This can be overcome

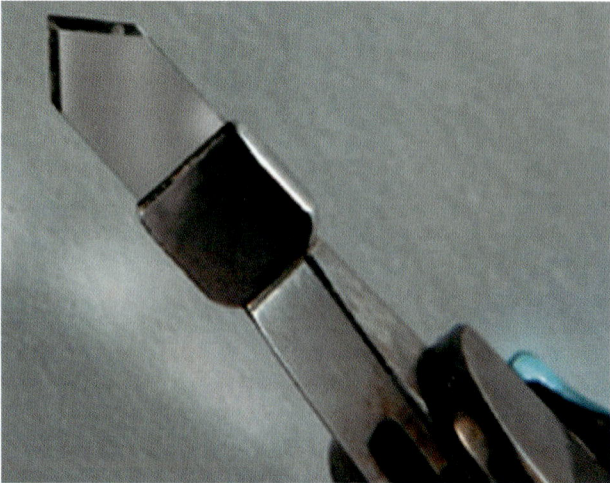

Fig. 1.9 Diamond blade with blunt parallel sides affords protection from inadvertent lateral extension of the wound.

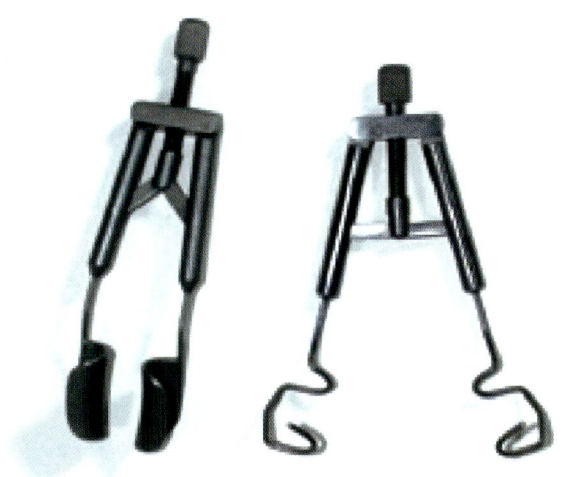

Fig. 1.10 The Lieberman speculum can be placed in the closed position and gradually opened to produce the optimal amount of lid separation.

by using an adjustable speculum such as the Lieberman design (**Fig. 1.10**), which incorporates an adjustable thumbscrew that can be gradually opened against the lid margins. Initially the speculum is opened to the minimum lid aperture needed to expose that required for surgery. However, if the patient continues to squeeze against the speculum, it should be opened as wide as necessary, as this gradual opening will ultimately ablate the patient's squeezing. Perhaps counterintuitively, then, wider opening of the speculum produces less orbicularis oculi contraction; the orbicularis muscle is extended to the end of its length/tension curve. Therefore, there is the least overlap of myosin and actin filaments. This will result in weakening of the patient's ability to squeeze.

Additionally, when RDTNBA is employed, and although it has less motor neuron effect than retrobulbar anesthesia, some globe and lid "hypokinesia" is seen with this technique.

Light sensitivity must be considered during topical anesthesia surgery. Topical anesthesia does not cause amaurosis. Consequently, excessive intensity of the microscope light will be uncomfortable for the patient. For that reason, the microscope light intensity must be turned to a low setting initially, and then gradually increased only to the level necessary for visualization. In so doing, the surgeon soon will realize that much less light is needed to perform surgery than originally believed.

Light sensitivity may have an important protective benefit as well. It can be implied that a light too bright to look at with the nonamaurotic eye is, in all probability, also too bright for the amaurotic eye (e.g., after injectable block). A lower microscope light will result in decreased light toxicity from the operating microscope.[129]

Conjunctival Ballooning

This problem is unique to subconjunctival or sub-Tenon's anesthetic techniques. The conjunctiva, upon injection with the anesthetic mixture, may become tumescent and interfere with surgical access and visualization. The fluid increases over time. Eventually the trapped fluid over the cornea forms a minus lens interfering with visualization. This problem is often avoided by the use of a Greenbaum-style cannula,[130,131] which features an enlarged hub. This hub can be used to engage and seal the conjunctival opening, directing fluid posteriorly.

Toxicity of Topical Agents

The availability of relatively nontoxic, effective topical and intracameral drugs has resulted in an acceptable risk/benefit ratio. However, all routes of administration carry some potential risks.

Intracameral Toxicity

Intracameral concentrations of anesthetics may reach as much as 250 times the concentration in the anterior chamber as may be achieved with topical administration. This gives rise to concerns about potential toxicity. Systemic absorption and toxicity of the drug given intracamerally is insignificant.[132] Garcia et al,[133] Elvira et al,[134] Masket and Gokmen,[135] and Gills[136] report no change in endothelial cell counts in humans with 1% lidocaine MPF. Sun et al [137] studied the effects of both lidocaine and bupivacaine and found no toxic corneal effects. However, a study by Anderson et al[138] in the rabbit model found that endothelial cell damage can occur with instillation of bupivacaine 0.5% unless diluted 1:1 with glutathione bicarbonate Ringer's solution. The same study compared clinical pain scores in humans with lidocaine versus bupivacaine and found the drugs to be similar in efficacy, suggesting therefore that lidocaine is the preferred drug for intracameral use.

Studies by Judge et al[139] found that bupivacaine 0.75%, lidocaine 4%, and proparacaine all caused corneal clouding and increased corneal thickness for up to 7 weeks in an animal model. Therefore, lidocaine 1% MPF is the ideal agent for intracameral use. Lidocaine instilled intravitreally will temporarily affect visual acuity,[140] and electroretinographic activity; however, no permanent functional or histological changes occur.[141] These findings confirm the clinical occurrence of transient but reversible loss of vision after intracameral instillation of lidocaine in the presence of a broken capsule. The demonstration that intracameral agents may be toxic to the endothelium may suggest a narrow therapeutic/toxic ratio of which the surgeon should be cognizant.

Topical Toxicity
Anesthetic Agents

Of the topical agents in use, tetracaine has the most potential for causing superficial punctate keratitis. However, this problem has been associated with almost all topical anesthetics (D. Davis, personal communication) (**Fig. 1.11**). Repeated or excessive administration of topical agents can produce superficial punctate keratitis (SPK) sufficiently severe to interfere with visualization of the anterior chamber structures during surgery.[141,142] The substitution of lidocaine gel 2% MPF may be considered as an acceptable alternative and may obviate this problem. Marcaine 0.75% may be mucogenic in susceptible patients, thus interfering with visualization as well (S. Masket, personal communication).

Hyaluronidase

A potential hazard of working in a surgical suite where a variety of anesthetic and surgical techniques are employed is that of confusion regarding anesthetic mixtures. I have reported three consecutive cases of moderately severe epithelial keratitis.[143] The diffuse nature of the clinical presentation led me to suspect, and later confirm, that sodium hyaluronidase had been mixed with the usual unpreserved lidocaine and bupivacaine and was intended for another surgeon who was using retrobulbar anesthetic. A first-day postoperative photograph (**Fig. 1.12**) of one of these patients shows the sloughing epithelium and keratitis,

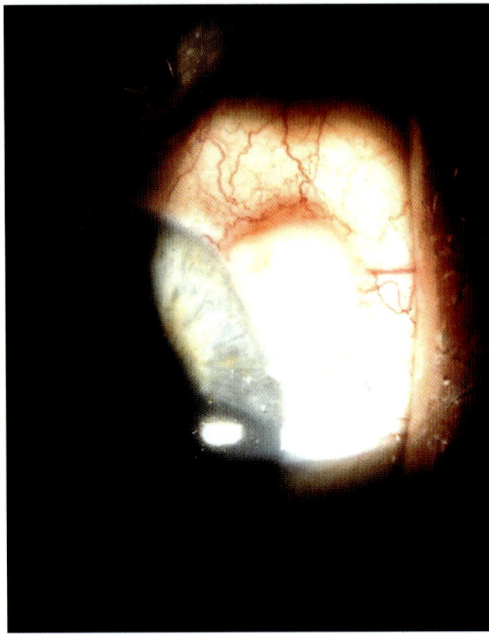

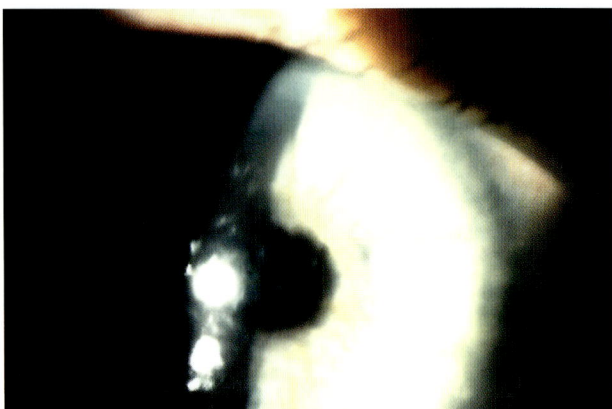

Fig. 1.12 Corneal epithelial sloughing on the first postoperative day following inadvertent administration of hyaluronidase.

Fig. 1.11 Presumed corneal and conjunctival toxicity from lidocaine.

which resolved in about a week with judicious debridement of loose epithelium, bandage contact lenses, topical NSAID, and antibiotic (**Fig. 1.12**).

Conclusion

The evolution of less invasive methods of cataract surgery has been successfully coupled with less invasive and safer methods of anesthesia. The result is less risk to the patient, more rapid visual recovery, and consequently earlier return to normal daily activities. A proper respect for, and understanding of, the limitations and requirements of these techniques will provide satisfactory results.

References

1. Eke T, Thompson JR. National survey of Local Anaesthesia for Ocular Surgery: early report. London: Audit Committee, Royal College of Ophthalmologists; 1997

2. Eke T, Thompson JR. National survey of Local Anaesthesia for Ocular Surgery. II. Safety profiles of local anaesthesia techniques. Eye (Lond) 1999; 13(Pt 2):196–204

3. Kamath G, Prasad S, Clearkin L. The national survey of local anaesthesia for ocular surgery: early report (letter). Eye (Lond) 1998;12(Pt 3a):489

4. Gillow JT, Kirkby GR. Ophthalmic local anesthesia. (letter) Ophthalmology 1999;106:858

5. Yashar AG. Teamwork, rapport keep surgeons out of court. Ophthalmology Times, March 1, 1999

6. Wong DHW. Ophthalmic anaesthesia in the 21st century. Lecture at the inaugural meeting of the British Ophthalmic Anaesthesia Society, Middlesbrough, UK, June 1999

7. Hustead RF, Hamilton RC, Loken RG. Periocular local anesthesia: medial orbital as an alternative to superior nasal injection. J Cataract Refract Surg 1994;20:197–201

8. Gillow JT, Aggarwal RK, Kirkby GR. Ocular perforation during peribulbar anaesthesia. Eye (Lond) 1996;10(Pt 5):533–536

9. Schein OD, Katz J, Bass EB, et al; Study of Medical Testing for Cataract Surgery. The value of routine preoperative medical testing before cataract surgery. N Engl J Med 2000;342:168–175

10. Rosenfeld SI, Litinsky SM, Snyder DA, Plosker H, Astrove AW, Schiffman J. Effectiveness of monitored anesthesia care in cataract surgery. Ophthalmology 1999;106:1256–1260, discussion 1261

11. Walters G, McKibbin M. The value of pre-operative investigations in local anaesthetic ophthalmic surgery. Eye (Lond) 1997;11(Pt 6):847–849

12. Eke T, Thompson JR. The National Survey of Local Anaesthesia for Ocular Surgery. Eye (Lond) 1998;12(Pt 4):750

13. Rubin AP. Complications of local anaesthesia for ophthalmic surgery. Br J Anaesth 1995;75:93–96

14. Barry P, moderator. Anaesthesia revisited. Symposium at the annual meeting of the European Society of Cataract and Refractive Surgeons, Nice, France, September 1998

15. Hamilton RH, Grizzard WS. Complications. In: Gills JP, Hustead RF, Sanders, DR, eds. Ophthalmic Anesthesia. Thorofare, NJ: Slack; 1993:187–202

16. Wilson RP. Complications associated with local and general ophthalmic anesthesia. Int Ophthalmol Clin 1992;32:1–22

17. Rosen E. Editorial review: anesthesia for cataract surgery. Eur J Implant Ref Surg 1993;5:1

18. O'Brien HD. Anesthesia for cataract surgery. Am J Ophthalmol 1964;57: 751–760

19. Pearce JL. General and local anaesthesia in eye surgery. Trans Ophthalmol Soc U K 1982;102(Pt 1):31–34

20. Adams AK, Jones RM. Anaesthesia for eye surgery: general considerations. Br J Anaesth 1980;52:663–669

21. Smith DC, Crul JF. Oxygen desaturation following sedation for regional analgesia. Br J Anaesth 1989;62:206–209

22. Neima D, Ramsey MS. Systemic illnesses in cataract patients: 1. Incidence. Can J Ophthalmol 1987;22:165–167

23. Backer CL, Tinker JH, Robertson DM, Vlietstra RE. Myocardial reinfarction following local anesthesia for ophthalmic surgery. Anesth Analg 1980;59: 257–262

24. Rao TLK, Jacobs KH, El-Etr AA. Reinfarction following anesthesia in patients with myocardial infarction. Anesthesiology 1983;59:499–505

25. Petruscak J, Smith RB, Breslin P. Mortality related to ophthalmological surgery. Arch Ophthalmol 1973;89:106–109

26. Quigley HA. Mortality associated wit ophthalmic surgery:a twenty year experience. Am J Ophthalmol 1974;77:517

27. Watson D. Hyaluronidase. Br J Anaesth 1993;71:422–425

28. Prosser DP, Rodney GE, Mian T, Jones HM, Khan MY. Re-evaluation of hyaluronidase in peribulbar anaesthesia. Br J Ophthalmol 1996;80:827–830

29. Gillow JT, Aggarwal RK, Kirkby GR. A survey of ocular perforation during ophthalmic local anaesthesia in the United Kingdom. Eye (Lond) 1996; 10(Pt 5):537–538

30. Jindra LF. Blindness following retrobulbar anesthesia for astigmatic keratotomy. Ophthalmic Surg 1989;20:433–435

31. Jackson PW. In support of general anesthesia for cataract surgery. Eur J Implant Refract Surg 1994;5:17–19

32. Ramsay RC, Knobloch WH. Ocular perforation following retrobulbar anesthesia for retinal detachment surgery. Am J Ophthalmol 1978;86:61–64

33. Davis DB 2nd, Mandel MR. Efficacy and complication rate of 16,24 consecutive peribulbar blocks. A prospective multicenter study. J Cataract Refract Surg 1994;20:327–337

34. David DB, Mandel MR. Anterior peribulbar. Ophthal Clin NA 1998;11(1):123–124

35. Teichmann KD, Uthoff D. Retrobulbar (intraconal) anesthesia with a curved needle: technique and results. J Cataract Refract Surg 1994;20:54–60

36. Honan PR. New safety valve for Honan balloon. J Am Intraocul Implant Soc 1982;8:163

37. Honan PR. New single-use Honan balloon. J Am Intraocul Implant Soc 1985;11:496–497

38. Honan PR. Preoperative ocular compression. (letter) J Cataract Refract Surg 1999;25:607

39. Duker JS, Belmont JB, Benson WE, et al. Inadvertent globe perforation during retrobulbar and peribulbar anesthesia. Patient characteristics, surgical management, and visual outcome. Ophthalmology 1991;98:519–526

40. Curtin BJ. The Myopias: Basic Science and Clinical Management. Philadelphia: Harper and Row; 1987:247–251

41. Cheng HM, Singh OS, Kwong KK, Xiong J, Woods BT, Brady TJ. Shape of the myopic eye as seen with high-resolution magnetic resonance imaging. Optom Vis Sci 1992;69:698–701

42. Edge R, Navon S. Scleral perforation during retrobulbar and peribulbar anesthesia: risk factors and outcome in 50,000 consecutive injections. J Cataract Refract Surg 1999;25:1237–1244

43. Fanning GL. Ocular perforation: causes, consequences and strategies for prevention. Presented at the annual meeting of the Ophthalmic Anesthesia Society, Chicago, October 1999

44. Hustead RF. The Wichita technique. In: Gills JP, Hustead RF, Sanders DR, eds. Ophthalmic Anesthesia. Thorofare, NJ: Slack; 1993:141–145

45. Bullock JD, Warwar RE, Green WR. Ocular explosion during cataract surgery: a clinical, histopathological, experimental, and biophysical study. Trans Am Ophthalmol Soc 1998;96:243–276, discussion 276–281

46. Waller SG, Taboada J, O'Connor P. Retrobulbar anesthesia risk. Ophthalmology 1993;100(4):506–510

47. Morgan CM, Schatz H, Vine AK, et al. Ocular complications associated with retrobulbar injections. Ophthalmology 1988;95:660–665

48. Edge KR, Nicoll JMV. Retrobulbar hemorrhage after 12,500 retrobulbar blocks. Anesth Analg 1993;76:1019–1022

49. Goldsmith MO. Occlusion of the central retinal artery following retrobulbar hemorrhage. Ophthalmologica 1967;153:191–196

50. Kraushar MF, Seelenfreund MH, Freilich DB. Central retinal artery closure during orbital hemorrhage from retrobulbar injection. Trans Am Acad Ophtalmol Otolaryngol 1974;78:OP65–70

51. Katsev DA, Drews RC, Rose BT. An anatomic study of retrobulbar needle path length. Ophthalmology 1989;96:1221–1224

52. Hamilton RC. Complications of ophthalmic regional anesthesia. Ophthalmol Clin North Am 1998;11:99–114

53. Huha T, Ala-Kokko TI, Salomäki T, Alahuhta S. Clinical efficacy and pharmacokinetics of 1% ropivacaine and 0.75% bupivacaine in peribulbar anaesthesia for cataract surgery. Anaesthesia 1999;54:137–141

54. Hamed LM. Strabismus presenting after cataract surgery. Ophthalmology 1991;98:247–252

55. Brown SM, Brooks SE, Mazow ML, et al. Cluster of diplopia cases after periocular anesthesia without hyaluronidase. J Cataract Refract Surg 1999;25:1245–1249

56. Hamed LM, Mancuso A. Inferior rectus muscle contracture syndrome after retrobulbar anesthesia. Ophthalmology 1991;98:1506–1512

57. Ong-Tone L, Pearce WG. Inferior rectus muscle restriction after retrobulbar anesthesia for cataract extraction. Can J Ophthalmol 1989;24:162–165

58. Carlson BM, Emerick S, Komorowski TE, Rainin EA, Shepard BM. Extraocular muscle regeneration in primates. Local anesthetic-induced lesions. Ophthalmology 1992;99:582–589

59. Porter JD, Edney DP, McMahon EJ, Burns LA. Extraocular myotoxicity of the retrobulbar anesthetic bupivacaine hydrochloride. Invest Ophthalmol Vis Sci 1988;29:163–174

60. Rosenblatt RM, May DR, Barsoumian K. Cardiopulmonary arrest after retrobulbar block. Am J Ophthalmol 1980;90:425–427

61. Javitt JC, Addiego R, Friedberg HL, Libonati MM, Leahy JJ. Brain stem anesthesia after retrobulbar block. Ophthalmology 1987;94:718–724

62. Rosen WJ. Brainstem anesthesia presenting as dysarthria. J Cataract Refract Surg 1999;25:1170–1171

63. Hamilton RC, Gimbel HV, Strunin L. Regional anaesthesia for 12,000 cataract extraction and intraocular lens implantation procedures. Can J Anaesth 1988;35:615–623

64. Hamilton RC. Brain-stem anesthesia as a complication of regional anesthesia for ophthalmic surgery. Can J Ophthalmol 1992;27:323–325

65. Hamilton RC. Brain stem anesthesia following retrobulbar blockade. Anesthesiology 1985;63:688–690

66. Antoszyk AN, Buckley EG. Contralateral decreased visual acuity and extraocular muscle palsies following retrobulbar anesthesia. Ophthalmology 1986;93:462–465

67. Pautler SE, Grizzard WS, Thompson LN, Wing GL. Blindness from retrobulbar injection into the optic nerve. Ophthalmic Surg 1986;17:334–337

68. Findl O, Dallinger S, Menapace R, et al. Effects of peribulbar anesthesia on ocular blood flow in patients undergoing cataract surgery. Am J Ophthalmol 1999;127:645–649

69. Buys NS. Mercury balloon reducer for vitreous and orbital volume control. In: Emery J, ed. Current Concepts in Cataract Surgery. St. Louis: CV Mosby; 1980:258

70. Davidson B, Kratz RP, Mazzocco TR, Maloney WF. An evaluation of the Honan intraocular pressure reducer. J Am Intraocul Implant Soc 1979;5:237

71. Drews RC. The Nerf ball for preoperative reduction of intraocular pressure. Ophthalmic Surg 1982;13:761

72. Palay DA, Stulting RD. The effect of external ocular compression on intraocular pressure following retrobulbar anesthesia. Ophthalmic Surg 1990;21:503–507

73. Zabel RW, Clarke WN, Shirley SY, Rock W. Intraocular pressure reduction prior to retrobulbar injection of anesthetic. Ophthalmic Surg 1988;19:868–871

74. Carl JR. Optic neuropathy following cataract extraction. Semin Ophthalmol 1993;8:144

75. Sugin SL, Yannuzzi LA. Choroidal ischemia following intraocular surgery. Semin Ophthalmol 1993;8:149,150

76. Hørven I. Ophthalmic artery pressure during retrobulbar anaesthesia. Acta Ophthalmol (Copenh) 1978;56:574–586

77. Jedeikin RJ, Hoffman S. The oculocardiac reflex in eye-surgery anesthesia. Anesth Analg 1977;56:333–334

78. Katz RL, Bigger JT Jr. Cardiac arrhythmias during anesthesia and operation. Anesthesiology 1970;33:193–213

79. Lindquist TD, Kopietz LA, Spigelman AV, Nichols BD, Lindstrom RL. Complications of Nadbath facial nerve block and a review of the literature. Ophthalmic Surg 1988;19:271–273

80. Nadbath RP, Rehmani. Facial nerve block. Am J Ophthalmol 1963;55:143–146

81. Kaplan LJ, Jaffe NS, Clayman HM. Ptosis and cataract surgery. A multivariant computer analysis of a prospective study. Ophthalmology 1985;92:237–242

82. Laws DE, Watts MT, Kirkby GR, Lawson J. Is padding necessary after cataract extraction? Br J Ophthalmol 1989;73:699–701

83. Friedberg HL. Use shorter needle behind globe to avoid persistent mydriasis. Ophthalmol Times 1988; 13:16,39

84. Lam S, Beck RW, Hall D, Creighton JB. Atonic pupil after cataract surgery. Ophthalmology 1989;96:589–590

85. Leaming DV. Practice styles and preferences of ASCRS members—1998 survey. J Cataract Refract Surg 1999;25:851–859

86. Claoué C, Lanigan C. Topical anaesthesia for cataract surgery. Aust N Z J Ophthalmol 1997;25:265–268

87. Claoué C. Simplicity and complexity in topical anesthesia for cataract surgery. [comment] J Cataract Refract Surg 1998;24:1546–1547

88. Jayamanne DG, Allen ED, Wood CM, Currie S. Correlation between early, measurable improvement in quality of life and speed of visual rehabilitation after phacoemulsification. J Cataract Refract Surg 1999;25:1135–1139

89. Dinsmore SC. Drop, then decide approach to topical anesthesia. [see comments] J Cataract Refract Surg 1995;21:666–671

90. Brain AI. The laryngeal mask—a new concept in airway management. Br J Anaesth 1983;55:801–805

91. Bernstein RM. Topical anesthesia in patients with communication deficits. [letter] J Cataract Refract Surg 1995;21:487–488

92. Herschfeld JJ. Carl Koller and the discovery of local anesthesia. Bull Hist Dent 1986;34:122–127

93. Liljestrand G. Carl Koller and the development of local anesthesia. Acta Physiol Scand Suppl 1967;299:1–30

94. Moore DC, Bridenbaugh LD, Bridenbaugh PO, Tucker GT. Bupivacaine. A review of 2,077 cases. JAMA 1970;214:713–718

95. Koller C. Ueber die Verwendung des Cocain zur Anas thesirung am Auge. Wien Med Wochenschr 1884;34:1276–1278, 1309–1311

96. Breathnach CS. Biographical sketches—45. Koller. Ir Med J 1984;77:335

97. Fine IH, Fichman RA, Grabow HB. Patient selection in topical anesthesia. In: Fine IH, Fichman RA, Grabow HB, eds. Clear Corneal Cataract Surgery and Topical Anesthesia. Thorofare, NJ: Slack; 1993:101–105

98. Fichman R. Topical anesthesia in cataract surgery. Presented at the annual meeting of the American Society of Cataract and Refractive Surgery, 1992

99. Leaming DV. Practice style and preferences of ESCRS members: 2013 survey. Eurotimes, September 2014

100. Gills JP, Cherchio M, Raanan MG. Unpreserved lidocaine to control discomfort during cataract surgery using topical anesthesia. J Cataract Refract Surg 1997;23:545–550

101. Shugar JK. Use of epinephrine for IFIS prophylaxis. J Cataract Refract Surg 2006;32:1074–1075

102. Shugar JK. Intracameral epinephrine for IFIS prophylaxis. Cataract & Refractive Surgery Today. 2006;6:7274

103. Shugar JK. Prophylaxis for IFIS. J Cataract Refract Surg 2007;33:942–943

104. Rosenthal KJ. Rosenthal deep topical, pressurized, fornix applied "nerve block" anesthesia. In: Video Textbook of Viscosurgery, vol 4. Piscataway, NJ: Kabi Pharmacia; 1995

105. Rosenthal KJ. Deep, topical, nerve-block anesthesia. [see comments] J Cataract Refract Surg 1995;21:499–503

106. Rosenthal KJ. Rosenthal deep topical, fornix applied, pressurized, "nerve block" anesthesia. Ophthalmol Clin North Am 1998;11:137–143

107. Rosenthal KJ. Four ways to approach topical anesthesia. Rev Ophthalmol 3:82–84

108. Hustead RF, Kornneef L, Zonneveld FW. Anatomy. In: Gills JP, Hustead RF, Sanders DR, eds. Ophthalmic Anesthesia. Thorofare, NJ: Slack; 1993:63

109. Srinivasan BD, Jakobiec FA, Iwamoto T. Conjunctival anatomy. In: Duane TD, Jaeger EA, eds. Biomedical Foundations of Ophthalmology, vol 1. Philadelphia: Harper and Row; 1985:23

110. Reeh MJ. The globe. In: Jones LT, Reeh MJ, Wirtschafter JD, eds. Ophthalmic Anatomy: A Manual with Some Clinical Applications. Rochester, MN: American Academy of Ophthalmology and Otolaryngology; 1970:105

111. Ahmed I, Patton TF. Importance of the noncorneal absorption route in topical ophthalmic drug delivery. Invest Ophthalmol Vis Sci 1985;26:584–587

112. Aziz ES, Samra A. Prospective evaluation of deep topical fornix nerve block anesthesia versus peribulbar nerve block anesthesia in patients undergoing cataract surgery using phacoemulsification. Presented at the inaugural meeting of the British Ophthalmic Anaesthesia Society, Middlesbrough, England, June 1999

113. Rosenthal KJ. A North American approach to topical anesthesia. Presented at the inaugural meeting of the British Ophthalmic Anaesthesia Society, Middlesbrough, England, June 1999

114. Fukasaku H. Sub-tenon's pinpoint anesthesia. Ophthal Clin NA 1998; 11(1):127–129

115. Fukasaku H, Marron JA. Pinpoint anesthesia: a new approach to local ocular anesthesia. J Cataract Refract Surg 1994;20:468–471

116. Assia EI, Pras E, Yehezkel M, Rotenstreich Y, Jager-Roshu S. Topical anesthesia using lidocaine gel for cataract surgery. J Cataract Refract Surg 1999;25:635–639

117. Barequet IS, Soriano ES, Green WR, O'Brien TP. Provision of anesthesia with single application of lidocaine 2% gel. J Cataract Refract Surg 1999; 25:626–631

118. Koch PS. Efficacy of lidocaine 2% jelly as a topical agent in cataract surgery. J Cataract Refract Surg 1999;25:632–634

119. Fichman RA. Use of topical anesthesia alone in cataract surgery. J Cataract Refract Surg 1996;22:612–614

120. LoMonaco EA, et al. Dexmedetomidine versus propofol in older adults having cataract surgery. Proceedings of the annual meeting of the American Society of Anesthesiologists, 2009

121. Brain AI. The laryngeal mask for intraocular surgery. [Letter; comment] Br J Anaesth 1993;71:772

122. Poloch A, Romaniuk W, Jałowiecki P, Krawczyk L, Wylegała E, Dyaczyńska-Herman A. [Evaluation of the usefulness of the laryngeal mask for general anesthesia in eye microsurgery—preliminary results]. Klin Oczna 1996; 98:45–49

123. Allen K. Effects of music on patients undergoing cataract surgery. Presented at the annual meeting of the American Psychosomatic Society, 1998

124. Allen K, Blascovich J. Effects of music on cardiovascular reactivity among surgeons. [Published erratum appears in JAMA 1994;272:1724] [see comments] JAMA 1994;272:882–884

125. Strobel I, Hühnermann M. [Eyedrop anesthesia in cataract surgery]. Ophthalmologe 1996;93:68–72

126. Rosenthal K. Use of virtual reality device for patient regulation during eye surgery. Presented at the annual meeting of the American Society of Cataract and Refractive Surgery, Boston, May 1997

127. Piovella M, Camesasca FI, Gratton I. Six years of phacoemulsfication with topical anesthesia: long term results and frequency of complications. Presented at the annual meeting of the American Society of Cataract and Refractive Surgery, Seattle, April 1999

128. Uusitalo RJ, Maunuksela EL, Paloheimo M, Kallio H, Laatikainen L. Converting to topical anesthesia in cataract surgery. J Cataract Refract Surg 1999;25:432–440

129. Byrnes GA, Chang B, Loose I, Miller SA, Benson WE. Prospective incidence of photic maculopathy after cataract surgery. Am J Ophthalmol 1995; 119:231–232

130. Greenbaum S. Parabulbar anesthesia. Am J Ophthalmol 1992;114:776

131. Greenbaum S. Parabulbar anesthesia. Ophthalmol Clin North Am 1998; 2:131–132

132. Wirbelauer C, Iven H, Bastian C, Laqua H. Systemic levels of lidocaine after intracameral injection during cataract surgery. J Cataract Refract Surg 1999;25:648–651

133. Garcia A, Loureiro F, Limão A, Sampaio A, Ilharco J. Preservative-free lidocaine 1% anterior chamber irrigation as an adjunct to topical anesthesia. J Cataract Refract Surg 1998;24:403–406

134. Elvira JC, Hueso JR, Martínez-Toldos J, Mengual E, Artola A. Induced endothelial cell loss in phacoemulsification using topical anesthesia plus intracameral lidocaine. J Cataract Refract Surg 1999;25:640–642

135. Masket S, Gokmen F. Efficacy and safety of intracameral lidocaine as a supplement to topical anesthesia. J Cataract Refract Surg 1998;24:956–960

136. Gills JP. Corneal endothelial toxicity of topical anesthesia. [Letter; comment] Ophthalmology 1998;105:1126–1127

137. Sun R, Hamilton RC, Gimbel HV. Comparison of 4 topical anesthetic agents for effect and corneal toxicity in rabbits. J Cataract Refract Surg 1999; 25:1232–1236

138. Anderson NJ, Nath R, Anderson CJ, Edelhauser HF. Comparison of preservative-free bupivacaine vs. lidocaine for intracameral anesthesia: a randomized clinical trial and in vitro analysis. Am J Ophthalmol 1999;127: 393–402

139. Judge AJ, Najafi K, Lee DA, Miller KM. Corneal endothelial toxicity of topical anesthesia. [see comments] Ophthalmology 1997;104:1373–1379

140. Hoffman RS, Fine IH. Transient no light perception visual acuity after intracameral lidocaine injection. J Cataract Refract Surg 1997;23:957–958

141. Liang C, Peyman GA, Sun G. Toxicity of intraocular lidocaine and bupivacaine. Am J Ophthalmol 1998;125:191–196

142. Koyama T. Lidocaine keratopathy. Video J Cataract Refract Surg 1999;15

143. Rosenthal KJ. Presumed hyaluronidase (Wydase) toxicity following cataract surgery with Rosenthal deep topical anesthesia. Video J Cataract Refract Surg 1999;15

2 Systemic Complications of Ophthalmic Anesthesia

Marc L. Leib

Although there has been significant growth in the use of topical anesthesia for cataract surgery, the role of anesthesia providers has not diminished.[1] Even under topical anesthesia, the proper preoperative evaluation of the patient, sedation before and during the procedure, and intraoperative monitoring all contribute to the prevention of systemic complications from ophthalmic anesthesia. A full discussion of anesthesia is beyond the scope of this chapter, but a brief overview of systemic complications is presented.

According to several studies, ~ 90% of cataract patients are over 50 years of age and two thirds are over 65. It is not uncommon to perform such operations on patients over 80 years of age. Therefore, many of the anesthesia considerations are those found in any procedure involving elderly patients. Older patients undergoing ophthalmic surgery frequently have concomitant conditions that should be evaluated preoperatively to determine whether those coexisting conditions are reasonably well controlled prior to surgery.[2]

Preoperative Evaluation

The preoperative evaluation fulfills several functions. The most important is the medical evaluation of the patient prior to anesthesia and surgery. Another is reducing anxiety by informing the patient about the procedure and administering preoperative medications. Both the medical evaluation and preoperative sedation contribute to preventing systemic complications in patients having ophthalmic surgery.

The requirements of the preoperative history and physical examination are variable. The history includes the major anatomic and physiological systems, all medications, drug allergies, previous surgical procedures, and any complications related to prior anesthetics. The cardiovascular history, including previous myocardial infarction, congestive heart failure, strokes, or hypertension, is particularly important. A history of pulmonary diseases, including asthma or severe chronic obstructive pulmonary disease (COPD), diabetes mellitus, hepatic insufficiency, or renal disease is also important. Each of these has implications for the administration of the anesthesia or potential complications that may occur.

It is also important that the anesthesia provider conduct a preanesthesia physical exam. This does not substitute for a complete physical exam by the patient's internist or other primary care provider, but can be used to assess whether the patient may safely undergo the anesthesia provided for the surgical procedure. The physical exam includes auscultation of the heart and lungs, an evaluation of the airway, and any abnormal system suggested by the patient's history.

Unlike in the past, there is no prescribed list of laboratory tests that all patients undergo prior to surgery. Testing is now individualized to the patient's underlying medical history. Diabetics should have a finger-stick blood sugar level performed immediately prior to surgery to determine the patient's current blood sugar levels. A hemoglobin A1$_c$ level is very useful to assess the long-term control, but this does not provide information on the current blood sugar level and should not substitute for a finger-stick test on the day of surgery. Patients on digitalis or diuretics should have a recent potassium level, and Coumadin users should have a prothrombin time/partial thromboplastin time (PT/PTT) done prior to surgery, especially if a peri/retrobulbar block is used as the anesthesia. Other tests may be indicated depending on the patient's history.

A recent electrocardiogram (ECG) is indispensable in patients with a known history of cardiac disease or diabetes mellitus, which may mask the existence of severe cardiac disease. Studies vary widely as to what percentage of patients have unknown cardiac disease discovered on a routine preoperative ECG, and some anesthesia providers obtain a recent ECG in all patients over 50 years of age. Others take a slightly different approach. They obtain a preoperative ECG on patients with a cardiac history or asymptomatic patients with at least one risk factor on the Revised Cardiac Risk Index (RCRI), but forgo ECG exams in asymptomatic patients with no RCRI risk factors. RCRI risk factors include cerebrovascular disease, congestive heart failure, ischemic cardiac disease, diabetes mellitus, or a creatinine level greater than 2.0 mg/dL.

Once the preoperative evaluation is complete, an intravenous (IV) line is started and the patient is placed on monitors, including an ECG, blood pressure cuff, and pulse oximeter. These monitors are sufficient in the freestanding ambulatory surgery center or hospital outpatient surgery department. If the patient requires more extensive monitoring, the surgery should be done in a hospital setting.

The patient is given preoperative antianxiety medications, most commonly a combination of fentanyl (narcotic) and midazolam (benzodiazepine). The usual dose is 1 cc fentanyl (50 µg) and 1 mg midazolam, although this should be reduced by half in frail, elderly patients. This combination produces a relaxed, but not overly sedated patient within 2 to 3 minutes. If a patient remains anxious, a second dose may be given after ~ 5 minutes. Antiemetics are not usually necessary for outpatient ophthalmic surgery. However, if a patient has a history of severe nausea and vomiting after surgery, an antiemetic medication can be added.

Occasionally a patient will have elevated blood pressure even after the premedications are given. This can be treated with a rapid-acting antihypertensive agent. Commonly used agents include IV labetalol, hydralazine, esmolol, or sublingual nifedipine. The blood pressure should be closely monitored, but surgery can proceed safely once the blood pressure is controlled.

Topical Anesthesia

The use of topical anesthesia has greatly expanded over the last two decades to the point where this is now the predominant form of anesthesia for cataract surgeries. Topical anesthesia is simple and quick. In addition, it avoids the potential complications associated with anesthetics involving injections around the eye.

Topical anesthesia provides corneal anesthesia that is sufficient for most routine phacoemulsification procedures. Surgeons who routinely use topical anesthesia prefer this to other techniques for an overwhelming percentage of their surgical cases. However, topical anesthesia has its drawbacks. It does not produce akinesia, allowing ophthalmic movements during the surgical procedure. In additions, it appears that patients do not experience the same level of comfort or satisfaction with topical anesthesia alone when compared with various injection techniques. Many surgeons and anesthesia providers have found that the addition of minimal sedation to the topical techniques alleviates many of these disadvantages.

General Anesthesia and Orbital Block

Some cataract surgeons still utilize retrobulbar or peribulbar blocks, although not to the same extent as in previous decades. Some surgeons administer the block to an awake or only slightly sedated patient. Although the block is more uncomfortable than painful, it produces anxiety in awake patients. This anxiety and discomfort increase the patient's heart rate and blood pressure, resulting in a potentially higher incidence of cardiac complications. Alternatively, the block can be safely performed under a brief general anesthetic to eliminate patient awareness and decrease the incidence of cardiac problems.

A short-duration anesthetic, lasting only 2 or 3 minutes, is ideal for administration of the block. The anesthetic should maintain cardiovascular stability and spontaneous respiration. There are several agents or combinations of agents that will produce this.

The most commonly used agent for this brief anesthetic is propofol. One downside of propofol is that it can produce a burning sensation at the injection site. As a result, several providers inject a small amount of lidocaine through the IV just prior to injecting the propofol. Patients administered propofol must be monitored for respiratory depression and hypotension, but these are not usually severe and can be easily managed. On rare occasions a patient will move slightly or groan during the block. This is usually an involuntary reaction and most patients have no memory of the block once they are awake. Other medications used for a brief general anesthetic during block administration are alfentanil or remifentanil, which are extremely potent but very short-acting narcotics.

The patients are fully awake within several minutes. Akinesia of the eye provides an assessment of the block. Even if some motion remains, the eye is usually insensate. If not, a few drops of topical anesthetic will eliminate any remaining sensation. Only rarely must a block be repeated or supplemented with a subconjunctival injection of local anesthesia.

Intraoperative Monitoring and Treatment

Proper monitoring during surgery helps prevent or reduce the severity of systemic complications. Because patients' faces are usually partially or completely covered by sterile drapes, they are given supplemental oxygen by nasal cannula. Although most patients are comfortable during surgery, a few apprehensive patients require additional medications for relaxation. A small dose of propofol or repetition of the preoperative medications is usually sufficient.

With the above regimen, most patients are awake during surgery. They are able to eat and drink right afterward and are ready for discharge within 30 minutes. Rarely do patients require any further treatment in the postoperative period.

Topical anesthetics, blocks, and general anesthetics each have specific considerations. If the surgeon prefers to operate under topical anesthesia, the patient must be sedated enough to feel relaxed, yet awake enough to cooperate with the surgeon. Patients with retrobulbar or other injection anesthetics are often more comfortable and require less intraoperative sedation. In rare circumstances a general anesthetic may be necessary for the entire surgical procedure, such as in children or adults with severe developmental delays that make their cooperation with the surgeon difficult or nearly impossible. Coughing and "bucking" on the endotracheal tube, either during or after the procedure, can cause injury to the eye. Using a laryngeal mask airway (see Chapter 1) instead of an endotracheal tube usually prevents this problem.

Complications

Anesthetic complications during surgery range from minor to life-threatening.[3] Fortunately, serious complications are rare. In one unpublished series of over 8,000 ophthalmic surgical patients treated by a single anesthesiologist, the serious complication rate was less than 0.2%. Minor complications occur more frequently, but are of little consequence. **Table 2.1** lists systemic complications of ophthalmic anesthesia seen in that series and other potentially serious complications that were not observed.

The systemic complications of ophthalmic anesthesia generally fall into several broad categories: airway obstruction and respiratory complications, cardiac complications, injuries associated with the block, and reactions to general anesthetics. Most airway difficulties are easily relieved with minimal airway support such as a jaw lift maneuver. Propofol and other agents used for brief general anesthesia cause relaxation of the airway musculature, allowing the patient's tongue to obstruct the airway. Gentle airway support lifts the tongue away from the hypopharynx, relieving the obstruction. Rarely does this require more than lifting the patient's mandible or chin. In the above series of 8,000 patients, none needed any other airway intervention such as placing an oral airway or intubation with an endotracheal tube. One patient with a history of asthma developed acute bronchospasm in the postoperative period that required treatment.

Potential cardiac anomalies include hyper- or hypotension, minor or severe arrhythmias, angina, myocardial infarction, or cardiac arrest.[4] These anomalies should be treated according to standard protocols. Severe cardiac complications are rare. In the above series there were no cardiac arrests in the operative or immediate postoperative period. One patient developed severe bradycardia during surgery but responded to atropine, and the surgery continued without complication. Although the patient had initially denied any history of cardiac problems, he admitted that he had had several such episodes in the past. A pacemaker was placed 6 hours later and the patient was discharged from the hospital within 18 hours.

Traumatic injuries can occur during the retro/peribulbar needle placement. Injuries to the intraorbital structures have been discussed, but systemic complications can also occur from the needle placement. If the needle tip penetrates the neural

Table 2.1 Systemic Complications of Ophthalmic Anesthesia in Approximately 8,000 Patients

Complication	Percentage
Minor, non–life-threatening	
Minor airway obstruction (easy to relieve with manual airway support, less than 5% decrease in SaO$_2$)	8
Hiccups	3
Breath holding	1
Nausea and/or vomiting	< 1
Disorientation requiring intraoperative sedation	< 1
Potentially life-threatening	
Moderate airway obstruction (difficult to relieve with manual support, greater than 10% drop in SaO$_2$)	< 2
Severe airway obstruction (not relieved with manual support, requiring artificial airway or intubation)	0
Cardiac arrhythmia requiring further treatment	< 0.05
Respiratory difficulties requiring treatment	< 0.05
Cardiac or respiratory arrest	0
Midbrain block, resulting in cardiopulmonary collapse	0
Malignant hyperthermia	0

Source: author's unpublished series.

sheath surrounding the optic nerve, local anesthetic can travel within the nerve sheath into the midbrain.[5] This produces a complete respiratory arrest. Both tachycardia and bradycardia have been reported. The process is self-limiting, but requires immediate cardiopulmonary support. Intubation and ventilation are required until the respiratory effects have resolved, usually within 1 to 4 hours. Cardiac support consists of treating the underlying rate and pressure abnormalities. Usually all treatment can be discontinued within several hours. Prompt supportive treatment of these events usually avoids permanent damage or other severe complications.

Malignant hyperthermia (MH) is a rare, potentially fatal reaction to general anesthesia. This is a hereditary disorder of calcium uptake and release at the cellular level. Certain anesthetics, such as the inhaled volatile agents or succinylcholine, trigger this disorder. It is manifested by marked tachycardia, tachypnea, increased carbon dioxide production, and a rapid rise in body temperature. Because anesthesia techniques for cataract surgery do not typically involve agents that trigger MH, this is rarely encountered during cataract procedures. Should this occur, however, treatment must be initiated promptly. Dantrolene is administered and mechanical ventilation provided as necessary. If this occurs in a freestanding ambulatory surgical center, the patient should be transferred by ambulance to the nearest hospital equipped to handle this emergency.

Conclusion

Anesthesia complications during ophthalmic surgery are not common. However, vigilance is necessary to recognize and treat complications when they do occur. Anesthesia personnel should monitor each patient during the critical portions of the procedure, such as during the block and the surgery. During other times, such as the pre- and postoperative periods, they should be immediately available for consultation and treatment should the need arise.

References

1. Leaming DV. Practice styles and preferences of ASCRS members—1997 survey. J Cataract Refract Surg 1998;24:552–561
2. Ripart J, Mehrige K, Rocca RD. Local and regional anesthesia for the eye. New York School of Regional Anesthesia. http://www.nysora.com/mobile/regional-anesthesia/sub-specialties/3029-local-regional-anesthesia-for-eye-surgery.html
3. Hamilton RC, Gimbel HV, Strunin L. Regional anaesthesia for 12,000 cataract extraction and intraocular lens implantation procedures. Can J Anaesth 1988;35:615–623
4. Rosenblatt RM, May DR, Barsoumian K. Cardiopulmonary arrest after retrobulbar block. Am J Ophthalmol 1980;90:425–427
5. Rosen WJ. Brainstem anesthesia presenting as dysarthria. J Cataract Refract Surg 1999;25:1170–1171

Section II   Wound Construction and Complications

3 Wound Construction and Complications

Patricia Ann Ple-plakon, William J. Fishkind, and Mitchell P. Weikert

As incisions in cataract surgery have evolved alongside improvements in intraocular lens (IOL) design, phacoemulsification systems, and surgical instrumentation, the incisions have become smaller. Both scleral tunnel incisions and clear corneal incisions are widely used today and have varying advantages and disadvantages. Ideal incisions minimize surgically induced astigmatism and are self-sealing to reduce the risks of hypotony and endophthalmitis. As technology continues to advance, femtosecond lasers have aided surgeons in creating more reproducible and customizable incisions while tissue adhesives provide alternative means for creating watertight closure with ease of use.

Vision outcomes in cataract surgery rely on wound size and architecture. Problems in wound construction are not uncommon, but the creation of proper wounds is crucial in wound healing and avoidance of potential complications. Surgeons should be able to quickly recognize inaccuracy in wound construction and be prepared to manage complications that may stem from the changes in surgical technique needed to adapt to poorly constructed incisions.

Incisions in Cataract Surgery

Proper design and construction of incisions used in cataract surgery are crucial in achieving successful surgical results. Cataract surgical incisions have evolved greatly overtime. With innovations in IOL design, phacoemulsification, and instrumentation, incision size has been reduced and has enabled improved outcomes in cataract surgery. The most common incision types include scleral tunnels, clear cornea, and femtosecond laser–assisted clear cornea; each type has advantages, disadvantages, and keys to success. Understanding the anterior segment architecture and structural relationships (**Fig. 3.1**) can aid in the successful creation of surgical incisions.

Scleral Tunnel Incisions

The scleral tunnel incision was introduced in 1977 by Richard Kratz. Incisions are created 2 mm posterior to the limbus. A scleral partial-thickness incision is made, tunneled through sclera into clear cornea parallel to the corneal surface, and Descemet's membrane is incised to enter the anterior chamber (**Figs. 3.2 and 3.3**). These incisions are up to 7 mm in length to enable the insertion of large, nonfoldable polymethylmethacrylate (PMMA) IOLs and require closure with multiple sutures.

In 1989, the Food and Drug Administration (FDA) approved the first foldable IOL (AMO PhacoFlex model SI-18, Allergan Medical Optics, Santa Ana, CA), which enabled making smaller incisions of 4 mm in width. These incisions could be closed with a single interrupted suture, providing greater wound stability, more astigmatic neutrality, and faster vision rehabilitation.

Another innovation in scleral tunnel design is the sclerocorneal frown incision, which is oriented with the curvature away from the limbus. The more anterior portion of the incision is 2 mm posterior to the limbus, and the incision varies in width depending on the size of IOL to be inserted. The internal lip of the incision is parallel to and positioned 1 mm anterior to the limbus. The external portion of the incision enables greater stretch for implantation of the IOL optic. As with tangential scleral tunnels, sutures are generally used to ensure watertight closure. In all incisions, sutures should be trimmed short and rotated to bury the knot and avoid postoperative patient discomfort.

Scleral tunnel incisions have the advantages of increased wound strength and a self-sealing nature (**Table 3.1**). To achieve watertight closure, the tunneled portion of the scleral and corneal stroma must be in a consistent plane aligned with the most posterior portion of the incision. Due to their greater distance from the visual axis, scleral tunnels induce minimal astigmatism. Potential disadvantages of scleral tunnel incisions include wound leaks, inadvertent creation of filtering blebs, tunnel hemorrhages leading to hyphema, and difficulty with manipulation of the phacoemulsification handpiece and instruments within the incision.

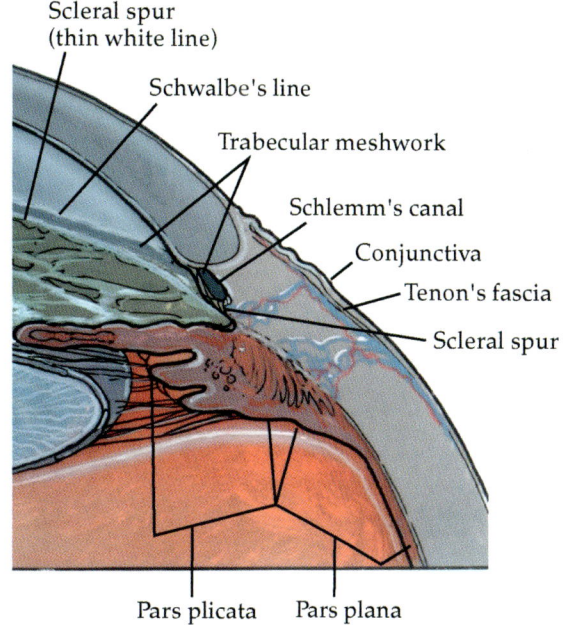

Fig. 3.1 Anatomic relationships. This cross-sectional image of the anterior segment shows the relationship between the peripheral cornea, corneoscleral junction, and anterior chamber angle in a phakic eye.

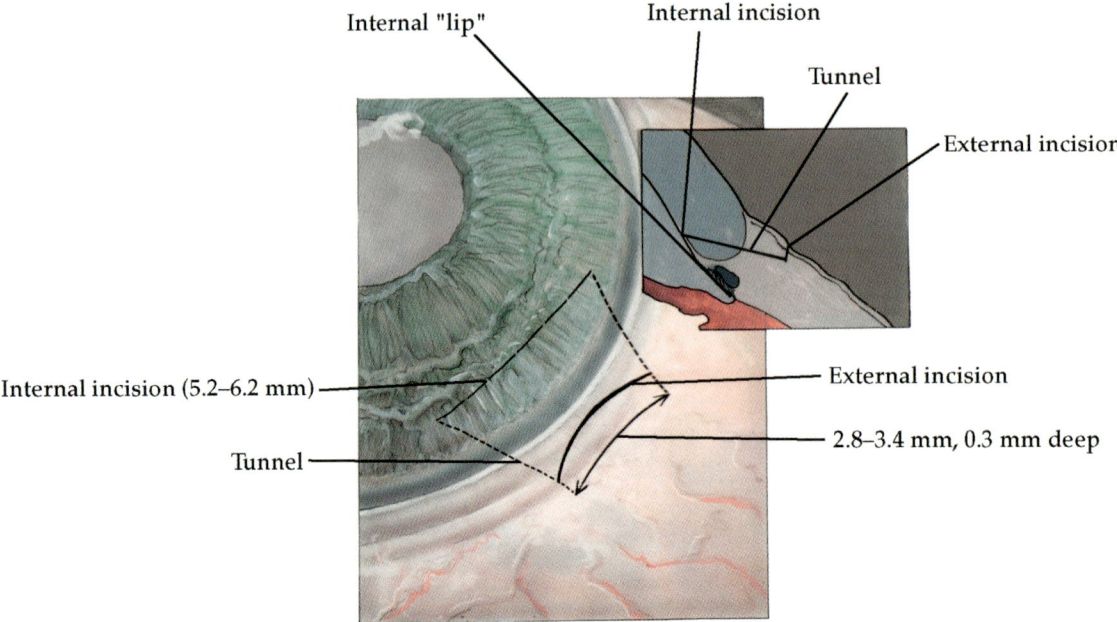

Internal "lip"

Internal incision

Tunnel

External incision

Internal incision (5.2–6.2 mm)

Tunnel

External incision

2.8–3.4 mm, 0.3 mm deep

Fig. 3.2 Scleral tunnel incision. The external incision is curved away from the limbus. The internal incision is 1 mm anterior to the limbus.

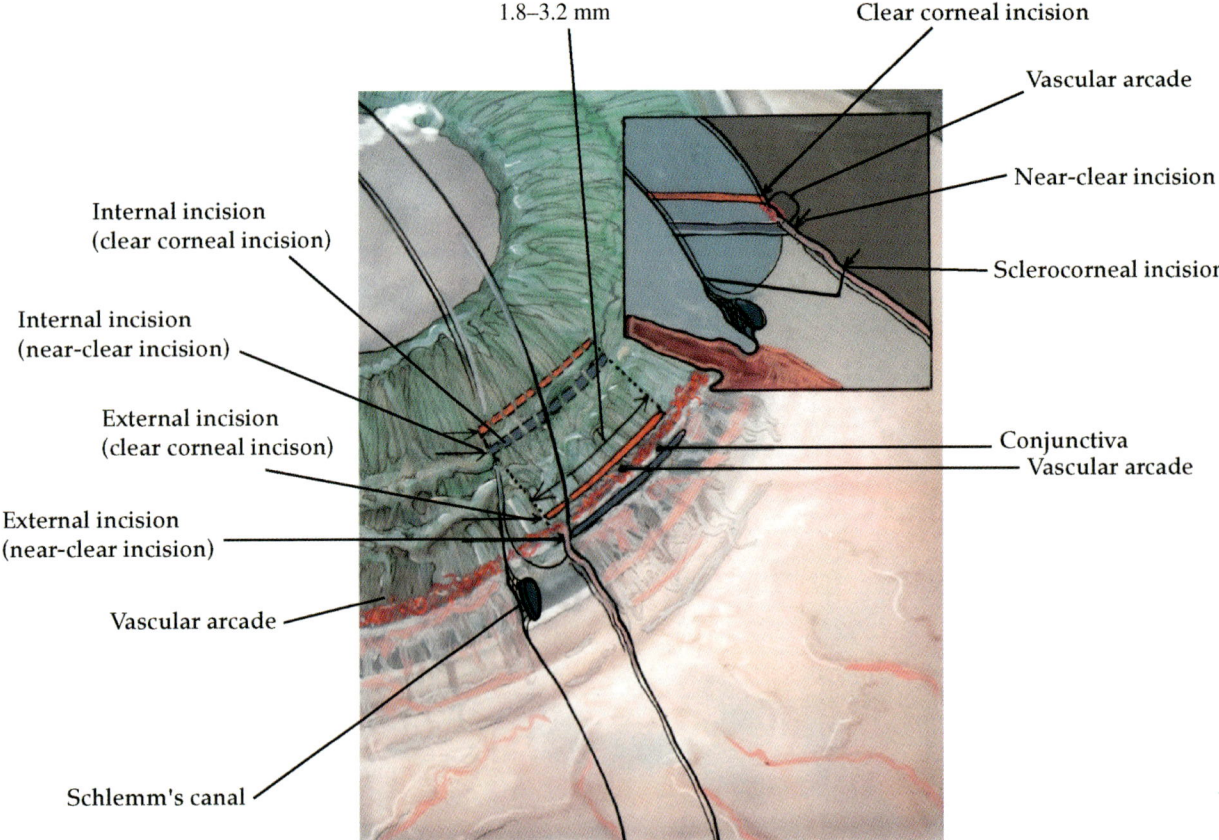

1.8–3.2 mm

Clear corneal incision

Vascular arcade

Near-clear incision

Sclerocorneal incision

Internal incision (clear corneal incision)

Internal incision (near-clear incision)

External incision (clear corneal incison)

External incision (near-clear incision)

Vascular arcade

Schlemm's canal

Conjunctiva
Vascular arcade

Fig. 3.3 Clear corneal, near-clear corneal, and sclera-corneal incisions. This diagram illustrates the locations of the different corneal and corneoscleral incisions, and their three-dimensional relationship to the anterior segment anatomy.

Table 3.1 Scleral Tunnel Incisions

Advantages	Disadvantages
More resistant to stretch and mechanical trauma	Time-consuming
Less surgically induced astigmatism	Often require sutures for closure
Self-sealing over longer lengths	Inadvertent creation of filtering blebs

Clear Corneal Incisions

Multiple surgical innovations led to the development of suture-less clear corneal incisions. First introduced by Howard Fine[1] in 1991, these incisions were initially 1.75 mm in length and 4 mm in width to enable IOL insertion. Watertight construction was difficult, leading to potential bacterial contamination and endophthalmitis. As IOL technology advanced, incision size decreased, and Fine later introduced stromal hydration to aid in wound sealing. These incisions were 2.8 to 3.2 mm in width at the limbus and 1.75 mm in length. The incision size has continued to decrease to 2.2 mm in width or even less. Smaller incisions have led to less surgically induced astigmatism and improved sealing.

The most posterior portion of the clear corneal incision is constructed just anterior to limbal arcades of conjunctival blood vessels (**Figs. 3.3** and **3.4**). A hinge of variable depth is created to provide a more watertight closure. Multiplanar incisions, incorporating both vertical and horizontal elements, provide stability at a wide range of intraocular pressure ranges. Although longer incisions may be more resistant to wound leakage, this benefit must be weighed against potential induction of corneal striae and poor visualization caused by the increased length.

The temporal clear corneal incision has become the most predominant incision used in cataract surgery.[2] The advantages include efficiency of wound creation, self-sealing nature, minimal astigmatism induction, rapid visual recovery, wound stability, and lack of conjunctival manipulation and trauma (**Table 3.2**). The temporal location has the advantage of accessibility, and due to the greater horizontal diameter of the cornea, temporal incisions are less likely to invade the visual axis. Additionally, temporal incisions may partially neutralize the against-the-rule astigmatism present in many patients undergoing cataract surgery. Disadvantages of clear corneal incisions include potential thermal damage or mechanical trauma during surgery, as well as the potential for bacterial contamination and subsequent endophthalmitis.

Femtosecond Laser Clear Corneal Incisions

Femtosecond laser technology is commonly used in laser-assisted in situ keratomileusis (LASIK) flap creation and has certain advantages over traditional microkeratomes for flap creation, including safety and reproducibility. More recently, it

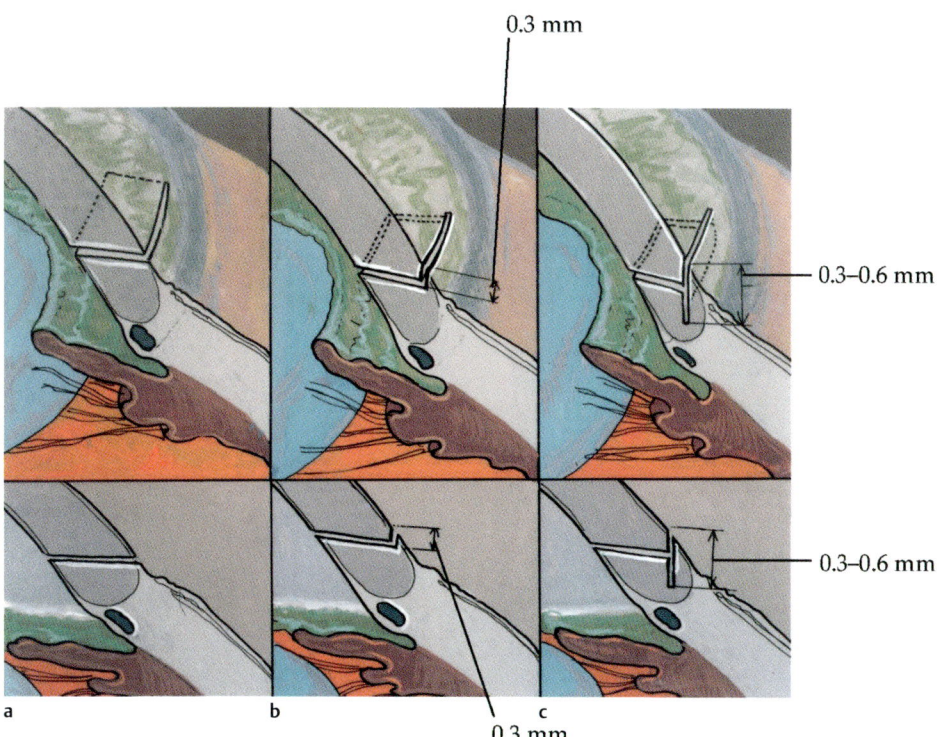

Fig. 3.4 Clear corneal incision. The external incision is just inside the conjunctival arcade. The internal incision is no wider than the tunnel length. (**a**) No hinge. (**b**) Small hinge. (**c**) Deep hinge.

Table 3.2 Clear Corneal Incisions

Advantages	Disadvantages
Ease of creation	Possible increased risk of endophthalmitis
Minimal astigmatic effect	Less wound strength
Sutureless watertight closure	
Lack of conjunctival manipulation and trauma	
Rapid visual recovery	

has been used in cataract surgery for clear corneal incisions as well as paracenteses. This new technology enables customization of the length, angles, and shape of incisions with excellent reproducibility. Grewal and Basti[3] used spectral-domain anterior-segment optical coherence tomography (AS-OCT) to evaluate the morphology of clear corneal incisions created by a femtosecond laser and compared them with those made by traditional steel keratomes. They found that femtosecond laser incisions had less endothelial wound gape and misalignment, as well as fewer Descemet's membrane detachments.

It is expected that laser-created incisions will improve in reliability with further technological advances in lasers and OCT. Although the clinical advantages over traditional incision construction remain to be proven, technological advances may enable improved refractive outcomes in the future.

Tissue Adhesives

Liquid adhesive ocular bandages, including OcuSeal (Beaver-Visitec, Waltham, MA) and ReSure sealant (Ocular Therapeutix, Inc., Bedford, MA) have been created for topical application to seal cataract wounds. These transparent polymerizing hydrogels may be applied topically and polymerize on the ocular surface to form an adhesive coating **(Fig. 3.5)**. Although OcuSeal is not yet available in the United States, the ReSure sealant is an available hydrogel composed of polyethylene glycol, trilysine, buffering salts, and 90% water.[4] Recent studies have demonstrated less

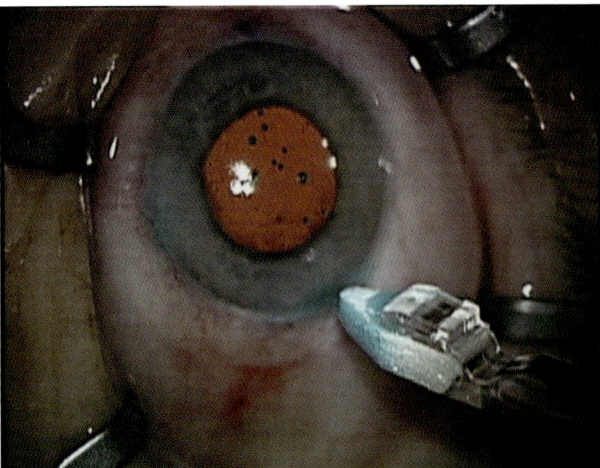

Fig. 3.5 ReSure hydrogel sealant. Application of ReSure sealant is shown at the temporal incision and inferior paracentesis. The tissue glue has a blue tint upon initial application.

surgically induced astigmatism with tissue adhesives in comparison with sutured wounds, and similar astigmatism in comparison with controls.[5] Although common side effects include foreign-body sensation and hyperemia, a study reported less foreign-body sensation in comparison with both sutured wounds and patients without any sutures.[5] Hydrogel sealants have been shown to be both safe and effective in preventing wound leakage after cataract surgery.[6]

Wound Healing

Studies using AS-OCT have enabled morphological evaluation of incisions and wound healing. Wang et al[7] used Fourier-domain AS-OCT to evaluate long-term architectural changes of clear corneal incisions in cataract surgery. They found that early postoperative changes, which persisted for up to 3 months, included Descemet's membrane detachment and posterior wound gape **(Fig. 3.6)**. Posterior wound gape was not affected by placement of corneal sutures. Posterior wound retraction was noted at 2 to 3 weeks postoperatively and was seen in 90% of eyes after 3 years, indicating long-term tissue remodeling.

Surgically Induced Astigmatism

Current techniques in smaller incision phacoemulsification lead to surgically induced astigmatism (SIA) that varies from 0.30 to 1.00 diopters depending on variables including incision location, length, and distance from central visual axis.[8–11] Larger incisions and more anterior incision placement increase the astigmatic effect. Superior incisions produce greater astigmatic changes, followed by superotemporal, nasal, superonasal, and finally temporal incisions.[12] Clear corneal incisions produce more SIA than scleral tunnels, and thinner corneas and stromal hydration may also increase SIA.[13] Square incisions create less SIA than rectangular incisions and are also less prone to wound leakage at a wider range of intraocular pressures. The astigmatism noted postoperatively decreases over time, and appears to stabilize at 3 months after cataract surgery.[14]

Problems in Wound Construction

Poorly constructed wounds may lead to wound leakage and poor visualization during surgery. These issues may cause further adverse events including hypotony, anterior chamber collapse, influx of bacteria or toxic materials, movement of the IOL, and intraoperative complications such as posterior capsular tears and vitreous loss. Early recognition of problems is crucial, and surgeons should be prepared to adjust their surgical approach to minimize complications.

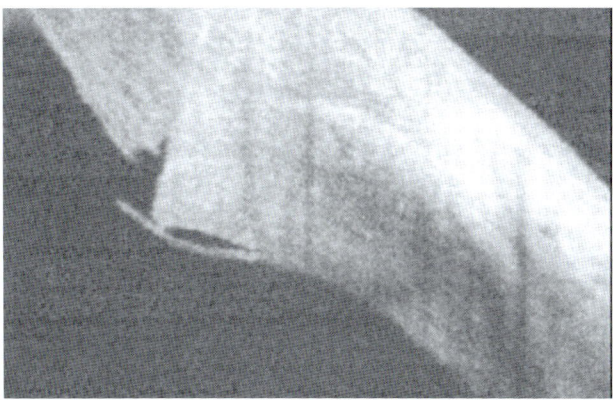

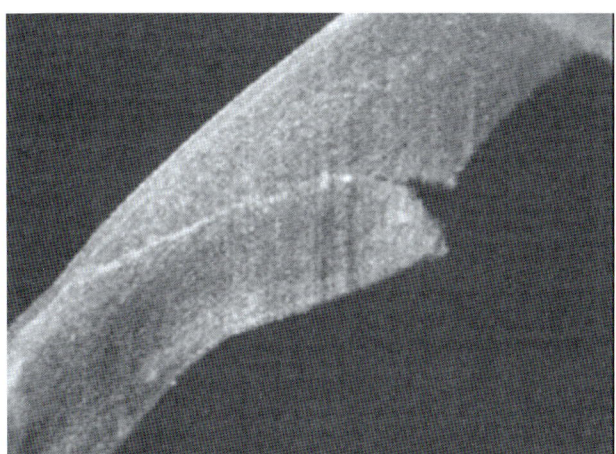

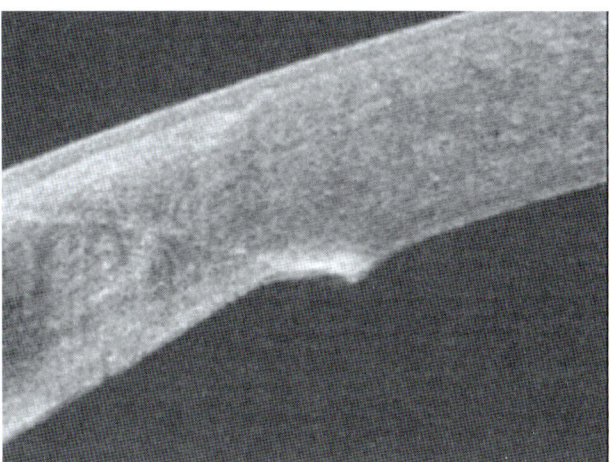

Fig. 3.6 Anterior-segment optical coherence tomography (AS-OCT) demonstrating **(a)** Descemet's membrane detachment, **(b)** posterior wound gape, and **(c)** posterior wound retraction of clear corneal incisions after cataract surgery.

Anterior Chamber Entry Too Anterior

Longer incisions may be more self-sealing, but incisions made too anterior can lead to corneal striae, which may impair visualization of the anterior chamber during surgery. Additionally, a central incision location may make manipulation of surgical instruments more difficult and cause mechanical trauma to the incisions.

Anterior Chamber Entry Too Posterior

When incisions enter the anterior chamber prematurely, balanced salt solution (BSS) may flow out of the wound, capturing iris tissue, and lead to iris prolapse. Iris trauma can cause iris dialysis and potential hyphema from trauma to blood vessels in the angle and iris root. This may be managed with a small peripheral iridotomy. If difficulty is encountered from posterior wounds, a surgeon may elect to suture the wound and create a new incision.

Long Incisions

Long incisions may enter the anterior chamber too anterior, and, as mentioned previously, cause corneal striae and poor visualization during surgery. If these incisions are in the visual axis, postoperative corneal edema and astigmatism may affect vision. Alternatively, excessively long incisions due to the external portion of the incision being made too posterior can make manipulation of instruments and the phacoemulsification handpiece more challenging. This increases the risk of complications such as posterior capsular tears.

Longer incisions may also increase the risk of fluid inflow obstruction and subsequent wound burns in coaxial phacoemulsification, especially in long eyes with deep anterior chambers. Surgeons may elect to abandon these incisions and create new incisions to avoid potential problems.

Short Incisions

Incisions of inadequate length may seal poorly and lead to iris prolapse as mentioned above. Placement of radial 10-0 nylon sutures may improve wound integrity. In sclerocorneal incisions, additional conjunctiva may be closed over the wound to address further fluid leaks, and subsequent filtering blebs may limit fluid egress and prevent postoperative hypotony.

Narrow Incisions

Incisions that are too narrow may cause difficulty with insertion of instruments and the phacoemulsification handpiece. The phacoemulsification tip may catch Descemet's membrane, leading to detachment. These incisions can be exposed to prolonged phacoemulsification, which may lead to excessive heat and wound burn. This may be compounded by narrow incisions that crimp irrigation sleeves and further impede inflow of BSS.

Wide Incisions

Wide incisions may lead to constant efflux of fluid from the incision and subsequent anterior chamber shallowing and instability. Surgeons may attempt to mitigate the shallowing chamber through placement of sutures to partially close the incision.

Shallow Incisions

Incisions that are too shallow can lead to tears or buttonholes. This may lead to wound leakage, and X-configuration sutures may be utilized. Conjunctival suturing over buttonholes may also limit fluid leakage, and subsequent filtering bleb formation may prevent possible hypotony. If this fails, scleral patch grafts may be necessary.

Deep Incisions

Scleral tunnel incisions that are too deep may expose the ciliary body or choroid. If this occurs, the incision should be sutured and a new incision made elsewhere. In clear corneal incisions, deep incisions can lead to short incisions due to premature entry in to the anterior chamber.

Conjunctival Chemosis

If the external portion of the incision is too posterior, fluid may flow into Tenon's fascia and cause fluid to collect underneath the conjunctiva and impair visualization. In these situations, the phacoemulsification handpiece should be removed from the eye. A conjunctival incision should be created with Westcott scissors to enable egress of fluid.

Managing Wound Complications

Wound Burn

As mentioned previously, wound burn may be caused by incisions that are too narrow, too long, or too tight, which may lead to poor BSS inflow, resulting in the phacoemulsification handpiece overheating. Incidence of thermal injury in phacoemulsification has been reported as 1 in 1,000.[15] Risk factors for wound burn include use of continuous ultrasound and the divide-and-conquer technique. Wound burn, if not detected and managed early, can lead to distortion of wound architecture. Surgeons may observe whitening and contracture of the wound as a sign of wound burn (**Fig. 3.7**). Additionally, bubbles may be observed along the length of the phacoemulsification tip. To enable watertight closure, multiple tight sutures are necessary. Sometimes limbus parallel sutures close the wound more effectively and reduce postoperative astigmatism. Also, new wound glues are available to glue the incision, with or without sutures. They impede wound leak without adding as much astigmatism as tight radial sutures. Wound burns typically require several weeks to heal, with suture removal occurring over several visits.

When primary closure with sutures is not feasible due to excessive wound gape, a scleral patch graft may be necessary. Patch grafts may be autologous or obtained from the eye bank. If

an autologous graft is utilized, a fornix-based peritomy is created and the sclera should be incised to a depth of 0.3 mm. A lamellar dissection is performed, and partial-thickness sclera of appropriate size is removed and placed over the area of wound gape. If sclera is obtained from the eye bank, it should be cut to appropriate size and be half-scleral thickness. The scleral graft can be positioned with the placement of four cardinal 10-0 nylon sutures followed by a single running 10-0 nylon suture.

Wound Leak

Wound leaks may lead to hypotony, IOL dislocation, or influx of bacterial contaminants, causing endophthalmitis. These problems should be managed with 10-0 nylon sutures to improve wound strength. Additionally, stromal hydration should be utilized to ensure watertight closure.

Descemet's Detachment

Descemet's detachments may occur in both scleral tunnel and clear corneal incisions. Trauma from insertion and removal of surgical instruments may also lead to detachment. Smaller Descemet's detachments may heal spontaneously, whereas larger detachments may require injection of air into the anterior chamber with patient positioning to maintain apposition of the bubble with the posterior cornea.

Stromal Hydration

Stromal hydration is effective in sealing wounds and has the advantages of efficiency, ease of technique, and no need for additional instrumentation. However, in some cases the hydrated incisions may not have enough strength to withstand external pressures and may lead to poorly sealing wounds. Studies have demonstrated the inflow of extraocular fluid into the anterior chamber through sutureless corneal incisions after phacoemulsification.[16,17] Other studies have reported that higher intraocular pressure in the initial postoperative period may lead to less microleakage and less hypotony.[18] Research utilizing high-resolution Fourier-domain OCT demonstrated that the effect of stromal hydration was present at 1 week postoperatively,[19] but also showed distortion of wounds with an increase in Descemet's detachment.[20]

Sutures

Studies utilizing OCT showed no differences in wound architecture between incisions with and those without sutures in the initial 1 month postoperative period.[7] Although sutures may be placed if wound leaks are noted intraoperatively, the literature does not demonstrate that suture placement is associated with a reduced risk of endophthalmitis. Additionally, the advantages of suture placement in reducing wound leakage must be weighed against increased operating time, surgically induced astigmatism, and potential suture-related complications, such as neovascularization and suture abscesses.

Conclusion

The key to avoiding wound complications is proper wound construction. When difficulties in incision construction are encountered, it is important to recognize issues early and adjust surgical techniques to avoid complications. As technology continues to evolve, including the refinement in femtosecond lasers and ocular tissue adhesives, incisions will improve, with the ultimate goal of improving patients' vision and refractive outcomes.

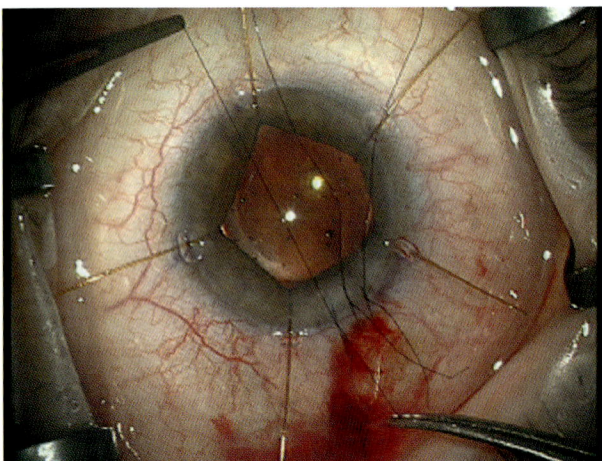

Fig. 3.7 Wound burn. The circular area of whitening shows the area of the wound burn. If the tissue is significantly contracted, it can be difficult to close the wound with a single suture because of the excessive tension required. Multiple sutures with slip knots are placed and they are adjusted gradually before locking.

References

1. Fine IH. Architecture and construction of a self-sealing incision for cataract surgery. J Cataract Refract Surg 1991;17(Suppl):672–676

2. Leaming DV. Practice styles and preferences of ASCRS members—1997 survey. J Cataract Refract Surg 1998;24:552–561

3. Grewal DS, Basti S. Comparison of morphologic features of clear corneal incisions created with a femtosecond laser or a keratome. J Cataract Refract Surg 2014;40:521–530

4. Dell SJ, Hovanesian JA, Raizman MB, et al; Ocular Bandage Study Group. Randomized comparison of postoperative use of hydrogel ocular bandage and collagen corneal shield for wound protection and patient tolerability after cataract surgery. J Cataract Refract Surg 2011;37:113–121

5. Uy HS, Kenyon KR. Surgical outcomes after application of a liquid adhesive ocular bandage to clear corneal incisions during cataract surgery. J Cataract Refract Surg 2013;39:1668–1674

6. Masket S, Hovanesian JA, Levenson J, et al. Hydrogel sealant versus sutures to prevent fluid egress after cataract surgery. J Cataract Refract Surg 2014;40:2057–2066

7. Wang L, Dixit L, Weikert MP, Jenkins RB, Koch DD. Healing changes in clear corneal cataract incisions evaluated using Fourier-domain optical coherence tomography. J Cataract Refract Surg 2012;38:660–665

8. Moon SC, Mohamed T, Fine IH. Comparison of surgically induced astigmatisms after clear corneal incisions of different sizes. Korean J Ophthalmol 2007;21:1–5

9. Altan-Yaycioglu R, Akova YA, Akca S, Gur S, Oktem C. Effect on astigmatism of the location of clear corneal incision in phacoemulsification of cataract. J Refract Surg 2007;23:515–518

10. Altan-Yaycioglu R, Pelit A, Evyapan O, Akova YA. Astigmatism induced by oblique clear corneal incision: right vs. left eyes. Can J Ophthalmol 2007; 42:557–561

11. Tejedor J, Murube J. Choosing the location of corneal incision based on preexisting astigmatism in phacoemulsification. Am J Ophthalmol 2005; 139:767–776

12. Park CY, Chuck RS, Channa P, Lim C-Y, Ahn B-J. The effect of corneal anterior surface eccentricity on astigmatism after cataract surgery. Ophthalmic Surg Lasers Imaging 2011;42:408–415

13. Scaltrini G, Piovella M. Hydrogel ocular bandages to protect and increase watertight properties of corneal incisions after cataract surgery: 4-year experience. Presented at the American Society of Cataract and Refractive Surgery Symposium on Cataract, Intraocular Lens, and Refractive Surgery, Boston, April 2010

14. Kadowaki H, Mizoguchi T, Kuroda S, Terauchi H, Nagata M. Surgically-induced astigmatism following single-site phacotrabeculectomy, phacotrabeculotomy and advanced non-penetrating phacotrabeculectomy. Semin Ophthalmol 2001;16:158–161

15. Bradley MJ, Olson RJ. A survey about phacoemulsification incision thermal contraction incidence and causal relationships. Am J Ophthalmol 2006;141:222–224

16. Sarayba MA, Taban M, Ignacio TS, Behrens A, McDonnell PJ. Inflow of ocular surface fluid through clear corneal cataract incisions: a laboratory model. Am J Ophthalmol 2004;138:206–210

17. Herretes S, Stark WJ, Pirouzmanesh A, Reyes JM, McDonnell PJ, Behrens A. Inflow of ocular surface fluid into the anterior chamber after phacoemulsification through sutureless corneal cataract wounds. Am J Ophthalmol 2005;140:737–740

18. Calladine D, Tanner V. Optical coherence tomography of the effects of stromal hydration on clear corneal incision architecture. J Cataract Refract Surg 2009;35:1367–1371

19. Fukuda S, Kawana K, Yasuno Y, Oshika T. Wound architecture of clear corneal incision with or without stromal hydration observed with 3-dimensional optical coherence tomography. Am J Ophthalmol 2011;151:413–9. e1

20. Walters TR. The effect of stromal hydration on surgical outcomes for cataract patients who received a hydrogel ocular bandage. Clin Ophthalmol 2011;5:385–391

Section III   Management of the Small Pupil

4   Small Pupil Recognition and Management

Fani Segev, Yokrat Ton, and Ehud I. Assia

The prevalence of visual impairment secondary to cataract increases with age and is expected to grow dramatically in the coming decades due to increased life expectancy and population growth. Intraoperative lens replacement for cataract extraction and intraocular lens (IOL) implantation are the most common surgical procedures performed worldwide.

Sufficient mydriasis during cataract surgery is imperative for a favorable outcome, thus providing good visualization of the lens structures, adequate space for surgical instruments and manipulations, and good red reflex. Pupil dilation is usually achieved by preoperative topical application of mydriatic agents.[1,2]

Many patients who present for cataract removal surgery have small pupils that do not adequately dilate despite several pharmacological attempts with topical mydriatic agents. Additionally, in some patients the initial mydriatic effect achieved may not last throughout the surgery, especially in patients who are treated with systemic α_1-adrenergic antagonist medications and in cases of surgical trauma that may induce intraoperative miosis through prostaglandin-related stimulation of the iris.[2–4]

Inadequately dilated pupil might complicate and challenge surgery. The causes of small pupil are numerous and include iris sphincter sclerosis from aging, pseudoexfoliation, posterior synechiae, previous trauma or surgery, diabetes, chronic syphilis, iridoschisis, uveitis, chronic miotic therapy, and systemic α_1-adrenergic antagonists medications for the treatment of lower urinary tract symptoms of benign prostatic hyperplasia (BPH).[3]

There is no strict definition of what is considered a small pupil. In practice, for the inexperienced surgeon a 4.0 to 5.0 mm is considered small, whereas an experienced surgeon may consider a pupil as being constricted only if the diameter is 3.5 to 4.0 mm or smaller.

Small pupils may entail risks at any step of surgery, from capsulorrhexis and lens particle removal to cortical aspiration and IOL implantation. If the pupil is not adequately dilated, surgeons tend to create a capsulorrhexis smaller than desired, which may further complicate surgery due to intraoperative difficulty in extracting nuclear fragments from within the capsular bag, and increased risk of postoperative capsule phimosis.

Pseudoexfoliation (PXF) is the most common cause of small pupil during cataract surgery. PXF is an age-related abnormal fibrillopathy that has been linked to the lysyl oxidase-like 1 *(LOXL1)* gene. It is characterized by the gradual synthesis, accumulation, and deposition of exfoliation material in the anterior segment of the eye and other tissues in the body.[5] PXF is associated with an increased incidence of cataract formation, including nuclear and subcapsular opacities.[6–8] It is estimated that 60 to 70 million people worldwide are affected by PXF. Prevalence of PXF increases with older age,[9] and it varies among geographic regions. In cataract surgery patients, the PXF prevalence ranges from 0.4% in the Chinese[10] up to 30.2% in the Estonian population.[11] Besides a nondilating pupil, PXF is often associated with weakened zonules and phacodonesis, which may further com-

plicate surgery. The influence of PXF on cataract surgery has been considerably documented. Earlier studies report a five- to 10-fold increased risk for surgical complications in eyes with PXF versus non-PXF eyes undergoing cataract surgery.[5,12,13] However, more recent studies report this difference to be smaller using technique modifications and devices.[14,15] Favorable outcomes can be achieved in cataract surgery in PXF syndrome as reviewed by Shingleton et al.[16]

Another common cause of small pupil or miosis during cataract surgery is intraoperative floppy iris syndrome (IFIS). Chang and Campbell[3] first described it in 2005 as occurring in 2% of cataract surgery patients, and Chang et al[17] further reviewed the topic in 2008. The syndrome is characterized by the following intraoperative triad: (1) a floppy iris that billows in response to normal irrigation in the anterior chamber; (2) a marked propensity for the floppy iris stroma to prolapse toward and into the corneal incisions; and (3) a progressive pupillary constriction during surgery. The syndrome has been documented to occur in patients with BPH treated with systemic α-antagonists in general and tamsulosin (Flomax, Boehringer-Ingelheim Pharmaceuticals, Ridgefield, CT) in particular. A recent retrospective study reported that 86% of the patients using tamsulosin had IFIS compared with 15% of those using alfuzosin (Uroxatral; Sanofi-Aventis, Bridgewater, NJ).[18] These findings are supported by those of a recent meta-analysis that found the risk of IFIS to be 16.5- to 40-fold higher in cases of previous tamsulosin use when compared with alfuzosin.[19]

During cataract surgery, IFIS can lead to many complications such as significant progressive pupil miosis, iris stromal atrophy, iris prolapse, capsulorrhexis tear, rupture of the posterior capsule, loss of lens material into the vitreous cavity, and others.[1,19–21] Patients with poor pupillary dilation should be questioned about the use of α_{1a}-adrenergic antagonists. Cessation of the drug before surgery may reduce the risk of IFIS. However, IFIS may still develop after patients discontinue systemic α_{1a}-adrenergic antagonist medications.[22] Overall, it appears that discontinuation of tamsulosin preoperatively is of unpredictable value and does not reliably prevent IFIS or reduce its severity.

Small pupil was reported in 1 to 11% of cataract operations, and varies by location and by definition of the term. IFIS was shown to occur in ~ 2% of men, and much less in women.

The overall incidence of small pupil is probably around 3 to 5% of cataract operations. This may sum up to an annual rate of 150,000 cases in North America or Europe and probably more than 500,000 operations per year worldwide.

Managing the Small Pupil

The small pupil can be dilated pharmacologically or mechanically. Preoperative topical nonsteroidal anti-inflammatory drugs (NSAIDs) in combination with mydriatic agents may help to reduce intraoperative miosis.[4,23,24] Srinivasan and Madhavaranga[4]

37

compared the effect of preoperative treatment of topical ketorolac tromethamine 0.5% solution and topical diclofenac sodium 0.1% solution on the inhibition of surgically induced miosis. Topical ketorolac was found to be a more effective inhibitor of miosis than topical diclofenac during extracapsular cataract extraction and IOL implantation. It also provided a more stable mydriatic effect throughout surgery.

A recent prospective study evaluated intracameral phenylephrine and ketorolac injection (*Overutilization Monitoring System* [OMS]302) for maintenance of intraoperative pupil diameter compared with placebo during IOL replacement.[25] OMS302 was superior to placebo in maintaining mydriasis and preventing pupil miosis.

Experienced surgeons often opt to perform surgery through a relatively small pupil in spite of limited visualization. However, the challenging surgery is often associated with an increased risk of iris and sphincter tears, bleeding, iris emulsification, ruptured posterior capsule, dropped nucleus or lens particles, and vitreous prolapse. Alternatively, surgeons may mechanically dilate the constricted pupil using a variety of instruments such as iris dilators and spatula. This is especially useful in cases of fibrotic pupillary membrane or posterior synechiae in posttraumatic or postuveitic constricted pupil. A fibrotic band at the pupillary margin may occasionally be stripped off using intraocular forceps to enable the pupil to properly dilate, but the sphincter function of the pupil is typically lost.

The Beehler pupil dilator has three microfingers with iris hooks and an additional hook on the tube. It is inserted into the anterior chamber through the main clear corneal incision, and the pupil is stretched in four quadrants. After the pupil is fully stretched, the prongs of the Beehler instrument are retracted, and the instrument is removed from the eye (**Fig. 4.1**).

Multiple iris sphincter tears with scissors, creating partial-thickness sphincterotomies, is effective in cases of fibrotic pupil. Many surgeons abandoned this technique because of postoperative aesthetically and functionally unacceptable iris irregularities. This technique is not effective in functional miosis such as IFIS and may actually aggravate pupil constriction.

Ophthalmic viscosurgical devices (OVDs) play an important role in managing the small pupil. An OVD with dispersive qualities is helpful to adequately coat the cornea during surgical maneuvers to protect the corneal endothelium. It may also help to create compartmentalization and prevent sucking a flail iris into the phacoemulsification tip. On the other hand, highly cohesive OVDs are very important for space maintenance, separation of posterior synechiae, and viscodilation of the pupillary margin. A combination of both cohesive and dispersive OVDs, such as the "soft shell" technique or using a "viscoadaptive" OVD, provides the advantages of both materials (see Chapter 33).

Intraoperative Floppy Iris Syndrome Management

As initially reported by Chang and Campbell,[3] partial-thickness sphincterotomies and mechanical pupil stretching are ineffective for IFIS and may exacerbate the condition and therefore are not recommended. Many surgical strategies have been proposed to minimize the occurrence and the severity of IFIS with variable success. Among them are the use of atropine,[26,27] intracameral epinephrine,[27,28] iris retractors,[29] dilator rings,[30–32] and OVDs.[32,33] Employment of highly retentive OVDs such as Healon 5 (Abbott Medical Optics, Abbott Park, IL) to viscodilate the pupil and maintain a concave iris near the incisions without preventing egress of irrigating fluid and use of low-flow settings and lens removal techniques can minimize anterior chamber turbulence (see Chapter 23).

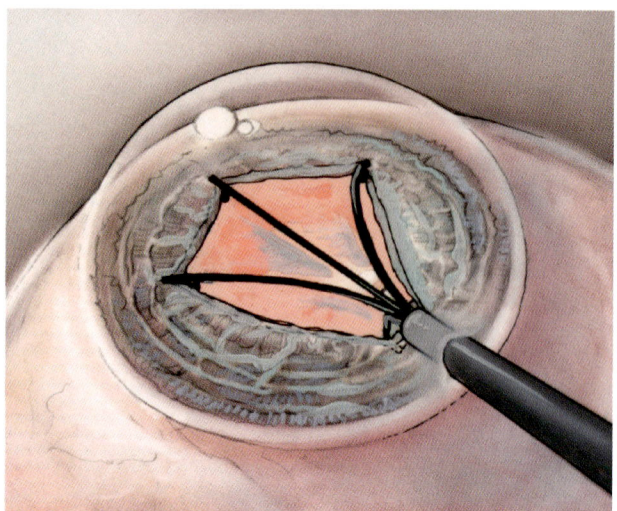

Fig. 4.1 Beehler pupil dilator is utilized to stretch the pupil. Each of the splines is engaged at the pupil margin opposite the wound. The hook on the barrel engages the iris near the wound. The splines are then gently wiggled to and fro to increase the micro-sphincter tears, resulting in more effective pupil dilation.

A simple technique that involves anterior elongated corneal incisions has been described to reduce the incidence and severity of IFIS and related complications.[33] The elongated incisions are performed ~ 1 mm anterior to the limbus and with a relatively long tunnel (~ 1.5- to 2.0-fold of the standard tunnel), distant from the peripheral iris to avoid iris billowing and eventual prolapse. This technique can be combined with any of the other surgical strategies and devices.

Pupil Expanders

There are generally three types of iris retractors: iris hooks, iris rings (open and closed loops), and the novel APX expander.

Iris retractors are simple and effective means to dilate the small pupil. Each hook is inserted through an individual stab incision, and usually three to five corneal incisions are required. The hooks can be placed in a variety of positions; thus, the pupil shape and dimension is determined by the surgeon (**Fig. 4.2a,b**). The hooks may occasionally be utilized to support the unstable capsular bag in cases such as PXF or subluxated crystalline lens. The disadvantages of the iris hooks include multiple stab incisions; time-consuming placement and removal; extension of the hook shafts beyond the surgical field, which may interfere with surgery; and permanent irregular pupil shape postoperatively.

A variety of pupillary rings were developed in recent years. These pupil expanders protect the iris sphincter during surgery and enable the pupil to return to its normal size, shape, and function after cataract surgery.

Open rings include the Perfect pupil device (**Fig. 4.3a**) (Milvella, Sydney, Australia) and the Morcher pupil dilator (**Fig. 4.3b**) (Morcher GMBH, Stuttgart, Germany). The Perfect pupil device is a disposable polyurethane ring with an internal diameter of 7.0 mm. The ring is open for 45 degrees (1.5 clock hour positions) to enable the passage of instruments. The Morcher pupil dilator is made of polymethylmethacrylate (PMMA) with an internal diameter of 6.0 mm. Kershner[32] reported a series of patients using the Perfect pupil device. The mean pupil was 3.2 mm preoperatively, 7.8 mm after device insertion, and 4.3 mm postremoval. No intraoperative or postoperative complications occurred. This device was effective also in cases of floppy iris.[33]

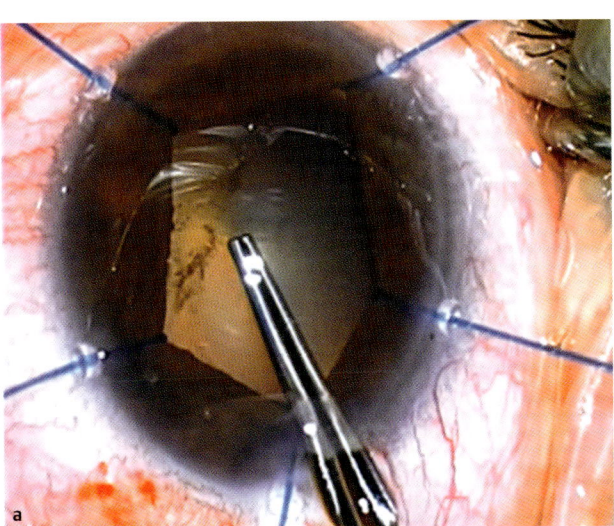

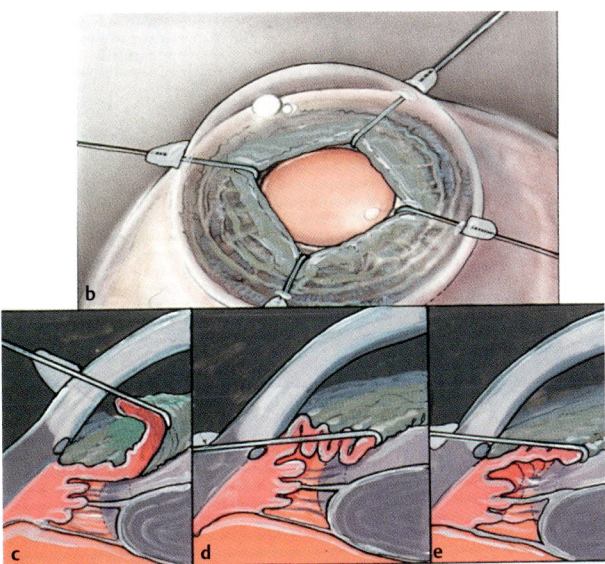

Fig. 4.2 **(a)** Iris hooks. The size and shape of the pupil are determined by the surgeon. **(b)** Micro-iris retractors shown with the appropriate amount of pupillary retraction. **(c)** The paracentesis is too high in the cornea. The iris is folded toward the cornea, making it impossible to pass the phaco tip into the anterior chamber without damaging the iris. **(d)** The paracentesis is too low. The iris is bunched up as the retractor is retracted. Passage of the phaco tip without iris damage is unlikely. **(e)** The correct placement of the paracentesis is demonstrated. Note the iris is retracted, and there is adequate space for the passage of the phaco tip.

Closed rings include the Graether 2000 pupil expander (**Fig. 4.3c**) (Eagle Vision, Inc., Memphis, TN), the Malyugin ring (**Fig. 4.3d**) (MicroSurgical Technology [MST], Redmond, WA), the Oasis iris expander (**Fig. 4.3e**) (Oasis Medical, Glendora, CA), and Xpand NT Iris Speculum (**Fig. 4.3f**) (Diamatrix, Woodlands, TX).

The Graether 2000 pupil expander is made of silicone and opens to 7.0 mm. The Malyugin ring is a disposable device made of PMMA with an internal diameter of 6.25 or 7.0 mm. The Oasis iris expander is also a disposable, a 6.25- or 7.0-mm ring made of polypropylene. The Xpand NT Iris Speculum is made of titanium-nickel alloy and is reusable for up to 20 repeated uses. The main advantage of the rings is that they are inserted through the main incision and no additional openings are required. However, placement of the rings, as well as their removal, require multiple

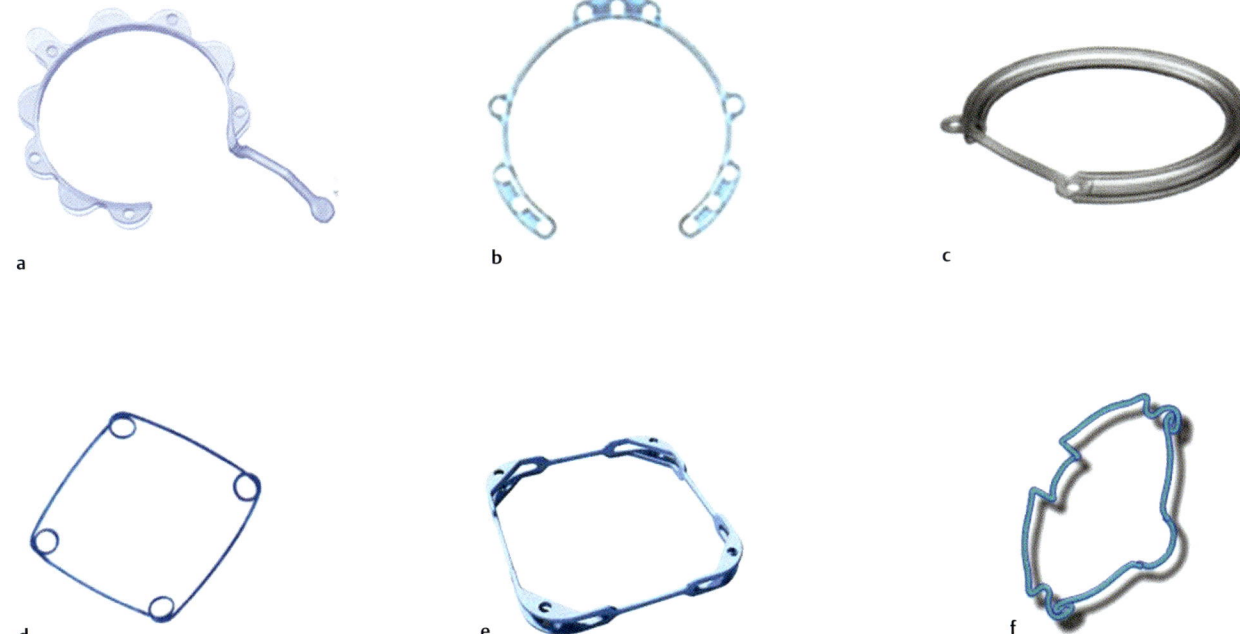

Fig. 4.3 Pupillary rings. Open rings: **(a)** Perfect pupil; **(b)** Morcher pupil dilator. Closed rings: **(c)** Graether 2000; **(d)** Malyugin ring; **(e)** Oasis iris expander; **(f)** Xpand NT Iris Speculum.

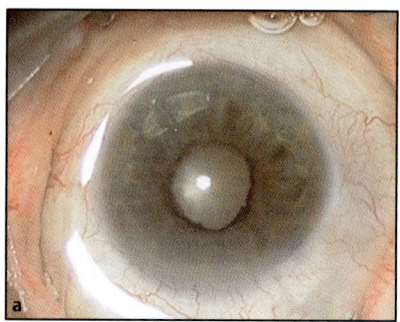
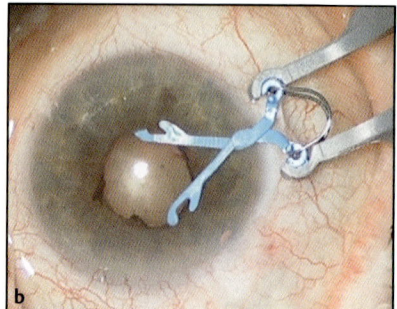
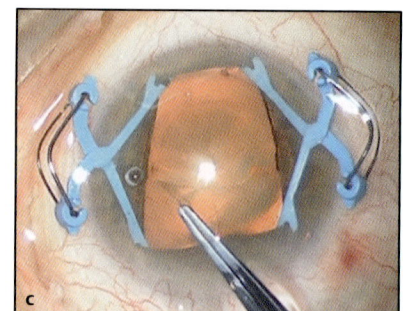
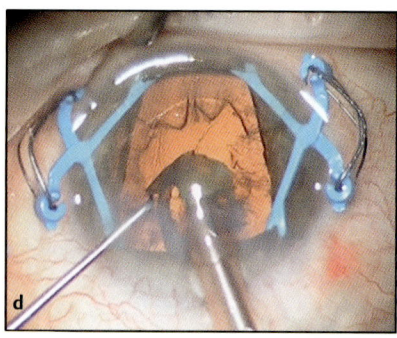
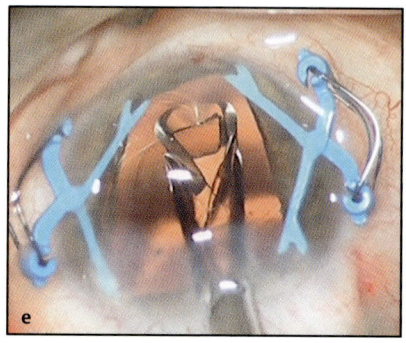
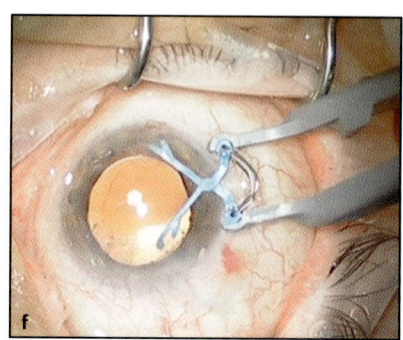

Fig. 4.4 The Assia Pupil Expander (APX). **(a)** Small pupil and posterior synechia in an eye with uveitic cataract. **(b)** The APX is inserted through a 19-gauge side-port incision. The terminal tips are positioned behind the iris. **(c)** Anterior continuous curvilinear capsulorrhexis (CCC) is performed under direct visualization. **(d)** Asymmetrical positioning of the two devices crates a trapezoidal opening. The wider base, facing the surgeon, provides a more "device-free" area for a convenient phacoemulsification. **(e)** A posterior-chamber intraocular lens is inserted though the visible anterior CCC. **(f)** Removal of the APX using the designated forceps. No intraocular maneuvers are required to position or remove the pupil expander.

intraocular manipulations and is time-consuming. The Malyugin ring is currently the most popular device in North America and is discussed in Chapter 5.

A novel device based on a different concept was recently developed by Assia—the APX (Assia Pupil Expander, APX Ophthalmology, Haifa, Israel). Two devices are inserted through opposite 19-gauge stab incisions using designated forceps. The terminal blunt tips are positioned behind the iris and the forceps are slowly released to allow the scissors-like miniature device to open to its full dimension. A 6-mm × 6-mm quadrangular or trapezoidal shaped pupillary opening is thus created (**Fig. 4.4**). No intraocular manipulations are needed for the insertion, positioning, or removal of the APX device. Removal of the pupil expanders is done by using the same designated forceps. The device is simply closed and pulled out in a matter of a few seconds. The plastic, single-use model APX-200 was used in a variety of cases including PXF syndrome, posttrauma, uveitic cataract, post–filtration surgery, lens coloboma, mature and hypermature dense cataract, and patients with clinical IFIS. Posterior-chamber IOLs were implanted as secondary procedures in aphakic eyes into the ciliary sulcus or "glued" to the sclera. The APX was also used in four cases of pars plana vitrectomy and did not interfere with the insertion and maneuvering of the vitreoretinal instruments. In all cases the operations were successfully performed with effective pupil dilation throughout surgery, and no intraoperative or postoperative device-related complications were noted. Surgeries were done in superior, lateral, or oblique approaches according to the surgeon's preference.

Conclusion

Small pupil is a major challenge in intraocular surgery, most commonly cataract surgery. A variety of pre- and perioperative medications, surgical instruments and techniques, and an arsenal of pupil dilators help perform a safe and successful operation in most cases.

References

1. Levine L. Mydriatic effectiveness of dilute combinations of phenylephrine and tropicamide. Am J Optom Physiol Opt 1982;59:580–594

2. Eyeson-Annan ML, Hirst LW, Battistutta D, Green A. Comparative pupil dilation using phenylephrine alone or in combination with tropicamide. Ophthalmology 1998;105:726–732

3. Chang DF, Campbell JR. Intraoperative floppy iris syndrome associated with tamsulosin. J Cataract Refract Surg 2005;31:664–673

4. Srinivasan R, Madhavaranga. Topical ketorolac tromethamine 0.5% versus diclofenac sodium 0.1% to inhibit miosis during cataract surgery. J Cataract Refract Surg 2002;28:517–520

5. Ritch R, Schlötzer-Schrehardt U. Exfoliation syndrome. Surv Ophthalmol 2001;45:265–315

6. Hiller R, Sperduto RD, Krueger DE. Pseudoexfoliation, intraocular pressure, and senile lens changes in a population-based survey. Arch Ophthalmol 1982;100:1080–1082

7. Puska P, Tarkkanen A. Exfoliation syndrome as a risk factor for cataract development: five-year follow-up of lens opacities in exfoliation syndrome. J Cataract Refract Surg 2001;27:1992–1998

8. Ritch R. Exfoliation syndrome. Curr Opin Ophthalmol 2001;12:124–130

9. Ritch R. Exfoliation syndrome and occludable angles. Trans Am Ophthalmol Soc 1994;92:845–944

10. Young AL, Tang WWT, Lam DSC. The prevalence of pseudoexfoliation syndrome in Chinese people. Br J Ophthalmol 2004;88:193–195

11. Kaljurand K, Puska P. Exfoliation syndrome in Estonian patients scheduled for cataract surgery. Acta Ophthalmol Scand 2004;82(3 Pt 1):259–263

12. Guzek JP, Holm M, Cotter JB, et al. Risk factors for intraoperative complications in 1000 extracapsular cataract cases. Ophthalmology 1987;94:461–466

13. Lumme P, Laatikainen L. Exfoliation syndrome and cataract extraction. Am J Ophthalmol 1993;116:51–55

14. Shingleton BJ, Heltzer J, O'Donoghue MW. Outcomes of phacoemulsification in patients with and without pseudoexfoliation syndrome. J Cataract Refract Surg 2003;29:1080–1086

15. Hyams M, Mathalone N, Herskovitz M, Hod Y, Israeli D, Geyer O. Intraoperative complications of phacoemulsification in eyes with and without pseudoexfoliation. J Cataract Refract Surg 2005;31:1002–1005

16. Shingleton BJ, Crandall AS, Ahmed II. Pseudoexfoliation and the cataract surgeon: preoperative, intraoperative, and postoperative issues related to intraocular pressure, cataract, and intraocular lenses. J Cataract Refract Surg 2009;35:1101–1120

17. Chang DF, Braga-Mele R, Mamalis N, et al; ASCRS Cataract Clinical Committee. ASCRS White Paper: clinical review of intraoperative floppy-iris syndrome. J Cataract Refract Surg 2008;34:2153–2162

18. Blouin MC, Blouin J, Perreault S, Lapointe A, Dragomir A. Intraoperative floppy-iris syndrome associated with alpha1-adrenoreceptors: comparison of tamsulosin and alfuzosin. J Cataract Refract Surg 2007;33:1227–1234

19. Chatziralli IP, Sergentanis TN. Risk factors for intraoperative floppy iris syndrome: a meta-analysis. Ophthalmology 2011;118:730–735

20. Takmaz T, Can I. Intraoperative floppy-iris syndrome: do we know everything about it? J Cataract Refract Surg 2007;33:1110–1112

21. Handzel DM, Briesen S, Rausch S, Kälble T. Cataract surgery in patients taking alpha-1 antagonists: know the risks, avoid the complications. Dtsch Arztebl Int 2012;109:379–384

22. Chang DF, Osher RH, Wang L, Koch DD. Prospective multicenter evaluation of cataract surgery in patients taking tamsulosin (Flomax). Ophthalmology 2007;114:957–964

23. Keates RH, McGowan KA. The effect of topical indomethacin ophthalmic solution in maintaining mydriasis during cataract surgery. Ann Ophthalmol 1984;16:1116–1121

24. Stewart R, Grosserode R, Cheetham JK, Rosenthal A. Efficacy and safety profile of ketorolac 0.5% ophthalmic solution in the prevention of surgically induced miosis during cataract surgery. Clin Ther 1999;21:723–732

25. Lindstrom RL, Loden JC, Walters TR, et al. Intracameral phenylephrine and ketorolac injection (OMS302) for maintenance of intraoperative pupil diameter and reduction of postoperative pain in intraocular lens replacement with phacoemulsification. Clin Ophthalmol 2014;8:1735–1744

26. Bendel RE, Phillips MB. Preoperative use of atropine to prevent intraoperative floppy-iris syndrome in patients taking tamsulosin. J Cataract Refract Surg 2006;32:1603–1605

27. Masket S, Belani S. Combined preoperative topical atropine sulfate 1% and intracameral nonpreserved epinephrine hydrochloride 1:4000 [corrected] for management of intraoperative floppy-iris syndrome. J Cataract Refract Surg 2007;33:580–582

28. Gurbaxani A, Packard R. Intracameral phenylephrine to prevent floppy iris syndrome during cataract surgery in patients on tamsulosin. Eye (Lond) 2007;21:331–332

29. Oetting TA, Omphroy LC. Modified technique using flexible iris retractors in clear corneal cataract surgery. J Cataract Refract Surg 2002;28:596–598

30. Graether JM. Graether pupil expander for managing the small pupil during surgery. J Cataract Refract Surg 1996;22:530–535

31. Chang DF. Use of Malyugin pupil expansion device for intraoperative floppy-iris syndrome: results in 30 consecutive cases. J Cataract Refract Surg 2008;34:835–841

32. Kershner RM. Management of the small pupil for clear corneal cataract surgery. J Cataract Refract Surg 2002;28:1826–1831

33. Segev F, Armarnic S, Rosen E, Assia EI. Anterior elongated corneal incisions to avoid surgical complications in IFIS (Intraoperative Floppy Iris Syndrome) prone patients. Presented at the 29th Congress of the European Society of Cataract and Refractive Surgery (ESCRS), Vienna, Austria, 2011

5 Malyugin Ring

Boris Malyugin

Despite the different treatments available to expand the iris during cataract extraction, performing surgery on an eye with a small pupil remains technically challenging. Complications that can occur during small pupil phacoemulsification surgery include iris damage and bleeding, iris prolapse through the paracentesis or the main wound, anterior capsule damage, incomplete evacuation of the cortical material, and difficulties with placing and aligning the intraocular lens (IOL) in the capsular bag.

Various pupil expansion devices are currently available, such as iris hooks, rings, and expanders. Among them, the Malyugin ring (MicroSurgical Technologies [MST], Redmond, WA) is currently one of the most popular. It was developed to give surgeons a reliable device that is easy to use, expands the pupil up to 7.0 mm, and protects the iris from damage.[1,2]

This chapter describes the technique of implantation and removal of the Malyugin ring in patients with small pupils or intraoperative floppy iris syndrome (IFIS) through various size incisions. Tips on how to better manipulate the device in and out of the eye and to avoid complications are provided. Special attention is paid to the use of the Malyugin ring pupil issues in femtosecond laser–assisted cataract surgery (FLACS).

Malyugin Ring Design and Characteristics

The Malyugin ring is made of 4/0 polypropylene, and has a one-piece design with a square shape and four equidistantly located circular loops (**Fig. 5.1**). The loops located at each corner have a wedge-shaped gap used to accommodate the iris tissue. The thin scroll design has eight points of fixation, providing the surgeon with a round pupil instead of the square one that is formed after using four iris hooks (**Fig. 5.2**).

The Malyugin ring comes in two sizes: 6.25 mm and 7.0 mm. The advantage of the smaller ring is that it is easier to insert and to remove. It is better for eyes with a small white-to-white diameter. The advantage of the 7.0-mm ring is that one can use it if the pupil is larger at the start of the procedure, as occurs often in IFIS cases. The Malyugin Ring System produced by MST consists of a presterilized single-use holder containing the ring and injector. The hook of the injection device is used to catch the proximal loops of the Malyugin ring and retract it inside the tube as well as expel it from the injector.

Surgical Technique with the Malyugin Ring

A stepwise approach to manage small pupils is preferable. It is recommended to start with an intracameral injection of phenylephrine or epinephrine and eventually work up to mechanical pupil expansion.

Surgical steps of the Malyugin ring implantation are as follows. After topical anesthesia is applied, a clear corneal incision is performed and anesthetic solution and ophthalmic viscosurgical device (OVD) are both injected into the anterior chamber in a sequential manner. It may be helpful to inject a small amount of OVD under the iris, at the pupillary margin, to slightly elevate the pupillary margin. This will facilitate the positioning of the ring loops. The Malyugin ring is loaded into the injector. The injector tip is inserted through a 2.2-mm or wider clear corneal incision. The tip of the injector is passed through the anterior chamber toward the pupillary margin (**Fig. 5.3**).

While slowly pushing on the injector plunger, the ring is released from the tip ~ 1.0 to 2.0 mm forward, and the distal scroll is engaged in the distal iris. Continued pressure on the injector plunger, while simultaneously slowly withdrawing the injector, permits injection of the remainder of the ring. The lateral scrolls emerge from the injector tube and one (or both) of them simultaneously catches the iris margins. If the lateral scrolls do not engage the pupillary margin, they are positioned with the Osher/Malyugin ring manipulator as noted below. When the proximal scroll is expelled from the injector, the injector hook is moved forward to the point when it is no longer holding the ring (**Fig. 5.4**). At this moment the scroll is usually lying on top of the injector platform. The injector is withdrawn from the eye, and the Osher/Malyugin ring manipulator is used to engage the proximal ring scroll (**Fig. 5.5**).

In some cases the ring manipulator is inserted through the paracentesis, which helps to disengage the proximal scroll from the injector hook by displacing the scroll to the side and away from injector tip.

The next steps of the surgical procedure are straightforward and are mostly specific to the lens capsule properties and nucleus hardness. These steps include anterior curvilinear capsulorrhexis, hydrodissection and hydrodelineation, ultrasonic nucleus fragmentation, evacuation of the cortical material, and IOL implantation (**Figs. 5.6, 5.7, 5.8**).

The Malyugin ring is removed from the eye in reverse order of its implantation. The anterior chamber should be re-formed with cohesive OVD. The Malyugin ring manipulator inserted through the main incision catches the distal scroll and moves it toward the center of the pupil and up until it disengages. Then this scroll is moved back toward the iris periphery to displace the ring downward. This maneuver helps to expose the proximal scroll, which is then disengaged by the manipulator from the iris and placed onto the anterior iris surface. Then the injector's platform is positioned under the proximal scroll, with the hook fully deployed from the tube. The proximal scroll catches with the hook and the plunger is moved backward (**Fig. 5.9**). The ring is retracted inside the injector tube. Being retracted halfway inside the injector, one of the side scrolls sits on top of the injector tube and does not allow the ring to go inside the injector completely. To fully retract the ring, I recommend pressing with the side-port

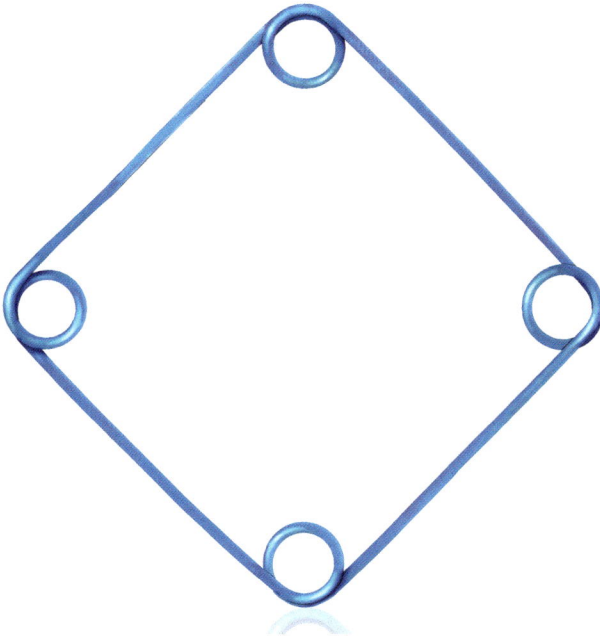

Fig. 5.1   The general view of the Malyugin ring.

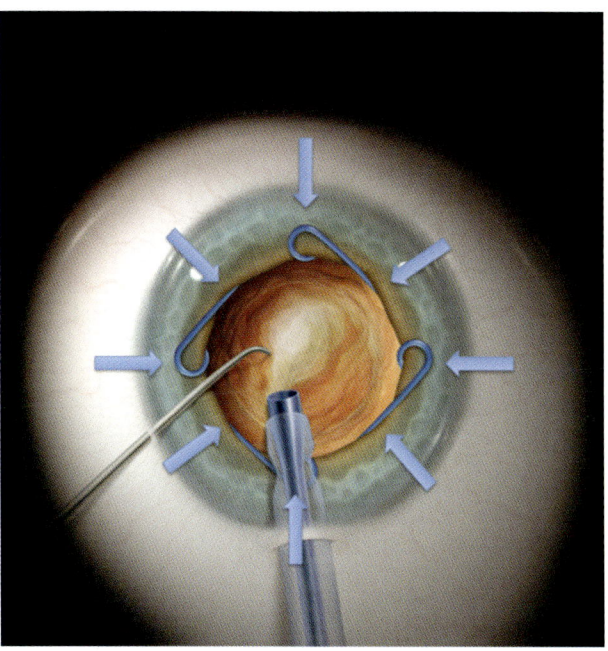

Fig. 5.2   Eight-point pupil fixation mechanism with the Malyugin ring.

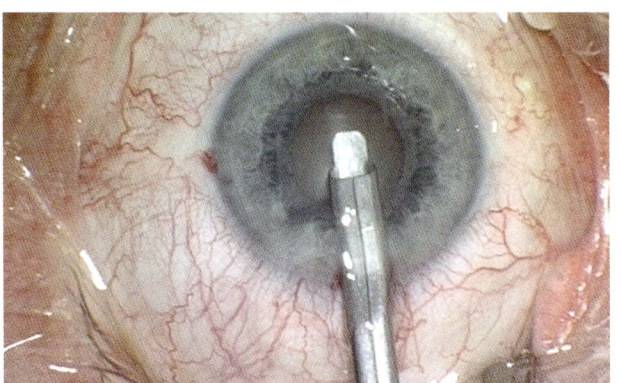

Fig. 5.3   Positioning of the injector close to the iris margin helps to control its engagement with the distal scroll.

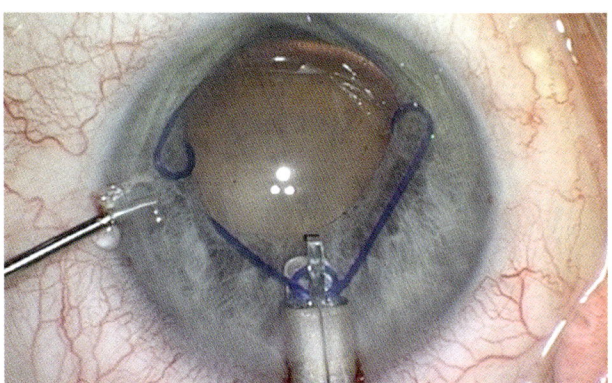

Fig. 5.4   Lateral scrolls emerge from the injector and both of them simultaneously catch the iris margins.

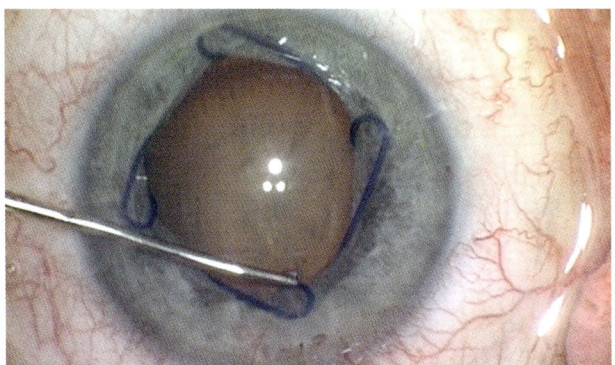

Fig. 5.5   The Osher/Malyugin ring manipulator is used to engage the last (proximal scroll) with the iris margin.

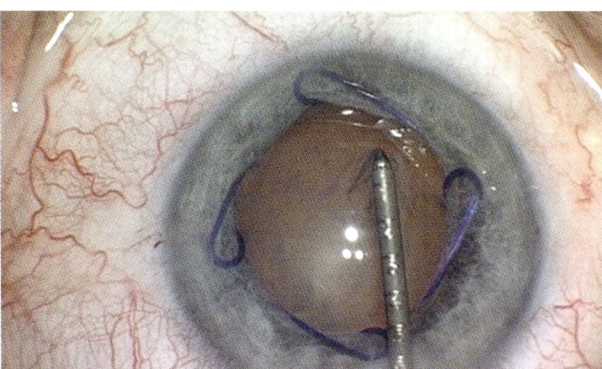

Fig. 5.6   The Malyugin ring is in place. Anterior curvilinear capsulorrhexis is performed with the forceps.

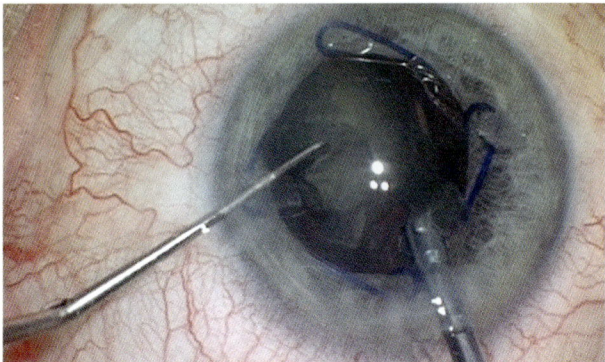

Fig. 5.7 Nucleus fragmentation is in progress.

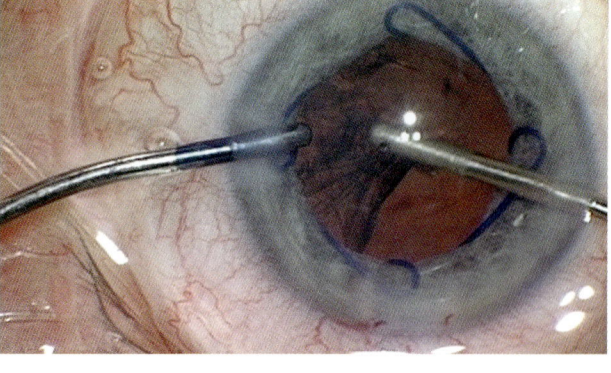

Fig. 5.8 Irrigation-aspiration of cortical material.

instrument on both lateral scrolls simultaneously when they merge together near the tip of the injector. With this maneuver the surgeon guides the scrolls inside the injector. With a 2.75-mm main incision, it is possible to stop retracting the ring when one of the lateral scrolls rides above the cannula and then remove the whole assembly.

Alternatively, each of the scrolls can be disengaged from the pupil with the Osher/Malyugin manipulator, and the ring is removed with it or with a Kuglen hook by engaging the proximal scroll and slowly extracting it through the incision.

After ring removal, the pupil usually constricts spontaneously (**Fig. 5.10**). Finally, OVD is aspirated from the anterior chamber and corneal wounds are checked for the self-sealing properties.

Because the Malyugin ring can be placed through a main incision that is 2.2 mm or larger, it eliminates the need for extra incisions or additional paracentesis for iris hooks. By using a wound-assisted technique for insertion and removal, the ring can be used in microincisional (1.8 mm) cataract surgery.

The latest version of the device, Malyugin ring 2.0, is made of 5/0 polypropylene. While maintaining the same geometrical dimensions and size, this ring can go through the smaller bore cannula because of its slimmer thread. It is now possible to implant and to remove this ring version through the 2.0-mm incision without enlarging it.

Malyugin Ring in Femtosecond Laser–Assisted Cataract Surgery

Having a wide, well-dilated pupil is a prerequisite for successful FLACS.[3] There are two ways of using the Malyugin ring in FLACS:

(1) Create the incision, insert the ring, remove OVD, make the incision watertight, and place the patient under the laser for docking and subsequent steps.[4,5] (2) Use the ring only at the surgical step of the procedure to expand the pupil for effective lens evacuation and IOL implantation.

The surgeon performing the laser step in the operating room may prefer using the first option. There is no waste of time moving the patient back and forth, and there is reduced risk of contamination when docking is performed on the eye with a preplaced incision.[6,7]

The second option is beneficial when the pupil unexpectedly constricts after the laser step. When implanting the Malyugin ring after the anterior capsulorrhexis have been created, there is a high risk of the surgeon catching the capsular edge with one or more of the scrolls. To prevent this, I recommend using highly viscous OVD, for instance Healon 5 (Abbott Medical Optics, Abbott Park, IL), and injecting it behind the iris at four points corresponding to the future position of the scrolls on the iris margin. Note that the regular cohesive OVD (1% sodium hyaluronate) usually does not provide sustainable iris lifting. While injecting the leading scroll, it is good to position the injector tip very close to the iris margin. This maneuver facilitates controlling the moment of engaging the scroll with the iris. The scrolls that are not in place after the ring is completely injected into the eye are positioned with the ring manipulator.

The next step is critical, as the surgeon must ensure that the ring is not engaging the anterior capsulorrhexis margin. For this step, a "picture frame" maneuver is very useful. With the side-port instrument, it is easy to displace the ring in any direction, very much like a picture frame. Restrictions to movement in certain directions usually correspond to the scroll that is catching the anterior capsule. After this is recognized, it is quite easy to

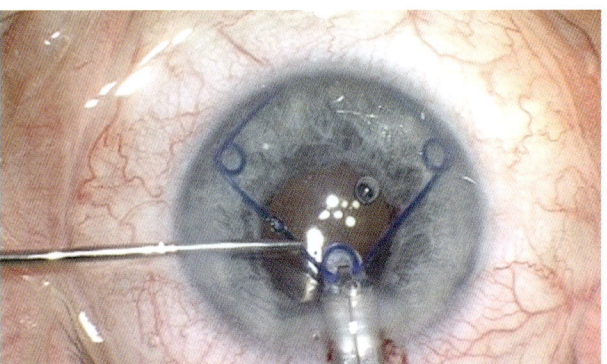

Fig. 5.9 Malyugin ring removal.

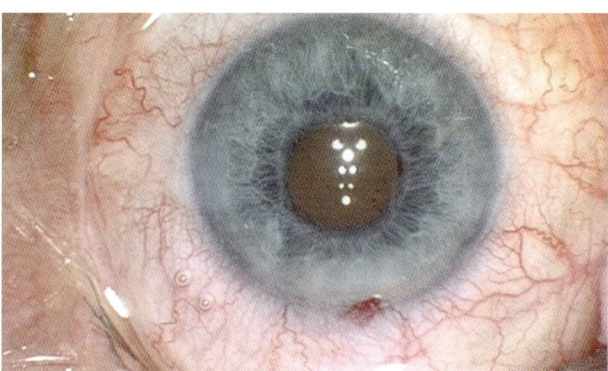

Fig. 5.10 The eye at the end of the procedure.

insert the ring manipulator, catch the scroll, retract it toward the center of the anterior chamber, disengage the scroll from the iris (and capsule), and then lift it a bit and reposition it back in contact with the pupillary edge. This step can be repeated if more ring scrolls are catching the anterior capsule. Finally, the "picture frame" maneuver is repeated to ensure the free movement and correct positioning of the Malyugin ring.

Typically in femtosecond laser–created capsulorrhexis the anterior capsular rim has a specific gray-whitish color. This is helpful for the surgeon to identify and visualize the capsular edge, in contrast to cases with manually created capsulorrhexis.

Complications

When the proper technique of Malyugin ring handling is applied, complications are uncommon. Careful intraoperative manipulation and insertion of the ring with liberal use of an OVD can help prevent problems in the majority of cases. If the pupil is fibrotic, one may expect to have sphincter micro-tears or bleeding from the iris margin vessels. The latter can also happen if a small pupil is associated with iris neovascularization. If the ring is disengaged too aggressively, it is possible to loosen the pigment epithelium from the posterior iris surface. Nevertheless, after surgery, most patients have pupils that are almost indistinguishable from their appearance before surgery, with functional activity well preserved. The use of the Malyugin ring greatly reduces postoperative abnormalities in pupil size and function that are a frequent finding with iris hooks.

Conclusion

With the advent of new medications and devices, performing cataract surgery on small pupils carries much lesser risk than in the past. The Malyugin ring is an important tool in phacoemulsification surgery armamentarium, and it has the following advantages:

- The instrument is inserted through the main incision, and thus multiple additional incisions are not necessary.
- It has no sharp or pointed ends that can damage the eye.

- Compared with other iris retractors, it is friendlier to the eye due to the well-distributed and well-controlled iris stretching, the gentle holding of delicate iris tissue, and easier and less traumatic handling.
- It is easy to insert the instrument into the eye and to remove it with a help of the inserter, thus reducing the risk of contamination and disturbance of the incision's architecture and wound integrity.
- Eight equidistant points of iris margin fixation ensure correct positioning of the iris and prevent the effects and consequences of pupil overstretching.
- The instrument provides sufficient room for nucleus fragmentation and removal.
- The instrument is more convenient than hooks in cases with narrow lid fissures because it does not involve additional external manipulations.
- The instrument works very well in patients who are on α1-adrenergic blocking agents (such as Flomax), which is a known risk factor for IFIS.

References

1. Malyugin B. Small pupil phaco surgery: a new technique. Ann Ophthalmol (Skokie) 2007;39:185–193
2. Chang DF. Use of Malyugin pupil expansion device for intraoperative floppy-iris syndrome: results in 30 consecutive cases. J Cataract Refract Surg 2008;34:835–841
3. Hatch KM, Talamo JH. Laser-assisted cataract surgery: Barriers of the femtosecond laser. Curr Opin Ophthalmol 2014;25:54–61
4. Donaldson KE, Braga-Mele R, Cabot F, et al; ASCRS Refractive Cataract Surgery Subcommittee. Femtosecond laser-assisted cataract surgery. J Cataract Refract Surg 2013;39:1753–1763
5. Jirasková N, Rozsíval P, Lešták L. Use of Malyugin pupil expansion ring in femtosecond laser-assisted cataract surgery. J Clin Exp Ophthalmol 2013;4: doi: 10.4172/2155-9570.1000312
6. Conrad-Hengerer I, Hengerer FH, Schultz T, Dick HB. Femtosecond laser-assisted cataract surgery in eyes with a small pupil. J Cataract Refract Surg 2013;39:1314–1320
7. Dick HB, Schultz T. Laser-assisted cataract surgery in small pupils using mechanical dilation devices. J Refract Surg 2013;29:858–862

Section IV Management of Capsulorhexis and Complications

6 Anterior and Posterior Capsulorhexis

Howard V. Gimbel and Anika Amritanand

The development of continuous-tear curvilinear capsulorhexis (CCC) by Gimbel and Neuhann in the 1990s was essential for the development of modern phacoemulsification techniques such as divide and conquer. The CCC technique has stood the test of time, and the tear-resistance and subsequent lens stability it provides has made it a standard in phacoemulsification surgery. The advantages of these qualities can also be utilized in planned extracapsular cataract extraction as well manual small-incision cataract surgery.[1-6]

Creating a tear-resistant CCC provides the basis for complication–free phacoemulsification. An intact capsular bag is critical for safe and complete removal of the native lens, cortex stripping, and vacuum polishing the capsule as well as for implant centration and stability. Even in cases with zonular dehiscence, an intact capsular bag may enable placement of a capsular tension ring and an in-the-bag posterior chamber lens implant.

Although intra- and postoperative complications of CCC are not common, there is the potential for vision loss as a direct result of mismanagement of complications. Thus, should a problem occur during the creation of the CCC, the surgeon should immediately attempt to rectify it so as to prevent further compromise to the surgery and minimize the risk of postoperative complications. In our experience, properly performed CCC with in-the-bag intraocular lens (IOL) placement has reduced the incidence of intra- and postoperative complications.[7-21]

Capsular Anatomy

It is helpful to consider the key anatomic features of the lens capsule and to keep them in mind while performing both CCC and phacoemulsification. The capsule is an elastic basement membrane made up of type IV collagen (**Fig. 6.1**). This basement membrane is laid down by the lens epithelial cells, which reside just inside the capsule; residual lens epithelial cells are responsible for the postoperative capsular opacification and capsular contraction. This may result in the need for neodymium:yttrium-aluminum-garnet (Nd:YAG) laser treatment following cataract extraction.[22-25] The zonules insert on the anterior capsule over an area 2 to 2.5 mm in breadth. Therefore, if the crystalline lens is on average 10.5 mm, and the anterior zonules insert 2.5 mm from the equator, a capsulorhexis greater than 5.25 mm may tear some of the more anterior zonules. Occasionally, a zonular fiber may insert more anteriorly than usual. This can redirect the progressing circular capsule tear toward the equator. The capsule may be as thin as 2 to 4 µm at the posterior pole. It is thickest (17 to 23 µm) near the anterior and posterior equator where the zonular fibers attach.[26] The anterior capsule can be as thick as 14 µm in adults and continues to increase in thickness with age. The posterior capsule may be particularly fragile in cases with congenital posterior lenticonus and posterior polar cataract. Age-related or corticosteroid-related posterior subcapsular (PSC) cataracts involve migration and enlargement of the lens epithelial cells posteriorly where the capsule is thinnest.[27]

The surgeon must also be aware of such patient factors as age, disease (e.g., pseudoexfoliation or Marfan's syndrome), or a history of ocular trauma, which may predispose the patient to zonular weakness or dehiscence. Zonular dehiscence is discussed in Chapter 25.

Surgical Technique of Continuous Curvilinear Capsulorhexis

There are a variety of methods described for performing CCC.[1,28-31] One technique is to puncture the anterior capsule centrally with a sharp needle or instrument. This is then exchanged for a capsulorhexis forceps, and the CCC is completed as described below.

Gimbel and Kaye[1] described their currently preferred method of forceps-puncture CCC in 1997. This technique has the advantage of using only a single instrument but does require the use of an ophthalmic viscoelastic device (OVD).

This technique begins with OVD injection into the anterior chamber (AC) following a corneal paracentesis or after the creation of a scleral tunnel or clear corneal incision. An OVD filling of the AC before the CCC is performed is important, as it flattens the anterior capsule and provides both resistance to forward pressure of the vitreous against the lens and protection to the corneal endothelium. Forward pressure that is not neutralized leaves the anterior capsule convex, which creates a vector force that will tend to drive the tear peripherally. The OVD minimizes the anteriorly directed force of the lens against the tearing anterior capsule. Thus, the tendency for the capsular tear to extend toward the equator is minimized. Some eyes, such as pediatric eyes and short eyes, require a highly cohesive OVD to flatten the anterior capsule.

To create the initial central anterior capsular puncture, the capsule forceps should have sharp tips and be held with the tips together and with the tips pointing toward the center of the lens. Assuming a superior incision to describe the clock hour positions, the capsulotomy is started just proximal to the center by applying downward and forward pressure to puncture the capsule (**Fig. 6.2a**). After the initial puncture is made, the tip of the forceps is lifted and extended forward a bit to create either a short linear or triangular tear toward the 6 o'clock position. The left arm of the triangular or linear tear is then grasped and gently guided to the 3 o'clock position by pulling slightly and moving the tip of the forceps toward the left (**Fig. 6.2b**). Without

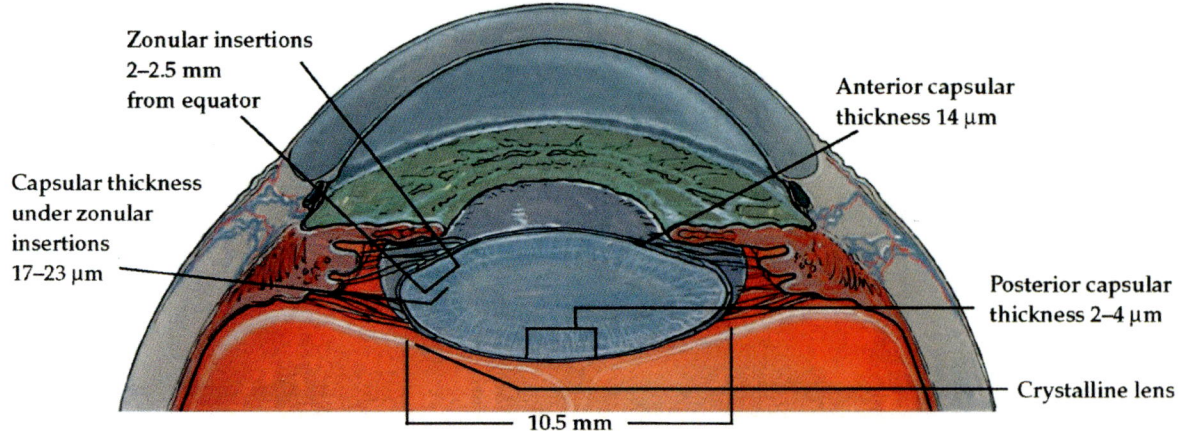

Fig. 6.1 The lens capsule is made up of type IV collagen. It is a basement membrane laid down by the lens epithelial cells residing just inside the capsule.

releasing the forceps, if possible, the tear is continued around to approximately the 12 o'clock position, where it can be easily re-grasped closer to the point of tearing for better control. The continuous tear can then proceed counterclockwise with two or three more re-grasps near the point of tearing to complete the CCC using a shearing technique (**Fig. 6.2c**). The capsule should be re-grasped as often as necessary to direct the tear in the direction desired.

The CCC can also be achieved using a bent needle or cystotome.[32] Under OVD cover the bent needle or cystotome is used to make an initial puncture at the planned center of the CCC. The opening is then extended to make a linear or triangular tear of the desired length. The flap is then turned over, and tearing forces are applied to the tearing edge to create a circular capsulorhexis. Similar to the forceps capsulorhexis, the CCC is completed by drawing the tear inward for the two torn ends to join with the ending tear joining the initial tear from the outside to avoid a triangular break in the circle.

Avoidance of Peripheral Extension of the Tear

To avoid the tendency for the tear to proceed peripherally, the tip of the forceps may have to be just behind the advancing tear. The tip of the forceps should then be directed such that the force of the movement is in anticipation of the intended direction of the tear. At times, the required vector force of the tear is such that the force needs to be directed centrally or even almost opposite to the advancing tear direction as the circular tear is created. If a tear begins to extend peripherally in spite of the above techniques, the surgeon should stop immediately. The possibility of positive posterior pressure should be entertained (**Fig. 6.3a**). This pressure will cause the lens to move anteriorly and create a vector force toward the periphery. This force will drive the tear relentlessly into the equator. Causes of increased posterior pressure should be minimized. The speculum may have to be loosened, the drapes relaxed, and if topical anesthesia is being

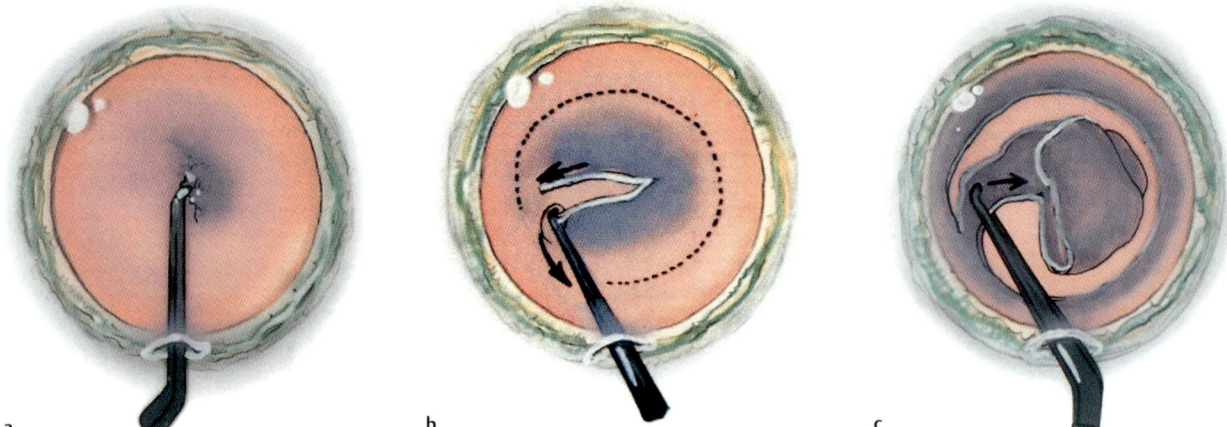

a **b** **c**

Fig. 6.2 **(a)** The Gimbel-modified Kraff-Utrata forceps is used to create the initial anterior capsular tear as well as to perform the continuous-tear capsulorhexis **(b,c)**. **(b)** The edge of the capsule is regrasped and guided in a controlled fashion to complete the capsulorhexis at the 3 o'clock position by drawing the tear inward **(c)**.

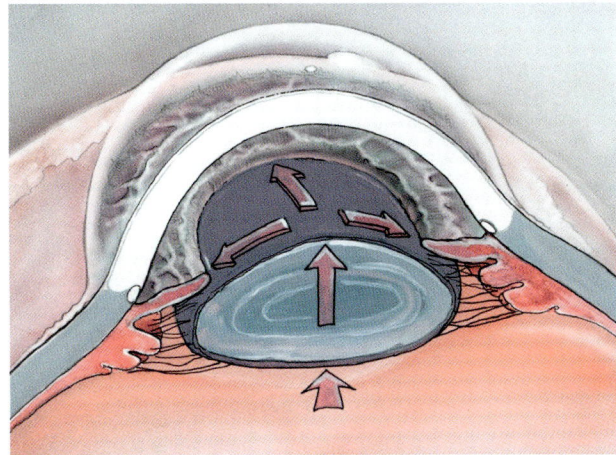

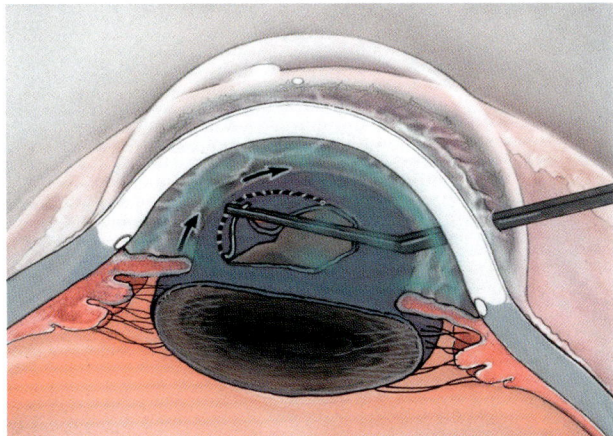

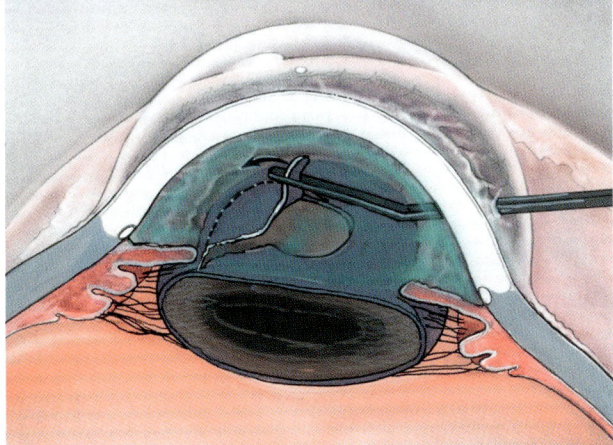

Fig. 6.3 **(a)** Positive pressure from behind the lens creates a vector force that directs the tear to extend toward the equator. **(b)** Deepening the anterior chamber with dispersive viscoelastic flattens the anterior lens surface and counteracts these vector forces. The tear can then be redirected toward the center of the nucleus. *Step 1:* Fold the flap over the anterior capsule. *Step 2:* Re-grasp the flap near the tear. *Step 3:* Pull the flap in the opposite direction and toward the center to redirect it. *Step 4:* Once redirected, continue the capsulorhexis. **(c)** The tear cannot be redirected. It is therefore completed from the opposite direction.

utilized and the patient is squeezing the eyelids, additional sedation may be necessary. Once these problems are remedied, additional OVD, preferably a highly cohesive one, should be added to further deepen the AC and flatten the anterior capsule/lens surface (**Fig. 6.3b**). This will reduce the tendency for the capsular tear to extend peripherally, and the rhexus can be completed. Then the capsular edge should be gently grasped immediately adjacent to the tear, and guided back with a careful movement directed centrally or against the extending tear (**Fig. 6.4a**).

Sometimes it is helpful to fold the tearing part of the capsule over on itself and then grasp it near the tear and tear it firmly toward the anatomic center of the lens as described by Little et al[33] (**Fig. 6.4b-d**). If an anterior tear cannot be turned back toward the center using the forceps, a small area of the can-opener technique can be utilized to remove this section of the capsule. A small strip of capsule encompassing a short tear can be created to avoid radial extension of the tear.[2,22] If the tear cannot be turned back, and it extends well into the equator, the capsulorhexis can be completed from the opposite direction (**Fig. 6.3c**). This type of rhexis is obviously not continuous. Therefore, in this situation, or anytime a capsule tear disappears under the iris such that its peripheral extent cannot be visualized, the surgeon must expend due care to prevent the extension of the tear around the equator and into the posterior capsule. In this circumstance, hydrodissection may have to be omitted, excess pressure during phacoemulsification avoided, and cortex removal performed carefully to avoid extension of the radialized tear. Additional principles of management in these cases are discussed below.

Capsulorhexis Technique for Patients with Small Pupils

In patients with small pupils, the use of a centrally directed tearing motion may move the side of the lens into view and enhance the visibility of a capsulorhexis edge that is larger than the pupil opening. In this setting, extreme care must be taken to ensure that, at the completion of the rhexis, the ends of the tear overlap, that is, the tear is completed from the outside toward the inside of the capsule edge. This will ensure that there are no nicks or triangular edges in the capsule. During later steps in the procedure, the angled edge has the potential to extend peripherally. It may be helpful, in addition, to use a second instrument through the paracentesis to gently push the iris aside for better visibility. The use of additional OVD between the iris and anterior capsule is another method to lift and help enlarge the pupillary aperature.[34] Although some surgeons may be able to accurately assess the location of the tear by noting the location of the folding of the anterior capsule as the CCC proceeds, even if it is hidden by the iris, direct visualization of the CCC as it is being performed is recommended.

If the pupil is too small for these measures, it should be enlarged with one of the methods described in Chapters 4 and 5. Devices such as iris retractors or other pupil expansion devices such as the Malyugin ring can also be used to stretch the pupil to achieve an optimal-sized CCC.[35,36] If the resulting CCC is too small, it can be enlarged by using Gills-Welsh/Vannas scissors or microscissors directed in a tangential counterclockwise direction to begin a slightly more peripheral tear (**Fig. 6.5a**). Care should be taken not to close the scissors completely, as the tips closing will create a jagged end to the snip. The new flap edge created in this way can then be directed using a forceps (**Figs. 6.5b–e**).

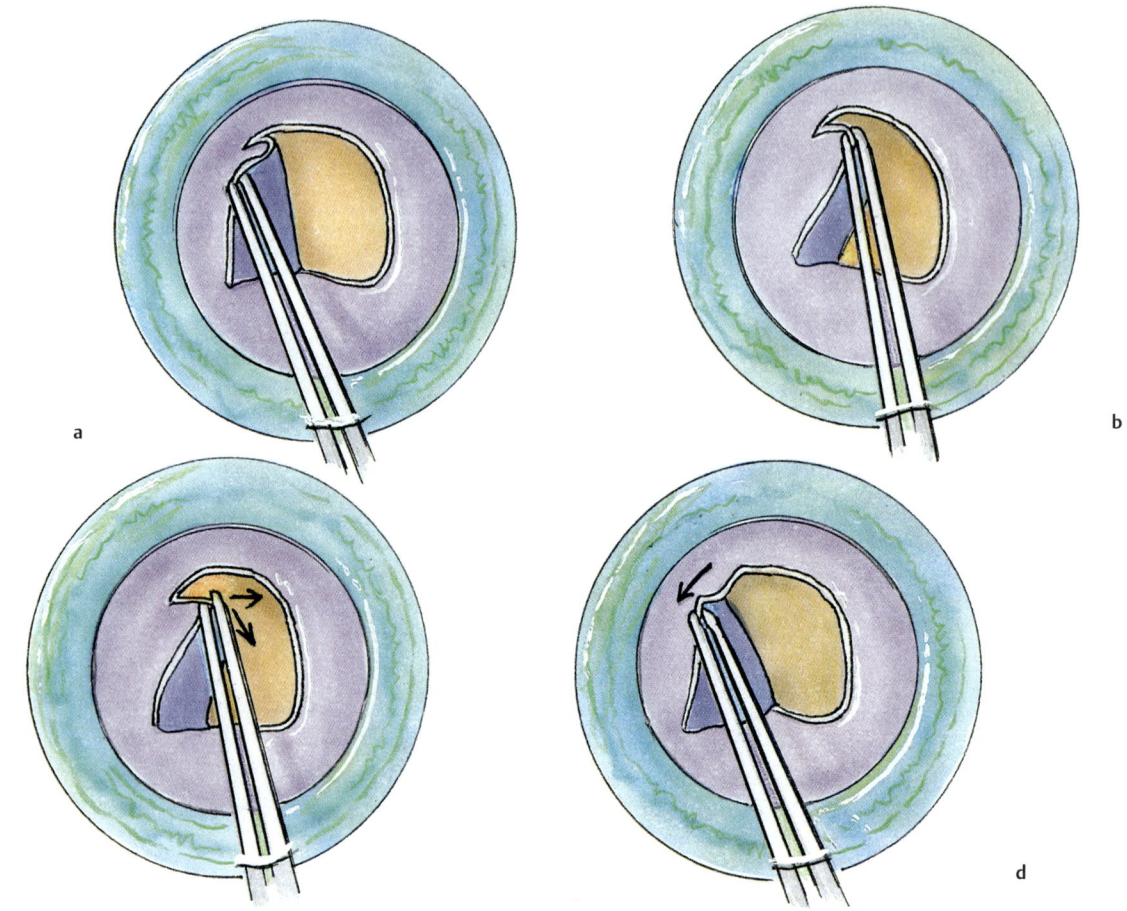

Fig. 6.4 Little Rescue Technique **(a)** Step 1: Fold the flap over the anterior capsule. **(b)** Step 2: Regrasp the flap near the tear. **(c)** Step 3: Pull the flap in the opposite direction and toward the center to redirect it. **(d)** Step 4: Once redirected, continue the capsulorhexis.

Capsulorhexis Size

There is debate regarding the optimum size for the capsulorhexis. Three significant factors determine CCC size: (1) the relationship of the capsular opening to the size and maturity of the cataract, and the expected lens removal procedure to be performed; (2) the size of the optic of the anticipated IOL; and (3) anatomic abnormalities of the zonules.

Cataract Size and Type

The capsule opening must provide adequate access to the cataract. In cases of nuclear mature, hard brown cataracts, too small a rhexis predisposes to rupture of the posterior capsule during the hydrodissection (see Chapter 7). Nuclear manipulation is facilitated by the creation of a large enough CCC. The likelihood of creating a tear in the anterior capsule during phacoemulsification is minimized as well as providing for more maneuvering. Should a tear occur, however, the risk of more significant complications exists. The tear does not have to extend very far to progress to or through to the equator, which would destabilize the remaining anterior capsular support for a sulcus-placed IOL.

In the case of white, cortically mature cataracts, an initially small CCC to be enlarged later in the procedure may be considered. This is discussed in greater detail below.

Intraocular Lens Optic Size

We recommend that the final CCC should be only about a millimeter smaller and concentric with the IOL so that no portion of the anterior capsule CCC edge can fuse to the posterior capsule. The IOL edge is held more posteriorly by the intact CCC and therefore creates a mechanical barrier to lens epithelial cell migration behind the IOL. This theory is confirmed by the decreased incidence of Nd:YAG capsulotomy seen in association with the thick angular edge of acrylic IOLs. In addition, a CCC that is concentric with the optic edge balances the forces of the contracting capsular bag, hence minimizing the tendency for tilting postoperative IOL movement. In a randomized controlled study, Hollick et al[37] reported a significantly higher incidence of posterior capsule wrinkling and opacification with a larger capsulorhexis that lay completely off the optic surface.

An asymmetrical CCC will result in part of the CCC being over the IOL and part being larger than the IOL and therefore against the posterior capsule. This may lead to subsequent asymmetrical fibrosis, which can nudge the lens to an eccentric position. In addition, where the anterior and posterior capsule is in contact, there will be fusion of the capsule. This often results in folds or a fibrous thickening and opacification of the posterior capsule.

A second reason that we favor a CCC smaller than, and concentric with, the optic is to maintain the compartmentalization of the eye even after Nd:YAG laser posterior capsulotomy. In a

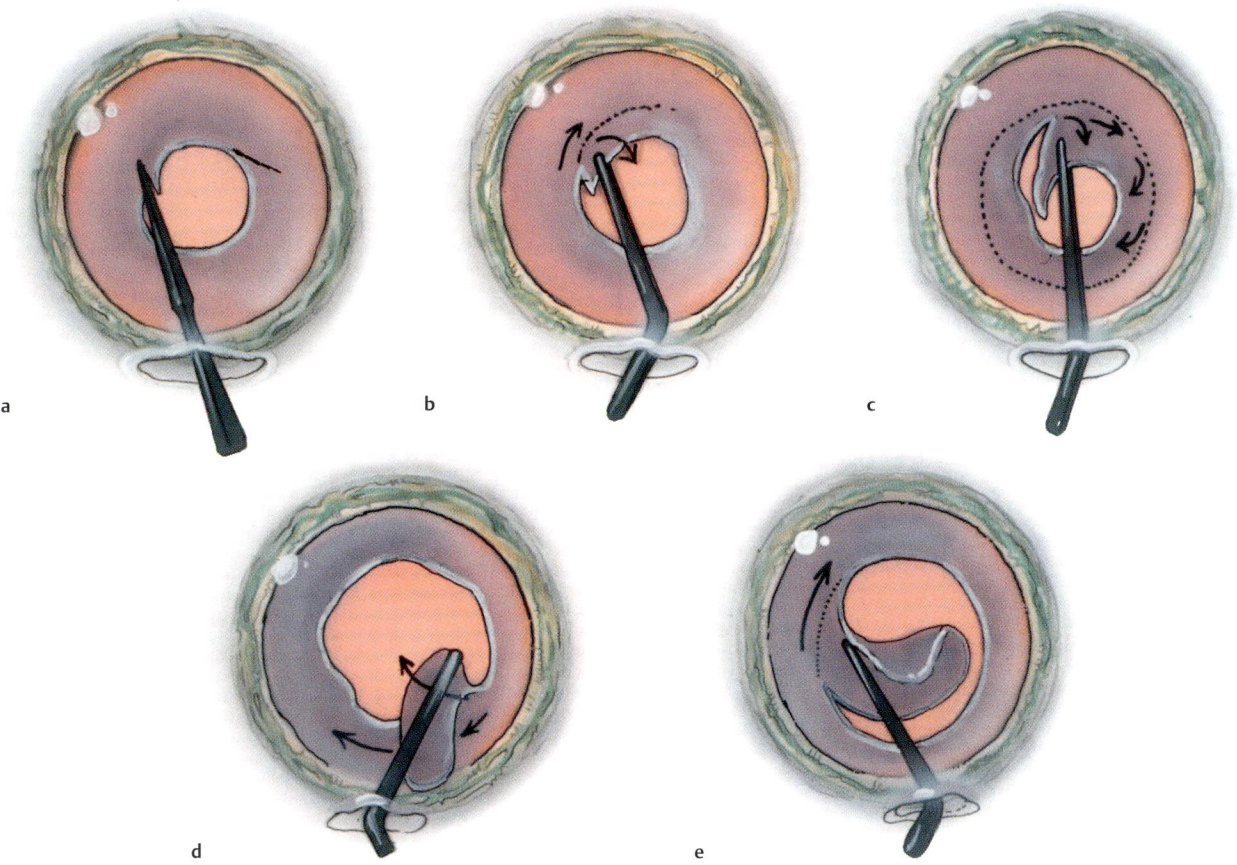

a   b   c

d   e

Fig. 6.5 **(a)** A small continuous-tear curvilinear capsulorhexis (CCC) can be enlarged using Gills-Walsh Vannas scissors to begin a slightly more peripheral tear. **(b,c)** A forceps can then be used with the same technique as described for the primary CCC to gently guide the direction of the tear to create a larger CCC. **(d,e)** The new CCC is then carefully finished in an inward direction. This method may be used intentionally in a two-staged capsulorhexis technique in cases of mature cataract or in cases with a small traumatic opening in the anterior capsule.

study that we conducted, we found that the initial pressure spike after Nd:YAG laser capsulotomy did not occur when the lens was completely sequestered in the capsular bag.[8] There was a significant pressure spike when the lens was in the sulcus or when the IOL optic was partly in the bag and partly out of the bag. We postulate that the sequestering of the AC by the seal created when the optic of the IOL is completely covered by the capsulorhexis becomes a barrier against liquefied vitreous elements coming into the AC. This barrier may reduce the possibility of pseudophakic glaucoma.

A third reason to advocate a CCC smaller than the optic is that in the event of a posterior capsule tear, the technique of sulcus placement of the loops and optic capture through the CCC, as proposed by Neuhann[38] can be utilized. If the capsulorhexis is larger than the IOL optic, this technique cannot be utilized. Additionally, the more remaining capsule existing for sulcus IOL support, the easier sulcus placement becomes.

The ideal CCC size therefore, would allow a ¼- to ½-mm overlap of the capsule over the IOL edge. For a 5.5-mm optic IOL, this would be a rhexis of 4.5 to 5.0 mm, and for a 6-mm IOL the size would be 5.0 to 5.5 mm.

Anatomic Abnormalities of the Zonule

Postoperatively, in cases of pseudoexfoliation, weak zonules, and excessive inflammation, the anterior capsular edge may fibrose and contract, creating the capsular contraction syndrome. This may necessitate the use of the Nd:YAG laser to incise the thickened capsular rim.[39]

In addition, Davison[40] has described the capsular block syndrome. It can occur intraoperatively or in the early or late postoperative period. Depending on the time of the capsular block, different materials accumulating behind the lens have been described.[41,42] It occurs in the presence of a small capsulorhexis and with implantation of silicone or acrylic IOLs. The material accumulates enough volume and pressure to eventually push the posterior capsule posteriorly and the IOL anteriorly, resulting in induced myopia. The syndrome is treated by Nd:YAG capsulotomy of the posterior capsule. The resultant equalization of pressure permits the posterior capsule and IOL to return to their normal pseudophakic configuration.[40]

Continuous Tear Capsulorhexis with the Intumescent Cataract

Mature cataracts pose a challenge for performing a complication-free capsulorhexis due to the difficulties encountered in visualizing the edge of the tear. Visualization can be limited due to a poor or no red reflex and may be further compromised by liquefied cortex, which may flow into the AC as soon as the initial puncture is made.

Methods of improving visualization if capsule staining material is not available include slowing the microscope focus to obtain precise control, dimming the operating room lights, and using high magnification and non-coaxial lighting. A small-gauge cannula may be helpful in removing the opaque liquefied cortex to further enhance visualization during CCC. A method of turning off the microscope and room lights and then using a light pipe to provide side light to illuminate the tearing capsular edge has been described by Gills[21] and Masket.[24]

Trypan blue ophthalmic solution (VisionBlue®, D.O.R.C. International, Zuidland, The Netherlands) is most commonly used to stain and visualize the anterior capsule. It is available in 1-cc dose vials of 0.1% solution in phosphate-buffered sodium chloride. Trypan blue provides better visualization of the anterior capsule during both capsulorhexis and phacoemulsification.[43–45]

Not infrequently in white, mature cataract cases a small capsulotomy may be more safely achieved than a large one. The nucleus with liquefied cortex may be under pressure. The initial entry into the capsule may be followed by the egress through the capsular opening of the liquefied cortical material. This may occur with sufficient pressure to extend the small penetration to a radial tear. Therefore, before penetrating the capsule the AC must be adequately filled with a retentive OVD. Once liquefied cortex has been removed, the intracapsular volume is decreased and the capsular edge can be visualized and the CCC can be enlarged. This is performed as described above after filling the capsular bag and AC with OVD and using a capsule scissors to create a tangential cut. This can then be enlarged to the desired size with capsulorhexis forceps (**Fig. 6.5**). Enlargement of the capsulotomy may be necessary for cortex removal and lens implantation. This two-stage CCC technique can also be used in cases with a small traumatic opening in the anterior capsule and for corneal endothelial protection in endocapsular cataract extraction.[9,22]

A more thorough discussion of the intumescent cataract is found in Chapter 14 in the discussion of the mature cataract.

Intraoperative Capsular Complications

Anterior Capsular Tears

Anterior capsular tears can be avoided by using the techniques described above. In some cases, such as a small pupil or a mature cataract as noted earlier, a planned two-staged capsulorhexis may be indicated. This technique provides control and visualization during CCC and enables enlargement of the capsulorhexis as needed either before or after lens implantation. By purposefully creating an initially small capsular opening, tears resulting from loss of control during CCC may be reduced. However, tears or the creation of a zonular dehiscence during phacoemulsification becomes a greater risk by contacting the CCC edge with the phaco tip, or by puncturing, tearing, or pulling on the anterior capsule with a second instrument.

Anterior capsule tears may also occur during cortex removal. This is of particular concern when removing the subincisional cortex. With a one-handed technique using the standard rigid irrigation and aspiration (I/A) tip in an effort to reach the cortex, the aspiration port must often be placed out of view under the iris. Often, the tip is rotated such that the aspiration port is facing superiorly or posteriorly. These maneuvers, while necessary to engage the cortex, cause distortion to the incision, creating poor visibility and increasing the risk of inadvertently engaging the capsular edge and creating a tear. In an effort to prevent this problem, some surgeons advocate the use of a two-handed I/A technique, with one cannula in one hand for balanced salt solution (BSS) inflow and the other cannula in the other hand

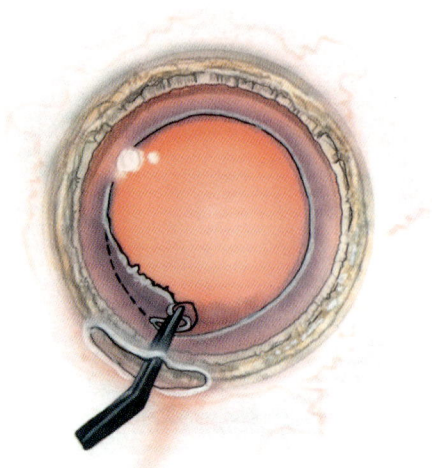

Fig. 6.6 Tearing a band of anterior capsule, including a short tear or area of can-opener capsulorhexis, will prevent extension of the tear. Alternatively, a scissors is used to start a larger CCC that is then taken around, or outside, the small tear. A continuous, though not necessarily circular, tear opening in the capsule is then still achieved.

for aspiration. The cannulas are placed through two paracenteses openings. This improves visibility and control for aspiration of the subincisional cortex. Alternatively, the angled, soft silicone I/A probe is well suited to removal of subincisional cortical material. The maneuverability combined with the softer tip in this type of I/A handpiece provides better visibility and protection against anterior and posterior capsule tears. Finally, it should be noted that subincisional cortex, when present, is more easily removed if a cortical cleaving hydrodissection has been performed.

Should a short anterior capsule tear occur during phacoemulsification or I/A, one method of management would be to inject OVD above and below the tear to support it. Using capsular forceps, the torn capsule is grasped at its furthest extent and redirected centrally, converting it into a rounded outgrowth of the capsulorhexis. Alternatively, employing a scissors to start a larger CCC which is then directed to go around the short tear thus eliminating the tear. These techniques result in an eccentric capsulorhexis. However, in this setting the maintenance of capsular integrity and prevention of further complications that may result from extension of an anterior capsular tear are of primary importance (**Fig. 6.6**).

Noncontinuous Capsulorhexis

If during the capsulorhexis the tear is lost toward the equator and must be completed from the opposite direction, or if the tear is not completed from the outside in leaving a notch, or if the tearing edge is lost due to disturbance of the underlying cortex from excessive manipulation while searching for the tearing edge, or if an anterior tear occurs during phacoemulsification and cannot be turned back into the CCC, extreme care must be taken throughout the remainder of the procedure. Pressure on the posterior capsule must be avoided. Any pressure on the capsule could cause radial extension of the tear through the equator and into the posterior capsule. If the tear occurs prior to hydrodissection, the hydrodissection should be omitted or carefully performed with gentle injection of small bursts of fluid. If the surgeon is concerned about the integrity of the posterior capsule, the capsulorhexis should be enlarged enough to enable the unimpeded prolapse of the nucleus into the AC. The lens is prolapsed into the AC and dispersive OVD is placed above and below the nucleus. This isolates the nucleus and prevents the possibility of its subsequently falling into the vitreous through a large posterior capsular tear during phacoemulsification (see **Fig. 36.13**). Emulsification can then be performed in the AC in between the layers of OVD. The OVD should be refreshed as is necessary. Some surgeons advocate converting to a can-opener style capsulotomy in the presence of radial extension of an anterior capsular tear.[26] However, with a gentle touch and careful technique, conversion to a can-opener capsulotomy is not necessary.

Intraoperative Lens Selection

When the capsulorhexis is not continuous, silicone plate-haptic lens implantation is contraindicated as these IOLs may subluxate into the anterior or posterior chamber as the capsule contracts postoperatively.

A one piece acrylic IOL may still be implanted in the capsular bag if the surgeon feels the IOL will not rotate and dislocate into the AC. Otherwise, a three-piece intraocular lens with a C-loop design with loops not longer than 11.5 and a rounded anterior edge may be carefully implanted in the capsular bag. A bimanual technique and adequate OVD to fill and stabilize the bag is necessary to minimize pressure on the weakened bag. This will help to avoid extension of the tear. The haptics should be placed so that their maximum pressure is perpendicular to the tear. Sometimes a matched tear (created with the Vannas scissors) created 180 degrees away from the initial tear will equalize forces created by postoperative capsule contraction and prevent postoperative lens decentration (**Fig. 6.7**). A further discussion of IOL selection after vitrectomy can be found in Chapter 21.

Posterior Capsule Tears

Posterior capsule tears, if managed properly, may not result in a poor visual outcome. However, any case in which the posterior capsule is ruptured has a higher risk of vitreous loss, cystoid macular edema (CME), retinal detachment (RD), and loss of nuclear fragments posteriorly.[10,22,26] As discussed previously, the surgeon must keep in mind the anatomic features of the lens capsule during phacoemulsification and aspiration; at the posterior pole the capsule may be as thin as 2 to 4 µm. Avoidance of posterior capsular tears requires judicious use of phacoemulsification settings that are tailored to both the surgical technique and the type of cataract being removed. For example, in younger patients in whom the nucleus is soft, lower power settings are appropriate. The posterior capsule can be aspirated by the phaco tip. If only suction has been engaged and the suction is immediately released and, if necessary, refluxed, a tear may not occur. If the phaco tip has burs or it is moved while the capsule is occluded on the phaco tip, it will tear. The vitreous face, however, often will remain intact. Care must be taken during all phacoemulsification and cracking maneuvers to avoid contacting the capsule with simultaneous vacuum and ultrasound. This will immediately tear the posterior capsule and rupture the vitreous face with instantaneous prolapse of vitreous into the AC. Obviously, care must also be taken to avoid contact of sharp second instruments with the posterior capsule. Blunt second instruments held steady under the phaco tip will not tear the posterior capsule if touched by the posterior capsule during nuclear fragment removal.

If the posterior capsule is vacuum polished, a vacuum setting of 5 mm Hg or less vacuum and 5 cc per minute of aspiration flow rate (if available) are helpful to prevent inadvertent tears. During this maneuver, when the capsule is engaged by the tip with vacuum and is within the 0.3-mm tip orifice, very slow

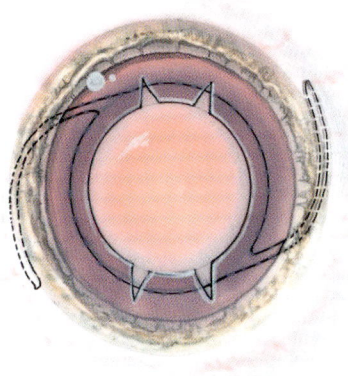

Fig. 6.7 In the event of anterior capsular tears, haptics should be oriented so that their point of maximal force, as may be seen by a fold in the posterior capsule, is perpendicular to the tear and a matched tear created 180 degrees away from the initial tear to neutralize forces.

movements of the tip are necessary to avoid snagging and tearing the capsule. Use only an I/A tip that has no sharp burs. Even if well polished the walls of the aspiration hole on stainless steel tips may have burs that easily snag and tear the capsule. Silicone or other nonmetallic tips are much safer than stainless steel and should be the only ones used for capsule polishing the posterior capsule.

The posterior capsule, despite being incredibly thin, does have remarkable elasticity and structural integrity. It will withstand blunt pressure. Therefore, although a gentle touch is advisable, blunt-tipped chopping instruments do not pose a high risk of posterior capsular rupture.

Posterior Capsulorhexis

In the event that a small tear occurs in the posterior capsule, it may be converted to a posterior CCC to prevent it from enlarging radially and further compromising capsular integrity.[11,12,22] The creation of this posterior CCC is similar in technique to the anterior CCC (**Fig. 6.8**). After adding a dispersive OVD to stabilize the capsule, to push the intact vitreous face back or prevent further vitreous herniation through the tear, one edge of the advancing tear is grasped with a forceps and directed in a curvilinear manner such that the entire tear is contained in the opening. To complete the tear, it is blended from the periphery. The posterior opening thus created should be kept as small as possible to ensure support for the IOL. This technique may not be feasible if the end of the posterior capsular tear cannot be visualized because it is too far peripheral or has a subincisional location. Sometimes only one end of a long tear can be reached. With courage and skill, it can be turned back and rounded off. This may then still allow for in-the-bag IOL placement. If both ends of a linear tear can be reached, they may be blunted individually rather than encircling the tear with the CCC.

This method of posterior CCC can be employed intentionally[46] to avoid the possible necessity of a Nd:YAG posterior capsulotomy such as for disabled patients unable to sit for the laser procedure or for patients for whom traveling back for the laser procedure would be a hardship or impossible. It may also be used for removal of posterior plaques and in young pediatric cataract cases for primary posterior capsulectomy.[13–15] Posterior CCC with optic capture has been used successfully to prevent secondary opacification of the visual axis in pediatric cataract cases; with this technique the haptics remain in the capsular bag

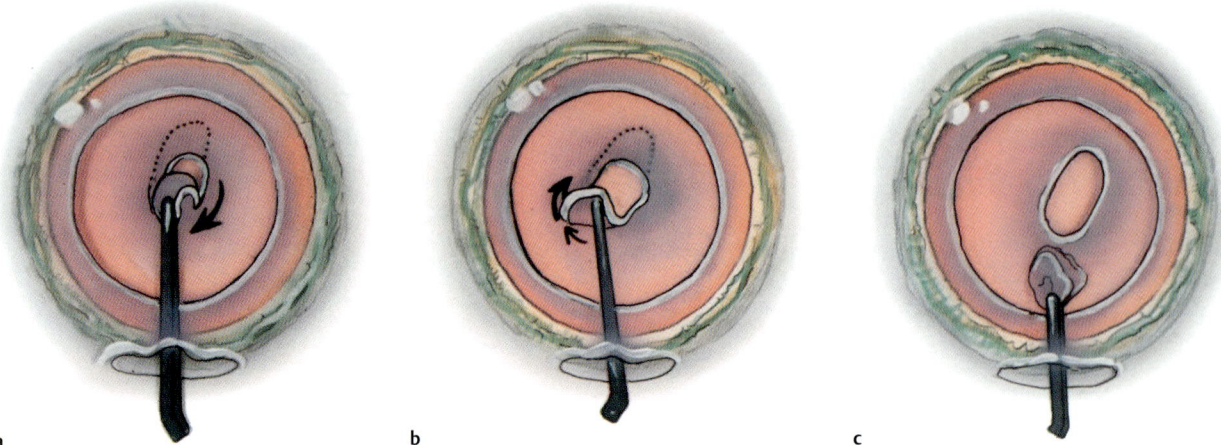

a   b   c

Fig. 6.8 **(a)** The creation of a posterior CCC is similar in technique to the anterior CCC. **(b)** The leading tear of a posterior CCC is controlled using abundant viscoelastic. Using vector principles of CCC, the posterior CCC is completed **(c)**. This technique is useful in pediatric patients to prevent posterior capsular opacification and may also be employed in the event that a small tear occurs in the posterior capsule to prevent it from radial extension.

and the optic is gently guided through the posterior CCC such that the optic is captured.[13–16] This requires that the size of the posterior opening be carefully controlled such that the optic is ~ 1 or 2 mm larger than the posterior CCC and will be captured when in proper position. The posterior CCC is performed either before or after IOL implantation but after inflating the capsular bag with viscoelastic.[24] Alternatively, the haptics may be left in the sulcus and the optic captured by the CCC and the posterior CCC (**Fig. 6.9**).[47] After IOL implantation the OVD is aspirated from in front of the IOL but is left to remain posterior to the IOL to avoid aspiration of vitreous requiring subsequent vitrectomy.

Anterior Capsular Intraocular Lens Optic Capture

The technique of anterior capsular optic capture developed by Neuhann (personal communication) may be employed in cases in which a posterior capsular rupture cannot be converted to a posterior CCC. In these cases an intact anterior CCC of a diameter

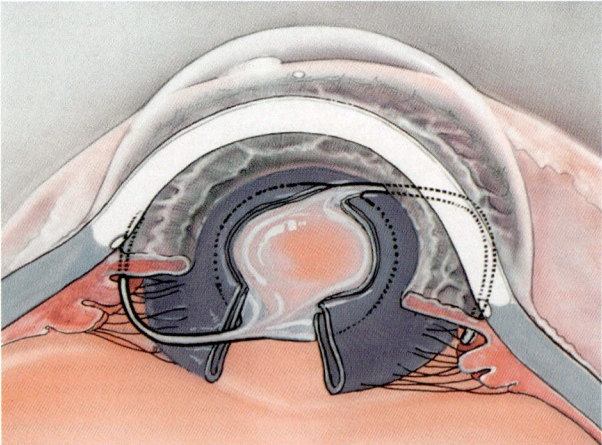

Fig. 6.9 Posterior CCC with IOL haptic fixation in the sulcus and optic fixation behind the posterior ccc. The IOL is equally well fixated with IOL haptic fixation in the capsular bag.

smaller than the IOL optic is required. The haptics of the IOL are placed in the sulcus. The optic is then pushed through the anterior capsular opening and is captured by the intact CCC.[13,22]

In any case in which complications occur, the surgeon must make the decision as to which of these methods to use to optimize the vision outcome and minimize associated risks. Larger posterior capsule tears with vitreous loss or loss of nuclear material into the vitreous is discussed further in subsequent chapters.

Zonular Dialysis

Zonular integrity can be compromised by a variety of conditions including prior trauma and pseudoexfoliation. These cases pose a challenge for phacoemulsification and for safe and stable placement of the IOL in the bag. Stability and centration of the implant may not be achieved or maintained because of zonular dehiscence and the postoperative contraction of the capsular bag. If zonular weakness is noted preoperatively, then, utilizing the proper techniques, a CCC can be performed without further disruption of the zonules. In a location away from the dehiscence, the rhexis should be initiated with a sharp needle. Thus, the capsule is incised without pulling on the area of weak or absent zonules. A vigilant shearing rhexis is then performed. In the area near the absent or weakened zonules, the tearing forces are performed tangential to the weakened capsular edge. The capsular tension ring may then be placed in the capsular bag prior to phacoemulsification. This serves to enhance safety and stability during nuclear and cortex removal.

We have found that the use of capsular tension rings (CTRs) after the CCC is performed guards against capsular collapse and vitreous presentation during phacoemulsification when zonular support is compromised. In addition, they stabilize the contour of the capsular bag such that the IOL can be placed securely within the bag and with excellent centration (**Fig. 6.10**).[16,48]

When placing a CTR in the presence of very loose zonules, the entering tip should be held with a Sinskey or similar hook to bend the ring as it is extruded from the injector to enable a broad segment of the ring to first engage the capsule rather than the tip alone, which could tear the capsule or tear more of the zonules because of the direct force of the tip. This technique also enables the ring to engage the weakened area of the capsule

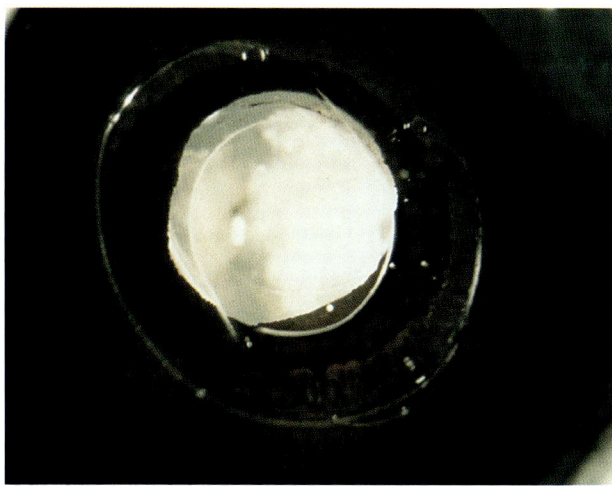

Fig. 6.10 Posterior view of a CTR implanted in a cadaver eye.

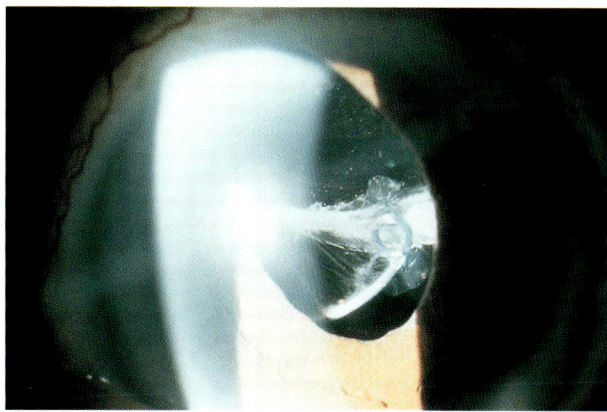

Fig. 6.11 Postoperative intraocular lens (IOL) and capsule decentration with posterior capsule opacification postoperatively. The risk of decentration postoperatively can be decreased by using an endocapsular tension ring and ensuring that the original CCC is centered and symmetric.

with the force applied 90 degrees against the zone of strong zonules rather than against the already weak or missing zone.

Unexpected excessive movement of the lens during CCC, hydrodissection, nuclear rotation, or phacoemulsification may indicate intraoperative zonular weakness. Excessively aggressive lens maneuvers will cause further disruption of the zonules. Aspirating the equatorial capsular bag with the phaco tip or I/A tip may tear the bag away from the zonule. Other signs of zonular weakness may include vitreous herniation around the bag with resultant iris bulge, and/or decentration of the crystalline lens. An endocapsular tension ring should be placed immediately after the CCC if these signs are noted. This will prevent collapse of the capsular bag and further zonular dehiscence. Capsular tension rings may also prevent migration and proliferation of lens epithelial cells and the attendant capsular contraction and opacification through compression inhibition. This has been described by Hara et al[17] in the rabbit model.

In cases with loose or broken zonules, the endocapsular tension ring with in-the-bag IOL placement offers an alternative to sutured posterior or anterior chamber IOLs. Zonular problems are discussed in greater detail in later chapters.

Postoperative Capsular Complications

Migration, proliferation, and fibrous metaplasia of residual lens epithelial cells following phacoemulsification and planned extracapsular cataract extraction (ECCE) are responsible for posterior capsular opacification, asymmetric capsular contraction with optic decentration, Soemmering's ring, capsular phimosis, and anterior inflammatory membranes (**Fig. 6.11**).[22–26]

Anterior capsular contraction syndromes and capsular block syndromes may occur months after the initial surgery. Anterior capsular contraction requires Nd:YAG incision of the fibrotic and phimotic anterior capsular ring. If the fibrotic ring again develops, it may require surgical excision by making a larger CCC around the fibrotic element. Capsular block syndrome requires a Nd:YAG posterior capsulotomy.

In pediatric patients, creation of an anterior and primary posterior CCC with or without anterior vitrectomy and then optic capture by the posterior CCC or both CCC and posterior CCC has been found to both provide stable support for lens implantation and reduce secondary visual axis opacification (**Fig. 6.9**).[13–15] As noted previously, to minimize the risk of decentration result-

ing from capsular contraction, the CCC should be symmetric and well centered (**Fig. 6.10**). If the capsulorhexis is asymmetric or irregular, the haptics should be aligned parallel to the irregularity in an attempt to provide a counterforce to capsular contraction.[22] In addition, as mentioned previously, anterior tears may be matched at 180 degrees and the IOL haptics placed so that their force is perpendicular to the tears (**Fig. 6.7**).

Nd:YAG Capsulotomy

Posterior capsular fibrosis/haze occurs in 10% of postoperative cataract cases per year. Over time treatment may be required in up to 50% of patients undergoing cataract extraction with an intact posterior capsule.[20] Certain lens designs and materials may reduce this incidence. Pediatric patients are at particularly high risk for this complication. It has become standard to treat posterior capsular opacification with Nd:YAG laser. Silicone plate haptic lenses, however, represent a special circumstance. Improper capsulotomy techniques in these cases may pose a risk for posterior subluxation of the lens implant. It is recommended that the anterior capsule be released and posterior capsulotomy be performed in a circumferential manner such that asymmetric contraction forces are neutralized and tears do not extend posteriorly, squeezing the IOL into the vitreous.[22] Although the Nd:YAG capsulotomy is commonly performed and yields excellent results, there are risks associated with its use. Transient intraocular pressure (IOP) spikes, iris hemorrhage, damage to the lens implant, CME, and an increased risk of retinal detachments have been reported following Nd:YAG capsulotomy.[49–51] Therefore, every effort should be made, using the operative techniques described above, to minimize the risk of developing postoperative complications related to capsular contraction and opacification.

We found that eyes with the CCC intact and smaller than the optic had a statistically significant lower incidence of IOP spikes, AC flare, and particulate matter in the AC after Nd:YAG capsulotomy, as compared with eyes with sulcus fixated lenses.[7] Our review of 218 consecutive Nd:YAG cases found a 1% rate of RD over 49.5 months of follow-up as compared with 0.5% of 198 matched controls who underwent phacoemulsification but required no Nd:YAG capsulotomy.[7] Our published results were lower than previously reported rates.[49–51] This decreased incidence of RD was thought to be related to the techniques of CCC and in-the-bag IOL placement, which were used during cataract surgery.

Conclusion

Avoidance of capsular complications during cataract surgery and postoperatively begins with proper CCC techniques. In the majority of cases, an excellent vision outcome may be obtained if the complications are managed appropriately.

References

1. Gimbel HV, Kaye GB. Forceps-puncture continuous curvilinear capsulorhexis. J Cataract Refract Surg 1997;23:473–475

2. Gimbel HV, Neuhann T. Development, advantages, and methods of the continuous circular capsulorhexis technique. J Cataract Refract Surg 1990;16:31–37

3. Arshinoff S. Mechanics of capsulorhexis. J Cataract Refract Surg 1992;18:623–628

4. Pande M. Continuous curvilinear (circular) capsulorhexis and planned extracapsular cataract extraction—are they compatible? Br J Ophthalmol 1993;77:152–157

5. Thim K, Krag S, Corydon L. Stretching capacity of capsulorhexis and nucleus delivery. J Cataract Refract Surg 1991;17:27–31

6. Venkatesh R, Veena K, Ravindran RD. Capsulotomy and hydroprocedures for nucleus prolapse in manual small incision cataract surgery. Indian J Ophthalmol 2009;57:15–18

7. Gimbel HV, Van Westenbrugge JA, Sanders DR, Raanan MG. Effect of sulcus vs capsular fixation on YAG-induced pressure rises following posterior capsulotomy. Arch Ophthalmol 1990;108:1126–1129

8. Gimbel HV. Two-stage capsulorhexis for endocapsular phacoemulsification. J Cataract Refract Surg 1990;16:246–249

9. Jaffe N. Cataract Surgery and Its Complications, 3rd ed. St. Louis: CV Mosby; 1981:368, 576–579

10. Gimbel HV. Posterior capsule tears using phacoemulsification: causes, prevention and management. Eur J Implant Refract Surg 1990;2:63–69

11. Gimbel HV. The prevention and management of capsule complications. Asia-Pac J Ophthalmol 1995;7:5–8

12. Gimbel HV, DeBroff BM. Posterior capsulorhexis with optic capture: maintaining a clear visual axis after pediatric cataract surgery. J Cataract Refract Surg 1994;20:658–664

13. Gimbel HV. Posterior capsulorhexis with optic capture in pediatric cataract and intraocular lens surgery. Ophthalmology 1996;103:1871–1875

14. Gimbel HV. Posterior continuous curvilinear capsulorhexis and optic capture of the intraocular lens to prevent secondary opacification in pediatric cataract surgery. J Cataract Refract Surg 1997;23(Suppl 1):652–656

15. Gimbel HV, DeBroff BM. Management of lens implant and posterior capsule with respect to prevention of secondary cataract. Oper Tech Cataract Refract Surg 1998;1:185–190

16. Gimbel HV, Sun R, Heston JP. Management of zonular dialysis in phacoemulsification and IOL implantation using the capsular tension ring. Ophthalmic Surg Lasers 1997;28:273–281

17. Hara T, Hara T, Sakanishi K, Yamada Y. Efficacy of equator rings in an experimental rabbit study. Arch Ophthalmol 1995;113:1060–1065

18. Cionni RJ, Osher RH. Endocapsular ring approach to the subluxed cataractous lens. J Cataract Refract Surg 1995;21:245–249

19. American Academy of Ophthalmology. Nd:YAG laser capsulotomy. In: Lens and Cataract: Basic and Clinical Science Course, 1996–1997. San Francisco: American Academy of Ophthalmology; 1996:135–136

20. Van Westenbrugge JA, Gimbel HV, Souchek J, Chow D. Incidence of retinal detachment following Nd:YAG capsulotomy after cataract surgery. J Cataract Refract Surg 1992;18:352–355

21. Gills JP. Cataract Surgery: The State of the Art. Thorofare, NJ: Slack; 1998

22. Apple DJ, Solomon KD, Tetz MR, et al. Posterior capsule opacification. Surv Ophthalmol 1992;37:73–116

23. Apple DJ, Kincaid MC, Mamalis N, et al. Intraocular Lenses. Baltimore: Williams & Wilkins; 1989

24. Masket S. Postoperative complications of capsulorhexis. J Cataract Refract Surg 1993;19:721–724

25. American Academy of Ophthalmology. Lens and Cataract: Basic and Clinical Science Course, 1996–1997. San Francisco: American Academy of Ophthalmology; 1996

26. Kuszak JR, Deutsch TA, Brown HG. Anatomy of aged and senile cataractous lenses. In: Albert DM, Jakobiec FA, eds. Principles and Practice of Ophthalmology: Clinical Practice. Philadelphia: WB Saunders; 1994:564–575

27. Brierley L. Vacuum capsulorhexis. J Cataract Refract Surg 1995;21:13–15

28. Luck J, Brahma AK, Noble BA. A comparative study of the elastic properties of continuous tear curvilinear capsulorhexis versus capsulorhexis produced by radiofrequency endodiathermy. Br J Ophthalmol 1994;78:392–396

29. Wilson ME, Bluestein EC, Wang X-H, Apple DJ. Comparison of mechanized anterior capsulectomy and manual continuous capsulorhexis in pediatric eyes. J Cataract Refract Surg 1994;20:602–606

30. Koch PS. Forceps capsulotomy. In: Koch PS, Davison JA, eds. Textbook of Advanced Phacoemulsification Techniques. Thorofare, NJ: Slack; 1991:49–56

31. Gimbel HV. Continuous curvilinear capsulorrhexis and nucleus fracturing: evolution, technique and complications. Ophthalmology Clinics of North America 1991;4:235–249

32. Neuhann T. [Theory and surgical technic of capsulorhexis]. [Article in German] Klin Monatsbl Augenheilkd 1987;190:542–545

33. Little BC, Smith JH, Packer M. Little capsulorhexis tear-out rescue. J Cataract Refract Surg 2006;32:1420–1422

34. Chen V, Shochot Y, Blumenthal M. Anterior capsulotomy through a small pupil. Am J Ophthalmol 1987;104:666–667

35. Akman A, Yilmaz G, Oto S, Akova YA. Comparison of various pupil dilatation methods for phacoemulsification in eyes with a small pupil secondary to pseudoexfoliation. Ophthalmology 2004;111:1693–1698

36. Wilczynski M, Wierzchowski T, Synder A, Omulecki W. Results of phacoemulsification with Malyugin Ring in comparison with manual iris stretching with hooks in eyes with narrow pupil. Eur J Ophthalmol 2013;23:196–201

37. Hollick EJ, Spalton DJ, Meacock WR. The effect of capsulorhexis size on posterior capsular opacification: one-year results of a randomized prospective trial. Am J Ophthalmol 1999;128:271–279

38. Neuhann T. The Rhexis-Fixated Lens. Film presented at the American Society of Cataract and Refractive Surgery Symposium on Cataract, Intraocular Lens, and Refractive Surgery, Boston, April 1991

39. Davison JA. Capsule contraction syndrome. J Cataract Refract Surg 1993;19:582–589

40. Davison JA. Capsular bag distension after endophacoemulsification and posterior chamber intraocular lens implantation. J Cataract Refract Surg 1990;16:99–108

41. Miyake K, Ota I, Ichihashi S, Miyake S, Tanaka Y, Terasaki H. New classification of capsular block syndrome. J Cataract Refract Surg 1998;24:1230–1234

42. Kim HK, Shin JP. Capsular block syndrome after cataract surgery: clinical analysis and classification. J Cataract Refract Surg 2008;34:357–363

43. Horiguchi M, Miyake K, Ohta I, Ito Y. Staining of the lens capsule for circular continuous capsulorrhexis in eyes with white cataract. Arch Ophthalmol 1998;116:535–537

44. Melles GRJ, de Waard PWT, Pameyer JH, Houdijn Beekhuis W. Trypan blue capsule staining to visualize the capsulorhexis in cataract surgery. J Cataract Refract Surg 1999;25:7–9

45. Rodrigues EB, Costa EF, Penha FM, et al. The use of vital dyes in ocular surgery. Surv Ophthalmol 2009;54:576–617

46. Menapace R. Posterior capsulorhexis combined with optic buttonholing: an alternative to standard in-the-bag implantation of sharp-edged intraocular lenses? A critical analysis of 1000 consecutive cases. Graefes Arch Clin Exp Ophthalmol 2008;246:787–801

47. DeBroff BM, Nihalani BR. Double optic capture with capsular bag fusion: A new technique for pediatric intraocular lens implantation. Techniques in Ophthalmology 2008;6:31–34

48. Gimbel HV, Sun R. Clinical applications of capsular tension rings in cataract surgery. Ophthalmic Surg Lasers 2002;33:44–53

49. Smith PW, Stark WJ, Maumenee AE, et al. Retinal detachment after extracapsular cataract extraction with posterior chamber intraocular lens. Ophthalmology 1987;94:495–504

50. Dardenne M-U, Gerten G-J, Kokkas K, Kermani O. Retrospective study of retinal detachment following neodymium:YAG laser posterior capsulotomy. J Cataract Refract Surg 1989;15:676–680

51. Rickman-Barger L, Florine CW, Larson RS, Lindstrom RL. Retinal detachment after neodymium:YAG laser posterior capsulotomy. Am J Ophthalmol 1989;107:531–536

Section V Management of the Hydrosteps and Complications

7 Complications of the Hydrosteps: How to Recognize and Avoid Them

William J. Fishkind

The hydrosteps consist of hydrodissection and hydrodelineation. Hydrodissection is defined as the separation of cortex from adjacent cortex or from the capsular bag. It is of two types—cortical cleaving and standard. Hydrodelineation is defined as the separation of the endonucleus from the epinucleus.

Anatomy

The capsular bag is an elastic transparent basement membrane made up of type IV collagen. This basement membrane is laid down by the lens epithelial cells, which reside just inside the capsule. The zonules insert on the anterior capsule over an area 2 to 2.5 mm anterior to the equator. They insert on the posterior capsule 1 mm posterior to the equator. The capsule may be as thin as 2 to 4 µm at the posterior pole. It is thickest (17 to 23 µm) near the anterior and posterior equator where the zonular fibers attach. The anterior capsule can be as thick as 14 µm in adults.[1] The posterior capsule may be particularly fragile in cases with congenital posterior lenticonus and posterior polar cataract; age-related or corticosteroid-related posterior subcapsular (PSC) cataracts involve migration and enlargement of the lens epithelial cells posteriorly where the capsule is thinnest.[2]

The lens is a crystalline structure with an obvious lamellar pattern containing 65% water. The 35% protein matrix is composed of soluble crystalline and insoluble albuminoid portions. It is ~ 10.5 mm in diameter and 4.5 mm thick. Anatomically it is composed of an embryonic nucleus, a fetal nucleus, an adult nucleus, and cortex. The Y-sutures demarcate the fetal and adult nucleus. With age, the lens increases in size due to continuous formation of new lens fibers. This causes the older fibers to become compressed and dehydrated. Water content decreases and the lens density increases. In addition, the accumulation of brown pigment within the lens causes discoloration[1] (**Fig. 7.1**).

Surgically, the adult cataractous lens can be separated into the endonucleus, epinucleus, and cortex. The endonucleus is connected to the epinucleus, cortex, and capsular bag by condensations of nuclear material, which are not evident on pathological examination. These can be termed nuclear-capsular connections.

Hydrodissection

Decompression of the Anterior Capsule

If the anterior chamber is filled with ophthalmic viscosurgical device (OVD) after the capsulorrhexis, the residual OVD will block fluid egress from the hydrodissection, creating posterior pressure. This can result in inadequate hydrodissection, as the surgeon is afraid to be more aggressive with fluid. Additionally, the lack of egress may cause a tear of the posterior capsule due to the inability of the fluid to escape during injection. Finally, the zonule may be disrupted.

It is therefore desirable to aspirate some OVD prior to initiating hydrosteps.

If Healon GV (Abbott Medical Optics [AMO], Abbott Park, IL) is used, its cohesive character permits straightforward irrigation out the manually depressed incision. However, when dispersive OVDs such as Viscoat (AMO) are used, an intensive effort is required to aspirate it. This is especially important with the visco-adaptive Healon 5 (AMO) as it will not irrigate from the anterior segment.[3]

In cortical cleaving hydrodissection, a cannula is placed between the cortex and anterior capsule. The tip of a 27-gauge cannula is attached to a 3-cc syringe filled with balanced salt solution (BSS) and is advanced under the anterior capsule until it is halfway between the anterior capsular rim and the capsular bag equator. The tip of the cannula is elevated until the anterior capsule is actually tented. A slow, steady, and firm stream of BSS is then injected. The stream of BSS will then advance anteriorly toward the anterior capsule and around the proximate equator. From there it passes behind the posterior pole of the nucleus and cortex and around to the opposite equator. It then progresses around the opposite equator emerging from the capsulorrhexis edge into the anterior chamber. Excess fluid then passes out of the incision, thus relieving excessive pressure in the anterior chamber (**Fig. 7.2a**).[4]

If the nucleus floats anteriorly, a common occurrence, the surgeon should cautiously push the nucleus posteriorly. This will effectively push fluid sequestered behind the nucleus around the equator (**Fig. 7.2b**). The surgeon is usually able to visualize the fluid flow as a wave passing around the posterior pole and then the equator. The anterior chamber is then perceived to deepen momentarily as it fills with fluid. The anterior chamber then becomes shallow as the fluid is seen to exit through the incision. Alternately, the nucleus floats forward, stretching the capsulorrhexis. The nucleus is then pushed posteriorly with the hydrodissection cannula. The chamber deepens, and fluid and viscoelastic escape through the incision. If performed adequately, the cortex is separated or cleaved from the capsule, allowing free rotation of the endonucleus, epinucleus, and cortex as a unit, within the capsular bag.

Standard hydrodissection is performed in a similar manner, except that the cannula is placed within the substance of the cortex. This produces a cleavage plane within the cortex. Consequently, part of the cortex remains attached to the capsular bag and part remains attached to the endonucleus (**Fig. 7.3**).

Cortical cleaving hydrodissection appears to have certain benefits over standard hydrodissection. First, if the cortex is

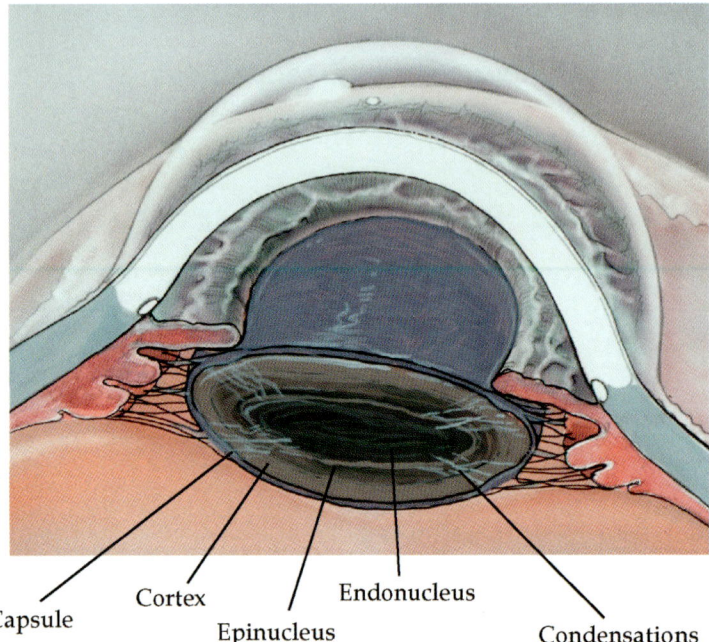

Fig. 7.1 Surgical anatomy of the lens and zonules. Capsule is thinnest (2 to 4 μm) at the posterior pole and thickest (17 to 23 μm) at the insertion of the zonules. The nuclear-cortical-capsular bag condensations of cortex can be seen to entirely surround the nucleus.

Capsule   Cortex   Endonucleus   Condensations
Epinucleus

cleaved from the capsular bag for 360 degrees, it is separated from the capsular bag but remains fused with the epinucleus. Therefore, the cortex is entirely removed during emulsification of the epinucleus. No irrigation and aspiration (I/A) is necessary. This eliminates the risk of ruptured posterior capsules during I/A. If the cortex is not entirely cleaved, it is usually significantly loosened from its capsular bag attachments. Hence, I/A is more easily performed. With cortical separation there is less traction on the zonules as cortex is pulled from the capsular bag during cortical aspiration. Subincisional cortex aspiration is enhanced, as it is less adherent to the capsular bag. Facilitated cortical aspiration minimizes the risk of capsular rupture during I/A. Second, less anterior segment manipulation is necessary if the capsular bag should be ruptured. This is due to the lack of need for I/A or to the necessity of minimal I/A. The risk of enlarging the tear or causing the need of increased vitrectomy is consequently decreased.

Hydrodelineation

Hydrodelineation is defined as the separation of the endonucleus from the epinucleus. It is generally performed immediately after hydrodissection.[5] The same cannula is moved to the paracentral zone of the nucleus. It is then embedded within the nuclear substance. The cannula tip is moved forward and backward two or three times to create a track within the nuclear material. BSS is then injected slowly and firmly into the bulk of the nucleus. The BSS will find the surgical plane at the junction of the epi- and endonucleus, thus creating the separation of these two entities. During the injection of BSS, the surgeon will view the fluid as it separates the endonucleus from the surrounding epinucleus, creating a "ring" around the endonucleus (**Fig. 7.4**). The anterior chamber will deepen momentarily as BSS passes around the endonucleus and into the anterior chamber. It then becomes shallow as the fluid advances out of the anterior chamber through

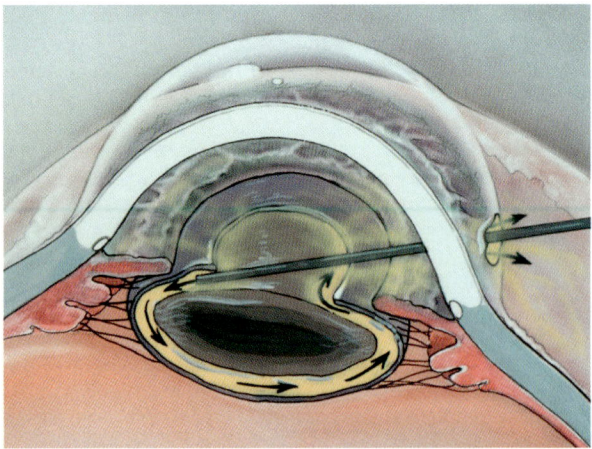

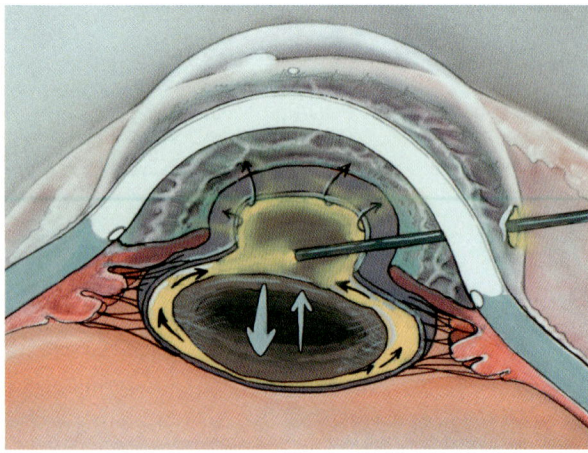

Fig. 7.2 **(a)** Cortical cleaving hydrodissection. The cannula elevates the anterior capsule. The fluid wave dissects cortex from the capsular bag. The nuclear-capsular bag condensations of cortex are disrupted. **(b)** Fluid deep to the nucleus will cause it to "float" anteriorly. Gentle pressure will displace fluid trapped behind the nucleus around the equator. Further disruption of cortex–bag connections occurs.

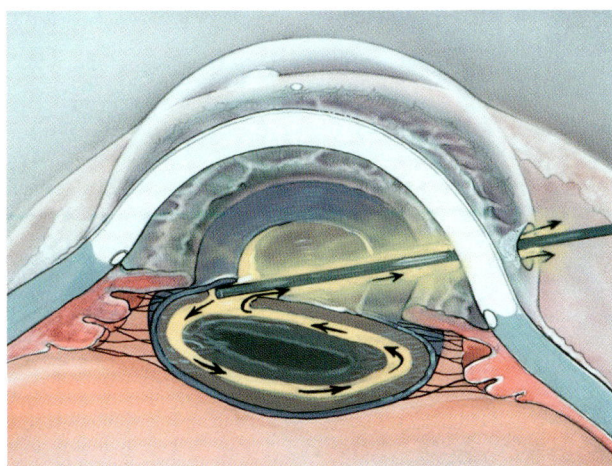

Fig. 7.3 Standard hydrodissection. Fluid wave passes between the epinucleus and cortex. Cortex is not cleaved from the capsular bag. The necessity for extensive irrigation and aspiration (I/A) with zonular traction is consequently necessary.

the incision. Even after adequate hydrodelineation the endonucleus will not rotate independently of adjacent epinucleus and cortex.

Hydrodelineation is necessary in performing those phaco procedures requiring lens disassembly methodology.

Complications

Complications that can occur during the hydrosteps include inadequate cortical-capsular bag separation, misdirection of the fluid flow, zonular damage, tears of the anterior capsule, and tears of the posterior capsule (see list below).

Most Common Causes of Capsular Tears During Hydrosteps

- Noncontinuous capsulorrhexis—visible or occult
- Pseudoexfoliation with friable capsule and weak zonules
- Mature cataract with poor view of the anterior capsule

- Relatively small rhexis in relation to maturity of the cataract
- Overzealous hydrodissection
- Viscodissection
- Calcified posterior polar cataracts

Inadequate Cortex-Capsular Bag Separation

If hydrodissection is inadequate, some areas of cortex will remain attached to the capsular bag (**Fig. 7.5**). Nucleus rotation will be difficult. Further hydrodissection in each quadrant for 360 degrees combined with gentle bimanual rotational forces on the nucleus, or even gentle viscodissection, will remedy this situation. Although not particularly serious a problem in routine cases, with zonular weakness, such as in pseudoexfoliation, adherence of cortex combined with rotational maneuvers may lead to further compromise of the zonules.

One reason this occurs is that there is inadequate fluid injection force. This results in inadequate hydrostatic pressure to separate the cortex from the capsule. Short, firm bursts of injection pressure, utilizing a 25-gauge cannula and a 3-cc syringe, provide enough force and back pressure for a stable injection. David Chang suggests that a right-angled irrigation cannula makes it easier to direct fluid injection anteriorly along the peripheral cortex to improve cortical-capsular bag separation. His cannula, manufactured by Katena (Denville, NJ), Mastel (Rapid City, SD), and Rhein (St. Petersburg, FL), is 27 gauge with a short, 1-mm right-angled tip.[3]

It is reasonable to persist in achieving nucleus rotation. Rotation of the nucleus suggests that there is thorough cortical cleavage. Rotation of the nucleus makes phacoemulsification easier, and safer. It also makes I/A significantly easier.

Finally, if there is an anterior capsular tear, good rotation and cortical cleavage allow for less traction of the cortex on the capsular bag, preventing tear extension.

Fluid Misdirection Syndromes

Misdirection of the fluid flow and tears of the zonules may occur separately or simultaneously. If the hydrodissection cannula is incorrectly placed deep to the iris but superior to the anterior capsule, the injection of BSS may pass through the zonules into the vitreous body (**Fig. 7.6**). Instantaneous increase of posterior

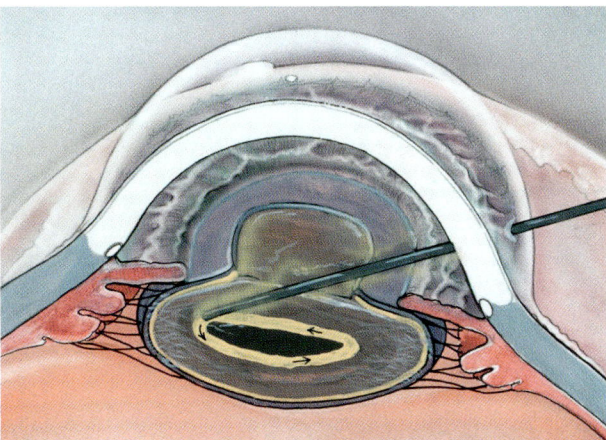

Fig. 7.4 Hydrodelineation. The endonucleus is separated from the epinucleus and cortex.

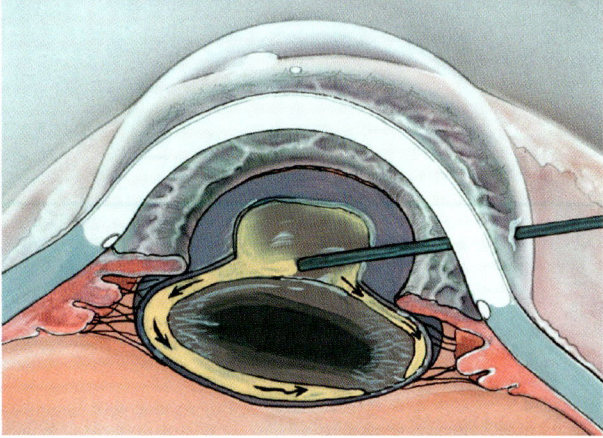

Fig. 7.5 Incomplete hydrodissection. Part of the nucleus remains adherent to the capsule. The nucleus will be difficult to, or may not, rotate.

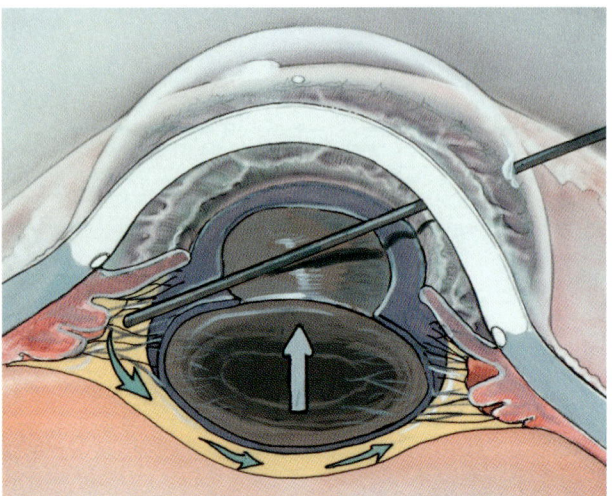

Fig. 7.6 A cannula inadvertently placed under the iris but over, rather than under, the anterior capsule. Injected fluid passes into, and is trapped within, the retrolental space. As the anterior chamber becomes shallow, intraocular pressure is significantly increased.

segment volume, and vitreous hydration, will then cause shallowing of the anterior chamber. Subsequent hydrodelineation and phacoemulsification may become impossible. Treatment plans for this complication are discussed in Chapter 8. The placement of the cannula or passage of BSS into the zonules may result in the severing of zonules. This may lead to unzipping of a small or large number of zonules. The ultimate outcome could be a small to large zonular dehiscence. Depending on the size and position of the zonular rent, a capsular tension ring (CTR) might be desirable (see Chapter 26).

A second cause of both fluid misdirection and zonular damage may rarely occur. If a highly dispersive viscoelastic, such as Viscoat (Alcon, Fort Worth, TX), or a viscoadaptive, such as Healon GV (AMO), is utilized, the viscoelastic may impede egress of surplus hydrodissection or hydrodelineation fluid from the anterior chamber. This fluid, unable to leave the anterior chamber and under pressure, has the potential to pass through the zonules, or rupture them, causing chamber shallowing or zonular dehiscence as noted immediately above.[6]

Capsular Block Syndromes[7]

In certain circumstances, the lens can float anteriorly and form a seal against the capsular bag, trapping fluid, creating pressure, and tearing the anterior or posterior capsule. This is most likely to occur when the capsulorrhexis is too small for a mature cataract and, in addition, hydrodissection fluid is injected too vigorously. Fluid inflow exceeds the ability for fluid to egress. There is, therefore, a buildup of fluid behind the lens, which, under pressure, is pushed anteriorly and seals the anterior capsular rim against the nucleus. With continued hydrodissection, fluid pressure builds behind the lens until either the anterior capsule or posterior capsule ruptures (**Figs. 7.7** and **7.8**).[8]

Using dispersive viscoelastic, there is one report of the development of instantaneous pupillary block due to retained viscoelastic between the lens, capsule, and iris, acting like glue and thereupon sealing the lens to the iris.[9] In this report, unenlarged miosis was noted to be a causative factor. Lack of recognition of this occurrence could lead to fluid misdirection syndromes when accompanied by continued irrigation of BSS into the anterior chamber.

Avoiding Fluid Misdirection and Capsular Block Syndromes

These two syndromes may be avoided if the surgeon does the following:

1. Decompresses the anterior segment by removing some OVD
2. Creates an adequately sized capsulorrhexis in relationship to the size and consistency of the nucleus
3. Injects fluid slowly, in bursts, with a 25-gauge cannula mounted on a 3-cc syringe
4. Depresses the central nucleus after hydrodissection to force fluid trapped behind the nucleus, around the

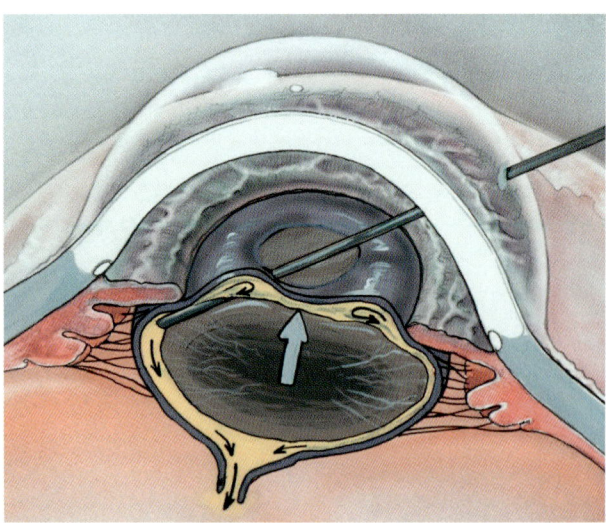

Fig. 7.7 A small rhexis large cataract. The nucleus seals against the anterior capsule. Fluid egress is blocked. Increased fluid pressure causes rupture of the posterior capsule.

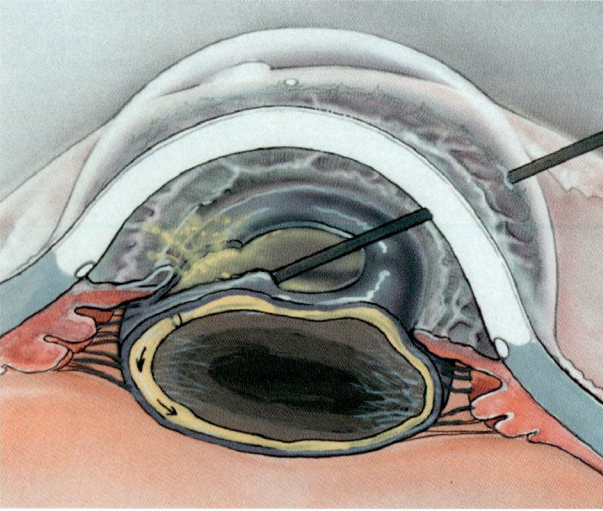

Fig. 7.8 Capsular block. A small rhexus and large cataract. The cataract seals against the cataract. Continued infusion results in a tear of the anterior capsule.

equator, and into the anterior chamber, so that the posterior capsule is decompressed

5. Depresses the posterior lip of the incision to release excess BSS and viscoelastic[10]

Noncontinuous Capsulorrhexis

Tears of the anterior capsule, either visible or occult, occur when the capsulorrhexis is not continuous. If recognized, after infusion of viscoelastic, one edge of the discontinuity can be grasped with capsulorrhexis forceps, folded on itself, and redirected centrally, bringing the tear back into the capsulorrhexis to make it continuous. Predisposing factors include the following:

1. Small pupils making visibility of the capsulorrhexis difficult
2. Positive posterior pressure from all causes, creating the vector forces that encourage the capsule to tear peripherally
3. Long axial length with excessively deep anterior chambers and weak zonules
4. Short axial length with crowded anterior chambers and the tendency for centripetal tearing
5. Pseudoexfoliation with fragile capsules and weak zonules
6. Mature white or black nucleus with poor capsular visibility and thin fragile capsules
7. Advanced patient age with thin, fragile capsules
8. Femtosecond laser–assisted cataract surgery (FLACS) in which occult tags become focal points for tearing peripherally

Small notches or tears in the rhexis act as weak points and focus the vector force of the expanding capsule during the hydrosteps. With the force of the fluid stream filling the bag and pushing the nucleus superiorly, the defect at the notch or tear will split outward toward the equator, stopping at the equator 50% of the time. However, 50% of the time it extends through the equator and into the posterior capsule. The surgeon will see the nucleus "pop up" into the anterior chamber. The new rent in the anterior capsule will be visible. Unfortunately, it is impossible at this juncture to know whether the tear has extended through the equator, compromising the posterior capsule. Even if the tear does not presently extend into the posterior capsule, it perhaps could extend during the ensuing phaco steps. The surgeon must therefore react to preserve the capsule and prevent enlargement of the tear.

The continuance of the procedure is performed in a manner that will enable emulsification without creating undue force on the ruptured capsule. In addition, if the vitreous face is exposed, it should be sequestered from the emulsification so as not to produce its disruption. This is accomplished by installation of a dispersive OVD (Viscoat) beneath the nucleus, gently elevating it to the plane of the iris. The same OVD is then placed above the nucleus to shield the endothelium. Emulsification is then accomplished within the layers of OVD. OVD is replenished as necessary to sequester the posterior capsule/vitreous face and the endothelium from the phaco procedure. Alternatively, the clear corneal wound can be sutured and a new corneal-scleral wound created for the extracapsular removal of the nucleus.

Posterior Capsule Rupture

Rupture of the posterior capsule during hydrosteps occurs infrequently in the absence of the extension of an anterior capsular tear. It is reported to occur in 0.04% to 2.7% of cases with the average around 1%.[11,12] Predisposing factors include the following:

1. Small pupils, making visibility of the capsulorrhexis difficult
2. Long axial length with excessively deep anterior chambers and weak zonules
3. Short axial length with crowded anterior chambers and the tendency for fluid pooling collection behind the nucleus
4. Pseudoexfoliation with fragile capsules and weak zonules
5. Mature white or black nucleus with poor capsular visibility associated with thin, fragile capsules
6. Advanced patient age with thin, fragile capsules
7. The proportional relationship of the size of the capsulorrhexis to the size of the nucleus

This last factor may be of particular importance. If the capsulorrhexis diameter is too small to allow egress of hydrodissection fluid trapped deep to the nucleus, progressive expansion of the posterior capsule and eventual capsular rupture may occur.

Three unique circumstances may give rise to posterior capsular tears during hydrosteps:

1. Posterior polar cataracts: Patients who have dense or calcified posterior subcapsular cataracts may have invasion of the posterior capsule with lens epithelial cells. Hydrodissection will tear the posterior capsule around the central plaque, creating a central defect in the posterior capsule.
2. Patients who have undergone previous vitrectomy may have an iatrogenic preexistent defect in the posterior capsule created inadvertently by the retinal surgeon.
3. The surgeon may inadvertently pass the hydrodissection cannula too far peripherally during the hydrodissection. This will result in the cannula passing through the equatorial capsular bag, splitting it. This tear may propagate into the posterior capsule at any time throughout the remainder of the procedure.

When the posterior capsule tears there may be a subtle deepening of the anterior chamber as the posterior capsule no longer supports the lens and the lens settles into the capsular rent. When detected, the nucleus should be immediately elevated within the anterior chamber and secured at the iris plane. This is accomplished by installation of a dispersive OVD (Viscoat) beneath the nucleus, and then following the procedure as specified above for noncontinuous capsulorrhexis.

Unfortunately, tears of the posterior capsule often remain occult until the anterior chamber is pressurized on initiating the phaco segment of the procedure. With the influx of irrigation fluid, the nucleus is thrust through the capsular rent and to a greater or lesser degree drops into the vitreous cavity. If it is recoverable, it should be stabilized with viscoelastic and promptly elevated into the anterior chamber. Alternately, it may be levered into the anterior chamber through pars plana posterior levitation.[13] It may then be emulsified beneath viscoelastic and over a Sheets' glide, creating a pseudo–posterior capsule as described by Marc Michelson.[14]

Conclusion

The hydrosteps occur early in the continuum of the phacoemulsification procedure. Complications are rare, especially if the principles enumerated above are observed. However, when they do occur they may lead to, at best, a more difficult procedure or termination of the procedure. At worst, a sudden nuclear loss is the result. In the performance of all surgical procedures, attention to detail and prudent skillful surgery will minimize the risk of adverse surgical outcomes.

References

1. Streeten BW. Pathology of the lens. In: Albert DM, Jakobiec FA, eds. Principles and Practice of Ophthalmology. Philadelphia: WB Saunders; 1994: 2182–2183

2. Brierley L. Vacuum capsulorhexis. J Cataract Refract Surg 1995;21:13–15

3. Chang DF, ed. Phaco Chop and Advanced Phaco Techniques, 2nd ed. Thorofare NJ: Slack; 2013:195–207

4. Fine IH. Cortical cleaving hydrodissection. J Cataract Refract Surg 1992; 18:508–512

5. Anis A. Understanding hydrodelineation: the term and related procedures. Ocular Surg News 1991;9:134–137

6. Anderson CJ. Pupillary block during cataract surgery. [letter; comment] Am J Ophthalmol 1994;118:265–267

7. Miyake K, Ota I, Ichihashi S, Miyake S, Tanaka Y, Terasaki H. New classification of capsular block syndrome. J Cataract Refract Surg 1998;24:1230–1234

8. Miyake K. A Japanese study of cases with the dislocation of the lens nucleus into the vitreous cavity after standard hydrodissection. Presented at the Hawaiian Eye Meeting, Kona, Hawaii, January 26, 1999

9. Updegraff SA, Peyman GA, McDonald MB. Pupillary block during cataract surgery. Am J Ophthalmol 1994;117:328–332

10. Koch DD, Novak KD, Liu JF. Pupillary block during cataract surgery. Am J Ophthalmol 1994;118:678–680

11. Ota I, Miyake S, Miyake K. Dislocation of the lens nucleus into the vitreous cavity after standard hydrodissection. Am J Ophthalmol 1996;121:706–708

12. Chang DF, ed. Phaco Chop and Advanced Phaco Techniques. 2nd ed. Thorofare NJ: Slack; 2013:288

13. Kelman C. PAL Technique. Audiovisual J Cataract Refract Surg 1996;12

14. Michelson MA. Use of a Sheets' glide as a pseudo- posterior capsule in phacoemulsification complicated by posterior capsule rupture. Eur J Implant Refract Surg 1993;5:70–72

Section VI Phacoemulsification Techniques and Complications

8 Divide-and-Conquer Technique and Complications

Thomas D. Bailey and James C. Loden

The term *divide and conquer* was first used to describe a technique for removal of the cataractous lens nucleus using phacoemulsification by Gimbel in 1986. When applied in a thoughtful and careful manner (while keeping in mind the anatomy of the cataractous lens), this technique, which involves dividing the hard lens nucleus in half and then typically into quarters, enables the safe and efficient disassembly and removal of the cataract while preparing for lens implant insertion. The goal of the surgeon is to remove the cataract and be left with an intact lens capsule that is well supported by the lenticular zonules and that is without compromise of the capsulorrhexis edge. This gives us the opportunity to place the lens implant in the ideal location—the capsular bag. Even if there is a defect of the capsulorrhexis edge, the lens can still be removed safely with the divide-and-conquer technique as long as the surgeon is careful in applying forces within the lens in such a way as to minimize the risk that a tear of the anterior capsule will extend into the posterior capsule, necessitating additional procedures such as anterior vitrectomy and alternate methods of placement and fixation of the implant.[1–3]

The first step in successful divide-and-conquer lens removal is the creation of an adequate capsulorrhexis. The capsulorrhexis should be no larger than 5.0 to 6.0 mm, as round as possible, and centered on the visual axis. Having the patient look at the microscope light will help the surgeon determine the visual axis. The visual axis is not usually perfectly centered in the cornea or within the edges of the pupil. If a round capsulorrhexis is nicely centered around the visual axis, the lens implant will usually also tend to be well centered on the visual axis when implanted in an intact capsular bag. Keeping the capsulorrhexis diameter at 5.0 to 6.0 mm leads to easier cortical removal from under the anterior capsule, including the portion under the incision. Problems with forming too large a capsulorrhexis include tears into the periphery, which occur when the leading edge of the tear encounters anterior zonules and then tears into the periphery.

When the capsulorrhexis tear is showing signs of extending into the periphery, it can often be salvaged with careful redirection of the tearing force being applied to the anterior capsule. Folding the edge of the capsule being removed and then directing the force applied with the forceps toward the center, or even backward from the center of the tear with a slow, steady movement, can often redirect the edge of the tear back toward the center of the lens. If the edge extends too far, and cannot be brought back, a scissors can be used to cut the edge of the capsule and the forceps used to restart the edge tear in the desired direction. This may help salvage the integrity of the capsule and prevent extension of the tear into the posterior capsule.

As long as the posterior capsule is intact and there is no vitreous prolapse, a three-piece posterior chamber lens implant can usually be placed in the posterior chamber with the haptics in the ciliary sulcus without the need for additional means of fixation. If there is compromise of the posterior capsule, but an intact anterior capsule with intact zonular support remains, the three-piece implant can again be safely placed in the posterior chamber, with the haptics anterior to the capsule, and with no additional fixation after ensuring no vitreous is prolapsed anteriorly. This may necessitate anterior vitrectomy prior to placement. If sulcus fixation is necessary, a one-piece intraocular lens (IOL) with square edged haptics should definitely not be used. It can result in several problems, including secondary glaucoma from pigment loss from chafing of the posterior surface of the iris, also resulting in late transillumination defects, inflammation, and sometimes hemorrhage, which can be recurrent, from erosion of the haptics into blood vessels and decentering of the optic due to its short length. If the anterior capsule edge is not intact, divide-and-conquer dismantling of the nucleus can still be accomplished, as described below, but care should be taken not to apply forces in a direction that will promote the further extension of a tear beyond the equator of the capsule; the forces should be applied only perpendicular to the axis of the tear.

It is useful to think about the substance of the crystalline lens as actually being composed of three portions, or structures, of differing consistency, each of which is handled in a different way. The innermost and hardest portion of the cataractous lens is the nucleus. Depending on the grade of nuclear sclerosis, this can be smaller in a softer, less advanced cataract or represent a much greater portion of the lens in advanced nuclear sclerosis. The nucleus is the main target of the divide-and-conquer technique, as it requires phacoemulsification to be dismantled and removed. The next portion of the lens is the epinucleus, which surrounds the nucleus. This layer is not as hard as the nucleus but is best removed through the larger port of the phaco tip with irrigation and aspiration (I/A). It requires little or no phacoemulsification energy to facilitate its removal. Finally, the outermost portion of the lens is composed of the newest and softest fibers of the lens cortex. These fibers can be removed without phaco power, most safely using the smooth-tipped I/A handpiece (**Fig. 8.1**).

In performing the divide-and-conquer technique, the surgeon needs to be cognizant of how his tools work together to safely remove the cataract. To protect the cornea and to maintain stability of intraocular structures, the anterior chamber is filled with a dispersive viscoelastic. The viscoelastic can be washed out and aspirated prematurely if the surgeon is not careful about the application of aspiration (foot pedal position 2 of 3). The surgeon should try to avoid application of aspiration (determined by the preset aspiration rate and maximum vacuum generated) unless there is lenticular material next to or in the tip of either the phaco or I/A handpiece and should be ready to back off to position 1 (irrigation only) once a given piece has been aspirated. Despite these precautions, it is likely that most of the viscoelastic will be aspirated along with the lens segments in the case of a relatively hard nucleus. For this reason, it is helpful to stop and add viscoelastic to continue to protect the corneal endothelium and minimize postoperative corneal edema in cases with denser nuclei.

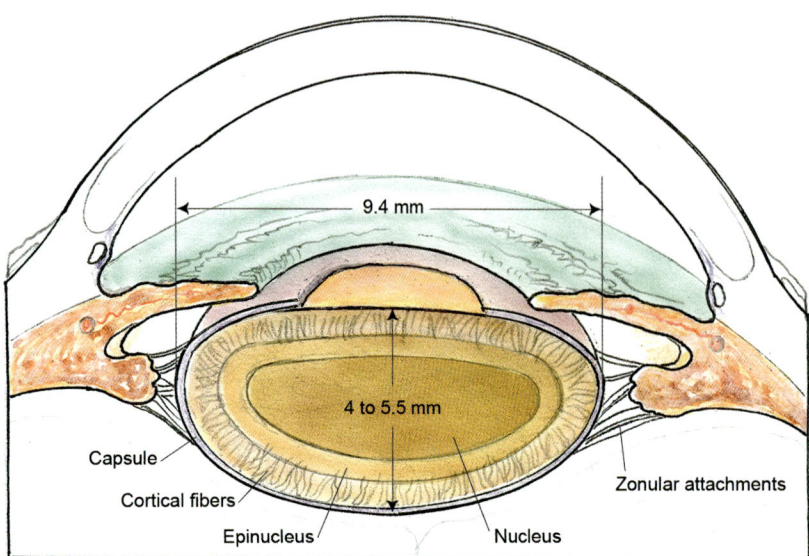

Fig. 8.1 Surgical anatomy of the crystalline lens.

9.4 mm

4 to 5.5 mm

Capsule

Cortical fibers

Epinucleus

Zonular attachments

Nucleus

The next tool vital to lens removal has already been mentioned: the phacoemulsification handpiece. Early phacoemulsification (phaco) was often technically very difficult, especially in the case of an advanced, hard, nuclear sclerotic cataract. Because of the back-and-forth vibration path of the original straight-tip needles, nuclear segments were often pushed away from the tip even when varying levels of vacuum and aspiration (e.g., off/on cycles, higher vacuum and aspiration rates) were used. Strategies involving intermittent aspiration and vacuum were developed to make it easier and safer to remove the nucleus and worked well except in particularly hard nuclei. The development of the Kelman-style tip, bent at the end, significantly improved the ability to remove a hard nucleus. Later, the introduction of nonlongitudinal tip movement, combined with a bent-tip phaco needle, greatly improved the surgeon's ability to safely remove a hard nucleus without having to resort to a large-incision extracapsular procedure. When presented with an advanced, hard nuclear sclerotic cataract, the surgeon should not hesitate to stop periodically during removal to add additional viscoelastic while also using techniques to minimize turbulence and avoid other complications such as wound burns by using only brief bursts of phaco energy and only when lens pieces are engaged by the tip of the handpiece.

The next important tool is the second instrument. There are many types of manipulators and "choppers" available. These are designed to help divide the nucleus and bring the pieces to the phaco tip. To protect the posterior capsule from rupture, the tip of the chopper should not be sharp. We prefer a Rosen-type chopper, which is shaped like a hockey stick on the end, with rounded outside edges and tip. It also has a wedge-shaped edge on the inside distal end that can be used to further divide the pieces of the nucleus when they are between the phaco tip and the Rosen chopper or other manipulator. It also is useful to help feed nuclear pieces to the tip of the phaco handpiece quickly and efficiently in the center of the pupil away from the lens capsule and iris. In this case the phaco tip also serves the additional function of an "anvil" against which the chopper can be used to break up large nuclear pieces with the inner wedge-shaped edge (**Fig. 8.2**).

There are additional intraocular aids for safe and efficient nuclear extraction. The epinucleus and the cortex both provide a barrier between the nucleus and the lens capsule. If possible, the epinucleus should not be removed until the entire nuclear portion

of the lens has been emulsified and aspirated. The chopper can be used to hold the softer epinucleus away from the phaco tip, and it in turn serves as a scaffold to hold the lens capsule away and safe from engagement and damage from the sharp phaco tip. Additionally, the lens capsule and iris can be used as a counterforce to divide pieces of a relatively soft nucleus with a gentle upward movement of the chopper through the nucleus toward the lens–iris diaphragm, after which the pieces can easily be brought into the center of the eye for phacoemulsification with minimal power and duration of phaco energy.

The pieces of the nucleus itself also work as barriers to forward prolapse and rupture of the capsule. Removing the pieces in front of remaining portions of the nucleus, in addition to maintaining a light foot on the pedal, keeps things from happening too quickly in the eye. As the surgeon approaches the last pieces of the nucleus for removal, it is also a good idea to slow down a bit and utilize only short, light bursts of phaco energy. This helps prevent collapsing of the chamber and forward bowing of the capsule when the aspiration rate increases as the pieces are aspirated. The chopper/manipulator should also be kept behind the phaco tip to hold the capsule gently back as the epinucleus is removed and to prevent rapid increases in the aspiration rate from drawing the capsule into the tip.

After capsulorrhexis, the first step to prepare for removal of the nucleus is adequate hydrodelineation/hydrodissection. Using a cannula placed under the anterior edge of the capsulorrhexis, balanced salt solution (BSS) is directed toward the equator of the lens. The best clue to loosening of the lens is visualization of a fluid wave crossing behind the nucleus. To ensure loosening of the lens in the capsule, it is helpful to attempt to achieve dissection with fluid at multiple levels in the lens, indicated by viewing

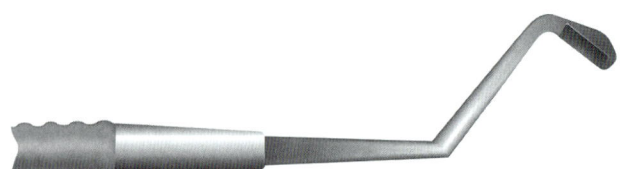

Fig. 8.2 The Rosen chopper is shaped like a hockey stick; the outside edges and tip are rounded. It also has a wedge-shaped edge on the inside distal end. (Courtesy of Bausch and Lomb Storz, Rochester, NY.)

multiple fluid waves. Multiple waves can be obtained by infusing fluid not only close to the anterior capsule but also at deeper levels to separate the nucleus from the epinucleus and also the outermost cortex. It can also be helpful to irrigate from multiple locations around the lens. Gentle movement of the cannula tip anteriorly and posteriorly can facilitate the separation of those layers. However, irrigation with the hydrodissection cannula should not be initiated until the cannula is in position. Problems that can occur if the fluid is infused with too much pressure include rupture of the capsule posteriorly or premature delivery of the nucleus and epinucleus into the anterior chamber when pushed forward by the hydraulic effect of the posteriorly directed fluid in the presence of a large capsulorrhexis. The goal is to achieve easy rotation of the nucleus with the tip of the cannula within the capsular bag to facilitate its removal and to minimize stress on the zonules, which can occur when the connections between the different layers of the lens are not disrupted adequately.

Sometimes, despite adequate hydrodissection, the nucleus and epinucleus will still not easily rotate. Additional hydrodissection will often help achieve adequate separation of the nucleus from the epinucleus, but sometimes free rotation is not achieved without excess manipulation and risk of complications. This is usually not a significant problem; adequate loosening of the nucleus can be achieved as the nucleus is dismantled. The tip of the cannula should not be extended more than 1.0 or 2.0 mm behind the anterior capsule edge because the equator is usually no more than 2.0 mm peripheral to the edge. With a well-centered 6-mm opening, there will be no more the 2 mm of anterior capsule until the equator of the 9.4 mm average diameter lens is encountered (see Chapter 7).

Once the viscoelastic is infused and the capsulorrhexis and hydrodissection have been performed, it is time to divide and conquer the lens nucleus. At this stage the surgeon does not want to risk drawing unwanted structures into the phaco tip. Low aspiration and vacuum settings help to sculpt out a central groove in the nucleus. Any epinucleus and cortical fibers overlying the nucleus anteriorly should be cleared first with irrigation and aspiration under viscoelastic with the phaco handpiece as the only instrument introduced into the eye. This can be done in foot position 2 alone or with very minimal applications of phaco power in position 3 as one moves the tip across the surface of the lens, being careful not to contact the edge of the capsule. At least three passes are needed to create a wide enough opening to easily see and access the nucleus.

The next step is to sculpt a groove down the middle of the nucleus. The surgeon should first do a central groove across the center of the nucleus. This need not be done all in one motion but can be divided into two or more sections starting under the incision. At this point, the lens, if loosened adequately by hydrodissection, may start to rotate. This can be avoided by taking care to groove directly down the center of the nucleus rather than to one side. The limits of the groove can be kept within the capsulorrhexis opening. During sculpting, one should not push against the substance of the nucleus but rather allow the application of ultrasound energy to remove the nucleus. Because the infusion sleeve can cause a drag on the nucleus as it is sculpted deeper, the initial groove should be widened on each side without pushing (**Fig. 8.3**), but by gently advancing across the nucleus halves as the phaco power dissolves it.

The nucleus does not extend all the way to the edge of the lens, so it is not necessary to sculpt all the way out. During sculpting it is important to remember that the lens is only on average 9.4 mm across and 4.0 mm in maximal thickness in the center, and rapidly thins toward the periphery. As the surgeon sculpts deeper, it is advisable to continue to widen the groove on each side to allow for the width of the sleeve and avoid pushing

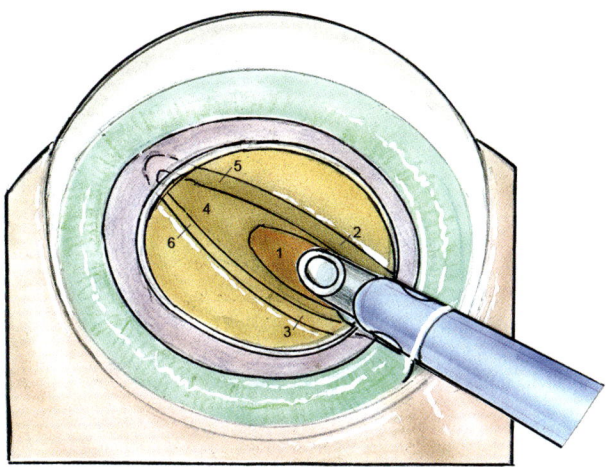

Fig. 8.3   Division of the nucleus by creating a progressively deeper groove using low vacuum and aspiration and by "sculpting" deeper with each pass while also widening the groove to provide room for the phaco tip and sleeve. By carefully limiting the deepest part to the center of the nucleus and lifting the tip as it progresses toward the periphery, damage to the posterior capsule can be avoided. In addition to stereoptic clues to depth, a brightening of the orange-red light reflex will be noted and will help indicate when adequate depth for splitting or dividing the nucleus in half has been achieved. The numbers 1 to 6 represent a suggested sequence of phacoemulsification applications to create and also widen a central nuclear groove to allow room for the tip and sleeve.

on the lens. In a very hard lens, smaller "bites" of the nucleus should be taken and the tip should be lifted anteriorly to parallel the curve of the posterior capsule as it is advanced toward the periphery. On the distal side, the nucleus can be sculpted slightly further toward the periphery; under the site of the entry wound, however, the groove cannot extend as far peripherally due to the edge of the capsule and the angle of the phaco handpiece as it enters the eye. A hard nucleus can be rotated 180 degrees with the tip and the chopper to allow slightly more peripheral extension of the groove. This is usually not needed in softer nuclei. In sculpting posteriorly, it is sometimes helpful to focus the microscope deeper to improve visualization. During hydrodissection, especially in the case of a fairly dense nucleus, the light reflex may be dim or difficult to see. But as sculpting proceeds, approaching the back surface of the nucleus, the surgeon should look for the return of a bright orange-red light reflex. At this point, the nucleus may be ready to split or divide. Once again, if the nucleus is quite dense, rotating it 180 degrees to extend the groove more peripherally on the side that was initially proximal and subincisional will make it easier to split.

Once it is adequately grooved, the nucleus can be separated in two before further dividing it into quarters. The chopper or manipulator is introduced through the paracentesis tract, and both it and the phaco tip are placed as deep as possible in the central groove. This will usually cause some rotation of the nucleus so that the two sides are perpendicular to the path of the instruments. When the two instruments are separated, the nucleus should split (**Fig. 8.4**). If it fails to split completely, the surgeon can move the instruments toward the unsplit side and repeat the maneuver. If the split does not go all the way through the depth of the nucleus, the groove may need to be further deepened to complete the split. One may, however, wish to first attempt to place the instruments deeper in the groove and repeat moving them apart (**Fig. 8.5**).

After splitting the nucleus into two halves, the next step is to rotate it 90 degrees so the phaco tip is perpendicular to the first

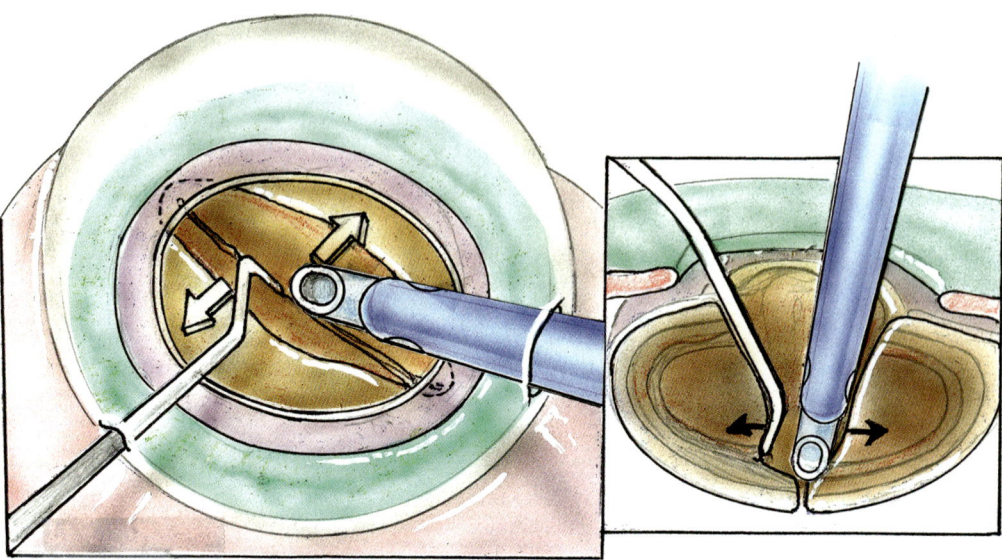

Fig. 8.4 The phacoemulsifier tip and the chopper are placed as deeply as possible into the groove and then pushed away from each other causing the nucleus to split and be divided in half. If the surgeon encounters difficulty in creating a complete division under the phaco incision, the nucleus can be rotated 180 degrees with the instruments, the groove lengthened, and the splitting maneuver repeated to complete the creation of two nuclear halves. The arrows indicate the direction of movement and hence the direction of force application of the instruments.

split, and then carefully sculpt again to divide the first half into quarters. This groove does not need to be as wide or as deep as the first; as soon as both instruments fit into the groove, one can attempt to separate them. The lens capsule is surprisingly elastic and can safely accommodate significant separation of the segments during these maneuvers (**Fig. 8.6**). After the first half is divided, the nucleus can be rotated 180 degrees and the same maneuver repeated on the other side. With experience, one might elect to wait to divide the second half until the first two quarters have been removed. There will be more room at that point to potentially move the second half into the center of the capsular opening, impale it on the phaco tip, and divide it into quarters by moving the inner edge of the chopper toward the tip.

Once the nucleus has been divided into quarters, the aspiration rate and maximum vacuum can be increased to better draw the nuclear segments into the tip. To avoid damage to the iris or capsule, the surgeon should bring each piece to the center of the capsulorrhexis for emulsification. Because the quarters have 90-degree angles, they may resist coming to the center even when engaged by the phaco tip. Particularly with the initial segment, it may be necessary to use the chopper to assist in moving the segment to the center. It may be necessary to move the

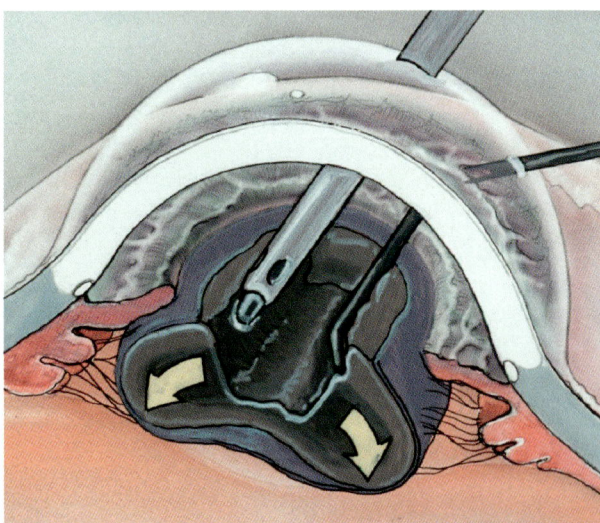

Fig. 8.5 In this illustration the cracking instruments are incorrectly placed too high in the trough. Separation bends the fragments but does not create a crack. The remedy is more phaco to deepen the trough or, if adequate depth is present, placing the instruments deeper into the trough.

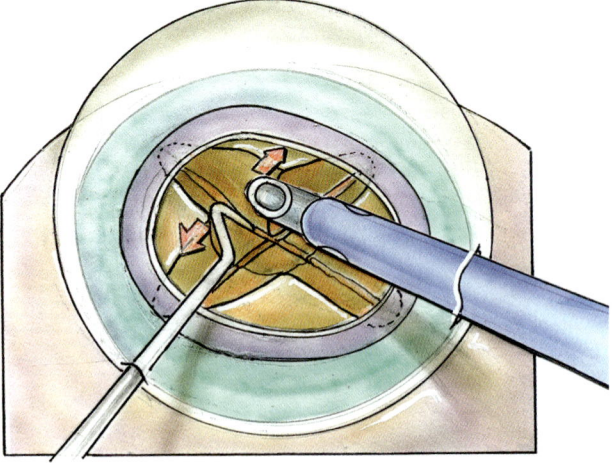

Fig. 8.6 The divided nucleus is rotated 90 degrees and then sculpted to divide the first half into quarters using the same maneuver. If the nucleus is not too hard, the two quarters can be removed prior to quartering the second half. If the nucleus is very hard, the second half can be divided with the "sculpt" setting by rotating the nucleus 180 degrees and dividing it into quarters prior to removal of the nucleus.

chopper peripherally under the edge of the capsule, rotate the tip down to reach around the edge of the nucleus, and pull the segment into the center and against the phaco tip. Or, the chopper can be placed underneath the segment to wedge it anteriorly and centrally. At this point the chopper should be kept between the nucleus and the epinucleus, and care should be taken not to move the chopper either too deeply or beyond the edge of the segment. As soon as one gains purchase on the segment, the chopper should be drawn back inward and if possible, behind the segment to protect the posterior capsule. Once the segment is in the central area, it can be safely emulsified.

If a nucleus is very soft, as in the case of a younger patient with a posterior subcapsular cataract, only the first groove and division of the nucleus may be needed, and from there the halves can be brought to the tip and moved to the center and aspirated with very little need for phacoemulsification. In a very hard nucleus, smaller sections of each half may need to be removed using a combination of grooving, cracking, and engagement of large pieces and use of the tip as an anvil against which to divide the large pieces into smaller ones with the sharp inner edge of the chopper. Complications such as posterior capsular rupture, compromise of the anterior capsule edge, aspiration of the capsule, and disruptions of the zonules can all occur if the surgeon operates in a rushed manner or is too aggressive with the instruments, such as reaching too far in the periphery, not keeping the tips in full view, or applying too much phaco for too long.

Although the divide-and-conquer technique was originally described as a way to remove the nucleus within the capsular bag and away from the corneal endothelium, it may be safest for emulsification to be performed in the capsule–iris plane. If phaco power is used as sparingly as possible, and aspiration and emulsification are performed only when lens material is in or near the tip, turbulence and premature removal of viscoelastic can be minimized. This maximizes protection of the endothelium, and clear corneas on postoperative day 1 will generally be the rule (**Fig. 8.7**).

Once the first segment has been emulsified, the remaining segments will be easier to centralize and emulsify. The remaining segments should be kept behind the segment being emulsified. As noted previously, the epinucleus can also provide a buffer between the tip and the capsule. After "conquering" the nucleus, the phacoemulsification handpiece should be used to remove the epinucleus. If adequately mobilized, the epinucleus should easily be drawn into the tip and can be removed with I/A and little to no phaco power. During this portion of the procedure, the chopper should be carefully maintained behind the tip to keep the posterior capsule from coming forward. The epinucleus can be rotated and fed into the tip in a limited fashion if needed, but great care should be taken not to reach too far under the anterior capsule or iris and compromise the capsule or zonules (**Fig. 8.8**). Once aspiration of the epinucleus has begun, it will often flip over and be easily drawn to the center and aspirated.

If the entire epinucleus resists coming into the center, it may be removed more safely with the smooth-tipped I/A handpiece, although this can take more time. Occasionally, it is helpful to use the chopper to crush a particularly firm piece of epinucleus or even a nuclear fragment into the port on the tip rather than reintroduce the phaco tip into the eye.

Finally, the cortical fibers can be quickly and safely stripped from the inside of the capsule with the I/A handpiece. The cortex is most easily removed by aspirating the anterior ends of the fibers. Then, applying aspiration and vacuum will draw the rest of the fibers into the center. With a 5.0- to 6.0-mm capsulorrhexis, even the fibers under the wound can be easily removed. If some

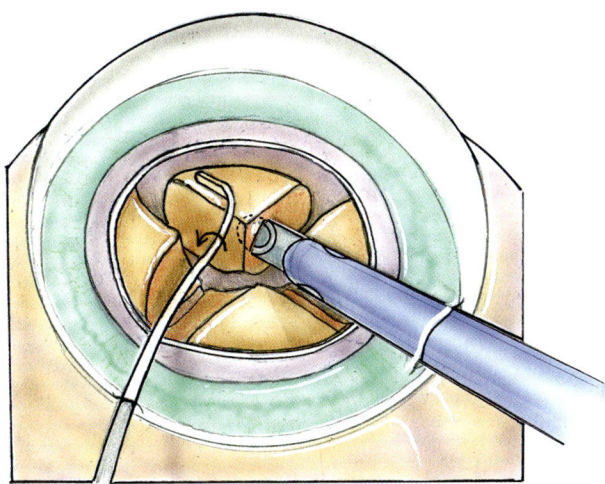

Fig. 8.7 Switching to the "quadrant" setting (high vacuum and aspiration rate), the first nuclear quadrant is drawn into the tip, engaged, and held while it is brought into the center of the capsule opening. The second instrument is used to reach around the edge and help bring the quadrant to the center. The inner edge of the chopper can also be used to further divide the segment into smaller pieces as it is fed into the phaco tip. The phacoemulsification is performed in short, controlled bursts while keeping the remaining nuclear pieces behind the quadrant being removed. As the last of the nucleus is removed, the capsule is shielded by the epinucleus and by keeping the second instrument turned to present a flat side to the capsule, behind the phaco tip. Only very short bursts of phaco power are applied. Foot position 3, irrigation, aspiration and phaco-emulsification, is applied only when a piece to be engaged is next to the tip, thereby limiting turbulence and premature removal of protective viscoelastic.

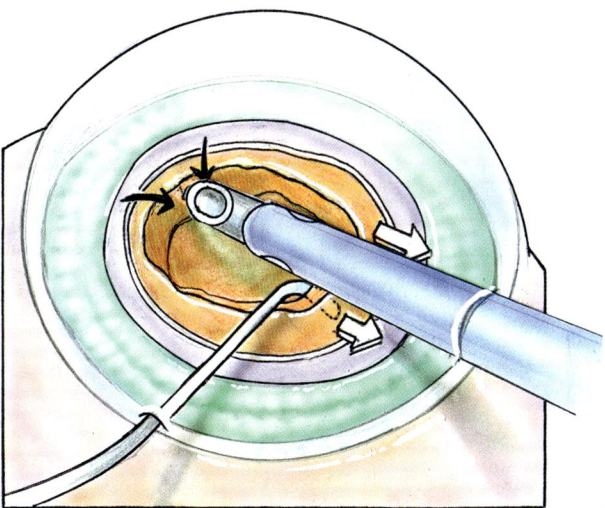

Fig. 8.8 The edge of the epinucleus is engaged in the tip of the phaco handpiece, drawn into the center, and aspirated in foot pedal position 2. If phaco power is needed, it should be applied only in very short bursts to avoid anterior movement of the posterior capsule, collapse of the anterior chamber, and possible posterior capsule rupture. The chopper can be used carefully to help bring the epinucleus to the center and should be behind the tip at all times when aspiration, vacuum, or phaco energy is applied, to protect the capsule.

of the cortical fibers are unusually difficult to aspirate without significant effort, it may be safer to first inject the lens implant. With some rotation of the implant, its haptics will help loosen the remaining fibers, enabling complete removal with coaxial or bimanual I/A. The IOL optic can act as a shield to keep the capsule from being aspirated into the port. In cases in which there is a very large, dense nucleus with little or no cortex, it can also be helpful to insert the IOL in the bag behind the partially debulked nucleus to help shield the capsule while the remainder of the nucleus is removed.

References

1. Tasman W, Jaeger EA, eds. Duane's Foundations of Clinical Ophthalmology, Vol 1. Philadelphia: Lippincott Williams & Wilkins; 1992:1–39
2. hyperphysics.phy-astr.gsu.edu/hbase/vision/eyescal.html
3. Gimbel HV. Divide and conquer nucleofractis phacoemulsification: development and variations. J Cataract Refract Surg 1991;17:281–291

9 Stop-and-Chop Phacoemulsification

Paul S. Koch

Technique Overview

The stop-and-chop phacoemulsification technique entails several simple steps and is a very efficient method for emulsifying the nucleus of any density. Thorough hydrodissection is performed to loosen the nucleus within the bag. Sculpting is performed to prepare space in the middle of the cataract, where the nucleus can be manipulated later on in the procedure. The sculpting should produce a trench in soft and medium-density cataracts and a large crater in dense cataracts. The posterior plate is split, producing two nucleus halves that are free-floating and capable of being manipulated into the space prepared by creating the trench or crater.

At this point, nucleus preparation stops and the emphasis shifts to the chop. The nucleus is rotated 90 degrees and the phaco tip is buried deeply into the hemi-nucleus about one third of the way from right to left. The chopper is placed in the periphery of the nucleus and pulled toward the phaco tip. As the instruments reach each other, they are separated, chopping off the nucleus segment. That chopped segment is already impaled on the phaco tip and can easily be emulsified without further manipulation. This step is repeated around the rest of the nucleus, chopping off segments and emulsifying them.

Problems During the Procedure

Damaging the Sides of the Corneal Incision

The temporal corneal incision should be as square as possible. If the incision is between 2.5 and 3 mm wide, it should also be ~ 2 mm in length. There are many excellent keratomes designed to make an incision of this proportion. The keratome is designed to be moved in a straight line from external to internal. If the blade is wiggled slightly to the left or to the right during incision construction, the sides of the incision can be nipped and "winged." When this happens, the central length of the incision could still be the full 2 mm, but the effective side length might be only 1 mm. This is an inadequate incision, and it is a source of fluid leakage and unsatisfactory incision closure. Stromal hydration could be enough to seal this part of the incision, but sometimes a suture is required to make it secure.

Controlling the Capsulorrhexis

A persistent and vexing problem is the capsulotomy that has a mind of its own and insists on going where it is not supposed to go. To avoid this problem, we must understand the anatomy of the anterior lens and capsule. The anterior capsule is convex. The center of the capsule is an apex surrounded by down-sloping sides. When the capsulorrhexis is being made, there is a tendency for the tear to extend down toward the periphery. That is a normal reaction in a curved surface—things go downhill. This tendency is avoided by adequately filling the anterior chamber with viscoelastic to flatten the anterior capsule. This eliminates the tendency for the downward/outward movement of the tear because it eliminates the "down." When a capsulotomy starts to drift toward the periphery, the treatment is the same: add viscoelastic and increase the pressure in the anterior chamber to flatten the capsule so that the tear can be redirected.

Hydrodissection

Phacoemulsification is performed more easily and safely when the nucleus is free to rotate within the capsular bag. Firm cortical capsular adhesions restrict this rotation and can stress the zonules or the bag itself when rotation is attempted. Avoidance of zonulysis and capsule rupture is facilitated by reliable means of nucleus capsule dissection. Fluid hydrodissection is the first and most reliable way to loosen the nucleus. There are many cannulas that permit hydrodissection by injecting a stream of fluid across the posterior capsule. In most patients, these fluid waves are predictable and provide thorough hydrodissection. In some instances, however, dissection does not occur under the incision. What appeared to be a strong fluid wave did not achieve total dissection so that the nucleus is reluctant to rotate.

One solution to this problem is to slip a cannula under the anterior capsule from the side port and irrigate more fluid directly under the incision.

Another solution to avoid this situation is to begin hydrodissection directly under the incision. This could be performed with a J-shaped cannula, but in my experience the cannula is sometimes difficult to remove because the tip can get caught on the lip of the incision. A better option is the cannula designed by Leif Corydon for viscoexpression of the nucleus. This cannula was designed for hydrodissection, viscodissection, manual dissection between the nucleus and the posterior capsule, and even to hook the underside of the nucleus and pull it from the eye.

The Corydon cannula can also be used for hydrodissection of a nucleus within the bag. Its tip is angled back ~ 150 degrees so it is easy to pass under the subincisional capsule and it is also easily removed from the anterior capsule without getting caught on the lip of the incision. To perform subincisional hydrodissection, the cannula is first directed under the subincisional capsule. It can be lifted slightly to tent the capsule off the nucleus. With firm but gentle injection, a fluid wave will be generated that will pass around the equator of the nucleus from near to far. After passage of the fluid wave, the cannula can be placed on the top of the nucleus and pressed down against it. This pushes the nucleus posteriorly, against the posterior capsule, squeezing the excess fluid around the equator, thus facilitating cortical cleavage.

The cannula can then be rotated so its tip is buried in the nucleus, just inside the capsulorrhexis. The embedded tip can then rotate the nucleus. This effectively completes total separation of the nucleus from the bag. The disruptions of the nucleus/cortical/capsular adhesions make aspiration of cortex during irrigation and aspiration (I/A) easier. The rotation of the nucleus within the capsular bag is a visual check that the hydrodissection is complete.

Maneuvers to Elevate the Nucleus Out of the Bag

At times it is necessary to elevate the nucleus out of the capsular bag. An example is significant zonulysis with poor bag integrity. The Corydon cannula is excellent for lifting the nucleus into the anterior chamber without turning it over. This technique requires a capsulorrhexis that is at least 5 mm in size for soft cataracts; slightly larger is better. If the cataract is very dense, the largest capsulotomy possible is suggested, even a can-opener capsulotomy if needed. The Corydon cannula is placed under the subincisional capsule and a fluid wave is generated as described above (**Fig. 9.1a**). Irrigation is continued slowly until the superior pole of the nucleus lifts out of the bag. Once this occurs, the Corydon cannula is rotated so that the curve is horizontal and parallel to the posterior capsule. Irrigation is continued while the smooth curve of the cannula is gently pushed between the posterior capsule and the nucleus. This manually hydrodissects the nucleus from the capsule. Throughout this maneuver the cannula is slightly lifted to prevent it from catching on the capsule (**Fig. 9.1b**). When the cannula reaches a position more than halfway across the posterior aspect of the nucleus, it is rotated once again so that the tip of the cannula is now lifted up and impaled into the underside of the nucleus. The cannula is gently lifted and tugged toward the incision. The nucleus, now hooked by the cannula, will lift out of the capsular bag (**Fig. 9.1c**). The cannula tip is then freed with the application of a little irrigation. Disengaged, it is slipped out from under the nucleus and removed from the eye.

This one-step maneuver for hydrodissection and for lifting the nucleus into the anterior chamber is safe when used with an adequate capsulotomy. The constant irrigation pushes the posterior capsule rearward, separating it from the nucleus, and creating sufficient room for the cannula to fit between them. The smooth, rounded curve of the cannula advancing under the nucleus tends to move freely without catching either the nucleus or the bag.

Manual Dissection

There are situations in which hydrodissection is inadequate or should not be performed, such as in a posterior polar cataract with capsular involvement. In these conditions, manual dissection is an alternative method for nucleus loosening. The Minami M-hook is an ingenious device for this. This instrument has a rounded distal tip designed to rub against the posterior capsule without breaking it. The various curves of the tip are designed so that the surgeon, by moving fingers or wrist, can direct the hook in almost any orientation within the eye. It can be placed around the lens equator and rotated 270 degrees, giving effective manual dissection of the nucleus from cortex and capsule. The M-hook can also be simultaneously lifted to enhance nucleus separation. This hook is also shaped for dividing the nucleus and for holding the capsular fornix stable in the axis of a zonulysis. I use the M-hook as an adjunct to hydrodissection. Minami uses it instead of hydrodissection (**Fig. 9.2**).

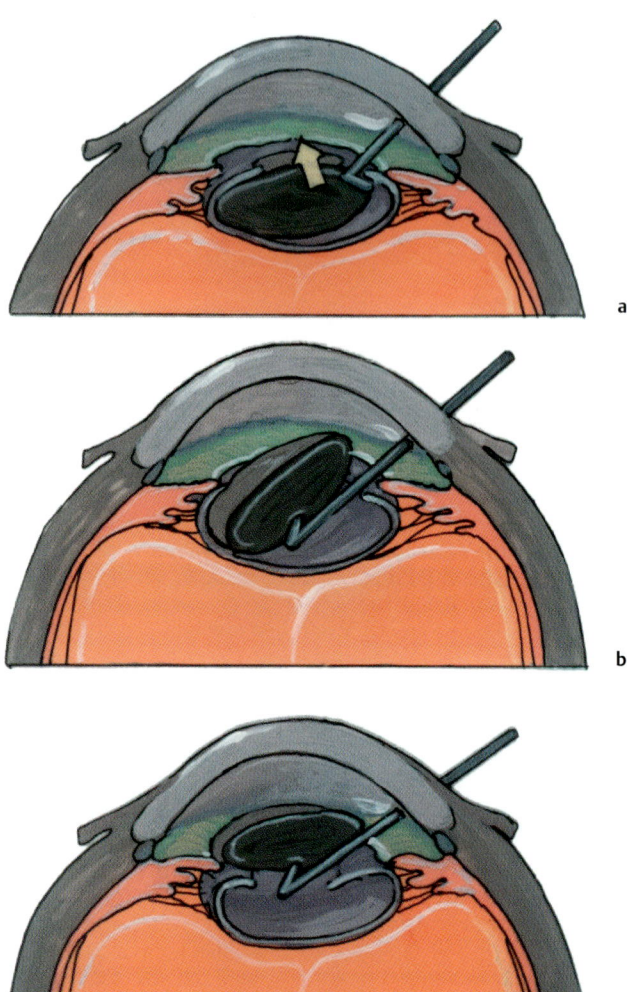

Fig. 9.1 Lifting the nucleus out of the bag. The surgeon may want to get the nucleus out of the bag electively or because the integrity of the bag support is compromised. One way to do this without placing much stress on the bag is a modified hydroexpression technique. **(a)** Subincisional hydrodissection is performed with a Corydon cannula until the superior pole of the nucleus lifts. **(b)** The cannula is rotated so that its flat surface is against the posterior capsule. Irrigation keeps the capsule away from the cannula as it is advanced under the nucleus. **(c)** The cannula is lifted, either in the flat orientation or "hooked" in the bottom of the nucleus, and the nucleus is brought out of the bag.

Stop and Chop in the Dense Nucleus

The traditional stop-and-chop phacoemulsification technique works best for medium-density cataracts. Very dense cataracts are a challenge. The ability to break and separate a dense nucleus is reduced as it becomes more leathery.

Therefore, for a very dense cataract, the concept remains the same but the technique changes. First, a crater is sculpted; this will remove the hard, central core of the cataract. Left behind is the softer peripheral cataract. The sculpting transforms the cataract from a very hard one to a dense but softer one (**Fig. 9.3**). Next, two relaxing nucleotomies are created. This is done by first sculpting a piece of the nuclear rim about two tip widths wide

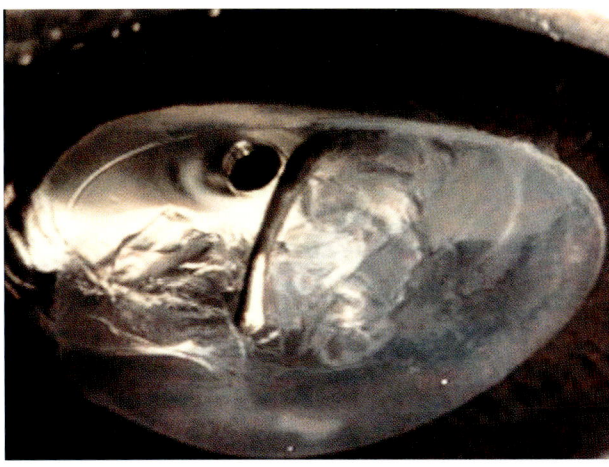

Fig. 9.2 Manual dissection. The M-hook (Minami) is designed to slip between the capsular fornix and the nucleus. Sweeping the hook through several clock hour positions separates adhesions and loosens the nucleus.

opposite the incision. Then the nucleus is rotated and a second one is sculpted 180 degrees away. The posterior plate between these two nucleotomies is sculpted for a few more passes to make a thin fault line along which the posterior plate can now be split.

There are now two very dense, very firm, crescent-shaped nuclear segments. At this point it is tempting to begin to remove the segments in the usual way, beginning one third of the way from right to left. Unfortunately, this technique does not work well for very dense cataracts because hard cataracts do not chop easily unless the nucleus is balanced on the phaco tip. If the chop is attempted when there is asymmetry of the nucleus on the tip, the segment will rotate using the tip as a fulcrum. Without a balance of forces, the segment will twist, tilting toward the side with more of the nuclear segment. This can then create pressure on other pieces of the nucleus, pressing it into the capsular fornix, leading to rupture of the capsule or zonules.

The technique must therefore be modified into what can be termed "repeated bisection." The phaco tip is placed exactly in the middle of the hemi-nucleus and the chop is performed. Now the forces are balanced on the tip. The chop is efficient. Each of

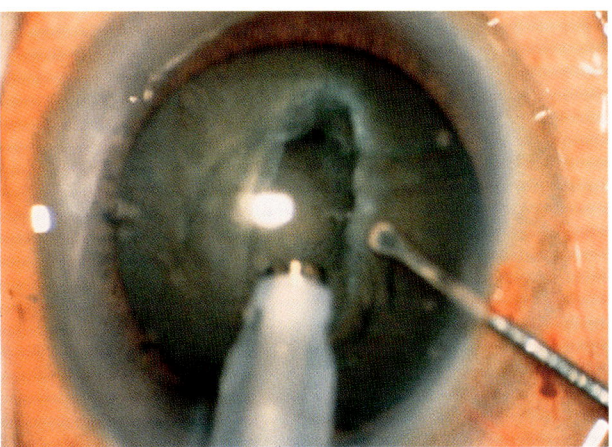

Fig. 9.3 Mature nuclear cataract. Brown or black nucleus with little or no epinucleus.

the segment halves can then be bisected into quarters, and so on, until the nucleus is chopped into appropriately small sizes. Very dense nuclear fragments tend to chatter. The phaco power needed to emulsify them is greater than the aspiration used to hold the nucleus to the tip. It is helpful, in these cases, to use the chopper to pull the pieces of nucleus to the phaco tip and to gently hold them there, improving the efficiency of the emulsification.

Stop and Chop in the Presence of a Small Pupil

The easiest way to deal with a small pupil is to enlarge it, as discussed in Chapter 6. However, if desired, the technique can be modified for phaco of the cataract behind a small pupil. In this situation there are significant hazards. The first is emulsifying the distal pupil, which can cause problems such as a frayed iris or even an iris dialysis The second is increased miosis, further limiting visibility. Finally, excessive iris manipulation will cause release of prostaglandins, with subsequent postoperative inflammation.

A technical difficulty that may occur when working through a small pupil is the over-sculpting and removal of easily visualized central nucleus. This causes an intact posterior plate surrounded by a hidden nucleus rim. The intact plate prevents the nucleus rim from being pulled into the pupillary space where it can be easily visualized and removed. The phaco tip should be kept above an imaginary line halfway across the pupil, so that it never is in a position where it could accidentally aspirate and damage the distal pupil. The phaco tip is used to sculpt a fan-shaped zone, with the narrow portion of the fan just below the incision and the wider portion extending across the nucleus from left to right. Sculpting is continued downward, making this zone as deep as possible and bringing the phaco tip as close to the posterior plate as is feasible.

These steps are performed with the machine at "low flow," a nebulous term that varies from machine to machine. The purpose of the low flow is to prevent the iris from being caught in a fluid stream that would propel it toward the phaco tip where it could be aspirated.

Once the sculpted area in the nucleus is considered deep enough, the next step is to create a trench in the distal nuclear rim. However, if the phaco tip is placed on the surface of the nucleus, as is normally done, the distal iris will quickly be damaged. Therefore, the strategy is to dig a tunnel deep in the body of the cataract. The tunnel is like a trench, except that, initially at least, some tissue is maintained between the phaco tip and the anterior capsule. To accomplish this, the phaco tip is placed deep in the sculpted area and worked out distally deep within the body of the nucleus. Once the tunnel is partially prepared, it can be unroofed, creating the trench. By applying emulsification power under a roof of protective tissue, hard material can be removed while minimizing the risk of aspirating the iris.

Once the trench has been created, the nucleus should be rotated 180 degrees. This ensures that the lens will rotate easily prior to attempting removal of the peripheral nucleus. If the nucleus does not rotate, further hydrodissection should be performed, until rotation is obtained.

Once the nucleus has been rotated 180 degrees, the two sides of the trench should be separated, just as in the traditional stop-and-chop technique. This will break apart the posterior plate. Once the posterior plate is broken, there is no risk of the nucleus being trapped in the peripheral fornix. The nucleus can now be rotated another 90 degrees and the nuclear halves removed by the traditional chop technique.

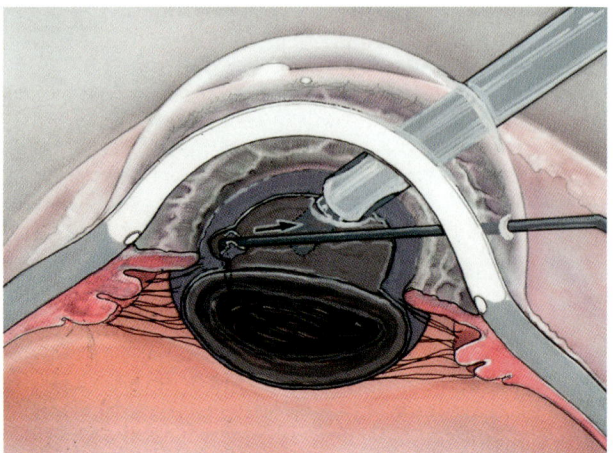

Fig. 9.4 The chopper is positioned over the anterior capsule and tears its edge.

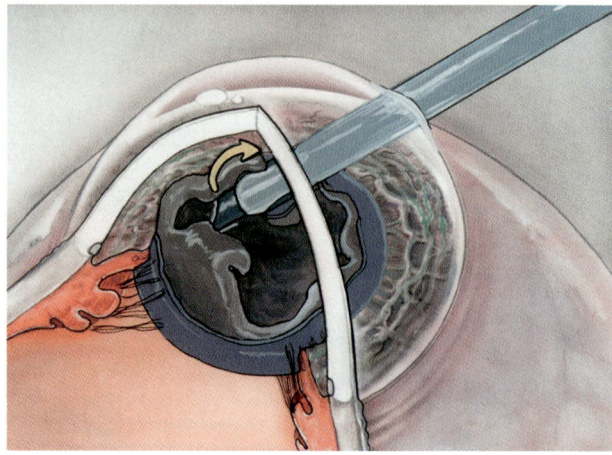

Fig. 9.5 The phaco tip can be used to aspirate the epinucleus and even thick cortex, too.

Stop and Chop When the Chopper Splits the Anterior Capsule

When the chopper is placed in the nucleus, it should be placed just inside the capsulorrhexis. Sometimes, if visualization is poor and the capsulorrhexis is not easily seen, a decision about chopper placement becomes mandatory. One choice, the conservative one, is to place it well within the area where the capsulotomy ought to be. Another choice is to place the chopper on top of the nucleus, and then push it out toward the periphery, retracting the capsule in the process. Either way, sometimes the anterior capsule is caught and ripped. Fortunately, due to the shape of the chopper, the distal end of the tear is usually slightly rounded and so it is unusual for this tear to be extended **(Fig. 9.4)**. The surgery can still be performed routinely with pieces of the nucleus being brought to the center of the capsular bag for chopping and removal. This is the appropriate tactic if the remaining nucleus is small. If, on the other hand, the remaining nucleus is large, and there is danger that the tear in the anterior capsule could be extended, an alternative technique is to bring the remainder of the nucleus into the anterior chamber. If the nucleus is intact, it can be raised with gentle hydrodissection or viscodissection. If the nucleus has already been broken into two separate pieces and the posterior plate has been separated, only half a nucleus at a time has to be brought into the anterior chamber. The chopper can be slipped under the anterior capsule and brought around to the nucleus equator where it can gently tug the equator of the lens away from the fornix while lifting gently. At least one portion of the nucleus will come up above the capsule where the chopper, combined with the aspiration of the phaco tip, and assisted as necessary with viscoelastic, can bring the piece rest of the way out of the bag. Once in the anterior chamber, the nucleus can be sandwiched in viscoelastic and emulsified directly. The same steps should be repeated for the remaining half of the nucleus.

Removing Thick Epinucleus

The removal of thick epinucleus may be a challenge, as aspiration instruments have certain limitations, chief among them the small aspiration port. There are several options to help in this case.

Most modern phaco machines can be programmed with an "epinucleus" setting. Generally these settings limit the power to 2 or 3%, so the epinucleus can be removed slowly and carefully. In the absence of such a setting the machine can be advanced to the irrigation and aspiration (I/A) mode where, although there is no power, the surgeon has delicate control of the vacuum. In this mode the surgeon can slowly aspirate the epinucleus similarly to using a wide-bore I/A tip.

The phaco tip can be used to remove not only epinucleus in the I/A mode but thick cortex as well **(Fig. 9.5)**. However, thin cortex is always better removed with the small port of the I/A tip. If all of the cortex is removed with the phaco tip, the phaco handpiece can be set aside and used later to remove the viscoelastic after lens implantation. The wide bore facilitates the aspiration and evacuation of the viscoelastic from the anterior chamber with remarkable efficiency and thoroughness. It also saves the scrub nurse the necessity of switching the tubing prior to viscoelastic removal.

Conclusion

The stop-and-chop technique, as with cataract surgery in general, can entail complications, but if the situations described in this chapter are mastered, there will be few occasions when the surgeon will be struck with a surprise situation.

10   Vacuum Hemi-Flip Phacoemulsification

R. Bruce Wallace III

Background

Over 30 years ago, surgeons like myself were excited about the evolution of the anterior capsulotomy from the can-opener capsulotomy to the continuous curvilinear capsulorrhexis (CCC) method of Thomas Neuhann and Howard Gimbel. At the advent of the CCC, existing methods of nuclear removal were fine for can-opener capsulotomies, but not for the CCC.

At that time, I was fortunate to be a program participant at a cataract surgery session of the Contact Lens Association of Ophthalmologists (CLAO) meeting at which John Shepherd[1] first described his divide-and-conquer phacoemulsification procedure. (Interesting that the most popular method for nuclear removal was introduced at a contact lens meeting.) Every phaco surgeon in the room knew this was a groundbreaking and important step for preserving the CCC. Four-quadrant divide and conquer appears to still be the preferred technique for phaco surgeons worldwide.

Soon after this event, I became an investigator for the Staar foldable intraocular lens, the "Mazzaco Taco," a welcome addition to small-incision cataract surgery. But what really inspired me to modify four-quadrant divide and conquer was the prediction in some circles that lens extraction and implantation of presbyopic intraocular lenses (IOLs) would become popular for precataract presbyopes as we became more familiar with multifocal IOLs and their benefit to cataract patients. Many of these younger, softer lens nuclei could be prolapsed through a standard 5.0-mm CCC, but there existed a subset in 50- to 60-year-old patients in whom the nuclei were firmer and full nuclear prolapse less predictable. The time period was the early 1990s, and phaco fluidics were continuing to be improved. I began trying to perform hemi-flip phaco on standard cataractous nuclei to feel proficient with hemi-flips for younger patients. At this time, Allergan (Parsippany, NJ) added the "Burst Mode" to its Sovereign phaco unit and I was finally able to consistently perform phacoemulsification of the hemi-nuclei.[2–4]

More recently, I have converted from peristaltic (flow based) phaco to venturi (vacuum) fluidics with the Bausch and Lomb (Rochester, NY) Stellaris and the AMO Signature (Abbott Medical Optics [AMO], Abbott Park, IL). Vacuum fluidics, more common for posterior segment surgeons, offer a welcome improvement for removing the hemi-nuclei.[5] Now I routinely perform what I term vacuum hemi-flip procedures on most cataract and presbyopic lens cases.

Surgical Technique

For standard nuclear removal without femtosecond CCC, I mark the centration and size of the CCC by placing a 6.0-mm optic zone marker on the central cornea.[6]

Cortical cleaving hydrodissection of the nucleus and cortex with balanced salt solution is performed through a 25-gauge cannula. A deep central nuclear groove is created with the 30-degree phaco tip (**Fig. 10.1a**). My second instrument, entered through the sideport incision, is a blunt "chopper," not used for chopping but for nuclear manipulation and posterior capsular bag protection (**Fig. 10.1b**). It is called the Wallace Guardian (Storz, Bausch and Lomb) (**Fig. 10.2**). This instrument can be helpful when grooving the nucleus with a small pupil. Simply pulling the proximal edge of the groove toward the surgeon allows the distal groove to be visualized and phacoemulsified. Splitting the nucleus in half is more predictable with a deep groove that is near both nuclear equators (**Fig. 10.1b**).

After separating the nuclear halves with the phaco tip and the Guardian, the halves are rotated 90 degrees. To avoid corneal endothelial trauma from streaming fluids and phaco energy, I adjust the irrigation ports in line with the phaco tip (**Fig. 10.3**). (I made this adjustment after learning about the significant phaco energy emanating from the phaco tip from a video presentation by William Fishkind.[7])

The first nuclear half is removed by using the Guardian to lift the left edge of the distal half and bringing it to the center of the pupil (**Fig. 10.4**). Modern vacuum fluidics enable the rapid nuclear removal of this first half. The second half is then rotated around in the capsular bag and the same method is employed for removal. The Wallace Guardian is placed posterior to the remaining nuclear material to protect the posterior capsule (**Fig. 10.5**). If significant phaco energy was needed to remove the first half, a dispersive viscoelastic (Viscoat, Alcon, Fort Worth, TX) is reinjected over the second nuclear half prior to phaco. Thanks to Howard Fine's cortical cleaving hydrodissection, there are cases where the cortex and nucleus are now removed and IOL implantation is performed without additional cortical irrigation and aspiration.

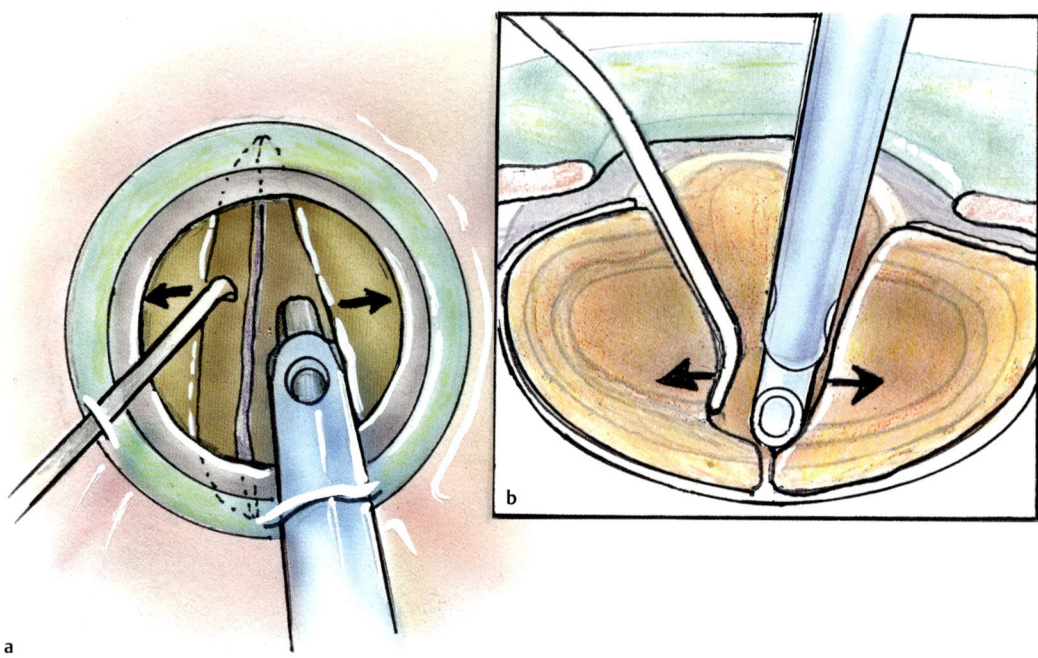

Fig. 10.1 **(a)** A deep central nuclear groove is created with a 30-degree phaco needle. **(b)** The Wallace Guardian instrument is used to create a crack in the nucleus. Splitting the nucleus is easier with a deep groove that extends to near the nuclear equator.

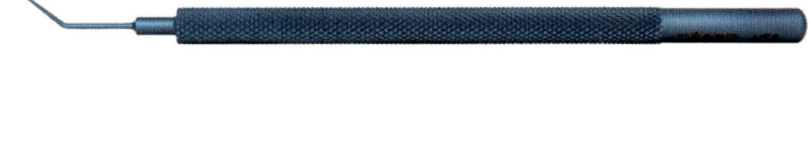

Fig. 10.2 The Wallace Guardian instrument. (Courtesy of Bausch and Lomb Storz, Rochester, NY.)

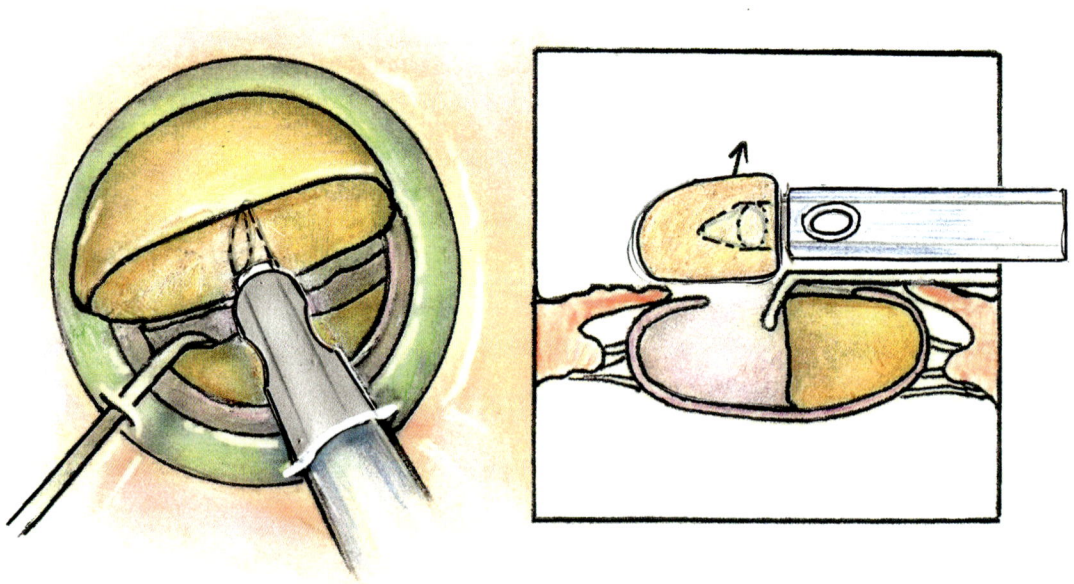

Fig. 10.3 The irrigation port is adjusted to be perpendicular to the phaco tip bevel to decrease physical damage from the irrigation inflow. The nucleus is rotated 90 degrees. The subincisional hemi-nucleus is separated from the distil hemi-nucleus, which is elevated.

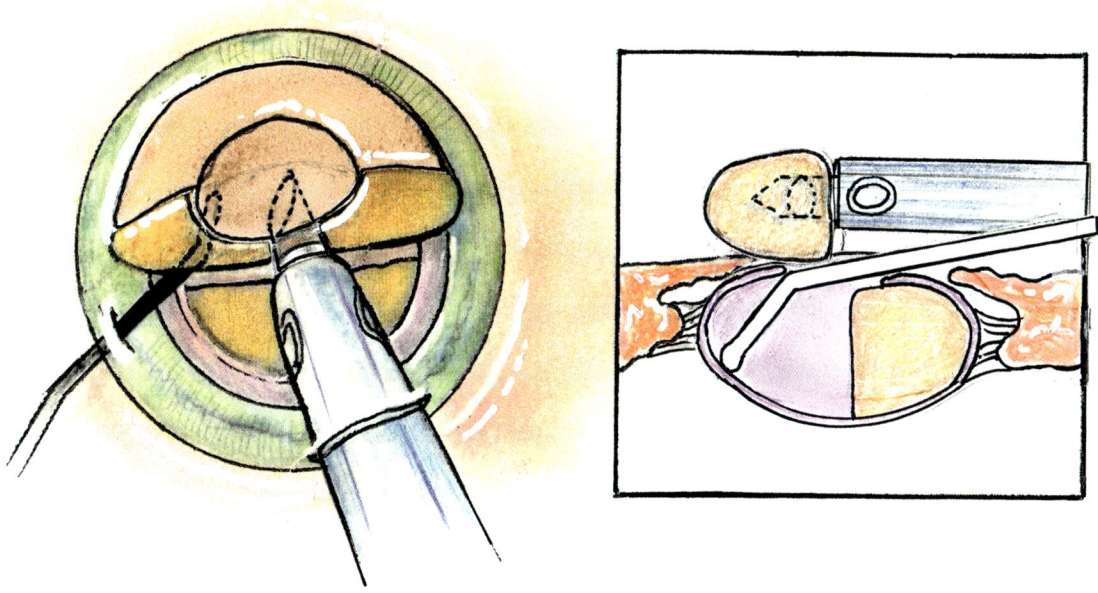

Fig. 10.4   The Guardian is used to lift the left side of the distil hemi-nucleus, bringing it to the center of the pupil, where it is emulsified in the plane of the iris.

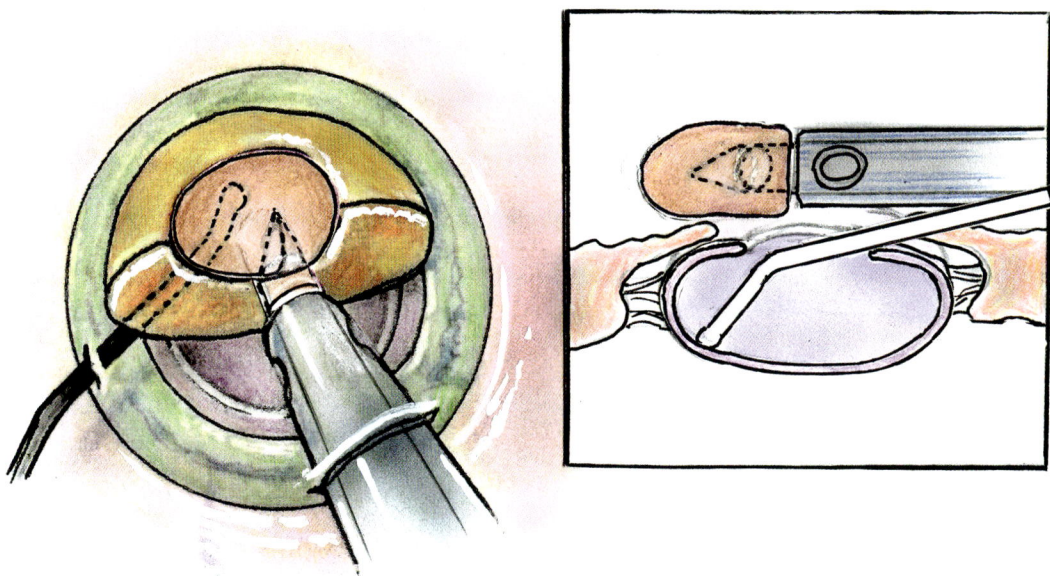

Fig. 10.5   The second hemi-nucleus is rotated and lifted. The guardian is repositioned to protect the posterior capsule, and the nucleus is emulsified.

Conclusion

As refractive cataract surgery continues to evolve and presbyopic IOLs become more popular, nuclear removal of cataractous and precataractous lenses remains an important procedure for successful outcomes for patients with high levels of expectation for spectacle-free vision. I have found vacuum hemi-flip phacoemulsification to be an efficient and dependable method for nuclear removal for modern lens surgery.

References

1. Shepherd JR. In situ fracture. J Cataract Refract Surg 1990;16:436–440
2. Olson RJ, Kumar R. White Star technology. Curr Opin Ophthalmol 2003; 14:20–23
3. Osher RH, Injev VP. Thermal study of bare tips with various system parameters and incision sizes. J Cataract Refract Surg 2006;32:867–872
4. Fishkind W, Bakewell B, Donnenfeld ED, Rose AD, Watkins LA, Olson RJ. Comparative clinical trial of ultrasound phacoemulsification with and without the WhiteStar system. J Cataract Refract Surg 2006;32:45–49
5. Wallace RB. Gravity feed gets upgraded. Ophthalmology Times 2010;35: SU6249
6. Wallace RB, Capsulotomy Diameter Mark. J Cataract Refract Surg 2003; 29:1866–1868
7. Fishkind WJ. Pop goes the microbubbles. Video presentation at the American Society of Cataract and Refractive Surgery 1997 meeting. Grand Prize Winning Video at the European Society of Cataract and Refractive Surgeons

11 Phaco-Chop Procedure: Management and Complications

Brian A. Hunter

The age- and sex-adjusted rates of cataract surgery between 1980 and 2011 have increased fivefold, to over 1,200 cases per 100,000 people.[1] These rates are expected to rise with the aging of the baby-boomer population and increases in second eye cataract surgery due to improved outcomes.[2] Given this increase in surgical rates, one may assume that the most efficient and effective means of performing cataract surgery would be clearly understood, and teaching it would be streamlined throughout residency programs. But this is not the case. Graduating from ophthalmology residency, many surgeons are comfortable with conventional techniques like divide and conquer[3] or stop and chop,[4] but they have little or no experience in phaco chop.[5]

There are numerous advantages to using the phaco-chop technique, but few surgeons employ this technique.[6] I assert that one answer may be simply the fear of the unknown. Anyone practicing the phaco-chop technique should be familiar with the management of several seen and unseen complications that arise frequently[7]; the ten most common complications that may occur during phaco-chop surgery for beginning surgeons are the following, and they are addressed in this chapter: (1) small capsulorrhexis; (2) inadequate hydrosteps; (3) a lens that does not spin; (4) poor control of the foot pedal, resulting in capsular damage; (5) the use of too much phaco energy in a soft nucleus; (6) not using enough phaco energy in a hard nucleus; (7) failure to remove the anterior epinucleus and delineate the capsulorrhexis edge; (8) the phaco tip placed too far off the center of the nucleus, resulting in tipping or flipping of the nucleus; (9) incorrect placement of the horizontal chopper (such as Seibel) anterior to the capsular bag; and (10) not knowing when to use a vertical, horizontal or hybrid, chopping technique.

This chapter: (1) provides some simple strategies for the beginning phaco surgeon to recognize, avoid, and manage common complications; (2) discusses how to minimize risks for complications, specifically in very soft and in very hard and leathery cataracts; (3) addresses additional complications associated with femtosecond laser–assisted cataract surgery (FLACS); and (4) presents alternatives to techniques previously discussed in the management of anterior chamber (AC) tears or zonular dialysis.

Small Capsulorrhexis

The ideal size of an anterior capsulotomy has been debated extensively, and it depends on a multitude of factors. But creating a consistently round and continuous anterior capsulotomy is a critically important early step in preventing complications from the phaco-chop procedure. Broadly speaking, the continuous curvilinear capsulorrhexis (CCC) should be between 5 and 6 mm

in diameter, with most phaco-chop surgeons preferring 5 to 5.25 mm for most cases.[8] There may be situations where a larger rhexis of up to 6 mm is needed in extremely dense nuclear sclerotic lenses, or smaller than 5 mm in white mature cortical cataracts under pressure. A CCC less than 4 mm usually necessitates avoidance of horizontal chop techniques and requires enlargement after placement of the intraocular lens (IOL). With the advent of FLACS, there is significantly more control not only of the size of the rhexis (often around 5 to 5.25 mm) but also of the location of the rhexis, which can be chosen to be centered over either the visual or the pupillary (anatomic) axis. This has some obvious benefits to the cataract and refractive surgeon in lens choice, but does not significantly affect the process of nuclear disassembly by the phaco-chop technique. The stability and integrity of the anterior rhexis is critical to good outcomes using phaco chop, and any weakness or irregularity can force the phaco-chop surgeon to change course and use another technique (e.g., changing from horizontal to vertical chopping) to avoid tears and resultant complications.[9] Management of AC tears will be discussed separately.

Inadequate or Incomplete Hydrosteps

Hydrosteps were discussed in great detail in Chapter 7, but I cannot stress enough the importance of adequate hydrodissection and hydrodelineation to the phaco-chop surgeon. Inadequate hydrodissection can result in inadvertent zonular dialysis during lens rotation.[10] Poor or incomplete hydrodelineation can result in improper positioning of the chopper proximal to the epinuclear–nuclear plane, resulting in posterior displacement of the lens and possible posterior chamber (PC) rupture or zonular dialysis. Positioning the chopper distal to this plane can lead to peripheral capsular puncture and vitreous loss.

A Cataractous Lens that Does Not Spin

Many surgeons are easily frustrated when they are unable to obtain an adequate hydrodissection and rotation of the phakic lens. Repeated attempts using large volumes of balanced salt solution (BSS) is not always successful and is often counterproductive. (We all know the adage that doing the same thing over and over again but expecting different results is the definition of insanity.) Incomplete hydrosteps may be due to the surgeon's inexperience or overabundance of caution, but may also be a result of certain lenticular pathologies, such as in patients with zonular laxity or dehiscence, a soft nucleus, highly myopic eyes, or pseudoexfoliation.[10] Often these conditions, if not diagnosed preoperatively, will only become evident during hydrodissection,

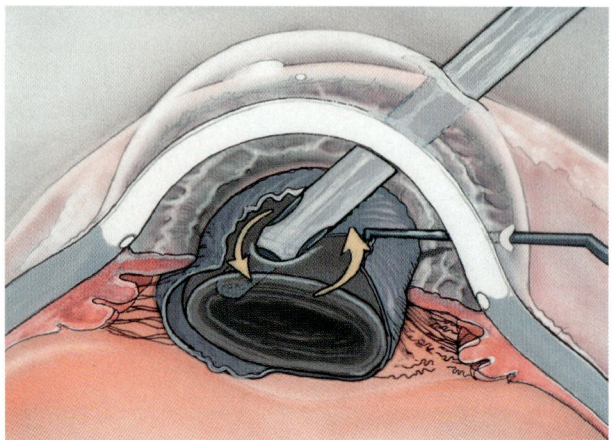

Fig. 11.1 Inadequate hydrodissection. In the presence of weak zonules, overt zonular dialysis is created during rotation of the nucleus.

but many times more significant zonular compromise may not become clear until after initial chopping (**Fig. 11.1**). What should the surgeon do if the lens still does not rotate even after the first piece has been removed? Two techniques can make a big difference: The first is manual chopping of pieces with the second instrument and subsequent phacoemulsification to increase space within the capsular bag. The goal is to methodically remove the first hemi-nucleus segment by segment. Alteration of the fluidics and the increased amount of irrigation of the remaining segment as a result of achieving this goal will often produce enough separation to enable the remaining hemi-nuclear segment to rotate. But what if it still won't rotate? In this circumstance, it is advisable to take a deep breath and proceed with plan B: hemi-nuclear lift and carry. Leaving quadrant removal mode and returning to the phaco-chop setting, the phaco tip is impaled into the subincisional nucleus, which is subsequently lifted and carried into the desired position. The lift is a move in which the segment is impaled and then elevated anteriorly and centrally. The carry is accomplished by carefully pushing the impaled segment in a direction opposite the main incision while concomitantly rotating in a clockwise direction (**Fig. 11.2**). This lift-and-carry technique often creates sufficient movement to break the few adhesions to the capsular bag and allow the hemi-nucleus to rotate in a desired position directly opposed to the main phaco incision. Aggressive hydration or even viscodissection can be employed if the above techniques fail.

Phaco Chop in a Soft Nucleus: The "Manual-Chop" Technique

How should the dreaded soft nucleus be managed? Once a horizontal chop technique is mastered, it is possible to remove a very soft cataract or, in the case of a refractive patient, a clear lens, without significant trouble. Most beginning choppers dread the soft nucleus because the usual techniques of chopping in a 2 to 3+ nuclear sclerotic cataract (NSC) no longer apply. In very soft cataracts, overuse of the aspiration or phaco ultrasound mode will easily "eat" through a soft nucleus and risk perforating the capsular bag.[11] In these cases, its possible to avoid using any aspiration or vacuum during the phaco chop maneuver. By positioning the phaco tip against the nuclear segment to produce sufficient countertraction, the nucleus is stable enough to enable correct placement of the second instrument into the epinuclear–nuclear plane. This manual chop technique enables efficient disassembly of the nucleus and epinucleus.

Failure to Delineate the Anterior Chamber Rhexis Edge, and Removal of the Central Anterior Epinuclear Shell

In most cases, after completing the capsulorrhexis, it is advisable to delineate the borders of the capsulorrhexis by aspirating the central anterior epinuclear shell using the phaco needle. This can be performed using either the sculpt or chop settings with a phaco tip of any angle. Usually a modest application of aspiration is required to complete this step. Of course, this step should be skipped in white mature cataracts, not only because of the scarcity of epinucleus in this setting, but also because attempting the maneuver may lead to excessive posterior pressure, resulting in submarining of the nucleus or the releasing of counterpressure that may induce anterior displacement of the nucleus, in turn resulting in the dreaded Argentinian flag sign.[12]

Information about the cataract density and zonular stability is gained during proper performance of this initial epinuclear cleanup and can help determine the most desirable chopping technique and phaco power requirements. The density of the cataract can be assessed either by the color (white, brown, or black) or by manual depression of the phaco tip into the anterior nucleus 3+ to 4+ NSC lenses that leave "ice skate marks" on the hard surface, whereas softer lenses leave "knife in jello"–like stab wounds.

Choosing Between Horizontal and Vertical Phaco-Chop Techniques and Common Pitfalls of Each

Horizontal Chop Phacoemulsification

Horizontal chop requires a small amount of horizontal displacement of the lens centrally during chopping and quadrant removal. To minimize the amount of displacement, each quadrant should be removed immediately after it is created. After a few pieces have been removed, there will be more space in the capsular bag to enable the remaining nuclear remnants to be removed without having to blindly chop in the peripheral capsular bag. In certain phacoemulsification platforms, settings can be maximized to increase the efficiency of the phaco-chop technique by obviating the need to select between chop and quadrant removal settings on the foot peddle during nuclear disassembly.

Horizontal Chopping Technique

In horizontal chopping, the chopper is placed at the epinuclear–endonuclear junction and repositioned horizontally to perform the chop.

In all chopping procedures the superficial nuclear cortex is removed immediately after entry of the phaco tip into the AC.

The maneuver is initiated by introducing the phaco tip, in position 1 (irrigation only), bevel down, to position it over the middle third of the subincisional nucleus. Phaco power is commenced introducing the needle into the body of the nucleus paracentrally. Foot pedal position 3 is employed to ensure that the phaco tip is completely plunged into the lens nucleus. Prior to entering the eye, the irrigation sleeve should be withdrawn 1 to 1.5 mm from the bottom of the bevel to enable the needle to adequately impale the nucleus. Phaco power is used until the needle is buried within the nucleus. Immediately upon passing the tip into the nucleus up to the sleeve, phaco power is terminated and the needle holds the nucleus with vacuum only (foot pedal position 2).

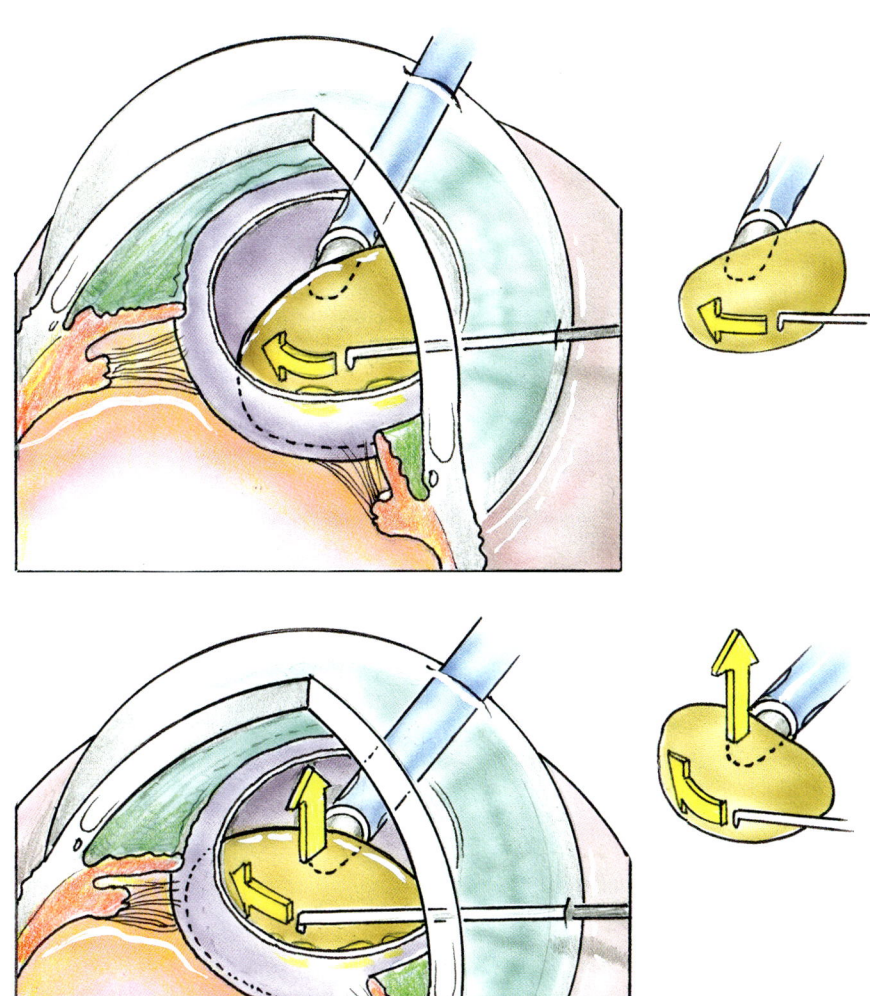

a

b

Fig. 11.2   (a,b) Lift and carry. The nucleus is almost simultaneously lifted anteriorly and centrally by the phaco tip and rotated in a clockwise direction.

The chopper is passed through the side port, rotated so that the chopping tip is iris parallel, and is placed at the anterior capsulorrhexis margin (**Fig. 11.3**). The phaco tip is pulled horizontally toward the incision, continuing to hold vacuum in foot pedal position 2. This predictably will split the endonucleus from the epinucleus, creating a cleavage plane. When this plane is sufficiently visualized, the chopper is rotated to vertical and positioned into the plane (**Fig. 11.4**).

The two instruments are, at this point, positioned for chopping (**Fig. 11.5**). Maintaining vacuum in the phaco tip, the tip is pushed up and to the right, thus elevating the endonucleus and moving it right.

The chopper is pulled toward the wound slightly and then moved down and to the left. The shearing force thus produced will crack the nucleus. The crack may or may not extend partway through the nucleus toward the incision. The chopper can be repositioned more centrally to enlarge the crack toward the incision, if preferred (**Fig. 11.6**).

The vacuum is released (foot pedal position 0), and the chopper and phaco tip are used to rotate the nucleus counterclockwise 10 to 30 degrees, depending on the density of the nucleus.

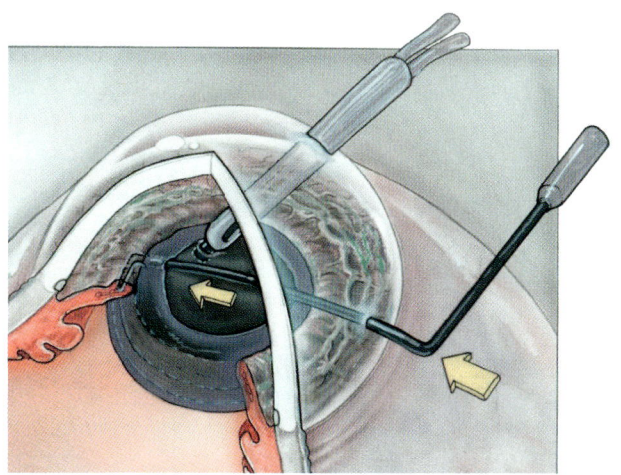

Fig. 11.3   The handle of the chopping instrument is rotated to the right until horizontal, resulting in rotation of the tip so that it is parallel to the nucleus and can be easily passed under the anterior capsule.

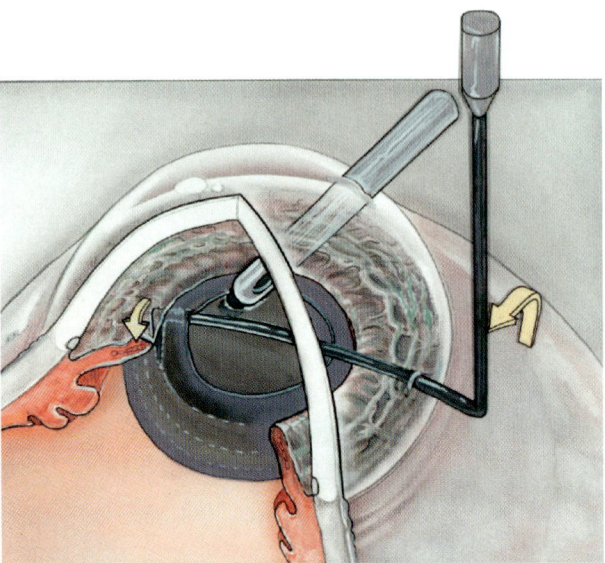

Fig. 11.4 Once past the junction of the epinucleus/cortex junction with the endonucleus, the handle is rotated back to vertical, which allows the tip to pass around the nucleus equator in preparation for the horizontal chop.

Generally, smaller rotations for a harder nucleus and larger rotation for a softer nucleus are indicated.

It is now straightforward to visualize the thickness of the endonucleus. Using position 3 with phaco power, once again the phaco tip is buried into the nucleus. The minute the phaco tip impales the nucleus solidly, and the tip is buried to the depth of the irrigation sleeve, the ultrasonic energy is turned off and vacuum is used exclusively to hold the nucleus. Once again the chopper is placed horizontally at the rhexus edge and then rotated to vertical and dropped into the endonuclear–epinuclear cleavage plane created by withdrawing the phaco tip toward the incision, with adherent nucleus affixed. Just as previously described, the phaco tip, in position 2, vacuum only, is pushed up and to the right and the chopper pulled down and to the left,

producing another crack and resulting in formation of a pie-shaped segment (**Fig. 11.7**).

In a soft or moderate nucleus, the pie-shaped segment can be mobilized, elevated to the pupillary plane, and emulsified (**Fig. 11.7**). In a hard nucleus, it is advantageous to continue rotating and chopping for 360 degrees. This will create multiple small pie-shaped segments, until the nucleus loses its inflexibility. At this point removal of the segments is expedited.

Vertical Chopping

Vertical chopping by definition minimizes the risks of peripheral capsular tears that can occur during horizontal chopping, by keeping the vertical chopper at or near the anterior rhexis edge during each chop. In contrast to the horizontal chop technique, during vertical chopping it is recommended to leave each piece in place until the entire nucleus has been chopped. Then each piece can be removed with minimal movement of the capsular bag or stress on the zonules.

Vertical Chopping Technique

The major principles previously explained are utilized with vertical chopping. The foremost difference in technique is that the creation of the endonuclear–epinuclear cleavage plane is unnecessary. Additionally, it is not necessary to place the chopper in the plane where the nucleus is thinner and the posterior capsule closer to the chopping instrument. Even more important is that it may be difficult to visualize the endonuclear–epinuclear plane when the pupil is small. This is not necessary with vertical chopping, making this variation of the procedure stress-free and safe.

In vertical chopping the phaco tip is prepared comparably to horizontal chopping and passed into the paracentral nucleus in the same way. Again, once solidly within the substance of the nucleus, position 2, vacuum only, is used to hold the nucleus on the phaco tip. The major difference in technique occurs at this point, as the chopper, passed through the side port is positioned vertically and hovers over the nucleus near the phaco tip. The phaco tip is now gently elevated vertically, remaining in position 2. The chopper is driven downward, into the nucleus adjacent

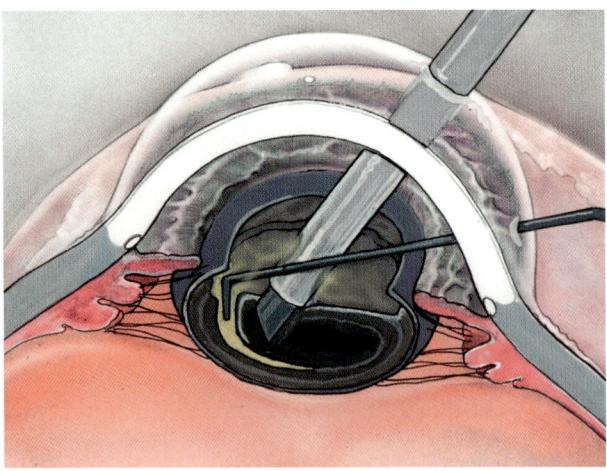

Fig. 11.5 The chopper is properly positioned below the anterior capsule in the space created by the hydrodelineation. The need to place the chopper under the iris where it cannot be visualized is therefore avoided.

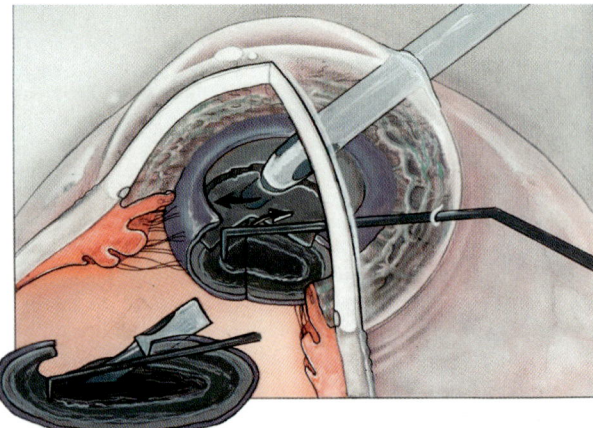

Fig. 11.6 First horizontal chop. The chopper passes beneath the anterior capsule edge to hook the nucleus equator. The phaco tip impales the nucleus proximally. The phaco tip will move rightward with a slight lifting motion. The chopper will move leftward with slight depression.

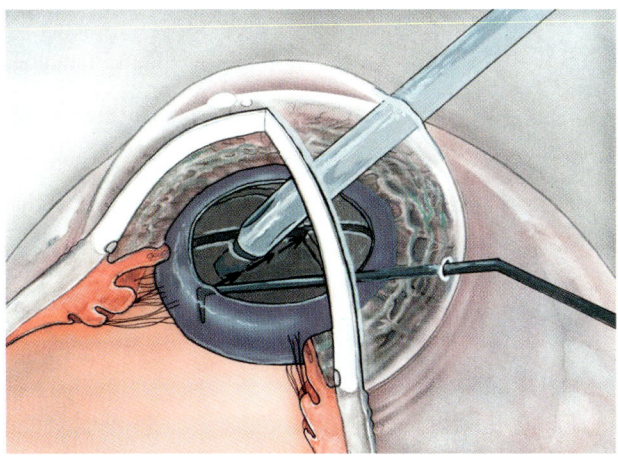

Fig. 11.7 Second horizontal chop. The above steps are repeated after slight nucleus rotation.

to the phaco tip. Once the chopper is entirely embedded within the nuclear substance, the phaco tip is moved up and to the right and the chopper down and to the left, thus cracking the nucleus (**Fig. 11.8**).

The chopper is then lifted from the crack, vacuum is released, and the two instruments are employed to rotate the nucleus as noted above, contingent on the density of the nucleus. Once rotated the nucleus is again impaled by the phaco tip in position 3 utilizing ultrasonic energy and vacuum. Then, again, when the tip is buried to the sleeve within the nuclear substance, position 2 and vacuum only is used to hold the nucleus. The chopper is then placed 1 mm lateral and 1 mm down from the phaco tip. Using vacuum only, the tip is elevated and repositioned to the right while the chopper impales the nucleus and is drawn down and to the left. A second crack ensues.

Once again dependent on density of the nucleus the first pie-shaped segment is mobilized to the pupillary plane where it

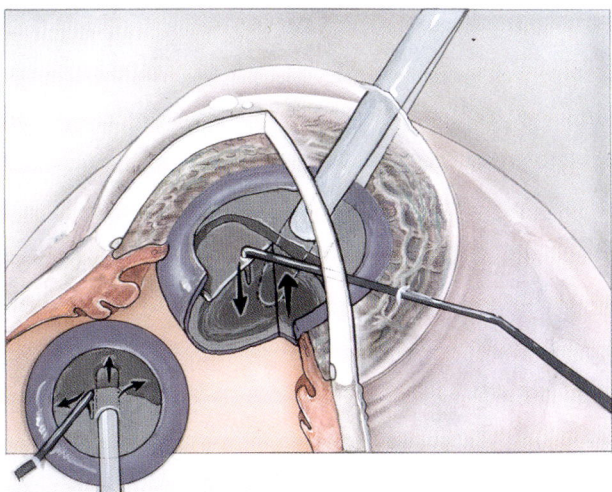

Fig. 11.8 Vertical chopping. The phaco tip is placed into the middle of the nucleus, impaling it. The sharp chopper is placed adjacent to the tip and driven into the nucleus. Once both instruments are stable, the phaco tip is pushed and lifted up and rightward and the chopper is pulled down and pressed inferiorly.

is emulsified. If the nucleus is firm, again, multiple small pie-shaped segments are created until nuclear rigidity is neutralized. Then each small segment is mobilized, in turn, and emulsified in the pupillary plane.

Hybrid Chop

Once both vertical and horizontal chopping is mastered, the two types of chopper–phaco needle interaction can be used interchangeably during nuclear emulsification. Therefore, in a moderate nucleus, a vertical chop might be most effective for the two chops creating the first pie segment. The remaining nucleus may then be easily elevated and mobilized, leading to further removal by horizontal chopping employed at the level of the anterior capsule in the center of the pupil.

When femtosecond laser pre-chopping is used, the hybrid chopping method is preferred. The pre-chopped nuclear fissures are used as planes of division of the nuclear material.

Hybrid chopping is perhaps the most common approach to phaco chopping.

Maximizing Machine Settings for Phaco Chop

Machine settings are relatively variable dependent on the machine and the phaco tip size and morphology chosen. Commonly, for chopping, higher vacuums (300–400 mm Hg) with very low flow (2–4 cc/min) are specified. To impale the tip, power is usually between 20 and 50%. A slow burst setting enables the surgeon to observe and enhance control of the tip as it passes into the nucleus. Turning the bevel down during impaling maneuvers more easily holds the nucleus. Any type of ultrasound energy, longitudinal (Bausch and Lomb, Rochester, NY), Elliptical (Abbott Medical Optics [AMO], Abbott Park, IL) or OZil (Alcon, Fort Worth, TX), is appropriate. However, it is imperative to stop utilizing power the moment the tip is buried within the substance of the nucleus. If this is not done, the continued ultrasonic energy will emulsify the wall of the trough the needle has created. This is the result of the sleeve preventing the needle from passing further into the endonuclear mass. The ultrasonic energy in the absence of forward movement of the tip will create a space between the phaco needle wall and the side of the nucleus trough. This permits fluid inflow to fill this space and hinder the phaco tip's ability to hold tightly to the nuclear material. The result is drastically reduced holding power when the chop is attempted (**Fig. 11.9**). This error and too little retraction of the sleeve before entering the eye are the most common causes of failed holding ability of the nucleus for the chop. With this error the tip exposure is inadequate to hold the nucleus. With poor holding power, the posterior vertical pressure of the chopper on the nucleus will push the nucleus off the phaco tip rather than chopping it.

Complications often arise when the wrong chop technique is used in the wrong setting. This is especially true in dense lenses. If little or no epinucleus is present and "ice skate marks" are visible on the nuclear surface, then the vertical chopping technique is usually required. In these circumstances, there is no plane into which the horizontal chopper can be placed to horizontally divide the lens because the epinucleus and cortex is fused to the endonucleus, essentially creating a large nuclear mass surrounding by a thin cortical shell; in very dense cataracts, even the cortex is subsumed by the nucleus. Using a horizontal chop method in this circumstance could lead to peripheral capsular rupture, zonular dialysis, or both. Thus, a vertical or hybrid technique, in

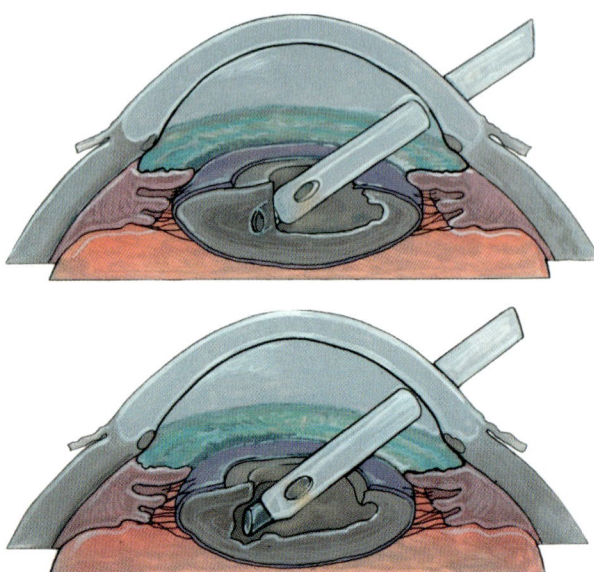

Fig. 11.9 Excessive vacuum in relation to nucleus density leads to removal of excess nuclear material contiguous with the tip. This disrupts the vacuum seal. There is resultant poor holding power.

which both vertical and horizontal chopping is used depending on what is needed at the time, is optimal in very dense nuclear sclerotic lens. Conversely, using a vertical chopping method in too soft of a cataract can lead to poor cleavage of the nucleus and potential compromise of the posterior capsular bag.

Mastering Foot Pedal Control

Mastering foot pedal control is an essential part of the beginning phaco-chop surgeon's technical goals.[13] By using the techniques described above, one can quickly estimate the cataract density and quality (e.g., fibrous, layered, or sticky) and adjust the amount of phaco power to maximize efficiency without risking capsular perforation. In most instances, the beginning phaco-chop surgeon will struggle more with the very soft lens than intumescent ones, because in the very soft lenses excessive ultrasound energy or aspiration will quickly and easily emulsify the tissue before the surgeon can reflexively withdraw his or her foot from the phaco peddle and possibly creating a peripheral rupture. In these cases, one can either avoid the chop or quadrant removal setting altogether and start with the epinuclear removal mode available in most platforms, or adjust downward the linear power and proceed with the "manual chop" technique described above. It helps to hydrodissect the nucleus into the anterior chamber where emulsification can be performed with the low aspiration and vacuum setting and low power or often with aspiration only.

Complications: Avoidance and Management in Special Situations

Extension of Anterior Capsular Tear During FLACS

Preventing extension of AC tears is a basic requirement for successful nuclear disassembly using the phaco-chop technique, pre-

viously described in detail by Dillman's group.[8] Studies on the use of the FLACS platforms (LensAR, LenSx, Catalys, and VICTUS) for anterior capsulotomy and nuclear fragmentation have shown significantly increased rates of AC tags (10.5%), AC tears (4%), posterior extension of AC tears (50%), and posterior lens dislocation (2%) when compared with manual CCC.[14]

But FLACS does has an advantage over manual capsulorrhexis techniques in that it can provide real-time centration of the capsulorrhexis either over the visual axis or the pupil center. However, the frequency of AC tears (1.87%) and posterior extension of AC tears (0.87%) has been reportedly by Abell et al[15] to be significantly increased compared with manual CCC (0.12%). Although in some studies these numbers have not reached statistical significance, comprehensive literature reviews still suggest a higher incidence of this in FLACS versus conventional techniques.[16] In my experience, anterior capsulorrhexis tags or strands are a more common occurrence than with CCC, and caution is advised when removing the AC cap, as it cannot be ensured to be free floating. Additional strands or wisps of duplicate rhexis may also occur, but these are not often easily recognized until during irrigation and aspiration (I/A). Care should be taken to avoid aspiration of these wisps in the capsular bag (**Fig. 11.10**). Due to the construction of the rhexis, which has a scalloped border microscopically, similar to a postage stamp edge, there appears to be an architectural weakness that could lead to peripheral AC tears.[17] The femtosecond laser energy applied to the region around the scalloped border may also further decreases the elasticity of the capsule and lead to posterior extension early during nuclear disassembly and cautioned is advised.

FLACS: The Bubble Factor

Anyone familiar with FLACS surgery is aware of the bubble factor—the large amount of air produced during femtosecond nuclear disassembly (**Fig. 11.11**). Significant care should be taken when removing this bubble, especially in special cases of suspected AC rent or possible posterior disruption in a postvitrectomized eye. For most phaco-chop surgeons, release of the air bubble, although time-consuming, is a relatively straightforward technique requiring the second instrument (e.g., Seibel chopper) to work with the phaco tip to rock the lens along its z-axis while simultaneously allowing the air to escape (**Fig. 11.12**). One could also consider using a Nagahara pre-chopper to displace the central nuclear pieces[18] to allow controlled release of the air centrally through the diced nuclear tissue. An Akahoshi irrigating cannula can also be useful to gently tilt the cataract in a region beneath the AC tear or opposite the PC tear to enable

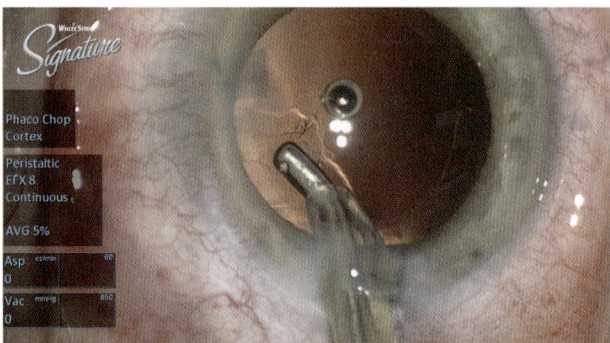

Fig. 11.10 Wisps of rhexis at 3 the o'clock position. These are easily aspirated and can lead to tears of the anterior capsule during phaco or irrigation and aspiration (I/A). (Courtesy of Brian A. Hunter, MD.)

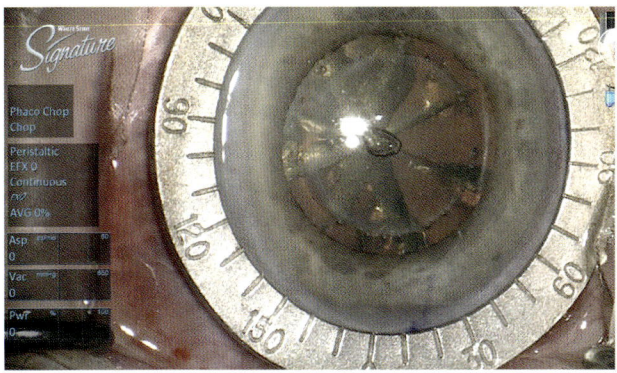

Fig. 11.11 Gas bubbles collecting behind the cataractous lens from the laser energy. (Courtesy of Brian A. Hunter, MD.)

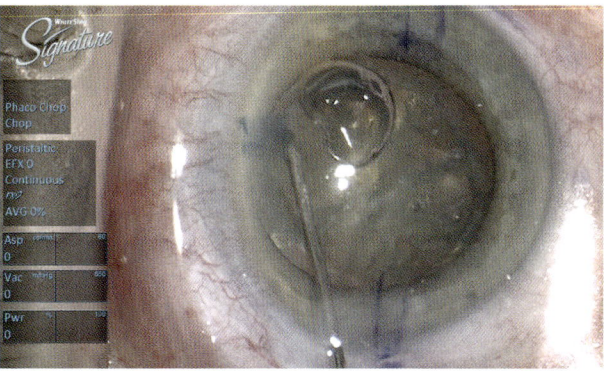

Fig. 11.12 Release of gas bubbles with the irrigating cannula. (Courtesy of Brian A. Hunter, MD.)

the air to gently escape prior to more extensive hydrodissection, hydrodelineation, or especially viscodissection.[19]

Managing an Incomplete Nuclear Cleavage in Very Dense Cataracts with a Leathery Nucleus

This decapitation technique can be employed in cases involving a thick fibrous posterior plate, when the cleavage plane produced during vertical chopping is incomplete. During application of this hybrid chop technique, a slightly larger than average capsulorrhexis is performed (5.75 to 6 mm) after staining the capsule with vision blue. The larger than normal rhexis may necessitate use of an intracameral Miochol (Ciba Vision, Duluth. GA) at the conclusion of the procedure to prevent anterior displacement of the lens, especially if there is any posterior pressure (and there often is). A vertical chopping technique such as the Nagahara karate-chop technique[11] or the Dillman crack and flip[20] is employed to disassemble the nucleus into eight or more pie-shaped anterior nuclear segments, leaving behind a small posterior plate that can then be easily visco-elevated, divided, and removed. Using the Seibel chopper, which is a combination horizontal ball-type chopper and a Chang vertical safety chopper on the opposite end, each nuclear segment is grasped by the phaco needle in the quadrant removal mode and pulled centrally away from the capsular bag. At this point the horizontal chopper is placed peripheral to the nuclear segment and the anterior two thirds or so of the nuclear segment is decapitated between the horizontal chopper and the phaco needle tip. In some instances, it may be necessary to debulk the central portion of the nucleus, using the sculpt mode, taking great care to remove as much tissue centrally as possible. This is repeated until all the nuclear pieces are cleaved, leaving behind the stumps of nucleus adherent to the leathery posterior plate. By elevating this plate of tissue with a cohesive ophthalmic viscosurgical device (OVD) or by using the horizontal chopper to manually flip it into the AC, the remaining tissue can be disassembled without concern for damage to the posterior capsule. Going into foot pedal position 0 enables the AC to become shallow. The vitreous actually supports the capsular bag. This phaco tip can then engage the epinuclear/cortical plate in the subincisional area. Gentle force on the phaco tip will push the plate opposite the incision so that it scrolls around the equator and presents in the plane of the anterior capsule for emulsification (**Fig. 11.13**). Maximizing phaco settings, and employing Arshinoff's soft shell technique,[21] this technique can be used for even the hardest of cataracts (4–5+).

Phaco-Chop Settings in the Rock-Hard Nucleus

What if the nucleus does not crack? You have just performed epinuclear cleanup to expose the underlying nucleus but find that you cannot bite into the rock-hard nucleus. Every phaco-chop surgeon needs both a routine and a rock-hard setting. For rock-hard cases, increasing your power settings will make all the difference in the world. My settings for general use with the AMO Signature phaco platform (AMO, Abbott Park, IL) using elliptical ultrasound energy with a 45-degree Kelman tip and peristaltic vacuum are linear aspiration 36 cc/min (20–60 cc/min); linear vacuum 385 mm Hg (300–650 mm Hg), and linear power 35% (0–100%). Hard-rock settings are linear aspiration 36 cc/min (26–60 cc/min); linear vacuum 385 mm Hg (335–650 mm Hg), and linear power 45% (0–100%). Note that a modest increase in linear power and increased baseline vacuum enables the phaco to bite into even a 5+ hard rock. During sculpting, it may be advantageous to use panel rather than linear power. In this mode the power is instantaneously at its preset level, thereby reducing the need for pushing the nucleus ahead of the phaco tip while waiting for maximum power to develop. This will reduce stress

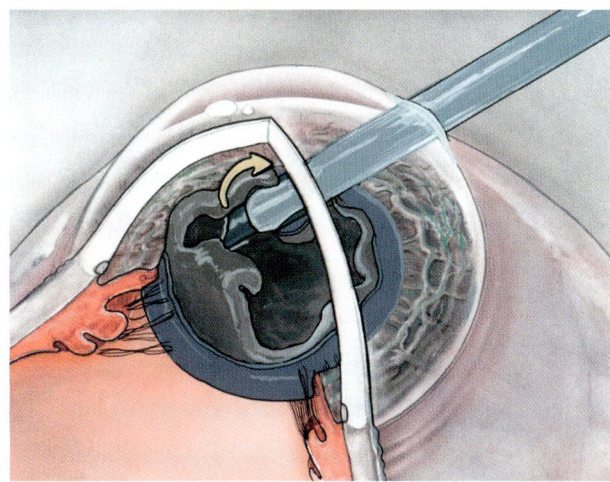

Fig. 11.13 Flipping of the epinucleus. The phaco chopper can be used to push the floor of the epinucleus distally to assist in flipping the epinucleus. This enables phacoemulsification of the distal plate in the plane of the anterior capsule.

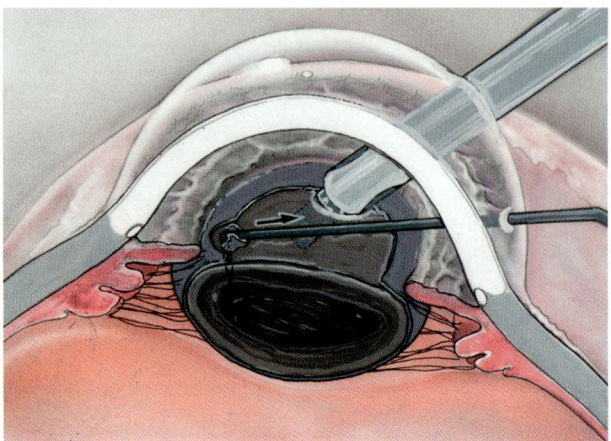

Fig. 11.14 The chopper is positioned over the anterior capsule and tears its edge.

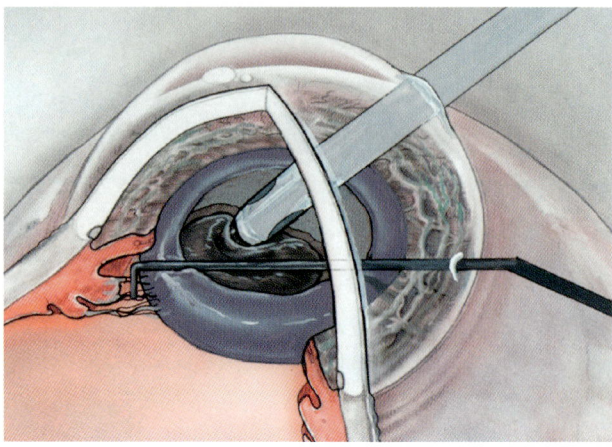

Fig. 11.15 The chopper is placed outside the capsular bag, which will create a zonular dialysis on attempted chopping.

on the zonule. Settings for epinuclear and I/A are typically unchanged between routine and hard-rock settings.

Anterior Chamber tears

The Seibel nucleus horizontal chopper (Rhein Medical, St. Petersburg, FL) has a sharp nape that is beneficial for horizontal chopping but does increase the risk of AC tears within 30 degrees of the paracentesis subincisional zone. Use of the horizontal chopper should be avoided during nuclear rotation in the subincisional area. While learning the horizontal chopping technique, a common complication is to mistakenly tear the AC during nuclear disassembly by reaching anterior to the capsular bag rather than through the epinucleus resulting in a large AC rent (**Fig. 11.14**) or zonular dehiscence (**Fig. 11.15**). Rotating the instrument horizontally, ensuring that the instrument is placed into the bag centrally, and observing the instrument as it displaces the epinucleus will ensure that the risk of this complication is minimized.

If an AC tear occurs, its important to first establish the extent of the tear. A Kuglen hook to displace the iris can be used to visualize the extent of the tear. If the tear does not extend beyond the equator, careful nuclear disassembly can be performed. If there is concomitant zonular instability or dehiscence, careful application of dispersive viscoelastic into the sulcus anterior to the area of weakness as described previously, or use of a capsular tension ring (CTR) or Ahmed segment may be required.[22] Further nuclear disassembly should be performed either in the AC overlying a dispersive OVD or by using a vertical chopping technique, with care being taken to minimize lens rotation and exacerbating zonular weakness.

Ophthalmic Viscosurgical Device

Choosing the right viscoelastic is essential. I routinely use the cohesive Healon GV (AMO), for routine cases. This permits faster cleanup at the end of the case and minimizes heat transfer to the wound (see Chapter 35). Most importantly, a viscoadaptive OVD minimizes how much time one spends removing OVD posterior to the implanted IOL and limits time spent retrieving nuclear debris from the AC. Using a highly dispersive OVD like Viscoat (Alcon) will often result in pieces of nucleus getting stuck in the AC and decrease the efficiency of the chopping technique. Remember, overinflation of the capsular bag with viscoelastic can easily result in extension of either AC rent or PC holes or tears.

Dispersive viscoelastic should be placed to avoid influx of vitreous in case of a PC rupture or to avoid vitreous from coming around through the weekend zonules (**Fig. 11.16**).

Phaco Chop Through Meiotic Pupils

Small pupil chopping can be done, but the first step is avoidance by increasing the pupil size. This is commonly due to intraoperative floppy iris syndrome (IFIS), and it occurs in patients using certain psychotropic medications, in patients with a history of uveitis or trauma, and in patients with posterior synechiae. There are multiple pharmaceutical or mechanical options to induce

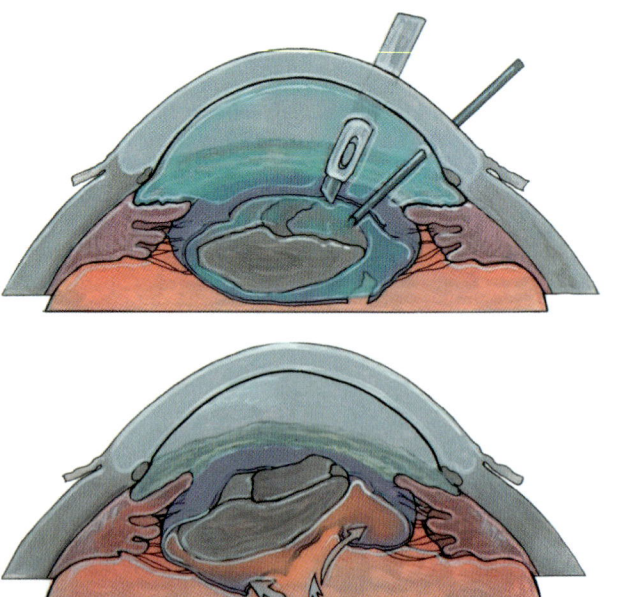

Fig. 11.16 **(a)** If a posterior capsular break or zonular dehiscence is suspected, viscoelastic should be injected through the paracentesis before withdrawing the phaco tip, and infusion should be performed to prevent shallowing of the anterior chamber. **(b)** If the anterior chamber becomes shallow, vitreous will herniate through the posterior capsular tear, often extending the tear.

mydriasis in patients with mitotic pupils.[23] It is still possible to perform vertical chopping in a very small pupil when employing one of many common modalities such as intracameral dilute preservative-free epinephrine or a pupil expander like Malyugin (MicroSurgical Technologies [MST], Redmond, WA) or I-Ring (Beaver Visitec, Waltham, MA). Vertical chopping works best in these circumstances. If these devices are not available or unsafe to use as in the case of a patient on multiple blood thinners, a patient with significant iris atrophy, a patient with prior partial iridectomy, or a patient posttrabeculectomy or with a tube shunt, then relying on a solid understanding of capsular anatomy will allow one to operate even on the smallest pupil.

Phaco Chop After Prior Vitrectomy

Any previous vitrectomy surgery can result in damage or weakening of the posterior capsular bag. In some instances, perforation of the posterior or peripheral capsular bag with or without Elschnig pearls present (depending on the age of the perforation) may be found during removal of the nucleus, resulting in significant complications.[24] This is a potential complication in any patient with previous retinal surgery, and possible risks during cataract surgery should be discussed with the patient preoperatively. As in most patients with increased risks for complications, most of these risks can be avoided or minimized through recognition and preparation. If the retinal surgery occurred in the distant past, any posterior capsular disruption will have had sufficient time to scar, thus making it less susceptible to complications during cataract surgery. Limited hydrodissection with focused hydrodelineation in combination with a hybrid chopping technique should be employed to reduce the risk of tearing, and early use of dispersive viscoelastic should be considered, similar to the treatment of a posterior polar cataract.[24]

Conclusion

There are many surgical techniques that can be used when performing cataract surgery in an ever-expanding population of patients requiring safe and effective cataract surgery. Phaco chop, with a horizontal, vertical, or hybrid technique, can be a safe, efficient, and effective means for nuclear disassembly in the majority of patients undergoing cataract surgery. By maximizing phaco-chop settings on your preferred phacoemulsification platform; utilizing situational awareness to identify risk factors such as small pupil, zonular instability, or very soft or hard nuclei; and understanding the risks associated with FLACS, one can master the phaco-chop technique and yield efficient and improved outcomes.

References

1. Erie JC, Baratz KH, Hodge DO, Schleck CD, Burke JP. Incidence of cataract surgery from 1980 through 2004: 25-year population-based study. J Cataract Refract Surg 2007;33:1273–1277
2. Congdon N, Vingerling JR, Klein BE, et al; Eye Diseases Prevalence Research Group. Prevalence of cataract and pseudophakia/aphakia among adults in the United States. Arch Ophthalmol 2004;122:487–494
3. Gimbel HV. Divide and conquer nucleofractis phacoemulsification: development and variations. J Cataract Refract Surg 1991;17:281–291
4. Koch PS. Stop and chop. In: Buratto L, Werner L, Zanini M, Apple D, eds. Phacoemulsification Principles and Techniques, 2nd ed. Thorofare, NJ: Slack; 2003:140–141
5. Randleman JB, Wolfe JD, Woodward M, Lynn MJ, Cherwek DH, Srivastava SK. The resident surgeon phacoemulsification learning curve. Arch Ophthalmol 2007;125:1215–1219
6. Cremers SL, Ciolino JB, Ferrufino-Ponce ZK, Henderson BA. Objective Assessment of Skills in Intraocular Surgery (OASIS). Ophthalmology 2005; 112:1236–1241
7. Chang DF. Phaco Chop: Mastering Techniques, Optimizing Technology, and Avoiding Complications, 1st ed. Thorofare, NJ: Slack; 2004
8. Maloney WF, Dillman DM, Nichamin LD. Supracapsular phacoemulsification: a capsule-free posterior chamber approach. J Cataract Refract Surg 1997;23:323–328
9. Gimbel HV, Neuhann T. Development, advantages, and methods of the continuous circular capsulorhexis technique. J Cataract Refract Surg 1990;16:31–37
10. Fishkind WJ. Avoiding and managing complications from hydrodissection—careful technique and a watchful eye can avert a capsular blowout. Cataract and Refract. Surg Today 2003; 66
11. Nagahara K. Personal phacoemulsification technique. Endocapsular phaco—techniques of pure nucleofracture. In: Buratto L, Werner L, Zanini M, Apple D, eds. Phacoemulsification Principles and Techniques, 2nd ed. Thorofare, NJ: Slack; 2003:303–308
12. Perrone DM. Argentininean flag sign is most common complication for intumescent cataracts. Ocular Surgery New, December 15, 2000
13. Hennig A, Schroeder B, Kumar J. Learning phacoemulsification. Results of different teaching methods. Indian J Ophthalmol 2004;52:233–234
14. Trikha S, Turnbull AMJ, Morris RJ, Anderson DF, Hossain P. Comprehensive review. The journey to FLACS: new beginnings or a false dawn. Eye (Lond) 2013;27:461–473
15. Abell RG, Davies PE, Phelan D, Goemann K, McPherson ZE, Vote BJ. Anterior capsulotomy integrity after femtosecond laser-assisted cataract surgery. Ophthalmology 2014;121:17–24
16. Grewal DS, Schultz T, Basti S, Dick HB. Femtosecond laser-assisted cataract surgery-current status and future directions. Surv Ophthalmol 2016; 61:103–131
17. Nagy Z, Takacs A, Filkorn T, Sarayba M. Initial clinical evaluation of an intraocular femtosecond laser in cataract surgery. J Refract Surg 2009; 25:1053–1060
18. Masket S, Sarayba M, Ignacio T, Fram N. Femtosecond laser-assisted cataract incisions: architectural stability and reproducibility. J Cataract Refract Surg 2010;36:1048–1049
19. Akahoshi T. Phaco prechop. In: Buratto L, Werner L, Zanini M, Apple D, eds. Phacoemulsification Principles and Techniques, 2nd ed. Thorofare, NJ: Slack; 2003:333–346
20. Fine H, Maloney WF, Dillman DM. Crack and flip phacoemulsification technique. Presented at the Symposium on Cataract, Intraocular Lens, and Refractive Surgery, San Diego, April 1992
21. Arshinoff SA. Dispersive-cohesive viscoelastic soft shell technique. J Cataract Refract Surg 1999;25:167–173
22. Carifi G, Miller MH, Pitsas C, et al. Complications and outcomes of phacoemulsification cataract surgery complicated by anterior capsule tear. Am J Ophthalmol 2015;159:463–469
23. Chang DF, Braga-Mele R, Mamalis N, et al; ASCRS Cataract Clinical Committee. ASCRS White Paper: clinical review of intraoperative floppy-iris syndrome. J Cataract Refract Surg 2008;34:2153–2162
24. Pardo-Muñoz A, Muriel-Herrero A, Abraira V, Muriel A, Muñoz-Negrete FJ, Murube J. Phacoemulsification in previously vitrectomized patients: an analysis of the surgical results in 100 eyes as well as the factors contributing to the cataract formation. Eur J Ophthalmol 2006;16:52–59

12 Phaco Prechop Procedure

Arthur J. Weinstein

The phaco prechop procedure is a very effective way to dismantle the nucleus prior to removal. Prechopping is utilized to achieve a split of the nucleus within the capsular bag without the use of phacoemulsification energy. Takayuki Akahoshi[1] first introduced this technique in 1993, and he has been instrumental in pioneering the prechop technique and in developing instrumentation for it.

Equipment

Several variations of the prechopper instrument are available. The prechopper is a cross-action forceps, and most are designed with a sharper-edged blade on one side and a rounded or blunted edge on the back. The rounded edge can be used to divide a softer nucleus, or to finish the split after the sharper edge has been employed (**Fig. 12.1**).

Technique

Prechopping provides the benefit of nucleus division without ultrasound energy or fluid. This technique is ideal for moderate nucleus densities (grades 2 and 3). To perform prechopping safely, thorough hydrodissection is imperative. In addition to hydrodissection (**Fig. 12.2**), hydrodelineation should be performed to improve safety and assist with nucleus quadrant removal. Hydrodelineation is accomplished by injecting fluid at the midperipheral nucleus to separate the epinuclear and endonuclear layers (**Fig. 12.3**). Hydrodelineation provides an additional cushion of protection prior to dividing the nucleus with the prechopper (**Fig. 12.4**).

Following hydrodissection and hydrodelineation, the surgeon should inject a dispersive viscoelastic agent to blow away the loose cortical material and provide a well-pressurized anterior chamber. This is essential. A cohesive viscoelastic is not ideal, as it can be inadvertently expressed out of the wound with the introduction of the prechopper. This will cause a loss of anterior chamber pressure, which significantly reduces the effectiveness of the prechop maneuver.

The technique for successful application of the prechopper involves placing the sharp end of the blades ~ 1 mm to the distal side of the center nucleus and applying gently downward pressure (**Fig. 12.5**). Once the nucleus is entered (to ~ 1½ mm depth or half the depth of the nucleus), the cross-action prechopper is then opened to achieve a split (**Fig. 12.6**). Maintaining the prechopper in the open position for a few seconds helps to effectuate the split across the nucleus. If the nucleus does not fully split, the instrument is placed in the same groove, slightly more posterior, and the maneuver is repeated. This should complete the split. The nucleus should then be rotated 90 degrees using the prechopper blades in the closed position. The prechopper is again placed slightly distal to the central nucleus to divide the distal hemi-nucleus). This placement often achieves a split of both hemi-nuclei; if not, the instrument is moved proximally and the maneuver repeated to split the proximal hemi-nucleus (**Fig. 12.7**).

Once the prechop has been accomplished, the surgeon performs phacoemulsification using nucleus quadrant removal settings. A second instrument can be utilized; however, phacoemulsification is often easily performed using a single-handed technique, particularly if the nucleus quadrants are already nicely delineated and divided.

Indications

Cataracts of grades 2 and 3 are optimal for prechopping. Prechopping the nucleus is a good technique to apply when pupil dilation is limited, as it obviates the need for grooving with phacoemulsification when visualization is compromised. It is also a good technique for the patient with a compromised endothelium, as it will significantly reduce phaco energy and the amount of fluid used.

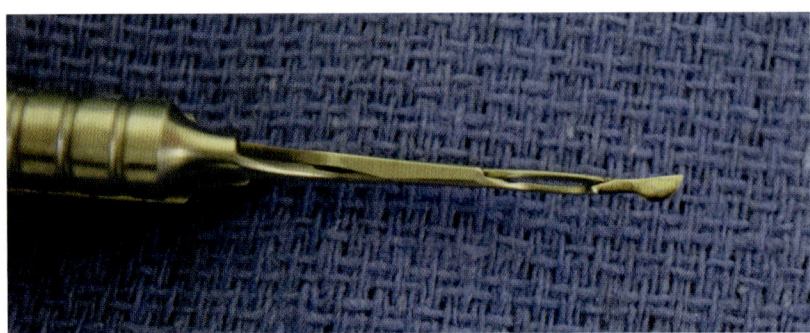

Fig. 12.1 The Akahoshi Combo Prechopper (Asico, Westmont, IL).

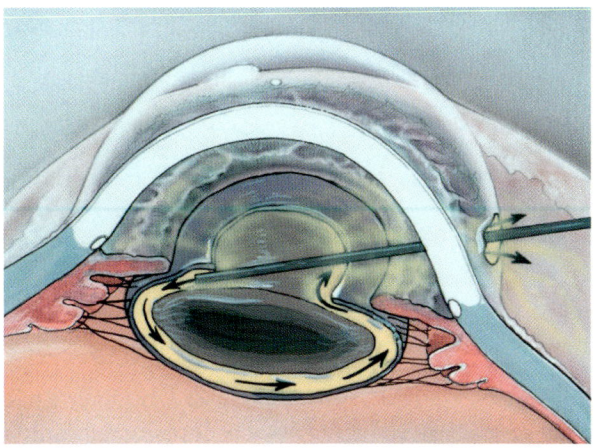

a

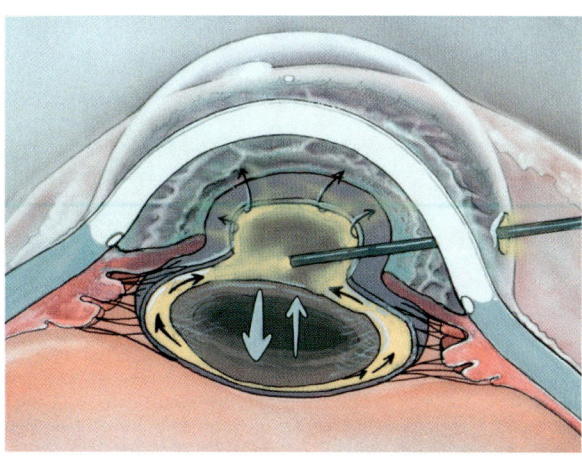

b

Fig. 12.2 **(a)** Hydrodissection. The cannula is placed just under the capsulorrhexis edge, tenting up the capsule while fluid is injected to separate the cortex from the lens capsule. Fluid follows the path of least resistance, allowing a fluid wave behind the nucleus with egress of fluid through the wound. **(b)** Fluid injected at the center of the capsulorrhexis opening. A fluid wave is not achieved, as fluid forces downward displacement of the nucleus. The path of least resistance is into the anterior chamber.

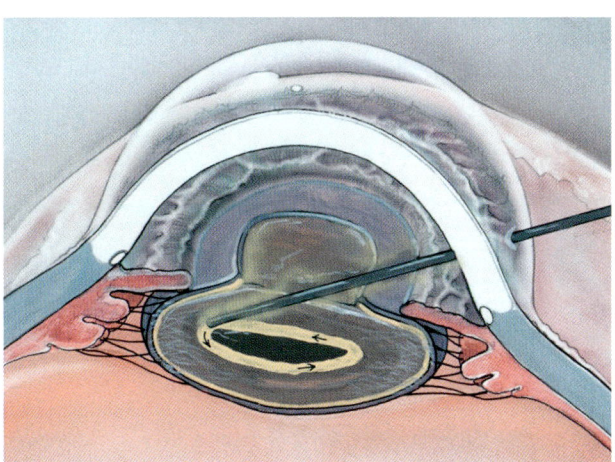

Fig. 12.3 Placement of the hydrodissection cannula in the midperiphery of the lens. Fluid is injected to achieve hydrodelineation of the nucleus from the surrounding epinuclear layer.

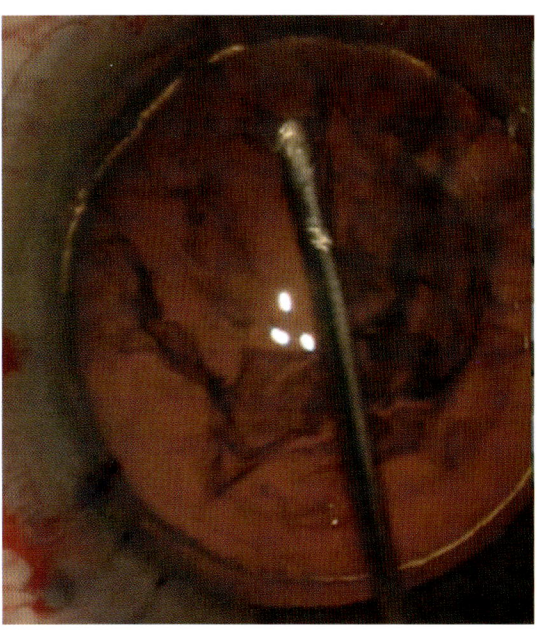

Fig. 12.4 The presence of a "golden ring" as hydrodelineation occurs.

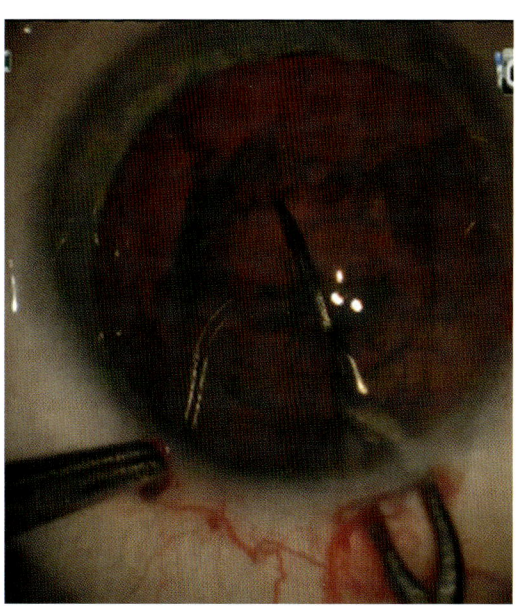

Fig. 12.5 The prechopper is placed just distal to the central nucleus with the blades closed.

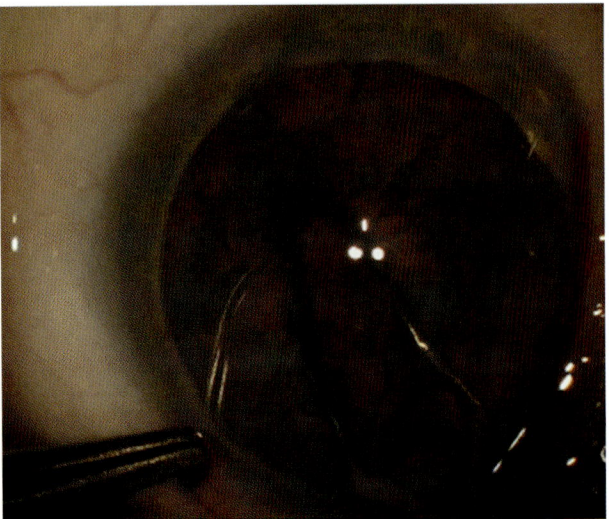

Fig. 12.6 Cross-action prechopper blades are open and held for a few seconds to achieve the first split.

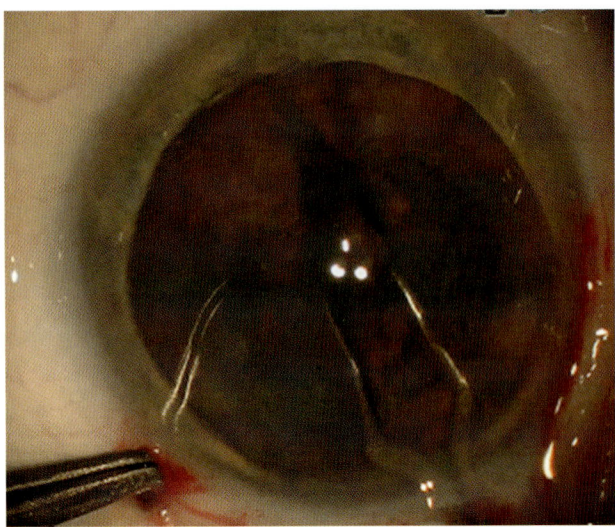

Fig. 12.7 The nucleus is rotated 90 degrees and a split of the distal and proximal hemi-nucleus is performed to divide the nucleus into quadrants.

Relative Contraindications

The prechop technique is not ideal in certain situations. Applying the pressure of the prechopper can further loosen a lens with already compromised zonules. The surgeon should be alert for zonular laxity when performing the capsulorrhexis, particularly in an eye with pseudoexfoliation or past trauma. A continuous capsulorrhexis is also imperative, and prechopping the nucleus should not be attempted if the anterior capsule is in any way compromised.

A previously vitrectomized eye can be more difficult to prechop, due to the lack of posterior pressure from normal vitreous. Although it is possible to prechop the nucleus in these eyes, the surgeon should avoid the tendency to apply too much downward pressure with the prechopper instrument.

Both soft and dense cataracts can be prechopped, but the surgeon should be aware of some potential pitfalls. It is possible to inadvertently penetrate the posterior capsule when prechopping a very soft nucleus. In these cases, the surgeon should consider using the blunted edge of the prechopper instead of the sharp edge, which will reduce the risk of a posterior capsule split. Alternatively, the surgeon can employ the phaco flip technique for softer lens densities. Splitting a very dense nucleus should not be attempted without the assistance of a nucleus stabilizer, as the additional downward force required to prechop a dense nucleus can weaken zonules.

Managing Problems

In the event that prechopping fails to achieve a good nucleus split, surgeons should revert back to their normal phaco technique. Stop and chop or divide and conquer can still be applied following unsuccessful prechopping.

An inadvertent posterior capsule split is the most significant complication of the prechop technique. However, with proper technique, this complication should be extremely rare. When it occurs, an opening is present in the posterior capsule with the entire nucleus still in place. Vitreous may or may not prolapse as a result of the split, and this will be a factor in determining the appropriate method for nucleus removal. The surgeon can inject a dispersive viscoelastic agent beneath the lens particles and perform phacoemulsification with very slow and controlled fluidics.

Reference

1. Akahoshi T. The karate prechop technique. Cataract and Refractive Surgery Today 2002; http://bmctoday.net/crstoday/2002/09/article.asp?f=0902/crst0902_161.html

Section VII   Soft and Mature Cataract Management and Complications

13 Management of the Soft Nucleus

William J. Fishkind

The human crystalline lens is a unique structure. It is a cellular structure that loses its innervation and vascularity during fetal development. It derives its nutrition from the surrounding aqueous and vitreous humor. A disturbance in these fluids or in the substance of the lens may lead to metabolic abnormalities, culminating in the development of a cataract.

Anatomy and Pathophysiology

The soft nucleus is usually cortical or subcapsular in nature. Cortical cataracts usually begin as water vacuoles and progress to transparent water clefts between cortical lamellae. The clefts become cloudy as they expand and imbibe water. They may begin peripherally and spread centrally or as discrete water vacuoles, which proliferate throughout the substance of the nucleus. Histopathologically, water clefts are areas where the cortical lamellae are separated by swollen, degenerate lens fiber debris appearing as anuclear, pink, globular aggregates surrounded by paler pink, granular material. When the whole lens is involved, it appears white and is classified as mature. At any point in the maturational process the lens may develop an osmotic gradient as a result of the increase in molecules due to breakdown of proteins. The resultant swelling is termed an intumescent cataract. When the brown endonucleus remains present, the cataract is classified as morgagnian.

Subcapsular cataracts begin as a subtle sheen on the anterior or posterior capsule. They progress to white granular opacities and then enlarge to form a plaque of vacuoles and crystals. The plaque may thicken. Histopathologically, this type of cataract is associated with posterior migration of lens epithelial cells. The cells then become larger, more spindled, and fibroblast-like. These cells then surround the liquefying posterior cortex in a ring.[1] The abnormal lens epithelial cells may then grow into the posterior capsule, causing a ring-like posterior capsular fibrotic plaque. The plaque is fused to the posterior capsule and cannot be removed surgically without tearing the capsule. When it is present, rather than attempt operative removal, the plaque should be polished intraoperatively as best as possible, and the procedure completed. Yttrium-aluminum-garnet (YAG) capsulotomy can then be performed as early as 2 weeks postoperatively, although a longer period of observation is advantageous to allow stabilization of the blood–aqueous barrier prior to the use of the laser. Posterior subcapsular cataracts are associated with diabetes mellitus, topical or systemic steroid use, trauma, inflammation, and irradiation.[2,3]

A unique type of posterior subcapsular cataract is the posterior polar cataract (**Fig. 13.1**). This cataract is often inherited as autosomal dominant.[4,5] In this type of cataract a dense white opacity occurs adjacent to the central posterior capsule. The opacity may be stationary or progressive, with cortical extensions. Concentric thickened rings around the central opacity give the impression of a bull's-eye.[6]

The posterior capsule beneath the opacity is reportedly thin and prone to rupture. Osher et al[7] report that one quarter of these cataracts are associated with capsular rupture. Dense white satellite opacities adjacent to the bull's-eye may indicate a preexisting capsular dehiscence.[8] Calcification is an almost sure sign of posterior capsular involvement and of the likelihood of capsular rupture during cataract surgery.

Surgical Technique

Surgically, soft cataracts are characterized by a minimally dense endonucleus with abundant sticky soft cortical material. The nuclear cortical bag adhesions are usually well developed. Removal of this type of cataract is therefore dependent on separating the sticky cortex from the capsular bag. If this is thoroughly performed, soft cataracts are usually easy to remove. Removal, therefore, begins with thorough cortical cleaving hydrodissection. Often, beneficially, the hydrodissection pushes the cataract through the capsulorrhexis and into the anterior chamber (**Fig. 13.2**). There, the epinucleus and endonucleus are aspirated, with only short bursts of low-power pulsed phaco. No specific divide-and-conquer or chop technique is required. In Chapter 16, Drs. Abhay R. Vasavada and Vaishali Vasavada provide a complete description of the use of the femtosecond laser in this unique cataract type.

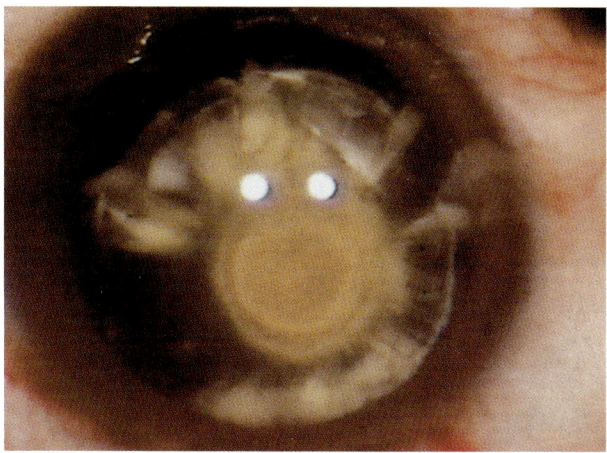

Fig. 13.1 Photograph of a dense, long-standing posterior polar cataract. The bull's-eye appearance and cortical extensions are observed. (From Lu LW, Fine IH, eds. Phacoemulsification in Difficult and Challenging Cases. New York: Thieme; 1999:122.)

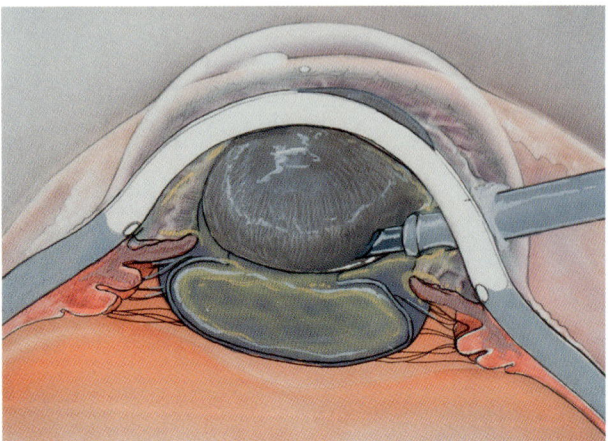

Fig. 13.2 Complete hydrodissection. The nucleus is in the anterior chamber.

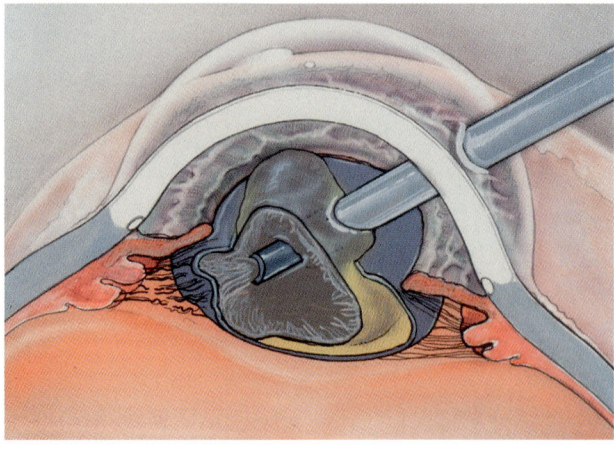

Fig. 13.3 Incomplete hydrodissection. The nuclear cortical bag connections pull the equator into the phaco tip.

Complications

Incomplete Hydrodissection

Complete and thorough hydrodissection is the most important step in removal of the soft cataract. Incomplete hydrodissection leads to small amounts of cortex adherent to the posterior capsule or in the fornices. This cortex is most easily removed with further hydrodissection or viscodissection prior to or after intraocular lens (IOL) insertion. The cortex can then be removed with the phaco tip in phaco mode or irrigation and aspiration (I/A) mode, or with the I/A tip.

Difficulty mobilizing a large amount of the nucleus is also due to inadequate hydrodissection. When this becomes apparent, the surgeon phacoemulsifies the nucleus and cortex that is easily accessible. This results in a large amount of cortex adherent to the capsule. The tendency is to perform phaco near the capsule to remove the sticky cortex. However, phaco near the capsule should be avoided. The sticky cortex often momentarily occludes the phaco tip and is then aspirated with a distinct surge. Due to the dense capsular cortical adhesions, the capsule is pulled into the phaco tip by the cortical-bag connections, essentially caught in the surge. It is instantaneously aspirated and emulsified. The result is a torn posterior capsule with immediate rupture of the vitreous face (**Fig. 13.3**).

If the cortex appears resistant to removal with the phaco tip, the I/A tip should be substituted. The case may proceed more slowly, due to slow aspiration of the cortex. The anterior chamber is more stable, however, and tears in the posterior capsule are less likely.

Posterior Subcapsular Cataract

One element of the histopathology of a posterior subcapsular cataract (PSC) is posterior migration and fibrosis of lens epithelial cells. When this occurs, a plaque of varying density remains on the posterior capsule after nucleus removal. Occasionally, it can be removed with a posterior capsular polishing instrument. However, if it is recalcitrant, the plaque should be left intact, rather than risk a rupture of the posterior capsule in attempts to remove it. YAG capsulotomy can be performed after an appropriate postoperative period.

Posterior Polar Cataract

When performing surgery on any patient with a dense posterior polar cataract, the possibility of posterior capsular thinning or potential capsular rupture must be considered. The patient, therefore, should be counseled preoperatively that there is an increased incidence of complications and should be given an explanation of the anticipated outcomes.

The capsulorrhexis should be made smaller than the diameter of the intended IOL optic. This enables the capture of the optic by the anterior capsule, should posterior capsular rupture be encountered.

Hydrodissection should be performed in all quadrants. However, rather than forcing fluid around the posterior pole to the opposite equator, the fluid wave should be carefully observed and allowed to pass only as far as the posterior polar opacity (**Fig. 13.4**). No attempt should be made to rotate the nucleus. Phaco should proceed without nuclear rotation, removing as much endonucleus and epinucleus as possible without disturbing the posterior pole of the nucleus. After removal of as much nucleus as possible, essentially "debulking" the capsular bag,

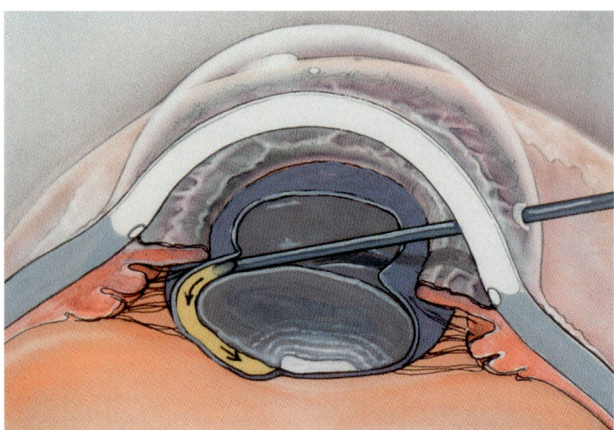

Fig. 13.4 Posterior polar cataract. Hydrodissection is allowed to proceed only as far as the posterior polar opacity.

gentle viscodissection with a dispersive viscoelastic agent should be accomplished. The viscoelastic passes behind the opacity. It lifts the cataract off the posterior capsule into the space created by the nuclear debulking. If the capsule is intact, the remainder of the nucleus may be gently emulsified. If the capsule is torn, the remainder of the nucleus is emulsified employing low-flow fluidics. It is hoped that the viscoelastic will protect the vitreous face and prevent vitreous loss. I/A may then be performed with the addition of viscoelastic as necessary.

If irregular, the posterior capsular tear can then be converted to a round tear with posterior capsulorrhexis (see Chapter 6). The IOL can then be inserted into the capsular bag.

If the posterior tear cannot be converted, or if there is vitreous loss requiring vitrectomy, the IOL can be inserted with the haptics in the sulcus and the optic captured within the anterior capsulotomy.

Conclusion

Phacoemulsification of the soft cataract is usually not a challenge after methodical hydrodissection. Phaco is then often performed in the anterior chamber. Posterior subcapsular and posterior polar cataracts need special treatment.

References

1. Eshaghian J, Streeten BW. Human posterior subcapsular cataract. An ultrastructural study of the posteriorly migrating cells. Arch Ophthalmol 1980;98:134–143

2. Streeten BW. Pathology of the lens. In: Albert DM, Jakobiec FA, eds. Principles and Practice of Ophthalmology. Philadelphia: WB Saunders; 1994: 2198–2207

3. American Academy of Ophthalmology. Basic and Clinical Science Course, 1996–1997. San Francisco: AAO; 1996:43–53

4. Tulloh CG. Hereditary posterior polar cataract with report of a pedigree. Br J Ophthalmol 1955;39:374–379

5. Nettlership E, Ogilvie FM. A peculiar form of hereditary congenital cataract. Trans Ophthalmol Soc U K 1996;26:19–20

6. Vasavada AR, Singh R. Phacoemulsification in posterior polar developmental cataracts. In: Lu LW, Fine IH, eds. Phacoemulsification in Difficult and Challenging Cases. New York: Thieme; 1999:121–123

7. Osher RH, Yu BC, Koch DD. Posterior polar cataracts: a predisposition to intraoperative posterior capsular rupture. J Cataract Refract Surg 1990; 16:157–162

8. Singh D, Worst J, Singh R, Singh IR. Cataract and IOL. New Delhi: Jaypee Brothers Medical Publishers; 1995:163–165

14 Cortically Mature Lens: White Cataract

Brock K. Bakewell

Cataract surgery performed for a cortically mature lens can be challenging even in the hands of an experienced surgeon. Therefore, having an established preoperative and operative routine for this type of cataract helps to ensure a successful case outcome. Prior to describing the actual surgical technique, it is important to consider the various types of white cataracts and their differentiating slit-lamp characteristics. Having a good idea of the type of white cataract that exists in a patient preoperatively enables the surgeon to anticipate what may be required at the time of surgery.

There are two basic types of white cataracts that are distinguishable at the slit lamp: pearly white and homogeneously white. The pearly white variety is characterized by having some degree of variegation in its white appearance and can vary on a spectrum from being mostly white with a tinge of an amber hue (**Fig. 14.1a**), to stark white with significant variegation (**Fig. 14.2a**), to being all white with only trace variegation (**Fig. 14.3**). A pearly white cataract variety may be nonliquefied (**Fig. 14.1b**), or may be somewhat liquefied (**Fig. 14.2b**). It is this latter variety that has increased intralenticular pressure, hence its description as being intumescent. The intumescent white cataract is always at risk for a tear out of the continuous curvilinear capsulotomy during its creation, resulting in an Argentinean flag sign (**Fig. 14.4a**); the seminal article postulating the cause of this was published in 2012 by Fiqueiredo et al.[1]

Figueiredo et al explain that within the capsular bag of an intumescent cataract is liquefied cortex that is located both anteriorly and posteriorly to the nucleus. They postulate that these two liquid compartments do not connect with each other due to the large nucleus making contact with the equatorial capsule, causing relative nuclear block (**Fig. 14.2b**). Consequently, after puncturing the anterior capsule when initiating a capsulotomy, the anterior intralenticular compartment decompresses but not the posterior compartment (**Fig. 14.4b**). As the performance of the capsulotomy proceeds, the posterior intralenticular compartment, which is still pressurized, causes the nucleus to move anteriorly, and this force, in turn, causes the incomplete capsulorrhexis to radialize toward the periphery so quickly that retrieval is not possible.

The homogeneously white cataract is confluently pale white in color without any variegation (**Fig. 14.5a**). It appears this way due to significant liquefaction of the lens, causing the nucleus to be free floating (**Fig. 14.6a**). This type of cataract is also termed a Morgagnian. Some authors call this type of cataract "intumescent," and it is under pressure, but there is low risk of an Argentinean flag sign occurring as long as the anterior chamber is well pressurized with an ophthalmic viscosurgical device (OVD), preferably a dispersive OVD or heavy cohesive such as Healon 5® (Abbott Medical Optics [AMO], Abbott Park, IL), when the tense anterior capsule is punctured with a 30-gauge needle at the time of capsulotomy creation. Figueiredo shows diagrammatically (**Fig. 14.5b**) that in a Morgagnian cataract, the anterior and posterior intralenticular compartments freely communicate. Hence, capsular puncture, at the initiation of the capsulotomy, effectively decompresses both the anterior and posterior spaces, thus averting the capsulotomy from tearing out during its creation. The capsular bag may decompress so significantly that it may be necessary to firm up the bag with an OVD prior to proceeding with a continuous curvilinear capsulotomy creation.

Brazitikos et al[2] classified white cataracts using A-scan echography. In their series of 100 consecutive white cataracts, the cataracts with liquid cortex had high internal acoustic reflections compared with the ones with a solid cortex that showed low internal acoustic reflectivity (**Fig. 14.7**). Thus, close examination of preoperative A-scans of white cataracts may alert the surgeon to the presence of liquid cortex and the need for following Figueiredo's intumescent cataract surgical protocol to prevent an Argentinean flag sign complication.

Schultz and Dick[3] and Steinert and Dick[4] have commented on the ability of the spectral-domain optical coherence tomography system in the Catalys Femtosecond Laser System (Abbott Medical Optics) to identify intralenticular fluid spaces within intumescent white cataracts (**Fig. 14.8**). They follow a specific femtosecond laser protocol for intumescent cataracts that is discussed later in this chapter.

Surgical Technique

The ideal surgical approach to a mature cortical cataract can be delineated as follows: (1) minimize posterior pressure, (2) use Trypan blue dye, (3) create a 3-mm capsulotomy and enlarge it to 5 mm after decompression of the anterior and posterior cortical spaces, and (4) perform phacoemulsification and intraocular lens (IOL) placement.

Minimize Posterior Pressure

Even though intralenticular pressure in the intumescent cataract is the main cause of radialization of a capsulotomy tear, minimization of any other source of posterior pressure is advisable to further optimize conditions for a successful case outcome. Figueiredo et al[1] recommend 250 cc of 20% intravenous (IV) mannitol 50 minutes prior to surgery. Also, if the surgeon is using a retro- or peribulbar anesthetic block, I recommend the use of a Honan balloon or Mercury bag to soften the orbit and reduce the posterior pressure. It is important to always ensure that the lid speculum is loosely opened so that it does not cause pressure on the eyelids that, in turn, can cause posterior pressure. Gorovoy and Jeng[5] recommend a prophylactic peripheral

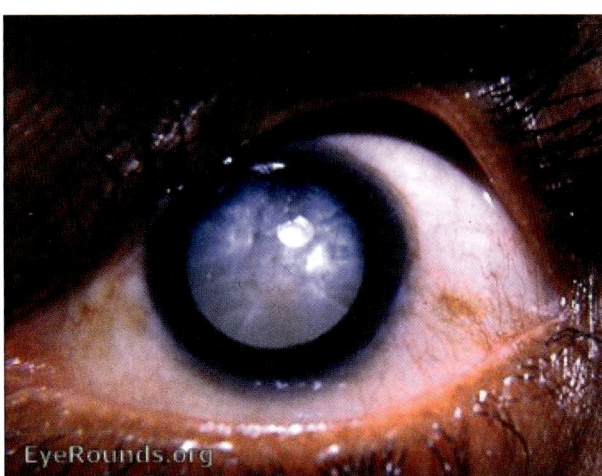

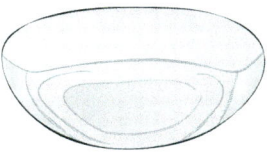
Healthy lens

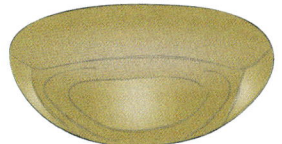
Cataract lens

b

Fig. 14.1 White cataract with no liquid cortex. (**a**) Photograph. (**b**) Illustration. (From EyeRounds.org. Reprinted by permission.)

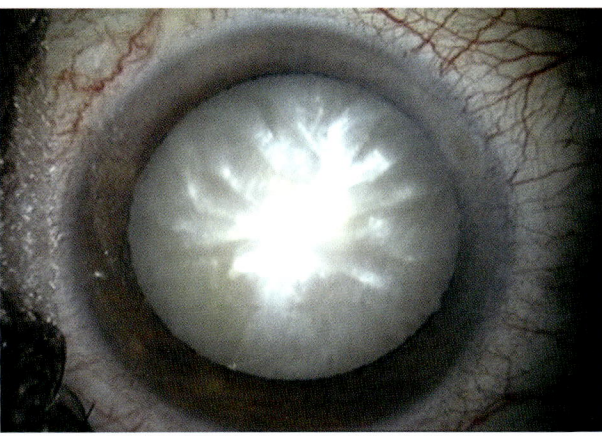

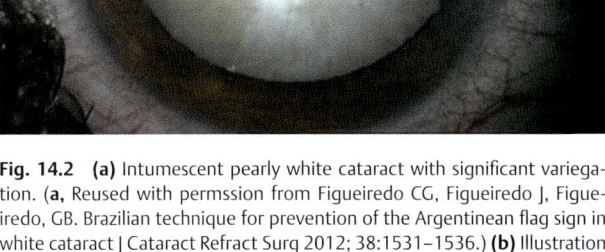

a

b

Fig. 14.2 (**a**) Intumescent pearly white cataract with significant variegation. (**a,** Reused with permssion from Figueiredo CG, Figueiredo J, Figueiredo, GB. Brazilian technique for prevention of the Argentinean flag sign in white cataract J Cataract Refract Surg 2012; 38:1531–1536.) (**b**) Illustration of a liquefied cortex under pressure, both anterior and posterior to the nucleus. Figueiredo postulates that these two liquefied, pressurized compartments do not communicate due to nuclear block. A is the anterior intralenticular pressurized cortical compartment; B is the posterior intralenticular pressurized cortical compartment. (**b,** Adapted from Figueiredo CG, Figueiredo J, Figueiredo, GB. Brazilian technique for prevention of the Argentinean flag sign in white cataract J Cataract Refract Surg 2012;38: 1531–1536.)

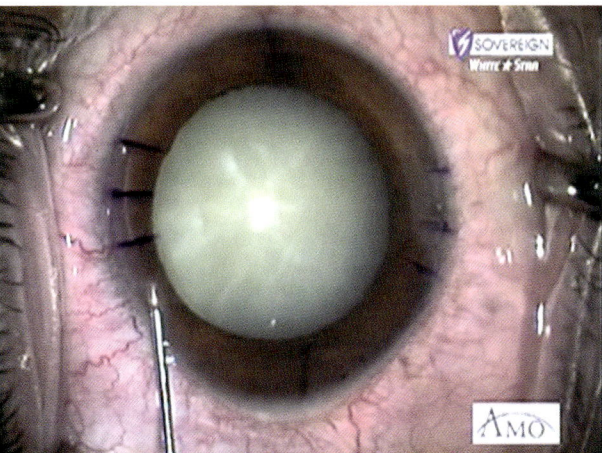

Fig. 14.3 Intumescent pearly white cataract with trace variegation.

iridotomy prior to intumescent white cataract surgery, theorizing that this will minimize pressure in the posterior chamber that can in a minor way help to reduce the chance of an Argentinean flag sign from occurring.

Staining of the Anterior Capsule

Use Trypan Blue Dye

The use of indocyanine green capsular (ICG) dye to facilitate capsulorrhexis creation was initially reported by Horiguchi et al[6] in 1998 and was a monumental advancement in the treatment of white cataracts. Melles et al[7] reported on the usage of trypan blue dye (Vision Blue®, DORC, Zuidland, The Netherlands) in 1999. Even though both ICG dye and trypan blue dye adequately stain the anterior capsule of a white cataract, Chang[8] compared the two dyes and found that trypan blue provides a significantly darker, more intense and persistent staining of the anterior capsule. This may be especially beneficial in improving visualization

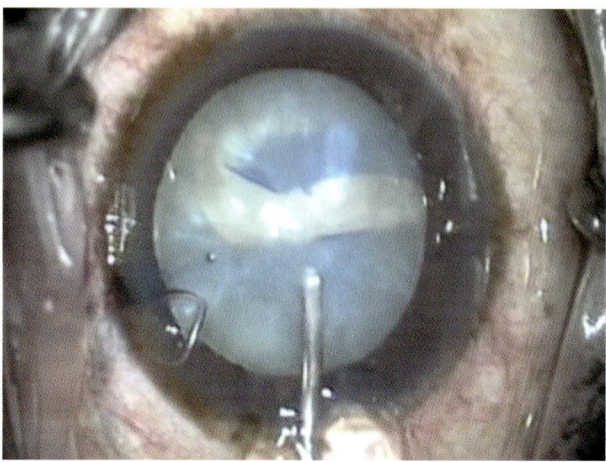

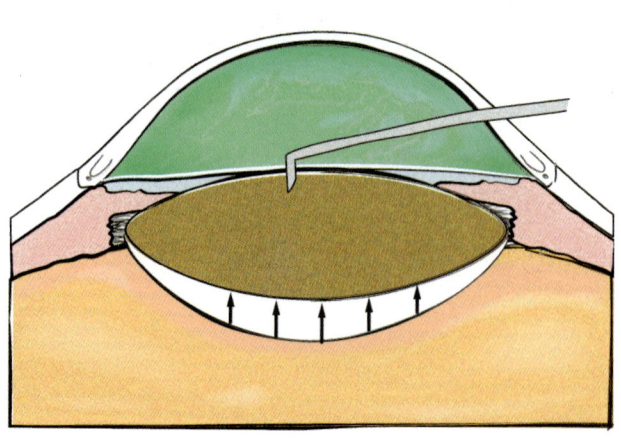

a

b

Fig. 14.4 **(a)** Argentinean flag sign occurring at the initiation of the capsulorrhexis. **(b)** Illustration of the proposed mechanism by which the Argentinean flag sign occurs. After decompression of the anterior cortical space, the pressurized posterior liquefied cortex pushes the nucleus anteriorly, causing the initial capsular tear to extend toward the equator. (**b,** Adapted from Figueiredo CG, Figueiredo J, Figueiredo, GB. Brazilian technique for prevention of the Argentinean flag sign in white cataract J Cataract Refract Surg 2012;38:1531–1536.)

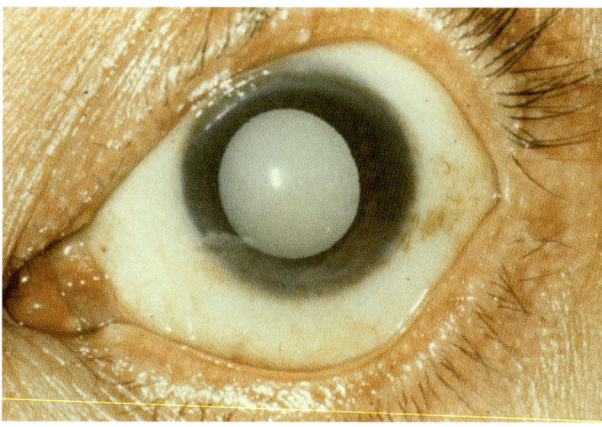

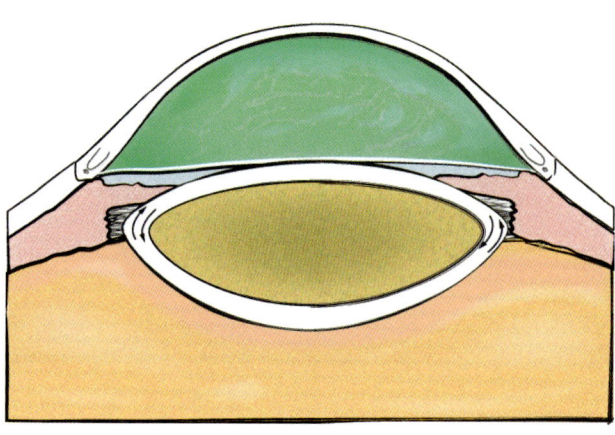

a

b

Fig. 14.5 **(a)** Homogeneously white cataract without variegation. (From EyeRounds.org. Reprinted by permission.) **(b)** Illustration of the homogeneously white cataract. There is communication between the anterior and posterior cortical spaces. Due to the communication, both liquefied cortical spaces will decompress simultaneously, when the anterior capsule is punctured, at initiation of the capsulotomy. (**b,** Adapted from Figueiredo CG, Figueiredo J, Figueiredo, GB. Brazilian technique for prevention of the Argentinean flag sign in white cataract J Cataract Refract Surg 2012;38:1531–1536.)

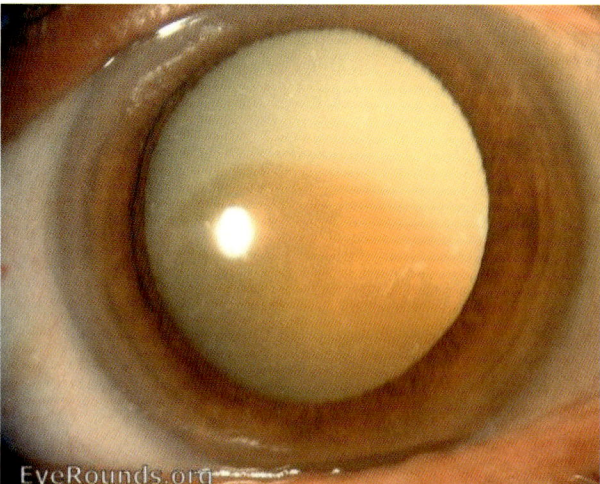

Fig. 14.6 Homogeneously white cataract with free-floating nucleus (Morgagnian). (From EyeRounds.org. Reprinted by permission.)

during phacoemulsification in a patient with preexisting corneal edema, prominent arcus senilis, or corneal scarring. Being able to see the edge of the continuous curvilinear capsulotomy helps the surgeon avoid damaging the capsule during phacoemulsification in difficult cases where there is no red reflex.

There have been reports of decreased lens epithelial cell density and viability[9] of capsules stained with trypan blue dye, as well as a report of an electron microscopy study showing that the basement membrane of a trypan blue stained capsule was focally ragged and irregular.[10] These reports infer that trypan blue may structurally weaken the capsule. A study comparing capsulorrhexis resistance to tearing with and without trypan blue dye using a mechanized tensile strength model was performed by Jaber et al[11] and showed that staining with trypan blue did not reduce continuous curvilinear capsulotomy strength.

Trypan blue may be applied to the anterior capsule in several ways: direct injection into the aqueous, injection or painting the capsule under air, injection mixed with viscoelastic, and painting the capsule under viscoelastic. The safest way, in my opinion, is to paint the anterior capsule under viscoelastic. Some blotching of dye on the capsule with this latter technique can be

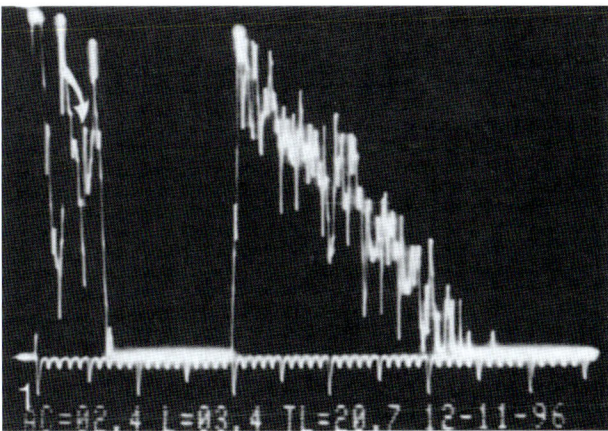

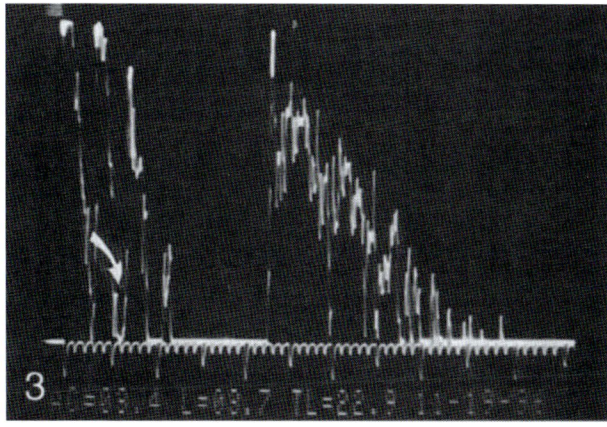

a

b

Fig. 14.7   (a) Scan of the high internal reflectivity *(arrow)* due to liquid cortex. **(b)** Scan of the low reflectivity *(arrow)* due to lack of liquid cortex. (From Brazitikos PD, Tsinopoulos IT, Papadopoulos NT, Fotiadis K, Stangos NT.

Ultrasonographic classification and phacoemulsification of white senile cataracts. Ophthalmology 1999;106;2178–2183. Reprinted by permission.)

made more homogeneous by rinsing with balanced salt solution (BSS) and then re-pressurizing the anterior chamber (AC) with OVD before starting the capsulotomy. This technique prevents inadvertent staining of the posterior capsule that can occur if a patient has a zonular dialysis. Posterior capsular staining greatly impairs observation of the red reflex while the nucleus is debulked, and therefore worsens its visualization, thus increasing the risk of complications.

Capsulotomy

Creating a 3-mm Capsulotomy and Enlarging it to 5 mm After Decompressing the Anterior and Posterior Cortical Spaces

After first staining the anterior capsule with trypan blue dye and pressurizing the AC with an OVD, the most reliable method for creating a capsulotomy in a mature white cataract is to begin by making a central anterior capsular puncture with a 30-gauge needle introduced bevel down through a 1-mm side port incision[1] (**Fig. 14.9a**). A dispersive OVD (Viscoat®, Alcon, Fort Worth, TX; or Endocoat®, AMO) is preferable, because it will allow the liquid white cortex of an intumescent cataract to seep into the

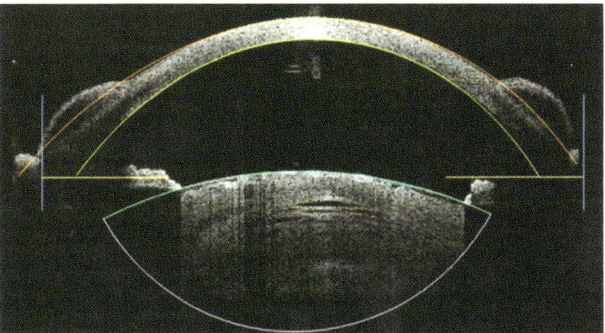

Fig. 14.8   Three-dimensional optical coherence tomography (OCT) (Catalys Laser) of an intumescent white cataract demonstrating intralenticular fluid spaces. (From Schultz T, Dick HB. Laser-assisted mini-capsulotomy: a new technique for intumescent white cataracts. J Refract Surg 2014;30:742–745. Reprinted by permission.)

AC. If there is no seepage of cortex into the AC after capsular puncture and using a dispersive OVD, then the white lens is not pressurized and a standard 5-mm capsulorrhexis may be performed with either a needle or forceps, through the main cataract incision, without concern for development of the Argentinean flag sign.

If liquid cortex does seep into the AC using a dispersive OVD, the white lens at hand is pressurized, indicating either an intumescent cataract, or a Morgagnian cataract. A Morgagnian lens will seep copious liquefied cortex into the AC, frequently collapsing the bag to such a degree that refilling the bag with a dispersive OVD is necessary to be able to complete a continuous curvilinear capsulotomy.

If the AC cortical seepage is mild to moderate, the lens is most likely intumescent. As Figueiredo et al[1] explained, this type of cataract has both an anterior and posterior liquefied cortical compartment under pressure and the two compartments do not connect due to relative nuclear block. Consequently, after anterior capsular puncture with a needle, only the anterior compartment decompresses, and therefore the posterior pressurized compartment can still push the nucleus anteriorly during continuous curvilinear capsulotomy creation, causing an Argentinean flag sign. Although gentle retropulsion of the nucleus with a 30-gauge needle may break the nuclear block and decompress the posterior compartment, this may not be 100% effective. Therefore, after first clearing the turbid AC by injecting additional dispersive OVD through the cataract incision into the angle opposite the incision, which forces the cloudy admixture of cortex and OVD out of the eye through the cataract incision, it is wise to create a 3-mm continuous curvilinear capsulotomy with a coaxial forceps through a side port incision (**Fig. 14.9b**). Bimanual irrigation and aspiration (I/A) (**Fig. 14.10a**) may then be used in the capsular bag to definitively decompress the posterior compartment of the capsular bag, after which the continuous curvilinear capsulotomy may be enlarged to 5 mm (**Fig. 14.10b**) before proceeding with phacoemulsification.

Some surgeons advocate using the cohesive OVD Healon 5 to assist with capsulotomy creation in white cataracts. However, Healon 5 is so heavy that it prevents any significant cortical seepage into the AC after capsular puncture, making it difficult to determine if the white cataract at hand is really intumescent. Therefore, if using this OVD, it is prudent to attempt aspiration of liquefied cortex within the bag, using either a 27- or 30-gauge needle (through the side-port incision) attached to a 3-cc syringe,

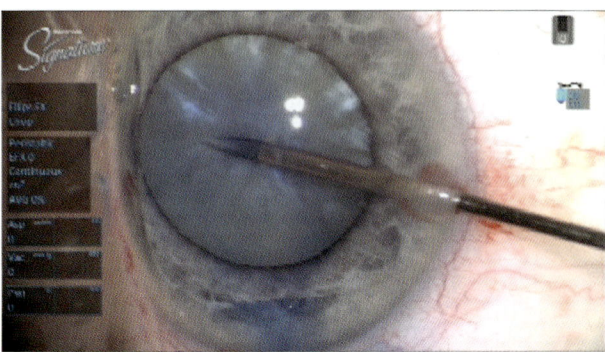

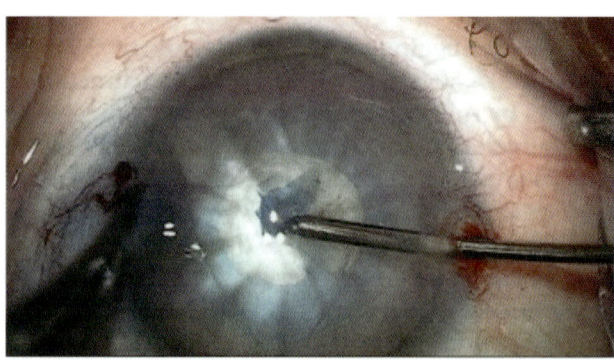

Fig. 14.9 **(a)** Anterior capsular puncture with a 27- or 30-gauge needle through a side-port incision allowing liquid cortex to seep into the anterior chamber. Gentle retropulsion with the bevel-down needle may be performed to attempt decompression of the posterior pressurized cortical compartment. **(b)** A 3-mm capsulotomy created with a coaxial forceps through a side-port incision. (**b**, From Figueiredo CG, Figueiredo J, Figueiredo, GB. Brazilian technique for prevention of the Argentinean flag sign in white cataract J Cataract Refract Surg 2012;38:1531–1536. Reprinted by permission.)

prior to proceeding with a continuous curvilinear capsulotomy. This maneuver is performed with the needle being bevel down within the capsular bag. If liquid cortex is forthcoming, then it is also advisable to gently retropulse the nucleus to break the relative nuclear block, which in turn will enable decompression of the posterior pressurized cortical compartment. The surgeon may then proceed with a continuous curvilinear capsulotomy, although a 3-mm size is still advisable in case the posterior compartment is not entirely decompressed. After confirmation of decompression of the posterior cortical compartment with bimanual I/A, the continuous curvilinear capsulotomy may be enlarged to 5 mm before commencing with phacoemulsification. This same principle of making a small capsulotomy followed by a larger capsulotomy after decompression of the capsular bag has been used with the Catalys Femtosecond Laser.[3]

Femtosecond Laser–Assisted Capsulotomy

Femtosecond laser–assisted capsulotomy in intumescent white cataracts has recently been reported by Conrad-Hengerer et al.[12] This prospective study involved 25 eyes, and in all eyes it was possible to create a capsulotomy with the laser. However, two eyes developed anterior capsular tears during phacoemulsification, nine eyes had an adherent tongue-like capsule adhesion, and three eyes had an incomplete capsulotomy button. A posterior chamber (PC) IOL was successfully placed into the capsular bag in all eyes. So, as the laser algorithm is refined with faster laser spot repetition rates, the femtosecond laser may become as safe as Figueiredo's technique for capsulotomy creation in intumescent white cataracts. At the point in time when the anterior capsule of an intumescent cataract is punctured with the femtosecond laser, cortex starts to seep into the AC and the physical position of the capsule may shift before the several-second laser capsulotomy is completed. This can result in more than the desired single circular row of laser spots as illustrated in **Fig. 14.11**. Consequently this aberrant laser pattern can result in the capsulotomy edge being weakened and this, in turn, can result in an anterior capsular tear during phacoemulsification or I/A. Sometimes a capsular tag can result, and if this occurs, the surgeon should avoid pulling on the tag because this may cause a radial tear.

Phacoemulsification

Because the liquid cortex has been mostly removed from the capsular bag of an intumescent cataract prior to phacoemulsification, the nucleus may be more mobile than in a cataract with intact nonliquid cortex. Consequently, in my opinion, vertical chopping techniques are more desirable for the ease and safety of lens disassembly than divide-and-conquer techniques or horizontal chopping techniques. For added safety and to stabilize a mobile nucleus, dispersive OVD may be injected behind and around the nucleus.

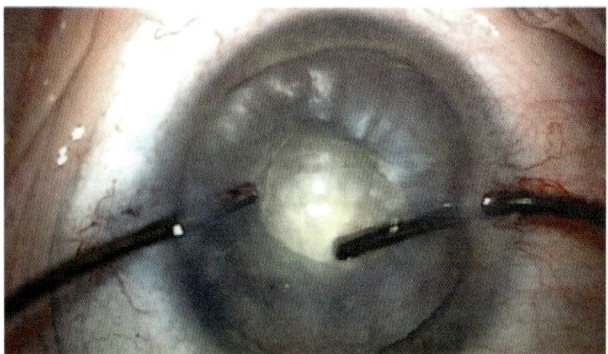

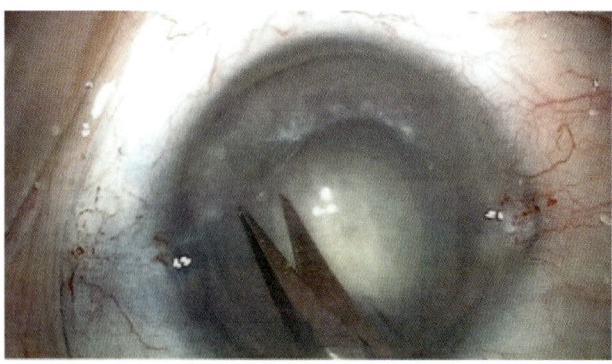

Fig. 14.10 **(a)** Bimanual irrigation and aspiration (I/A) performed to definitively decompress the posterior cortical compartment. **(b)** Use of intraocular scissors to initiate enlargement of the capsulotomy to 5 mm. (From Figueiredo CG, Figueiredo J, Figueiredo, GB. Brazilian technique for prevention of the Argentinean flag sign in white cataract J Cataract Refract Surg 2012;38:1531–1536. Reprinted by permission.)

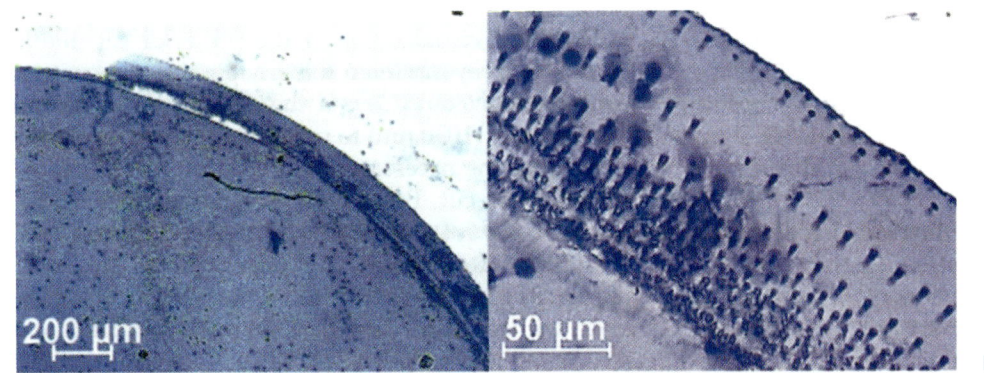

Fig. 14.11 **(a)** Capsulotomy tag that occurred with femtosecond laser–assisted treatment in an intumescent white cataract. **(b)** High magnification of the capsulotomy edge showing aberrant intracapsular laser shots due to capsule disk movement during femtosecond laser–assisted treatment in an intumescent white cataract. (From Conrad-Hengerer I, Hengerer FH, Joachim SC, Schultz T, Dick HB. Femtosecond laser-assisted cataract surgery in intumescent white cataracts. J Cataract Refract Surg 2014;40:44–50. Reprinted by permission.)

Salvaging an Argentinean Flag Sign Case

Once a tear has occurred in the anterior capsule during capsulotomy creation, it is important to proceed cautiously. Chances are that in a case like this, the tear or tears have extended to near the equator of the crystalline lens and it is unlikely that Brian Little's rescue maneuver[13] will retrieve the radialized capsular edge. Aspiration of some of the liquid cortex with a 27-gauge cannula is advisable prior to gently flattening the peripheral anterior capsule with additional dispersive viscoelastic. Then, use either intraocular scissors or a cystotome (**Fig. 14.12**) to incise the anterior capsule perpendicular to and within the radial tear

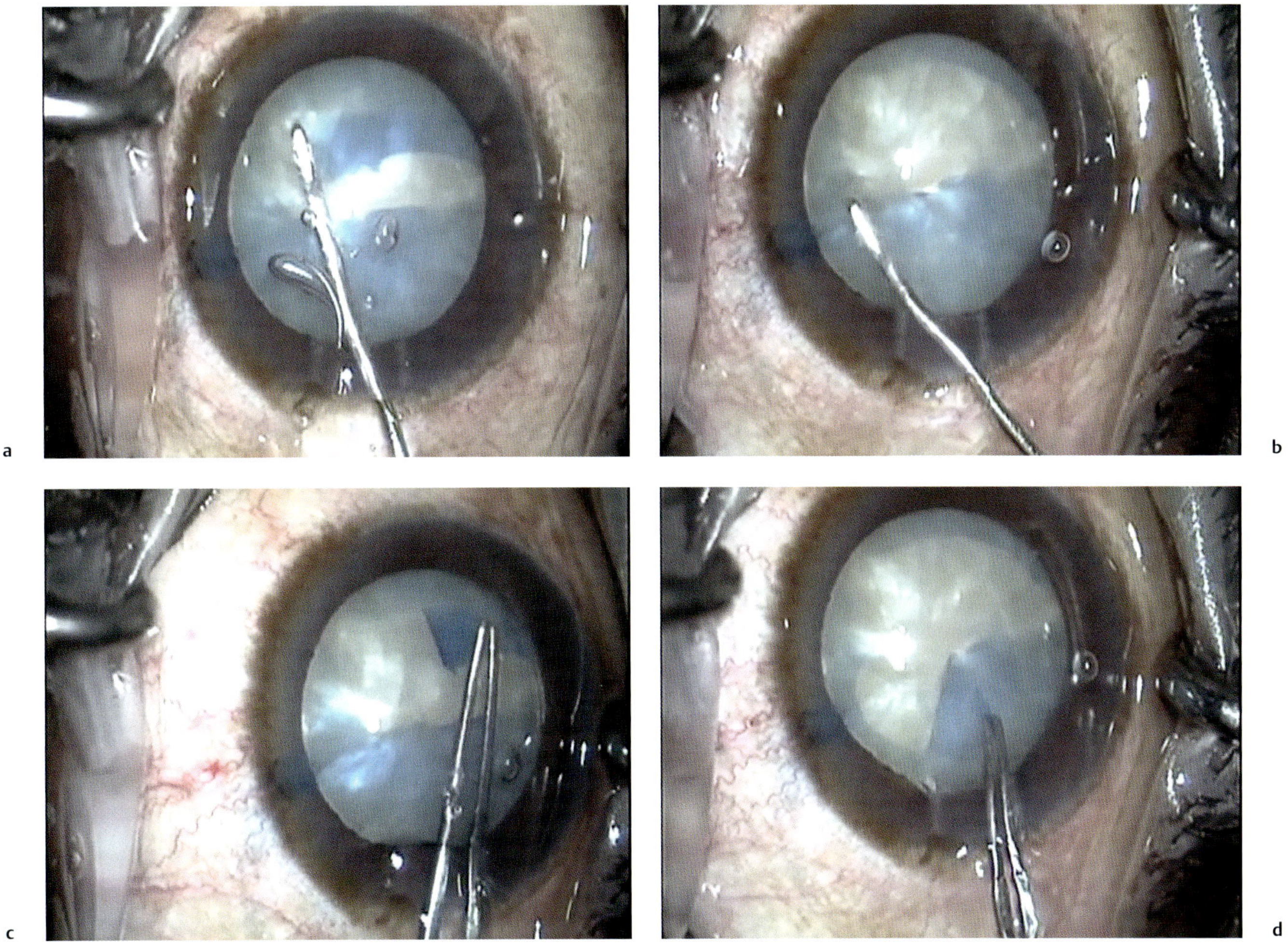

Fig. 14.12 Use of a cystotome **(a,b)** and Utrata forceps **(c,d)** to create a capsulotomy (discontinuous) after an Argentinean flag sign has occurred.

at the specific location required to create a 5- to 5.5-mm opening (obviously this capsulotomy will be discontinuous). This maneuver will have to be repeated twice if two radial tears exist. Once a capsulotomy is achieved, proceed with "slow-motion phacoemulsification." This term, coined by Robert Osher,[14] means to lower the aspiration flow rate so that movement of the nucleus toward the phaco tip happens slowly, and also to lower the bottle height so that the inflow of BSS into the eye is reduced. This latter step prevents the initial inflow of BSS into the eye from dramatically deepening the anterior chamber and stressing the zonules and the peripheral bag, thereby helping to prevent extension of the radial tear(s).

A vertical chop technique is favored. This prevents the nucleus from being directed posteriorly. Posterior pressure is a common trigger of anterior extension of the capsular tear around the equator and into the posterior capsule. To accomplish this technique, the nucleus is impaled with the phaco tip, after which the nucleus is elevated slightly toward the iris plane while simultaneously using a vertical chopper to impale and delicately push posteriorly, producing a split the nucleus. The nucleus is gently rotated 90 degrees and the same technique is repeated to create another split in the lens. Once the lens is split into four to eight pieces, gentle emulsification proceeds. Automated irrigation and aspiration is performed by first stripping the cortex from beneath the intact capsule, and then by stripping the cortex that is adjacent to the radial tears. Bimanual I/A is the safest procedure for cortical removal. Even though a single-piece IOL may sometimes be safely placed into the capsular bag in these cases, a safer option may be to place a three-piece IOL in the ciliary sulcus.

Conclusion

By following the thought patterns and techniques outlined in this chapter, white intumescent cataract surgery should be more straightforward, less stressful, and more successful than in the past. It is always best to assume that any white cataract may be intumescent, and therefore the surgeon is always prepared to handle the toughest of cases.

References

1. Figueiredo CG, Figueiredo J, Figueiredo GB. Brazilian technique for prevention of the Argentinean flag sign in white cataract. J Cataract Refract Surg 2012;38:1531–1536

2. Brazitikos PD, Tsinopoulos IT, Papadopoulos NT, Fotiadis K, Stangos NT. Ultrasonographic classification and phacoemulsification of white senile cataracts. Ophthalmology 1999;106:2178–2183

3. Schultz T, Dick HB. Laser-assisted mini-capsulotomy: a new technique for intumescent white cataracts. J Refract Surg 2014;30:742–745

4. Steinert RF, Dick HB. Femtosecond laser: why we need it for cataract surgery. Interview at the 2013 American Academy of Ophthalmology annual meeting. www.medscape.com/viewarticle/814732_6

5. Gorovoy IR, Jeng BH. Peripheral iridotomy to prevent Argentinian flag sign during capsulorhexis in the white cataract. J Cataract Refract Surg 2014;40:335–336

6. Horiguchi M, Miyake K, Ohta I, Ito Y. Staining of the lens capsule for circular continuous capsulorrhexis in eyes with white cataract. Arch Ophthalmol 1998;116:535–537

7. Melles GR, de Waard PW, Pameyer JH, Houdijn Beekhuis W. Trypan blue capsule staining to visualize the capsulorhexis in cataract surgery. J Cataract Refract Surg 1999;25:7–9

8. Chang DF. Capsule staining and mature cataracts: a comparison of indocyanine green and trypan blue dyes. Br J Ophthalmol 2000;84:video report. Available at http://bjo.bmjjournals.com/cgi/content/full/84/8/DC1

9. Nanavaty MA, Johar K, Sivasankaran MA, Vasavada AR, Praveen MR, Zetterström C. Effect of trypan blue staining on the density and viability of lens epithelial cells in white cataract. J Cataract Refract Surg 2006; 32:1483–1488

10. Rangaraj NR, Ariga M, Thomas J. Comparison of anterior capsule electron microscopy findings with and without trypan blue stain. J Cataract Refract Surg 2004;30:2241–2242

11. Jaber R, Werner L, Fuller S, et al. Comparison of capsulorhexis resistance to tearing with and without trypan blue dye using a mechanized tensile strength model. J Cataract Refract Surg 2012;38:507–512

12. Conrad-Hengerer I, Hengerer FH, Joachim SC, Schultz T, Dick HB. Femtosecond laser-assisted cataract surgery in intumescent white cataracts. J Cataract Refract Surg 2014;40:44–50

13. Little BC, Smith JH, Packer M. Little capsulorhexis tear-out rescue. J Cataract Refract Surg 2006;32:1420–1422

14. Osher RH, Marques FF, Marques DM, et al. Slow motion phacoemulsification technique. Tech Ophthalmol 2003;1(2):73–78

15 Dense Brunescent Cataract

Stephen S. Lane

Phacoemulsification of the extremely dense cataract poses challenges for even the most experienced cataract surgeon. The absence of a protective epinuclear layer, the paucity of cortex, the fragility of the capsule, and the potential laxity of zonules all increase the risk to the supportive structures of the lens during surgery. Most often, longer phaco times at higher energy levels increase not only the risk of corneal endothelial damage, but also the risks of mechanical or thermal injury to the iris or corneal incision. Successful surgical management of these cases requires planning and careful attention to detail. Although these patients are at a higher risk for complications, they are among the most grateful for the treatment because they go from legally blind back to normal vision, assuming the retina is normal, and are usually able to resume their normal activities of daily living. This chapter addresses some of the specific considerations presented by the rock-hard cataract, characterized by a darkly brunescent nucleus with the color of a cola soft drink.

Preoperative Examination

Patients with dense brunescent cataracts often present with a long-standing history of markedly decreased vision that has slowly deteriorated over the years. These patients typically have visual acuities worse than 20/200, and both eyes tend to be affected relatively equally. The patients are often older and may have coexisting ocular pathology or conditions that can affect the final visual outcome. Unilateral brunescent cataracts with minimal to no cataract in the opposite eye should alert the surgeon to the potential of previous trauma in the cataractous eye.

A careful slit-lamp microscopy examination can detect corneal endothelial compromise, a shallow anterior chamber, and signs of lens zonular laxity. The density and opacity of the nucleus may preclude a clear view of the posterior segment of the eye, and an ultrasonic examination may be required to rule out a retinal detachment or choroidal tumor. Patients with very dense cataracts often have not received medical eye care for years, and there can be occult comorbidities, such as glaucoma, macular degeneration, or retinal disease; as best as these comorbidities can be visualized, attempts should be made to determine the status of the retina.

Biometry can be a challenge as well because optical methods of axial length determination may not be able to penetrate the dense cataract. Similarly, the patient may have trouble fixating on a target during keratometry evaluation. Because of the severe visual deficit, these patients tend to be very forgiving of any residual refractive error, and we can further enhance useful vision by leaning toward a myopic result should there be any issues with lens calculations.

The following section describes the step-by-step management of the challenges presented by these cases.

Intraoperative Techniques and Considerations

Consider a Scleral Incision

The phacoemulsification primary incision can be made in either the sclera or the cornea. Wound construction and location are critical as there is an increased risk of corneal incisional burns as the result of higher amounts of ultrasound energy used in removing a dense cataract. A clear corneal incision most often enables the balanced salt solution to keep the incision cooled. However, a scleral tunnel incision has the benefit of potential enlargement should the surgeon wish to convert to a manual extraction method. The advantages of starting with a scleral incision is that if the surgeon should encounter a nucleus that is simply too dense to be emulsified or if the procedure is proceeding poorly, a larger incision is much more easily accomplished from a scleral approach than if the incision was purely clear corneal.

Enhanced Visualization of the Capsule

Visualization of the anterior capsule is often a problem with highly dense cataracts.[1] Staining the capsule with trypan blue provides far better visualization, enabling the surgeon to perform the capsulorrhexis with greater safety and much more confidence.[2] If a femtosecond laser is available, an anterior capsulorrhexis using femtosecond technology ensures a properly sized and precisely placed capsulorrhexis while enhancing the safety of these usually fragile capsules.

Avoid Capsular/Lenticular Block

Care must be taken to avoid capsular block during hydrodissection of brunescent dense nuclei. When there is very little cortex, the large dense nucleus can act as a block, as it lifts up during hydrodissection, occluding the anterior capsulotomy and completely blocking egress of balanced salt solution from the posterior to the anterior chamber. The posterior capsule in these mature cataracts is often very fragile and can be broken easily with increased posterior pressure. For this reason, it is important to generally tap the nucleus down after every hydrodissection bolus injection to allow the balanced salt solution to slip around the nucleus and decompress the posterior chamber (**Fig. 15.1**).

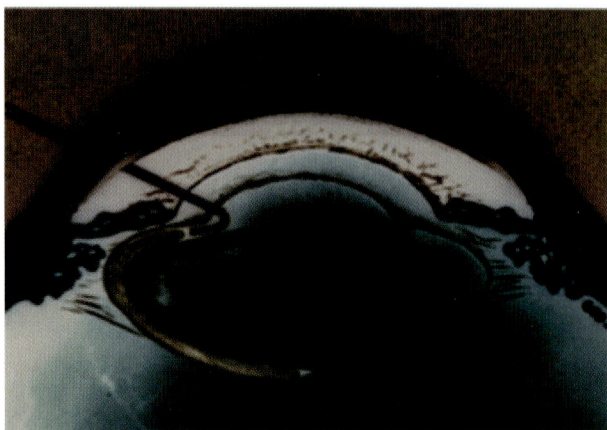

Fig. 15.1 Hydrodissection in a nuclear mature cataract. The absence of an epinucleus and cortex requires careful hydrodissection to prevent inadvertent rupture of the anterior or posterior capsule or capsular block.

Create a Posterior Capsular Buffer Zone with an Ophthalmic Viscosurgical Device

Dispersive, retentive viscoadaptive agents can be used to create an artificial epinucleus to protect the posterior capsule. A dense brunescent cataract usually has little to no epinucleus, as the epinucleus has stiffened and become part of the nucleus. The posterior capsule, therefore, has no protective layer to guard against laceration from the sharp and bulky nuclear fragments. In addition, the posterior capsule is usually thinner and more vulnerable because the advanced cataract has stretched the capsule as the cataract has expanded. Although the large nucleus tends to hold back the posterior capsule early in the procedure, as more and more nucleus is removed, there is increased propensity to injure the posterior capsule with the phaco tip. The capsular bag in these cases tends to be large and somewhat floppy that can easily be drawn into the tip. Toward the end of the phaco procedure, further dispersive ophthalmic viscosurgical device (OVD) may be used to inflate the posterior chamber and push back the posterior capsule, again protecting it from the potentially sharp edges of the nucleus and from the phacoemulsification tip. The dispersive OVD resists aspiration, and maintains the distance between the nuclear material and the posterior capsule, and helps to prevent injury to the capsule during the final part of the phaco procedure. This maneuver has been termed the "visco vault" by Roger Steinert, because the OVD acts like a protective wall, or "vault," to protect the posterior capsule.[3]

Beware of Incisional Wound Burn

Special care must be taken to avoid corneal wound burns. Always make sure that the OVD is flowing readily into the phaco tip during aspiration, before even beginning to use phaco power, and watch carefully for "phaco smoke" during phaco, suggesting that there is impairment of outflow. Dense lens material can easily clog the phaco tip and result in excessive heating, which can occur very quickly.[4] At the first hint of obstruction, phaco ultrasound power must be stopped immediately. This can be identified by any evidence of whitening of the phaco tip. Similarly, any sign of "lens milk" with a whitening of the lens material should indicate to the surgeon obstruction of flow; the use of ultrasound power should be immediately

stopped, and the surgeon should come off of position 3 on the foot pedal. It is imperative at the first sign of obstruction that phacoemulsification be stopped instantly and the obstruction be cleared. If there is any evidence of thermal injury to the phaco entry site, the surgeon should consider moving the incision to another location to finish the procedure and close the wound with either sutures or tissue glue.

Protect the Endothelium

Phacoemulsification of the dense nucleus requires longer phaco times and higher energy levels. An endothelial protective dispersive OVD is desirable in these cases to help prevent endothelial injury.[5] Care should be taken, however, to perform as much of the phacoemulsification procedure as possible in the pupillary plane or below. Special care should be taken in hyperopic patients and others with shallow anterior chambers to avoid endothelial damage. It is often necessary and prudent to replenish the dispersive OVD during the phacoemulsification process, as this material may be aspirated or lost through the incision site.

Disassembly of the Nucleus

Chopping of a very dense nucleus can be difficult to accomplish because of the leathery nature of the lens material. A frequent surgical observation during phacoemulsification of a dense brunescent nucleus, whether by quadrant cracking or phaco-chop technique, is that the split fragments will resist being drawn into the mid-anterior chamber for complete emulsification and aspiration by the ultrasound needle. This problem occurs because the tough elastic strands have a "leathery" quality and they span across and connect the split nuclear segments on their posterior surface. These leathery strands emanate from the epinuclear layer, which in advanced brunescence become stiff and are more tightly adherent to the nucleus. These strands on the posterior surface will challenge the surgeon trying to mobilize nuclear pieces in a controlled manner. It is important in these cases to carry grooves deeply through the nuclear material to see the fundus reflex at the bottom of the groove. Creating a central bowl assists in facilitating deeper sculpting of the central groove to make cracking the nucleus more successful **(Fig. 15.2)**. This allows

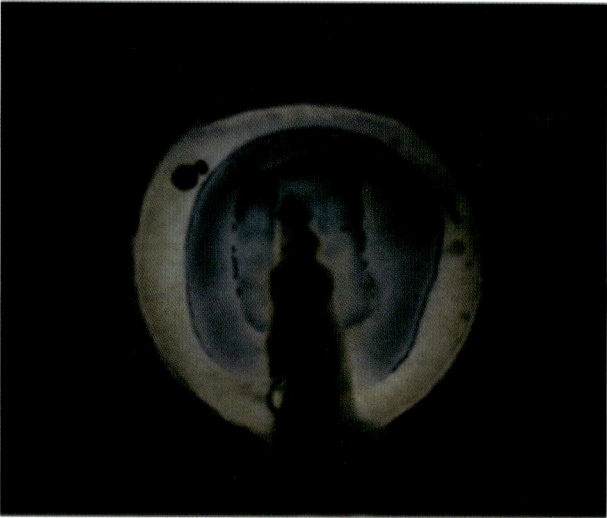

Fig. 15.2 Creating a central bowl in a nuclear mature cataract facilitates deeper sculpting of the first trough to perform a hemi-nuclear chop.

the surgeon to make deep cracks through the entire thickness of the nucleus, which are necessary to help divide the nucleus completely.

When the strands prevent splitting of the lens, it is easiest to address the strands by breaking them with a blunt instrument, often directed posteriorly to anteriorly. As long as a blunt chopper-type instrument is parallel to the posterior capsule, and the surgeon maintains proper infusion of balanced salt solution, the posterior capsule will not be endangered. It is critical that the surgeon be patient in dealing with these strands, as they most often need to be broken one at a time, dissecting the lens into many segments in more of a tearing motion than a splitting/cracking motion. Once again, dispersive OVD is helpful in creating a cushion behind the leathery lens nuclear material and the posterior capsule, providing space for instrumentation to break and tear these leathery bands. Once the segments of the nucleus are freely mobile, removal techniques can be employed utilizing ultrasonic energy.

If accessible, the femtosecond laser is a noteworthy improvement on nuclear emulsification. Reportedly, using it to soften a rock hard nucleus will reduce phaco energy by 46%[6] and render nuclear removal more straightforward. Therefore, the risk of tearing the anterior or posterior capsule is diminished. Thus, the procedure is appreciably safer.

Watch Carefully for "Lost" Chips

Very dense nuclei often break into many tiny particles that can get trapped in the eye during the phaco procedure. Care should be taken to look for and remove all small chips that may be "hiding" in the anterior chamber, in the primary incision, in the paracentesis, under the incision site, or behind the iris. It is wise to reenter the phaco incision with the phaco tip and to irrigate the side ports at the end of the case to free, identify, and aspirate chips that may be trapped in the incision sites themselves.

Special Instruments

The removal of dense nuclei is very challenging, and the surgeon should be prepared with several different instruments at hand to aid in the removal of these brunescent lenses. The capsule and supporting structures of dense, mature cataracts are always fragile. Even with the greatest care, these structures can become compromised during the procedure, and it is important that the surgeon have capsular tension rings, capsular hooks, vitrectomy instrumentation, and other special choppers and hooks available and readily at hand.

Conclusion

Phacoemulsification of a very dense cataract presents the surgeon with a series of specific and difficult challenges. Successful management of these cases requires a thoughtful step-by-step approach that anticipates these challenges and enables the surgeon to complete the procedure successfully.

References

1. Mansour AM. Anterior capsulorhexis in hypermature cataracts. [letter] J Cataract Refract Surg 1993;19:116–117

2. Melles GRJ, de Waard PWT, Pameyer JH, Houdijn Beekhuis W. Trypan blue capsule staining to visualize the capsulorhexis in cataract surgery. J Cataract Refract Surg 1999;25:7–9

3. Steinert RF. Dense brunescent cataract. In: Steinert RF, ed. Cataract Surgery, 3rd ed. Philadelphia: Saunders Elsevier; 2010:339–341

4. Ernest P, Rhem M, McDermott M, Lavery K, Sensoli A. Phacoemulsification conditions resulting in thermal wound injury. J Cataract Refract Surg 2001;27:1829–1839

5. Koch DD, Liu JF, Glasser DB, Merin LM, Haft E. A comparison of corneal endothelial changes after use of Healon or Viscoat during phacoemulsification. Am J Ophthalmol 1993;115:188–201

6. Uy H. 48 cases performed in Philippines by Harvey Uy: Clear benefits emerge. Presented at the American Society of Cataract and Refractive Surgery meeting, March 2012

16 Posterior Polar Cataract

Abhay R. Vasavada and Vaishali Vasavada

Posterior polar cataracts (PPCs) are a challenge for every cataract surgeon due to their propensity for posterior capsule dehiscence and weakness. Although the initial reported incidence of posterior capsule rupture (PCR) ranged from 26 to 36%,[1,2] subsequent improvements in understanding of techniques[2–17] and technology have led to a reduction in the rates of PCR to 6 to 7%.[8,9]

Depending on the clinical presentation, PPCs can be divided into three categories: (1) polar cataracts without evident posterior capsule dehiscence (**Fig. 16.1**); (2) polar cataracts with preexisting posterior capsule dehiscence (**Fig. 16.2**); and (3) spontaneous dislocation. PPCs without evident dehiscence account for 97% of all polar cases and are the most common presentation in patients under 40 years of age.

This chapter describes the difficulties associated with PPC emulsification and different surgical strategies to improve safety, reduce posterior capsule rupture, and enhance the predictability of outcomes in emulsifying PPCs. It also discusses the role of femtosecond laser–assisted cataract surgery to improve safety in these cataracts. Both the novice and the experienced surgeons will find useful practical tips that they can use when faced with PPCs. The discussion addresses the clinical presentation, the principles for safe removal of PPCs, as well as the different surgical approaches to deal with PPCs.

Clinical Presentation

Most commonly, PPCs present with glare disability in bright light conditions. Two types of PPCs have been described in literature: stationary and progressive.[18] The stationary type is characterized by a central, dense, disk-shaped opacity located on the posterior capsule with concentric rings around the central plaque opacity that look like a bull's-eye. It has a cone-shaped projection in the subcapsular region or central posterior cortex. This type of PPC is compatible with good vision. In the progressive type of PPC (**Fig. 16.3**), changes take place in the posterior cortex in the form of radiating rider opacities. Patients with progressive opacity become more symptomatic as the peripheral extensions enlarge.

Normally the patient seeks help in the third or the fourth decade of life. PPCs are present bilaterally in 90% of our cases in adults and 70% in a study conducted by Gavriş and colleagues.[19]

Risk Factors for Posterior Capsule Dehiscence in Posterior Polar Cataracts

Often, a posterior capsule defect is observed as an elliptical-shaped defect (**Fig. 16.2**), which is generally vertically oriented with a central bull's eye–shaped opacity. Coexisting anomalies have not been reported in the literature, except for a report of coexisting retinitis pigmentosa in the Siatiri and Moghimi[10] study.

It has been suggested that the size of the polar opacity has a significant impact on the risk of posterior capsule rupture.[16] In the same study, in eyes with polar opacities of 4 mm or more, seven eyes (30.43%) had posterior capsule rupture, whereas in eyes with polar opacities of less than 4 mm, two eyes (5.71%), had PCR.[16] Further, PCR was found to be more common in patients younger than 40 years and in the eyes that underwent extracapsular cataract extraction as compared with phacoemulsification.[15]

Surgical Strategies in Posterior Cataract Emulsification

The final surgical goal for every surgeon is to be able to safely remove the entire cataract and implant an intraocular lens (IOL), preferably in the capsular bag. To protect the inherently weak posterior capsule, the strategy for posterior polar emulsification involves the following:

- Avoiding rapid buildup of hydraulic pressure within the capsular bag
- Creating a mechanical cushion above the weak capsule
- Adhering to the principles of closed-chamber technique

Several surgical approaches have been proposed for emulsification of PPCs. Our preferred approach is usually a temporal, clear corneal incision. The smallest size of the incision compatible with the surgeon's phaco tip, sleeve, and comfort level should be selected. We prefer a 2.2-mm incision, as it facilitates maintenance of a closed chamber during surgery. High molecular cohesive ophthalmic viscosurgical devices (OVDs) should be used during capsulorrhexis. While making the capsulorrhexis, a moderate size should be aimed at so that in the eventuality of inadequate posterior capsule support, a sulcus IOL can be placed.

Cortical cleaving hydrodissection should be avoided in PPCs, as it can lead to a rapid buildup in hydraulic pressure and blowout of the posterior capsule.[1,2,6] Instead, several authors have recommended performing hydrodelineation to create a mechanical cushion of the epinucleus.[2,5,8,10,20] The rationale is to create a mechanical cushion that separates the nucleus from the fragile posterior capsule and thereby prevents transmission of mechanical and fluidic forces to the weakest part of the capsule.

Similarly, viscodissection has also been performed to protect the posterior capsule.[5,6] A dispersive OVD is injected between the epinucleus and the posterior capsule to create a plane of separation and generate space that cordons off the polar opacity during phacoemulsification, and reduces transmission of mechanical forces to the potentially weak capsule.

In addition to hydrodelineation, Fine and coauthors[6] also perform hydrodissection in multiple quadrants injecting tiny

a

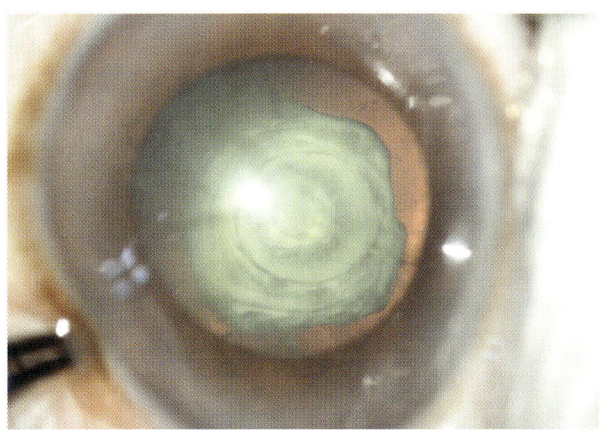

b

Fig. 16.1 **(a,b)** Posterior polar cataract (PPC) characterized by a central, dense, disk-shaped opacity located on the posterior capsule with concentric rings around the central plaque opacity that look like a bull's-eye.

quantities of fluid gently, such that the fluid wave is not allowed to spread across the posterior capsule.

Inside-Out Delineation

We published the inside-out delineation in PPCs,[9] in which a central trench is sculpted. Then, specially designed right- and left-angled cannulae are placed at a chosen depth in the trench, and fluid is injected (**Fig. 16.4**). A golden ring within the lens is evidence of successful delineation (**Fig. 16.5**). Fluid injection is performed in both right and left walls of the trench. The advantage of this technique is that as fluid is injected at a desired depth, under direct vision, a desired thickness of epinucleus cushion can be achieved, and inadvertent subcapsular fluid passage is prevented, which can often happen with conventional hydrodelineation (**Fig. 16.6**).

Nucleus Removal

Nucleus removal should be performed within the cushion of the epinucleus, so that there is a mechanical so that there is a mechanical layer that protects the posterior capsule. Whatever the nucleus division technique, the surgeon should ensure that

a closed chamber is maintained at all times. OVD should be injected into the anterior chamber before withdrawal of any instrument to prevent collapse of the anterior chamber.[2] Low aspiration flow rate (AFR) and bottle height (BH) should be used in accordance with the slow-motion technique.[21] The collapse of the anterior chamber and forward bulge of the PC is prevented throughout the procedure by injecting a viscoelastic before the instrument is withdrawn (**Fig. 16.7**).

In dense nuclear sclerosis, Lim and Goh[22] suggest performing a pre-chop of the anterior epinucleus prior to mobilizing, segmenting, and emulsifying the dense endonucleus. Lee and Lee[7] use the lambda technique to sculpt the nucleus, followed by cracking along both arms and removal of the central piece.

Epinucleus Removal

Perhaps one of the most crucial steps during which PCR occurs is removal of the epinucleus. The epinucleus should first be stripped off the capsule using the phaco tip with minimal AFR (14 to 16 cc/min) and vacuum (around 100 mm Hg). At this point, no attempt should be made to completely remove the epinucleus, and the central area is left attached.[2,4,6] Then, multiquadrant hydrodissection is performed using special angled

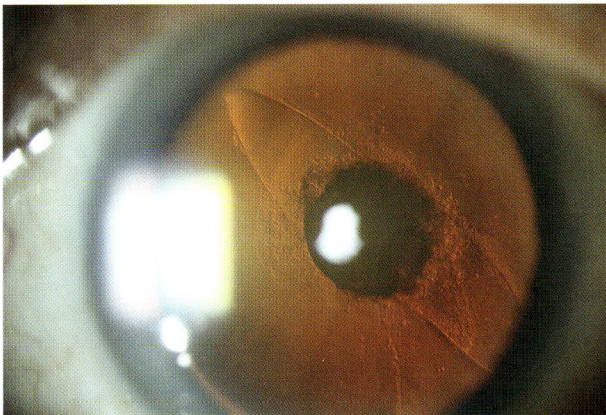

Fig. 16.2 Posterior polar cataract with a preexisting posterior capsule dehiscence.

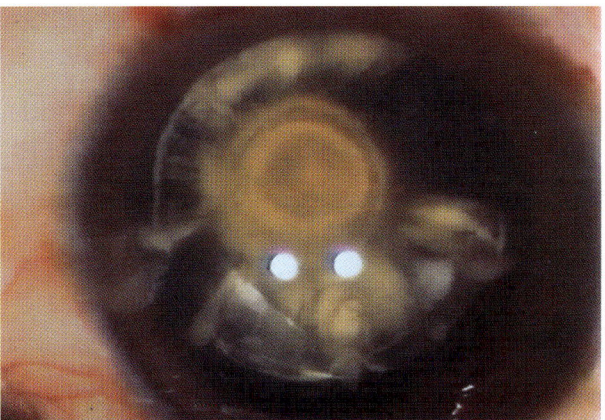

Fig. 16.3 Progressive type of PPC. Changes take place in the posterior cortex in the form of radiating rider opacities.

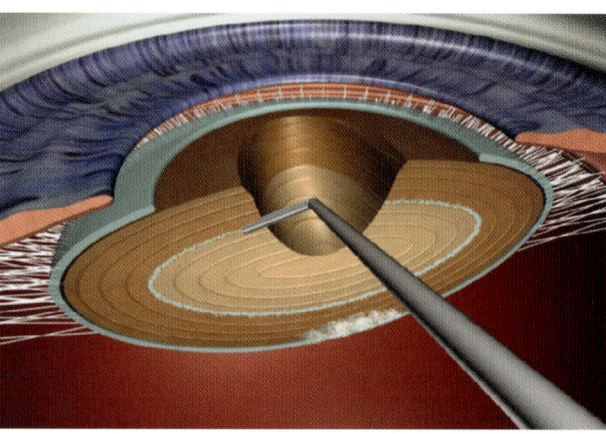

a

b

Fig. 16.4 **(a)** The technique of inside-out delineation, wherein a bent cannula is inserted at the desired depth in the trench to achieve a delineation from within outside. **(b)** Illustration of the concept of inside-out delineation.

cannulae (**Fig. 16.8**). Because separating the epinucleus from the fornices creates a cleavage plane, passage of fluid does not cause buildup of hydraulic pressure. Therefore, even if there is a pre-existing or intraoperative PCR, there is minimal enlargement of this rupture. The epinucleus is then completely aspirated. We prefer bimanual irrigation and aspiration (I/A), as it provides access to cortex all around without causing incision distortion or anterior chamber shallowing. Posterior capsule polishing should be avoided due to the possibility of a fragile capsule.

Femtodelineation: Femtosecond Laser–Assisted Delineation of the Nucleus in Posterior Polar Cataracts

As the femtosecond laser technology promises to enhance the precision and the outcomes of cataract surgery, we have recently explored the application of this technology to enhance safety in PPCs.[23] Using the femtosecond laser platform for cataract surgery, the cylindrical pattern of lens division is chosen to create multiple cylinders within the lens. This leads to creation of sharply demarcated layers within the nucleus (**Fig. 16.9**). The number, size, and depth of these cylinders can be controlled by

the surgeon using the live anterior segment optical coherence tomography view (**Fig. 16.10**). The multiple layers act as mechanical cushions that allow removal of each layer within the protection of the other (**Fig. 16.11**). Finally, the last epinuclear layer that is left behind can be easily stripped off using a combination of phaco probe and bimanual I/A due to its sharp demarcation. This approach eliminates the need for any kind of hydroprocedure in PPCs. It reduces PCR rates and enhances safety in PPC emulsification. Our PCR rates have dropped from 8%[9] to 4.4% after having adopted the femtodelineation approach.[23]

Surgical Approach in Eyes with a Preexisting Defect in the Posterior Capsule

We follow the same paradigms as those used in eyes with an intact posterior capsule. The aim here is to prevent enlargement of the existing defect and vitreous prolapse in the anterior chamber. Maintaining a closed chamber at all times and liberal use of dispersive OVD before withdrawing any instruments from the eye is important. Further, in such cases, minimal possible BH, AFR, and vacuum should be used. In cases where vitreous prolapses into the anterior chamber, we prefer to perform a

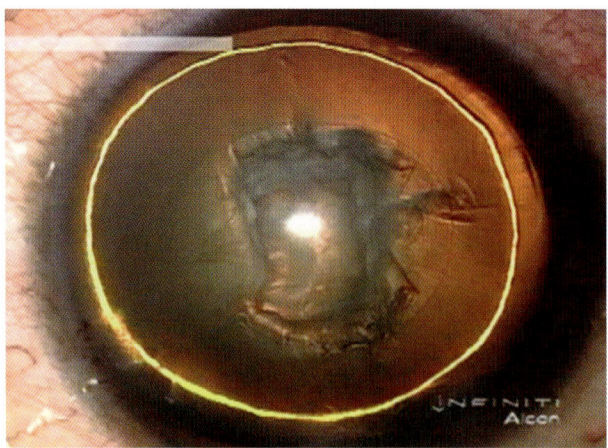

Fig. 16.5 A golden ring within the lens is evidence of successful delineation.

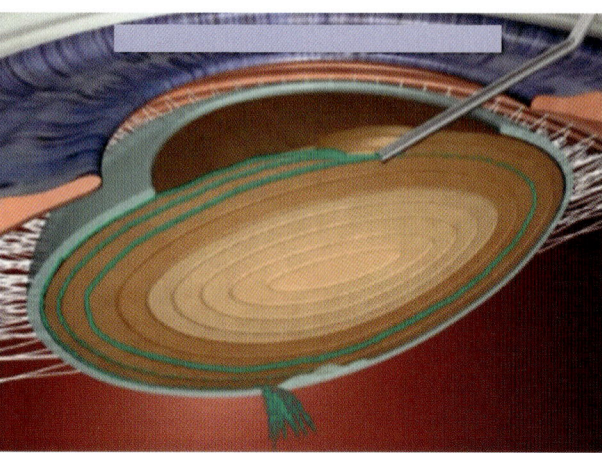

Fig. 16.6 Illustration showing how inadvertent subcapsular injection of fluid can occur in conventional hydrodelineation.

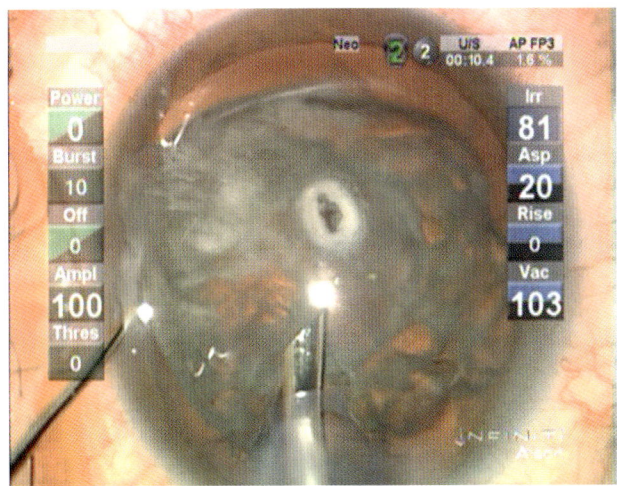

Fig. 16.7 Dispersive ophthalmic viscosurgical device (OVD) being injected through the paracentesis before withdrawing the phaco probe.

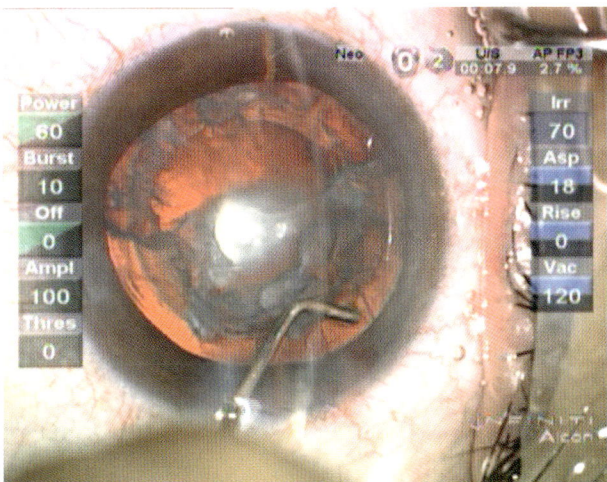

Fig. 16.8 Focal and multiquadrant hydrodissection using bent cannulae to cleave apart the subincisional epinucleus from the capsule.

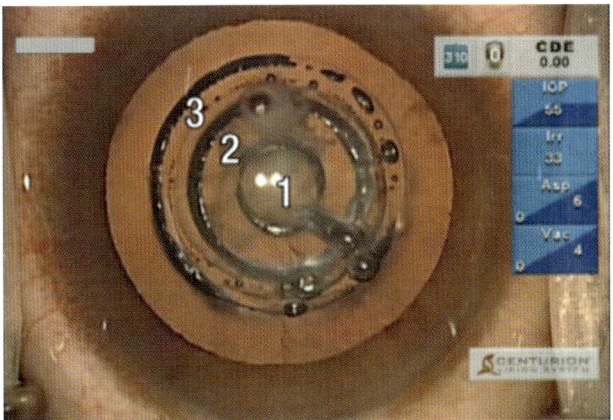

Fig. 16.9 Multiple concentric layers with sharp demarcation borders are created within the lens using femtosecond laser.

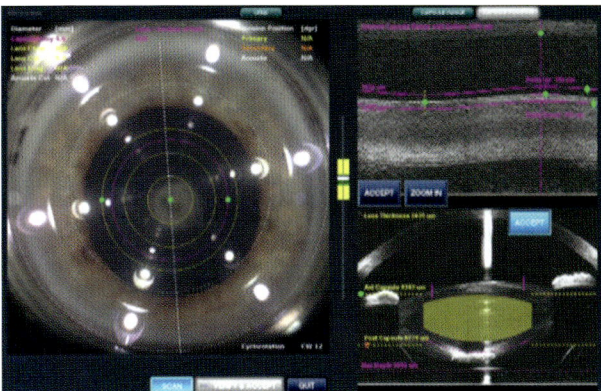

Fig. 16.10 View of the LenSx® (Alcon Laboratories, Fort Worth, TX) femtosecond laser in which the number and depth of cylinders can be customized based on surgeon preference.

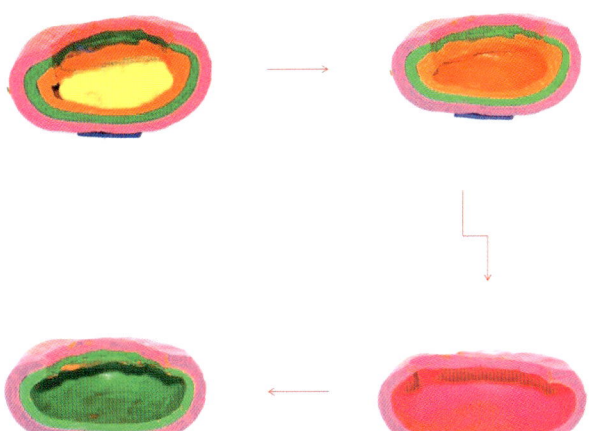

Fig. 16.11 Clay models showing how, in femtodelineation, each demarcated layer is removed one by one, with the cushion of the other layer, until the very end. At the end, a thick, uniform epinuclear cushion still protects the area of potential weakness.

bimanual, pars plana vitrectomy with irrigation probe through the corneal paracentesis and vitrector introduced through the pars plana. Using the highest possible cut rate, and moderate vacuum, AFR, and BH settings, anterior vitrectomy is performed. The advantage of pars plana approach over a limbal approach for vitrectomy is that there is minimal enlargement of the original PCR, as there is no upward traction on the vitreous body. On the other hand, when limbal anterior vitrectomy is performed, the entire vitreous body attached to the prolapsed strand is pulled upward, causing traction, and thereby enlargement of the PCR. Intracameral use of preservative-free triamcinolone acetonide helps in identifying vitreous strands in the anterior chamber to confirm adequate vitrectomy. A posterior continuous curvilinear capsulorrhexis (PCCC) may be performed if the rupture is confined to a small central area.

Conclusion

Posterior polar cataracts pose a surgical challenge to cataract surgeons. The surgical steps include performing some form of hydrodelineation or femtosecond laser–assisted delineation, thus creating a cushion to protect the posterior capsule. Adhering to the closed chamber technique, adopting the slow motion technique for lens removal, and using focal and multiquadrant hydrodissection after nucleus removal to achieve adequate cleavage of the subincisional epinucleus from the capsule can help successfully navigate this potentially complicating situation. In the event of a breach in the posterior capsule in these eyes, a periodic evaluation for retinal break, cystoid macular edema, and raised intraocular pressure is necessary.

References

1. Osher RH, Yu BC, Koch DD. Posterior polar cataracts: a predisposition to intraoperative posterior capsular rupture. J Cataract Refract Surg 1990;16:157–162

2. Vasavada A, Singh R. Phacoemulsification in eyes with posterior polar cataract. J Cataract Refract Surg 1999;25:238–245

3. Fine IH. Cortical cleaving hydrodissection. J Cataract Refract Surg 1992;18:508–512

4. Masket S. Consultation section. Cataract surgical problem. J Cataract Refract Surg 1997;23:819–824

5. Allen D, Wood C. Minimizing risk to the capsule during surgery for posterior polar cataract. J Cataract Refract Surg 2002;28:742–744

6. Fine IH, Packer M, Hoffman RS. Management of posterior polar cataract. J Cataract Refract Surg 2003;29:16–19

7. Lee MW, Lee YC. Phacoemulsification of posterior polar cataracts—a surgical challenge. Br J Ophthalmol 2003;87:1426–1427

8. Hayashi K, Hayashi H, Nakao F, Hayashi F. Outcomes of surgery for posterior polar cataract. J Cataract Refract Surg 2003;29:45–49

9. Vasavada AR, Raj SM. Inside-out delineation. J Cataract Refract Surg 2004;30:1167–1169

10. Siatiri H, Moghimi S. Posterior polar cataract: minimizing risk of posterior capsule rupture. Eye (Lond) 2006;20:814–816

11. Haripriya A, Aravind S, Vadi K, Natchiar G. Bimanual microphaco for posterior polar cataracts. J Cataract Refract Surg 2006;32:914–917

12. Chee SP. Management of the hard posterior polar cataract. J Cataract Refract Surg 2007;33:1509–1514

13. Vajpayee RB, Sinha R, Singhvi A, Sharma N, Titiyal JS, Tandon R. "Layer by layer" phacoemulsification in posterior polar cataract with pre-existing posterior capsular rent. Eye (Lond) 2008;22:1008–1010

14. Ghosh YK, Kirkby GR. Posterior polar cataract surgery—a posterior segment approach. Eye (Lond) 2008;22:844–848

15. Das S, Khanna R, Mohiuddin SM, Ramamurthy B. Surgical and visual outcomes for posterior polar cataract. Br J Ophthalmol 2008;92:1476–1478

16. Kumar S, Ram J, Sukhija J, Severia S. Phacoemulsification in posterior polar cataract: does size of lens opacity affect surgical outcome? Clin Experiment Ophthalmol 2010;38:857–861

17. Nagappa S, Das S, Kurian M, Braganza A, Shetty R, Shetty B. Modified technique for epinucleus removal in posterior polar cataract. Ophthalmic Surg Lasers Imaging 2011;42:78–80

18. Duke-Elder S. Posterior polar cataract. In: Duke-Elder S, ed. System of Ophthalmology, vol 3, pt 2: Normal and Abnormal Development, Congenital Deformities. St. Louis: CV Mosby; 1964:723–726

19. Gavriş M, Popa D, Cărăuş C, et al. [Phacoemulsification in posterior polar cataract]. Oftalmologia 2004;48:36–40

20. Anis AY. Understanding hydrodelineation: the term and the procedure. Doc Ophthalmol 1994;87:123–137

21. Osher RH. Slow motion phacoemulsification approach. J Cataract Refract Surg 1993;19:667

22. Lim Z, Goh J. Modified epinucleus pre-chop for the dense posterior polar cataract. Ophthalmic Surg Lasers Imaging 2008;39:171–173

23. Vasavada AR, Vasavada V, Vasavada S, Srivastava S, Vasavada V, Raj S. Femtodelineation to enhance safety in posterior polar cataracts. J Cataract Refract Surg 2015;41:702–707

17 Femtosecond Laser–Assisted Cataract Surgery

Ronald Yeoh

Femtosecond laser–assisted cataract surgery (FLACS) is rapidly gaining momentum, and I estimate that one thousand of these lasers have been installed worldwide. If cost was not an issue, I believe that most cataract surgeons would adopt this new technology, as it makes the surgery simpler and arguably safer. Proof of improved refractive precision is awaited.

The procedure itself is similar, whichever FLACS platform a surgeon selects. It involves the "femto" step followed by the "phaco" step. This chapter describes both steps, in particular the modifications in technique needed when changing from phaco to femtophaco, and discusses the potential complications and their management and prevention.

Preoperative Preparations

One hour before surgery, I administer my standard pre-phaco dilatation regime: Guttae tropicamide 1% ×4 and Guttae phenylephrine ×2, both an hour prior to surgery. For FLACS, I add a topical nonsteroidal anti-inflammatory drug (NSAID), typically G nepafenac × 2.

The Femto Step

All FLACS machines do the same three steps: continuous curvilinear capsulorrhexis (CCC), nuclear fragmentation, and corneal incisions. They all require that the eye be docked into a patient interface (PI) to stabilize the eye, and this enables precise delivery of laser energy as needed to the anterior capsule, lens nucleus, and cornea. There are variations in the type of docking between the major platforms, the most obvious being the single-piece docking device of the Lensx system (Alcon, Fort Worth, TX) (versus the two-piece docking devices of Catalys, Victus, Lensar, and the Ziemer Z8.

The Lensx PI has a proprietary contact lens inserted into the suction cup and this is lowered directly onto the eye, and suction is then applied. The other two-piece designs require that a suction ring or cup is first applied to the patient's eye and suction applied prior to the docking of the laser PI into this ring or cup.

Good, secure docking without tilt generally yields good femtolaser outcomes. But if there is significant tilt or inadequate suction, poor capsulorrhexis, nuclear fragmentation, or incision may result. One of the most important determinants of how easy or difficult a dock may be is the size of the palpebral aperture.

> ### Femto Tip 1
>
> - Avoid patients with narrow palpebral apertures and poorly dilating pupils, which may challenge the beginning FLACS surgeon.

Docking

The docking process is a critical step, as it stabilizes the eye and enables delivery of the femtolaser pulses in a controlled and precise manner. All the major FLACS platforms require docking, and there are two fundamentally different ways of docking: the single-piece patient interface, and the two-piece interface.

The Lensx utilizes a single-piece docking system in which no suction ring or cup is used; a speculum is used to open the palpebral aperture widely and the PI is lowered directly onto the patient's eye under direct visualization (**Fig. 17.1**).

The single-piece docking is very simple and intuitive to use, and even the surgeon who has no prior experience with laser-assisted in situ keratomileusis (LASIK) docking should find it straightforward. Viewing, centration, and applying suction on single-piece PIs is easy, as there is an unblocked view of the limbus (**Fig. 17.2**).

The patient who exhibits a strong Bell's reflex at the time of suction may end up with a decentered or tilted dock, and the surgeon needs to recognize this so that a re-dock can be performed.

The other FLACS platforms all utilize a two-piece patient interface in which a suction ring or cup is first applied to the patient's eye, usually without a speculum, and then approximated to the laser head (**Figs. 17.3** and **17.4**).

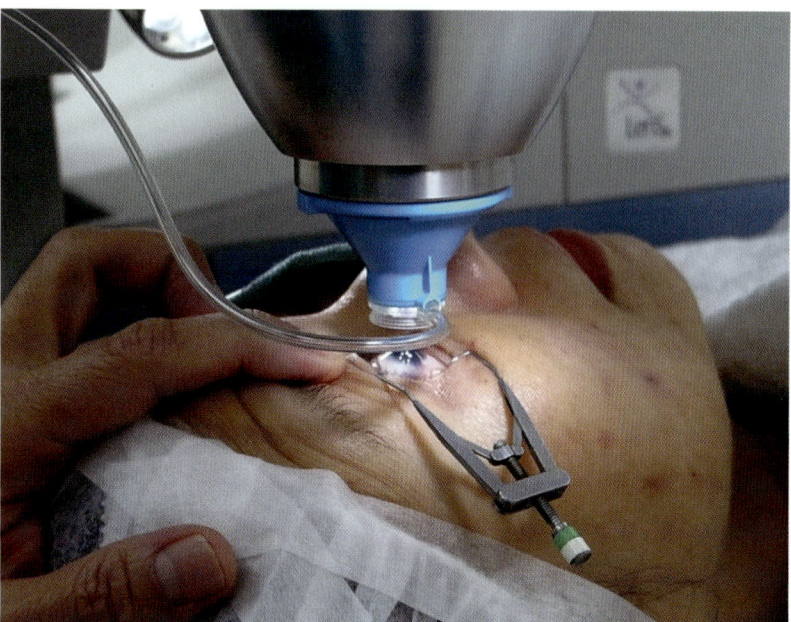

Fig. 17.1 The patient interface is lowered directly onto the eye.

Experienced LASIK surgeons who are familiar with placing a suction ring on the eye and then docking the PI will find the transition to two–piece docking extremely easy. Centration in two–piece docking systems is based on aligning the superior portion of the PI with the already applied suction ring or cup, and not the limbus (**Figs. 17.5** and **17.6**).

Certain femtolaser parameters are preset before docking, such as CCC size, nucleus fragmentation pattern and size, and incision size. Laser power and spot and layer separations are all designated at this stage. The placement of the CCC outline, the fragmentation depth, and the incision location for a particular

eye are then determined after docking. Some systems feature automated planning of these parameters, and some require manual input. Preferred CCC sizes average 5 mm. Nuclear fragmentation diameters are often 1 to 2 mm larger than the CCC size, and the posterior offset from the posterior capsule ranges from 500 to 700 µm. Incision widths are ~ 2.3 mm for main incisions and vary from 0.8 to 1.2 mm for the side port. Checking and confirming that all the above parameters are correct is vital, similar to the preflight checks that pilots perform prior to takeoff. Because even automated planning systems can have problems (e.g., a small pupil), it is good practice for the surgeon to know how to input and control these variables rather than relying on a technician.

The final stage of the femto step is the actual firing of the femtosecond laser itself, usually controlled by a foot pedal. Treatment starts with the CCC, continues with the nuclear fragmentation, and ends with corneal incisions and astigmatic keratotomies. Suction or vacuum is then turned off and the eye undocked.

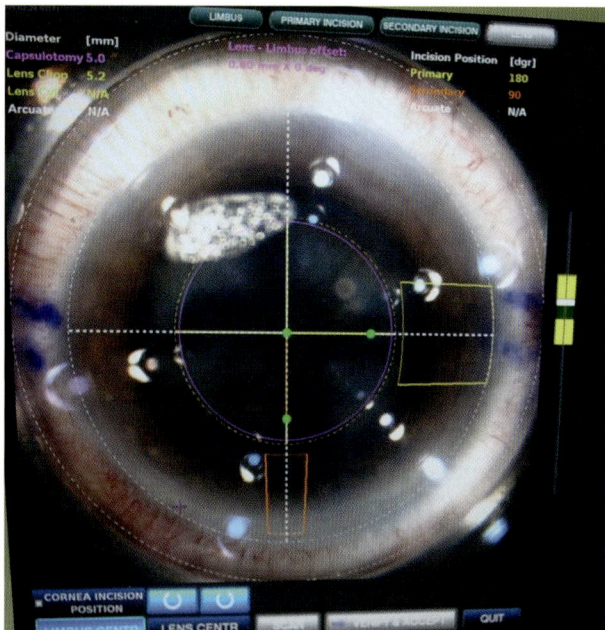

Fig. 17.2 A clear view of the limbus and landmarks with single-piece docking.

> **Femto Tip 2**
>
> • Once the femtolaser pedal is depressed, do not lift your foot or let it slip off the pedal, as some systems may not allow the treatment to continue. The eye then needs to be undocked and re-docked and the procedure started again.

Outcomes with the Femto Step

The FLACS procedure has been in clinical usage since 2011; in the first 3 years, the few systems available issued numerous software and hardware upgrades, all for the betterment of our patient outcomes. Patient interfaces have become smaller, treatment planning and delivery protocols have become quicker, and nuclear fragmentation patterns have become more sophisticated.

One concern when the eye is docked is the elevation in intraocular pressure (IOP), but the new-generation machines only raise the IOP between 10 and 17 mm Hg.[1] Another consideration is the amount of time that the patient's eye is subjected to this elevated pressure; this varies widely between the different

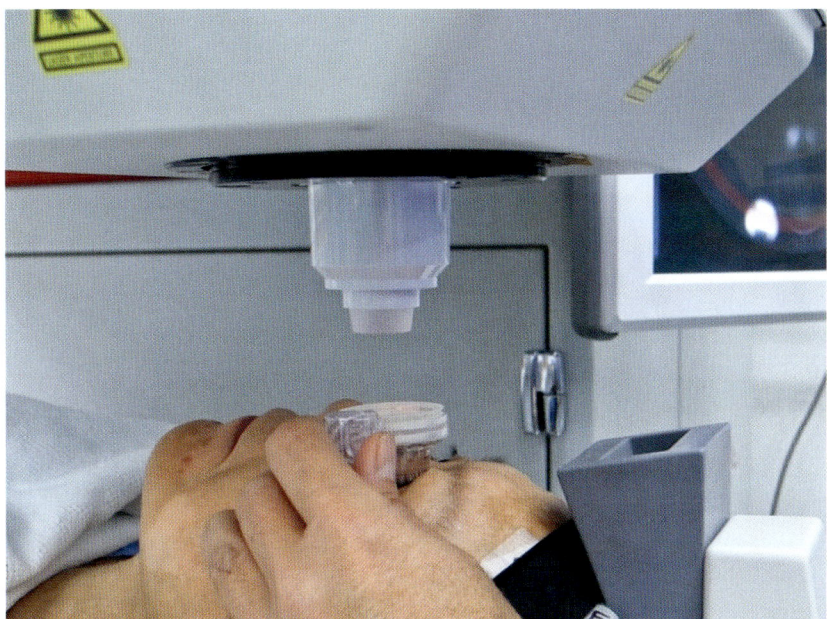

Fig. 17.3 The two-piece docking system with a suction cup.

platforms (1.5 to 3.5 minutes) and some platforms can take twice as long.[2] Although there is little danger to the optic nerve with such small elevations of IOP, prolonged suction-on times lead to greater patient discomfort and bruising, and may increase the risk of suction loss.

The Phaco Step

Although the femto step includes three main steps of CCC, nuclear fragmentation, and incisions, it would be naive to expect that the phaco step of the procedure would be simple. With any change in instrumentation, surgeons also needs to adapt their surgical technique, and so it is with FLACS.

First, the eye after the femto step is different in several ways (**Fig. 17.7**):

1. The pupil may be constricted.
2. Incisions are present.
3. There is a perfectly round but white-edged CCC.
4. The fragmentation pattern is visible.
5. Gas is present anteriorly and deep within the lens.

The Pupil with Miosis

About 20 to 25% of all eyes show a constricted pupil (likely prostaglandin mediated) to some extent after the femto step.[3] This is

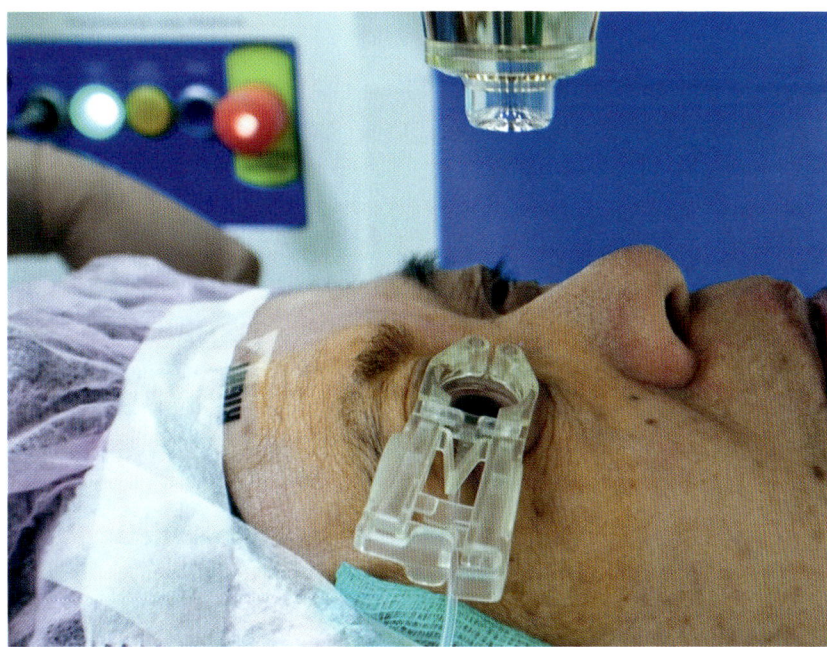

Fig. 17.4 The two-piece docking system with a suction ring.

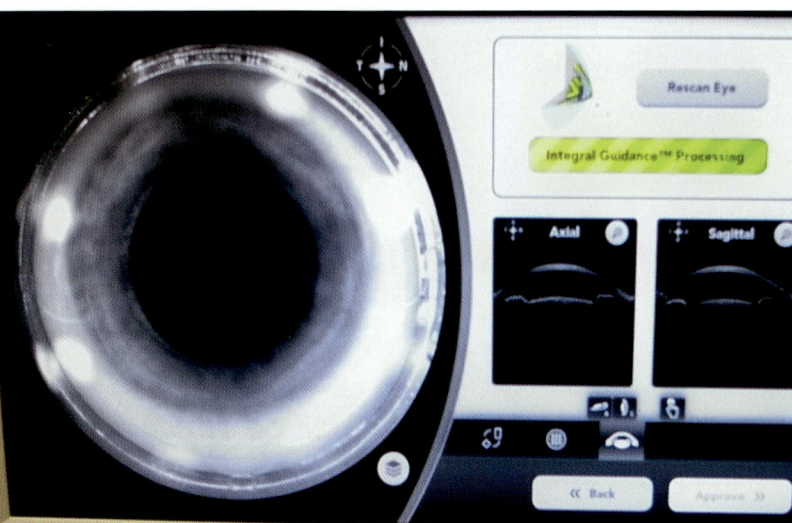

Fig. 17.5 The view of the eye after docking with a water bath in the suction cup.

obviously disconcerting, especially if a 2- to 3-mm pupil results, making it difficult to assess the completeness of the CCC and to fragment the nucleus **(Fig. 17.8)**. If this happens, use an ophthalmic viscosurgical device (OVD) to enlarge the pupil or a Kuglen hook to push aside the iris so that the quality of the CCC can be ascertained before proceeding. It is much better to prevent this situation, and the use of a preoperative drop of NSAID with the dilating drops is most useful in eradicating this problem.[4]

Femto Tip 3

- Apply your preferred NSAID with the dilating drops in your preoperative medication.

Femtolaser Incisions

One of the three fundamental capabilities of FLACS is the creation of the main and side-port incisions as well as astigmatic keratotomies (AK). Femtolaser-created incisions are similar to femtolaser-created LASIK flaps; they can be adherent and require some effort to open. Two problems that may be encountered by the beginning FLACS surgeon are (1) imprecise placement of incisions, and (2) difficulty in opening FLACS incisions. With better sizing of suction cups and rings and software improvements in incision placement, FLACS incision creation is now a routine part of the procedure.

Undoubtedly, the most important point about opening a FLACS incision is to have the right spatula with the right profile and bevel for that particular incision. It is worth noting that most side-port incisions angle slightly downward at about 10 degrees, whereas many main-port configurations angle downward at about 40 degrees for the first plane before flattening out to about 10 degrees. I therefore designed a double-ended spatula taking into consideration these angles (AE2332, Asico, Westmont, IL; I have no financial interest in this product). I usually perform 0.9-mm-wide side-port incision and a 2.3-mm-wide main-port incision. Some surgeons favor bimanual irrigation and aspiration (I/A), and they require a much larger side port of 1.2 mm. The

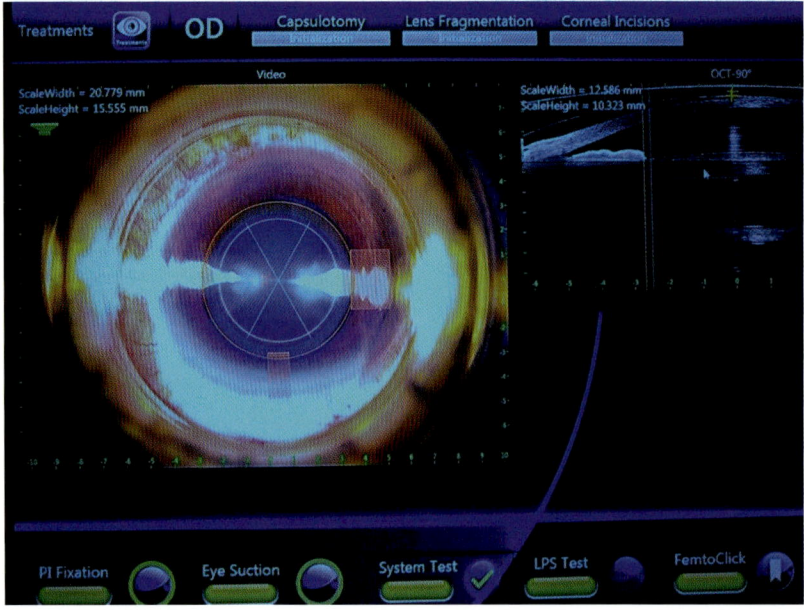

Fig. 17.6 Another view of the eye after docking in the two-piece docking system with a suction ring.

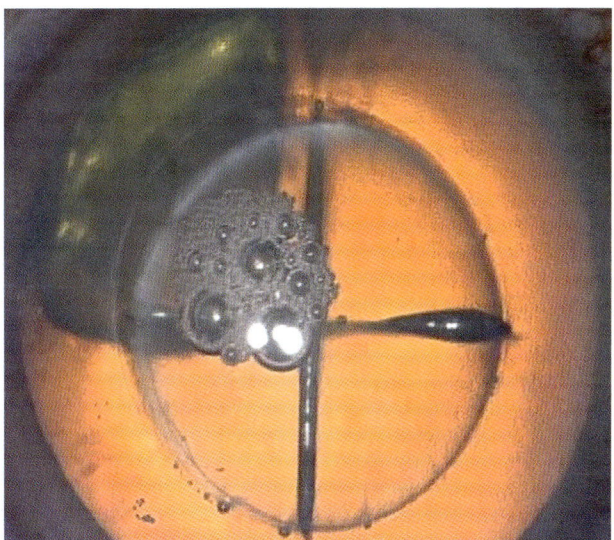

Fig. 17.7   The femtolasered eye looks different.

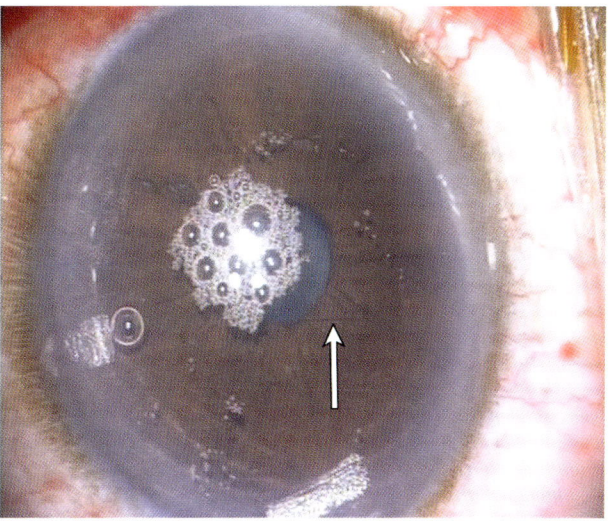

Fig. 17.8   Miosis after the femto step. Note the edge of the lifted capsule at the 4 o'clock position (*arrow*).

more difficult incision to open is always the smaller side-port incision, so I invariably start with this. Place the spatula just proximal to the external opening of the incision, press downward and forward while moving the spatula tip left and right, and entry is usually easily effected (**Figs. 17.9** and **17.10**).

Some surgeons advocate injecting OVD through this side port prior to opening the main port; I have found it difficult achieving a good OVD fill by injecting through the side port, as the eye is watertight at this stage, and I prefer to go ahead with opening the main incision next in the same way, using the other end of the spatula I designed. When this is open, I then inject OVD to re-form the chamber, prior to removing the free anterior capsular disk.

Femto Tip 4

- Use appropriate femto-phaco–designed spatulae to open the FLACS incisions.

Femtolaser Incisional Issues

If the FLACS incisions are badly positioned, usually too central, it is best not to use them and to create new surgical incisions using a blade. FLACS incisions will also not be patent if positioned within areas of white arcus senilis or over a pterygium!

Some surgeons like to "flare" the internal opening of the main incision such that the external opening is 2.3 mm and the internal may be 2.5 mm. I have found that this can lead to excessive wound hydration, and so I no longer flare my incisions internally (**Fig. 17.11**).

Femtolaser Continuous Curvilinear Capsulorhexis

The circularity and precise positioning of the capsulorhexis is the main raison d'être for the interest in FLACS. Depending on the surgeon's preference, the CCC may be designated as 4.5 to 5.5 mm in diameter, with 5 mm being a popular choice. Ideally,

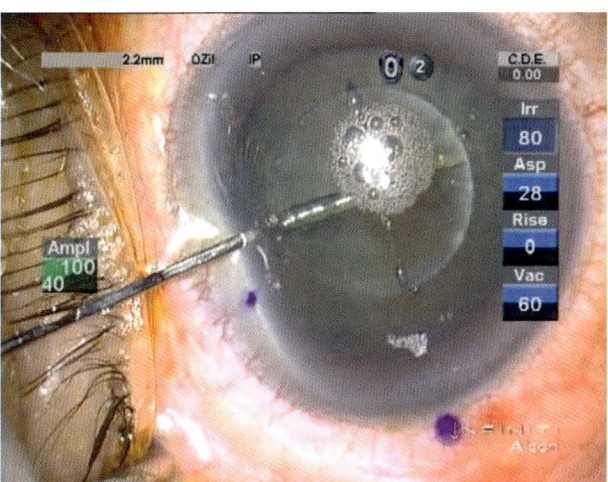

Fig. 17.9   Downward and forward pressure with slight side-to-side movement.

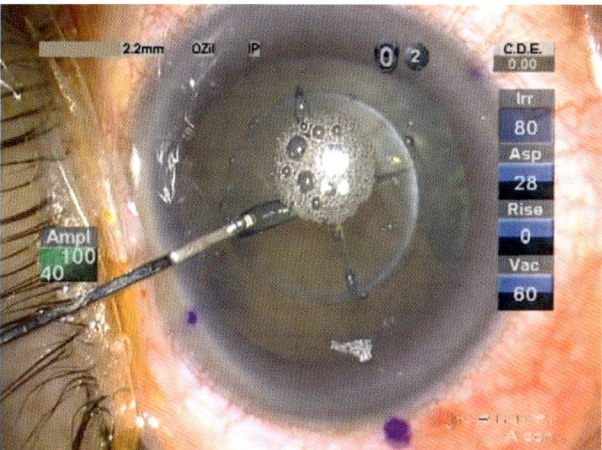

Fig. 17.10   Entry into the anterior chamber. Note how the surgeon's fingers do not obstruct the surgical field of view due to the optimal angled design of the spatula.

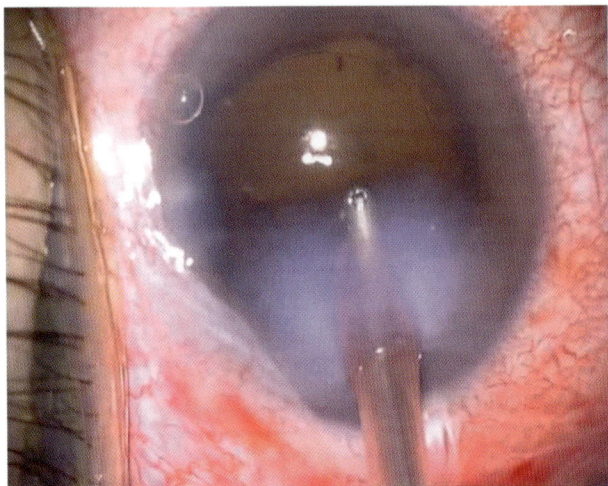

Fig. 17.11 Excessive wound hydration with too flared an internal opening.

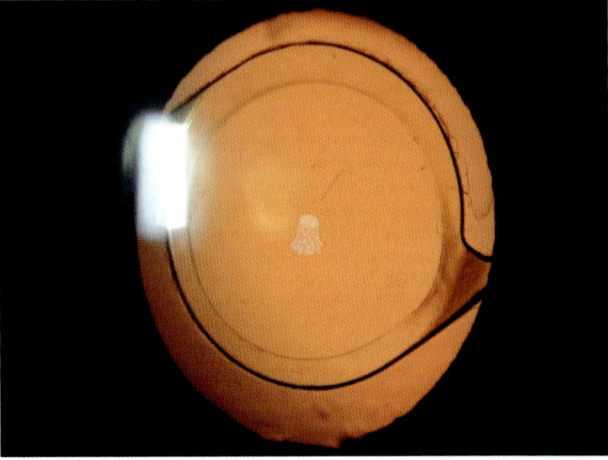

Fig. 17.12 A round continuous curvilinear capsulorrhexis (CCC) with ideal overlap of the lens optic.

the size chosen should enable the lens implant to have symmetrical capsular cover of the edge for 360 degrees, resulting in better effective lens positions (**Fig. 17.12**).

What the CCC should be centered on, though, is a matter of some debate—pupil centered, scanned capsule, or limbus?

In the early days of FLACS, there was some concern about the integrity and strength of the femtolasered CCC. This was because some platforms applanated the cornea, resulting in corneal folds and consequent obstruction of the laser beam. This in turn led to unlasered portions of the anterior capsule with capsular tags and bridges being present. Inadvertent aspiration and traction of these tags and bridges occasionally led to anterior radial tears, which became a potentially serious problem if they extended to the posterior capsule. Thankfully, with improved software and hardware, the incidence of incomplete femtolaser CCCs is now very low, and many surgeons report completely free and round anterior capsules after a femtolaser CCC in 95 to 97% of all cases.[5] Nevertheless, there are a few modifications in technique that the beginning FLACS surgeon needs to be aware of.

When the femtolaser is cutting the capsule, the surgeon can assess the completeness of the CCC. If there is any area where the femtolaser might not have cut the capsule, then under the operating microscope the surgeon should examine the CCC outline more carefully at that point and exercise more care in removing the capsule.

If the capsule looks to be well cut by the femtolaser, then the "dimple-down" technique as described by Dick's group[6] is useful. In this technique, downward pressure on the center of the anterior capsular flap pulls the edge of the circular flap away from the remaining capsule, like an umbrella closing (**Fig. 17.13**).

Complications of Femtolaser Continuous Curvilinear Capsulorrhexis

The completeness of the femtolaser CCC is arguably the most important issue regarding the FLACS procedure, failing which there may be problems such as radial tears with posterior extension and poor lens position.

In an obvious case of a large uncut segment of capsule (**Fig. 17.14**), management is straightforward; just grasp the edge of the cut capsular flap and complete a manual capsulorrhexis, ideally describing a larger diameter arc than originally intended so that when it joins back with the cut capsule, a smooth joint results without a linear tag.

For smaller uncut segments, one can easily leave a tag behind; the tag is easily removed later (**Figs. 17.15, 17.16, 17.17**). Careful attention to these tags will reduce the likelihood of anterior radial tears.

Problems arise when there may be hidden tags at the edge of the CCC. Aspiration of these hidden tags or excessive force on the subincisional CCC edge may lead to anterior capsular radial tears (**Fig. 17.18**).

An anterior radial capsular tear is undesirable, but in itself, if managed properly, does not necessarily lead to posterior extension and difficulty implanting an intraocular lens (IOL). Awareness of the radial tear having occurred necessitates the use of gentler surgical parameters and preservation of anterior chamber stability; these steps will reduce the likelihood of posterior extension.

Femto Tip 5

- Be mindful of areas where there may be uncut capsule after the femtolaser step, and, when doing I/A of cortex, aspirate a little beyond the edge of the CCC to avoid catching unseen tags.

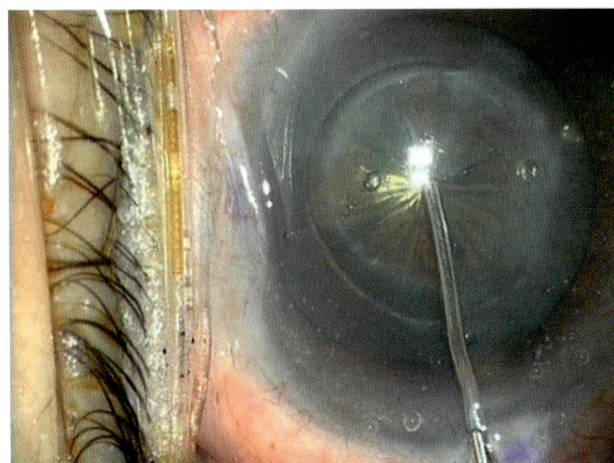

Fig. 17.13 The dimple-down technique of Dick.

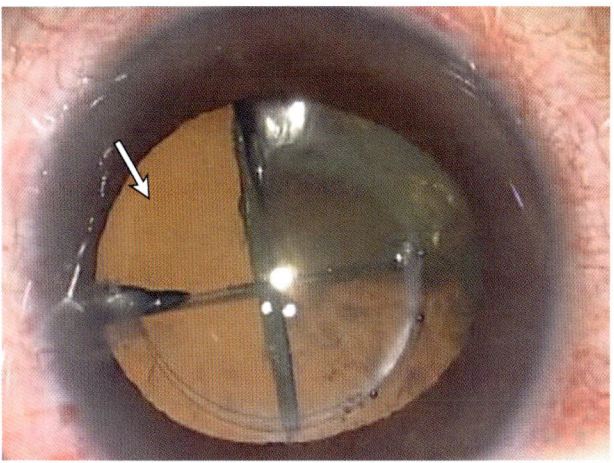

Fig. 17.14 An obvious area of at least 25% uncut capsule *(arrow)*.

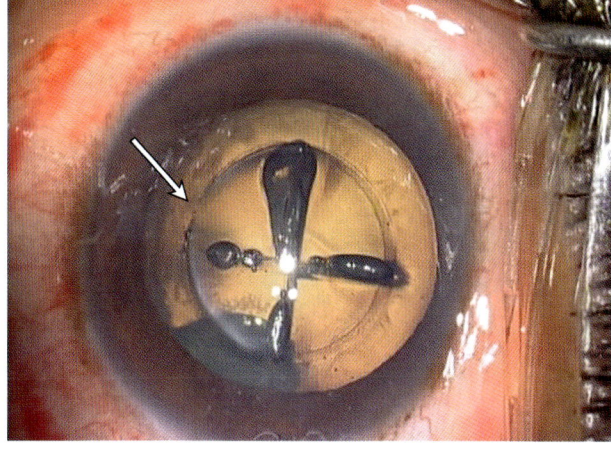

Fig. 17.15 A small uncut segment at the 10 o'clock position *(arrow)*.

The strength of the femtolaser CCC is the subject of controversy, with some authors claiming weakness compared with conventional manual CCCs, and others claiming greater strength. Whatever the truth is, the beginning FLACS surgeon needs to be mindful of the CCC as described above and consider using bimanual I/A to reduce stressing the edge of the subincisional capsule. There are, however, reports emerging of surgeons using capsular hooks successfully on femtolaser-created CCCs.[7]

Hydrodissection

A freely mobile nucleus is desirable during the phaco step. Hence, hydrodissection is still an important step in FLACS. Hydrodissection is arguably easier to perform after the femto step, as there is usually an element of pneumo-dissection caused by gas formation. However, the very presence of this gas is also a reason for being extra cautious when performing hydrodissection in FLACS, as one of the first major FLACS complications reported was that of dropped nuclei related to hydrorupture of the posterior capsule, in two cases.[8] The hydrorupture occurred as the presence of gas in the perinuclear area increased the pressure within the capsular bag such that even normal hydrodissection forces resulted in hydrorupture of the posterior capsule. With

greater understanding of the forces within the lens after the femto step, we now know that it is important to burp some gas out from behind the nucleus, creating space for the hydrodissecting fluid (**Fig. 17.19**). There have been no further reports of dropped nuclei since then.

Femto Tip 6

- Depress the nucleus to release gas into the anterior chamber prior to hydrodissection

Nucleus Management

It may be erroneously assumed that the femtolaser having fragmented the nucleus would make the nucleus removal quicker and safer when compared with standard phaco. What is often not appreciated is that although the nucleus has been femtolaser fragmented, this fragmentation is incomplete, particularly with regard to the posterior part of the nucleus. This is because all FLACS platforms have an anterior safety offset of between 500 and 700 µm from the posterior capsule. So what we are left with is a fairly anterior pattern of a quadrant or cylinders or grids

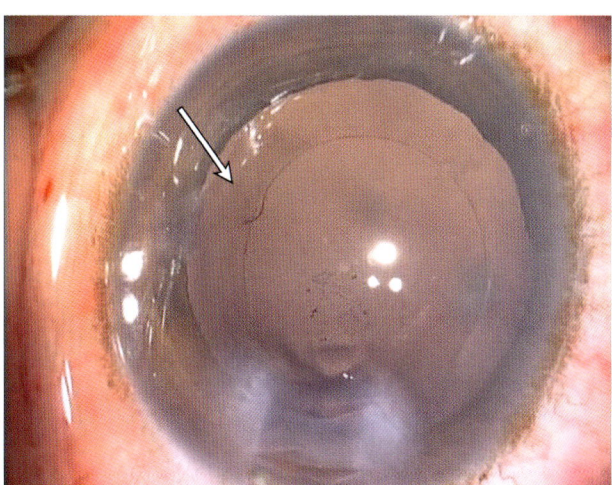

Fig. 17.16 An obvious tag *(arrow)* after removal of the central capsule.

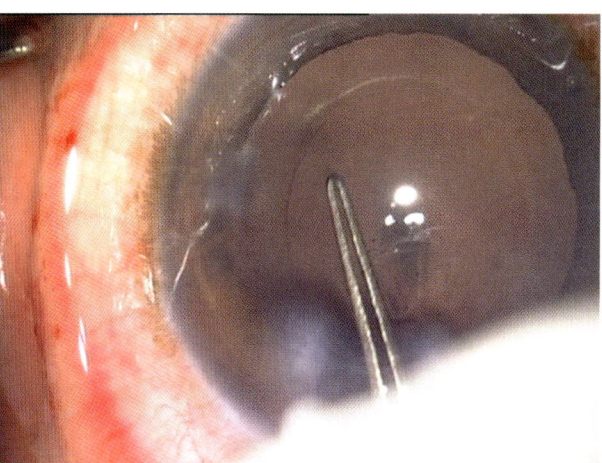

Fig. 17.17 Gently tearing off the tag restores the smoothness of the capsulotomy.

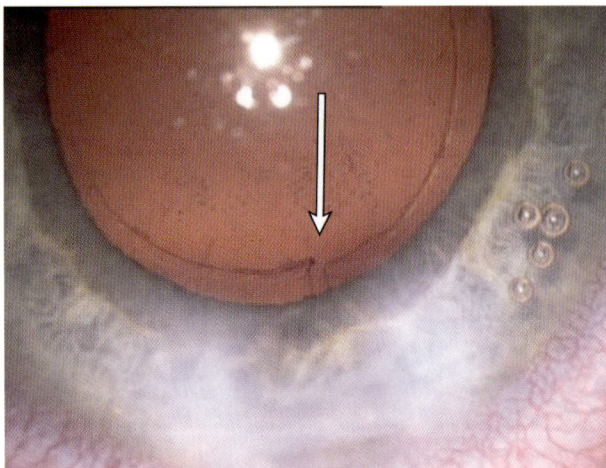

Fig. 17.18   An anterior radial capsular tear *(arrow)*.

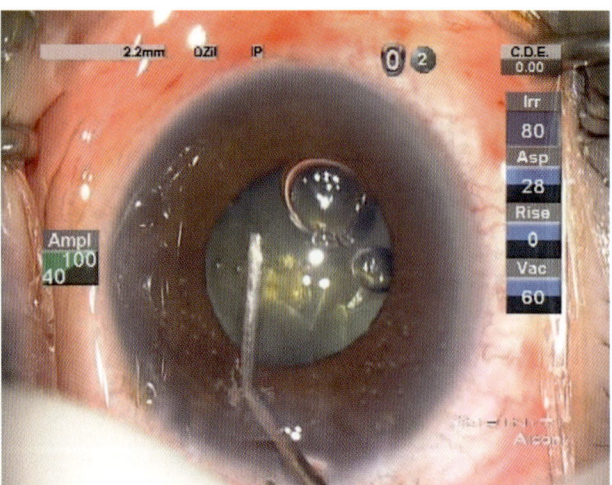

Fig. 17.19   Depressing the nucleus to burp gas out.

with the common denominator of an unfragmented posterior nuclear plate. This can lead to problems, especially with softer nuclei.

A fundamental principle of standard phacoemulsification is that chopping reduces the size of the nucleus to manageable, bite-sized pieces of nucleus that are then easily emulsified. This is no less true in FLACS. One of the most important maneuvers when removing the nucleus, therefore, is to ensure complete separation of the nuclear quadrants.

The simplest way of doing this is to phaco a little bit into the heart of the nucleus and then chop along the femtolasered lines with a chopper or to phaco a groove as in a stop-and-chop procedure and then just pushing the hemi-nuclei apart. This still expends ultrasonic energy, which begs the question of why an expensive laser was purchased in the first place!

The principle of prechopping an intact nucleus was introduced by Takayuki Akahoshi of Japan in 1994, when he won a prize at the American Society of Cataract and Refractive Surgery (ASCRS) film festival for his film "Phaco Prechop."[9] Prechopping and femtolaser fragmentation of the nucleus is a marriage made in heaven. One of the difficulties with prechopping an intact nucleus is that in denser cataracts, it is not possible to insert the prechopper into the heart of the nucleus without using a counter-prechopper. However, in the FLACS procedure, separation planes of cleavage have already been created by the laser, and it is much easier to insert a prechopper and then crack the nucleus. Although the standard prechopper designs (e.g., Combo prechopper) can be used, a new prechopper called the "paddle prechopper" (AE4294, Asico), which is specially designed for femto-prechopping, is easy to use and safe, as it takes away the sharp point of the combo prechopper. Femto-prechopping can be used in conjunction with the four-quadrant fragmentation pattern or with any of the newer grid or matrix patterns offered by the manufacturers (**Figs. 17.20** and **17.21**). When prechopping on a grid fragmentation pattern, the prechopper can be inserted into any of the linear grooves, although it is best to insert it into a groove as central as possible (**Figs. 17.22** and **17.23**).

To perform femto-prechopping, first hydrodissect adequately as described above, then inject OVD to gently push aside the lens cortex and expose the anterior surface of the nucleus. Insert the prechopper gently into the groove that is in alignment with the incision, and open the prechopper, which will crack the nucleus into two halves. Using the prechopper, the nucleus can then be rotated 90 degrees and the same maneuver done for the second crack, resulting in four free quadrants.

Using the paddle prechopper to divide the nucleus into four quadrants effectively addresses the issue of the intact posterior nuclear plate, and it is then very straightforward to pull each quadrant out of the bag using vacuum on the phaco tip. In very dense nuclei, it is sometimes difficult to insert the prechopper into the groove, and if resistance is encountered, the surgeon should desist and revert to grooving or chopping techniques.

Femto Tip 7

- Use a prechopper to divide the femto-fragmented nucleus into quadrants to facilitate phacoemulsification.

There are any number of fragmentation patterns that the different platforms can generate in femto-fragmenting the nucleus.

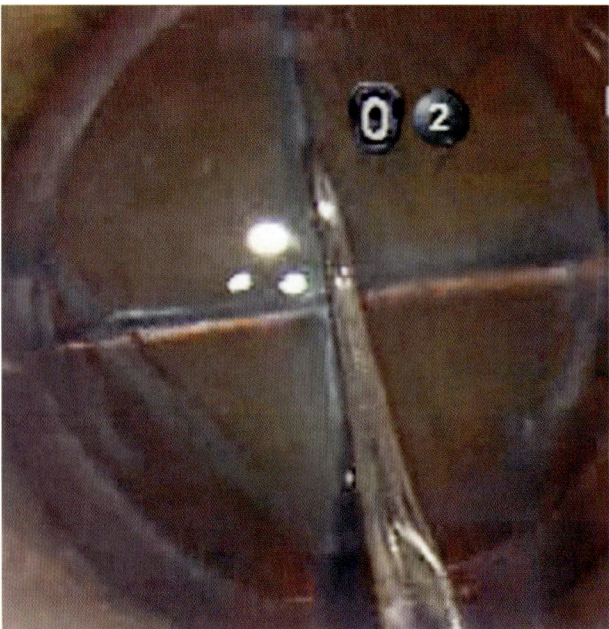

Fig. 17.20   Inserting a prechopper into the femto groove.

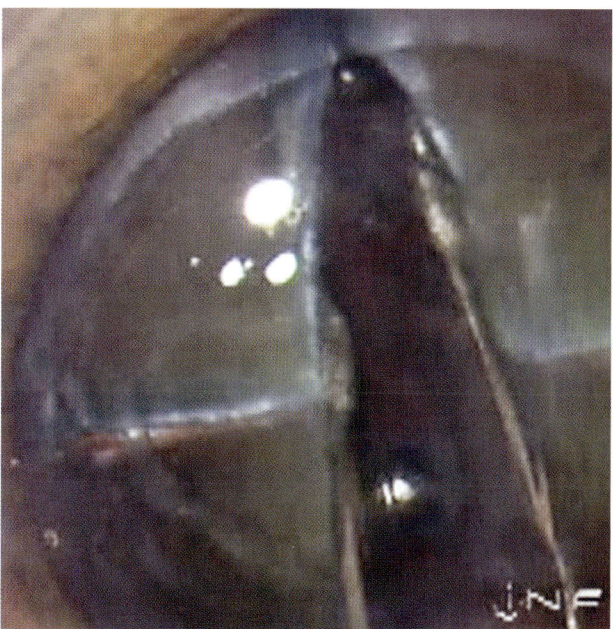

Fig. 17.21 Spreading a prechopper.

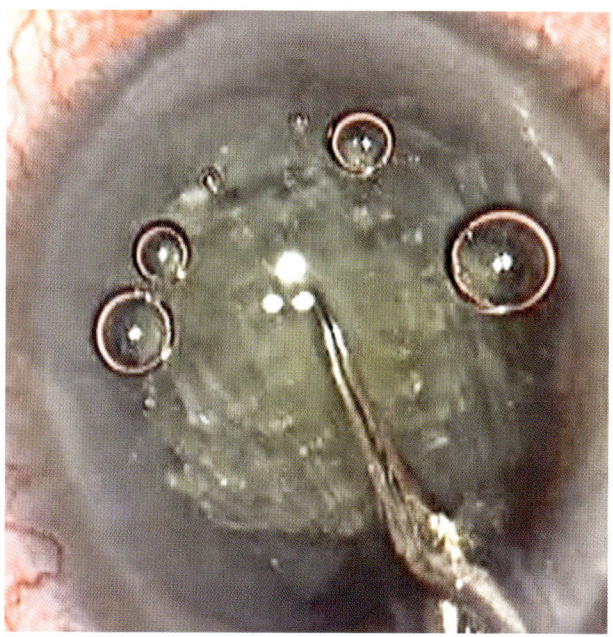

Fig. 17.22 Inserting a prechopper into grid.

The most popular are the four, six, or eight segment patterns with or without cylindrical patterns and a grid, a matrix, or "french-fry" patterns. Using the grid pattern to soften a nucleus may reduce the amount of energy needed to remove a harder nucleus, but for the softer nuclei, the surgeon needs to be mindful that the nucleus will be harder to grip and crack, as there is a tendency for the phaco tip to burrow through the cubes and only grip the peripheral rim. There is also less resistance to pushing apart and separating nuclear segments. The prechopping technique mentioned above addresses this issue very well. One other limitation of using the grid pattern is that the surgeon's view of the edge of the femtolasered CCC is often obscured by the pattern.

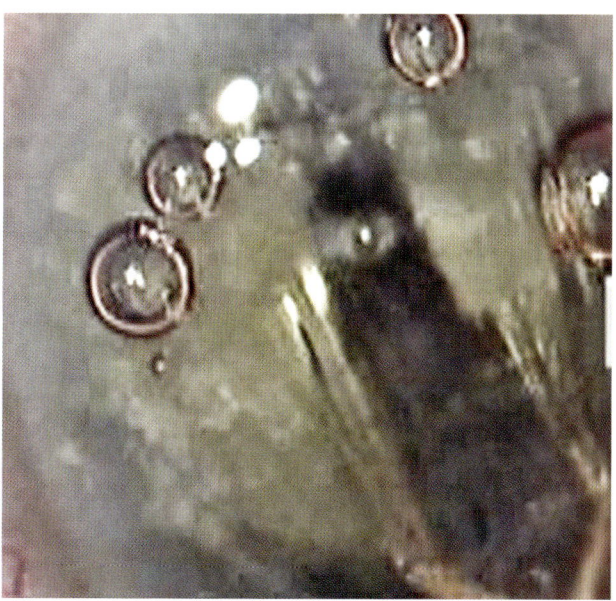

Fig. 17.23 Spreading a prechopper.

Irrigation and Aspiration of Cortex

In FLACS, I/A is often described as being difficult. I believe that it is different but not really any more difficult than I/A in phaco. The main difference is that there is some adhesion of the edge of the cut underlying cortex to the CCC edge, manifest as the whitened rim of the CCC. The surgeon, therefore, needs to aspirate cortex from the back of the anterior capsule in a sweeping side-to-side motion to free the cortex prior to aspiration. As mentioned previously, it is safer to aspirate a little beyond the very edge of the CCC so that the risk of aspirating a hidden tag is reduced (**Fig. 17.24**).

Finally, some surgeons prefer to use a bimanual I/A technique to remove subincisional cortex; this has the advantage of easier access to the subincisional area and arguably stressing the edge of the CCC less. The disadvantage is that two side ports, each ~ 1.2 mm wide, are needed for bimanual I/A. A "mini-I/A" cannula can also be used through the side port to free the subincisional cortex.

> **Femto Tip 8**
>
> • Aspirate a little beyond the edge of the femto CCC and sweep the cannula from side to side to engage and free the lens cortex from the back of the anterior capsular rim

Intraocular Lens implantation

This step is no different from standard phaco surgery except that the lens almost invariably is beautifully centered and covered symmetrically by the femto CCC.

Unique FLACS Complications

Apart from the complications mentioned in the individual sections above, there are several other complications unique to

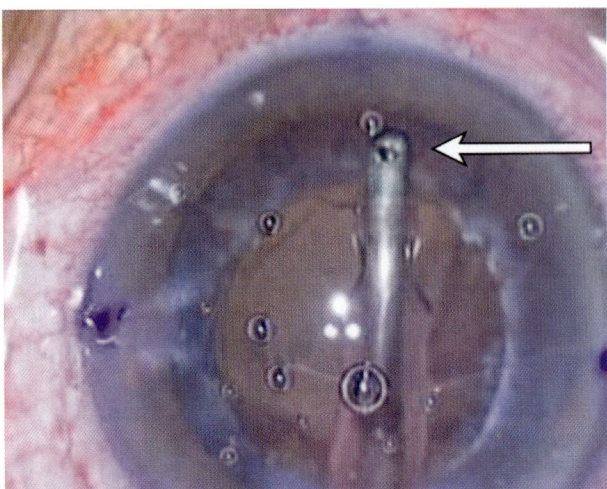

Fig. 17.24 Aspirating beyond the whitened edge of the femto CCC *(arrow)*.

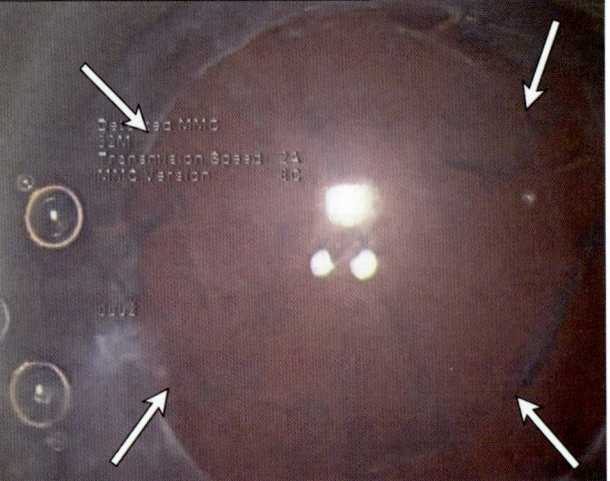

Fig. 17.25 Lost circular anterior cap found under the cornea *(arrows)*.

FLACS, such as the lost free anterior capsular cap. In one case, after opening the incisions, OVD was inadvertently injected under the free cap, which pushed it against the back of the cornea, and its presence there was only detected after the nucleus was removed (**Fig. 17.25**).

With cubing or grid fragmentation patterns, small cubes or "french fries" are created, and these small blocks of nucleus may nestle in the anterior chamber angle or in the ciliary sulcus, resulting in a higher risk of retained nuclear fragments, leading to chronic uveitis or localized corneal edema (**Fig. 17.26**).

Conclusion

As phacoemulsification replaced planned extracapsular cataract extraction, so I believe it will be with FLACS, as it assumes greater prominence over the next decade. In transiting from phacoemulsification to FLACS, the surgeon needs to be aware that some modifications in technique are needed to ensure smooth and safe surgery. It is still important for the FLACS surgeon to have acquired the manual skills of a phaco surgeon, for there are many situations in FLACS where these skills are needed.

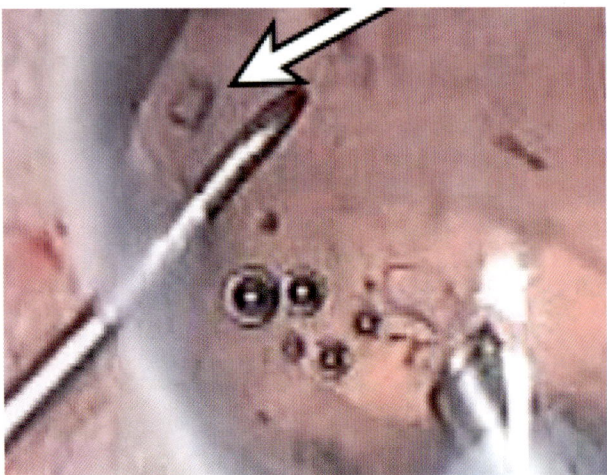

Fig. 17.26 A rectangular block of nucleus *(arrow)* after grid fragmentation.

References

1. Donaldson KE, Braga-Mele R, Cabot F, et al; ASCRS Refractive Cataract Surgery Subcommittee. Femtosecond laser-assisted cataract surgery. J Cataract Refract Surg 2013;39:1753–1763

2. Yeoh R. Practical differences between 3 femtosecond phaco laser platforms. J Cataract Refract Surg 2014;40:510

3. Nagy ZZ, Takacs AI, Filkorn T, et al. Complications of femtosecond laser-assisted cataract surgery. J Cataract Refract Surg 2014;40:20–28

4. Yeoh R. Intraoperative miosis in femtosecond laser-assisted cataract surgery. J Cataract Refract Surg 2014;40:852–853

5. Roberts TV, Lawless M, Bali SJ, Hodge C, Sutton G. Surgical outcomes and safety of femtosecond laser cataract surgery: a prospective study of 1500 consecutive cases. Ophthalmology 2013;120:227–233

6. Arbisser LB, Schultz T, Dick HB. Central dimple-down maneuver for consistent continuous femtosecond laser capsulotomy. J Cataract Refract Surg 2013;39:1796–1797

7. Grewal DS, Basti S, Singh Grewal SP. Femtosecond laser-assisted cataract surgery in a subluxated traumatic cataract. J Cataract Refract Surg 2014;40:1239–1240

8. Roberts TV, Sutton G, Lawless MA, Jindal-Bali S, Hodge C. Capsular block syndrome associated with femtosecond laser-assisted cataract surgery. J Cataract Refract Surg 2011;37:2068–2070

9. Akahoshi T. Phaco Prechop. 1994 American Society of Cataract and Refractive Surgery Film Festival, new techniques category, runner up prize

18 Conversion to Extracapsular Cataract Extraction

Anya Gushchin, Sanduk Ruit, and Geoffrey Tabin

Planned extracapsular cataract extraction (ECCE) is a technique that involves removal of an intact crystalline lens from the eye through a large incision without disturbing the integrity of the posterior capsule and zonules. It is also an important technique to master for cases in which a nucleus is not amenable to phacoemulsification or there is a need to convert from a small-incision phacoemulsification procedure to safely extract the lens. Manual small-incision cataract surgery (MSICS) is a low-cost, highly efficient, high-quality procedure first described in 1994; it is an excellent solution for black or brunescent cataracts. It does not have the same limitations as phaco surgery, with increased surgical time and ultrasound energy required to break the dense nuclear material typical of advanced cataracts. In cases of dense nuclei, this technique may be preferable to avoid endothelial damage and corneal edema. The advantages of MSICS over standard ECCE are that it entails a much smaller, self-sealing incision that essentially eliminates the need to suture the wound, and therefore decreases the surgically induced astigmatism, and improves the vision recovery and long-term wound stability.

Other situations where MSICS is preferable as a primary method of lens extraction is in cases of zonular laxity. In the divide-and-conquer technique, excessive stress may be placed on the bag-zonular complex, which can lead to capsular rupture. A thickened posterior plate of the lens can also be very difficult to disassemble in piecemeal lens extraction. These challenges can be avoided by MSICS. When performed by an experienced surgeon, the technique will take 5 minutes or less, and it treats the thickest and blackest cataracts with minimal zonular and endothelial stress.

When performing MSICS, fewer instruments are required (**Table 18.1**). The incision can be made from a temporal or superior approach, typically guided by keratometry measurements or by surgeon preference. A temporal tunnel is preferred over a superior tunnel due to the effective decrease in against-the-rule astigmatism. This position also minimizes the effect of a prominent brow or enophthalmos on proper instrument handling and improves intraoperative exposure and red reflex visualization.

Manual Sutureless Small-Incision Cataract Surgery Technique

To gain better surgical exposure and aid in the nucleus delivery step, a bridle suture may be helpful. If the surgeon elects a superior approach, a 4-0 silk bridle suture is placed beneath the superior rectus tendon, and for a temporal approach a bridle of the lateral rectus may be used. A bridle suture is not required in all cases where there is good surgical exposure.

The next step is wound construction—creation of a fornix-based conjunctival flap of ~ 7 mm in length, taking care to displace the Tenon's capsule. Light cautery may be used in this step to stop any bleeders. The external scleral incision is placed 1.5 mm from the limbus and at a 50% depth. A bevel-up crescent blade is then advanced parallel to the ocular surface to extend the tunnel 1.5 mm into clear cornea. The external incision should be 5.5 to 7.0 mm in length, depending on the size of nucleus. The internal portion fans out to 9.0 mm, yielding a trapezoidal incision with a wider base facing the anterior chamber and tapering narrower toward the external incision (**Fig. 18.1**). This conical, multiplanar tunnel construction enables a smooth delivery of a large, dense nucleus through a self-sealing wound. A larger nucleus will require a slightly larger tunnel profile. Avoid premature entry into the anterior chamber at this point. The depth of the tunnel is very important: too shallow and there is risk of button-holing and wound instability, but too deep and there is risk of premature entry and iris prolapse.

After creating a corneal tunnel, the anterior chamber is filled with viscoelastic and a large curvilinear capsulotomy is created with or without relaxing incisions. The size of the capsulorrhexis will need to have a minimum diameter of 5 to 6 mm up to 7 to 8 mm, depending on the size of the cataract. A capsulorrhexis that is too small for the size of the nucleus will need to be converted to a "can-opener" capsulotomy by adding four or more radial relaxing incisions to afford easy nucleus delivery into the anterior chamber. The capsulorrhexis is usually accomplished through a paracentesis incision. Alternatively, a small entry wound could be made through the sclerocorneal incision to accommodate a cystotome (**Fig. 18.2**). After an adequate capsulorrhexis is created, a 3.2-mm angled keratome is used to enter the anterior chamber and to extend the wound from side to side for the full extent of the internal tunnel. Care must be taken to keep the incision in one plane. The nucleus is prolapsed into the anterior chamber by hydrodissection, viscoelastic, Sinskey hook, or a Simcoe cannula (**Fig. 18.3**). One should preplace additional viscoelastic around the nucleus to protect the endothelium from injury in the nuclear expression step. At the conclusion, the nucleus is gently delivered through the tunnel using viscoelastic or fluid pressure.

After safely delivering the nucleus, a Simcoe cannula or another irrigation and aspiration (I/A) device can be used to remove cortex and epinucleus. After cortical cleanup, the bag is reinflated with viscoelastic, and a 6-mm lens can be placed through the tunnel without folding, taking care not to damage the endothelium. Occasionally, a surgeon may opt to preplace the lens at an earlier step in the surgery if the capsular bag is unstable. In that situation, the haptics of the rigid polymethylmethacrylate (PMMA) lens act as a capsular tension ring and protect the bag and zonules during cortical removal. If a V-capsulotomy was performed at the beginning of the surgery, the flap is severed with Vannas scissors to avoid obstruction of the visual axis. The viscoelastic is then removed with the use of a Simcoe or I/A cannula, and the anterior chamber reformed with balanced salt solution (BSS) on a 27-gauge cannula. If a watertight wound was created, no sutures are necessary. This is verified by pressing

Table 18.1 Instruments for Manual Sutureless Small-Incision Cataract Surgery

Tray	Toothed 0.12 Forceps	Cautery (Low-Temp or Wet-Field)
Gauze pads	Bevel-up crescent blade	25- to 27-gauge needle
5% betadine	Microkeratome blade	1-mL syringe
Eyelid speculum	Viscoelastic	3-mL syringe
4-0 silk	27-gauge cannula	Sinskey hook
Needle driver	Corrugated Simcoe irrigation and aspiration cannula	Posterior chamber intraocular lens
Superior rectus forceps	Tying forceps	Microscope
Westcott scissors	Long blade Vannas scissors	

down on the central cornea and noting no wound distortion or collapse of anterior chamber. At the conclusion of the procedure, the conjunctiva is replaced back to the limbus and reapposed either with cautery or a single interrupted suture.

In the following situations, MSICS should be considered as primary surgery:

1. Morgagnian and brown or black cataract
2. Pseudoexfoliation, weak zonules, poor pupil dilation
3. Subluxed lenses
4. Phacolytic glaucoma
5. Shallow anterior chamber
6. Poor visibility due to corneal scar or milky liquefied cortex

These scenarios are well suited for small-incision cataract surgery (SICS) with some additional precautions. In a morgagnian cataract with a fibrotic capsule and poor visibility, if a continuous curvilinear capsulotomy is not achievable, an envelope or V-capsulotomy could be performed instead (**Fig. 18.4**). This is accomplished by introducing a 27-gauge needle and making a linear cut with the bevel tip from the 4 to 12 o'clock positions and the 8 to 12 o'clock positions (if sitting superiorly) to create a triangular V-shaped flap with apex oriented toward the surgeon.

Place each point of the triangle ~ 3 mm from the center of the pupil. The flap is then lifted to verify that it is connected at the apex, and gentle hydrodissection is employed to hydro-rotate the nucleus out of the bag. Delivering the nucleus with a bimanual technique using a spatula can protect the bag or iris. Use the sweep below and a Sinskey hook from above. Another trick is to preplace the intraocular lens into the capsular bag under the viscoelastic to aid in nucleus expression while protecting the capsular bag from coming forward.

In cases of pseudoexfoliation, poor pupil dilation, posterior synechiae, shallow chamber, phacodonesis, or subluxed lenses, there is an increase in difficulty, but these patients are still very well suited for the SICS method. Small sphincterotomies can be made to facilitate nuclear expression and minimize zonular trauma. If the iris is poorly dilated and floppy, iris edges could be gently brought out through small, equally spaced paracentesis incisions with a Sinskey hook, effectively enlarging the pupil as a Malyugin ring would, without impeding fluidics of whole lens extraction.

In cases with phacolytic glaucoma, weakened zonules, and poor visibility from elevated pressure, the additional factors could be controlled by initially lowering the intraocular pressure with preoperative mannitol or by applying pressure on the globe for 10 minutes after peri/retrobulbar block. A Simcoe cannula is also

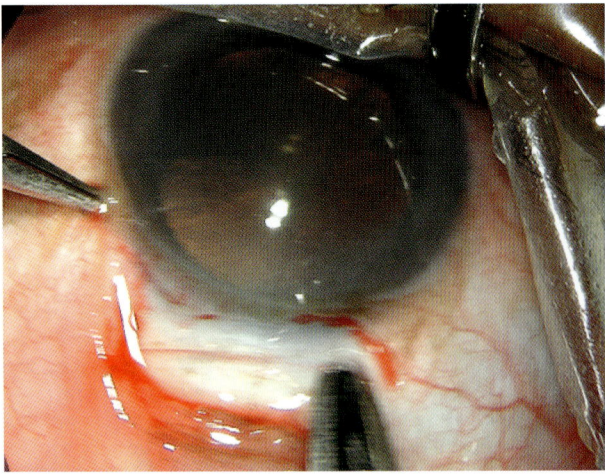

Fig. 18.1 An external scleral incision is made at 50% depth, 1.5 mm back from the limbus. Then turn the Beaver blade with the heel parallel to the surface of the globe to advance another 1.5 mm into clear cornea.

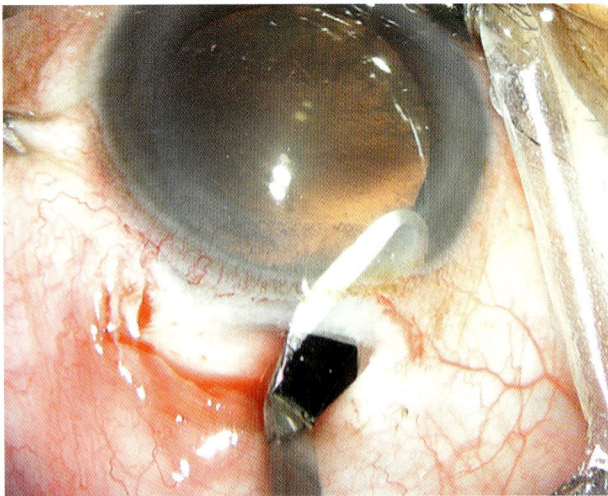

Fig. 18.2 The Beaver blade is advanced to the maximum internal diameter of the wound, forming a trapezoidal, self-sealing wound.

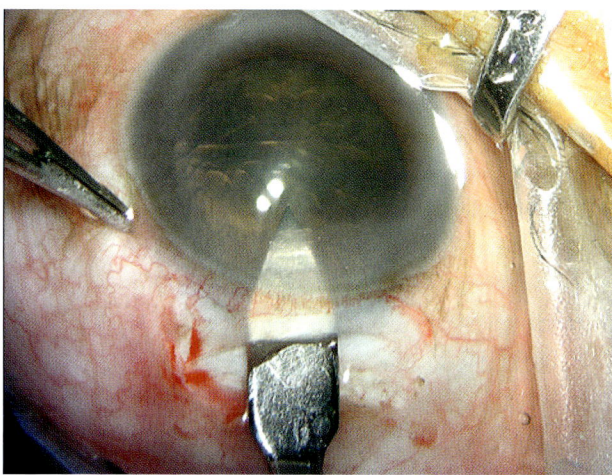

Fig. 18.3 Using a 3.2-mm keratome, the anterior chamber is entered and the wound extended in the same plane.

useful for clearing anterior chamber debris at any portion of the procedure.

In cases of shallow anterior chamber, SICS could avoid the difficulties with maneuvering a phaco tip and decrease the endothelial damage incurred with energy and fluid transmitted directly to the endothelial cells or the Descemet's membrane. In all of these advanced cases, small-incision cataract extraction, therefore, decreases instrumentation and improves safety.

Poor visibility is much less a problem in SICS than phacoemulsification because the former relies more on external wound construction and fluidics rather than depth perception in nucleus disassembly. The nucleus can be safely removed with SICS even in cases with corneal opacity or vascularization. If available,

0.1 mL of 0.06% trypan blue dye is helpful to improve anterior capsular visualization. In a hypermature cataract, one can use a 27-gauge needle to aspirate any liquid cortex to improve visualization and decompress the capsular bag.

Potential Problems and Their Management

Common pitfalls in starting MSICS procedure include making the tunnel too narrow, too posterior on the sclera, or too forward into clear cornea. The downside of making the internal tunnel opening too narrow is an inability to hydro-express a larger nucleus. If too much pressure is required to advance the nucleus, stop and enlarge the internal diameter of the wound. If it is still too forceful, the external diameter of the wound should be enlarged as well. It is best to place sutures later to close an enlarged wound rather than being too vigorous with hydroexpression in the setting of a narrow/short wound leading to a posterior capsular rupture and zonular damage.

Arguably, one of the more challenging steps in MSICS is rotating the lens out of the capsular bag into the anterior chamber. This requires a large enough capsulorrhexis and a good hydrodissection to mobilize the nucleus.

Too small of a capsulorrhexis becomes a hazard when trying to express a brown or black cataract. Aim to create a 6.0- to 7.5-mm rhexis and to avoid forceful hydrodissection.

In cases with highly mobile lenses, a bimanual prolapse technique is preferable using a cyclodialysis spatula below through a paracentesis incision and a Sinskey hook above via the sclerocorneal tunnel. The spatula serves as a fulcrum to rotate the lens out of the eye, minimizing downward forces on the capsular bag (**Fig. 18.5**).

If the lens still fails to be extracted, several alternative techniques are available: (1) irrigating vectis, (2) phaco sandwich, (3) phaco fracture technique, (4) fishhook technique, and (5) corrugated Simcoe technique.

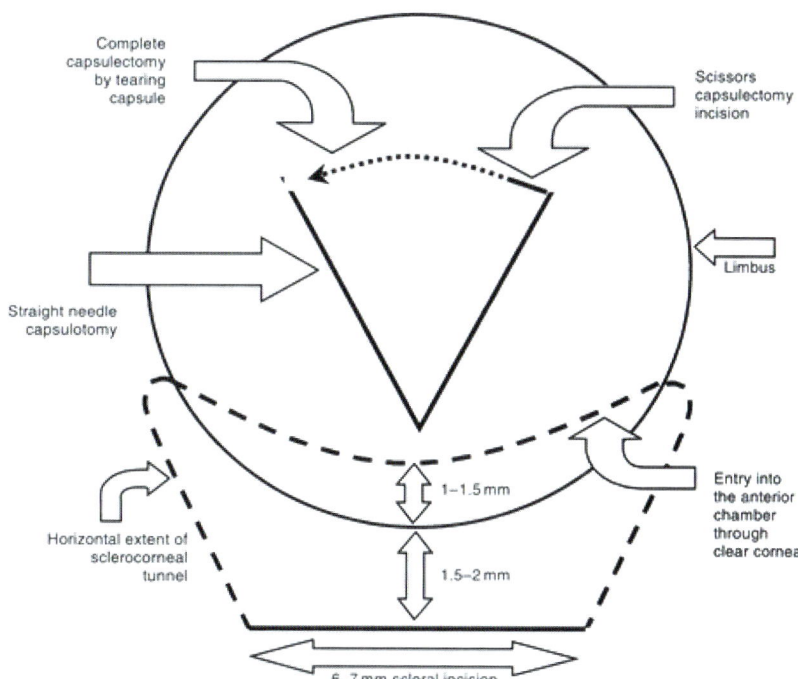

Fig. 18.4 Schematic of trapezoidal wound and the position of the V-capsulotomy.

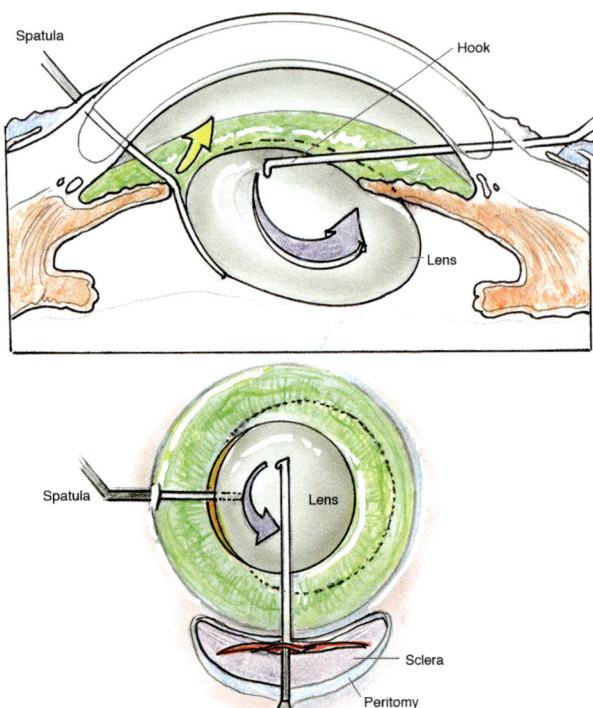

Fig. 18.5 Bimanual technique to help prolapse the nucleus. The left instrument is a spatula that supports the nucleus, and the right instrument is a Sinskey hook helping to draw the lens out into the anterior chamber.

Irrigating Vectis

An irrigating vectis uses mechanical and fluidic forces to extract the nucleus. The vectis is an 8-mm-long and 4-mm-wide loop, and it has a slight concavity anteriorly and three small 0.3-mm ports on the anterior end. The posterior end is continuous with a syringe that can be filled with lactated Ringer's solution or BSS. To use a vectis, liberally apply viscoelastic above, below, and in front of the nucleus. A superior bridle suture is necessary to rotate the globe away with the left hand; the vectis is introduced under the nucleus, taking care to position the anterior tip anterior to the iris. The vectis is slowly withdrawn without irrigation until the nucleus is engaged. Gentle pressure on the posterior lip of the wound with gentle irrigation will deliver the nucleus without sudden anterior chamber decompression. If sitting temporally, an assistant is required to gently pull on the nasal conjunctiva to aid in the extraction.

Potential pitfalls of this technique include placing the anterior edge of the vectis below the iris, causing an iridodialysis, and endothelial damage if metal comes in contact in an uncontrolled extraction. A posterior capsular rent or zonular dialysis can occur if the extrusion of too big of a nucleus through a small wound is performed too forcefully.

Phaco Sandwich

The vectis technique could be supplemented with a Sinskey hook to gently sandwich an otherwise gummy nucleus between the two instruments.

Phaco Fracture technique

Phaco fracture involves using a manual method of fragmentation to remove an overly large nucleus through the small incision. A bisector or trisector is used anteriorly instead of a Sinskey hook

to cleave the nuclear substance. The split fragments can then be individually hydro-expressed with an irrigating vectis.

Fishhook Technique

This involves fashioning a 30-gauge needle into the form of a fishhook, which is advanced into the anterior chamber sideways and maneuvered behind the lens, rotating it to engage the nucleus. Posterior pressure is applied to the lip of the wound, and the hook is used to maneuver the nucleus out of the eye.

Corrugated Simcoe Technique

The corrugated Simcoe technique involves using hydrostatic and mechanical forces to extract the nucleus. After rotating the globe away from the surgeon and introducing the cannula into the wound posterior to the lens and anterior to the iris, gentle irrigation is turned on and the cannula is slowly withdrawn at the same time, while placing gentle downward pressure on the external lip of the wound. The advantage of using a Simcoe extraction is that the cannula can then immediately be reintroduced to aid in the cortical cleanup step. This specially designed Simcoe cannula has an infusion bore of 21 gauge instead of the conventional 23 gauge. This enables a very large inflow of fluid through the infusion, maintaining the chamber depth during nucleus delivery. The corrugated surface gives a firm grip from the undersurface of the nucleus, facilitating its delivery through the wound.

Overall, SICS is a good method for extraction of a wide variety of complicated cataracts, is invaluable in resource-poor environments, and should be part of every surgeon's repertoire when phaco is not ideal for challenging nuclear disassembly.

Timing of Conversion to These Techniques

When a surgeon has initially opted for a clear corneal phacoemulsification approach, and finds the nucleus disassembly challenging or impractical, it is always best to avoid greatly enlarging the corneal wound to address the dense nuclear material. A small-incision surgery could still be performed in this case, with some modifications. It is important to ensure that the globe is normotensive when planning to create a new sclerocorneal tunnel, as hypo- or hypertensive globes will more likely lead to inaccurate wound construction. Ideally, avoid placement of the SICS tunnel in an area where the phaco wound could overlap, as this could lead to step-offs and subsequent wound leaks. After creation of an appropriate tunnel, the nucleus can be hydro-delivered or bimanually expressed just as in primary SICS surgery. If the capsular bag is not violated, a lens could be placed through the tunnel or through the clear corneal incision. Check the integrity of each wound at the completion of the surgery, and it is always best to place a suture if there is any question of wound integrity. Many times when there is large enough posterior capsular rupture involving more than one fourth of the surface, it is best to relocate to a small incision tunnel and do a good anterior vitrectomy and place a rigid single-piece PMMA intraocular lens through the scleral tunnel into the sulcus. Conversion to SICS could be undertaken if there is evidence of a larger zonular dehiscence, or posterior capsular rupture. Before nuclear fragmentation, the conversion to SICS and delivering the nucleus through the tunnel may be much safer and may avoid a dropped nucleus. During capsulorrhexis, if accidentally the rhexis runs out to the equator we can safely convert to SICS and put in a single-piece PMMA lens. At some stage during the rhexis or during nucleus management, if the chamber suddenly deepens it indicates a posterior rupture or zonular compromise and it is always safer to convert to SICS at that point to safely deliver the whole nucleus.

Section VIII   Vitrectomy

19 Torn Posterior Capsule and Anterior Vitrectomy

Mark H. Blecher and Charles M. Calvo

Rupture of the posterior capsule during phacoemulsification is a rare but serious intraoperative complication and carries the risk of precipitating problems such as retinal detachment that may lead to permanently decreased visual acuity.[1] Recent studies report that the rate of posterior capsular rupture, with or without vitreous loss, ranges from 0.45 to 7.9%.[2-5] In the event of a posterior capsular rupture, the outcome is heavily dependent on the surgeon's early recognition and management of the problem.

Capsular Anatomy

The lens capsule is an elastic, clear, basement membrane composed of type IV collagen produced by lens epithelial cells. The zonular fibers insert on the equatorial lens capsule, anteriorly 1.5 mm onto the anterior capsule and posteriorly 1.25 mm onto the posterior capsule.[6] The capsule has variable thickness. Although the capsule is thickest (17 to 23 μm) near the anterior and posterior equator where the zonular fibers attach, it is only 2 to 4 μm thick at the posterior pole. The anterior capsule is considerably thicker than the posterior pole (14 μm in adults), and it continues to increase in thickness with age. The posterior capsule may be particularly fragile in patients with congenital posterior lenticonus and posterior polar cataract[7] (**Fig. 19.1**).

Risk Factors for Capsular Rupture

Patient factors that increase the risk of capsular rupture have been well identified.[8,9] Eyes with long or short axial lengths, that is, with associated deep or shallow anterior chambers, respectively, present certain challenges. In high myopia, the anterior chamber is deeper, drawing the surgeon's instruments to a more vertical position. The posterior capsule may exhibit a "trampolining" motion due to the thinner, more pliant tissues. Lowering the bottle height and decreasing the vacuum and flow settings can help compensate for this movement. In high hyperopia, the anterior chamber is crowded, decreasing the area in which to work. Furthermore, the posterior capsule is more anterior and closer to the surgeon's instruments.

Dense, mature cataracts described as black or white cataracts present added risk. These lenses bring challenges to performing a capsulorrhexis, require increased phacoemulsification energy, and impede adequate visibility. Such dense cataracts are more prevalent in older patients, and advanced age is an independent risk factor. This risk is likely best explained as a combination of coexisting factors such as zonular weakness, small pupil, and dense lens.[10] Management of white cataracts and brunescent cataracts is discussed in Chapters 14 and 15, respectively.

Small pupils are a significant predisposing factor for violating the posterior capsule during surgery. Floppy iris syndrome, posterior synechiae, and pseudoexfoliation are some of the most common causes of inadequate pupil size. Small pupils may be a harbinger of further problems, as many causes of small pupils carry other risks such as zonular laxity and iris billowing.[11] These problems, and the techniques to address them, are discussed fully in Chapters 4, 5, and 23.

Other predisposing factors for capsular rupture may include (1) uncooperative, disoriented, or anxious patients with subsequent inadvertent movements; (2) poor visualization due to unclear media such as corneal disease; (3) preexisting trauma with unseen capsular rupture or zonular damage; (4) previous ocular surgery, especially vitrectomy with or without silicone oil; (5) a history of intravitreal injections, which may have violated the posterior capsule; and (6) an inexperienced surgeon (e.g., a resident).

Lastly, the surgeon can reduce the risks by proper positioning and management of the surgical field. Appropriate placement of the surgeon's hand position in relation to the patient's brow can improve visualization and decrease torsion of the globe. A temporal position, which is now favored by cataract surgeons, is particularly advantageous if the brow is prominent (e.g., a deepset eye). Pooling of fluid on the surgical field can be addressed by turning the head temporally to allow fluid to drain.

Signs of Capsule Rupture

During phacoemulsification the hydrostatic pressure in the anterior chamber is greater than physiological intraocular pressures (IOPs) but ideally is maintained in a constant state. This is the result of the balance of numerous factors: (1) hydrostatic pressure created by the height of the infusion bottle (11 mm for every 15 cm of bottle height) or a phacoemulsification platform with target IOP control, (2) the evacuation of fluid or lens material controlled by the surgeon through vacuum and aspiration, and (3) the egress of fluid through the wounds. When the posterior capsule unexpectedly ruptures, there is a sudden equalization of the hydrostatic pressure between the anterior chamber and the vitreous cavity. This causes an abrupt posterior displacement of the iris and dilation of the pupil as the posterior capsule opens. This is often the first warning of capsular rupture. Another indicator of capsular rupture is that the nucleus seems to "fall away" from the phaco tip. This phenomenon is due to the loss of the support of the posterior capsule and subsequent movement of lens material posteriorly. The apparent loss of the phaco effect and a sudden clear zone that appears near the phaco tip are indicators that vitreous may be caught in the phaco tip.

These warning signs are especially important when visualization of the posterior capsule is impaired in scenarios such as poor dilation or dense cataract. Generally, if the surgeon is suspicious that the posterior capsule has ruptured, it probably has. The surgeon is therefore justified in modifying the surgical plan on the suspicion of a tear of the posterior capsule.

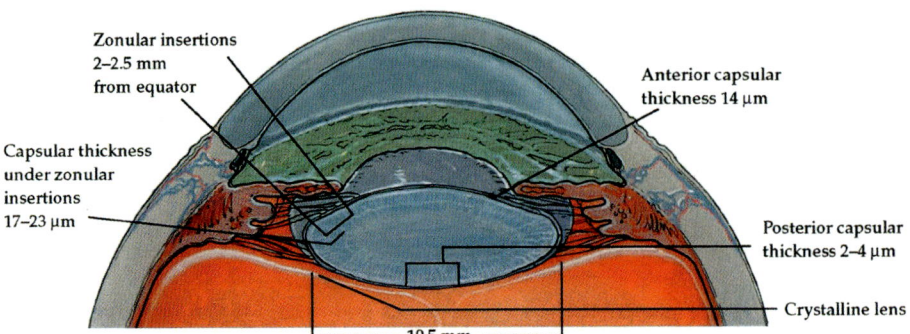

Fig. 19.1   Anterior segment: anatomic relationships.

These signs of posterior capsule rupture can occur not only during phacoemulsification or irrigation and aspiration (I/A), but may also occur during hydrodissection. Aggressive hydrodissection may result in a posterior capsular rupture, especially in the presence of a small or noncontinuous capsulorrhexis. If a posterior capsular rent that developed during hydrodissection is not identified before the infusion of fluid from the phaco handpiece, the lens may be driven into the vitreous.[12]

First Steps

To repeat, if the surgeon is suspicious that the posterior capsule may be torn, it probably has. Before any management decisions have been made, the first step should be to stabilize the anterior chamber. The phaco or infusion-aspiration tip should remain in the eye, aspiration should be immediately stopped, and infusion should continue to maintain positive pressure. The second instrument can then be carefully removed so that dispersive viscoelastic can be generously injected to aid in holding the vitreous behind the posterior capsule. After a liberal amount of viscoelastic has been injected, then the phaco tip can be cautiously removed from the eye and the surgeon can prepare for possible vitrectomy. After these steps have been taken, the surgeon can then develop a concise alternative surgical plan with the goal of minimizing the duration of surgery and decreasing the risk of injury to the cornea or retina (**Fig. 19.2**). The surgeon's alterna-

tive surgical plan hinges on two questions: First, has vitreous migrated into the anterior chamber? Second, does nucleus still remain in the eye?

Conversion to Extracapsular Cataract Extraction

When in doubt, it is prudent to convert to an extracapsular cataract extraction rather than proceed with phacoemulsification. A key factor in the determination as to whether to continue phaco or convert to extracapsular surgery might be the presence of vitreous in the anterior chamber combined with a large piece of nucleus. If vitreous is present immediately after a capsular tear, generally it indicates a large capsular tear combined with syneretic poor vitreous support.

Once a posterior capsular rupture is identified, it is of utmost importance to inject a dispersive ophthalmic viscoelastic device (OVD) beneath the lens material to tamponade the vitreous posteriorly and hold all lens fragments anteriorly (**Fig. 19.3**). The advantage of dispersive viscoelastic is that it resists egress through incisions or by aspiration.[13] Additionally, dispersive agents are well absorbed through the trabecular meshwork, which aids in decreasing a spike in postoperative IOP.

The clear corneal incision should be sutured and abandoned if large lens material is to be evacuated manually, and a shelved

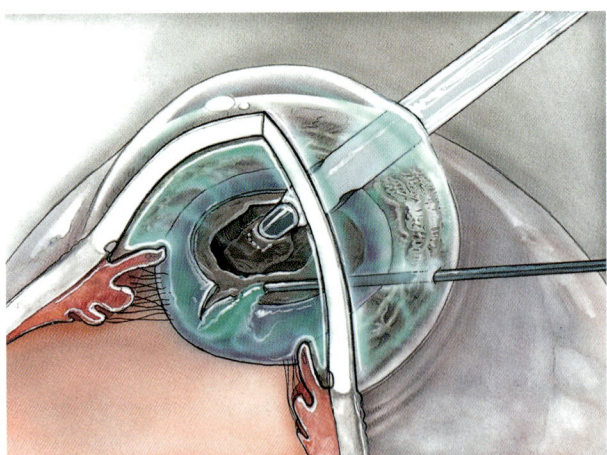

Fig. 19.2   Prevention of enlargement of a capsular tear. The phaco tip remains within the incision with minimal irrigation and no aspiration. The second instrument is removed and replaced with an ophthalmic viscoelastic device (OVD) cannula. Dispersive OVD is injected above and below the nucleus to stabilize the anterior chamber. Then the phaco tip can be removed.

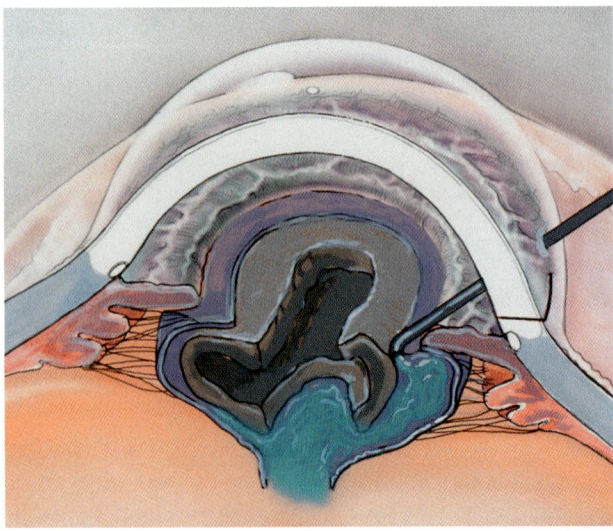

Fig. 19.3   Dispersive viscoelastic (teal) is injected below the lens fragments to prevent loss of fragments into the vitreous and to hold the vitreous back.

limbal incision should be created after conjunctival peritomy.[14] Expanding clear corneal incisions to 10 mm or greater to facilitate removal of large nuclear fragments will result in large amounts of irregular astigmatism that will be challenging to manage. Surgeons commonly underestimate the size of the limbal incision required to remove the largest nuclear remnant. Therefore, it is wise to create an incision larger than thought necessary. Extracting lens fragments using a lens loop, a Sinskey hook and spatula, or a Kansas forceps should be approached cautiously as it may pull the vitreous with it. As a result, much of the nuclear extraction should be attempted by viscoelastic prolapse. External pressure should be avoided, as vitreous will preferentially be expelled.

Continued Phacoemulsification

If a posterior capsular tear is found in the later stages of phacoemulsification, the surgeon may decide that continued phacoemulsification is appropriate. Dispersive viscoelastic should be injected initially before removal of the phaco or I/A handpiece. Additionally, dispersive viscoelastic should be injected below the lens nucleus to raise it into the anterior chamber. This may be injected through a side-port incision or through a pars plana incision to perform posterior assisted levitation of nuclear fragments.[13] Once nuclear fragments have been successfully floated into the anterior chamber with a layer of dispersive viscoelastic, cautious phacoemulsification may be continued with low vacuum and low irrigation. A second instrument should be used to deliver nuclear fragments into the phaco tip so as not to aspirate vitreous. Resist the temptation to further fragment the nucleus by cracking or other maneuvers, as these smaller fragments are difficult to chase and may then fall posteriorly. (For additional information on this topic, see Chapter 51.)

Removing cortex once a posterior capsular tear has been identified also entails special considerations. Low-flow I/A or using a Simcoe extraction cannula will minimize the turbulence that might enlarge the capsular rent and encourage movement of further vitreous anteriorly. If an inadequate amount of dispersive viscoelastic is remaining over the capsular rent, additional viscoelastic should be injected generously. The I/A tip should be brought into contact with the cortex before the initiation of vacuum to avoid aspirating the vitreous preferentially. Stripping the cortex should be performed in a motion toward the capsular tear, as stripping away from the rent will pull the tear further. Ultimately, if the surgeon is concerned that efforts to remove all the cortex are too dangerous, they should be abandoned. A small amount of cortex can be left behind if maneuvers needed to remove it put the patient at unnecessary risk. Alternatively, bimanual I/A can be utilized to provide exquisite control over I/A. This technique provides improved maneuverability and maintains a more stable anterior chamber. If the vitrector is in use, or going to be used, remaining cortex can be aspirated by bimanual vitrectomy with the cutting mode turned off.[15]

Posterior Capsule Capsulorrhexis

Some posterior capsular tears may present as round holes, usually as a result of damage by the phaco tip. If the rent is visible and size and location allow, it may be converted into a posterior capsule capsulorrhexis (PCC), which was first described by Gimbel et al[16] (**Fig. 19.4**). After creating some tension to the posterior capsule by injecting viscoelastic through the tear into Berger's space, coaxial microforceps are used to perform the capsulorrhexis. This technique decreases the likelihood of expanding of the tear during subsequent surgical steps. The creation of a PCC may enable the intraocular lens (IOL) to still be implanted in the

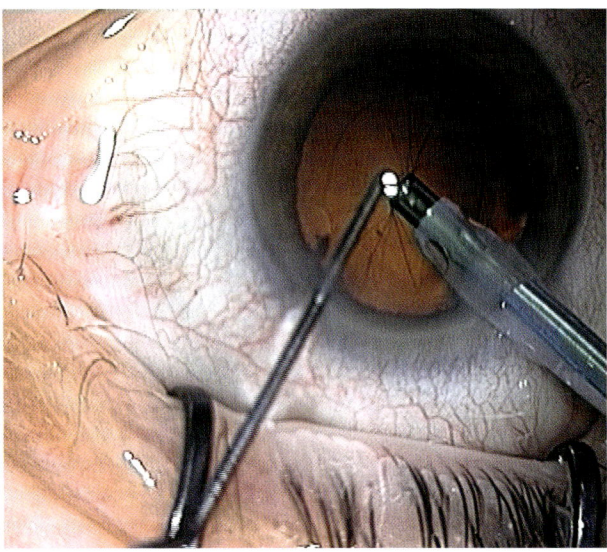
a

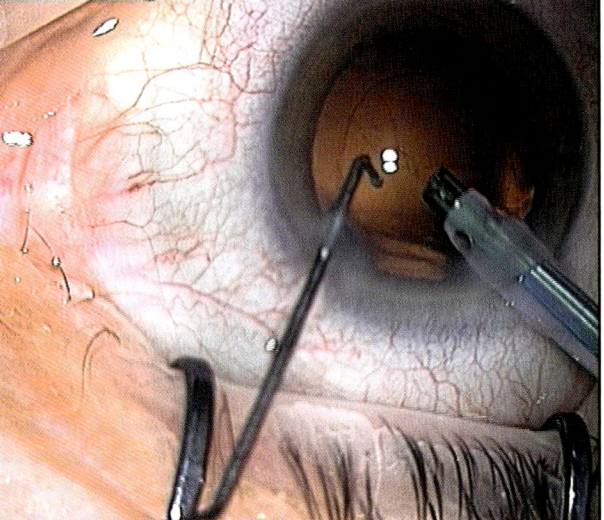
b

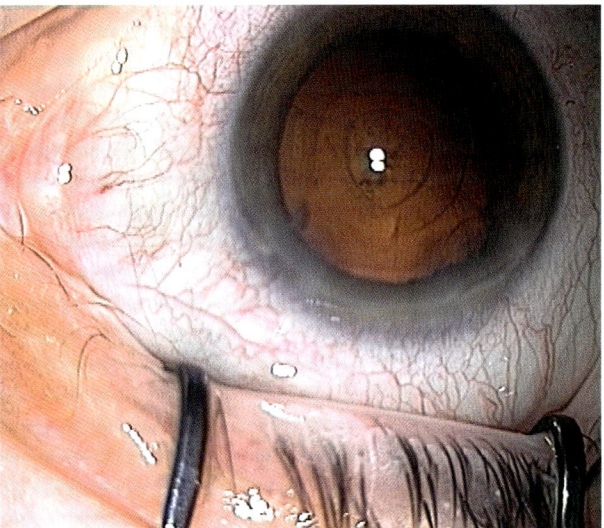
c

Fig. 19.4 **(a)** In the first image of this sequence, the posterior capsule is drawn into the phaco tip, **(b)** resulting in a posterior capsular tear. **(c)** The irregular break is converted into a posterior capsule capsulorrhexis. (Courtesy of Dr. Brian Little.)

capsular bag if anterior vitrectomy is performed sufficiently and without expanding the hole. If the decision is made to place a lens in the capsular bag, a single-piece implant may be preferred because it unfolds slowly and in a controlled manner. (Further information is found in Chapter 6.) For a larger capsular defect, a three-piece implant may be placed with capture of the optic through the anterior capsulorrhexis. Unfortunately, the feasibility of creating a PCC may be limited by residual cortex or peripheral location. The surgeon's ability to perform a PCC is dependent on obtaining good visibility of the torn posterior capsule's borders and requires a working coaxial microforceps.

Anterior Vitrectomy

Clearing the anterior chamber of vitreous is a crucial step in ensuring stable placement of an IOL and preventing further injury to the eye. Adherence of vitreous to the IOL or incarceration of vitreous in wounds can lead to retinal tears, retinal detachment, and cystoid macular edema. Vitreous to the wounds may also increase the risk of endophthalmitis, as these strands may act as a channel for ocular surface bacteria. Therefore, the surgeon's understanding of vitreous dynamics following posterior capsular rupture and its management is essential.

Vitreous Anatomy

The vitreous can be considered a transparent connective tissue surrounded by the posterior lens capsule anteriorly and the retina posteriorly. It is composed of a complicated arrangement of long, thin collagen fibrils suspended in a network of glycosaminoglycan (GAG) chains and hyaluronic acid (HA).[17] The organization of collagen fibrils, widely separated by hydrated GAG/HA chains, permits the transmission of light to the retina with minimal scattering. The vitreous base is the point of strongest attachment: a ring-like band extending 2 mm anterior and 3 mm posterior to the ora serrata. Posteriorly, the vitreous gel is also firmly adherent to the optic nerve, retinal vessels, and macula.

Although it is difficult to appreciate in vivo, the network of vitreous fibrils appears to be continuous from the anterior peripheral vitreous to the posterior vitreous. Therefore, traction on the anterior vitreous fibrils may eventually cause vitreoretinal traction.

Visualization of the Vitreous

The transparency of vitreous is a significant challenge to removing it from the anterior chamber. Burk et al[18] in 2003 first described the staining of vitreous with triamcinolone acetate in the context of anterior vitrectomy. A small volume of triamcinolone diluted 10:1 with balanced salt solution can be injected into the anterior chamber to effectively stain vitreous and aid its visualization. A preservative-free formulation, Triesence (Alcon Laboratories Inc., Fort Worth, TX), is also available and is recommended for safety. Triamcinolone acetate can also provide additional suppression of inflammation postoperatively. The small volume used during anterior vitrectomy is tolerated well, but larger volumes, as given as treatment for intraocular inflammation, can lead to ocular hypertension.[19] Insertion of an endoillumination cannula into the anterior chamber with dim microscope illumination is an another technique demonstrated to successfully visualize vitreous.[20]

Vitrectomy Basic Principles

Vitreous will always follow the path of least resistance. Vitreous will migrate into the anterior chamber if there is a pressure gradient between the anterior and posterior chambers. Therefore, the vitreous will only move anteriorly if there is inadequate anterior chamber pressure, or if the vitreous is drawn anteriorly by aspiration (**Fig. 19.5**). By this principle, maintaining the IOP in a constant state after the posterior capsule tears will hold the vitreous posteriorly and reduce the risk of vitreous loss. Applying these concepts will assist the surgeon in confining the vitreous to its correct anatomic location, and limit excessive and lengthy anterior vitrectomy.

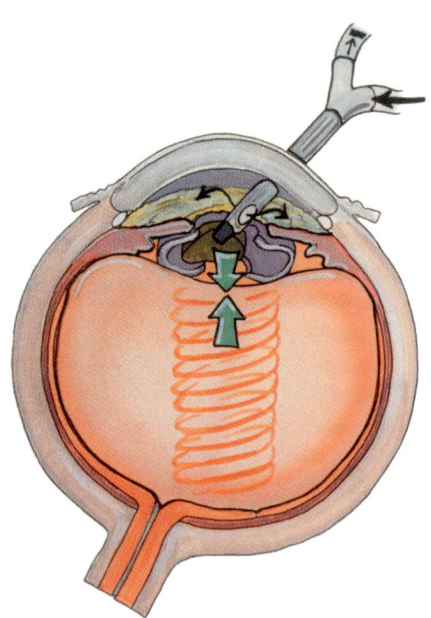
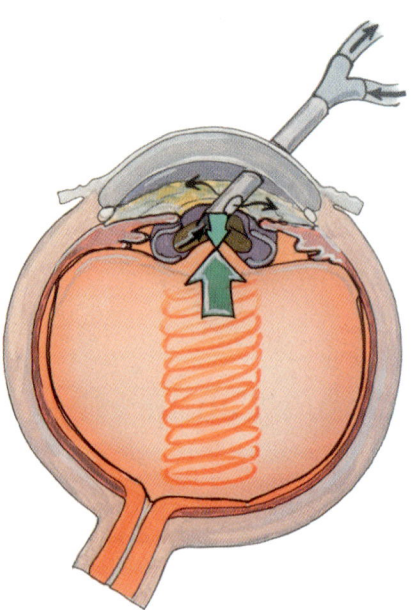

a   b

Fig. 19.5 **(a)** When the posterior capsule ruptures, the pressure in the anterior chamber holds the vitreous back, preventing vitreous prolapse. **(b)** Vitreous can come forward only if the pressure in the anterior chamber is low, as when aspiration continues. (Note the *dark, thicker arrow* on the aspiration line, indicating continued aspiration and phacoemulsification.)

Coaxial Anterior Vitrectomy

Numerous factors have led surgeons to favor a bimanual technique over the use of a coaxial handpiece.[14] The infusion port and vitreous cutter are positioned very closely to one another; therefore, the force from the infusion pressure will promote expansion of the capsular tear when the coaxial cannula is advanced posteriorly. Introduction of infusion pressure near the vitreous also increases hydration of the vitreous, increasing its volume. Lastly, it has been demonstrated that coaxial infusion of fluid causes significant vitreous turbulence, and subsequent prolapse of vitreous in the anterior chamber.[21] Therefore, do not use coaxial infusion!

Performing Anterior Vitrectomy

Once a posterior capsular tear is identified, the anterior chamber must be stabilized before beginning vitrectomy through the aforementioned first steps. If the surgeon is using the coaxial vitrectomy tip, the primary clear corneal or sclerocorneal incision may still be utilized, but shortening the incision should be considered. The vitrectomy tip without the infusion cannula should not be placed through the primary phaco incision because the instrument is too small and fluid will escape around it **(Fig. 19.6)**. Alternatively, a second paracentesis must be created for the vitrectomy tip. An oversized incision will enable fluid egress and invite vitreous to the wound. Vitreous incarceration discovered after vitrectomy has been reported to occur in as many as 33% of cases.[22]

Some surgeons may employ anterior vitrectomy without the use of an irrigating cannula or anterior chamber maintainer. Close attention must be given in this scenario to prevent loss of anterior chamber positive pressure. As a result, viscoelastic should be replaced frequently. Again, preserving positive pressure in the anterior chamber will assist in holding back vitreous and minimize the scale of required vitrectomy.

Utilizing an infusion cannula or anterior chamber maintainer provides continuous replacement of volume removed by vitrectomy. Although this technique may hydrate the vitreous, directing the infusion parallel to the iris will limit the hydration to only the vitreous in the anterior chamber. Any hydrated vitreous in the anterior chamber will be subsequently removed by vitrec-

tomy. With the vitrectomy tip positioned below the posterior capsule and the aspiration port directed up toward the cornea, fluid from the infusion will be aspirated before hydrating the vitreous body **(Fig. 19.7)**.

Vitrectomy should be performed thoroughly until all vitreous is cleared to below the level of the posterior capsule. At this point the vitrectomy can be stopped. If a sulcus lens is to be implanted, special attention should be given to clear the vitreous through the ciliary plane. Although vitrectomy should be thorough, overzealous vitrectomy should be avoided. Venturing too far into the anterior vitreous body can cause the same peripheral retinal injuries that the vitrectomy was designed to prevent.[21]

It should be stated that while anterior vitrectomy is a great technique, performing vitrectomy through the pars plana has many advantages over the anterior approach. This technique is discussed in Chapter 20.

Anterior Chamber Lens Fragments

Anterior chamber fragments occur rarely. They are more common when emulsifying a 4–5+ nucleus. The fragments are usually small and visible in the chamber angle inferiorly within the first week postoperatively. Any fragment of nucleus requires immediate removal. Prolonged contact with a nuclear fragment will cause uveitis, glaucoma, corneal edema, and endothelial cell loss. Cortex will be absorbed spontaneously and does not require intervention. It is helpful to use pilocarpine to create miosis so that the fragment does not migrate behind the iris, only later to reappear. The fragment is then easily removed in the operating room after trapping it with cohesive OVD and using the I/A tip with a second instrument to grind the fragment into the anterior chamber. In this way the fragment is visualized during removal and the surgeon can be assured it is totally eliminated. In the unusual case of a large fragment, the phaco tip my be utilized.

Posteriorly Retained Lens Fragments

Intravitreal retained lens fragments have an incidence of 0.1 to 1.6% and are a potential serious complication of cataract surgery.[23] Lens fragments sequestered in the anterior vitreous should be

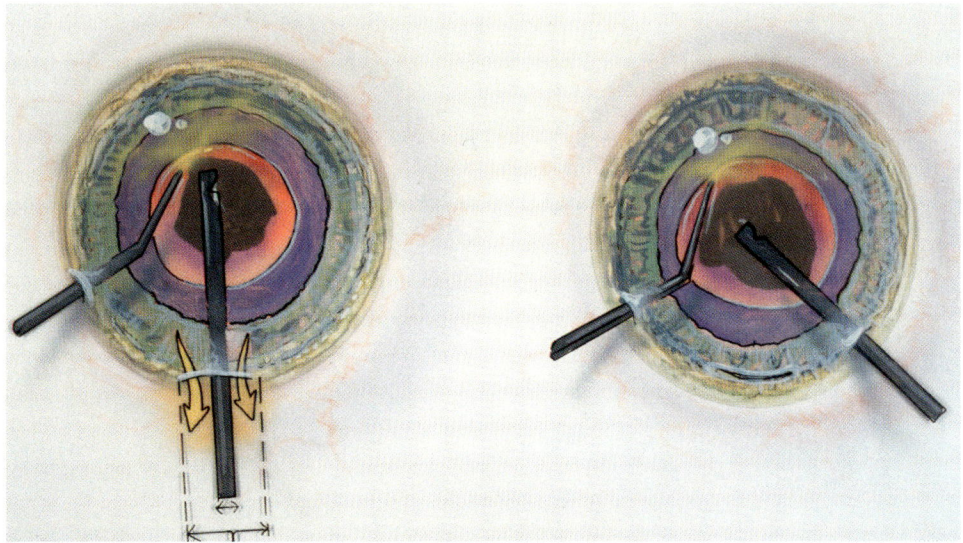

a   b

Fig. 19.6   **(a)** As the phaco incision is too large for the vitrectomy tip, fluid can leak around the instrument and bring vitreous to the wound. **(b)** A new incision should be made specifically for the vitrectomy tip to develop a closed, controlled system.

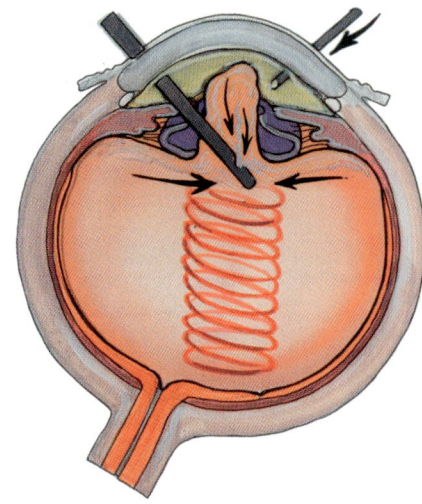
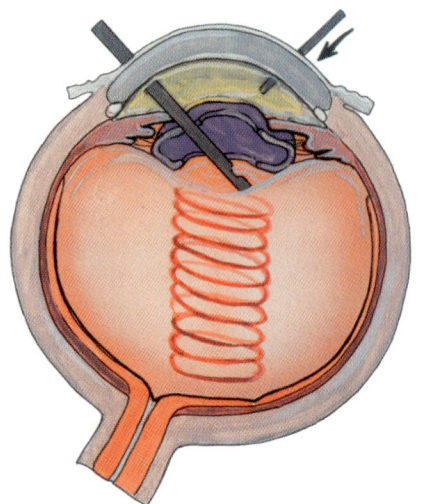

Fig. 19.7 **(a)** The vitrectomy tip should be placed below the posterior capsule, with the aspiration tip facing the cornea. The vitreous in the anterior chamber should be pulled down to the vitrectomy tip. **(b)** The procedure is finished when all of the vitreous has been removed from the anterior chamber and the edges of the posterior capsule.

retrieved by surgeons but only if the fragments are easily accessible. Injection of additional viscoelastic may aid the surgeon in trapping or securing the fragments. Anterior vitrectomy should not be performed until accessible lens fragments have been removed because the vitreous may act as a scaffolding to support the fragments from further posterior displacement. In the event that lens fragments do fall into the posterior vitreous cavity, the surgeon should perform a complete anterior vitrectomy without regard for the dropped nucleus; the surgeon should remove the cortex, and consider placement of an IOL. These patients will benefit from co-management with a vitreoretinal surgeon. In the event of a future pars plana vitrectomy (PPV), the phaco incision should be closed with a suture.

Cortical fragments are likely to be well tolerated and reabsorbed over time. However, nuclear remnants, particularly those larger than 2 mm, may incite severe inflammation and secondary glaucoma. Indications for PPV include uncontrolled IOP, phacoanaphylactic uveitis, and large nuclear fragments.[24] The ideal timing for PPV is unknown and controversial, but meta-analyses suggest that early PPV within 1 to 2 weeks is better than late.[23] Macrophage-mediated inflammation, found in inflamed eyes with retained lens, is reported to begin after day 3.[25] Therefore, this may explain why it is acceptable to give patients a few days to recover from complicated cataract surgery before PPV.

Conclusion

Just as Benjamin Franklin famously stated, "An ounce of prevention is worth a pound of cure," recognizing risk factors for posterior capsular tear preoperatively is the best method for achieving safe and successful cataract surgery. Likewise, timely identification of intraoperative problems and appropriate adjustment of the surgical plan will help prevent sight-threatening complications. If managed carefully and skillfully, patients with posterior capsular tears and vitreous loss can still achieve a great visual outcome.

References

1. Mearza AA, Ramanathan S, Bidgood P, Horgan S. Visual outcome in cataract surgery complicated by vitreous loss in a district general hospital. Int Ophthalmol 2009;29:157–160

2. Jaycock P, Johnston RL, Taylor H, et al; UK EPR user group. The Cataract National Dataset electronic multi-centre audit of 55,567 operations: updating benchmark standards of care in the United Kingdom and internationally. Eye (Lond) 2009;23:38–49

3. Greenberg PB, Tseng VL, Wu WC, et al. Prevalence and predictors of ocular complications associated with cataract surgery in United States veterans. Ophthalmology 2011;118:507–514

4. Haripriya A, Chang DF, Reena M, Shekhar M. Complication rates of phacoemulsification and manual small-incision cataract surgery at Aravind Eye Hospital. J Cataract Refract Surg 2012;38:1360–1369

5. Lee RM, Foot B, Eke T. Posterior capsule rupture rate with akinetic and kinetic block anesthetic techniques. J Cataract Refract Surg 2013;39:128–131

6. American Academy of Ophthalmology. Lens and Cataract: Basic and Clinical Science Course, 2013–2014. San Francisco: AAO; 2013

7. Kuszak JR, Deutsch TA, Brown HG. Anatomy of aged and senile cataractous lenses. In: Albert DM, Jakobiec FA, eds. Principles and Practice of Ophthalmology: Clinical Practice. Philadelphia: WB Saunders; 1994:564–575

8. Narendran N, Jaycock P, Johnston RL, et al. The Cataract National Dataset electronic multicentre audit of 55,567 operations: risk stratification for posterior capsule rupture and vitreous loss. Eye (Lond) 2009;23:31–37

9. Blomquist PH, Morales ME, Tong L, Ahn C. Risk factors for vitreous complications in resident-performed phacoemulsification surgery. J Cataract Refract Surg 2012;38:208–214

10. Zare M, Javadi MA, Einollahi B, Baradaran-Rafii AR, Feizi S, Kiavash V. Risk factors for posterior capsule rupture and vitreous loss during phacoemulsification. J Ophthalmic Vis Res 2009;4:208–212

11. Shingleton BJ, Crandall AS, Ahmed II. Pseudoexfoliation and the cataract surgeon: preoperative, intraoperative, and postoperative issues related to intraocular pressure, cataract, and intraocular lenses. J Cataract Refract Surg 2009;35:1101–1120

12. Gimbel HV. Posterior capsule tears using phacoemulsification-causes, prevention and management. Eur J Implant Refract Surg 1990;2:63–69

13. Chang DF, Packard RB. Posterior assisted levitation for nucleus retrieval using Viscoat after posterior capsule rupture. J Cataract Refract Surg 2003;29:1860–1865

14. Chiu CS. 2013 update on the management of posterior capsular rupture during cataract surgery. Curr Opin Ophthalmol 2014;25:26–34

15. Koch PS. Managing the torn posterior capsule and vitreous loss. [review] Int Ophthalmol Clin 1994;34:113–130

16. Gimbel HV, Sun R, Ferensowicz M, Anderson Penno E, Kamal A. Intraoperative management of posterior capsule tears in phacoemulsification and intraocular lens implantation. Ophthalmology 2001;108:2186–2189, discussion 2190–2192

17. American Academy of Ophthalmology. Retina and Vitreous: Basic and Clinical Science Course, 2013–2014. San Francisco: AAO; 2013

18. Burk SE, Da Mata AP, Snyder ME, Schneider S, Osher RH, Cionni RJ. Visualizing vitreous using Kenalog suspension. J Cataract Refract Surg 2003;29: 645–651

19. Jonas JB, Degenring RF, Kreissig I, Akkoyun I, Kamppeter BA. Intraocular pressure elevation after intravitreal triamcinolone acetonide injection. Ophthalmology 2005;112:593–598

20. Nichamin LD. Endoilluminated infusion cannula for anterior segment surgery. J Cataract Refract Surg 2012;38:1322–1324

21. Eller AW, Barad RF. Miyake analysis of anterior vitrectomy techniques. J Cataract Refract Surg 1996;22:213–217

22. Fishkind WJ. The torn PC mechanisms and outcomes. Presented at the American Society of Cataract and Refractive Surgeons annual meeting, Seattle, April 1999

23. Vanner EA, Stewart MW. Vitrectomy timing for retained lens fragments after surgery for age-related cataracts: a systematic review and meta-analysis. Am J Ophthalmol 2011;152:345–357.e3

24. Vilar NF, Flynn HW Jr, Smiddy WE, Murray TG, Davis JL, Rubsamen PE. Removal of retained lens fragments after phacoemulsification reverses secondary glaucoma and restores visual acuity. Ophthalmology 1997; 104:787–791, discussion 791–792

25. Wilkinson CP, Green WR. Vitrectomy for retained lens material after cataract extraction: the relationship between histopathologic findings and the time of vitreous surgery. Ophthalmology 2001;108:1633–1637

20 Pars Plana Anterior Vitrectomy

Lisa Brothers Arbisser

Every cataract surgeon encounters unplanned vitreous loss. Eyes respond differently, and surgeons are not automatons. Ideally, we would not lose vitreous the same way twice—a rarely achieved yet lofty goal. The incidence varies widely in the literature from 0.45%, reported years ago by Howard Gimbel, to reports that are logarithmically higher. A national registry measures it at 2.09%. A surgeon with a higher rate warrants remediation.[1] It behooves us all to have a plan in mind, tools with which to execute the plan at the ready, and to be prepared for contingencies for every case. The earlier a complication is recognized and the stage of complication limited, the better the result. Rarely do we breach the posterior capsule without rupturing the anterior hyaloid. When limited to this stage, optimal outcomes uniformly result, assuming implant stability is achieved. Rupture of the anterior hyaloid membrane with prolapse of vitreous into the anterior segment increases the risk of late complications. Once vitreous is lost through incisions there is a greater likelihood of retinal tear or detachment; another set of actions is indicated. Depending on the timing, this problem may be associated with residual lens remnants.

Benjamin Franklin's famous advice, as also cited in the previous chapter, bears repeating: "An ounce of prevention is worth a pound of cure." When the surgery is optimally managed, outcomes can rival those of uncomplicated surgery. This chapter, based on both experience and laboratory exploration, discusses a set of cardinal principles that cannot be violated, and describes the tools and techniques for this procedure. Anterior segment surgeons are most comfortable with anterior incisions. Regardless of the incision site, there are universal principles for success. Although this chapter is intended to fully describe the pars plana approach to anterior vitrectomy, gaining experience in skills-transfer wet laboratories, apprenticing for a day with a vitreoretinal surgeon, or acquiring other hands-on experience is recommended prior to attempting a new technique in the setting of a complicated cataract case.

Guiding Principles

Avoid intra- and postoperative vitreous traction. Vitrectomy itself need not result in significant visual disability. Visual function is impaired by sequelae of retinal detachment, hemorrhage, and macular edema resulting from suboptimal vitreous management. Strictly embracing proper technique almost universally avoids impaired visual outcomes.

Maintain a Normotensive Globe

Employ tight incisions for anterior vitrectomy. Complications prolong surgery and hypotony invites hemorrhage, choroidal effusion, and subsequent edema. Alternating high and low intraocular pressure (IOP) can cause shear where choroidal vessels are tethered by anatomy; sudden hemorrhage may result. Phacoemulsification can fail without a controlled and stable environment; our vitreoretinal colleagues would not dream of using leaky incisions. The anterior segment surgeon must follow suit in handling complications.

Vitreous Always Follows a Gradient from High to Low Pressure

Once a complication is recognized, maintenance of the anterior chamber (AC) and avoiding collapse are essential. Think of vitreous as egg white in a bowl; tilt the bowl and it will come streaming out, running downhill. Vitreous follows an instrument withdrawn from an incision and may convert vitreous prolapse into vitreous loss. Infusion may easily displace vitreous. This is the logic for a biaxial approach to vitrectomy for any incision. Always separate the irrigation sleeve from the vitrector shaft and always discontinue infusion before exiting the eye. Incisions exceeding the diameter of the vitrector facilitate vitreous's preferential egress through the leaky incision rather than into the vitrector port.

Never Fish Around the Complex and Wondrous Structure of Vitreous

Not typically visible in vivo, the vitreous body is composed of solid parts: cortex, septa, and cisternal walls. These surround and separate more liquid parts: canals, cisterns, and spaces. The equator-parallel and sagittal septa follow an incomplete spiral, which is mirror image in the left and right eye. The vitreous body resembles a snail shell in this way, as septa radiate between the 12 petal-like cisterns that surround the bursa premacularis and the cistern preoptica. In equator-parallel section, the vitreous body resembles a cut orange. Collagen fibrils and fibers interact with hyaluronic acid, as formed vitreous and the lamellae are interconnected by a loose mesh of fibers. The high water/low protein content is unique in the body. This complex structure we are manipulating acts like a toy slinky attached to wallpaper (the retina). It functions as both a filter and a barrier.[2] Cataract surgeons must respect the vitreous. In the setting of unplanned loss, remove only the prolapsed vitreous that may adhere to anterior structures or incisions; disturb the unoffending structure as minimally as possible. Placing instruments other than a vitrector into the vitreous body to retrieve lens fragments courts disaster. Robert Machemer irrigated into the vitreous to create an animal model for retinal detachment research. Although taught as an option, levitation of a descended nucleus with either a spatula or ophthalmic viscosurgical device (OVD) cannula through the pars plana is risky both for vision and medicolegal outcomes (**Fig. 20.1**).

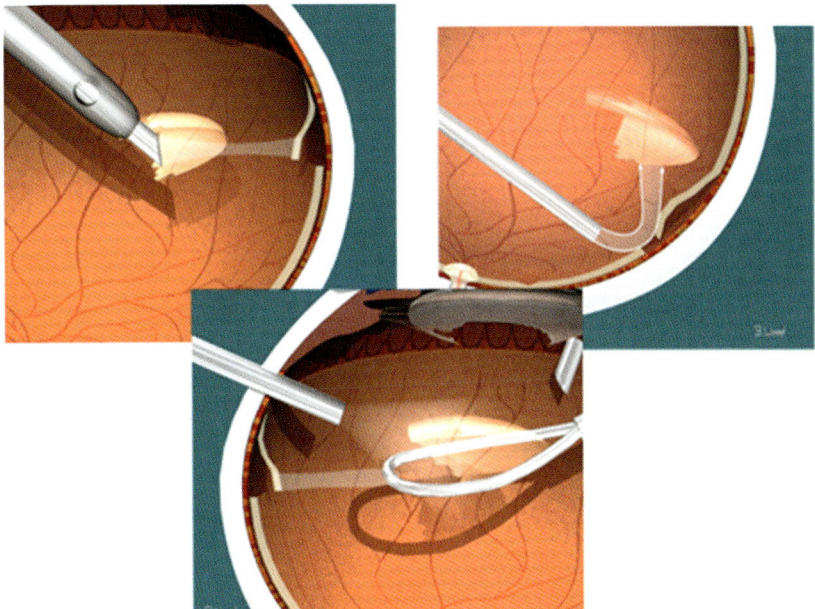

Fig. 20.1 Do not fish around in the vitreous. In the absence of total vitrectomy placing a phacoemulsification needle, an irrigating cannula or a vectus into the posterior segment risks a retinal tear. (Courtesy of Steve Charles, MD.)

Protect Other Tissues from Collateral Damage

Although we must deal with vitreous, there is no justification for losing much-needed capsule support, chewing up the iris, or causing corneal edema by failing to protect the endothelium. The thinnest part of the retina and likeliest to tear is located anteriorly near the vitreous base. This attachment must be respected. The anterior segment surgeon must leave a clean anterior segment with a stable implant whenever appropriate, and a clean bag and a clear visual axis for rapid visual rehabilitation or to allow further timely management. Avoid vitreous incarceration in the pars plana sclerotomy just as we would an anterior incision to prevent postoperative traction. Visualization of the incision site with indentation ophthalmoscopy is mandatory within the early postoperative period.

Endophthalmitis Prophylaxis Is Critical

The incidence of infection is a multiple of that of a standard case.

Be Prepared

Code red, code blue, and amber alerts are accepted random routine preparation in the medical environment. Consider establishing and practicing Code V at the end of a random surgical day. Have a reusable clean vitrectomy kit for practice available. Make sure the surgeon and the staff know where the equipment is kept, how to set it up, and the parameters to check, and that instruments, medications, and devices are at the ready. The higher the volume of cataract surgery, the lower the complication rate and the less prepared for contingency a center may be without this Code V practice routine (**Box 20.1**).

First Signs of Complication

A rupture in the posterior capsule and, in particular, the anterior hyaloid changes the pressure relationship between the anterior and posterior chambers and the posterior segment. This change in the distribution of fluid will in turn affect the AC's depth and, often, the pupil's size; the pupil may suddenly bounce or snap. An increase or decrease in the AC's depth during phacoemulsification or irrigation and aspiration (I/A) are both warning signs; unless there is a good explanation for the change, stabilize and explore.

Box 20.1 Vitrectomy Kit Items (Not Exhaustive)

- Vitrectomy pack for phaco
- Calipers
- Microvitreoretinal (MVR) blades
- Trocars
- 23-gauge angled infusion cannula if not included in the vitrectomy pack
- Triesence (Alcon, Fort Worth, TX)
- Arbisser nuclear spears (Epsilon USA Instruments)
- Scissors
- Nonirrigating vectis
- Rings and segments for zonular defects
- Intraocular instruments (helpful)
- Sutures: 8-0 polyglactin, 10-0 nylon, 9-0 and 10-0 polypropylene, CV-8 Gore-Tex (off-label)
- Backup implants [three-piece AC intraocular lens (IOL)]
- Extra OVD dispersive and cohesive
- Acetylcholine
- Preservative-free (PF) epinephrine
- Trypan blue
- 2% lidocaine for sub-Tenon's anesthesia
- 26-gauge straight and J-cannulas, syringes for dry cortex removal

A momentary spider of the posterior capsule is likely associated with a tear and must be inspected after stabilizing the chamber and protecting the hyaloid with OVD. An unusually clear appearance of the posterior capsule is usually a rent or hole.

Because vitreous follows a gradient from high to low pressure, it will always preferentially seek to flow into the phaco or I/A tip and obstruct its action. If lenticular material suddenly stops coming to the phaco tip, there is likely vitreous in the way. Vitreous cannot be refluxed out of an I/A tip but must be sharply cut to avoid traction.

The classic later signs of vitreous loss are an asymmetrically enlarged pupil and remote movement of the iris when touching the incision. Another ominous sign of vitreous loss is tilting of the nucleus's equator or loss of mobility in a previously rotatable nucleus. Seeing clear space beyond the equator or having the equator come into view after removing the nucleus are sure signs of zonular loss with possible vitreous prolapse through the defect. A subtle sign of the presence of a forward strand of vitreous may be the inability to seal a properly constructed incision.

Vitrectomy Options

To best avoid vitreous traction, consider the best approach based on the particular condition of the eye. We need not always use an automated vitrector. If a small wisp of vitreous presents around zonules, it can be amputated with a scissor and reposited to the posterior segment with OVD.

A simple wisp that can be controlled is rare when vitreous prolapses through a broken posterior capsule. In the face of prolapse, automated vitrectomy is almost universally needed. In all cases the clear corneal paracentesis will be used for the irrigation cannula. When there is a small amount of prolapse without vitreous loss through incisions, vitrectomy can be nicely handled with the vitrector inserted through a clear corneal incision sized to fit the bare vitrector shaft. This is always the right choice when there is no view through the pupil or there is extreme or abnormal dimensional anatomy (**Fig. 20.2**).

In my experience, both in a laboratory setting and in the operating room, in the presence of copious vitreous prolapse, with vitreous loss through incisions or significant herniation around the bag equator, a pars plana sclerotomy approach to anterior vitrectomy is most efficient and preferable. The irrigating cannula is still placed through the clear corneal paracentesis. A direct entry sclerotomy under a fornix-based conjunctival flap created with an MVR blade and subsequently sutured whatever the vitrector gauge is worth learning to do safely. Alternatively, and theoretically the safest, a trocar system that enables a trans-conjunctival sutureless entry is best when the globe is closable or intact at the time of sclerotomy, as it requires pressure to insert. Trocars have the advantage of enabling repeated entry without trauma to sclera or proximity to the scleral wall and choroid. It is least likely to result in vitreous traction associated with incarceration at the incision site, as long as self-sealing, limbus parallel scleral tunnel is performed prior to entry perpendicular to the sclera. Any incision, anterior or posterior, must be closed when not in use. Sclerotomies are closed with a temporarily tied suture, preferably 8-0 polyglactin suture, a scleral plug, or, when available, the use of a valved trocar to maintain a closed environment and pressurized globe upon withdrawal of the vitrector shaft and during subsequent maneuvers (**Fig. 20.3**).

Rationale for a Pars Plana Approach to Anterior Vitrectomy

Because vitreous follows a pressure gradient from high to low, ideally the lowest pressure will always be in the posterior seg-

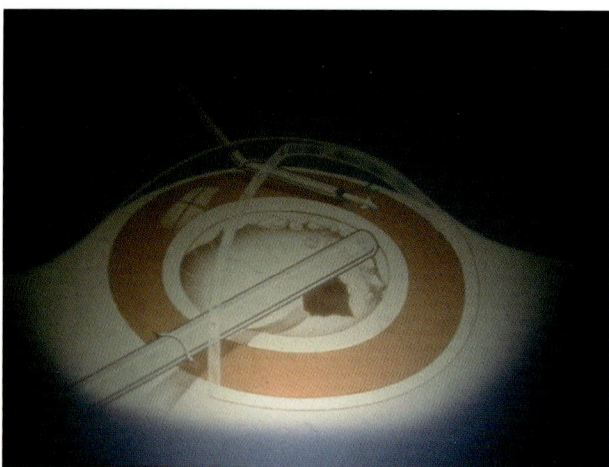

Fig. 20.2 Biaxial incisions with new anterior paracentesis to fit the vitrector—the simplest choice for minimal vitreous presentation and the only choice when the view behind the pupil is obscured.

ment relative to the anterior segment once the hyaloid is ruptured and during the remainder of a procedure after vitreous presentation. The best way to accomplish this is with a pars plana exit. We also want to minimize traction by removing the vitreous close to its base. As instruments exit the eye, vitreous will tend to follow. If any vitreous follows the instrument to the incision, it will be right near the vitreous base, where we can eliminate incarceration at the pars plana, rather than up at the corneal incision.

This technique is the most efficient, because it calls the vitreous home or amputates the anteroposterior attachment to prolapsed vitreous, immediately relieving traction without increasing the size of the posterior capsule rent. It is least likely to encourage more vitreous prolapse and removes only the offending vitreous, sparing the general vitreous body structure. With an anterior incision, and a downward angled vitrector through a rent in the posterior capsule, the view can be compromised. Also there is a tendency to remove nonprolapsed vitreous, encouraging more to come forward, which almost always enlarges the posterior capsular rent. It is also very challenging to clear sheets of vitreous in intimate contact with posterior capsule or iris

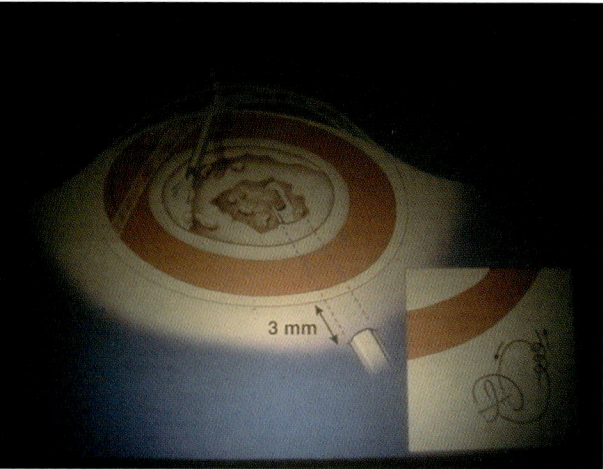

Fig. 20.3 Cadaver eye shows a Triesence-identified vitreous anterior/posterior connection severed after a pars plana anterior vitrectomy. The remaining anterior wisp can now be sponged away without fear of causing traction.

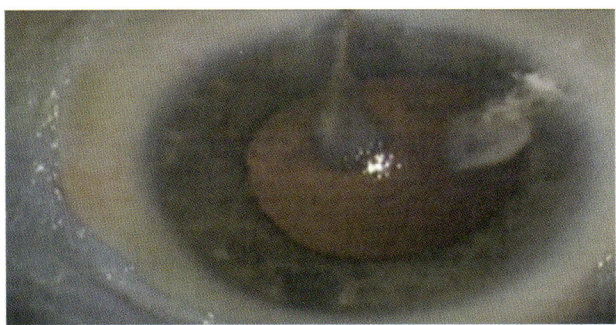

Fig. 20.4 The pars plana incision for anterior vitrectomy: irrigation through the side port with a vitrector through the pars plana 3 to 3.5 mm posterior to the limbus. Always suture the direct entry incision regardless of the gauge.

without damaging those structures from the anterior approach. The sheet tends to be broad, thin, and tightly adherent to these structures. Anteriorly placed irrigation and posteriorly located vitrector keeps a higher pressure in the AC. Multiple attempts in Liliana Werner's University of Utah laboratory with eye bank and porcine eyes with Kenalog delineation confirm the biaxial pars plana approach with the vitrector posteriorly and irrigation anteriorly is vastly superior to an anterior approach under a bubble, as recommended initially by Steve Charles or vitrectomy by standard anterior limbal approach.[3]

The pars plana technique maintains low pressure posteriorly. Subsequent manipulation to remove cortex and implant a lens is least likely to result in re-presentation of the vitreous so long as the AC is maintained. It will not unzip the zonules when vitreous presents around the lens equator by calling more vitreous forward through the defect or risking a posteriorly inserted vitrector near the retina! wall through zonules. Finally, the pars plana approach facilitates amputation of the vitreous within incisions (**Fig. 20.4**). The method if classically taught, using a sweep from the side-port incision to drag entrapped vitreous from the incision actually creates more traction on the connection through the pupil rather than efficiently freeing the vitreous from incarceration in the wound. This practice is strongly discouraged.

Nomenclature: Vitrectomy Mode (I/Cut/A) Versus Cortex Mode (I/A/Cut)

The nomenclature is confusing. The lack of standardization among manufacturers compounds the confusion. This chapter, therefore, refers to the order in which each function is engaged by the foot pedal. The best machine parameters for performing vitrectomy are the same regardless of what incision location is used for the vitrector needle. Employ the settings that most effectively reduce vitreoretinal traction and prevent followability. For the majority of phacoemulsification machines, bear in mind that foot position (FP) 1 is irrigation only, FP 2 engages both irrigation and cutting by activating the guillotine, and aspiration ensues only as FP 3 is entered, resulting in irrigating, cutting, and sucking simultaneously, ensuring that no vacuum is applied to the vitreous without chopping it off in tiny bites, minimizing traction in any part of the FP sequence.*

---

*The newest phaco machine at the time of this writing, the Alcon Centurion, employs only FP 1 and FP 2 in which cutting speed and vacuum magnitude is linear, somewhat different from other phaco machines and will not be discussed further in this chapter.

All machines have an alternate setting that is not the default, wherein FP 1 initiates irrigation as before, but FP 2 allows vacuum, and cutting mode only activates on FP 3. This setting, in this chapter's nomenclature I/A/Cut versus the default I/Cut/A, goes by different names on different platforms and is useful when followability is desired during removal of the residual cortex, once prolapsed vitreous is dispatched. This useful setting allows the surgeon to remain in FP 2 while removing lens material where followability is desirable but can allow near-instant activation of the cutter in the event vitreous presents.

Always employ the default setting when there is any likelihood that vitreous will be encountered.

Machine Settings

Cutting Rate and Flow

Steve Charles has coined the term *port-based flow limiting*. This describes the goal of achieving the highest cut rate possible, the lowest effective flow rate, and the lowest vacuum that generates the removal of vitreous. As the vitreous is engaged, the faster the guillotine opens and closes, the more traction is reduced because a lower volume of vitreous enters with less followability. The highest cut rate possible on some older phaco machines is 400 cuts per minute. Newer models achieve up to 16,000 cuts per minute. Faster cutting leads to less traction and a smoother removal of vitreous. Always use the available machine's fastest cut rate for vitrectomy. The higher rates are one of the reasons that three-port total planned vitrectomy has become safer over time. When close to the retinal surface the higher rates are critical. For anterior vitrectomy where we remain within the pupillary aperture, this speed is less critical and still acceptable with any phaco machine for the cataract surgeon's purpose. The technique, however, will vary slightly depending on the cut rate. At lower rates the episodic pull of the vitreous is almost visible, as is the opening and closing of the guillotine. With these lower cut rates it is very important not to drag vitreous around and critical to keep the vitrector handpiece steady in one place until the advantage of that location has concluded removing accessible prolapsed vitreous. The needle can then be moved to a new location in FP 2 to be certain no vitreous is dragged along by the flow, and then FP 3 is reengaged to remove prolapsed vitreous in this new location. Waving the needle around and rapidly moving its position is discouraged. With the higher cut rates the action of the guillotine is such a blur that only the sound provides the feedback of activity. The effect is more like erasing than aspirating vitreous and the activity at the vitrector tip can be more efficient and dynamic without causing traction. This simultaneously promotes safer and quicker surgery. The aspiration flow rate (for peristaltic pump platforms) is generally set at 15 to 20 cc/min depending on the vitrector gauge. The logic is simply to make things happen but not too fast.

Linear Versus Fixed Vacuum Setting

Vitreoretinal surgeons who frequently work in the posterior segment prefer to use linear vacuum for vitrectomy, and therefore this is usually the default for phaco machines as well. Familiarity leads to facility. Surgeons may adjust the vacuum on the fly based on how vitreous is behaving. They may wish to be more or less aggressive with vacuum, and the nuance of where they are in FP 3 is intuitively controllable. Anterior-segment surgeons who rarely perform vitrectomy are not usually as adept at these maneuvers and often get nowhere due to a light foot that may not even venture into FP 3. Staying in FP 2 accomplishes nothing because there will be continuous cutting without suction. For those with a heavy foot, the nuance of applying more or less vacuum during vitreous removal is lost, and they may use more vacuum than necessary and may cause more traction. Anterior-segment surgeons can consider a panel/fixed setting for vacuum instead of a linear vacuum setting for vitrectomy. Find and maintain the lowest level of vacuum that moves the vitreous; there is no reason to use higher or lower vacuum once vitreous removal is evident. The panel setting allows us to either go pedal-to-the-metal in FP 3 with suction, or come up into FP 2 without suction. The vacuum default settings on today's phaco machines are usually set at 150 mm Hg, ideal perhaps for primary three-port total vitrectomy. In unplanned vitrectomy, however, the anterior segment surgeon is almost always removing vitreous in a sea of dispersive viscoelastic, causing an effective level to be closer to 250 mm Hg for 20-gauge and 350 mm Hg for 23-gauge vitrectomy on average.

Adjusting Irrigation Inflow

The irrigation bottle must be kept moderately high to maintain a normotensive eye. If there is forced infusion, then a normotensive setting in the range of 25 mm Hg should be chosen. Most phaco machine's default settings place the bottle low. The appropriate bottle height depends on the size of cannula we use as well as the vacuum level. Most anterior-segment surgeons opt for a 23-gauge cannula, which is delivered with most newer vitrector kits. The port of the irrigation cannula should be held sideways, neither irrigating down into the vitreous nor directly up toward the endothelium. To control the IOP, have the scrub nurse stand with one hand on the bottle's button, ready to raise it as needed, and one hand on the vacuum button. Start the vacuum for 20-gauge vitrectomy at around 200 mm Hg, and ask the scrub nurse to progress by 10-mm increments to 250 mm Hg or stop once the vitreous begins to move. As soon as movement toward the vitrector port is seen, with a finger on the globe from the nondominant hand holding the irrigation cannula, the surgeon can instruct the scrub nurse to raise the bottle until homeostatic normotension is achieved. Ideally, just prior to removing the vitrector at the end point, when not aspirating any longer, the bottle would once again be lowered to reduce the IOP when there is no material being removed and just before irrigation is turned off and the vitrector exited from the incision to reduce pressure variation.

Visualization: Particulate Staining

Although slit or tangential illumination with a light pipe can help to visualize the invisible vitreous, nothing compares to triamcinolone acetonide as a tool to particulate stain the vitreous. Essentially we "throw a sheet over the ghost" (**Fig. 20.5**), as originally devised by Gholam Peyman,[4] and then popularized in the anterior segment by Scott Burk[5,6] using preserved Kenalog off-label. Kenalog must be washed of the preservative. However the commercially available nonpreserved Triesence (triamcinolone acetonide injectable suspension; Alcon Laboratories, Inc.) preparation is Food and Drug Administration (FDA)-approved and billable. When instilled intracamerally, the suspended particles are individually trapped in the vitreous matrix but will rinse out of aqueous. It will not adhere to OVD but can be blocked by it. Triesence is best diluted 10 to 1 with balanced salt solution (BSS) to prevent a whiteout effect within the AC, obscuring intraocular structures. The dilution also provides enough volume for repeated use during the procedure. The suspension can settle out of its diluent in the syringe, as there is no chemical to keep it suspended. A small pearl: have the scrub nurse introduce an air bubble into the syringe to facilitate shaking up and resuspending

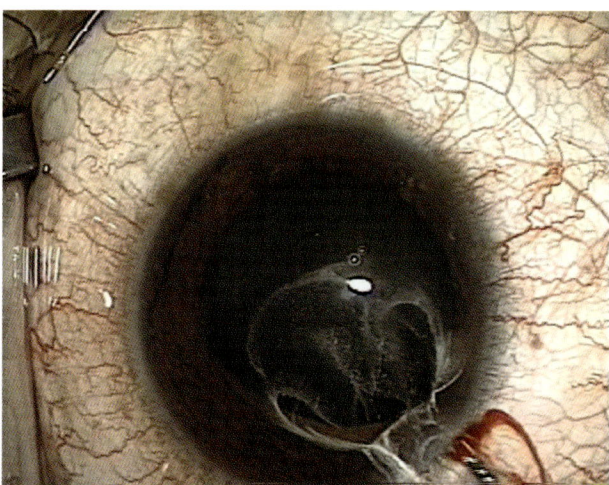

Fig. 20.5 Triamcinolone preferentially adheres to vitreous like "throwing a sheet over the ghost."

the particles. Of course, expel the air prior to handing it to the surgeon. In the best of all worlds, Triesence would be prepared preoperatively and kept on the back table, ready to be used immediately upon suspicion of a complication to be followed by OVD. However, as OVD is always at hand, it is preferentially used immediately to stabilize the environment when a complication is suspected. The Triesence then is usually used after initial vitrectomy, once the OVD is also removed, to provide a critical visual end point for vitrectomy. Triesence instillation into the AC of a minim or two should always be one of the last maneuvers in the complicated case to rule out any unsuspected vitreous representation. As an added benefit, the drug has the therapeutic effect of reducing postoperative inflammation.

Early Response

When danger threatens, the innate response is withdrawal. Control that natural response to pull out of the eye upon the recognition of a complication. The phaco or I/A tip between the lips of the wound controls the intraocular environment. Upon recognition of a problem, go to FP 1 to maintain irrigation in the AC but do not move the irrigating tip. Remove the nondominant hand instrument from the paracentesis, which will not result in chamber instability. Trade this for an OVD syringe. Once the cannula is past the internal Descemet's membrane, then go to FP 0 and instill OVD (dispersive ideally) through the paracentesis over the suspected rent and between the posterior capsule and any remaining lens fragments until the AC is normal depth. Only then can the phaco (I/A) tip be withdrawn from the eye without AC collapse. If the chamber is permitted to become shallow in the presence of a tear in the capsule, vitreous pressure will extend the tear and the stage of complication may progress from rupture to vitreous prolapse or from prolapse to vitreous loss. Vitreous always follows the path of lowest pressure. Now, with the incision effectively closed and the intraocular environment stabilized, it is time to assess the situation, inspect the result, relax, and think. Announce the delay to the operating room staff to avoid having the next patient, who may be on the table in the next room, prepped and draped prematurely. Remember, too, to relax yourself and your voice as the awake patient deserves to feel the surgeon is in calm control. Consider a code word for the staff such as "timing," which alerts them to spring into action with a prepared and well-rehearsed plan.

Anesthesia

In potentially difficult cases or for patients who cannot follow directions during an indirect retina exam, the surgeon may wish to consider peribulbar anesthesia preoperatively. For patients who cannot be relied on to remain still during the procedure (pediatric, disabled, or severely claustrophobic patients) the surgeon may consider general anesthesia. Topical anesthesia does not preclude managing complications.

Without pain receptors, the vitreous cannot "hurt." Topical and or intracameral anesthesia may not require supplementation for anterior incisions. When the pars plana incision is employed, or the wound needs to be significantly enlarged, a bleb of subconjunctival lidocaine 2% over the intended scleral incision prior to incising a fornix flap for sclerotomy incision is appropriate. A cellulose sponge soaked in anesthetic as a pledget held directly in contact with the sclera for 30 seconds may also suffice and is ideal for trocar placement.

Avoid reintroduction of intracameral unpreserved 1% lidocaine. Although there is evidence that there will be no permanent damage to the neuroretina, there will be a transient amaurosis as a result of contact of the anesthetic with the posterior segment through broken zonules or a capsule rupture.[7] This can be disconcerting or even frightening to both patient and surgeon, and is unlikely to be helpful regardless, as the lidocaine will not remain in contact with innervated structures as it would with a closed chamber. The availability of intravenous sedation is desirable to help the patient cooperate or to make the time pass more quickly during a prolonged case. Oversedation can cause sudden awakening and movement or agitation, further complicating the case. If the patient is uncomfortable, tiny aliquots of short-acting narcotics such as alfentanil hydrochloride injection (Alfenta; Akorn, Inc., Lake Forest, IL) or midazolam (Versed; Hoffmann-La Roche Inc., Branchburg, NJ) can be helpful. Of course, a calm voice (vocal local) and having an operating room team that can seamlessly prepare for a vitrectomy is extremely helpful in minimizing patient anxiety without sedation. If these measures fail and the patient loses the ability to cooperate, akinesia may be required. First be sure the incisions are closed to avoid loss of chamber. A snip down to bare sclera and use of a Greenbaum or Masket cannula to perform sub-Tenon's or parabulbar block resulting in akinesia without sharp injection is optimal. This obviates the risk of retrobulbar hemorrhage, particularly untimely in this setting.

Controlling the Damage

Once vitreous begins to prolapse, use a dispersive viscoelastic to separate the lens material from the vitreous as much as possible so they do not become entangled. True compartmentalization means first using a dispersive viscoelastic (such as Viscoat OVD, Alcon, Fort Worth, TX) over the area you want to isolate, such as a tear, and then barricading the dispersive agent by adding a cohesive viscoelastic such as Provisc OVD (Alcon) behind it. As the cohesive agent dissipates, you can work where that agent used to be while the remaining dispersive OVD keeps the eye compartmentalized. The goal is to convert any posterior capsular break or rent into a true posterior continuous curvilinear capsulorrhexis (CCC). Even when the rent appears round, minimal force can cause it to extend, because only a true CCC that finishes outside of where it began has full strength. When you recognize a break in the posterior capsule, first stabilize the AC with dispersive OVD, then gently irrigate a cohesive OVD into Berger's space through the tear to push back and stabilize the hyaloid. If the hyaloid is intact it should begin to take on the form of Berger's space filling into itself. If the hyaloid is broken, it will fall backward into the vitreous cavity—a diagnostic sign of vitreous pro-

lapse. This prolapse must be removed with the vitrector prior to attempting to convert the rent into a posterior CCC. Once free of any vitreous, the torn posterior capsule (PC) edge is grasped with a capsulorrhexis forceps (you may need to first create an edge with intraocular scissors) and, with a more centripetal vector due to the thin elastic nature, complete a true rhexis. This can be kept very small for bag implantation or made large enough for posterior optic capture into Berger's space.

If any nuclear fragments remain in the posterior capsule (not in the posterior segment below the PC, which may be best handled by referral for total vitrectomy), raise them up above the iris to separate them from vitreous for extraction. If the pupil is small and additional intracameral preservative-free 1:4,000 epinephrine does not enlarge it adequately, performing a two-point stretch pupilloplasty, microsphincterotomies, or iris hooks can be helpful. An intraocular device such as a Malyugin ring (MicroSurgical Technology, Redmond, WA) is not recommended in this complex setting.

Spare the intact anterior rhexis for optic capture from the sulcus. If it is impeding forward movement of fragments, rather than relaxing the edge with a radial cut, make a tangential cut, and spiral the flap around so that it is slightly smaller in diameter than the optic of the lens you plan to implant. Then dial, lift, cantilever, float with viscoelastic, or use Arbisser nuclear spears (Epsilon Ophthalmic Instruments, Ontario, CA; **Figs. 20.6** and **20.7**) from two opposing corneal paracenteses to elevate the fragment up above the iris plane. If prolapsed vitreous is compartmentalized, slow-motion phaco parameters can be used, taking care to establish flow before engaging ultrasound in an OVD-filled environment.[8] Some advocate placing an IOL as a scaffold to prevent nuclear drop.[9] If there is possible admixture of vitreous and lens, enlarge the incision for manual removal without pressure on the globe in a dispersive OVD sandwich protecting the endothelium.

Getting Started: Vitrectomy Mode and Incisions

The first step is to confirm the initial vitrectomy mode settings and then to prime the line by irrigating away any bubbles while the vitrector is outside the eye. If choosing an anterior approach, make a second paracentesis a little less than 180 degrees away from the original side port, large enough to fit the bare vitrector

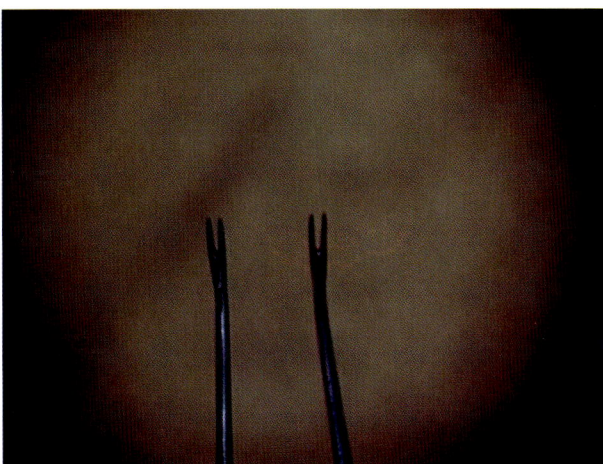

Fig. 20.6   Arbisser nuclear spears can be used through two opposing paracenteses to spear and elevate the descending nucleus, which is still in the posterior chamber without entering the pars plana.

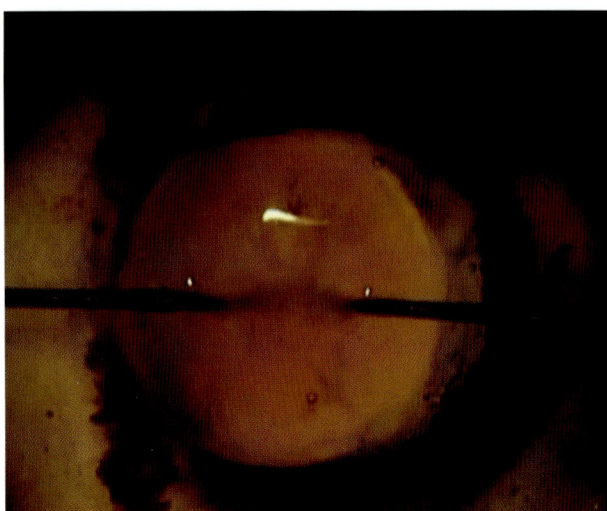

Fig. 20.7 Nuclear spears impaling the nucleus in a cadaver eye for easy elevation. They are curve-down spears to fit within the anterior capsulorrhexis and can be used for fragments as well.

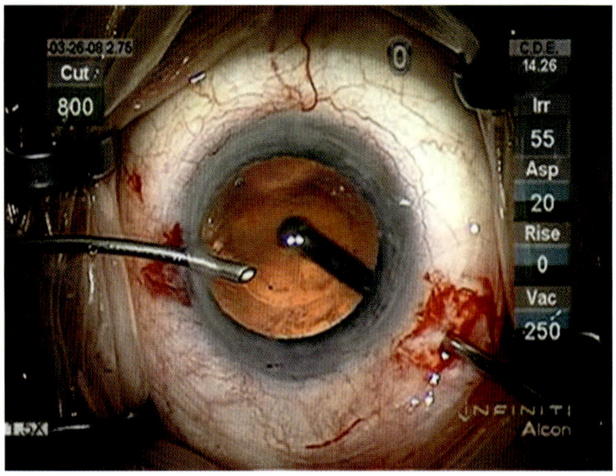

Fig. 20.8 An irrigating cannula is always placed through the anterior paracentesis and pointed sideways. A vitrector can be placed through a tight anterior paracentesis or, in this case, through a pars plana sclerotomy. Note that the vitrector is under the posterior capsule (PC) rent and the port is visible. Using the machine's highest available cut rate, irrigation balances the vacuum, which is the lowest effective setting.

needle. If planning a pars plana incision under topical anesthesia, first place a bleb of lidocaine with epinephrine sub-Tenon's over the intended area of the incision for the patient's comfort. This step permits a small, fornix-based peritomy to bare the sclera without cautery.

Next, secure the primary wound if there is no vitreous loss. If vitreous is incarcerated in the incision, blocking a watertight closure, fill the AC with OVD to approximate normal pressure.

Clear Corneal Anterior Incision

Any phaco incision, clear corneal or scleral tunnel, is too large to secure a closed system with the vitrector handpiece without a coaxial sleeve. Biaxial vitrectomy has become standard of care due to the reduced tendency to displace vitreous and promote further prolapse. The original clear corneal paracentesis becomes the port for irrigation through a chamber maintainer, butterfly needle, or other cannula of 20 or 23 gauge (**Fig. 20.8**). Consideration then needs to be given to the creation of the vitrectomy port incision. Just as we would never use a leaky incision safely for the rest of the procedure, so should the incision fit the vitrectomy handpiece snugly. A 20- or 23-gauge MVR blade or a keratome capable of creating this size opening can be employed.

Sutured Direct Pars Plana Sclerotomy Incision

Avoid the 3, 6, 9, and 12 o'clock positions for scleral incisions so as to avoid the ciliary vessels and nerves. Always use a caliper to measure 3.5 mm posterior to the limbus in the quadrant most convenient to the dominant hand, avoiding perforating vessels to obviate the need for cautery, which only invites inflammation and astigmatism. This measurement is optimal in all but pediatric, buphthalmic, and nanophthalmic eyes where sclerotomy may best be avoided by the anterior-segment surgeon (**Fig. 20.9**).

For a direct sclerotomy, while stabilizing the eye with a forceps 180 degrees away at the limbus, enter the pars plana at the caliper mark with an MVR blade of the gauge appropriate to the vitrector perpendicular to the sclera. Perforate until the blade is just visualized in the pupil, ensuring complete entry (**Fig. 20.10**). Withdraw the blade. Insert the irrigating 23-gauge chamber

maintainer or cannula through the original clear corneal incision paracentesis on FP 0 (not irrigating). Now insert the vitrector through the sclerotomy, advancing it until it is within view through the pupil. Step down to FP 2, which will be irrigating and cutting without allowing vacuum to build, and bring it under the capsular rent. Always make sure you can see the port during vitrectomy; the only exception is when performing a dry vitrectomy to make space in a crowded AC. In this scenario, make sure the port is sideways or backward to avoid engaging the posterior capsule while removing a small amount of vitreous.

No matter the gauge of the MVR blade or vitrector, a direct incision demands a suture. One bite for 23 or 25 g and a two-bite X or horizontal mattress suture for 20 g. Keep in mind we are not doing a total vitrectomy. This means that, unlike the vitreoretinal surgeon who risks minor transient hypotony, we risk vitreous incarceration, which can surely lead to retinal tears in the postoperative period. Endoscopy reveals a gaping hole at least briefly left by the round vitrector withdrawn from the sclerotomy site, which has little elasticity and no endothelial pump to close it. This invites vitreous incarceration. When the vitrector is with-

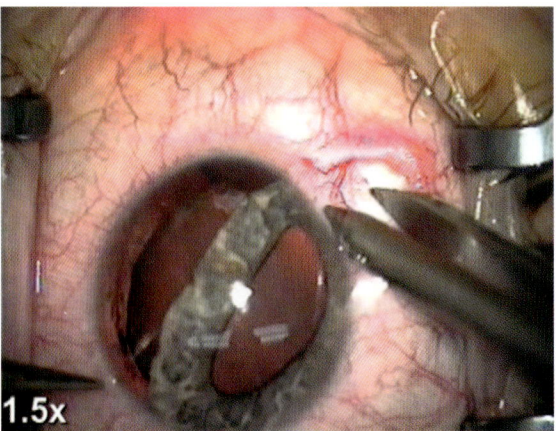

Fig. 20.9 Measuring 3.5 mm behind the limbus under the fornix-based flap for a pars plana sclerotomy.

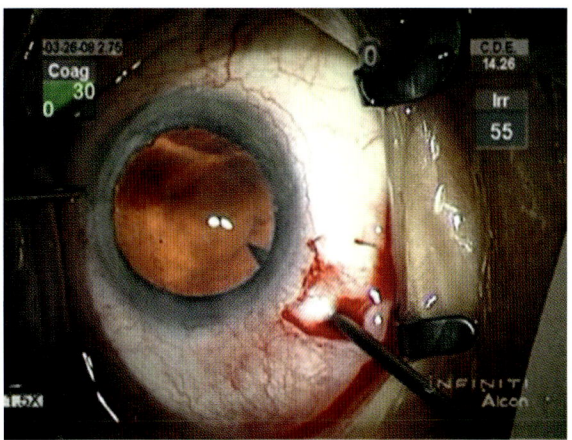

Fig. 20.10 A 20-gauge MVR blade enters through the pars plana until it is just visualized in the pupil to ensure complete perforation.

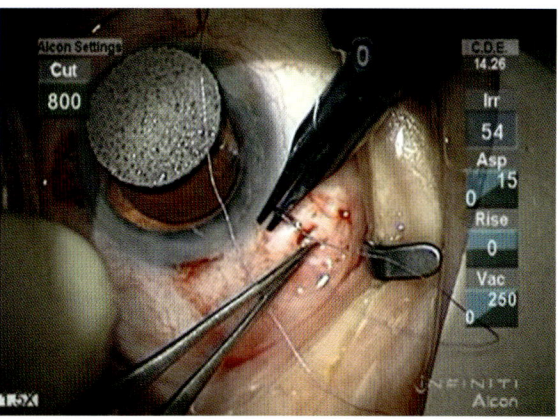

Fig. 20.11 Suturing a pars plana direct sclerotomy under a fornix-based flap. The flap can then be secured in place with the same absorbable suture. Protect the macula from light during a prolonged procedure.

drawn a scleral plug is temporarily placed in case of needed re-entry. Prior to suturing the sclerotomy, irrigate the lips of the incision while using the vitrector in FP 2 (cutting), with the port down against the scleral surface to clear any incarcerated strands of vitreous rather than using a cellulose sponge at a pars plana sclerotomy. A small amount of dispersive OVD can be insinuated between the sclerotomy edges to hold back any vitreous threatening to escape as an 8-0 polyglactin suture is secured, thereby not incarcerating vitreous (**Fig. 20.11**). It may be best to orient the needle from a posterior to anterior position when taking the half-thickness bite(s) to ensure that the needle's point does not come out too far posteriorly. It is not necessary to bury the knot, as it will be covered by the Tenons' and conjunctival fornix-based flap that should be secured in place with the same absorbable suture. Tie the knot on the inside of the flap for the patient's comfort (**Fig. 20.12**). The sclerotomy should be watertight, and no bleb should form from pressurizing the globe.

Sutureless Pars Plana Trocar System Insertion

The concept of a self-sealing pars plana sclerotomy is similar to a scleral tunnel cataract incision in concept, where a tunnel-like partial depth incision is created with a floor and ceiling that, when approximated, seal water- (or vitreous) tight. A noncoincident incision in the conjunctiva and the sclera is optimal, which is why it is difficult to make a sutureless incision without the help of a cannula to keep the two openings lined up. Finding the openings with the vitrector via an MVR blade–created shelved entry is very challenging. The trocar system is a hollow-tubed cannula that encases a sharp MVR blade. Once the incision is completed, the blade is withdrawn leaving the tube as a conduit for the vitrector needle, which can be repeatedly insert as needed until the procedure is completed. A trocar cannula system offers another advantage: it protrudes into the vitreous cavity so the vitrector probe never gets close to the retinal surface, as it does when inserted through a bare sclerotomy. This design provides a margin of safety upon entry and exit, and there is some evidence it decreases the risk of retinal tears. As they become sharper and require less pressure for entry, trocars will be the entry method of choice.

Using a trocar cannula system requires a firm, intact eye with closed incisions to handle the pressure applied to the globe upon entry. If incisions are already present, do not simply close them with hydration, but suture them closed, because the force of

inserting the trocar will likely cause iris prolapse if they are not entirely secure. A soft eye will risk choroidal detachment or hemorrhage due to incomplete penetration or choroidal detachment with this procedure. If vitreous has been lost, you will not be able to close the incisions, even with sutures, so a direct MVR entry with suturing would be safest.

Fill the eye with BSS or OVD until it is firm, while ascertaining that the cataract incisions are closed. Pull the conjunctiva away from the site of puncture 3.5 mm back from the limbus and initiate a partial-thickness scleral tunnel at an angle of 30 degrees to the sclera with the trocar parallel to the limbus (**Fig. 20.13**). Travel ~ 1 to 2 mm to make a tunnel until the cannula approximates the sclera, then elevate the heal to turn the device perpendicular to the sclera and puncture, driving the trocar cannula system through the eye wall (**Fig. 20.14**). Once the trocar cannula is in place, remove the MVR blade while holding the neck of the cannula still with a forceps, and leave the seated cannula for the vitrector's insertion. Due to the intrascleral travel of the cannula, the protruding lip should tilt sideways slightly rather than sitting perfectly flush at the scleral surface, providing assurance that an adequate tunnel has been made for self-sealing

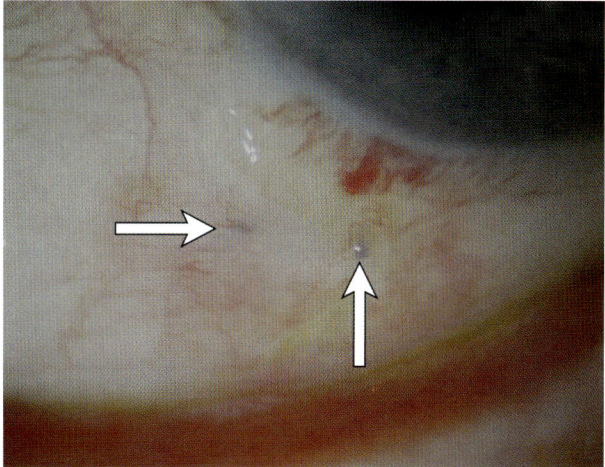

Fig. 20.12 One day postoperative: pars plana sclerotomy slit-lamp photographs. (**a**) Faint evidence of 8-0 polyglactin suture *(horizontal arrow)* in sclerotomy under a fornix-based conjunctival flap. (**b**) Buried suture holding a flap in place covering the sclerotomy *(vertical arrow)*.

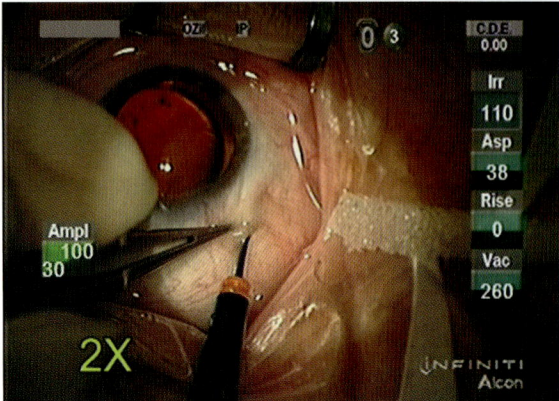

Fig. 20.13 Transconjunctival 23-gauge trocar system incision. The angle of attack of 30 degrees to the plane of the sclera 3.5 mm back from limbus and limbus-parallel makes a self-sealing scleral tunnel before angling the heal 90 degrees to the sclera and perforating through the pars plana.

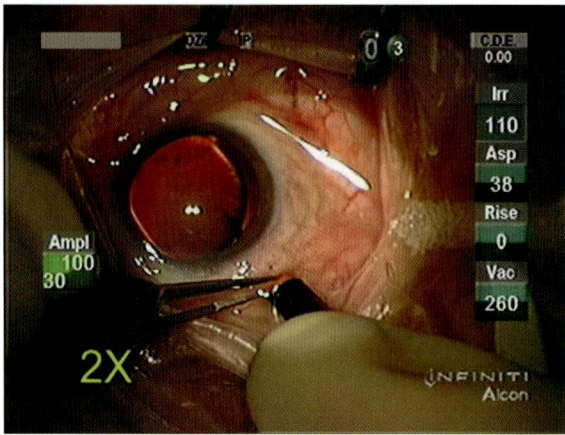

Fig. 20.14 The trocar collar is now seated against the sclera. A forceps holds the collar to permit withdrawal of the MVR blade, leaving the cannula through the eye wall into the vitreous cavity as a conduit for the vitrector.

upon removal. Some newer models have one-way valves. Others require a scleral plug (and the forceps to manipulate the plug) to ensure a closed system when the vitrector is not in working position inserted through the cannula into the eye. As with the direct-entry incision, the infusion cannula is placed through the anterior side port. The bare vitrector needle slides through the cannula into the position of action.

Upon completion of the procedure, immediately upon removing the trocar cannula, point pressure is applied on the surface of the conjunctiva over the opening with the point of the cannula or the wooden end of a cotton swab to crush the tunnel floor and ceiling together, assuring a secure seal. No bleb should form upon pressurizing the eye.

Process

Once the vitrector is visualized in the pupil and the irrigation cannula is positioned in the anterior side port, engage FP 3. Look for any small bubble or particle to confirm when the vacuum is high enough to move vitreous. If you have set the vacuum on panel or fixed rather than linear, now begin the process of finding the lowest effective vacuum level by asking the scrub nurse to raise the vacuum slowly until effective, usually at 200 mm Hg for 20-gauge or 300 mm Hg for 23-gauge vitrectomy. Once effective aspiration occurs, raise the bottle to achieve homeostasis for a normotensive globe. Normotension is often achieved at 70- to 80-cm bottle height while aspirating vitreous (above the default setting for most machines), depending on where the patient's head is relative to the machine's cassette and the gauge of the irrigation cannula. As noted, the flow rate on machines with a peristaltic pump usually stays at 20 cc/min for 20-gauge and 15 cc/min for 23-gauge vitrectomy, and it need not be adjusted.

Completing the Vitrectomy

Keep the pedal to the metal until it is evident that there is no more prolapsed vitreous flowing to the port. If the position of the vitrector must be moved to better advantage, change from FP 3 to FP 2 to cut with no suction, and then readjust the location of the port to address any other areas of vitreous prolapse. Do not move the vitrector around through vitreous without being in FP 2 to avoid inadvertent traction due to flow. The higher the cut rate, the smaller the sphere of influence of the cutter on vitreous

removal due to the reduced followability. The higher the cut rate, then the more movement of the tip may be necessary and the more important particulate identification becomes, as, without the drag on the vitreous seen with low cut rates, it is harder to determine the end point.

When the end point is likely achieved, hold the vitrector steady within view and come to FP 0. Remove the irrigation cannula, and irrigate some diluted Triesence into the AC. Again place the irrigator through the paracentesis to disperse the Triesence, thereby confirming the complete absence of prolapsed vitreous. Before extracting the vitrector from the eye, lower the bottle to 15 to 20 cm (Christopher Riemann, MD, personal communication). This maneuver prevents the eye from being overpressurized upon removal of the vitrector. Remain in cutting mode (FP 2) just until visualization is lost under the iris. Come up into FP 1 for the brief interval that the vitrector is between the edge of the iris and when it exits the sclera, but go to FP 0 right before exiting the incision, so as not to blow vitreous out of the incision, causing incarceration. Retinal surgeons continue irrigating until they are out of the eye, but that is because they have done a total vitrectomy, so only BSS exits, not vitreous. Immediately place a scleral plug or a temporary tie suture to close the sclerotomy. If an anterior approach was utilized, confirm that the clear corneal incision closes and that no strand of vitreous has followed withdrawal of the vitrector needle. The eye is now closed and ready for further maneuvers, and the vitrectomy site is available in case vitreous presents again.

Sponging and Sweeping Incisions

For decades, ophthalmic residents were told to use a cyclodialysis spatula to sweep from the paracentesis to just inside the main incision to identify, release, and remove incarcerated vitreous. This practice causes significant traction on the posterior vitreous and should be abandoned. The preferred technique is particulate identification and sharp cutting or, ideally, using a vitrector to amputate anteroposterior connections, thus obviating traction and the need to sweep. Once the vitreous sheet either retracts to the posterior segment or is severed from the vitreous within the wound, it is safe to remove residual vitreous from the incision with a cellulose sponge. Sponges should not be used to remove vitreous that is still attached posteriorly, however, because they absorb vitreous strands with capillary action and, more grossly,

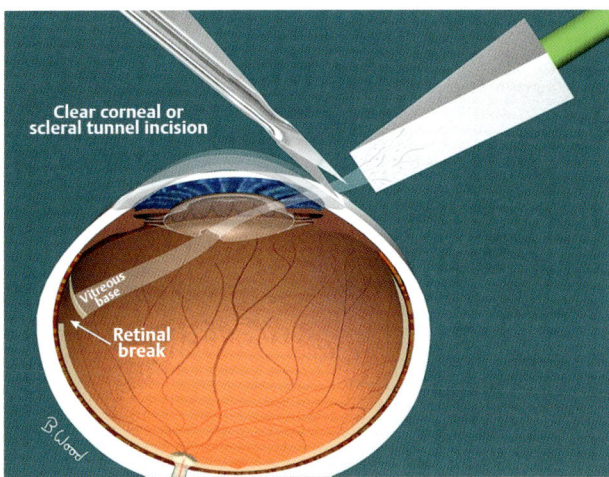

Fig. 20.15 Sponging vitreous at the incision causes dangerous traction. (Courtesy of Steve Charles, MD.)

when lifted to cut the strands. Additionally, they cause inflammation upon contact with iris tissue. If a sponge is touched to an incision, have scissors ready in the other hand so that, should vitreous be present, it can be cut without lifting or stretching the strands. Immediately cut off the vitreous at the plane of the sclera so it is not pulled forward out of the wound. Then address the vitreous in the optimal manner (**Fig. 20.15**).

Residual Cortex Removal

Residual cortex should be cleanly removed to avoid inflammation, prevent a poor-quality view with fluffed up cortex in the postoperative period, to reduce the risk of cystoid macular edema (CME), and even to reduce the media for bacterial growth leading to endophthalmitis. Regardless of the technique, compartmentalization with dispersive OVD over the capsule rent and then cohesive anteriorly under which to work is ideal. A "dry" technique, meaning aspirating with a syringe and 26-gauge cannula under cohesive OVD without irrigation, is safest, as there is no turbulence. It is time-consuming and can require extra OVD. Alternatively, the vitrector handpiece can be used set to vacuum before cutting to avoid damage to the capsule edge, to promote followability, and to minimize risk of vitreous traction as FP 3 can be engaged in the event of vitreous representation. For 20-gauge vitrectors, there is built-in inefficiency due to the need to occlude the 1-mm guillotine opening to build vacuum; smaller gauge vitrectors are far more efficient due to their size opening. Bimanual I/A is the most efficient method with the 0.3-mm port and, because irrigation remains anterior through the paracentesis and the aspiration targets cortex directly, is a safe choice. Coaxial I/A should be avoided, for it causes the most turbulence and encourages representation of vitreous. Incarcerating vitreous causes maximal traction. Remember to secure the pressurized AC during and after cortex removal.

Inspect Prior to Implantation

To make sure the anterior segment is cleaned of all cortex, retract the iris to fully view the bag fornix. Re-instill Triesence and then rinse it away to be sure there is no vitreous present. Check that the pupil is round and that the incisions are sealed. Verify the status and size of the capsulorrhexis, and evaluate the extent of the posterior capsular tear and whether there is a true continuous curvilinear tear. Be aware of any retained nuclear fragment

below the posterior capsule, and make certain no fragments are hiding anteriorly under the iris or subincisionally.

Intraocular Lens Selection and Placement

Vitreo-retinal surgeons prefer acrylic to silicone if a retinal procedure is anticipated. Plate haptic models are unwise in complicated cases, one-piece lenses should never be put in the sulcus, and, whenever possible, optic capture is optimal for long-term lens stability.[10] Unsecured pure sulcus placement often leads to late subluxation, and multifocals should never be placed if centration is not ensured. In the absence of capsule support, it remains controversial, with little long-term data to confirm the superiority of scleral-fixated, iris-fixated, or open loop AC IOLs (with peripheral iridectomy), but the trend is toward sutureless scleral fixation. Capsular tension rings are appropriate when zonular defects present but are contraindicated in the setting of a ruptured anterior or posterior capsule. Details are beyond the scope of this chapter.

Removing OVD and Closing the Eye

Only when the implant optic is effectively captured will the anterior and posterior segments be sealed and segregated. If uncaptured, beware aggressive removal of OVD at the end of the procedure for fear of encouraging vitreous to herniate around the implant. Manual removal by burping the incision, careful irrigation, and a push/pull technique through the paracenteses need not be thorough and are far safer than using automated methods of OVD removal. The AC pressure must remain higher than the PC pressure, or vitreous representation is invited at any point as even a captured lens can slip away and become uncaptured. Residual Healon 5 (Abbott Medical Optics Inc., Abbott Park, IL) can cause a severe rise in IOP in the postoperative period, whereas Viscoat is the most forgiving agent, because it is of a smaller molecular weight. Any OVD that remains behind a properly captured optic is of no concern, as it will not have access to the trabecular meshwork and will slowly be absorbed without incident.

Miochol E (acetylcholine) will provide miosis, protect the IOL's position, and ensure a round pupil with no peak, which would indicate a vitreous wick.

A final minim of Triesence and rigorously closed incisions with dry tunnels will confirm that no incarcerated vitreous lurks. Even if the clear corneal incision seals flawlessly, a suture is indicated if a follow-up retinal procedure may be needed due to retained lens material.

Postoperative Care

Endophthalmitis prophylaxis with intracameral Vigamox or compounded moxifloxacin (off-label) (off-label) should be considered.[11] Immediately postoperatively, consider one oral dose of Avelox (Bayer Corporation, Passaic, NJ), which is a systemic form of moxifloxacin (400 mg PO) that crosses the blood–retina barrier to achieve an appropriate minimally inhibitory concentration (MIC) in the vitreous.

Patients with an open hyaloid need an aggressive anti-inflammatory regimen, which can start in the immediate postoperative period.

Warn vitrectomy patients to expect floaters postoperatively and to call and identify themselves as surgical patients if they experience pain or decreasing vision at any time. Treat any IOP spikes aggressively and follow them closely, especially over the first 48 hours. Instruct patients to check their peripheral vision at home. Perform a scleral-indented retinal examination and/or refer for a retinal subspecialty consultation within 1 to 2 weeks after the surgery. Closely monitor these patients for CME with an Amsler grid at home, looking for decreased contrast not distortion centrally. Also, optical coherence tomography is indicated. A longer taper of topical steroids and remaining on topical non-steroidal anti-inflammatory drugs (NSAIDs) for a longer period than routine cases (off label) to prevent CME is indicated. Ocular hypertension prophylaxis is wise for residual OVD or lens fragments. If an eye has retained lens material, a timely referral of the patient to a retinal specialist for possible definitive treatment is needed. Meta-analysis of the literature shows patients fare best if the intervention is from 3 to 7 days after surgery that was complicated by retained lens material.[12] Every complicated cataract surgery patient deserves full disclosure, close follow-up, timely scleral depressed retinal evaluation, and appropriate specialty referral. It is critical to inform these patients of their increased risk of developing a retinal tear or detachment in the future, in addition to the increased risk of glaucoma and CME.

Conclusion

Although a pars plana vitrector incision proves to be more efficient and, when properly executed, superior in many ways, it is most important to have a bimanual approach to anterior vitrectomy with tight incisions and minimal pressure fluctuation. Preventing intraoperative and postoperative vitreous traction and leaving a clean anterior segment without collateral damage are the cataract surgeon's goal. With advance preparation for complications and a comprehensive strategy, optimal outcomes are the norm.

References

1. Lundström M, Behndig A, Kugelberg M, Montan P, Stenevi U, Thorburn W. Decreasing rate of capsule complications in cataract surgery: eight-year study of incidence, risk factors, and data validity by the Swedish National Cataract Register. J Cataract Refract Surg 2011;37:1762–1767
2. Worst JGF, Los LI. Cisternal Anatomy of the Vitreous. Amsterdam and New York: Kugler; 1995
3. Arbisser LB, Charles S, Howcroft M, Werner L. Management of vitreous loss and dropped nucleus during cataract surgery. Ophthalmol Clin North Am 2006;19:495–506
4. Peyman GA, Cheema R, Conway MD, Fang T. Triamcinolone acetonide as an aid to visualization of the vitreous and the posterior hyaloid during pars plana vitrectomy. Retina 2000;20:554–555
5. Burk SE, Da Mata AP, Snyder ME, Schneider S, Osher RH, Cionni RJ. Visualizing vitreous using Kenalog suspension. J Cataract Refract Surg 2003;29:645–651
6. Burk SE, Da Mata AP, Snyder ME, et al. Identifying the vile humor. Video J Cataract Surg 2002;18
7. Lincoff H, Zweifach P, Brodie S, et al. Intraocular injection of lidocaine. Ophthalmology 1985;92:1587–1591
8. Osher RH. Slow motion phacoemulsification approach. J Cataract Refract Surg 1993;19:667
9. Agarwal A, Jacob S, Agarwal A, Narasimhan S, Kumar DA, Agarwal A. Glued intraocular lens scaffolding to create an artificial posterior capsule for nucleus removal in eyes with posterior capsule tear and insufficient iris and sulcus support. J Cataract Refract Surg 2013;39:326–333
10. Gimbel HV, DeBroff BM. Intraocular lens optic capture. J Cataract Refract Surg 2004;30:200–206
11. Arbisser LB. Safety of intracameral moxifloxacin for prophylaxis of endophthalmitis after cataract surgery. J Cataract Refract Surg 2008;34:1114–1120
12. Vanner EA, Stewart MW. Vitrectomy timing for retained lens fragments after surgery for age-related cataracts: a systematic review and meta-analysis. Am J Ophthalmol 2011;152:345–357.e3

21 Postvitrectomy Considerations in Phacoemulsification

Alan S. Crandall, Hari Bodhireddy, Hreem N. Patel, and Kristin Ow Chapman

Pars plana vitrectomy (PPV) was first introduced by Machemer et al[1] in 1971, and it has since undergone many important advances in instrumentation and technique. Modern PPV is widely performed employing a microincisional transconjunctival sutureless technique. A few low-powered and short-term studies report a lower incidence of cataract formation after these surgeries, compared with older techniques, possibly due to reduced balanced salt solution (BSS) consumption, lower intravitreal flow, and reduced operative time.[2-5] However, it is well accepted that cataracts develop in up to 76% of eyes within 2 years after PPV, which makes them the most common complication of the procedure.[6,7]

Although there are no known causative factors, risk factors may include older age, preexisting nuclear sclerosis, light toxicity from operating microscope, intraoperative oxidation of lens proteins, intraoperative lens touch (mechanical trauma from surgical instruments), duration of exposure to irrigating solution, diabetic retinopathy, and injection of silicone oil or intravitreal expansile gas.[2,8-12]

As the indications for PPV expand due to improved surgical techniques and results, this patient population is more likely to present to the anterior-segment surgeon's clinic with increasing frequency. These patients are more likely than the general age-matched population to have associated ocular or systemic comorbidities and sequelae of prior surgery, including but not limited to conjunctival and episcleral scarring, corneal endothelial cell loss, poor pupillary dilation, zonular weakness, preexisting posterior capsular compromise, low scleral rigidity (high myopes), denser nuclear (brunescent) cataracts, and cystoid macular edema (CME).[2]

Phacoemulsification can be performed safely in this patient population, but there are important issues to consider preoperatively, intraoperatively, and postoperatively. There are no randomized clinical trials on outcomes of cataract surgery in eyes that previously underwent vitrectomy, but only retrospective case reports and nonrandomized prospective case series.[13] Effective management of the challenges presented by coexisting ocular pathology requires a thorough understanding of the potential complications.

Preoperative Discussion

The most important consideration in the process also happens to be the most basic, and that is the decision to perform the surgery. A comprehensive discussion with the patient of risks and benefits is of utmost importance. The surgeon should discuss the indications for the procedure as well as the chances of success. It is necessary for the cataract surgeon to be as familiar with the patient's retinopathy as the retinal specialist, allowing for a collaborative informed decision to be made by the surgeon and the patient.

Explain to the patient that removing the cataract will provide a better view into the eye for the ophthalmologists and may provide improved peripheral vision and color perception for the patient. Improved central visual acuity is not always probable, so knowing the patient's best corrected visual acuity prior to the development of the cataract is helpful. The potential acuity meter is a low-tech but highly effective tool in predicting post-surgical visual acuity.

Explain that even with an uncomplicated cataract surgery, visual potential will be limited by the underlying retinal disorder. In addition to describing the risks that are inherent to a standard phacoemulsification procedure, emphasize that the patient may experience postoperative diplopia, anisometropia, central scotoma, or metamorphopsia. Cataract surgery in eyes with retinal disease may increase the occurrence of neovascular events, such as neovascularization in age-related macular degeneration, and secondary glaucoma.

Preoperative Examination

To minimize intraoperative surprises and make an educated recommendation, the surgeon should perform a thorough preoperative exam that centers around slit-lamp biomicroscopy. This discussion addresses issues that are specific to the postvitrectomized eye, and assumes that findings pertinent to a standard candidate for phacoemulsification are screened for, such as corneal guttae and pseudoexfoliation material. The surgeon should obtain a baseline intraocular pressure reading by applanation tonometry.

Also, note the presence of silicone oil bubbles or vitreous strands in the anterior chamber or iridophacodonesis, which may represent posterior capsular compromise or zonular weakness or dehiscence. Remember that these eyes have been previously entered through the pars plana, which puts them at a higher risk for zonular trauma. Also look for inflammatory cells that may represent ongoing healing from PPV or an underlying uveitis. Preoperative topical or oral steroids and topical nonsteroidal anti-inflammatory drugs should be considered.

Allow ample time after dilating the patient in the clinic to assess maximal pupillary dilation. Some surgeons like to start long-acting preoperative topical cycloplegics several days before surgery, but intraoperative 1% preservative-free lidocaine with epinephrine, combined with viscomydriasis and slow-motion fluidics settings works well, employing an iris expansion device such as the Malyugin ring (MicroSurgical Technology [MST], Redmond, WA) as necessary.

Posterior capsular compromise should be suspected if a posterior capsular plaque is present or if a history of rapidly progressive postvitrectomy cataract exists.

The optic nerve and retinal status should be documented, with particular attention to the presence of optic disk cupping, CME, neovascularization, and retinal tears or detachments. These pathologies may need to be addressed before, in combination with, or immediately after cataract surgery.

If an advanced cataract precludes a satisfactory view to the retina, perform a B-scan. In addition to looking for retinal pathology, also look to see if there is an abnormally large lens thickness or an outpouching of the posterior lens surface, suggesting a defect in the posterior capsule and an intumescent lens.

Intraocular Lens (IOL) Selection

Optical biometry like the Zeiss IOL Master (Zeiss, San Diego, CA), which uses partial coherence interferometry and infrared light, has been shown to be more accurate than ultrasound biometry in vitrectomized eyes.[14] A high percentage of vitrectomized eyes are highly myopic or staphylomatous. Therefore, the true axial length (AL) through the visual axis of these eyes is best measured as the patient fixates on a laser target, as opposed to an operator holding an ultrasound probe against the eye.[15]

In silicone oil-filled eyes, the correction factor for AL calculations is smaller as infrared light travels through different media compared with ultrasound waves.[14] The AL is often overestimated using ultrasound biometry in a silicone oil-filled eye, and thus the patient is left with unintended postoperative hyperopia. To facilitate appropriate IOL power calculations, always consult with the retina specialist regarding the expected duration that silicone oil will remain in the eye.

No matter which method is used, alterations in the anatomy of vitrectomized eyes present challenges to biometry technologies. Ultrasound measures AL in reference to the retinal internal limiting membrane, whereas optical biometry measures AL in reference to the retinal pigment epithelium.[16] If there remains a question about the validity of one method after comparing the measurements to those in the fellow eye, for example, it may be a good idea to obtain both ultrasound and optical biometry for comparison.[2,17]

Avoid silicone IOLs due to the possibility of future air-fluid exchange or silicone oil fills, which can cause interface issues[18] (**Fig. 21.1**). These interface issues are less likely but still possible with polymethylmethacrylate (PMMA) lenses or hydrophobic and hydrophilic acrylic lenses.[19] Consider surface modified heparin-coated IOLs to prevent these interface issues.[20]

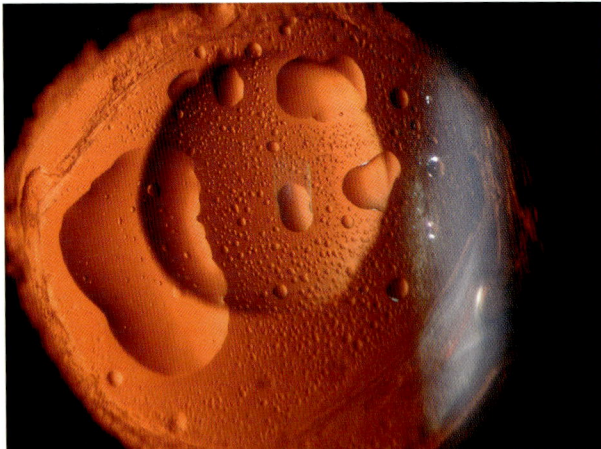

Fig. 21.1 Silicone oil emulsification on silicone intraoperative lens (IOL). (Courtesy of Paula F. Morris, CRA, FOPS, Moran Eye Center.)

Have IOL power calculations prepared for both single-piece monofocal acrylic lenses and three-piece monofocal acrylic lenses in the event that sulcus placement with or without optic capture in the bag is necessary. Consider an IOL with a 360-degree square edge design with at least a 6.0-mm optic diameter to maximize the viewing area. Postoperatively, this can make the difference between missing and catching a small peripheral retinal tear. The Alcon acrylic lenses (Alcon Laboratories, Fort Worth, TX) are particularly tacky and may enable a more transparent IOL–capsulotomy interface.

In silicone oil–filled eyes, consider plano-convex IOLs like the Duralens II DL60L (Abbott Laboratories, Abbott Park, IL) with the plano surface facing posteriorly to minimize postoperative refractive surprises.

Avoid multifocal optics, which can decrease contrast sensitivity in an eye that may already have impaired photoreceptor functionality.[21] They will also impair the ophthalmologist's view to the fundus for necessary peripheral retinal examination.[22] The Crystalens (Bausch & Lomb, Rochester, NY) is a multifocal silicone IOL, so this lens should be avoided for multiple reasons.

Intraoperative

A clear corneal incision is preferred due to the presence of conjunctival scarring that would make a scleral tunnel incision more difficult. However, a scleral tunnel may be preferred in particularly challenging cases requiring a rigid IOL or a larger incision and a nonphacoemulsification extracapsular lens extraction technique. Consider such a technique if posterior capsular compromise is noted preoperatively, as any fragments liberated during phacoemulsification will fall rapidly to the posterior segment due to lack of vitreous support. If this were to happen, cleanup is best left to a vitreoretinal surgeon using a pars plana approach.

Warn patients of temporary amaurosis from preservative-free intracameral lidocaine causing "retinal block" in postvitrectomized eyes, due to enhanced posterior diffusion through weakened zonules.[23] The decreased physiological barrier between the anterior and posterior segments is also why anterior-segment neovascularization and posterior-segment inflammation are more of a concern postoperatively. Intracameral lidocaine works well to minimize discomfort from excessive stretching of the iridozonular apparatus. This stretching may occur due to zonular weakness as the lens moves in the anterior-posterior direction as infusion is suddenly activated in the eye. Similarly, excess deepening of the anterior chamber when entering the eye with infusion may occur, due to loose zonules and a fluid-filled vitreous cavity instead of semi-solid viscous vitreous. Do not overinflate the anterior chamber with viscoelastic prior to capsulorrhexis. Increased posterior pressure may be provided by performing a retrobulbar or peribulbar block prior to the procedure.

Intraoperative miosis and posterior synechiae should be dealt with in such a way as to minimize intraocular manipulations. In a stepwise fashion, intracameral mydriatics, posterior synechialysis, viscomydriasis, and a Malyugin ring or iris hooks may be used.

Tightly sealing the main and side-port wounds is more important than in standard phacoemulsification surgery because of the lower threshold for instability of the anterior chamber from egress of fluid through the wounds. However, do not make them too long, and maintain the irrigation ports of the phacoemulsification and irrigation and aspiration (I/A) instruments well inside the anterior chamber and away from the wound. Corneal striations and premature wound hydration will prevent adequate visualization, which is particularly important if you are working in a deep anterior chamber.

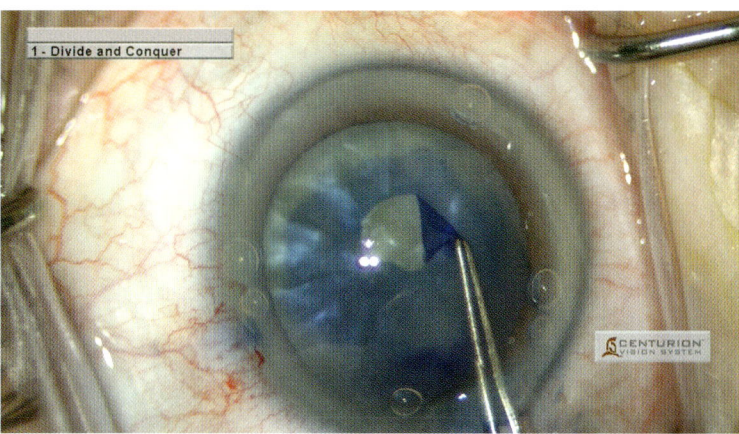
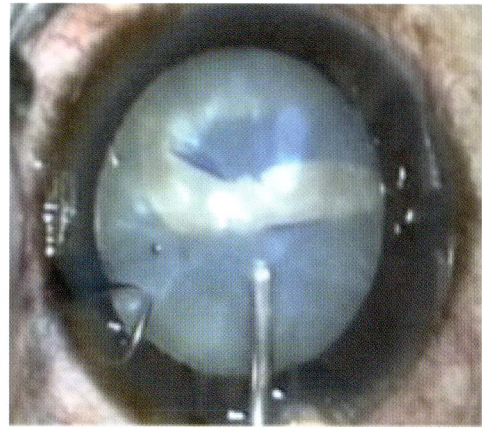

a

b

Fig. 21.2 **(a)** Initiation of capsulorrhexis with aid of trypan blue stain in intumescent cataract in post-vitrectomized eye. **(b)** Argentinean flag sign.

A compromised corneal endothelium, anterior capsular fibrosis, advanced cataract, and blunted red reflex from retinal pathology may also make visualization challenging, so consider trypan blue stain (Vision Blue, Dutch Ophthalmics, Exeter, NH) to enhance visibility of the anterior capsule.

If the cataract is intumescent (think rapidly progressive white cataract postvitrectomy), decompress the liquefied subcapsular component using a 30-gauge needle on a syringe with gentle manual aspiration at the center of the capsule prior to capsulorrhexis to avoid the Argentinian flag sign (**Fig. 21.2**). Do not hesitate to use a cystotome to initiate the capsulorrhexis, as well as retinal microscissors and microrhexis forceps to work around or incorporate an anterior subcapsular plaque, especially in eyes after long exposure to silicone oil. If there is a particularly dense anterior subcapsular plaque, a vitrector with the port facing posteriorly can be used through an anterior approach to create and complete the capsular opening. The capsulorrhexis should overlap the IOL by 0.5 to 1.0 mm. It needs to be big enough to provide adequate working space for nuclear disassembly but small enough to allow for potential sulcus placement of the IOL.

Watch for signs of zonular weakness or dehiscence. If moderate to severe, zonulopathy may be evidenced by phacodonesis on preoperative examination. If mild to moderate, it may manifest as early as during capsulorrhexis, when the lens–capsule complex is seen to be hypermobile within the zonular plane and countertraction is less than ideal. Similar hypermobility may be seen during rotation and sculpting.

Ocular hypotony due to decreased scleral rigidity, particularly in highly myopic eyes, may be encountered, and judicious use of an ophthalmic viscosurgical device (OVD) is recommended. Alternatively, a self-retaining infusion cannula may be inserted through a self-sealing transconjunctival sclerotomy using a 23-gauge trocar. Dispersive OVD (Viscoat, Alcon; component of DuoVisc, Alcon) protects the corneal endothelium the best, but it is not as effective at creating working space and it makes for a more difficult capsulorrhexis and OVD removal. The surgeon can use a softshell technique if working with nuclear fragments relatively anteriorly, which is often required to prevent posterior capsular rupture, or a very dense nucleus. This measure is to protect the corneal endothelium while providing ample working space during high-energy phacoemulsification in the anterior chamber. Cohesive OVD (ProVisc, Alcon; also a component of DuoVisc) is better at creating space in the anterior chamber and is more easily removed. An adaptive OVD like Healon 5 (Abbott) and DisCoVisc (Alcon) maintain cohesive qualities at low aspira-

tion flow rates and dispersive qualities at high aspiration flow rates like phacoemulsification. At aspiration flow rates of 25 cc or ML per minute and lower, given well-constructed wounds and avoidance of wound manipulation, any of these OVDs will stay in the eye until they are intentionally removed. Work with slower fluidics settings to allow more OVD to stay in the eye longer, but compensate for the lower aspiration flow rate by lowering the vacuum and infusion bottle height to steadily maintain the anterior chamber volume.[24]

Use a lower bottle height when entering the eye with infusion to avoid excess deepening of the anterior chamber, and to prevent the self-explanatory lens–iris diaphragm retropulsion syndrome or reverse pupillary block.[25] Lift up the iris at the pupillary margin or depress the anterior capsular surface with the second instrument or I/A tip to equalize pressures between the anterior and posterior chambers if reverse pupillary block occurs. This syndrome is not to be confused with fluid misdirection syndrome or infusion deviation syndrome,[26] where intact or compromised zonules act as a one-way valve for irrigation fluid and cause vitreous hydration, thus increasing posterior chamber pressure and *shallowing* the anterior chamber. Raising the bottle height has the paradoxical effect of further shallowing the anterior chamber in infusion deviation syndrome.

Hydrodissection should be gentle with frequent decompressions to avoid posterior capsular tension. Achieve enough separation to allow easy rotation of the nucleus so that zonular stress is minimized. If posterior capsular rupture is suspected either preoperatively or intraoperatively, perform hydrodelineation or viscodissection.

The posterior capsule is generally more mobile, and a trampolining effect during phacoemulsification may be encountered due to reduced vitreous support. The Alcon Centurion's Active Fluidics technology may minimize this effect. Regardless of the platform used, heightened awareness and measures to ensure a stable chamber are required to prevent iatrogenic posterior capsular rupture.

Be judicious in the use and timing of phacoemulsification power to avoid surge, but due to postvitrectomy cataracts generally being quite dense, more phacoemulsification energy may be necessary, so watch for thermal corneal wound burns. A simple way for the surgical technician or assistant to help is to periodically apply cold BSS at the main wound during phacoemulsification. Consider using the Alcon UltraChopper for sculpting dense nuclei to prevent undue zonular stress (**Fig. 21.3**).

Use a lower level of aspiration and vacuum when performing cortical cleanup, and employ circumferential or tangential,

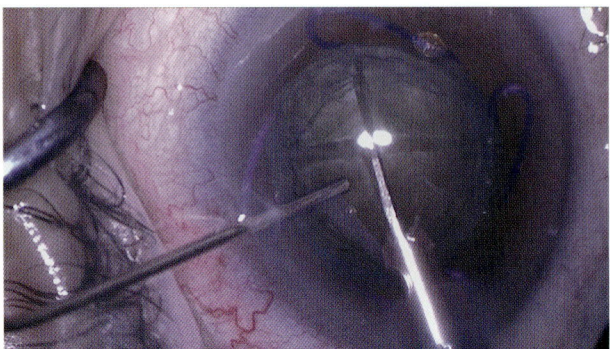

Fig. 21.3 Alcon UltraChopper sculpting dense nucleus with Malyugin ring (MST) already inserted.

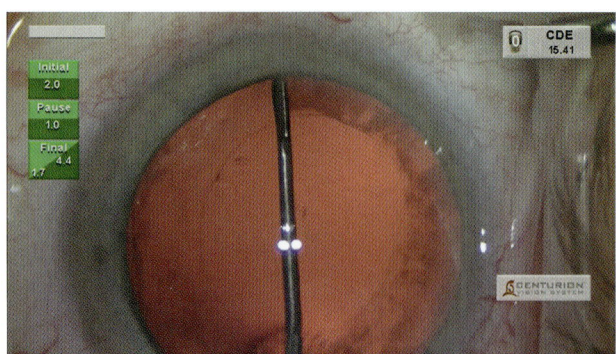

Fig. 21.4 Debridement of lens epithelial cells on the anterior capsule using a Singer sweep polisher.

versus radial, stripping to minimize zonular stress. Bimanual I/A is safe and allows for thorough cleanup, but one cannot perform the efficient "hurricane cortical aspiration technique" with bimanual instrumentation, because by definition, it requires maintaining occlusion for 360 degrees of cortex removal.[27]

Polishing an intact posterior capsule minimizes the chances of posterior capsular opacification (PCO) and is particularly helpful when silicone oil is present or planned, so as not to compound opacification and emulsification issues.

If a posterior capsular rent is encountered, viscodissect and prolapse the nucleus into the anterior chamber and disassemble it there, so as not to extend the rent. Posterior capsular plaques are common in silicone oil–filled eyes, and they can be addressed by polishing with the I/A tip or peeling with Utrata or microrhexis forceps. If the plaque is particularly dense, a cystotome may be used to initiate an edge to a posterior capsulorrhexis, which can then be completed with Utrata or microrhexis forceps. The plaque can be incorporated into the rhexis using microscissors, which can also be used to work around it. Similar to a dense anterior capsular plaque, a vitrector can be used to open the posterior capsule, and a postoperative neodymium:yttrium-aluminum-garnet (Nd:YAG) capsulotomy is also an option. Be sure to perform a thorough anterior vitrectomy, using triamcinolone stain as necessary to visualize elusive vitreous strands.

Take steps to maximize the view to the peripheral fundus, because this population is predisposed to retinal disease. A Singer-style sweep instrument to debride lens epithelial cells or thorough polishing of the undersurface of the anterior lip of the lens capsule by aspiration may be performed (**Fig. 21.4**). This step may also minimize capsular phimosis, which is important in preventing IOL subluxation in eyes with underlying zonulopathy.[28]

Implant the IOL gently, avoiding excessive rotational maneuvers so as not to stress zonules. In one study, 19% of 86 patients who had late in-the-bag spontaneous IOL dislocation had a history of PPV, occurring on average 8.5 years after implantation.[29] If even mild phacodonesis is observed, consider inserting a capsular tension ring (CTR), or implant the IOL in the ciliary sulcus, capturing the optic in the capsular bag when possible. Excessive phacodonesis may necessitate an anterior chamber, iris-fixated, or scleral-fixated IOL. In the event of zonular dialysis, definitely use a CTR or capsular tension segment to ensure even distention of the capsular bag, and place the IOL with one haptic in the area of dehiscence (our personal preference), or suture the IOL to the iris or sclera[30] (**Fig. 21.5**).

Our personal preference is always to use 10-0 nylon sutures to close the main and side-port wounds partly due to decreased scleral rigidity. In patients who have preoperative CME amenable

to treatment with intravitreal injection of triamcinolone acetonide or bevacizumab, consider combining injection with cataract surgery or work with the retinal specialist to arrange preoperative injection.

Postoperative

This population is predisposed to retinal disease, so nonsteroidal anti-inflammatory drops and steroid drops are a must, with reasonable variation in dosing as well as preoperative use. Always check postoperatively for new retinal tears or detachments. The timing for these checks is variable and based on symptoms and the surgeon's follow-up preferences.

Inform your patients about the symptoms of a retinal tear or detachment, and tell them to call immediately if they experience new floaters, photopsias, curtains, or a decrease in peripheral vision.

There are a few postoperative complications to keep in mind that are unique to postvitrectomized eyes that have undergone cataract surgery. Within the first week after surgery, silicone oil may enter the anterior chamber. This may also occur later, and the surgeon must watch for the development of PCO, which occurs with higher incidence in vitrectomized eyes, and occurs in up to 100% of silicone oil–filled eyes.[31] Other findings to note

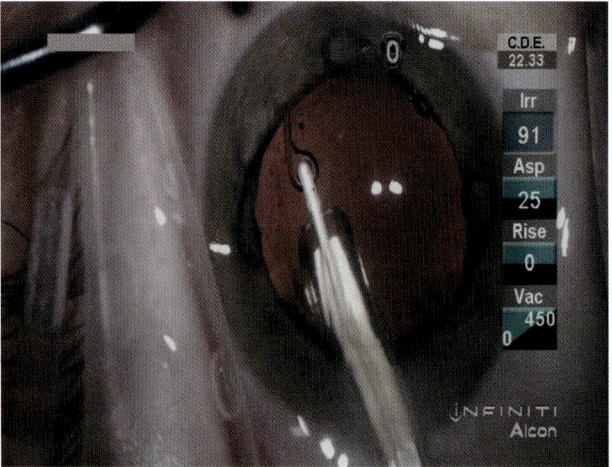

Fig. 21.5 Insertion of Morcher EyeJet preloaded size 14A capsular tension ring (CTR) (Morcher GmbH, Germany) with a Malyugin ring (MST) already inserted.

on postoperative exams include elevated intraocular pressure, CME, proliferative diabetic retinopathy, retinal tears or detachments, epiretinal membrane, recurrence of macular holes, and vitreous hemorrhage. Of note, a 5.2% rate of recurrent retinal detachments has been demonstrated in eyes that have undergone phacoemulsification after PPV.[32]

There is still some controversy with regard to the development of late-onset open-angle glaucoma (OAG) after post-PPV cataract extraction, but there is evidence to suggest that at the least, it is worth mentioning to the patient as a potential risk. Data presented at the LXII Edward Jackson Lecture in 2006[33] suggests that there is an increased risk of OAG after uncomplicated PPV, and the presence of a crystalline lens may be protective. Oxidative stress is hypothesized to have a role in the pathogenesis. Koreen et al[34] reached the same conclusion in 2012 with a better-powered study (285 vitrectomized eyes versus 68). However, a 5-year follow-up study by Yu et al[35] in 2010 included 441 patients, with 157 of them completing follow-up, and concluded that an increased incidence of late-onset OAG and ocular hypertension could not be observed. Also, the removal of the crystalline lens did not increase the risk of OAG or ocular hypertension in vitrectomized eyes.

Despite the increased risks and complication rate involved with phacoemulsification after PPV, it has been shown that 90% of patients can expect an improvement in best corrected visual acuity (BCVA).[32] By being mindful of the potential complications and taking measures to avoid them, the surgeon can strive to achieve even better success rates.

References

1. Machemer R, Buettner H, Norton EW, Parel JM. Vitrectomy: a pars plana approach. Trans Am Acad Ophthalmol Otolaryngol 1971;75:813–820

2. Shousha MA, Yoo SH. Cataract surgery after pars plana vitrectomy. Curr Opin Ophthalmol 2010;21:45–49

3. Rizzo S, Genovesi-Ebert F, Murri S, et al. 25-gauge, sutureless vitrectomy and standard 20-gauge pars plana vitrectomy in idiopathic epiretinal membrane surgery: a comparative pilot study. Graefes Arch Clin Exp Ophthalmol 2006;244:472–479

4. Lott MN, Manning MH, Singh J, Zhang H, Singh H, Marcus DM. 23-gauge vitrectomy in 100 eyes: short-term visual outcomes and complications. Retina 2008;28:1193–1200

5. Shah CP, Ho AC, Regillo CD, Fineman MS, Vander JF, Brown GC. Short-term outcomes of 25-gauge vitrectomy with silicone oil for repair of complicated retinal detachment. Retina 2008;28:723–728

6. Chang MA, Parides MK, Chang S, Braunstein RE. Outcome of phacoemulsification after pars plana vitrectomy. Ophthalmology 2002;109:948–954

7. Cherfan GM, Michels RG, de Bustros S, Enger C, Glaser BM. Nuclear sclerotic cataract after vitrectomy for idiopathic epiretinal membranes causing macular pucker. Am J Ophthalmol 1991;111:434–438

8. Hsuan JD, Brown NA, Bron AJ, Patel CK, Rosen PH. Posterior subcapsular and nuclear cataract after vitrectomy. J Cataract Refract Surg 2001;27:437–444

9. Melberg NS, Thomas MA. Nuclear sclerotic cataract after vitrectomy in patients younger than 50 years of age. Ophthalmology 1995;102:1466–1471

10. Cheng L, Azen SP, El-Bradey MH, et al. Duration of vitrectomy and postoperative cataract in the vitrectomy for macular hole study. Am J Ophthalmol 2001;132:881–887

11. Federman JL, Schubert HD. Complications associated with the use of silicone oil in 150 eyes after retina-vitreous surgery. Ophthalmology 1988;95:870–876

12. Hiscott P, Magee RM, Colthurst M, Lois N, Wong D. Clinicopathological correlation of epiretinal membranes and posterior lens opacification following perfluorohexyloctane tamponade. Br J Ophthalmol 2001;85:179–183

13. Do DV, Gichuhi S, Vedula SS, Hawkins BS. Surgery for post-vitrectomy cataract. Cochrane Database Syst Rev 2013;12:CD006366

14. Manvikar SR, Allen D, Steel DH. Optical biometry in combined phacovitrectomy. J Cataract Refract Surg 2009;35:64–69

15. Findl O, Drexler W, Menapace R, Heinzl H, Hitzenberger CK, Fercher AF. Improved prediction of intraocular lens power using partial coherence interferometry. J Cataract Refract Surg 2001;27:861–867

16. Hitzenberger CK, Drexler W, Dolezal C, et al. Measurement of the axial length of cataract eyes by laser Doppler interferometry. Invest Ophthalmol Vis Sci 1993;34:1886–1893

17. Braunstein RE, Airiani S. Cataract surgery results after pars plana vitrectomy. Curr Opin Ophthalmol 2003;14:150–154

18. Apple DJ, Federman JL, Krolicki TJ, et al. Irreversible silicone oil adhesion to silicone intraocular lenses. A clinicopathologic analysis. Ophthalmology 1996;103:1555–1561, discussion 1561–1562

19. Apple DJ, Isaacs RT, Kent DG, et al. Silicone oil adhesion to intraocular lenses: an experimental study comparing various biomaterials. J Cataract Refract Surg 1997;23:536–544

20. Arthur SN, Peng Q, Apple DJ, et al. Effect of heparin surface modification in reducing silicone oil adherence to various intraocular lenses. J Cataract Refract Surg 2001;27:1662–1669

21. Buznego C, Trattler WB. Presbyopia-correcting intraocular lenses. Curr Opin Ophthalmol 2009;20:13–18

22. Kumar A, Goyal M, Tewari HK. Posterior segment visualization problems with multifocal intraocular lenses. Acta Ophthalmol Scand 1996;74:415

23. Chia K, Teoh S. Transient amaurosis with intracameral lidocaine. Eye (Lond) 2009;23:1483

24. Osher RH, Marques FF, Marques DMV, et al. Slow-motion phacoemulsification technique. Tech Ophthalmol 2003;1:73–79

25. Ghosh S, Best K, Steel DH. Lens-iris diaphragm retropulsion syndrome during phacoemulsification in vitrectomized eyes. J Cataract Refract Surg 2013;39:1852–1858

26. Nichamin LD. Phacoemulsification following vitreoretinal surgery. In: Lu LW, Fine IH, eds. Phacoemulsification in Difficult and Challenging Cases. New York: Thieme; 1999:145–150

27. Nakano CT, Motta AFP, Hida WT, et al. Hurricane cortical aspiration technique: one-step continuous circular aspiration maneuver. J Cataract Refract Surg 2014;40:514–516

28. Tadros A, Bhatt UK, Abdul Karim MN, Zaheer A, Thomas PW. Removal of lens epithelial cells and the effect on capsulorhexis size. J Cataract Refract Surg 2005;31:1569–1574

29. Davis D, Brubaker J, Espandar L, et al. Late in-the-bag spontaneous intraocular lens dislocation: evaluation of 86 consecutive cases. Ophthalmology 2009;116:664–670

30. Crandall AS, Slade DS. Placement of endocapsular IOLs in eyes with zonular compromise. American Academy of Ophthalmology, Focal Points 2014;32:2–8

31. Pinter SM, Sugar A. Phacoemulsification in eyes with past pars plana vitrectomy: case-control study. J Cataract Refract Surg 1999;25:556–561

32. Cole CJ, Charteris DG. Cataract extraction after retinal detachment repair by vitrectomy: visual outcome and complications. Eye (Lond) 2009;23:1377–1381

33. Chang S. LXII Edward Jackson lecture: open angle glaucoma after vitrectomy. Am J Ophthalmol 2006;141:1033–1043

34. Koreen L, Yoshida N, Escariao P, et al. Incidence of, risk factors for, and combined mechanism of late-onset open-angle glaucoma after vitrectomy. Retina 2012;32:160–167

35. Yu AL, Brummeisl W, Schaumberger M, Kampik A, Welge-Lussen U. Vitrectomy does not increase the risk of open-angle glaucoma or ocular hypertension—a 5-year follow-up. Graefes Arch Clin Exp Ophthalmol 2010;248:1407–1414

22 Posterior-Segment Complications

Matthew J. Welch, Leonard Joffe, William E. Smiddy, and Harry W. Flynn, Jr.

Cataract surgery is one of the most common performed operations in the United States and has one of the highest success rate. Previous population surveys have reported up to 7.4% of the population undergoes cataract surgery annually.[1,2] Phacoemulsification techniques have revolutionized the field of cataract surgery, and have facilitated the development of innovations such as small incisions and foldable intraocular lens (IOL) implants. Sutureless clear corneal incision techniques have become the standard methodology of contemporary cataract surgery. Newer innovations related to micro-incisional surgery and laser-assisted surgery remain at the forefront of surgical technique advancement.

Advances in technology have led to equally remarkable refinements in the surgical skills of the ophthalmologist, operations of shorter duration, and higher surgical case loads. Expectations of patients have increased as a result of the rapid visual and physical rehabilitation of what has become a well-refined procedure, with reasonably predictable vision outcomes. Commercial advertising for cataract surgery has fueled this increase in expectations by minimizing the need for injections or patches, reducing postoperative pain, and emphasizing that return to normal activities may be possible within days.

The uncomplicated cataract operation with intraocular implant placement is indeed a refined operation with remarkable outcomes in the vast majority of cases. Although the complication rate is quite low, the consequences of these complications may cause significant vision loss. Awareness of these complications and appropriate management can minimize the vision impairment and enhance the outcome and recovery for the patient, thereby reducing the risk of litigation that so often arises when patients' expectations are not met.

The posterior-segment complications of cataract surgery are not specific to phacoemulsification. This chapter reviews the important clinical features and treatment options, with emphasis on phacoemulsification. The most serious posterior-segment complications include retained lens fragments, dislocated IOL implant, endophthalmitis, suprachoroidal hemorrhage, and needle penetration of the globe when periocular or retrobulbar anesthesia is used.

Retained Lens Fragments

The most common clinical situation leading to retained lens fragments in the vitreous is posterior capsular rupture, with loss of lens fragments posteriorly into the vitreous cavity during the fragmentation or chopping phase of phacoemulsification. The displaced lens fragment may encompass the entire nucleus or any segmented nuclear or cortical fraction. The best estimate of the incidence of posteriorly displaced lens fragments is 0.3% in both the United States and United Kingdom, but has been suggested possibly to be as frequent as 1.1% in published series.[3–5] Once posterior capsule rupture occurs, the surgeon must proceed with extreme caution in using a limbal approach to retrieve displaced lens fragments. Although in some instances converting to a larger incision and using a lens loop or forceps facilitate retrieval of a nuclear fragment before it migrates posterior through the capsule, once the fragment falls posteriorly a high risk of further complications ensues with limbal retrieval attempts.

Previously, surgeons have advocated vigorous attempts at retrieving the lost lens nucleus from the limbal cataract incision by probing posteriorly with a lens loop or other instrumentation, or by using high volumes of infusion fluid to create vortex currents to float the lens fragment anteriorly.[3,6] However, vigorous attempts at retrieving a posteriorly dislocated nucleus from the limbus with high volumes of intraocular fluid or posterior manipulation of the instrument has been associated with giant retinal tears that have a poor prognosis for visual acuity.[7] In a case managed by one of the authors, the nucleus was found underneath a giant-tear retinal detachment in the inferior nasal quadrant.

Furthermore, some anterior-segment surgeons have advocated placement of a vitrectomy probe through the pars plana with the use of a small irrigating handpiece to more safely remove lens material. This approach has also been suggested to be used in combination with elevation techniques involving the use of viscoelastic devices to elevate posteriorly dislocated lens material. It is important to note that this pars plana vitrectomy approach differs from the standard three-port system, vitrectomy probe, and vitrectomy machine commonly used by vitreoretinal surgeons.[8–10]

Clinical Features

Posterior displacement of lens fragments is usually recognized intraoperatively after posterior capsular rupture. Occasionally retained lens material may present with chronic intraocular inflammation and no visible fragments in the posterior pole. The degree of intraocular inflammation usually reflects the size of the retained lens fragment, the time interval since cataract surgery, individual inflammatory reactivity, and the extent of previous intraocular manipulations. Associated clinical signs include corneal edema, elevated intraocular pressure (IOP), uveitis, and vitreous opacities. Initially, these findings are frequently mild, especially in the immediate postoperative interval, but over time they may worsen and lead to other complications such as retinal detachment, causing profound vision loss. Published series have reported a retinal detachment rate ranging from 6.3 to 12.8% in patients presenting for management of IOL dislocation. Macular involvement has been reported to be found on presentation in up to 50% of cases.[5,11–19]

Surgical Indications

The size of the lens fragment, the extent of IOP control, the degree of corneal edema, and the severity of intraocular inflammation usually form the basis for surgical intervention. Proceeding with surgical intervention is often most necessary in the setting of large retained nuclear lens fragments in which clinical complications secondary to inflammatory response are highly probable.[8] Eyes with very small retained fragments have a better prognosis and can often be observed indefinitely. However, if inflammation has not subsided by 1 to 2 weeks, surgical intervention should be considered, regardless of how small the retained fragment is, because other occult fragments may be harbored behind the iris.

Chronic IOP elevation was reported to be more common when the subsequent vitrectomy was performed more than 3 weeks following surgery.[7] Other studies have not found any outcome differences between earlier and later intervention.[5,8,12,18,19] Published series have reported an incidence in the range of 25 to 37% of patients presenting with IOP greater than 30 mm Hg for vitrectomy following phacoemulsification, with resultant retained lens fragments. The IOP normalized in all but 2 to 3% of patients after vitrectomy.[8,12] The patient's overall clinical situation may influence the timing, but usually surgery to remove retained lens material is performed within 2 weeks of the original cataract surgery to expedite the vision rehabilitation, to break the cycle of progressive lens-induced inflammation, and to lessen risks of secondary lens-induced glaucoma. These goals may be logistically maximized when lens fragment retrieval and removal can be expertly performed during the original cataract operation. When this is not feasible, a delay of several days or even weeks may be equally effective, because the inflammation, corneal edema, and elevated IOP can improve with topical treatment over several days following cataract surgery.

Surgical Techniques

A variety of techniques have been described for use by the anterior-segment surgeon at the time of lens fragment loss. Although some cases may be satisfactorily managed through a limbal incision, pars plana vitrectomy techniques probably offer superior results in most cases.[5,9,10,17–24] The technique of removal is dependent in large part on the firmness of the lens material. Almost all material can be fragmented with contemporary ultrasonic instruments, whereas softer material such as cortex may be aspirated with the vitreous cutter. Rarely, nuclear or inspissated old lens material requires direct removal through an anterior incision.

There are three key elements in successful lens fragment removal technique. First, adequate initial vitrectomy avoids unintended vitreous traction during phacofragmentation (**Fig. 22.1**). Second, reducing fragmentation power as the remnants become smaller and softer, sometimes to as low as 10% of maximum, enables more efficient nuclear extraction by continuous occlusion of the suction port, minimizing the risk of mechanical retinal trauma from projectile fragments. This maneuver also minimizes the risk of fragments dropping back onto the retina even though these fragments rarely strike the retina with sufficient force to damage the retina. Third, fragments should be cautiously aspirated from the retinal surface and moved to the midvitreous before activating ultrasonic fragmentation to avoid suction or ultrasonic damage to the retina (**Fig. 22.2**).

Previously, perfluorocarbon (PFC) liquids have been described to float the nucleus anteriorly to facilitate removal,[24,25] but are most useful when retinal detachment coexists.[26] Techniques for reattaching the retina when associated with retained lens fragments are similar to those for other complex retinal detachments.[27,28] With modern developments in vitreoretinal surgical

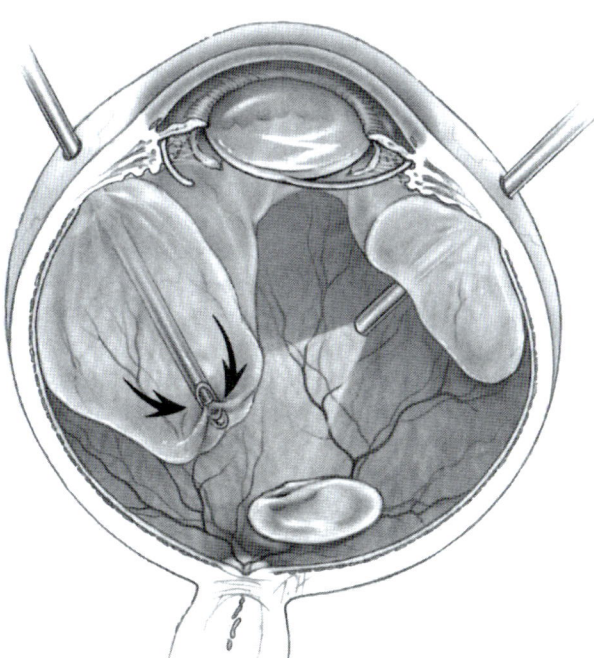

Fig. 22.1 Attention to complete central vitrectomy allows access to retained lens fragments. (From Regillo CD, Brown GC, Flynn HW Jr. Vitreoretinal Disease: The Essentials. New York: Thieme; 1999:568. Reprinted by permission.)

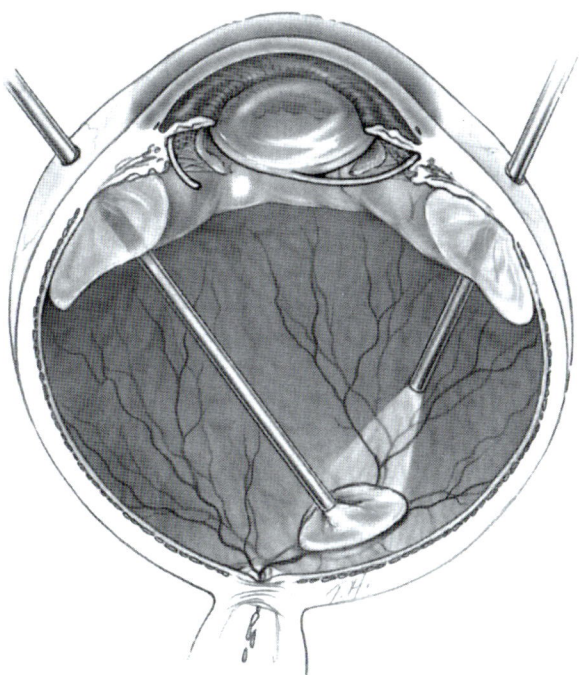

Fig. 22.2 Low ultrasonic fragmentation power allows more controlled removal of fragments. (From Regillo CD, Brown GC, Flynn HW Jr. Vitreoretinal Disease: The Essentials. New York: Thieme; 1999:569. Reprinted by permission.)

techniques and equipment, the routine use of PFC liquids in surgical treatment of retained lens fragments is uncommon.

Most anterior-segment surgeons proceed to IOL insertion at the time of the original cataract surgery, as is recommended by the majority of vitreous surgeons in spite of the intraoperative complication of posteriorly displaced lens fragments. If there is sufficient capsular support, a three-piece IOL is often placed in the ciliary sulcus, because a single-piece acrylic lens is not suitable for such anatomic positioning. If not, suture fixation or scleral fixation techniques may be used,[29–47] or an anterior chamber (AC) IOL may be placed. If the cataract surgeon is reluctant to insert the IOL primarily, it can be inserted at the time of the subsequent vitrectomy or later.

Outcomes of Vitrectomy for Retained Lens Fragments

The vision outcomes in these cases are generally good.[4,5,17–24,48,49] Published reports have suggested that final postoperative visual acuity equivalent to 20/40 is achievable in 60 to 82% of cases.[5,8,18–23,49] This apparent improvement may reflect changing patterns of cataract surgery technique, because a poorer prognosis (20/60 final acuity) has been suggested with dropped lens nuclei when extracapsular cataract extraction (ECCE) techniques are used compared with phacoemulsification extraction methods.[17]

Postoperative complications related to vitrectomy surgery may be difficult to differentiate from those attributable to complicated cataract surgery, and may include corneal edema, glaucoma, persistent intraocular inflammation, and new retinal detachment. Retinal detachment coexisted with retained lens material in 8.0 to 12.8% of reported series, and retinal detachment has been reported after vitrectomy for removal of retained lens fragments in 5.5 to 8.3% of reported series (**Table 22.1**).[12,14,50,51] Thus, it is of critical importance to evaluate the retina throughout the perioperative course in such patients.

Recommendations for Management of Retained Lens Fragments

Recommendations for the anterior-segment surgeon experiencing the complication of posterior dislocation of lens fragments

include the following: (1) confine the posterior migration of fragments by the immediate use of dispersive viscoelastic; (2) use a glide sheet or even extractor spoon to stabilize the nucleus in the presence of a large capsular tear; (3) attempt lens fragment retrieval *only* if the fragment is readily accessible (at or near the iris plane; (4) perform anterior vitrectomy as necessary to avoid vitreous prolapse into the surgical incision; (5) if possible, insert a posterior chamber (PC) IOL using a residual posterior capsule, or insert an AC IOL, as merited by the situation; (6) suture the closure of the cataract wound in a standard fashion and remove viscoelastic (sutures are indicated to ensure wound integrity during subsequent vitrectomy); (7) prescribe frequent postoperative topical anti-inflammatory treatment and IOP-reducing agents as clinically indicated; and (8) refer the patient for vitreoretinal consultation within a few days for consultation (**Box 22.1**). If the opportunity exists, perform the vitrectomy for retrieval of displaced lens fragments at the same operation.[52,53]

Recommendations for the vitreoretinal surgeon include the following: (1) consider recommending observation initially for eyes with minimal inflammation and a very small lens fragment; (2) reassess supportive treatment with topical corticosteroids and antiglaucoma agents as clinically indicated; (3) intervene surgically if inflammation or IOP is not controlled, or if the fragment is estimated be sizable; (4) time the surgical intervention to maximize the initial treatment of postoperative inflammation and corneal edema.

Box 22.1 Posterior Dislocation of Lens Fragments: Management by Cataract Surgeon

- Attempt retrieval only if the fragment is easily accessible.
- Do anterior vitrectomy to avoid vitreous prolapse.
- Insert an IOL if it is safe to do so and indicated.
- Do standard wound closure and viscoelastic removal.
- Use frequent topical postoperative anti-inflammatory and IOP-lowering agents.
- Request vitreoretinal consultation promptly.

Table 22.1 Incidence of Retinal Detachment (RD) Occurring Before and After Vitrectomy for Removal of Retained Lens Fragments

Series (Date)	Initial Coexisting RD	RD After Vitrectomy	Combined
Hutton[20] (1978)	5/26 (19%)	5/26 (19%)	10/26 (38%)
Fastenberg[22] (1991)	3/13 (23%)	2/13 (15.4%)	5/13 (38.5%)
Blodi[17] (1992)	4/36 (11%)	3/36 (8.3%)	7/36 (19%)
Gilliland[5] (1992)	4/56 (7%)	4/56 (7%)	8/56 (14%)
Kim[19] (1994)	2/57 (3.5%)	2/57 (3.5%)	4/57 (7%)
Borne[18] (1996)	8/121 (6.6%)	11/121 (9.1%)	19/121 (16%)
Vilar[8] (1997)	11/126 (8.7%)	11/126 (8.7%)	22/126 (17.5%)
Kapusta[23] (1996)	0/25 (0%)	0/25 (0%)	0/25 (0%)
Totals	37/460 (8.0%)	38/460 (8.3%)	75/460 (16.3%)

If surgery is undertaken: (1) perform adequate core vitrectomy and induce posterior vitreous detachment as necessary to maximally remove vitreous before attempting phacofragmentation; (2) use lower fragmentation power settings for more efficient removal of smaller fragments; (3) be prepared for secondary IOL insertion in aphakic eyes or IOL exchange in some pseudophakic eyes by having measured or retrieving IOL calculations; and (4) examine peripheral retina thoroughly with scleral depression for possible retinal tear or detachment (**Box 22.2**).

Intraocular Lens Dislocation

Postoperative decentration of PC IOLs occurs in 0.2 to 1.2% of cases and usually does not require treatment.[54,55] A less common but more significant complication is IOL dislocation into the vitreous cavity. A common element in all cases is insufficient posterior capsule support. This is typically due to posterior capsule rupture during cataract extraction. When dislocation occurs within the first few days or weeks after surgery, the cause may be less apparent and may be the result of unknowingly placing the IOL through a posterior capsule defect, or as a result of subsequent IOL haptic rotation out of a zone of residual capsule remnants. Late dislocation is less common and may be due to traumatic[56] or spontaneous loss of zonular support, such as in eyes with pseudoexfoliation syndrome.[57,58]

Clinical Characteristics

Dislocation of PC IOLs into the vitreous cavity is typically observed within the first week following surgery (26 of 32 cases in one series). Less commonly it occurs during surgery or several months after surgery.[57–59] The presenting visual acuity with aphakic correction may be very good, but is commonly decreased to a moderate degree despite the best spectacle correction. Patients with luxated or subluxated PC IOLs are usually symptomatic because of the variable position of the optic within the visual axis. In addition, a mobile PC IOL may also generate unique floater-like symptoms, or even lead to pupillary block glaucoma.

The presenting symptoms of patients with dislocated IOLs range from minimally symptomatic lens decentration to complete luxation into the vitreous cavity.[55] Decentration or subluxation refers to mild malposition with the optic still covering more than half of the pupillary space. In many cases of decentration, one haptic is in the ciliary sulcus and the other is in the capsular bag. Progressive decentration may become apparent with progressive capsular fibrosis. Patients at this milder end of the spectrum usually present several weeks after cataract extraction with good visual acuity and normal IOP, and without inflammation.

Visual symptoms usually are mild and may be related to glare from the edge of the optic.

Management Options

There are four general classes of management options for dislocated IOLs: observation, removal, exchange, or repositioning (which may incorporate suture fixation or sutureless scleral fixation).[13,29–47,59–65] The management plan and timing are formulated based on clinical factors such as the type of IOL and any observed secondary complications.

Patients presenting with substantial intraocular inflammation, vitreous hemorrhage with or without concomitant hyphema, retinal detachment, or cystoid macular edema (CME), especially when associated with vitreous to the cataract incision, most clearly constitute candidates for surgery. Another possible contributing factor to the development of such complications may include a malpositioned haptic causing posterior iris surface chafing and inflammation. When such clinical suspicion exists, ultrasound biomicroscopy (UBM) or anterior-segment optical coherence tomography (OCT) imaging may provide more definitive evaluation. Although a posteriorly dislocated IOL may be well tolerated in many patients, the difficulty in vision rehabilitation necessitates surgical intervention in most. For symptomatically subluxated IOLs, surgery may be performed via a limbal or a pars plana approach. Patients with less extensive subluxation can be managed through a limbal incision with minimal or no anterior vitrectomy if the posterior capsule is largely intact. However, if there is a large posterior capsular rent, vitrectomy using a pars plana approach may offer optimal control to achieve the goals of surgery and address unforeseeable intraoperative complications.

Observation

An IOL with limited decentration is usually minimally symptomatic, so it is satisfactorily managed by observation. Observation also may be recommended even for more extensive subluxation if other superseding medical or ophthalmic problems prohibit further surgery, or if the patient simply elects not to pursue further surgery. Occasionally, management with topical miotics can be visually beneficial, especially for minor subluxations. In a series of 15 patients with dislocated or subluxated anterior chamber or iris plane IOLs that were managed with observation, a visual acuity of ≥ 20/40 was reported in 60%, but retinal detachment occurred in two patients.[60]

Removal or Exchange

The IOL exchange is most commonly associated with the following: damage to the IOL (e.g., broken haptic); lack of available instrumentation to reposition; and certain IOL designs, such as those with highly flexible haptics (e.g., polypropylene) or plate haptic design, which make the IOL unsuitable for sulcus fixation unless the peripheral capsule is almost completely intact.

In patients for whom repositioning PC IOLs proves problematic, an intraoperative decision can be made to remove and exchange it with an AC IOL or scleral suture-fixated PC IOL (with or without the need for suture material). Exchange for a suture-fixated (PC) IOL was initially simplified by the availability of IOL designs that include holes (eyelets) in the haptics alone. Newer IOL design produced three-piece Prolene haptic IOLs, which may be readily amenable to scleral fixation by methods of scleral tunnel or pocket formation, scleral glue, or suture fixation.[13,29–47,61–67]

Explanting and reimplanting an IOL may risk more corneal endothelial cell trauma as compared with repositioning techniques.

Exchange for an AC IOL may be less traumatic to the corneal endothelium and may be easier and faster to accomplish. Newer AC IOL designs reportedly avoid complications caused by the mechanical side effects of earlier AC IOL designs compared with PC IOLs, and the results presumably can be extrapolated to dislocated IOL management.[68] In any case, it is important that the possibility of either PC IOL or AC IOL implantation should be anticipated with proper IOL power calculations, and IOL availability, before surgery.

An ancillary option is observation of the dislocated IOL, in which case visual rehabilitation is achieved with implantation of a second (usually AC) IOL.[69–71] This should be considered an option of last resort, however, as most patients are concerned about the presence of a dislocated lens implant.

Intraocular Lens Repositioning

Intraocular lens repositioning completes the initial surgical objectives of the cataract surgery and is the most commonly elected surgical approach. There are three basic approaches to IOL repositioning: (1) without sutures, using residual peripheral anterior or posterior capsule; (2) iris-sutured fixation; and (3) scleral fixation with or without the use of suture material.

Subluxated IOLs associated with an intact, or mostly intact, posterior capsule may be repositioned from an anterior approach if there is only moderate subluxation. Usually at least one haptic is posteriorly malpositioned—either protruding through an unseen zonular dehiscence in an area without posterior capsular support or posterior to the residual capsule. A pars plana approach is optimal for patients with large posterior capsule defects, for patients with IOL luxation into the vitreous cavity, and for patients with coexisting ocular complications such as retinal detachment.

Recognition and use of adequate capsular support are as important for repositioning the PC IOL as they are for primary placement. Generally, the IOL remains well supported if at least 180 degrees of peripheral capsular material is intact. More extensive support is necessary, however, when the inferior capsule is absent or if the margin of the residual capsule where IOL haptics are to be placed is of questionable integrity. Repositioning by capsular fixation is the most common management technique in reported series,[13,59–65] and is our first choice when technically possible and when the design of the PC IOL is appropriate for such positioning (i.e., not a one-piece acrylic IOL). Surgical success depends on accurate placement of the haptics into the ciliary sulcus, which requires visualization of the residual capsule.[72,73] Placement of iris hooks is useful in selected cases, but usually strategic local iris retraction with a hooked instrument allows confident visualization. The use of viscoelastic devices can serve as an additional measure to aid in visualization of the ciliary sulcus and provide mechanical opening of this space to facilitate IOL placement. A useful maneuver in a pars plana approach is to bring the IOL anteriorly and capture at least one haptic anterior to the iris **(Fig. 22.3)**. After the IOL is stabilized in the anterior chamber, the second haptic can be guided between the residual capsule and posterior iris surface either by rotating the lens or by grasping the haptic with an intraocular forceps via the pars plana. Because of the modern techniques related to capsulorrhexis creation, the peripheral anterior capsule is usually intact and serves as an effective interface for sulcus fixation. Repositioning a PC IOL permanently into the anterior chamber also has been reported, but is not recommended because of chronic chafing of the iris by the IOL and lens power considerations.[74]

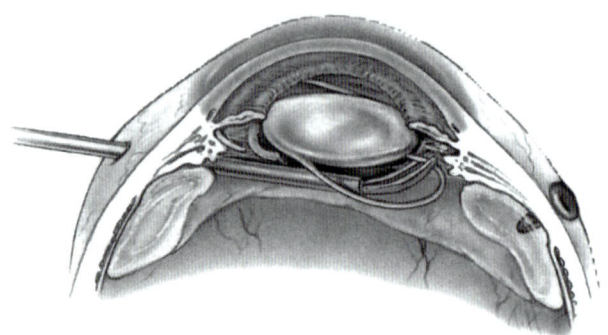

Fig. 22.3 When repositioning a posterior chamber (PC) intraocular lens (IOL) onto residual capsular remnants, it may be useful to bring one haptic anterior to the iris to facilitate accurate visualization of haptic placement over residual capsule. (From Regillo CD, Brown GC, Flynn HW Jr. Vitreoretinal Disease: The Essentials. New York: Thieme; 1999:572. Reprinted by permission.)

Intraocular Lens Fixation Techniques

Iris fixation sutures were initially described for the use of dislocated AC IOLs.[75] Their use has been modified for fixation of dislocated posterior chamber implants using a limbal or a pars plana approach.[72,76] Iris claw IOL implants are another option, with both anterior and posterior types available. This technique requires that a suture pass through the cornea and iris, around the IOL haptic, and back out through the iris and cornea. Because accurate placement of the needle is difficult, it is challenging to optimize IOL centration. In addition, concern regarding iris-mediated chronic inflammation, chronic pupillary miosis, chronic macular edema, and the technical difficulty encountered during suture placement have led to the development of other techniques.[29–47]

Scleral fixation sutures were first introduced for implantation of secondary IOLs and for primary IOL placement in the absence of satisfactory peripheral capsular support in a limbal or pars plana approach.[29–40] Early reports described pulling the haptic to or externally through[77–79] a sclerotomy to position a suture on the haptic before suturing to the deep part of the sclerotomy wound. Subsequently, IOL repositioning using transscleral fixation sutures via a pars plana approach mimicking the techniques of secondary IOL fixation was described. Components common to all scleral suture fixation techniques include (1) retrieving the IOL, (2) introducing a suture loop through the ciliary sulcus region into the vitreous cavity, (3) passing the suture loop around the IOL haptic, (4) securing the suture to the sclera, and (5) covering or burying the scleral suture knot. A wide variety of techniques have been described to achieve these goals.[29–47,76–79]

Most proposed techniques modify how the suture loop is introduced and attached to the IOL haptic. Such techniques have included imbricating the IOL haptic into the sutures used to close the sclerotomy, externalizing the haptics to attach a suture, using a needle guide to thread the suture around the haptic, introducing a small needle intraocularly to capture the haptic, suturing through IOL optic positioning holes, backing a large needle into the eye to introduce a suture loop, grasping a loop by intraocular forceps, and introducing the suture from a third sclerotomy. Other proposed variation techniques include achieving three- or four-point fixation to lessen lens torsion, using specially designed small-gauge forceps to aid in maneuvering the loop around the haptic, and using perfluorocarbon liquids to place the implant in a convenient position for suturing. Most posterior segment surgeons find the use of perfluorocarbon liquids unnecessary.[29–47,76–95]

Anatomy of Scleral Suture Fixation

Histopathological and ultrasound biomicroscopic studies have shown that little or no fibrosis occurs around sutured PC IOL haptics,[96] but one study has shown cicatrization around the haptics.[97] Either way, it is vital to use a nondissolving suture material because it may provide the sole means of support at the ciliary sulcus.

Intraocular lens torsion and decentration can be avoided by accurate ciliary sulcus placement and by adequate excision of bulky capsular and cortical remnants. It may be necessary to exchange some IOLs that are too short from haptic to haptic for sulcus fixation. Anatomic studies have located the sulcus ~ 1 mm posterior to the limbus.[98] Consequently, suture placement more posteriorly may cause IOL optic torsion by forcing the circumferentially oriented haptic over radially oriented ciliary processes. The sutures must be placed 180 degrees apart for proper centration. In addition, the IOL must be rotated minimally and cautiously to the center at the end of the operation.

Outcomes of Surgery for Dislocated Posterior Chamber Intraocular Lenses

The final visual acuity probably depends on not only preoperative macular function, but also complications from the original cataract surgery, such as CME and retinal detachment. Despite the possibility of complicating factors, a final visual acuity ≥ 20/40 in more than 90% of eyes has been reported in some series (**Table 22.2**). Surgical series are difficult to compare accurately due to nonhomogeneity and the variety of management techniques.

Table 22.2 Visual Acuity Outcomes of Pars Plana Vitrectomy for Dislocated Intraocular Lens

Series (Date)	No. of Patients	> 20/40 (%)
Campo[82] (1989)	17	59
Flynn[60] (1990)	25	68
Smiddy[59] (1991)	32	69
Chan[81] (1992)	12	92
Panton[62] (1993)	31	94
Smiddy[63] (1994)	46	50
Mello[13] (2000)	110	57

Postoperative Complications of the Sutured Intraocular Lens

An intraoperative or postoperative vitreous hemorrhage commonly occurs, given that sutures are placed through the vascular ciliary body, but are almost always self-limited and of little clinical significance. Bacterial migration along the transscleral suture tract has been described as being the possible route for infection in cases of delayed-onset endophthalmitis.[60,99,100] Rotating the suture knot or the use of a partial-thickness scleral flap to cover the scleral suture knot should reduce the risk of this complication. However, the suture knot can erode through the flap.

Other postoperative complications are difficult to separate from those that would be expected with complicated cataract surgery. Both CME and retinal detachment have been described after IOL repositioning surgery. Retinal detachment occurs in combination with dislocated PC IOL in ~ 2 to 3% of cases, and may be less frequent than with retained lens fragments[13,59,60,62,63,81] (**Table 22.3**). Possible reasons for the disparity include less inflammation with IOL dislocation relative to lens nuclear and cortical materials. Also, primary vitrectomy is often performed

Table 22.3 Incidence of Retinal Detachment (RD) Occurring Before and After Vitrectomy for Dislocated Posterior Chamber Intraocular Lens

Series (Date)	Initial Coexisting RD	RD After Vitrectomy	Combined
Flynn[60] (1990)*	1/20 (5%)	0/20 (0%)	1/20 (5%)
Smiddy[59] (1991)*	1/32 (3%)	1/32 (3%)	2/32 (6%)
Chan[81] (1992)	0/12 (0%)	0/12 (0%)	0/12 (0%)
Smiddy[63] (1994)*	0/59 (0%)	0/59 (0%)	0/59 (0%)
Panton[62] (1993)	0/31 (0%)	0/31 (0%)	0/31 (0%)
Mello[13] (2000)*	0/110 (0%)	7/110 (6.4%)	7/110 (6.4%)
Totals	2/264 (0.8%)	8/264 (3%)	10/264 (3.8%)

*These four series are from the same institution, but are listed here as consecutive series without overlap of cases.

from the limbus at the time the lens fragment is lost, whereas with the dislocated IOL this is usually less aggressively performed. The surgical approach typically involves standard vitreoretinal surgical techniques, but perfluorocarbon liquids may be useful in selected cases to better manipulate the IOL while avoiding retinal trauma. A final issue to consider in IOL suture fixation is the long-term stability of the suture material. Although published reports are limited, it has been shown that 10-0 polypropylene suture material can break down, resulting in the need for secondary intervention as early as 2 years following original surgery, and up to 16 years later within a pediatric study population. Although some surgeons prefer the use of 9-0 Prolene, there is limited published information as to the exact difference in breakdown as compared with a 10-0 Prolene suture.[101]

Recommendation for Management of Dislocated Intraocular Lens

For the anterior-segment surgeon, avoidance of PC IOL dislocation depends on accurate assessment of posterior capsule status intraoperatively. The anterior-segment surgeon must take care to evaluate the integrity of the peripheral capsule carefully before implanting a PC IOL in the presence of a posterior capsular rupture. Minimally, six clock hour positions (180 degrees) of peripheral capsular support (including the inferior meridians) are necessary to maintain IOL positioning, though this degree of support is by no means an absolute minimum and can prove insufficient for IOL support in many eyes. Retraction of the iris may be necessary to directly visualize the extent of peripheral capsular support before placing the PC IOL. Once it is determined that it is safe to proceed with IOL placement, it is vital that the haptics are placed precisely. As previously mentioned, viscoelastic devices and iris retraction (using iris hooks) may facilitate this placement.

Recommendations for the anterior-segment surgeon who encounters PC IOL dislocation intraoperatively include performing anterior vitrectomy to avoid vitreous incarceration in the wound. Postoperatively, frequent topical corticosteroids, nonsteroidal anti-inflammatory drugs (NSAIDs), and, as clinically indicated, IOP-reducing agents should be prescribed. For most cases, referral to a vitreoretinal surgeon for definitive management is advisable, although, as described previously, some cases are best observed, or may be amenable to management with limbal incisions. Careful attention is necessary to determine the presence of other complications such as retinal detachment.

Recommendations for the vitreoretinal surgeon include careful assessment of existing capsular anatomy and coexisting complications to formulate a treatment plan in terms of timing and technique options. Generally, allowing 1 week or longer for treatment and resolution of acute postoperative inflammation is advisable. The vitreoretinal surgeon should also be aware of IOL calculations from the cataract surgeon so that appropriate IOL power can be accurately selected if necessary.

Postoperative Endophthalmitis

Infectious endophthalmitis following ocular surgery is an uncommon clinical entity often causing severe vision loss.[102,103] As previous estimates have indicated that at least 1.35 million cataract operations are performed each year in the United States,[1] pseudophakic endophthalmitis is the most frequently encountered category in reported series. This complication is not specific to phacoemulsification or cataract surgery. Other categories of intraocular surgery may also lead to endophthalmitis but are

Table 22.4 Incidence of Endophthalmitis at the Bascom Palmer Eye Institute (1984–1994)[110] and (2002–2009)[111]

Cumulative Total Rate (in Percents) of Endophthalmitis*	1984–94 0.09	2002–09 0.025
Following cataract surgery	0.30	0.028
Following pars plana vitrectomy	0.05	0.011
Following penetrating keratoplasty	0.11	0.108

*Reported cumulative rate of endophthalmitis from 1995–2001 reported to be 0.05%.[111]

less frequent in reported clinical series. Endophthalmitis after secondary IOL implantation, corneal transplant, pars plana vitrectomy, and glaucoma filtering surgery is reported less often in large series.[104–109]

Incidence

In surveys of postoperative endophthalmitis at the Bascom Palmer Eye Institute from 1984 to 1994 and again from 2002 to 2009, the incidence of nosocomial endophthalmitis was reported to be low, with a continued trend toward a lower overall rate over a 25-year period[110,111] **(Table 22.4)**. The incidence of endophthalmitis after penetrating ocular trauma (3 to 30% of patients in reported trauma series) is much higher than in the postoperative categories.[112–115] Even in the era of advanced modern surgical techniques, prevention of postoperative endophthalmitis must be considered. In fact, some authors have provided study results suggesting that postoperative endophthalmitis may be a result of sutureless corneal wounds now commonly used in cataract surgery, thus making postoperative endophthalmitis a continuing concern.[103]

Clinical factors associated with a higher frequency of endophthalmitis include vitreous loss (cataract surgery), repeat incisions in the surgical limbus with potential poor wound healing (secondary IOL), and use of adjunctive antimetabolites (glaucoma filtering surgery).

Clinical Diagnosis and Microbiological Confirmation

The diagnosis of postoperative endophthalmitis is made by recognition of clinical features and by microbiological confirmation. The clinical features of post–cataract surgery endophthalmitis include marked intraocular inflammation and fibrin in the anterior chamber **(Fig. 22.4)** often with hypopyon.[102] In addition, conjunctival congestion, corneal edema, and lid edema are traditional signs associated with intraocular infection. Symptoms often include pain and marked loss of vision. Although endophthalmitis caused by less virulent organisms may have minimal or no pain, some degree of pain is still present in the majority of postoperative endophthalmitis patients. The loss of vision is usually profound and out of proportion to the typical postoperative vision measured during the first days or weeks after intraocular surgery.

An attempt is made to confirm the clinical diagnosis by microbiological growth from intraocular specimens. Vitreous specimens are more likely to yield a positive culture result than simultaneously obtained aqueous specimens.[116] Many different techniques have been described for obtaining these specimens. The anterior chamber specimen is typically obtained using a syringe with a 30-gauge needle. The vitreous specimen can be

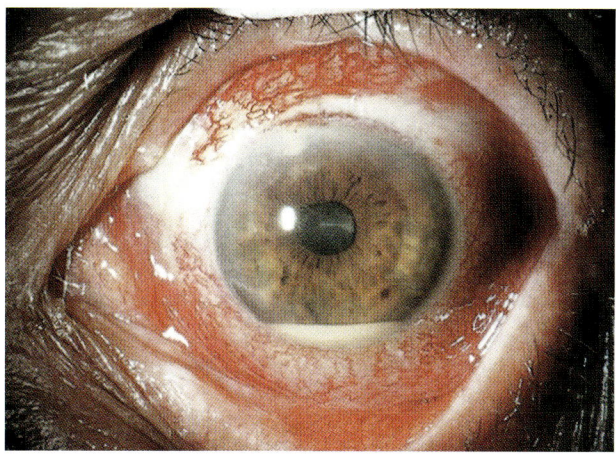

Fig. 22.4 Acute-onset endophthalmitis caused by *Staphylococcus aureus* presenting 3 days following cataract surgery with posterior chamber implant. (From Regillo CD, Brown GC, Flynn HW Jr. Vitreoretinal Disease: The Essentials. New York: Thieme; 1999:559. Reprinted by permission.)

obtained either by a needle tap or by a vitrectomy instrument. The needle tap technique generally employs a 23- or 25-gauge needle (although some surgeons may use a 27- or 30-gauge needle, such small bore needles may limit efficacy and sample yield) introduced through the pars plana and directed toward the midvitreous cavity. Neither a conjunctival incision nor a suture closure is necessary for the needle entry site. A small specimen (0.2 to 0.5 mL) is obtained and is directly inoculated into culture media or delivered to the laboratory without delay. If a vitrectomy instrument is utilized, the specimen may be passed through a membrane filter system to concentrate the microorganisms on the filter paper. Using sterile techniques, the filter paper sections are placed on appropriate culture media. Alternatively, freshly collected vitrectomy specimen can be injected directly into blood culture bottles for analysis by the microbiology department as growth occurs. In a reported study comparing membrane filter cultures versus blood culture bottles, similar rates of positive cultures were obtained from both culture techniques.[117] At night or on the weekends when the microbiological staff is not available to process the vitrectomy specimen, the blood culture bottles are particularly useful.

The source of the infecting organisms causing postoperative endophthalmitis is generally thought to be the patient's own flora from the lids, conjunctiva, and periocular tissues.[118] Molecular epidemiological techniques have demonstrated that the genetic identity of bacteria from vitreous aspirates is the same as those from eyelid or conjunctival isolates in 82% of cases in one study of endophthalmitis.[119] Similarly, in an analysis of 105 coagulase-negative *Staphylococcus* endophthalmitis cases with paired isolates from the individual patient's eyelid and intraocular compartments, pulsed-field gel electrophoresis demonstrated genetically identical organisms in 67.6%.[120] These results reinforce the necessity of following stringent surgical-site preparation prior to eye surgery. Ophthalmic surgeons now routinely instill povidone-iodine 5% solution at the beginning of an intraocular procedure to further reduce resident flora and, it is hoped, the risk of endophthalmitis.[121]

The Endophthalmitis Vitrectomy Study

The Endophthalmitis Vitrectomy Study (EVS) was a randomized prospective, clinical trial evaluating treatment strategies for acute-onset endophthalmitis following cataract surgery or secondary IOL surgery.[122–125] The EVS compared treatment outcomes between immediate three-port pars plana vitrectomy and immediate vitreous tap/biopsy, and between the use and nonuse of intravenous antibiotics. The systemic antibiotics selected by the EVS investigators were amikacin and ceftazidime for a minimum 5-day course. The EVS entry criteria were as follows:

- A clinical diagnosis of endophthalmitis was made within 6 weeks of cataract surgery or secondary IOL.
- Hypopyon or clouding of AC or vitreous media was sufficient to obscure clear visualization of second-order retinal arterioles.
- The cornea and AC were clear enough to visualize some part of iris.
- The cornea was clear enough to allow the possibility of pars plana vitrectomy.
- Visual acuity was worse than 20/50 but entailed at least light perception.
- The patient had no serious coexisting diseases that might compromise visual outcomes or performing immediate three-port pars plana vitrectomy.

A double-randomization scheme provided four groups for analysis: immediate three-port pars plana vitrectomy with intravenous antibiotics, immediate three-port pars plana vitrectomy without intravenous antibiotics, immediate tap/biopsy with intravenous antibiotics, and immediate tap/biopsy without intravenous antibiotics.[122]

The microbiological results of the EVS confirmed bacteria growth in 69.3% of intraocular cultures.[123–125] The coagulase-negative micrococci accounted for 70% of the EVS isolates. *Staphylococcus aureus* (9.9%), *Streptococcus* species (9.0%), *Enterococcus* species (2.2%), gram-negative organisms (5.9%), and miscellaneous gram-positive organisms (3.1%) occurred less often. All gram-positive organisms were sensitive to vancomycin, but two of the gram-negative organisms were resistant to both amikacin and ceftazidime.

The EVS results were as follows:

- No difference in final visual acuity or media clarity whether or not EVS systemic antibiotics were employed
- For patients with hand motion or better vision, no difference in outcomes between immediate three-port pars plana vitrectomy and tap/biopsy
- For patients with initial visual acuity of light perception (LP), better visual results occurred in only the immediate three-port pars plana vitrectomy group (versus tap/biopsy group)
  - Three times more likely to achieve ≥ 20/40 (33% versus 11%)
  - Two times more likely to achieve ≥ 20/100 (56% versus 30%)
  - Less likely to incur < 5/200 (20% versus 47%)

The EVS treatment outcomes demonstrated no difference in final visual acuity or media clarity outcomes whether or not systemic antibiotics were employed. Likewise, if the patient had hand motion or better visual acuity on the initial examination, the EVS showed no difference in these outcomes between the immediate three-port pars plana vitrectomy group and the immediate tap/biopsy group. For patients with initial vision of light perception only (26% of patients in the EVS), much better outcomes occurred in the immediate three-port pars plana vitrectomy group. Using multivariate analysis, the presenting visual acuity was the single most important factor in predicting EVS outcomes regardless of the treatment group.

Table 22.5 Endophthalmitis Vitrectomy Study Visual Acuity Outcomes by Microbiology Results

Visual Acuity Outcome	No or Equivocal Growth (*n* = 123)	Coagulase Negative Micrococci (*n* = 187)	Other Gram Positive (*n* = 56)	Gram Negative (*n* = 16)	Mixed Growth (*n* = 12)
≥ 20/40	55%	62%	29%	44%	25%
≥ 20/100	80%	84%	43%	56%	42%
≥ 5/200	92%	96%	63%	69%	92%

The EVS visual acuity outcomes can be stratified by microbiological results.[124,125] The best EVS outcomes occurred in the groups with either no or equivocal growth and in the coagulase-negative micrococci group (**Table 22.5**). EVS patients with gram-negative organisms had intermediate visual outcomes compared with the gram-positive category (composed mainly of *S. aureus* and *Streptococcus* species), which had the poorest outcomes. These outcomes stratified by microbiological isolates are similar to a previous report that showed visual acuity outcomes of 20/400 or better in more than 80% of endophthalmitis cases caused by the coagulase-negative staphylococci.[93] Less favorable outcomes occurred in the *S. aureus* and gram-negative groups, but the worst outcomes occurred in the *Streptococcus* species group.[126]

Because the EVS selected amikacin and ceftazidime for systemic use, some authors have questioned whether these EVS results can be extended to other systemic antibiotics.[127–129] Amikacin was selected for coverage of the gram-negative organisms, but the penetration of amikacin into the vitreous cavity has been shown to be poor in an experimental model.[130] Ceftazidime also has a broad coverage of gram-negative organisms but its effectiveness against gram-positive organisms is variable. Notably absent for systemic use in the EVS, vancomycin has excellent coverage of gram-positive organisms and has been shown in an experimental model to penetrate well into the vitreous cavity.[131] Orally administered antibiotics, such as ciprofloxacin, were also not evaluated in the EVS. Therefore, the EVS outcomes with systemically administered amikacin and ceftazidime may not reflect the outcomes obtained with other antibiotics currently available or potentially available in the future. Orally administered moxifloxacin and gatifloxacin have been previously evaluated and shown to achieve therapeutic levels within noninflamed eyes.[132,133] This has suggested that the use of such oral medication as an adjunct to additional measures taken in the treatment of endophthalmitis may confer further therapeutic benefit, though randomized-controlled studies are lacking. As such, no definitive recommendations can be made as to the routine use of these oral agents as part of a treatment regimen.

The drug dosages used in the EVS and alternative drugs recommended by the authors are listed in **Table 22.6**. When rapid-onset (≤ 2 days) endophthalmitis cases with very severe intraocular inflammation are encountered, the use of systemic vancomycin should be considered. However, no systemic antibiotics are recommended in the majority of postoperative endophthalmitis patients.

Systemic corticosteroids were used in all patients in the EVS. In the elderly post–cataract surgery population, the use of systemic corticosteroids may often be contraindicated because of the high prevalence of diabetes mellitus and other medical risks from the use of systemic corticosteroids. Intravitreal corticosteroids have been used as an adjunct to intraocular antibiotics in reported clinical series.[126,134] The authors currently recommend intravitreal dexamethasone 0.4 mg in 0.1 mL as a part of the initial treatment in postoperative endophthalmitis.

Ten patients among the 420 EVS patients developed acute postoperative endophthalmitis in spite of having received antibiotics in the irrigation solution during the cataract surgery. Because of the ineffectiveness of this approach, the risk of antibiotic toxicity, the tendency to foster the emergence of vancomycin-resistant organisms, and the increased risk of CME, the use of irrigating solution antibiotics for routine cataract surgery has been generally discouraged.[135–137] However, there has been more recent interest in the use of intracameral injection of antibiotics at the time of cataract surgery. In a review of 32,180 procedures, 22 cases of postoperative endophthalmitis were observed—a rate of 0.07%—when intracameral cefuroxime injection was performed at the time of surgery.[138] Additional, a European series evaluating 13,698 patients undergoing cataract surgery reported results suggesting that the incidence rate of postoperative endophthalmitis could be almost five times as high in a group of patients not receiving prophylactic cefuroxime treatment.[139] Similar results have been reported from France with comparative rates of endophthalmitis of 1.238% without intracameral cefuroxime injection and 0.044% when prophylaxis was given.[140] Intracameral moxifloxacin injection at the time of cataract surgery, as a means of endophthalmitis prophylaxis, has also been reported to produce lower endophthalmitis rates.[141] Although this is an emerging area of interest and study, the American Society of Cataract and Refractive Surgery has reported on member preferences for endophthalmitis prevention in association with cataract surgery; the members show a strong preference for topical pre- and postoperative antibiotic use, even with limited experience, and for the use of intracameral prophylaxis.[142] Certainly this is an area of continued interest, debate, and research, with far-reaching potential impacts that must be considered as the ophthalmic community continues to strive for even lower rates of cataract-associated endophthalmitis.[143]

The aminoglycosides have a narrow range of safety for intravitreal use during endophthalmitis treatment. Because vancomycin covers gram-positive organisms causing greater than 90% of postoperative endophthalmitis and because aminoglycosides add the risk of inadvertent retinal toxicity, we recommend intravitreal ceftazidime (instead of amikacin) for coverage of gram-negative organisms when treating clinically diagnosed endophthalmitis (**Table 22.6**).

Endophthalmitis may also occur following suture removal or late-onset keratitis involving the wound.[137,144,145] The removal of 10-0 nylon sutures may allow entry of organisms in sufficient quantity to cause intraocular infection. With the trend to sutureless cataract surgery, these cases are now becoming less common. Delayed-onset keratitis associated with a previous cataract wound may be associated with breakdown of the wound allowing entry of organisms. These keratitis-associated cases are often caused by more virulent organisms and generally have a poor visual prognosis.[137] Strictly speaking, the EVS results apply only to cataract and secondary IOL surgery, but the EVS antibiotic treatment regimen may be used for other postoperative endophthalmitis categories.

Table 22.6 Drugs Used in Endophthalmitis Vitrectomy Study (EVS) Compared with Authors' Recommended Antibiotics for Treatment of Acute Postoperative Endophthalmitis

Drug	EVS Medications		Authors' Recommendations*	
	Dose		Drug	Dose
Intravitreal				
Vancomycin	1 mg in 0.1 mL		Vancomycin	1 mg in 0.1 mL
Amikacin	0.4 mg in 0.1 mL		Ceftazidime	2.25 mg in 0.1 mL
No intravitreal steroids			Dexamethasone	0.4 mg in 0.1 mL
Subconjunctival				
Vancomycin	25 mg in 0.5 mL		Vancomycin	25 mg in 0.5 mL
Ceftazidime	100 mg in 0.5 mL		Ceftazidime	100 mg in 0.5 mL
Dexamethasone	6 mg		Dexamethasone	12 mg
Topical				
Vancomycin	50 mg/mL drops		Vancomycin	50 mg/mL drops
Amikacin	20 mg/mL drops		Ceftazidime	50 mg/mL drops
Cycloplegics	b.i.d.		Cycloplegics	b.i.d.
Prednisolone acetate	1% drops q2h		Prednisolone acetate	1% drops q2h
Systemic ceftazidime	2 g IV q8h (1.5 g if weight less than 50 kg; modify for abnormal renal function)		Ceftazidime	1.0 g IV q12h
Amikacin	7.5 mg/kg initially followed by 6 mg/kg		Vancomycin	1.0 g IV q12h (modify for abnormal function)
Prednisone	30 mg p.o. b.i.d. (5 to 10 days)		No systemic steroids	

*After EVS reports, the authors recommend systemic antibiotics *only* in rapid-onset cases with more severe intraocular inflammation. In mild or moderate inflammation cases, no systemic antibiotics are utilized.

Delayed-Onset Endophthalmitis

Delayed-onset or chronic postoperative endophthalmitis occurs weeks to months after cataract surgery and is not specific to phacoemulsification. These patients present with progressive intraocular inflammation and a chronic indolent course. The most frequent reported organisms include *Propionibacterium acnes, Staphylococcus epidermidis,* and fungi.

The clinical features of delayed-onset endophthalmitis observed on slit-lamp examination usually help to distinguish among these causative organisms. *P. acnes* cases are characterized by the presence of a large white intracapsular plaque associated with chronic granulomatous inflammation (**Fig. 22.5**).[146,147] These eyes may have large keratic precipitates on the corneal endothelium and beaded fibrin strands in the anterior chamber. One author (L.J.) has previously encountered a bilateral case, with earlier-onset iritis, eventually mimicking granulomatous uveitis, occurring 1 year after cataract surgery. In cases caused by *S. epidermidis,* chronic progressive vitreitis is a typical feature with no white intracapsular plaque. In cases caused by fungi, the anterior chamber may often be relatively quiet, but linear, white strands resembling "a string of pearls" may be present in the anterior vitreous indicating the presence of *Candida* organisms (**Fig. 22.6**). Because these organisms generally replicate more slowly, they are often resistant to medical therapy alone.[102,144–147]

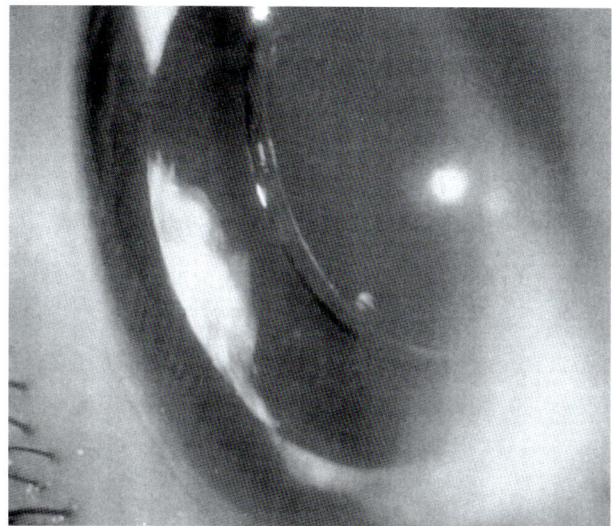

Fig. 22.5 Delayed-onset endophthalmitis caused by *Propionibacterium acnes* occurring 4 months after cataract surgery and showing a white intracapsular plaque with moderate intraocular inflammation. (From Regillo CD, Brown GC, Flynn HW Jr. Vitreoretinal Disease: The Essentials. New York: Thieme; 1999:564. Reprinted by permission.)

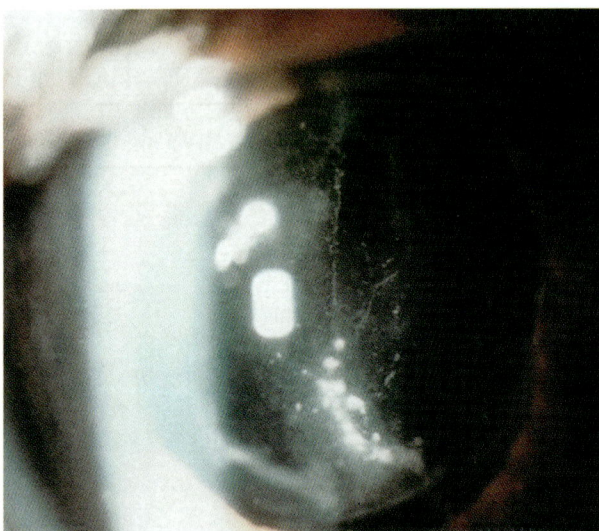

Fig. 22.6 Delayed-onset endophthalmitis caused by *Candida parapsilosis* occurring 6 weeks after cataract surgery and characterized by a string of pearls and white infiltrates in the anterior vitreous. (From Regillo CD, Brown GC, Flynn HW Jr. Vitreoretinal Disease: The Essentials. New York: Thieme; 1999:564. Reprinted by permission.)

In delayed-onset endophthalmitis, pars plana vitrectomy is commonly recommended to establish the correct diagnosis by culture, remove offending organisms, and remove areas of localized white intracapsular plaque when present. Recurrent or resistant infection despite vitrectomy may require removal of the entire capsular bag and the IOL.[144–147]

Suprachoroidal Effusion/ Hemorrhage

Suprachoroidal effusion/hemorrhage (SCH) may occur during or after any form of intraocular surgery (see also Chapter 24). Transient hypotony is a common feature during or after all intraocular surgery that may lead to a choroidal effusion followed by rupture of long or short posterior ciliary arteries with subsequent frank hemorrhage.[148] Obstruction of vortex veins during scleral buckling procedure is another mechanism that has been historically referenced to predispose to development of choroidal effusion and/or SCH.[149] SCH may be limited to one or two quadrants or can be massive (360 degrees), resulting in extrusion of intraocular contents or forcing retinal surfaces centrally into apposition (with each other). Reported risk factors for SCH include glaucoma, aphakia, myopia, advanced age, arteriosclerotic cardiovascular disease, hypertension, and intraoperative tachycardia.[150–157]

Management and Course of Suprachoroidal Effusion/ Hemorrhage

Intraoperative management strategies are controversial. Most authors recommend immediate closure of ocular incisions, removal of vitreous prolapse into the wound if possible, and drainage of SCH if continued high pressure is present.[150–153] Intraoperative SCH drainage is almost never complete but is usually successful in lowering IOP and creating a scleral opening for continued postoperative drainage.

In cases of suprachoroidal effusion due to hypotony, the hypotony must be managed to prevent continued effusion. If the effusions enlarge and touch, retinal apposition may occur. Although retinal apposition does not always equate with a poor vision outcome, it has been suggested to be a poor prognostic indicator in a reported series.[158] The effusions, therefore, should be drained when the effusions begin to "kiss." The timing of the secondary surgical intervention for SCH remains controversial, but most surgeons recommend observation for 7 to 14 days to allow liquefaction of the SCH. There are no randomized prospective clinical trials addressing this timing issue because of the multiple ocular diseases in these patients and the complex variables present prior to the occurrence of massive SCH. The surgical goals of secondary surgical intervention for massive SCH include drainage of liquefied SCH, removal of prolapsed vitreous by vitrectomy, and management of rhegmatogenous retinal detachment, if present, using a scleral buckle or intraocular gas tamponade **(Fig. 22.7)**.[150–155] Perfluorocarbon liquids have also been advocated and used by some authors.[159,160] Likewise, some authors have recommended high-dose systemic and topical corticosteroids during the immediate postoperative period.[153] Risk factors for poor vision outcome include concurrent retinal detachment and more than two quadrants of SCH involvement.[152]

We strongly prefer nonintervention in SCH, and follow patients closely, offering surgery when resolution is slow (> 3 weeks) or when secondary complications such as glaucoma, traction, rhegmatogenous retinal detachment, or vitreous hemorrhage occur.

Needle Penetration of the Globe

Cataract surgery today is usually performed under topical anesthesia, which obviates the concern about needle penetration during administration of retrobulbar or peribulbar anesthesia. However, some surgeons occasionally prefer traditional anesthesia, which may result in this rare complication.

The Atkinson retrobulbar block employs an elevated and adducted eye position to place the needle tip into the muscle cone adjacent to the optic nerve. Because of the risk of needle entry into either the globe or the optic nerve, many ophthalmologists switched to use of a peribulbar block with the eye position straight ahead and larger volumes of anesthetic to fill the orbit.[161]

Factors predisposing to needle penetration of the globe include axial high myopia, posterior staphyloma, previous scleral buckling surgery, and poor patient cooperation with the injection.[162–164] Additional consideration must be given to the experience of the other medical professionals (e.g., anesthesiologists, nurse anesthetists) who may have limited experience in providing this method of anesthesia, but can find themselves providing such anesthesia is certain surgical centers. Although no published studies report a clear difference in the complication rates of retrobulbar anesthesia between ophthalmologists and nonophthalmologists, the differences in training, techniques, and experience must be considered to optimize patient safety.

When needle entry is suspected, indirect ophthalmoscopy is recommended to evaluate the posterior segment. The visual acuity and IOP should be documented. If marked IOP elevation occurs, one should consider anterior chamber paracentesis. Ocular hypotony may also indicate that penetration has occurred.

Early management of posterior-segment needle entry wounds is controversial. Most authors recommend prompt laser treatment or cryopexy to visible retinal perforation sites, but blood or lens opacities may preclude a satisfactory view of the area. The patient can be followed with serial echography examination until clearing of vitreous hemorrhage occurs. If retinal detachment occurs, early intervention is recommended. Any elective surgery should be postponed.

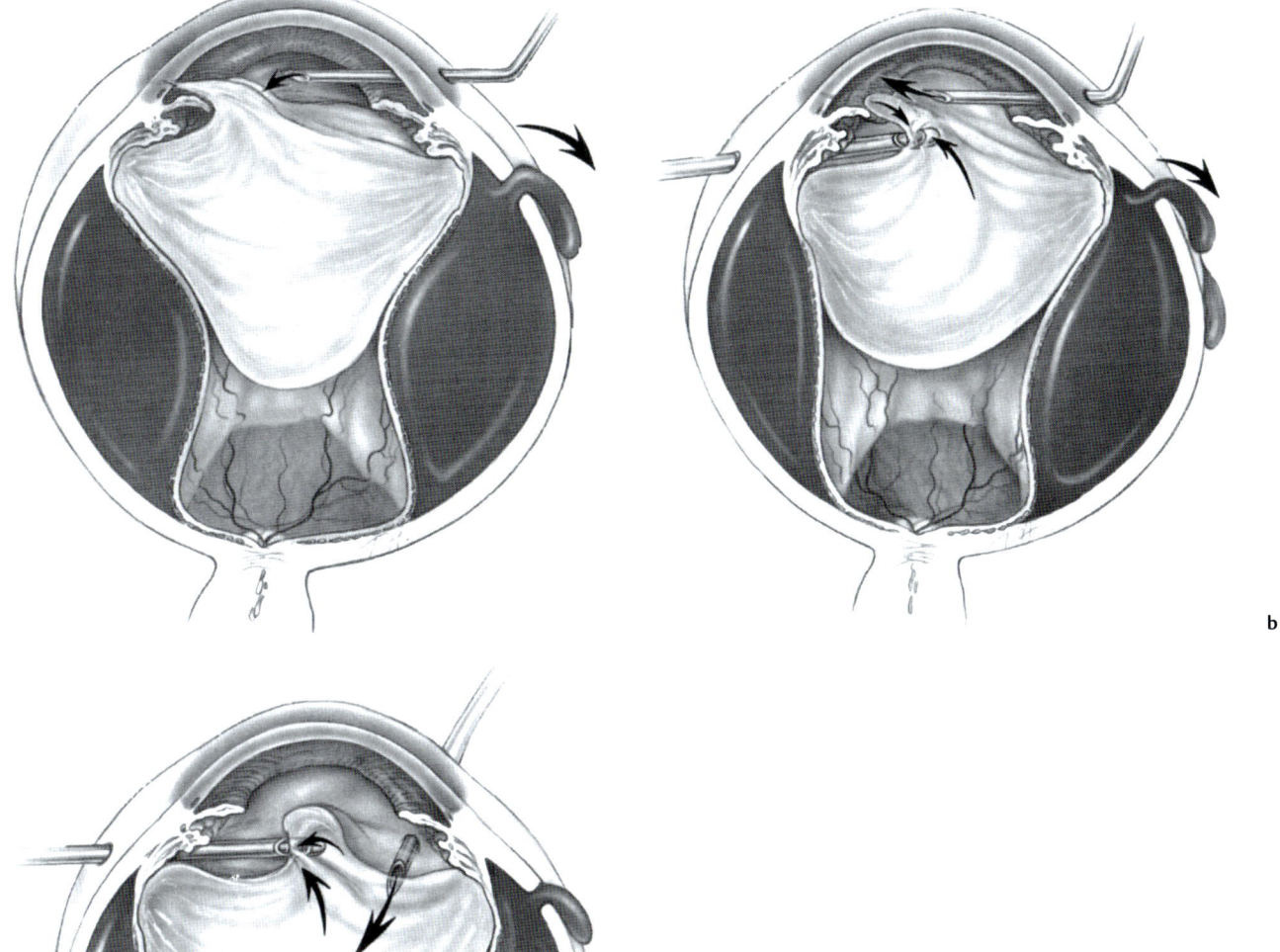

Fig. 22.7 Management of massive suprachoroidal hemorrhage. **(a)** Needle infusion into anterior chamber and scleral drainage of suprachoroidal hemorrhage. **(b)** Anterior vitrectomy and continued scleral drainage. **(c)** Posterior vitrectomy and continued scleral drainage. (From Regillo CD, Brown GC, Flynn HW Jr. Vitreoretinal Disease: The Essentials. New York: Thieme; 1999:565. Reprinted by permission.)

The vision prognosis is usually dependent on the presence or absence of retinal detachment and initial damage inflicted initially to the posterior pole.[160] In one report, retinal breaks without retinal detachment had a much better vision prognosis than eyes complicated by retinal detachment. In the former category, seven of nine cases without retinal detachment achieved 20/50 or better visual acuity, whereas in the latter category only two of 14 retinal detachment cases achieved 20/400 or better visual acuity.[162]

Role of the Posterior Segment Surgeon

Retina-vitreous specialists have a critical role in the management of many of the complications of phacoemulsification and cataract surgery. The final vision outcome is highly dependent on their judgment and surgical skills. A sympathetic and cooperative team approach with the anterior-segment surgeon will help alleviate patient anxiety during this phase of management.

Conclusion

The anterior-segment surgeon should have a good working relationship with the retina specialist. If serious intraoperative or postoperative complications occur, and the posterior segment has been violated, a retinal consult will add valued management options. Early referral and management may prevent sight-threatening outcomes.

Acknowledgments

Matthew J. Welch and Leonard Joffe acknowledge the remarkable work of coauthors William E. Smiddy, and Harry W. Flynn, Jr. in the publication of many original articles and several chapters in this field. They graciously permitted the reorientation of their published materials for this chapter under combined authorship.

References

1. Prevent Blindness America. Vision problems in the US. In: Prevent Blindness America. New York: Prevent Blindness America Publishers; 1994: 8–10

2. Williams A, Sloan FA, Lee PP. Longitudinal rates of cataract surgery. Arch Ophthalmol 2006;124:1308–1314

3. Leaming DV. Practice styles and preferences of ASCRS members—1994 survey. J Cataract Refract Surg 1995;21:378–385

4. Mahmood S, von Lany H, Cole MD, et al. Displacement of nuclear fragments into the vitreous complicating phacoemulsification surgery in the UK: incidence and risk factors. Br J Ophthalmol 2008;92:488–492

5. Gilliland GD, Hutton WL, Fuller DG. Retained intravitreal lens fragments after cataract surgery. Ophthalmology 1992;99:1263–1267, discussion 1268–1269

6. Weinstein GW, Charlton JF, Esmer E. The "lost lens": a new surgical technique using the Machemer lens. Ophthalmic Surg 1995;26:156–159

7. Aaberg TM Jr, Rubsamen PE, Flynn HW Jr, Chang S, Mieler WF, Smiddy WE. Dropped nuclei and giant retinal tears as a complication of cataract surgery. Am J Ophthalmol 1997;124:222–226

8. Vilar NF, Flynn HW Jr, Smiddy WE, Murray TG, Davis JL, Rubsamen PE. Removal of retained lens fragments after phacoemulsification reverses secondary glaucoma and restores visual acuity. Ophthalmology 1997; 104:787–791, discussion 791–792

9. Chang DF, Packard RB. Posterior assisted levitation for nucleus retrieval using Viscoat after posterior capsule rupture. J Cataract Refract Surg 2003;29:1860–1865

10. Chang DF. Strategies for managing posterior capsular rupture in phaco chop. In: Chang DF, ed. Phaco Chop: Mastering Techniques, Optimizing Technology, and Avoiding Complications. Thorofare, NJ: Slack; 2004

11. Lifshitz T, Levy J. Posterior assisted levitation: long-term follow-up data. J Cataract Refract Surg 2005;31:499–502

12. Moore JK, Scott IU, Flynn HW Jr, et al. Retinal detachment in eyes undergoing pars plana vitrectomy for removal of retained lens fragments. Ophthalmology 2003;110:709–713, discussion 713–714

13. Mello MO Jr, Scott IU, Smiddy WE, Flynn HW, Feuer W. Surgical management and outcomes of dislocated intraocular lenses. Ophthalmology 2000;107:62–67

14. Modi YS, Epstein A, Smiddy WE, Murray TG, Feuer W, Flynn HW Jr. Retained lens fragments after cataract surgery: outcomes of same-day versus later pars plana vitrectomy. Am J Ophthalmol 2013;156:454–9.e1

15. Irvine SR, Irvine AR. Lens-induced uveitis and glaucoma. Arch Ophthalmol 1958;60:829–840

16. Epstein DL. Diagnosis and management of lens-induced glaucoma. Ophthalmology 1982;89:227–230

17. Blodi BA, Flynn HW Jr, Blodi CF, Folk JC, Daily MJ. Retained nuclei after cataract surgery. Ophthalmology 1992;99:41–44

18. Borne MJ, Tasman W, Regillo C, Malecha M, Sarin L. Outcomes of vitrectomy for retained lens fragments. Ophthalmology 1996;103:971–976

19. Kim JE, Flynn HW Jr, Smiddy WE, et al. Retained lens fragments after phacoemulsification. Ophthalmology 1994;101:1827–1832

20. Hutton WL, Snyder WB, Vaiser A. Management of surgically dislocated intravitreal lens fragments by pars plana vitrectomy. Ophthalmology 1978;85:176–189

21. Lambrou FH Jr, Steward MW. Management of dislocated lens fragments after cataract surgery. Ophthalmology 1992;99:1260–1262

22. Fastenberg DM, Schwartz PL, Shakin JL, Golub BM. Management of dislocated nuclear fragments after phacoemulsification. Am J Ophthalmol 1991;112:535–539

23. Kapusta MA, Chen JC, Lam WC. Outcomes of dropped nucleus during phacoemulsification. Ophthalmology 1996;103:1184–1187

24. Liu KR, Peyman GA, Chen MS, Chang KB. Use of high-density vitreous substitutes in the removal of posteriorly dislocated lenses or intraocular lenses. Ophthalmic Surg 1991;22:503–507

25. Greve MDJ, Peyman GA, Mehta NJ, Millsap CM. Use of perfluoroperhydrophenanthrene in the management of posteriorly dislocated crystalline and intraocular lenses. Ophthalmic Surg 1993;24:593–597

26. Lewis H, Blumenkranz MS, Chang S. Treatment of dislocated crystalline lens and retinal detachment with perfluorocarbon liquids. Retina 1992; 12:299–304

27. Brod RD, Flynn HW Jr, Clarkson JG, Blankenship GW. Management options for retinal detachment in the presence of a posteriorly dislocated intraocular lens. Retina 1990;10:50–56

28. Smiddy WE, Flynn HW Jr, Kim JE. Retinal detachment in patients with retained lens fragments or dislocated posterior chamber intraocular lenses. Ophthalmic Surg Lasers 1996;27:856–861

29. Malbran ES, Malbran E Jr, Negri I. Lens guide suture for transport and fixation in secondary IOL implantation after intracapsular extraction. Int Ophthalmol 1986;9:151–160

30. Lindquist TD, Agapitos PJ, Lindstrom RL, Lane SS, Spigelman AV. Transscleral fixation of posterior chamber intraocular lenses in the absence of capsular support. Ophthalmic Surg 1989;20:769–775

31. Smiddy WE, Sawusch MR, O'Brien TP, Scott DR, Huang SS. Implantation of scleral-fixated posterior chamber intraocular lenses. J Cataract Refract Surg 1990;16:691–696

32. Grehn F, Sundmacher R. Fixation of posterior chamber lenses by transscleral sutures: technique and preliminary results. [letter] Arch Ophthalmol 1989;107:954–955

33. Lewis JS. Sulcus fixation without flaps. Ophthalmology 1993;100:1346–1350

34. McCluskey P, Harrisberg B. Long-term results using scleral-fixated posterior chamber intraocular lenses. J Cataract Refract Surg 1994;20:34–39

35. Teichmann KD. Pars plana fixation of posterior chamber intraocular lenses. Ophthalmic Surg 1994;25:549–553

36. Tomikawa S, Hara A. Simple approach to secondary posterior chamber intraocular lens implantation in patients without a complete posterior lens capsule support. Ophthalmic Surg 1995;26:160–163

37. Vajpayee RB, Angra SK, Sandramouli S, Rewari R. Direct scleral fixation of posterior chamber intraocular lenses using a special needle-holder. Ophthalmic Surg 1992;23:383–387

38. Mittelviefhaus H, Wiek J. A refined technique of transscleral suture fixation of posterior chamber lenses developed for cases of complicated cataract surgery with vitreous loss. Ophthalmic Surg 1993;24:698–701

39. Lyle WA, Jin JC. Secondary intraocular lens implantation: anterior chamber vs posterior chamber lenses. Ophthalmic Surg 1993;24:375–381

40. Regillo CD, Tidwell J. A small-incision technique for suturing a posterior chamber intraocular lens. Ophthalmic Surg Lasers 1996;27:473–475

41. Por YM, Lavin MJ. Techniques of intraocular lens suspension in the absence of capsular/zonular support. Surv Ophthalmol 2005;50:429–462

42. Wagoner MD, Cox TA, Ariyasu RG, Jacobs DS, Karp CL; American Academy of Ophthalmology. Intraocular lens implantation in the absence of capsular support: a report by the American Academy of Ophthalmology. Ophthalmology 2003;110:840–859

43. Gabor SG, Pavlidis MM. Sutureless intrascleral posterior chamber intraocular lens fixation. J Cataract Refract Surg 2007;33:1851–1854

44. Agarwal A, Kumar DA, Jacob S, Baid C, Agarwal A, Srinivasan S. Fibrin glue-assisted sutureless posterior chamber intraocular lens implantation in eyes with deficient posterior capsules. J Cataract Refract Surg 2008; 34:1433–1438

45. Mohr A, Hengerer F, Eckardt C. Retropupillare Fixation der Irisklauenlinse bei Aphakie. Einjahresergebnisse einer neuen Implantationstechnik. [Ret-

ropupillary fixation of the Iris claw lens In aphakia; 1 year outcome of a new Implantation technique.] Ophthalmologe 2002;99:580–583

46. Thach AB, Dugel PU, Sipperley JO, et al. Outcome of sulcus fixation of dislocated posterior chamber intraocular lenses using temporary externalization of the haptics. Ophthalmology 2000;107:480–484, discussion 485

47. Prenner JL, Feiner L, Wheatley HM, Connors D. A novel approach for posterior chamber intraocular lens placement or rescue via a sutureless scleral fixation technique. Retina 2012;32:853–855

48. Scott IU, Flynn HW Jr, Smiddy WE, et al. Clinical features and outcomes of pars plana vitrectomy in patients with retained lens fragments. Ophthalmology 2003;110:1567–1572

49. Hansson LJ, Larsson J. Vitrectomy for retained lens fragments in the vitreous after phacoemulsification. J Cataract Refract Surg 2002;28:1007–1011

50. Smiddy WE, Flynn HW Jr. Managing retained lens fragments and dislocated posterior chamber IOL's after cataract surgery. Focal Points 1996; 14:1–14

51. Ross WH. Management of dislocated lens fragments after phacoemulsification surgery. Can J Ophthalmol 1996;31:234–240

52. Kageyama T, Ayaki M, Ogasawara M, Asahiro C, Yaguchi S. Results of vitrectomy performed at the time of phacoemulsification complicated by intravitreal lens fragments. Br J Ophthalmol 2001;85:1038–1040

53. Lai TY, Kwok AK, Yeung YS, et al. Immediate pars plana vitrectomy for dislocated intravitreal lens fragments during cataract surgery. Eye (Lond) 2005;19:1157–1162

54. Stark WJ, Worthen DM, Holladay JT, et al. The FDA report on intraocular lenses. Ophthalmology 1983;90:311–317

55. Smith SG, Lindstrom RL. Malpositioned posterior chamber lenses: etiology, prevention, and management. J Am Intraocul Implant Soc 1985;11: 584–591

56. Murphy GE. Traumatic dislocation of a shearing lens 31 months after implantation. Ophthalmic Surg 1983;14:53–54

57. Jehan FS, Mamalis N, Crandall AS. Spontaneous late dislocation of intraocular lens within the capsular bag in pseudoexfoliation patients. Ophthalmology 2001;108:1727–1731

58. Gross JG, Kokame GT, Weinberg DV; Dislocated In-The-Bag Intraocular Lens Study Group. In-the-bag intraocular lens dislocation. Am J Ophthalmol 2004;137:630–635

59. Smiddy WE, Flynn HW Jr. Management of dislocated posterior chamber intraocular lenses. Ophthalmology 1991;98:889–894

60. Flynn HW Jr, Buus D, Culbertson WW. Management of subluxated and posteriorly dislocated intraocular lenses using pars plana vitrectomy instrumentation. J Cataract Refract Surg 1990;16:51–56

61. Capone A Jr, Mandell BA, Aaberg TM Sr, Sternberg P Jr, Lambert HM, Lopez PF. Contemporary vitreoretinal surgical management of posteriorly dislocated intraocular lenses. Proceedings of the Symposium on Retina and Vitreous, New Orleans Academy of Ophthalmology, 1993:271–281

62. Panton RW, Sulewski ME, Parker JS, Panton PJ, Stark WJ. Surgical management of subluxed posterior-chamber intraocular lenses. Arch Ophthalmol 1993;111:919–926

63. Smiddy WE, Flynn HW Jr. Management options for posteriorly dislocated intraocular lenses. Ophthalmic Practice 1994;12:72–77

64. Shakin EP, Carty JB Jr. Clinical management of posterior chamber intraocular lens implants dislocated in the vitreous cavity. Ophthalmic Surg Lasers 1995;26:529–534

65. Smiddy WE, Ibanez GV, Alfonso E, Flynn HW Jr. Surgical management of dislocated intraocular lenses. J Cataract Refract Surg 1995;21:64–69

66. Batlan SJ, Dodick JM. Explantation of a foldable silicone intraocular lens. Am J Ophthalmol 1996;122:270–272

67. Schneiderman TE, Johnson MW, Smiddy WE, Flynn HW Jr, Bennett SR, Central HL. Surgical management of dislocated plate haptic silicone posterior chamber intraocular lenses. Am J Ophthalmol 1997;123:629–635

68. Ellerton CR, Rattigan SM, Chapman FM, Chitkara DK, Smerdon DL. Secondary implantation of open-loop, flexible, anterior chamber intraocular lenses. J Cataract Refract Surg 1996;22:951–954

69. Jacobi KW, Krey H. Surgical management of intraocular lens dislocation into the vitreous: case report. J Am Intraocul Implant Soc 1983;9:58–59

70. Brockman EB, Franklin RM, Kaufman HE. Visual disability resulting from a dislocated intraocular lens. J Cataract Refract Surg 1993;19:312–313

71. Sinskey RM. Posterior chamber implant removal with or without replacement. Cataract 1983;1:8–10

72. Stark WJ, Bruner WE, Martin NF. Management of subluxed posterior-chamber intraocular lenses. Ophthalmic Surg 1982;13:130–133

73. Eifrig DE. Two principles for repositioning intraocular lenses. Ophthalmic Surg 1986;17:486–489

74. Allara RD, Weinstein GW. A new surgical technique for managing sunset syndrome. Ophthalmic Surg 1987;18:811–814

75. McCannel MA. A retrievable suture idea for anterior uveal problems. Ophthalmic Surg 1976;7:98–103

76. Sternberg P Jr, Michels RG. Treatment of dislocated posterior chamber intraocular lenses. Arch Ophthalmol 1986;104:1391–1393

77. Lyons CJ, Steele AD. Report of a repositioned posteriorly dislocated intraocular lens via pars plicata sclerotomy. J Cataract Refract Surg 1990;16: 509–511

78. Moretsky SL. Suture fixation technique for subluxated posterior chamber IOL through stab wound incision. J Am Intraocul Implant Soc 1984;10: 477–480

79. Insler MS, Mani H, Peyman GA. A new surgical technique for dislocated posterior chamber intraocular lenses. Ophthalmic Surg 1988;19:480–481

80. Girard LJ, Nino N, Wesson M, Maghraby A. Scleral fixation of a subluxated posterior chamber intraocular lens. J Cataract Refract Surg 1988;14:326–327

81. Chan CK. An improved technique for management of dislocated posterior chamber implants. Ophthalmology 1992;99:51–57

82. Campo RV, Chung KD, Oyakawa RT. Pars plana vitrectomy in the management of dislocated posterior chamber lenses. Am J Ophthalmol 1989; 108:529–534

83. Smiddy WE. Dislocated posterior chamber intraocular lens. A new technique of management. Arch Ophthalmol 1989;107:1678–1680

84. Koch DD. New optic hole configuration for iris fixation of posterior chamber lenses. Arch Ophthalmol 1988;106:163–164

85. Nabors G, Varley MP, Charles S. Ciliary sulcus suturing of a posterior chamber intraocular lens. Ophthalmic Surg 1990;21:263–265

86. Friedberg MA, Pilkerton AR. A new technique for repositioning and fixating a dislocated intraocular lens. Arch Ophthalmol 1992;110:413–415

87. Maguire AM, Blumenkranz MS, Ward TG, Winkelman JZ. Scleral loop fixation for posteriorly dislocated intraocular lenses. Operative technique and long-term results. Arch Ophthalmol 1991;109:1754–1758

88. Lawrence FC II, Hubbard WA. "Lens lasso" repositioning of dislocated posterior chamber intraocular lenses. Retina 1994;14:47–50

89. Bloom SM, Wyszynski RE, Brucker AJ. Scleral fixation suture for dislocated posterior chamber intraocular lens. Ophthalmic Surg 1990;21:851–854

90. Anand R, Bowman RW. Simplified technique for suturing dislocated posterior chamber intraocular lens to the ciliary sulcus. Arch Ophthalmol 1990;108:1205–1206

91. Chang S, Coll GE. Surgical techniques for repositioning a dislocated intraocular lens, repair of iridodialysis, and secondary intraocular lens implantation using innovative 25-gauge forceps. Am J Ophthalmol 1995; 119:165–174

92. Lewis H, Sanchez G. The use of perfluorocarbon liquids in the repositioning of posteriorly dislocated intraocular lenses. Ophthalmology 1993; 100:1055–1059

93. Fanous MM, Friedman SM. Ciliary sulcus fixation of a dislocated posterior chamber intraocular lens using liquid perfluorophenanthrene. Ophthalmic Surg 1992;23:551–552

94. Smiddy WE, Flynn HW Jr. Dislocated IOL repositioning technique. [letter] Arch Ophthalmol 1993;111:161–162

95. Murray TG, Abrams GW, Stanley J. Pars plana vitrectomy in the management of dislocated posterior chamber lenses. [letter] Am J Ophthalmol 1990;109:362

96. Pavlin CJ, Rootman D, Arshinoff S, Harasiewicz K, Foster FS. Determination of haptic position of transsclerally fixated posterior chamber intraocular lenses by ultrasound biomicroscopy. J Cataract Refract Surg 1993; 19:573–577

97. McDermott ML, Puklin JE. Pars plana cicatrization of sewn-in posterior chamber intraocular lens haptics. Ophthalmic Surg Lasers 1997;28:239–240

98. Duffey RJ, Holland EJ, Agapitos PJ, Lindstrom RL. Anatomic study of transsclerally sutured intraocular lens implantation. Am J Ophthalmol 1989; 108:300–309

99. Schechter RJ. Suture-wick endophthalmitis with sutured posterior chamber intraocular lenses. J Cataract Refract Surg 1990;16:755–756

100. Heilskov T, Joondeph BC, Olsen KR, Blankenship GW. Late endophthalmitis after transscleral fixation of a posterior chamber intraocular lens. Arch Ophthalmol 1989;107:1427

101. Buckley EG. Hanging by a thread: the long-term efficacy and safety of transscleral sutured intraocular lenses in children (an American Ophthalmology Society thesis). Trans Am Ophthalmol Soc 2007;105:294–311

102. Flynn HW Jr, Brod RD, Pflugfelder SC, Miller D. Endophthalmitis management. In: Tasman W, Jaeger E, eds. Duane's Clinical Ophthalmology, vol 6. St. Louis: CV Mosby; 1994:1–22

103. Taban M, Behrens A, Newcomb RL, et al. Acute endophthalmitis following cataract surgery: a systematic review of the literature. Arch Ophthalmol 2005;123:613–620

104. Scott IU, Flynn HW Jr, Feurer W. Endophthalmitis associated with secondary intraocular lenses. Ophthalmology 1995;102:1925–1931

105. Cohen SM, Flynn HW Jr, Murray TG, Smiddy WE; The Postvitrectomy Endophthalmitis Study Group. Endophthalmitis after pars plana vitrectomy. Ophthalmology 1995;102:705–712

106. Kangas TA, Greenfield DS, Flynn HW Jr, Parrish RK II, Palmberg P. Delayed-onset endophthalmitis associated with conjunctival filtering blebs. Ophthalmology 1997;104:746–752

107. Kunimoto DY, Kaiser RS; Wills Eye Retina Service. Incidence of endophthalmitis after 20- and 25-gauge vitrectomy. Ophthalmology 2007;114:2133–2137

108. Scott IU, Flynn HW Jr, Dev S, et al. Endophthalmitis after 25-gauge and 20-gauge pars plana vitrectomy: incidence and outcomes. Retina 2008;28:138–142

109. Parolini B, Romanelli F, Prigione G, Pertile G. Incidence of endophthalmitis in a large series of 23-gauge and 20-gauge transconjunctival pars plana vitrectomy. Graefes Arch Clin Exp Ophthalmol 2009;247:895–898

110. Aaberg TM Jr, Flynn HW Jr, Newton J. Nosocomial endophthalmitis survey: a 10-year review of incidence and outcomes. Ophthalmology 1998;105:1004–1010

111. Wykoff CC, Parrott MB, Flynn HW Jr, Shi W, Miller D, Alfonso EC. Nosocomial acute-onset postoperative endophthalmitis at a university teaching hospital (2002–2009). Am J Ophthalmol 2010;150:392–398.e2

112. Thompson WS, Rubsamen PE, Flynn HW Jr, Schiffman J, Cousins SW. Endophthalmitis after penetrating trauma. Risk factors and visual acuity outcomes. Ophthalmology 1995;102:1696–1701

113. Barr CC. Prognostic factors in corneoscleral lacerations. Arch Ophthalmol 1983;101:919–924

114. Boldt HC, Pulido JS, Blodi CF, Folk JC, Weingeist TA. Rural endophthalmitis. Ophthalmology 1989;96:1722–1726

115. Reynolds DS, Flynn HW Jr. Endophthalmitis after penetrating ocular trauma. Curr Opin Ophthalmol 1997;8:32–38

116. Donahue SP, Kowalski RP, Jewart BH, Friberg TR. Vitreous cultures in suspected endophthalmitis. Biopsy or vitrectomy? Ophthalmology 1993;100:452–455

117. Joondeph BC, Flynn HW Jr, Miller D, Joondeph HC. A new culture method for infectious endophthalmitis. Arch Ophthalmol 1989;107:1334–1337

118. Callegan MC, Engelbert M, Parke DW II, Jett BD, Gilmore MS. Bacterial endophthalmitis: epidemiology, therapeutics, and bacterium-host interactions. Clin Microbiol Rev 2002;15:111–124

119. Speaker MG, Milch FA, Shah MK, Eisner W, Kreiswirth BN. Role of external bacterial flora in the pathogenesis of acute postoperative endophthalmitis. Ophthalmology 1991;98:639–649, discussion 650

120. Bannerman TL, Rhoden DL, McAllister SK, Miller JM, Wilson LA. The source of coagulase-negative staphylococci in the Endophthalmitis Vitrectomy Study. A comparison of eyelid and intraocular isolates using pulsed-field gel electrophoresis. Arch Ophthalmol 1997;115:357–361

121. Aiello LP, Brucker AJ, Chang S, et al. Evolving guidelines for intravitreous injections. Retina 2004;24(5, Suppl):S3–S19

122. The Endophthalmitis Vitrectomy Study Group. A randomized trial of immediate vitrectomy and of intravenous antibiotics with treatment of postoperative bacterial endophthalmitis: results of the Endophthalmitis Vitrectomy Study. Arch Ophthalmol 1995;113:1479–1496

123. Han DP, Wisniewski SR, Wilson LA, et al. Spectrum and susceptibilities of microbiologic isolates in the Endophthalmitis Vitrectomy Study. Am J Ophthalmol 1996;122:1–17

124. The Endophthalmitis Vitrectomy Study Group. Microbiologic factors and visual outcome in the endophthalmitis vitrectomy study. Am J Ophthalmol 1996;122:830–846

125. Johnson MW, Doft BH, Kelsey SF, et al. Relationship between clinical presentation and microbiologic spectrum: the Endophthalmitis Vitrectomy Study. Ophthalmology 1997;104:261–272

126. Mao LK, Flynn HW Jr, Miller D, Pflugfelder SC. Endophthalmitis caused by Staphylococcus aureus. Am J Ophthalmol 1993;116:584–589

127. Flynn HW Jr, Meredith TA. Interpretation of EVS results. [letter] Arch Ophthalmol 1996;114:1027–1028

128. Peyman GA. The Endophthalmitis Vitrectomy Study: a different point of view [editorial]. Arch de la Sociedad Espanola de Oftalmologia 1996;3:205–207

129. Davis JL. Intravenous antibiotics for endophthalmitis. [editorial] Am J Ophthalmol 1996;122:724–726

130. el-Massry A, Meredith TA, Aguilar HE, et al. Aminoglycoside levels in the rabbit vitreous cavity after intravenous administration. Am J Ophthalmol 1996;122:684–689

131. Meredith TA, Aguilar HE, Shaarawy A, Kincaid M, Dick J, Niesman MR. Vancomycin levels in the vitreous cavity after intravenous administration. Am J Ophthalmol 1995;119:774–778

132. Hariprasad SM, Shah GK, Mieler WF, et al. Vitreous and aqueous penetration of orally administered moxifloxacin in humans. Arch Ophthalmol 2006;124:178–182

133. Hariprasad SM, Mieler WF, Holz ER. Vitreous and aqueous penetration of orally administered gatifloxacin in humans. Arch Ophthalmol 2003;121:345–350

134. Stonecipher KG, Ainbinder DI, Maxwell DP, et al. Infectious endophthalmitis: a review of 100 cases. Ann Ophthalmol 1994;26:108–115

135. Axer-Siegel R, Stiebel-Kalish H, Rosenblatt I, Strassmann E, Yassur Y, Weinberger D. Cystoid macular edema after cataract surgery with intraocular vancomycin. Ophthalmology 1999;106:1660–1664

136. Alfonso EC, Flynn HW Jr. Controversies in endophthalmitis prevention. The risk for emerging resistance to vancomycin. Arch Ophthalmol 1995;113:1369–1370

137. Gritz DC, Cevallos AV, Smolin G, Whitcher JP Jr. Antibiotic supplementation of intraocular irrigating solutions. An in vitro model of antibacterial action. Ophthalmology 1996;103:1204–1208, discussion 1208–1209

138. Montan PG, Wejde G, Koranyi G, Rylander M. Prophylactic intracameral cefuroxime. Efficacy in preventing endophthalmitis after cataract surgery. J Cataract Refract Surg 2002;28:977–981

139. Barreau G, Mounier M, Marin B, Adenis JP, Robert PY. Intracameral cefuroxime injection at the end of cataract surgery to reduce the incidence of endophthalmitis: French study. J Cataract Refract Surg 2012;38:1370–1375

140. Barry P, Seal DV, Gettinby G, Lees F, Peterson M, Revie CW; ESCRS Endophthalmitis Study Group. ESCRS study of prophylaxis of postoperative endophthalmitis after cataract surgery: Preliminary report of principal results from a European multicenter study. J Cataract Refract Surg 2006;32:407–410

141. Matsuura K, Miyoshi T, Suto C, Akura J, Inoue Y. Efficacy and safety of prophylactic intracameral moxifloxacin injection in Japan. J Cataract Refract Surg 2013;39:1702–1706

142. Chang DF, Braga-Mele R, Mamalis N, et al; ASCRS Cataract Clinical Committee. Prophylaxis of postoperative endophthalmitis after cataract surgery: results of the 2007 ASCRS member survey. J Cataract Refract Surg 2007;33:1801–1805

143. Schimel AM, Alfonso EC, Flynn HW Jr. Endophthalmitis prophylaxis for cataract surgery: are intracameral antibiotics necessary? JAMA Ophthalmol 2014;132:1269–1270 Epub ahead of print

144. Winward KE, Pflugfelder SC, Flynn HW Jr, Roussel TJ, Davis JL. Postoperative Propionibacterium endophthalmitis. Treatment strategies and long-term results. Ophthalmology 1993;100:447–451

145. Fox GM, Joondeph BC, Flynn HW Jr, Pflugfelder SC, Roussel TJ. Delayed-onset pseudophakic endophthalmitis. Am J Ophthalmol 1991;111:163–173

146. Clark WL, Kaiser PK, Flynn HW Jr, Belfort A, Miller D, Meisler DM. Treatment strategies and visual acuity outcomes in chronic postoperative Propionibacterium acnes endophthalmitis. Ophthalmology 1999;106:1665–1670

147. Deramo VA, Ting TD. Treatment of Propionibacterium acnes endophthalmitis. Curr Opin Ophthalmol 2001;12:225–229

148. Maumenee AE, Schwartz MF. Acute intraoperative choroidal effusion. Am J Ophthalmol 1985;100:147–154

149. Zauberman H. Expulsive choroidal haemorrhage: an experimental study. Br J Ophthalmol 1982;66:43–45

150. Speaker MG, Guerriero PN, Met JA, Coad CT, Berger A, Marmor M. A case-control study of risk factors for intraoperative suprachoroidal expulsive hemorrhage. Ophthalmology 1991;98:202–209, discussion 210

151. Welch JC, Spaeth GL, Benson WE. Massive suprachoroidal hemorrhage. Follow-up and outcome of 30 cases. Ophthalmology 1988;95:1202–1206

152. Reynolds MG, Haimovici R, Flynn HW Jr, DiBernardo C, Byrne SF, Feuer W. Suprachoroidal hemorrhage. Clinical features and results of secondary surgical management. Ophthalmology 1993;100:460–465

153. Lambrou FH Jr, Meredith TA, Kaplan HJ. Secondary surgical management of expulsive choroidal hemorrhage. Arch Ophthalmol 1987;105:1195–1198

154. Lakhanpal V, Schocket SS, Elman MJ, Dogra MR. Intraoperative massive suprachoroidal hemorrhage during pars plana vitrectomy. Ophthalmology 1990;97:1114–1119

155. Lakhanpal V, Schocket SS, Elman MJ, Nirankari VS. A new modified vitreoretinal surgical approach in the management of massive suprachoroidal hemorrhage. Ophthalmology 1989;96:793–800

156. Ingraham HJ, Donnenfeld ED, Perry HD. Massive suprachoroidal hemorrhage in penetrating keratoplasty. Am J Ophthalmol 1989;108:670–675

157. Cantor LB, Katz LJ, Spaeth GL. Complications of surgery in glaucoma. Suprachoroidal expulsive hemorrhage in glaucoma patients undergoing intraocular surgery. Ophthalmology 1985;92:1266–1270

158. Ling R, Cole M, James C, Kamalarajah S, Foot B, Shaw S. Suprachoroidal haemorrhage complicating cataract surgery in the UK: epidemiology, clinical features, management, and outcomes. Br J Ophthalmol 2004;88:478–480

159. Desai UR, Peyman GA, Chen CJ, et al. Use of perfluoroperhydrophenanthrene in the management of suprachoroidal hemorrhages. Ophthalmology 1992;99:1542–1547

160. Meier P, Wiedemann P. Massive suprachoroidal hemorrhage: secondary treatment and outcome. Graefes Arch Clin Exp Ophthalmol 2000;238:28–32

161. Grizzard WS. Ophthalmic anesthesia. In: Reineke R, ed. Ophthalmology Annual 1989. New York: Raven Press; 1989:265–294

162. Hay A, Flynn HW Jr, Hoffman JI, Rivera AH. Needle penetration of the globe during retrobulbar and peribulbar injections. Ophthalmology 1991;98:1017–1024

163. Duker JS, Belmont JB, Benson WE, et al. Inadvertent globe perforation during retrobulbar and peribulbar anesthesia. Patient characteristics, surgical management, and visual outcome. Ophthalmology 1991;98:519–526

164. Morgan CM, Schatz H, Vine AK, et al. Ocular complications associated with retrobulbar injections. Ophthalmology 1988;95:660–665

Section IX   Difficult Circumstances

23 Intraoperative Floppy Iris Syndrome

Steven H. Dewey

Board certification may be a nuisance, but some of the board questions surprisingly pop up in your everyday practice. Take this question, which "walked into my office" in the form of a patient with a damaged iris sphincter and another patient with a broken posterior capsule—issues that could not be resolved after problems were encountered during the patients' cataract surgery. Here is the question:

> *Which of the following statements best exemplifies your practice?*
> 1. Everyone in my practice receives the full benefit of my advanced surgical skills.
> 2. Men receive better treatment than women.
> 3. Men with large prostates receive better treatment.
> 4. Men with the largest prostates receive the best treatment.
> 5. Men with prostates of amazing size receive absolutely the best treatment.

As with any multiple choice question, I make certain I know what is being asked. It seems like a fairly subjective question, and I believe it is referring to intraoperative floppy iris syndrome (IFIS). Funny, I'd never seen it presented quite this way. How to answer this one? I'll take it step by step. What do we know about treating IFIS?

Since the description of IFIS by David Chang and John Campbell in 2005, IFIS has undoubtedly become the most frequently encountered condition to potentially complicate an otherwise routine cataract surgery. In its mild form, the iris simply billows. Moderate cases have the pupil shrinking. In severe cases, iris prolapse occurs. Potential problems range from iatrogenic capsule rupture to dropped nuclei to retained fragments with the risk of prolonged inflammation and corneal endothelial damage.

Any number of techniques have been described to decrease the complications associated with IFIS. Many of these steps have to be taken in anticipation of IFIS. To do this, we have to identify the patients at risk. But that's the catch—it is called *intraoperative* floppy iris syndrome because it is not easy to spot in the office. We can spot pseudoexfoliation or Fuchs's syndrome at the slit lamp, but not IFIS.

To go back to the question, I'll just answer with option 1, and be justifiably content. There is absolutely no reason in my practice that I would ever consciously restrict the application of my best skills for any patient requesting my services.

That little nagging voice bugs me as I try to move on. It reminds me that if I'm doing anything to separate out the IFIS patients, the correct answer might not be what I think it is.

How are we trying to identify patients at risk for IFIS? I'll start with men currently on Flomax. But the drug's effects may persist years after its discontinuation. So, then, we need to identify men who have ever taken Flomax. Generics being prevalent,

we ask specifically about tamsulosin as well. Did we get them all? No, we didn't get them all. Wives will point out their husband's fallibility when it comes to remembering his own medical history. Besides, doesn't having prostate surgery mean you don't have the problem any more?

I'll change the approach and ask men about trouble urinating due to prostate problems at any time at all in the past, and assume they've taken the drug at one point or another if they agree. Better results, but we're still going to miss the women with a history of off-label use of tamsulosin. And, of course, the various patients of either gender who may take any other of the dozen or so medications with α-blocking effects associated with IFIS.

So, let me reverse this and think about the patients who should *not* receive the special IFIS precautions. These are techniques incorporated proactively into the surgical procedure that improve the outcome of an individual patient's result, and certain patients will be excluded from the utility of these precautions because they could not be identified as being at risk for IFIS? These are steps that will admittedly reduce the risk of capsule or iris damage, and some patients won't be included.

Because we were so focused on tamsulosin as the primary risk factor for encountering IFIS, and yet still missing any number of cases, I was providing preferential treatment for patients with benign prostatic hypertrophy.

The magnitude of the IFIS issue predicates action to reduce its impact. If the goal is to reduce the complications of this highly sporadic condition, then everyone in my practice should be treated as if they are at risk for IFIS. Everyone: men, with or without prostates; those who remember their medication history, and those who don't; women, even if they have never heard of a prostate, let alone never had one.

Everyone then benefits from the special steps, and they no longer remain "special." Everyone shares the potential of a better result. The best part is that patients are no longer responsible for influencing their own surgical environment through no fault of their own. My staff has had a tremendous burden taken from them, and the unsuspected IFIS case blends into the background of a normal surgical day.

An Aside

Many of the topics discussed in this chapter to avoid complications associated with IFIS may have no obvious connection to the condition. Rather, this chapter includes many of the changes to the procedure that have taken place in my operating room, either as establishment of best practices or elimination of bad habits. The ultimate goal of these changes is to reduce the impact of the unexpected, unwanted event. IFIS just happened to be the catalyst in taking an organized approach to reducing risks, not just those one can identify in an individual patient.

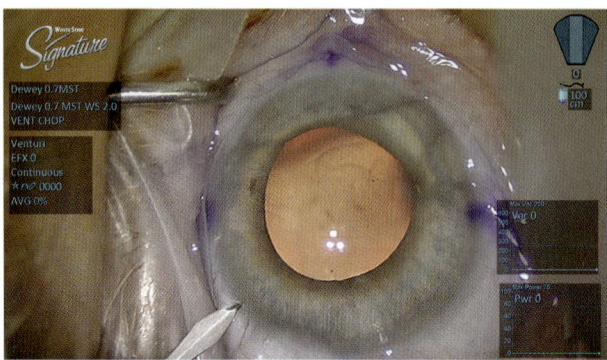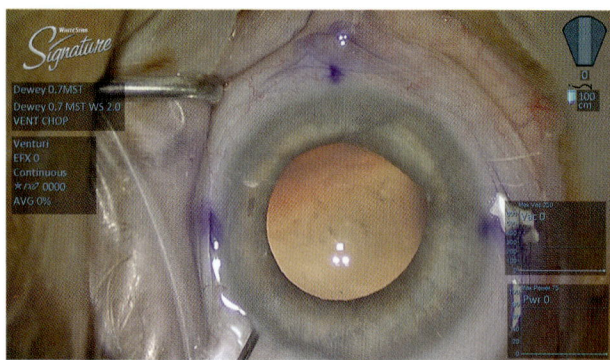

a   b

Fig. 23.1 **(a)** Preoperative tropicamide and phenylephrine were used to achieve a mid-dilated pupil for this patient on tamsulosin. Intracameral dilation is being administered through the side port. **(b)** A modest amount of dilation and additional tone are achieved with the intracameral solution. Figures 23.4 to 23.9 are video captures from the same case as Figure 23.1.

Preoperatively

The most obvious issue with IFIS is dilation. It has to be consistent and effective—quality and quantity. At the Pinnacle Surgery Center in Colorado Springs, we have adopted a regimen of spraying the open eye with a compounded formula of one part 1% tropicamide, one part 2.5% phenylephrine, and one part 0.5% ketorolac. The patient opens the eye, and the eye is spritzed (not unlike a fragrance associate at your local cosmetics establishment). The dilation is effective for both femtosecond cataract surgery and standard phacoemulsification (**Fig. 23.1a**).

The surprise about the spritz is that it is effective even with the patient closes the eye. Our original experience with this regimen was with the eye closed. Although that was successful, having the lids open certainly improves the efficacy of the regimen. Comparing this to three different agents delivered as drops 5 minutes apart for three different applications, it really is not surprising that this regimen is preferred by both patients and staff.

Intracameral Dilation

Is it the size of the pupil or the tone that will help in IFIS cases? Topical atropine starting 3 days prior to surgery was an accepted standard for improving dilation in those pesky miotic pupils. The problems with this approach are twofold. First, to whom is this approach offered? Second, the very patients in whom this regimen will work are those in whom atropine will induce acute urinary retention. (I know of two patients who ended up in the Emergency Department after successful cataract surgery for this very reason. That experience seemed to ruin the otherwise uneventful cataract surgery earlier in the day.)

This is a compounded solution of one part 4% nonpreserved lidocaine and one part 1:1,000 epinephrine in three parts balanced salt solution (BSS). Although the preoperative spritz is effective, intracameral dilation appears to substantially increase the iris's tone (**Fig. 23.1b**).

The advantage of the compounded intracameral formulation is simple: the exact specified concentration of each drug is administered directly to the target tissue. To avoid mixing errors, we do not create this solution on-site. As the solution is clear, it can be passed through a micropore filter under sterile conditions. It does, however, have a limited shelf life, so frequent reordering is necessary.

Encountering Small Pupils

In some patients a small pupil will remain small regardless of the pharmacological manipulations. Only the operating surgeon can determine whether a small pupil is large enough for cataract surgery.

Personally, I find that a 3-mm pupil in most cases is large enough, but this is with a highly stable chamber, excellent patient cooperation, a medium-density nucleus, and a specific phaco needle with a rounded edge. But these factors can fall apart at a moment's notice, requiring another step to regain the pupil dilation. Alternatively, we can infer that a small pupil phaco does not work with an excessively unstable chamber, a patient resistant to immobility, and denser cataracts.

One of the most common mistakes in dealing with an IFIS pupil is irritating it. If one intends to use a pupil expansion device, feel free to stretch the pupil to a degree if this will help with placement of the device. If one is trying to obtain a larger pupil without using mechanical support, forget the old teaching about stretching the pupil to enlarge it. Stretching will likely make this worse (**Fig. 23.2**).

In my experience, it does not take much to irritate an IFIS iris. Deliberate iris manipulation in the form of stretching will undoubtedly trigger pupillary miosis. I have personally experienced this with inadvertent engagement of the iris with the phaco needle during insertion, and with the mildest iris prolapse through either the main or side port.

Pupil Expansion Devices

Fundamentally, two styles of pupil expansion devices are available: hooks and rings.

Hooks are packaged as a set, and the typical deployment uses four to expand the small pupil. Each hook requires a paracentesis port, and the resulting pupil has a diamond configuration. Tom Oetting, MD, in Iowa City, places one of the hooks in the subincisional space to create a good point of access for performing phaco.

Hooks are easy to place, and easy to remove. The one problem with using hooks is the potential to stretch a sphincter beyond its capacity to recover. This can result in a postoperative mydriasis that can be both cosmetically and functionally unacceptable. Expanding the pupil to a 6-mm diamond should be well tolerated.

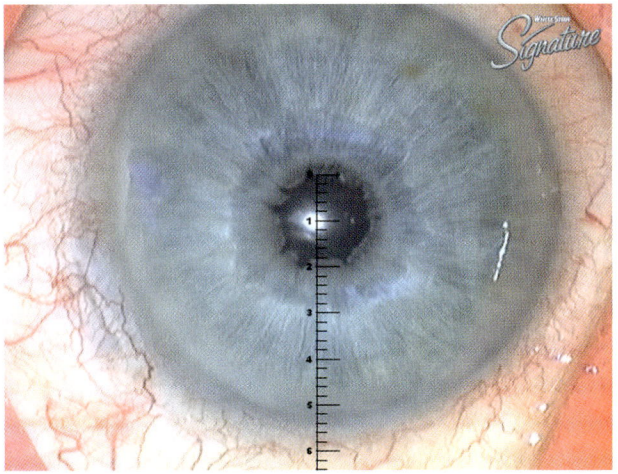

a

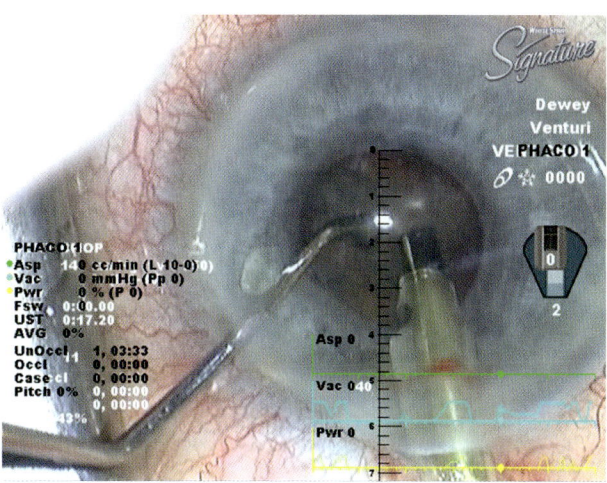

b

Fig. 23.2 The left and right eyes of a patient on Coumadin and tamsulosin. He presented with frustration after a prolonged cataract surgery involving bleeding during surgery. **(a)** The sphincterotomies are evidence of a surgical manipulation to achieve a larger pupil intraoperatively. The concomitant use of Coumadin only worsened the situation. **(b)** Using intracameral dilation and viscomydriasis, this pupil remained stable at just under 4 mm despite the tamsulosin use.

Rings are the class of expanders that support the pupil size internally. They do not require a paracentesis for external fixation. Several devices are available, and each has advantages and specific insertion techniques. These include the Malyugin ring (MicroSurgical Technologies [MST], Redmond, WA), the Perfect Pupil (Milvella, Savage, MN), the Pupil Dilator (Morcher, Stuttgart, Germany), and the Graether 2000 Pupil Expander (Eagle Vision, Memphis, TN).

I have the most experience with the Malyugin ring. The device comes with its own injector, and provides eight points of support. It comes in two sizes, 6.25 and 7 mm, but I have used only the 6.25. It is a single-use device and is inserted and removed with relative ease.

Regardless of whether hooks or rings are used, the stage of the surgery will determine the ease of application. Prior to performing the capsulorrhexis, these devices have only the iris to catch upon. Once the capsule is open, greater care should be taken to avoid catching the edge of the capsulorrhexis at the same time as the pupil margin.

In cases of dense or leathery nuclei, I use a pupil expansion device with little or no hesitancy. It is difficult to say which of the characteristics of these cases make the iris less well behaved. It could be the additional power, the additional manipulation, the increase in irrigation fluid, or any combination of these factors. In reviewing the videos of these cases, one can see that the pupil almost always ends up smaller, regardless of the initial size (**Fig. 23.3**).

Chamber Stability

Does the iris billow on its own due to lack of tone, or does it billow due to chamber instability? Probably the easiest way to create an IFIS case is (1) not to use an α-agonist for dilation and (2) create an unstable chamber.

Chamber stability begins with a comfortable patient, lying peacefully, not coughing and not moving. For my patients, the first step is Tessalon Perles in the preoperative area. This is 100 mg of sodium benzonatate, and effectively suppresses the cough reflex. It is not perfect, but it is good enough that patients have requested it for home use for the same reason.

Two other tricks we use to decrease coughing include punctal occlusion during administration of the topical anesthetic, and a touch of fentanyl when the situation warrants. Regarding the punctal occlusion, it is quite possibly the partial anesthesia of the nasopharynx that stimulates the cough reflex in some patients when assuming the supine position during surgery. The fentanyl is our anesthesia group's drug of choice, but the group will occasionally use intravenous lidocaine for the recalcitrant cougher.

To keep the patient from moving, the anesthesiologist has to be on board with your surgical plan. In an eye center with a dedicated sedation regimen, this is nearly a given. Regardless of the setting or the skill of the anesthesiologist, I highly recommend taping the patient's head, and strapping the chest and arms. Although the occasional gentle drift is annoying, it will likely cause you to need to remove the instruments from the eye. Once, no problem. Twice, annoying. By the third time, the change in anterior chamber dynamics may be enough to trigger billowing, miosis, or prolapse, even in low-risk patients. The restraint will slow a sudden movement enough to keep a disaster at bay.

Using the correct speculum for the situation is the next step. Simple wire specula may be useful for most cases, but pay particular attention to narrow lid fissures. Use a speculum with an active adjustable spreading mechanism. A wire speculum takes up less space in the lid fissure than a closed speculum, and appears to compress the eye less during surgery.

Sizing the Incision

Whether the patient is still or not, one often overlooked source of chamber instability is the fit of the incisions. During the crafting of the primary incision, the goals are to have it be both self-sealing and astigmatically neutral, and large enough to avoid binding during the procedure. Given the current size of our incisions (below 2.8 mm), even an imperfect incision will seal well, and induce very little astigmatism.

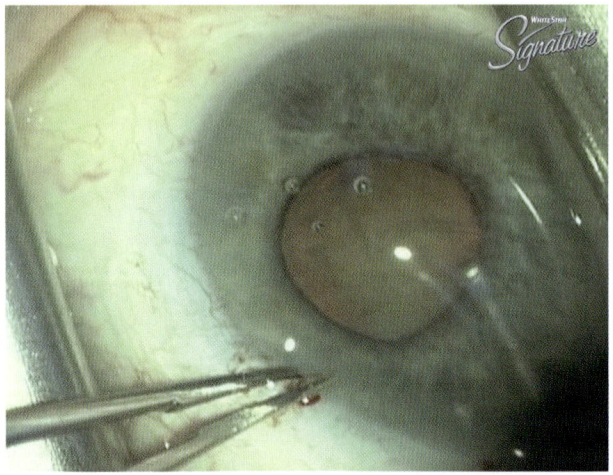

a

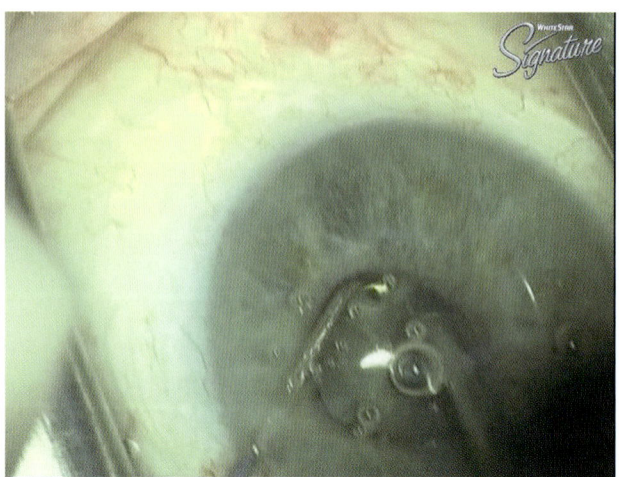

b

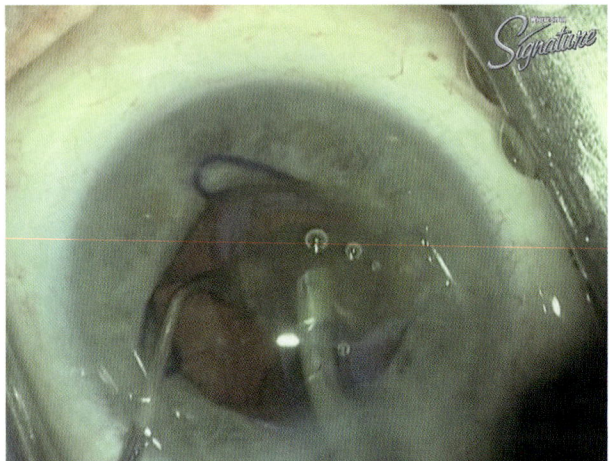

c

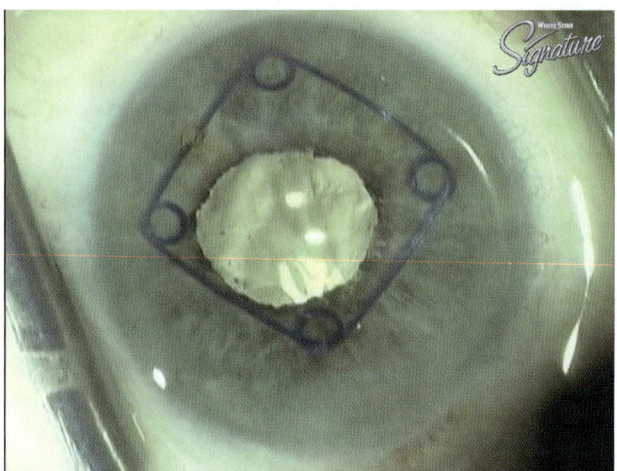

d

Fig. 23.3 **(a)** This pupil dilated to a reasonable size, but the exceptionally dense cataract is the result of a pars plana vitrectomy for a retinal detachment following brachytherapy for choroidal melanoma. This patient denied any risk factors for intraoperative floppy iris syndrome (IFIS). **(b)** With very little intraocular manipulation, the shrinking pupil was noted during phaco-emulsification. In addition, the iris prolapsed slightly with removal of the phaco handpiece. **(c)** With the Malyugin ring in place, the pupil is enlarged to a 6.25-mm working diameter. **(d)** The Malyugin ring is fully detached from the pupil, and shows the advantage in working size. The red reflex is obscured by intravitreal triamcinolone.

Properly sizing the incision depends on the manufacturer's recommendations for the preferred combination of phaco needle and irrigating sleeve, the style of preferred incision, and the design of the keratome.

First, regarding the variability in the manufacture of keratomes, the labeled size is typically close to the measured size, but it is not likely the exact size. This is typically trivial, but be skeptical of any claims of accuracy in size smaller than a tenth of a millimeter.

Second, regarding the normal pitch and yaw that occur during the insertion and removal of the blade, we like to think we go straight in and straight out. The slightest movement to either side will enlarge the incision as the keratome is removed. This effect is greater with a more challenging surgical approach, such as a large overhanging brow, or in the event of a sudden squirm.

Avoid the Superior Surgical Approach

To improve the consistency of incision creation, and to reduce the impact of patient movement during surgery, I have moved entirely away from using a superior surgical approach. The temporal aspect facilitates both access and easy withdrawal of

the instruments in cases of sudden movements. The superior approach compromises the situation in several ways, not the least of which is the brow becoming a fulcrum for instruments in the eye during sudden movements. Avoiding the superior approach has the secondary benefit of improving the ease of patient positioning, as the "chin to the ceiling" head tilt to access the superior limbus is no longer necessary.

On occasion, a nasal approach offers better access, and this is usually associated with pathology of the lateral orbital rim.

Viscomydriasis and Capsulorrhexis

By habit, many of us place the viscoelastic cannula completely across the anterior chamber from the incision, and fill the eye as we withdraw the cannula. This has the advantage of driving any bubbles out of the anterior chamber, and out of the incision. The iris becomes compressed against the anterior lens capsule, and with a nearly complete fill, there is a degree of iris stability conferred.

When performing viscomydriasis, the tip of the cannula is placed within a millimeter or so inside the pupil, and the viscoelastic is injected from here. The bolus of material accumulates,

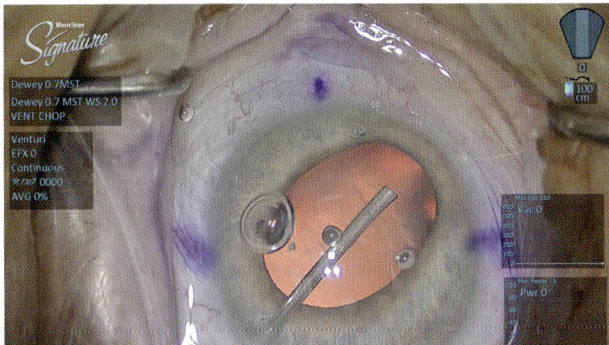
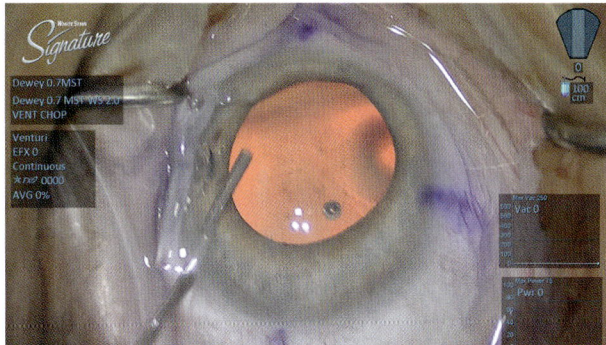

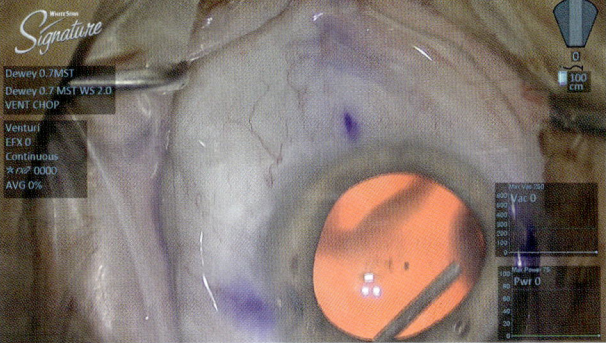
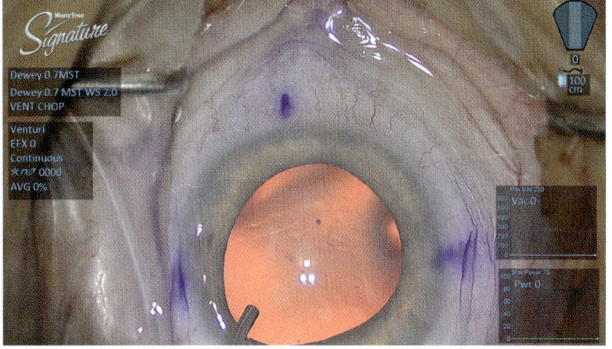

Fig. 23.4 **(a)** Through the side port, dispersive viscoelastic is injected adjacent to the iris across from the incision. **(b,c)** While retracting the cannula, the injection continues along the margins of the iris. **(d)** A final bolus is administered in the subincisional space. The iris is now stretched against the anterior capsule by the viscoelastic.

presses the iris against the lens, and slides it toward the periphery. This should be done slowly, and the cannula can be directed to the right and left as the viscoelastic fills the eye, finally directing it toward the most proximal portion inside the dilated pupil **(Fig. 23.4a–d)**.

For viscomydriasis, a retentive viscoelastic will work—either a dispersive, such as Viscoat (Alcon, Fort Worth, TX) or EndoCoat (Abbott Medical Optics [AMO], Abbott Park, IL), or a supercohesive, such as Healon V (AMO). Cohesives simply do not work to the same degree. [I do place a small bolus of cohesive, such as Healon, Amvisc (Bausch and Lomb, Rochester, NY), or Provisc (Alcon), across the anterior chamber in the area in which I am going to perform the viscomydriasis. Then I inflate this dollop with the retentive viscoelastic. This modification of the soft shell technique has the advantage of improving the ease of removal at the end of the procedure.]

The pupil is typically 1 mm larger that it was. Unlike stretching, this is a stable enlargement that does not induce miosis. It provides the largest visualized space for performing the capsulorrhexis, whether one uses forceps or a bent needle cystotome **(Fig. 23.5)**. Hydrodissection is much easier to observe as well **(Fig. 23.6)**. As one begins to perform phaco, a simple aspiration of the viscoelastic from the immediate surface of the lens will improve flow and decrease the risk for wound burns.

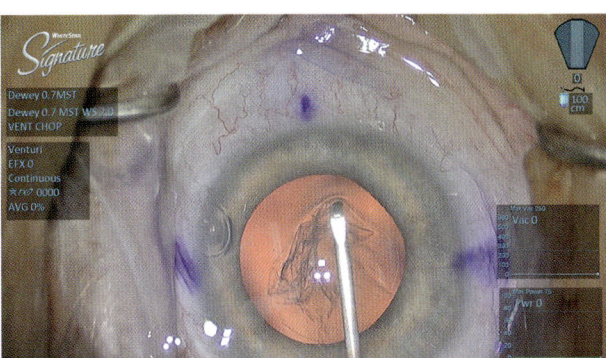

Fig. 23.5 The capsulorrhexis is performed with a bent needle, following the contour of the enlarged pupil.

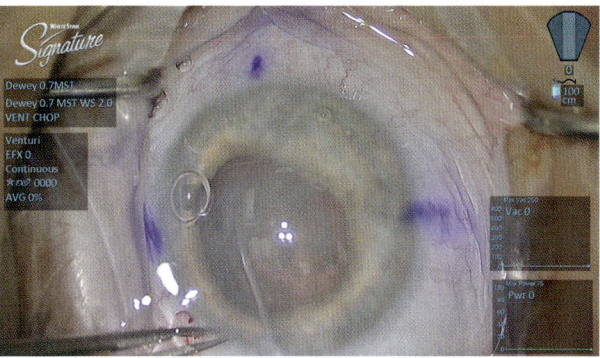

Fig. 23.6 Hydrodissection is performed with a minimal amount of irrigation. The nucleus is rotated simultaneously to free it from the capsule. The hydrodissection cannula is being pressed gently against the posterior lip of the incision to enable fluid egress and to maintain the iris position within the anterior chamber.

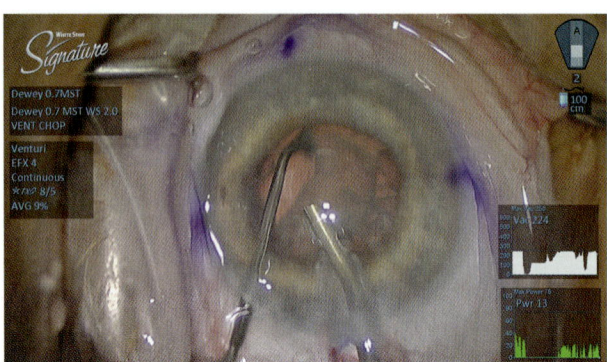

Fig. 23.7 During phacoemulsification, the pupil is already smaller, having lost the viscomydriatic effect (compare especially with **Fig. 23.3**).

At this point, the viscomydriasis effect will typically be lost (**Fig. 23.7**). The backward bowing of the iris that places the sphincter on increased stretch will be overcome by breaking the seal of the iris against the lens capsule. This alone does not increase the likelihood of worsening IFIS. Rather, the viscoelastic effect stabilizes the peripheral iris and decreases the potential billowing for at least part of the case.

Phaco Settings and Needle Characteristics

With the old cookie-cutter motion of longitudinal phaco, certain teachings to improve the safety of the surgery became entrenched. This included the promotion of low-flow, slow-mo phaco.

The origin of this teaching is found in the very nature of peristaltic vacuum itself. Larger bore needles, such as 19-gauge, were necessary to evacuate material. With peristaltic vacuum, flow is unimpeded until an occlusion is reached, and only with occlusion of the needle is vacuum created. The large nuclear plug was formed by the longitudinal motion, flow stopped, vacuum rose, and, with continued ultrasonic power, the plug would be dislodged and aspirated.

The problem arose when this break in occlusion resulted in the simultaneous evacuation and collapse of the anterior chamber. The structure closest to the tip of the needle then engaged the needle. This could be the capsule or the iris, and with the traditional sharp needle, the result of this interaction could result in significant complications.

The current nontraditional phaco modalities, from micropulse to torsional to transversal, enable the use of smaller gauge needles. Due to the asymmetry of these methods of power delivery, the typical plug is not formed. As a result, the typical postocclusion surge is not created, as flow never completely stops. Add to this the advances in software controlling the fluidics, and improved noncompliant tubing, and the chamber stays considerably more stable.

The Venturi vacuum offers another alternative to improving chamber stability. Most surgeons are familiar with the ebb and flow of peristaltic vacuum. The Venturi vacuum is different in that the vacuum level is always active, and not dependent on occlusion. Flow is not controlled independently, and is dependent on the level of vacuum being generated.

The advantage of the Venturi vacuum is the movement of material to the tip. Nuclear fragments mobilized and more or less free-floating will have a seemingly natural attraction to the tip of the needle. This is in contrast to peristaltic vacuum, where the fragments will remain in the periphery and will require moving the tip of the needle to acquire the fragment. This places the

iris at risk by moving the tip out of the safer zone of the central pupil.

With the newer phaco technology, and with the improved fluidics, nuclear material can be safely evacuated through smaller needles. Compared with the old standard 19-gauge needles, these smaller gauge phaco needles act as flow restrictors and have the benefit of reducing the potential for postocclusion surge.

The first reaction when observing a 20- or 21-gauge needle in action was that nothing was happening. I was accustomed to the "suddenness" of nuclear material disappearance with the 19-gauge needle, and my need to just as suddenly react by withdrawing my foot to avoid chamber collapse. In reviewing video after video, the cases took the same amount of time, but they simply lacked a "suddenness." This smooth nuclear evacuation preserves the pupil dilation by avoiding the cyclical chamber shallowing of the larger needle. The smaller needles do require 10 to 20% more power in denser nuclei to effect the removal, but this difference does not alter the clinical outcome.

The Phaco Needle's Edge and Finish

None of our precautions are so effective that complications will be eliminated. Patients cough even with Tessalon Perles. The iris will still constrict despite intracameral dilation. The chamber will still become shallow despite a small needle and new technology. Any unexpected, untoward event can jeopardize our surgical results.

Ultimately, the complications associated with IFIS are the result of contact of a sharp phaco needle with the iris or capsule. I cannot overemphasize the benefit of a phaco needle free from sharp edges. The ability of this needle to engage the iris or capsule and reduce the associated iatrogenic damage is invaluable. It can take a potential disaster of a case, and preserve the outcome for the patient under circumstances that would otherwise compromise the outcome (**Fig. 23.8**).

This technology is exceptionally easy to incorporate. There are no changes to the surgical procedure. It is the same needle, but with a highly polished, rounded edge, and it will perform as the old, sharp needle did. It will function on any current-generation phaco machine. The specific settings on the phaco machine may require some tweaking, and this is especially true if transitioning from a sharp needle with an aspiration bypass system (ABS) port.

Cortical Removal

Depending on the residual iris dilation and tone, there is no reason to switch from coaxial irrigation and aspiration (I/A). If the pupil is not as cooperative, biaxial I/A makes the most sense. Simply having the irrigation separate from the aspiration allows the infusion instrument to be used to retract the iris for easy aspiration.

Intraocular Lens Insertion

My preferred technique involves distending the posterior capsule with a cohesive viscoelastic for easy evacuation following implantation. In a normally dilating pupil, I distend the capsule at least half-full, taking care not to tightly distend the capsule. Intraocular lens (IOL) implantation is the point of highest intraocular pressure, and the increased volume from the IOL can rupture the capsule under the right circumstances.

To stabilize the chamber by preventing the cohesive viscoelastic from "burping" out of the incision, I plug the incision with

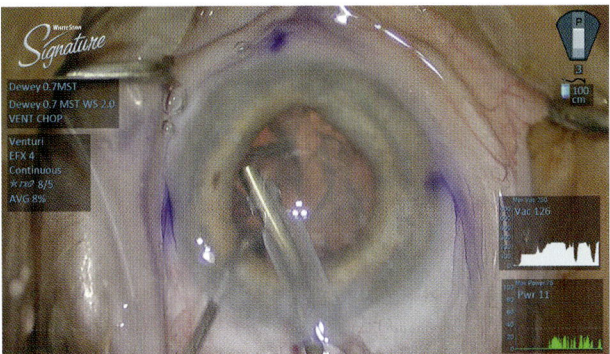
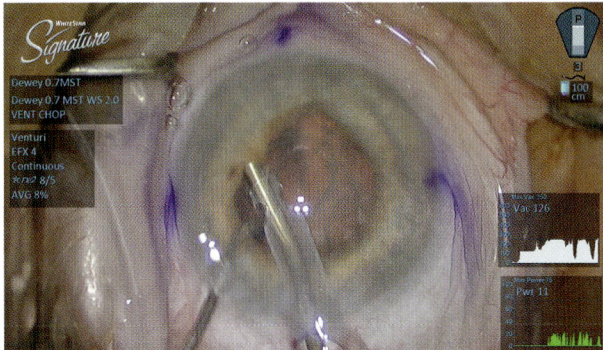
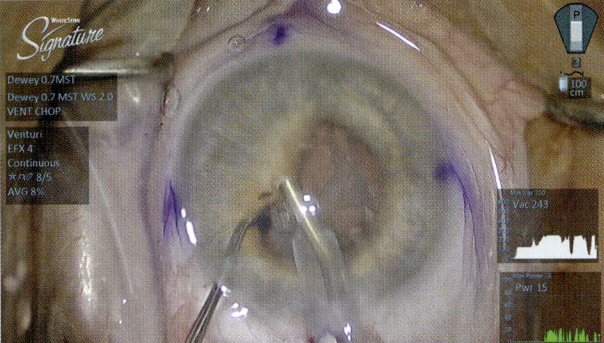
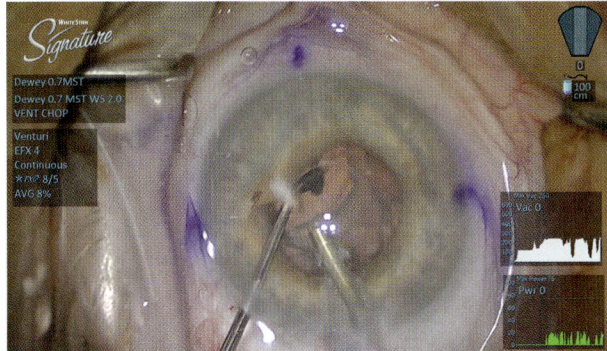
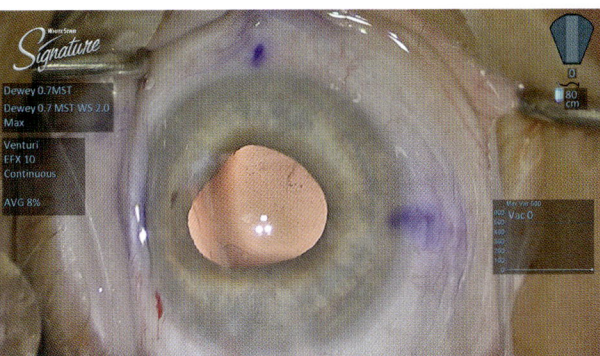

Fig. 23.8 This is a case from the author's practice and demonstrates the utility of the Dewey Radius Tip. **(a)** The surgeon attempts to engage the cortical shell. **(b)** Inadvertently, the iris is aspirated along with the cortical shell. **(c)** The phaco needle is drawn to the center of the field, attempting to draw the cortical shell centrally. **(d)** The surgeon releases the iris. The iris was engaged and released within 0.9 seconds. The maximum power was 22%, and the maximum vacuum 243 mm Hg during this interaction. **(e)** Although a small defect is visible at the slit lamp, the iris remains functionally and cosmetically intact. A sharp needle would have shredded the iris during the same timeframe.

a dispersive. If the pupil is small, I frequently place this small bolus prior to inflating the capsule in a fashion similar to visco-mydriasis. This helps position the iris posteriorly, as the cohesive viscoelastic filling the bag has the potential to push it forward.

Removing the viscoelastic after IOL insertion is most effectively achieved with much higher flow and vacuum settings than with cortical removal. My preference is to directly irrigate the viscoelastic from behind the IOL and chamber angle prior to I/A. With the small pupil, access to the space behind the optic is difficult, and there is the risk of flipping a partially folded IOL.

The "rock-and-roll" technique consists of placing the tip of the I/A handpiece directly on the IOL, and gently rocking the handpiece and IOL. This gentle posterior displacement drives the cohesive viscoelastic forward. The critical factor is keeping the active aspiration port away from the iris sphincter, or learning how to quickly kick the foot pedal into reflux mode.

Just as with cortical removal, this may be the best opportunity to switch to a biaxial system. Retracting the iris with the irrigating tip, and aiming the flow of irrigation into pockets of viscoelastic, provide the aspirating tip with better access than with coaxial alone.

Removing the I/A handpiece, or the phaco handpiece for that matter, can be challenging if the iris has previously fled the incision. Do not come out of the eye with vacuum active, but do not come out of the pressurized eye and allow the iris to follow. In some cases, lowering the bottle height to about half will keep the anterior chamber (AC) deep enough with irrigation to remove the instrument without the iris following. Otherwise, remove the instrument without irrigation and reform the AC through the side port. If the iris situation is tenuous, a new side port may be necessary far away from the primary incision.

Toric Intraocular Lenses

Although a small pupil typically constrains the size of the capsulorrhexis to one favorable for a toric IOL, the pupil size itself makes the rest of the situation more challenging. Thorough removal of the viscoelastic is just the first step, but it is critical to reduce the risk of toric rotation in the postoperative period.

Positioning the axis is obviously a problem if the margin of the pupil covers the alignment marks (**Fig. 23.9**). Although any number of methods can establish the position with normally

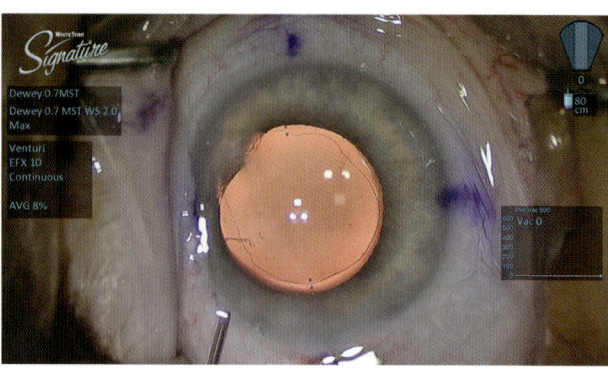

Fig. 23.9 **(a)** Although the toric intraocular lens (IOL) alignment marks are barely visible at the iris margin (6 o'clock position in the surgeon's orientation), the IOL is positioned by aligning it with the axis marker. **(b)** With great care to avoid inflating the capsule, the anterior chamber is distended to stretch the iris and confirm placement of the toric IOL.

dilating pupils, directly marking the axis either on the cornea or limbus is the best method for this situation. The closer the alignment mark is to the mark on the optic, the easier it is to align the two.

Start by attempting the best-guess alignment as the IOL is unfolding and the viscoelastic removal is completed. Using a blunt irrigating chopper in one hand, and an IOL manipulating hook in the other (Lester hook, Rhein Medical, St. Petersburg, FL; Graether Collar Button, multiple manufacturers), retract the iris with the chopper, manipulating the IOL with the other. Align the marks directly with the marks on the cornea, one side at a time.

Once the axis is as aligned as best possible, hyperinflating the anterior chamber may create a reverse pupillary block. The pressure in the eye will be above physiological, so efficiency is dictated in terms of speed. If the iris does bow backward and stretch along the surface of the optic, the alignment marks will become visible on both sides of the optic. Although this configuration will not enable manipulation, it will enable for confirmation of orientation.

Repositing the Iris

Regardless of how carefully these steps are followed, the iris will escape the incision, usually at the worst possible time. The strong inclination is to push the iris back into the eye. Resist this urge.

Instead, depressurize the eye. If the iris has escaped both the primary and side-port incisions, another paracentesis can be created in an area far from these incisions. Recheck the speculum to look for pressure on the globe. Have the anesthesiologist provide a bolus of sedation.

In an old technique recently revived by Daniel Chang, MD, Bakersfield, CA, gently stroke the cornea above the incision. Start close to the external aspect of the incision, and gently rub the cornea toward the center. With patience, this will enable the iris to reenter the anterior chamber without excessive damage.

Unfortunately, this technique does not always work. In this case, still avoid pushing the iris back into the eye. Instead, use a long, blunt iris sweep to stroke the iris back into the eye, but from the inside of the eye. This instrument can be introduced through the side port, or through a new side port created specifically to facilitate this maneuver (**Fig. 23.10a–c**).

The need to relocate the primary incision based on iris prolapse depends entirely on the timing and the extent. Severe prolapse occurring early in the procedure impedes the progress of the surgery, potentially compromising the outcome, and a new

primary incision should be created. Although the original incision may be perfectly watertight under normal circumstances, the dynamics of pressure that take place during routine phaco will require the first primary incision to be sutured to finish the procedure without further incident.

As an observation, if the iris is irreparably damaged before any corrective steps can be taken, consider surrendering. The anterior chamber will remain shallow until the chamber is made deeper. If this is associated with a particularly large nucleus in a particularly shallow anterior chamber, sculpt the central nucleus to create a large bowl. Without removing the phaco needle, reintroduce retentive viscoelastic through the side port to deepen the anterior chamber, and continue nuclear removal.

Through these steps, the damage to the iris will be limited. Provided the nucleus can be successfully removed, and the IOL successfully implanted, the damage to the iris will be limited to one to two clock hour positions. This typically will require two iris sutures to close the defect—one near the sphincter and one about mid-stroma.

Closing this defect does not have to take place during the primary surgery. Most patients are understanding that specific steps taken during surgery to make the best of a bad situation helped preserve the outcome, but surgeons should not expect that two clock hour positions of iris defect will be tolerated. (**Fig. 23.10d,e**).

Alternatively, if the iris prolapse is occurring due to posterior pressure, a quick check of the fundus should be made to look for a rare, but potentially devastating choroidal hemorrhage. In the case of choroidals, the incision should be stabilized, and the anterior chamber pressurized to minimize the extent of the problem.

If no choroidals are visible, this is likely due to aqueous misdirection. A medical approach would include stabilizing the incision, and administering gentle pressure and mannitol to medically decompress the vitreous. This process can be lengthy, and may involve removal of the patient from the operating room to be brought back once the intraocular pressure has been reduced.

The old standby for aqueous misdirection is the blind pars plana tap with virtually any gauge needle, withdrawing liquid vitreous until the AC deepens. This technique is wanting for those unaccustomed to the pars plana approach, and I have successfully created a posterior capsule split merely attempting to visualize the inserted needle.

Alternatively, a simple pars plana stab incision can be made, 3.5 mm posterior to the limbus, with the microvitreoretinal (MVR) blade directed posteriorly toward the optic nerve. Prepare

24 Positive Pressure

Paul N. Arnold and James A. Davison

Primarily because of the evolution of more gentle techniques with even fluidics and pressure control and secondarily because of lower intraoperative intraocular pressures (IOPs) and much more brief surgical times, positive pressure situations are very rarely seen in modern cataract surgery.

However rare, one of the most disconcerting problems faced by the anterior-segment surgeon in an open eye is progressive positive pressure. With this sudden rise in IOP, the cataract surgeon finds there is no room in which to work. The risk to the endothelium rises (as does the surgeon's heart rate and blood pressure), and the surgeon shudders to think of inadvertently tearing a convex posterior capsule. Raising the infusion bottle and instilling more viscoelastic only cause more iris prolapse. The situation gets worse by the minute! The more the surgeon does to ameliorate the situation, the worse it gets. This horrible cascade of events could lead to the worst outcome—an expulsive hemorrhage.

How should the cataract surgeon evaluate and deal with this awful scenario? It is necessary to understand the various risk factors leading to positive pressure in a given patient. This awareness should lead the surgeon to consider preventive measures. The surgeon must recognize positive pressure at the earliest moment to begin the evaluation process that will lead to the best therapeutic decisions. This is one of those intraoperative situations where old aphorisms ring true: an ounce of prevention is worth a pound of cure, and a stitch in time saves nine—literally!

Classification

Positive pressure during cataract surgery can be classified into three general groups: (1) mechanical or external forces applied to the eye, (2) intraocular fluid deviation or misdirection into the posterior segment, and (3) acute intraoperative suprachoroidal effusion or hemorrhage. Once an accurate categorical assessment has been made, the surgeon can perform the appropriate intervention.

Mechanical or External Causes

Lids and Speculum

Certain patients are more likely to demonstrate positive pressure because of their inherent periocular anatomy. Those with small palpebral fissures and tight orbits require special attention. The more forcefully the speculum is opened, the more eye pressure is created by forcing more orbital fat and tissue posteriorly. The surgeon must find the optimum speculum opening, perhaps accepting a less than ideal aperture. There is greater accessibility afforded by a temporal approach to the eye. A lateral canthotomy can be performed, although this is of marginal benefit.

The speculum itself can be a source of positive pressure. Specula with larger solid blades to sequester the lid margin can occupy enough space to exert external pressure on the eye. Modern open-bladed specula that are light and follow orbital contours help alleviate this problem. The surgical assistant can help by elevating the speculum and the offending lid (with a muscle hook or irrigating cannula) to alleviate this external force. The phaco tip or handpiece may inadvertently push on the speculum, transmitting this pressure to the eye (especially with closed-bladed specula). If using a bridle suture, overtightening may be a cause. Therefore, loosen the bridle suture. Better yet, don't use one!

In association with topical anesthesia, squeezing lids are the most likely source of positive pressure. In these circumstances, the wire speculum may not be forceful enough to keep the orbicularis muscles from squeezing the eye. A speculum that can hold the lids open a given amount, held by a screw mechanism, works well in this situation. One can always administer a facial nerve, orbicularis, or sub-Tenon's block, or increase the depth of the conscious sedation with systemic propofol.

In all of these lid/speculum-related situations, it is helpful to use the sterile drape or Steri-Strips to tape the lids open. This exerts no pressure on the globe and the speculum becomes merely an adjunct in opening the lids.

Regional Anesthesia

The regional anesthetic block given before cataract surgery can lead to positive posterior pressure. The fear of depositing too much fluid behind the eye may be one reason many surgeons still prefer the retrobulbar to the peribulbar block. An effective block can be achieved with as little as 3.0 mL given in a retrobulbar or peribulbar fashion; however, this type of block may require an additional seventh cranial nerve or lid block. The peribulbar is effective with as little as 3.0 mL of anesthetic, with the addition of topical lidocaine 2% gel for additional corneal anesthesia. Both methods are good. Both can "overfill" the orbit leading to positive pressure.[1] The best way to prevent overfill is to palpate the globe and orbit while administering the anesthetic. We have seen this problem occur infrequently once the surgeon or anesthetist develops a "feel" for the proper orbital volume. There is no single volume that is correct for every patient's eye.

The use of hyaluronidase (Wydase) in the anesthetic mixture is mandatory in promoting the distribution of the anesthetic throughout the periocular tissues. When clinical trials were performed without this protein enzyme in the peribulbar block, there was a much greater incidence of positive orbital pressure and postoperative muscle palsy. It could be concluded that the anesthetic acted more like a "space-occupying lesion" rather than absorbing into the interstitial space of the orbital tissues.

The surgeon should recognize excessive orbital volume when the lids are too tight to open adequately and chemosis is present. This can occur even when devices to soften the eye, such as the Honan balloon, are used. Once excessive orbital volume is recognized, the prudent surgeon will place the Honan balloon (assuming it is available and used originally) back on the eye and simply wait. If it is not available, steady firm manual pressure is a reasonable alternative. After an additional 30 minutes, the surgery can be completed with much greater ease than if the surgeon had pushed ahead with a tight orbit.

Retrobulbar hemorrhage is another complication of injection anesthesia leading to positive pressure. Any type of block and any type of needle can cause a periocular hemorrhage. Most of the time it can be controlled with external pressure applied for 15 to 30 minutes, and surgery can be completed. However, if the hemorrhage is severe, causing extremely elevated IOP, surgery should be postponed and the patient's pressure treated aggressively.

Fluid Dynamics

The surgeon must constantly consider the intraocular fluid dynamics at work during phacoemulsification. Excessive outflow or restricted inflow are common causes of pseudopositive pressure. If the phaco incision or the paracentesis are too large, the intracameral pressure cannot be maintained and the chamber will become shallow. The slightest external force on the eye will exacerbate the condition. Simply elevating the balanced salt solution (BSS) infusion bottle will not solve the problem of excessive outflow. The surgeon should maintain a constant, slightly elevated intracameral pressure. If excessive outflow is causing a shallow, dangerous anterior chamber, stop and place a suture or two to create a more watertight chamber. Remember that infusion bottle height is relative to patient eye height. Temporal incisions often require elevation of the patient to make room for the

surgeon's legs. If the patient's eye is higher, the bottle needs to be proportionately higher.

Fluid Deviation or Misdirection Syndrome

Etiology

In varying circumstances, this syndrome has gone by various names: aqueous misdirection, ciliary block, and malignant glaucoma (in the postoperative setting). The etiology is similar in all circumstances: the aqueous or BSS is diverted behind the zonulocapsular diaphragm into the vitreous and creates high pressure within the posterior segment. This can lead to pupillary block and angle closure as the lens and iris shift forward, exacerbating the IOP elevation. There is anterior rotation of the ciliary body, the chamber shallows, and during surgery the iris may prolapse. If the surgeon continues to infuse fluid, the eye gets harder and the surgeon becomes more frustrated. The zonulocapsular diaphragm acts like a one-way valve, assisted by an intact vitreous face; BSS gets into the posterior segment and it is blocked from reentry into the anterior chamber by the "vitreous valve" (**Fig. 24.1**).

Several risk factors are likely to give rise to this syndrome. Anything that disrupts the zonular apparatus—pseudoexfoliation syndrome, previous ocular trauma, a radial tear in the anterior capsule, zonulysis, and any opening in the posterior capsule—may allow fluid to pass through into the posterior segment. A small pupil and a narrow angle may hide these peripheral capsular defects, delaying the surgeon's recognition of this syndrome.

Common Environment for Fluid Misdirection

Fluid deviation can occur during any phase of the operation in which fluid is infused into the eye. The surgeon must be aware that hydrodissection, phacoemulsification, and irrigation and aspiration (I/A) can all cause fluid misdirection and positive pressure.

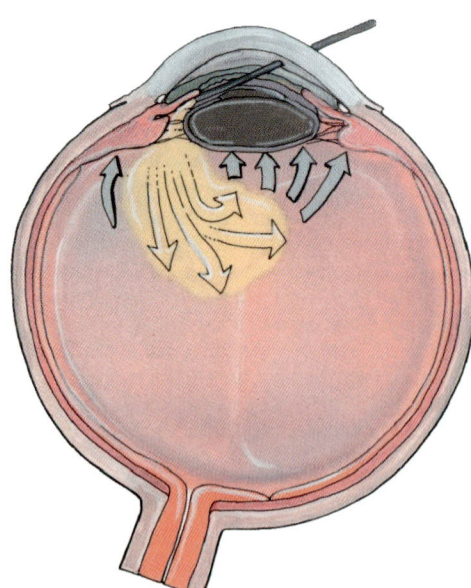
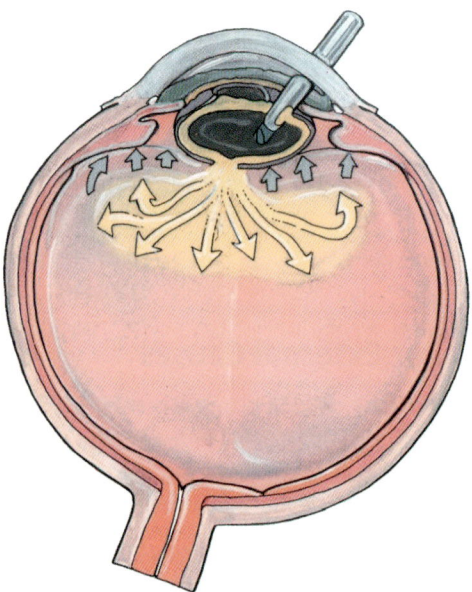

a

b

Fig. 24.1 Fluid misdirection. If fluid passes through **(a)** the zonules or **(b)** an opening in the posterior capsule, it can create an aqueous pocket behind the vitreous face. In turn, this may force the vitreous forward, closing the "vitreous valve." A ciliary block is created when this fluid cannot escape from the posterior segment.

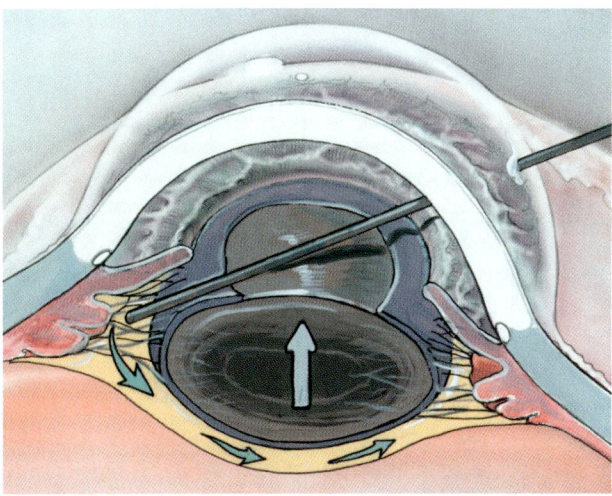

Fig. 24.2 A cannula inadvertently placed under the iris but over rather than under the anterior capsule. Injected fluid passes into, and is trapped within, the retrolental space. As the anterior chamber shallows, intraocular pressure (IOP) is significantly increased.

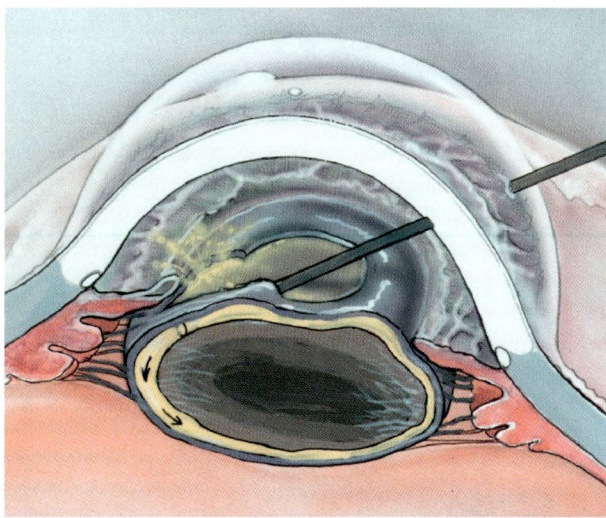

Fig. 24.3 Incomplete capsulorrhexis. Pressure of the hydrodissection causes extension of the torn anterior capsule. It is surgically observed as a "pop" when the capsule splits and the nucleus moves anteriorly.

During hydrodissection, the cannula may inadvertently not be placed under the anterior capsule. The injection forces fluid through the zonules into the vitreous. (**Fig. 24.2**) Updegraff et al[2] described another scenario in small pupil cases: the fluid is injected under the anterior capsule, but this leads to elevation of the capsule and lens, causing pupillary block (**Fig. 24.3**). They believe the viscoelastic may contribute to an iridocapsular seal by causing adhesion of the iris to the capsule, preventing fluid egress.

During phacoemulsification, the fluid may be forced posteriorly if a dense viscoelastic prevents good anterior fluid circulation and the bottle is quite high. This problem has been encountered when an occult radial capsular tear or small area of zonulysis occurs. An intact vitreous face closes the one-way valve that leads to elevated posterior pressure (**Fig. 24.4**).

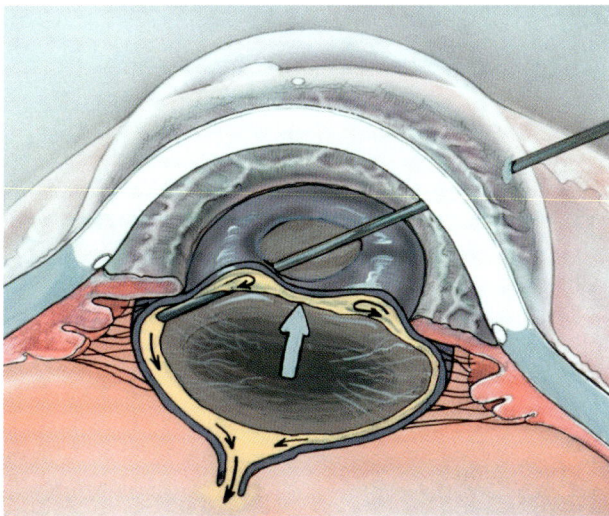

Fig. 24.4 A small rhexis large cataract. The nucleus seals against the anterior capsule. Fluid egress is blocked. Increased fluid pressure causes rupture of the posterior capsule.

During I/A, fluid misdirection has occurred by aggressively attempting to aspirate subincisional cortex. A small iatrogenic anterior capsular tear can allow the BSS to be infused into the vitreous. This usually forces the iris up into the incision with positive posterior pressure. Even aspirating the viscoelastic from the eye after lens placement can lead to BSS misdirection and shallowing of the anterior chamber. This can occur if the surgeon is intent on going behind the intraocular lens (IOL) to remove all traces of viscoelastic—if there is a small opening in the zonulo-capsular diaphragm.

Treatment of Fluid Deviation

At the first sign of positive pressure, the surgeon should remove the irrigating instrument from the eye and apply Q-tip or digital pressure over the incision. Q-tip pressure entails holding a cotton-tipped applicator like a pencil and pushing down on the anterior lip of the incision (**Fig. 24.5**). This simultaneously closes the incision and creates anterior pressure to counteract the posterior pressure—from whatever etiology. This maneuver stabilizes the eye while the surgeon assesses the situation. The surgeon then determines which of the three main causes of positive pressure applies in this episode: external forces, fluid misdirection, or acute intraoperative suprachoroidal effusion/hemorrhage.

Once the surgeon has concluded that the etiology is fluid misdirection, several options are available. One is to typically just continue to apply Q-tip pressure until the eye softens. The fluid eventually equilibrates by seeping back into the anterior chamber or by being absorbed. If an impatient surgeon chooses not to wait 5 to 15 minutes, the incision can be hydrated or sutured if necessary and the surgery delayed a few hours or a day.

After watchful waiting, the procedure can be completed using a "low-flow" technique. Lower the infusion bottle, use plenty of viscoelastic to maintain the anterior chamber, and avoid the area of zonulocapsular disruption. Use viscoelastic to seal off this area of disruption. Decreasing the aspiration/flow rate may also increase safety. The goal is to avoid pushing more fluid into the posterior segment.

More aggressive intervention may rarely be required and is not recommended. However, occasionally a circumstance forces assertive treatment. An acute intraoperative suprachoroidal

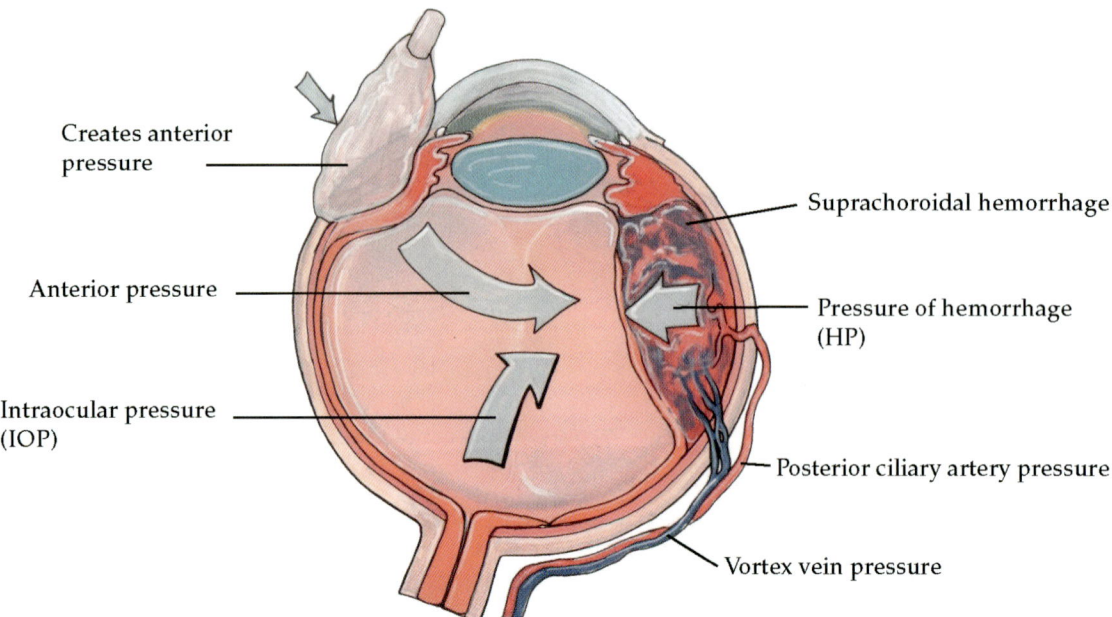

Creates anterior pressure

Anterior pressure

Intraocular pressure (IOP)

Suprachoroidal hemorrhage

Pressure of hemorrhage (HP)

Posterior ciliary artery pressure

Vortex vein pressure

Fig. 24.5 To tamponade the rising "posterior pressure" behind the retina during an acute intraoperative suprachoroidal hemorrhage (AISH), the surgeon must raise the "anterior pressure," the IOP. The posterior pressure is determined by the blood pressure in the ciliary arteries and the impedance to outflow in the vortex veins. The IOP is raised by Q-tip pressure on the globe.

hemorrhage (AISH) must be ruled out as the etiology of the increased IOP. This can be done by examination of the periphery with an indirect ophthalmoscope. Alternatively, Robert Osher[3] has developed a fundus lens for examination of the periphery that can be maintained sterile and utilized in just such an emergency. Once verified that an AISH has not occurred, the increased IOP can be alleviated by a pars plana vitreous tap. A 21-gauge needle on a tuberculin (TB) syringe is inserted 3.5 mm posterior to the limbus and directed toward the central anterior vitreous. Slowly withdraw 0.1 to 0.3 mL of liquid vitreous. If this is not effective, it may be necessary to use a mechanical vitrectomy instrument to perform a small vitrectomy through a pars plana incision. The vitreous behind the open zonulocapsular region must be removed or allowed to fall back from the affected area (**Fig. 24.6**) The one-way valve must be opened.

Work done on pseudophakic malignant glaucoma has shown that an intact posterior capsule and/or vitreous face can prevent resolution of the problem.[4] An evident opening in the posterior capsule requires a vitrectomy through this opening or through a pars plana incision. The aqueous must be able to circulate freely and not remain trapped behind cortical vitreous or an intact anterior hyaloid.

Acute Intraoperative Suprachoroidal Hemorrhage

Etiology

Acute intraoperative suprachoroidal hemorrhage is probably the best term to describe this continuum of conditions that may be as slight as swelling in the suprachoroidal space leading to positive pressure, or as severe as a blinding expulsive hemorrhage. The terminology in the literature is varied and confusing. Some authors refer to all such events as "expulsive hemorrhages," but this dread term should only be used when the contents of the posterior segment and blood are truly expulsed through the incision. AISH is an accurate general designation of this spectrum

of events that begin in the suprachoroidal space during intraocular surgery.

The sequence of events leading to an expulsive hemorrhage begins with transudation of fluid from the choriocapillaris. A uveal effusion occurs because of the pressure differential between the intravascular blood and the intraocular fluid[5] (**Fig. 24.7**). Once the eye is opened for surgery, the IOP falls. The effusion fills the spongy choroidal space between Bruch's membrane and the sclera. The larger choroidal vessels are stretched between the

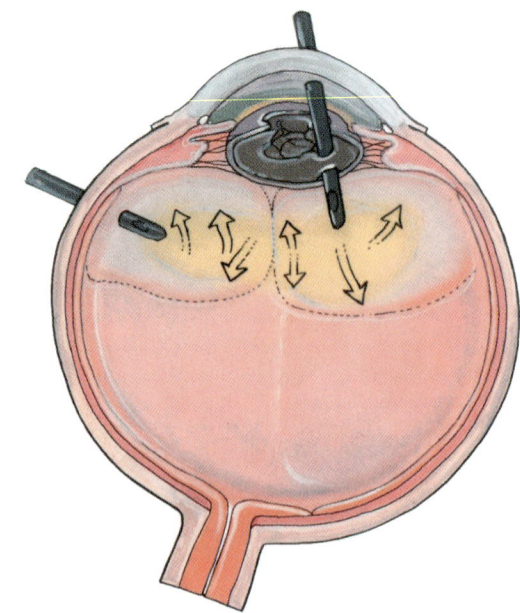

Fig. 24.6 To break the fluid misdirection block, the surgeon must remove the "vitreous valve." This is accomplished by vitrectomy in the area behind the open capsule or zonulysis.

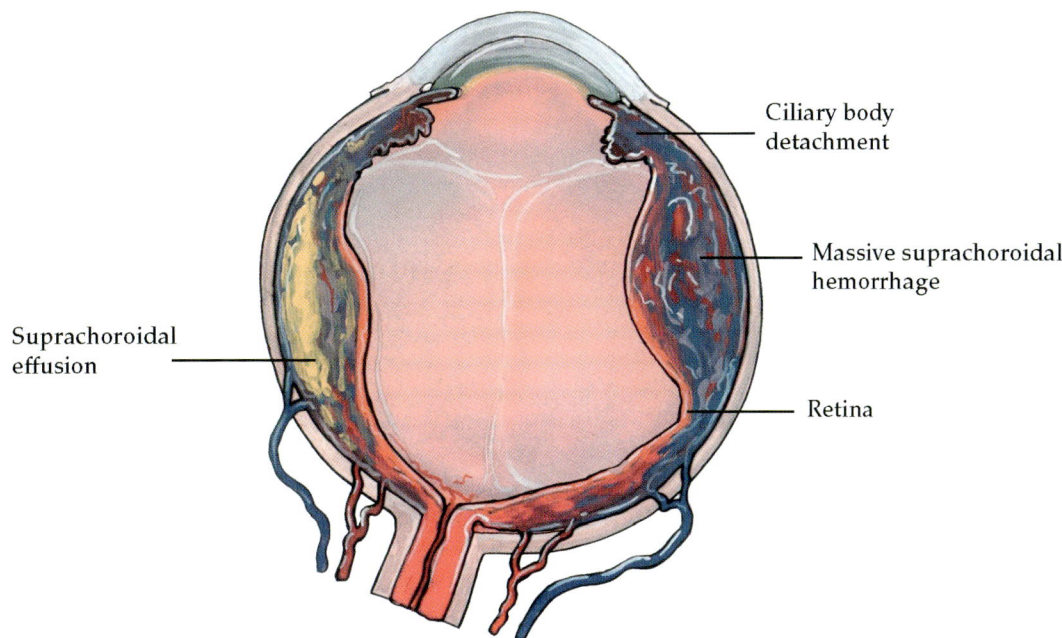

Fig. 24.7 Transudation of fluid *(left)* from the choriocapillaris fills the suprachoroidal space. Rupture of the short posterior ciliary vessels *(right)* causes hemorrhage to occur in the suprachoroidal space.

sclera and choriocapillaris until a rupture occurs in one of the short posterior ciliary vessels. The hemorrhage into the suprachoroidal space hastens the expansion and leads to more ruptured vessels. If nothing is done to stop this cascade, the hemorrhage will detach the ciliary body, tearing the higher-pressure ciliary vessels **(Fig. 24.7)**. This massive bleed near the pars plana will propel the iris, lens, vitreous, retina, and uvea out through the incision.[6] The event may begin relatively slowly only to end with the speed of an explosion.

The choroid has the highest blood flow per gram of tissue in the body, and its venous fenestrations are among the largest.[7] Hemorrhages were particularly common (10%) in patients 90 years of age or older.[8]

Although a drop in IOP is necessary to initiate the cascade of events from effusion to hemorrhage to expulsion, other factors must also be present. Fortunately, not everyone undergoing cataract surgery has an AISH. The three most important elements are the degree and duration of the pressure differential, and the degree of vascular fragility.

Pressure Differential

The intravascular pressure driving blood into the eye is essentially reflected by the systemic blood pressure; however, other vascular factors contribute. The health of the ipsilateral carotid and ophthalmic arteries affects the intraocular blood pressure. Impaired venous outflow through the vortex veins predisposes the patient to uveal effusion. This may be affected by a voluminous regional anesthetic injection, a Valsalva maneuver, or coughing. The position of the head relative to the body, and how massive that body is, will affect the ocular intravascular pressure.

On the other side of the equation is the IOP. In a closed eye, homeostasis is usually maintained unless the IOP drops below 5 mm Hg. However, the relationship between the two pressures, the IOP and the ocular intravascular pressure, over time is also a factor. An eye that is accustomed to a higher IOP that suddenly falls to 0 mm Hg is less likely to tolerate that change than an eye

with a chronically very low IOP. So if there is a precipitous drop in IOP from a very high level and the intravascular pressure remains constant, an effusion becomes more likely. Think of a long-term glaucoma patient who has filtering surgery. If the IOP is very low for several days, a suprachoroidal effusion is quite common (most are not clinically significant, but present nevertheless).

In the setting of cataract surgery, the two pressures can be thought of simplistically: the choroidal intravascular pressure is "posterior" and the IOP is "anterior." In this force equation, the anterior pressure must be in balance with the posterior pressure. If the anterior pressure drops suddenly to zero, there is nothing to hold back the posterior pressure, except the blood vessel wall (quite weak in the choriocapillaris), the retina, the gravitational pressure of the vitreous, and the zonulocapsular diaphragm.

The duration of decreased IOP is an important additional risk factor in developing AISH. In our study of AISH, patients undergoing phacoemulsification developed their intraocular positive pressure later in the procedure[9] **(Fig. 24.8)**. Those having extracapsular cataract extraction (ECCE) (9.0- to 10.0-mm incision) developed positive pressure soon after nucleus delivery in most cases. This phenomenon is presumably related to the greater time duration of relative maintenance of near-normal anterior pressure with phacoemulsification than with large-incision extracapsular surgery. Surgeons performing penetrating keratoplasty and glaucoma-filtering procedures confirm that the duration of hypotony correlates with the onset of positive pressure.

From a pressure differential point of view, the worst-case scenario consists of an obese patient with a bull neck lying with his head lower than his body, who also has a blood pressure of 210/120 in his ophthalmic arteries and has had an IOP of 40 mm Hg for years. His peribulbar block has been too voluminous, impairing venous outflow. He further complicates the pressure differential by coughing, accentuating this Valsalva nightmare. And you have to perform large incision cataract surgery on his only seeing eye!

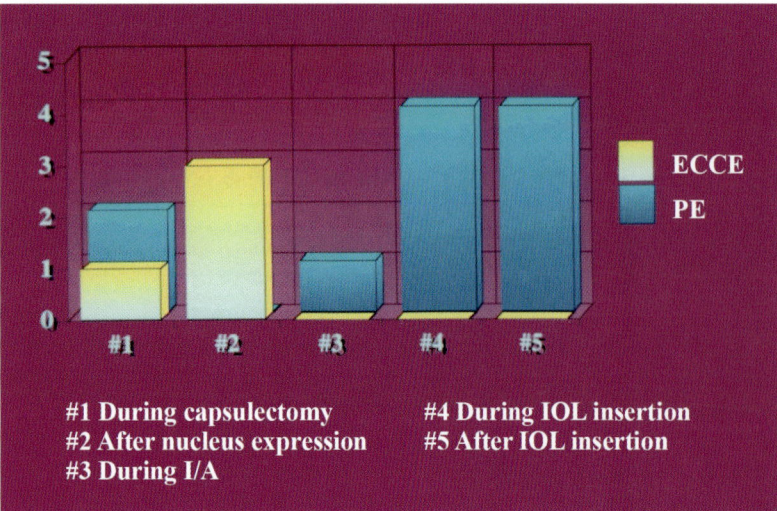

Fig. 24.8 Occurrence of AISH. The AISH had a tendency to occur earlier during extracapsular cataract extraction (ECCE) and later in the operation with phacoemulsification (PE). In our phacoemulsification series, the AISH occurred after the cataract had been removed in most cases. The y-axis represents the number of cases.

Now consider the factors affecting the barrier between the posterior and anterior pressures.

Choroidal Vascular Fragility

The innermost layer of the choroid is the choriocapillaris, made up of large, fenestrated capillaries without an elastic lamina. The lumina are large enough to allow red blood cells to pass easily through into the expandable choroidal space. Sattler's layer of medium-sized vessels is found between the choriocapillaris and the outermost Haller's layer of large vessels.

Two long posterior and 20 short posterior ciliary arteries must pierce the sclera to enter the choroid. Four vortex veins drain the blood from the choroid.

Anything that makes the thin choroidal vessel weaker, and more prone to leakage and rupture, will make an AISH more likely. The aging process, senescence, makes the vascular wall more brittle. Years of hypertension may contribute; diabetes certainly can lead to greater vascular leakage. A history of carotid occlusive disease or coronary artery disease suggests that the choroidal vessels are also affected by the arteriosclerotic process.

With fluctuation of the IOP, there is distortion of the soft tissues of the eye. In some cases, there is actual deformation of the globe, as in nucleus expression ECCE. These factors create a shearing force in the choroidal vascular space. This shear contributes to the likelihood of vascular leakage into the suprachoroidal space. Scleral rigidity in the senescent eye may contribute to the shearing force between the choroidal vessels and a less pliable scleral wall.

Anticoagulation with aspirin or warfarin would theoretically increase the likelihood that once a suprachoroidal hemorrhage occurred, it would be more likely to proceed rapidly.

Speaker et al[10] performed a case-control study of risk factors in 68 cases of what they called "suprachoroidal expulsive hemorrhage" from the 35,459 patients having intraocular surgery at their institution between 1981 and 1986. It is not clear what percentage of these cases had only sudden intraoperative hardening of the eye and not prolapse of intraocular contents because both groups met the patient inclusion criteria. We may conclude that these 68 cases covered the AISH spectrum, from mild to the more rare true expulsive hemorrhage. The authors found that the statistically significant risk factors were a history of glaucoma, axial length greater than 25.8 mm, elevated IOP greater than 18, generalized atherosclerosis, and intraoperative tachy-

cardia greater than 85 beats/minute (**Box 24.1**). They suggested an interesting correlation between an increased risk of AISH with increased intraoperative sympathetic tone and a decreased risk with antihypertensive agents that block sympathetic outflow from the central nervous system.

These factors may explain why we found in our prospective series of patients that AISH was more likely in senescent eyes (those with very brunescent nuclear cataracts, not necessarily in those patients who were older), which required ECCE rather than phacoemulsification,[9] and why we found AISH more likely in those with significant vascular disease, especially those requiring systemic anticoagulation. It is not possible to determine which are the preeminent factors. Is it senescence, the larger incision ECCE (with more hypotony and choroidal shear), the history of vascular disease, or the anticoagulation?

Incidence of Intraoperative Suprachoroidal Expulsive Hemorrhage

The reported incidence of AISH during cataract surgery has varied significantly, from 3.1% with intracapsular cataract extraction (ICCE) to 0.03% with phacoemulsification.[11,12] Some of this variation can be ascribed to the definition employed; some investigators included limited suprachoroidal effusions, whereas others studied only complete expulsive hemorrhages. Some have been very careful observers and included limited suprachoroidal effusions, whereas others may not have counted them. We also see a clear reduction in the incidence of AISH over time as our cataract

---

Box 24.1 Risk Factors for Intraoperative Suprachoroidal Expulsive Hemorrhage (A Case-Control Study)

- Glaucoma
- Increased axial length > 25.8 mm
- Elevated IOP > 18
- Elevated intraoperative pulse > 85 bpm
- Generalized atherosclerosis

Source: From Speaker et al.[10]

surgical techniques have improved, decreasing both the incision size and the intraoperative time.

Although the number of operations is low, Bukelman et al[11] reported a decrease in their incidence after they moved from ICCE in 521 cases (3.1%) to ECCE in 368 cases (2.2%). The next step in our surgical evolution and its relation to AISH was best evaluated by Eriksson et al.[12] They examined the records of 37,565 cases from 1990 to 1996; 14,352 had undergone ECCE and 23,213 had phacoemulsification. The incidence of AISH had dropped in a highly statistically significant manner from 0.13% with ECCE to 0.03% with phacoemulsification ($p = 0.0003$).

Davison's[7] experience details this evolutionary phenomenon with different phacoemulsification techniques. In his original study of AISH from 1986, he encountered an incidence of 0.81% with iris plane emulsification. By 1993, using a capsular bag phacoemulsification technique that reduced the amplitude of IOP swings; his incidence had dropped to 0.06%.[8] Arnold[9] has also seen this happen in his practice. By seeking to maintain an extremely watertight incision and reduce intracameral pressure fluctuations as much as possible, his incidence dropped from 0.45% of all phacoemulsification cases to 0.08%.

Preventive Measures

All of these risk factors are additive; that is, the patient with all five of the risk factors is more likely to develop AISH than the patient with only one. The surgeon must think about prevention in susceptible patients and be prepared to deal with an AISH in these cases.

Do phacoemulsification! The studies cited above demonstrate a lower incidence of AISH with phacoemulsification than any other cataract extraction technique. By employing the small, self-sealing incision, the surgeon accomplishes several goals: the intracameral pressure is more stable, the globe is not mechanically distorted, and the eye can be quickly closed if a choroidal effusion arises. It is very important to decrease the fluctuation of IOP during cataract extraction. A steady, somewhat elevated "anterior pressure" can be maintained with an elevated infusion bottle, a watertight incision, and the use of viscoelastic when an infusion instrument is not in the anterior chamber. It is not unusual for patients to have a coughing spell or spells during surgery. It is important to keep the anterior chamber pressure positive by keeping the phacoemulsification tip or I/A tip in the eye if it is being used while the coughing spell occurs. The scrub technician can stabilize the head. Try to keep your hands in contact with the patient's face so that their face, your hands, and the instruments are one solid unit. The anesthetist can give IV lidocaine to help reduce the tendency for cough. Blumenthal et al[13] have demonstrated a decreased incidence of AISH in eyes in which they used an anterior chamber maintainer.

In patients with glaucoma or ocular hypertension, try to get the IOP as controlled as possible before surgery. This may require carbonic anhydrase inhibitors in addition to topical agents. The goal is to prevent a great, sudden fall in IOP when the anterior chamber is entered. Remember that the duration as well as the degree of hypotony are risk factors. If a larger incision must be employed, it should be closed, with the anterior chamber maintained as much of the time as possible. Preplaced sutures are essential in eyes with AISH risk factors requiring larger incision surgery. In an eye with a 4+ brunescent nucleus in which I must perform ECCE, I will place three interrupted 9-0 nylon sutures after creating a posterior scleral shelved incision, but before entering the anterior chamber. Or perform small-incision ECCE but be ready for chamber shallowing.

Control the blood pressure and heart rate before surgery. We instruct our patients to take all of their normal medications the day of their eye surgery. We routinely give a benzodiazepam

to anxious patients before surgery. In patients with uncontrolled hypertension or preoperative tachycardia, we administer intravenous labetalol to block both α- and β-receptors. This medication is very effective at decreasing the overall sympathetic tone of the patient.

Intraoperative Diagnosis

The most important factor in achieving a successful resolution of AISH is the rapidity with which the surgeon recognizes the event. The diagnosis must be made at the earliest possible moment so the surgeon can perform the most efficacious treatment. If recognized early, the result will be a completely normal eye; if the warning signs are ignored, an expulsive hemorrhage may eventuate in evisceration. The difference between these two outcomes may be due to a diagnostic delay of only 1 to 2 minutes. That is as long as it takes for an eye to go from positive pressure to expulsive hemorrhage.

Be suspicious of patients and eyes exhibiting the risk factors mentioned above. During surgery, be constantly cognizant of the anterior chamber depth. If it seems to shallow progressively, check first for mechanical/external factors. If none are present, then evaluate the fluid inflow and outflow. Make sure the fluid leaving the eye through the incision or paracentesis is not excessive. This might require a suture to create a watertight system. If outflow is not a problem, check the inflow to see if the infusion tubing is kinked or the sleeve is too compressed within the incision (**Box 24.2**). Is the BSS bottle empty? If this quick checklist fails to uncover the problem, remove the infusion instrument from the eye and look for subtle signs of fluid misdirection.

This is an appropriate time to place a cellulose sponge, a Q-tip, or a finger over the incision to both seal the opening and qualitatively assess the IOP. Positive posterior pressure causes a convex posterior capsule, a shallow anterior chamber, and, eventually, iris prolapse. Applying several minutes of Q-tip pressure over the incision will gradually soften the eye if fluid misdirection is the problem; it may become even harder if an AISH is in progress. Don't waste time before applying Q-tip pressure! If a suprachoroidal effusion is occurring, the first step in effective management has taken place.

Management of Intraoperative Suprachoroidal Expulsive Hemorrhage

If the eye has become rock hard, an AISH is in progress. The patient may also complain of pain despite adequate anesthesia; there is a rich supply of ciliary nerves throughout the choroid. There is no need to waste time on other diagnostic tests at this juncture. The surgeon should immediately close the incision, with stromal hydration and even sutures if necessary. The suture

---

Box. 24.2   Positive Pressure Checklist

- Anterior chamber depth
- External factors
- Fluid inflow/outflow
  - Bottle height
  - Incision too small: crimping sleeve/too large: excessive outflow
  - Adjust machine parameters
- Fluid misdirection: apply Q-tip or digital pressure

material should have good tensile strength and be easily handled; 8-0 nylon is a good suture.

Apply significant digital or Q-tip pressure over the incision to the globe (**Fig. 24.5**). This external, anterior pressure will increase the IOP and tamponade the effusion or hemorrhage, thus limiting its extent. It is very important to limit the effusion or small hemorrhage to avoid stretching and rupturing the larger choroidal vessels in the suprachoroidal space. By maintaining the uveal anatomy, the tangential shearing force of the effusion is limited, preventing hemorrhage. This event occurs along a logarithmic time line; things move slowly at first, but erupt swiftly toward the end.

Stop the Surgery and Do Not Enlarge the Incision

If the eye remains hard after 5 to 10 minutes of Q-tip pressure, place a sterile gauze over the closed eyelids, and then, if one is available in the facility, place a Honan balloon over the eye (**Fig. 24.9**). The balloon can be inflated to 50 mm Hg and the eye checked every 10 to 15 minutes.

The surgeon may choose to confirm the diagnosis of AISH by performing indirect ophthalmoscopy or scleral transillumination at this point.

There is no doubt that the retinal circulation is threatened during episodes of AISH; however, applying significant anterior pressure is necessary to prevent an expulsive hemorrhage. This is the price we pay to save the eye. Hayreh and Weingeist[14] have shown that retinal ischemia is tolerated for 90 to 100 minutes with good recovery of visual evoked responses and retinal morphology; ischemia beyond this time results in irreparable retinal damage. They state, "The retinal tolerance time to acute ischemia is almost identical whether the ischemia is produced by clamping the central retinal artery alone or by raising the IOP to above the level of the arterial blood pressure (with arrest of both the retinal and choroidal circulations)." The additional benefit of controlling the AISH by raising the IOP is that it does slow or stop the choroidal circulation, aiding in the arrest of a choroidal hemorrhage.

Note that performing a sclerotomy is not recommended because it is counterproductive. The goal is to achieve tamponade rapidly; a sclerotomy takes precious moments and prevents tamponade by creating another opening through which blood may flow. Maumenee and Schwartz[15] also recommended simply suturing the corneal incision and not creating a sclerotomy: "Drainage of the choroid through a transscleral puncture is not necessary." Lakhanpal[16] has demonstrated experimentally in the rabbit eye that "immediate sclerotomy during the acute formation … resulted in further increase in the supra choroidal hemorrhage, with marked extension of the hemorrhage into the retina and vitreous."

Under no circumstances should the wound be opened in an attempt to perform an ECCE. The large wound and immediate anterior segment hypotony will lead to immediate expulsive hemorrhage and loss of the eye.

The surgeon may also choose to treat the inevitable postoperative pressure elevation by beginning systemic therapy at this time. We administer one or two ampules of intravenous mannitol and 500 mg of acetazolamide. We also administer 100 mg of intravenous (IV) hydrocortisone in an attempt to reduce vascular permeability and ocular inflammation.

If the patient is having cataract surgery under topical anesthesia, the pain may require a peribulbar injection and systemic sedation. Once the incision is stable a small volume of anesthetic is administered. In the setting of an AISH, this may seem counterintuitive, as it adds more "posterior pressure," but keep in mind the two different spaces affected—the periorbital and the suprachoroidal. Patients appreciate that the pain is diminished.

We have been able to complete all procedures within 60 minutes of the onset of the AISH using this technique. The procedure remains difficult, but manageable. Q-tip pressure is applied at intervals during the surgery to keep the effusion or hemorrhage in check and to keep the eye as soft as possible during surgery. The incision must be watertight and the infusion bottle as high as possible (if the posterior capsule is intact).

It is desirable to complete the surgery during the time frame provided by the regional block. There is psychological stress inflicted on the patient and the family by delay. However, if the surgeon is uncomfortable proceeding, or if the eye remains firm for an inordinate amount of time, there is no significant ocular morbidity involved in delaying the completion of the cataract extraction. Even after capsulotomy and/or partial phaco, treating aggressively for elevated IOP and inflammation and waiting a few days for the eye to stabilize is acceptable.

If surgery is continued, every prudent attempt must be made to remove the cataract, which is possible by following the management technique outlined here. Once the cataract has been

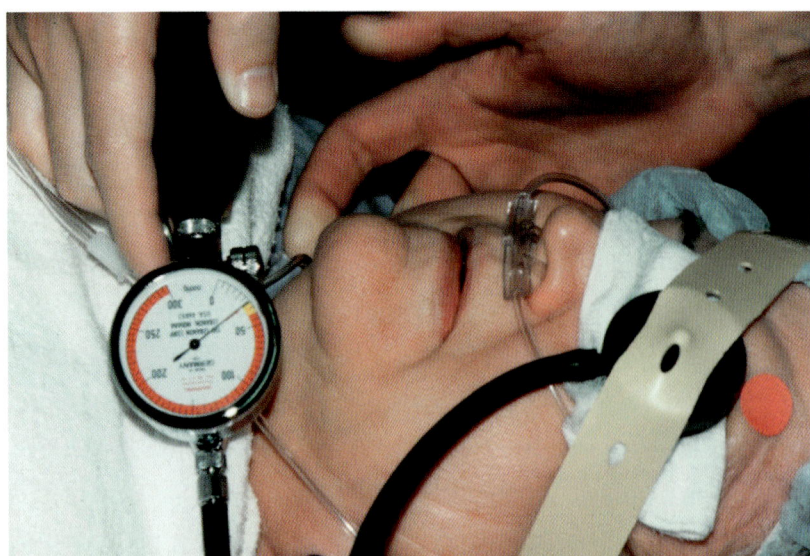

Fig. 24.9 In the event of extreme positive pressure from fluid misdirection or AISH, a sterile gauze is placed over the closed lids and the Honan balloon is applied. This aids in fluid redistribution or absorption in fluid misdirection syndrome and to tamponade a suprachoroidal hemorrhage.

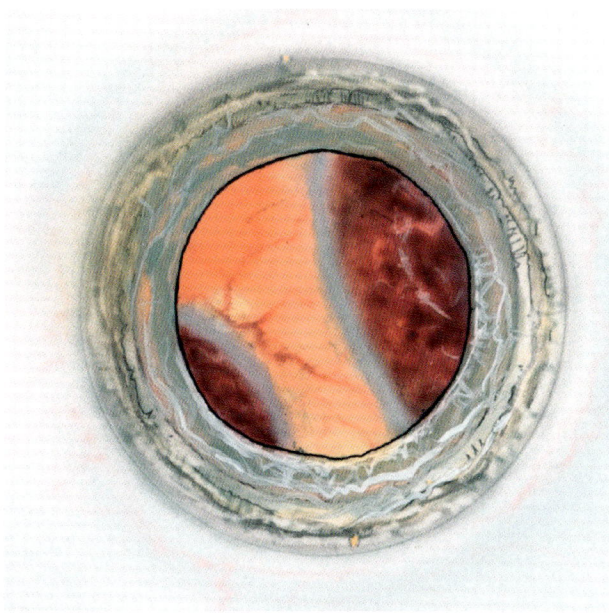

Fig. 24.10 A choroidal elevation may be evident on indirect examination.

removed, it is usually not too difficult to insert an IOL. The only exception to this guideline might be the secondary insertion of an IOL if the capsule has been severely compromised during the initial operation.[17]

These patients should be treated aggressively post operatively with topical steroids and ocular pressure lowering medications. We routinely use oral systemic carbonic anhydrase inhibitors until the IOP is controlled. The choroidal elevation is usually evident postoperatively by indirect ophthalmoscopy (**Fig. 24.10**) or B-scan ultrasonography (**Fig. 24.11**). Effusions usually resolve within 2 weeks, whereas suprachoroidal hemorrhages may require 1 to 2 months.

Expulsive Hemorrhage

In the unfortunate event that a true expulsive hemorrhage occurs, the same basic principle applies: Close the incision. Clean the incision as well as possible; there should be no vitreous or uvea

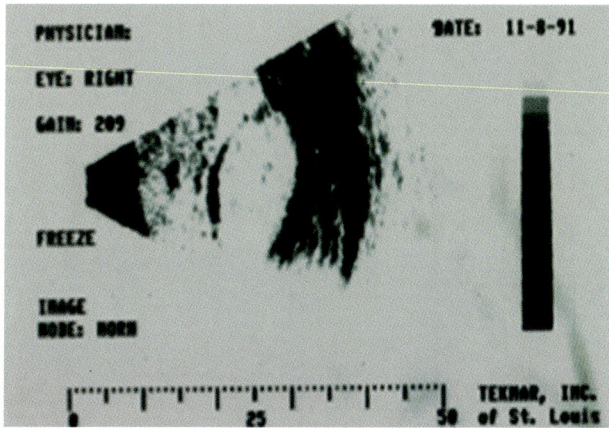

Fig. 24.11 This B-scan ultrasound demonstrates the mound-like elevation of an expulsive hemorrhage.

in or beyond the incision. A retina/vitreous specialist should be consulted within 24 hours. Repair of a true expulsive hemorrhage, or a severe AISH with "kissing choroidals," requires the help of an experienced posterior segment specialist.

Treatment of Massive Suprachoroidal Hemorrhage

Just because a patient has a massive suprachoroidal hemorrhage does not mean that a secondary surgery will be needed. Each case must be judged individually. If the eye has vitreous or uvea in the incision, secondary surgery is probably indicated. Drainage of the suprachoroidal space in the immediate surgical and postoperative period is probably not helpful. Most of the time, the hemorrhage will simply recur.[16,18] Massive kissing choroidals, in which there is apposition of the retinal surfaces, presents more of a dilemma. Experimental and clinical work indicates that a suprachoroidal hemorrhage begins to liquefy between 7 and 14 days; therefore, such a hemorrhage is optimally drained during this time.[16] Chu et al[18] used echography to follow these patients and noted that many cases resolved spontaneously without immediate retinal sequelae in spite of a mean period of retinal apposition of 15 days.

Reynolds et al[19] also concluded that secondary surgery was not indicated if a kissing choroidal was the only problem. If retinal detachment or vitreous incarceration was present, vitrectomy with air–fluid exchange, combined with drainage of the suprachoroidal blood, was indicated. Scott et al[20] evaluated visual acuity in eyes having appositional suprachoroidal hemorrhage and found significantly worse vision if the appositional choroidal was present for more than 14 days.

All patients having a massive suprachoroidal hemorrhage have a very guarded prognosis. Even in the best-case scenario, eyes requiring secondary surgery do not often see well. An acuity of 20/200 or better should be judged a success in these cases. Concurrent or delayed retinal detachment is always a risk, just one more reason an experienced retina/vitreous surgeon should be managing patients with complicated, massive suprachoroidal hemorrhage, and more reason than ever to understand the nature of positive pressure development during phacoemulsification and the management of AISH!

Conclusion

Treatment of AISH has as its primary goal the prevention of expulsive hemorrhage. This is achieved by intervening at the earliest possible recognition of a suprachoroidal effusion. Get as much of the surgery done as possible without risking trauma to essential structures, such as the cornea, iris, and posterior capsule. If positive pressure is occurring, never extend an incision, as more intraocular contents will present and catastrophic expulsive hemorrhage would be more likely. Discontinue surgery by closing incisions no matter what the stage of surgery, if necessary, and come back the next day to finish. Examine with the indirect ophthalmoscope to ascertain the localization and extent of hemorrhage. By the next day a natural equilibration will have been accomplished because the internal tamponade effect created by the positive pressure will have stopped the bleeding. The suprachoroidal space increase will have been accompanied by a commensurate vitreous volume reduction. More normal anterior chamber relationships will also have been created overnight. Rarely an increase in positive pressure can occur with secondary surgery the next day. In our experience, when using this method of management of positive posterior pressure, no eyes have developed and expulsive hemorrhage.[7]

References

1. Arnold PN. Prospective study of a single-injection peribulbar technique. J Cataract Refract Surg 1992;18:157–161

2. Updegraff SA, Peyman GA, McDonald MB. Pupillary block during cataract surgery. Am J Ophthalmol 1994;117:328–332

3. Osher MS. Emergency treatment of vitreous bulge and wound gaping; complicating cataract surgery. Am J Ophthalmol 1957;44:409–411

4. Tsai JC, Barton KA, Miller MH, Khaw PT, Hitchings RA. Surgical results in malignant glaucoma refractory to medical or laser therapy. Eye (Lond) 1997;11(Pt 5):677–681

5. Wolter JR, Garfinkel RA. Ciliochoroidal effusion as precursor of suprachoroidal hemorrhage: a pathologic study. Ophthalmic Surg 1988;19:344–349

6. Beyer CF, Peyman GA, Hill JM. Expulsive choroidal hemorrhage in rabbits. A histopathologic study. Arch Ophthalmol 1989;107:1648–1653

7. Davison JA. Acute intraoperative suprachoroidal hemorrhage in extracapsular cataract surgery. J Cataract Refract Surg 1986;12:606–622

8. Davison JA. Acute intraoperative suprachoroidal hemorrhage in capsular bag phacoemulsification. J Cataract Refract Surg 1993;19:534–537

9. Arnold PN. Study of acute intraoperative suprachoroidal hemorrhage. J Cataract Refract Surg 1992;18:489–494

10. Speaker MG, Guerriero PN, Met JA, Coad CT, Berger A, Marmor M. A case-control study of risk factors for intraoperative suprachoroidal expulsive hemorrhage. Ophthalmology 1991;98:202–209, discussion 210

11. Bukelman A, Hoffman P, Oliver M. Limited choroidal hemorrhage associated with extracapsular cataract extraction. Arch Ophthalmol 1987;105:338–341

12. Eriksson A, Koranyi G, Seregard S, Philipson B. Risk of acute suprachoroidal hemorrhage with phacoemulsification. J Cataract Refract Surg 1998;24:793–800

13. Blumenthal M, Grinbaum A, Assia EI. Preventing expulsive hemorrhage using an anterior chamber maintainer to eliminate hypotony. J Cataract Refract Surg 1997;23:476–479

14. Hayreh SS, Weingeist TA. Experimental occlusion of the central artery of the retina. IV: Retinal tolerance time to acute ischaemia. Br J Ophthalmol 1980;64:818–825

15. Maumenee AE, Schwartz MF. Acute intraoperative choroidal effusion. Am J Ophthalmol 1985;100:147–154

16. Lakhanpal V. Experimental and clinical observations on massive suprachoroidal hemorrhage. Trans Am Ophthalmol Soc 1993;91:545–652

17. Bryant WR. Secondary intraocular lens implantation in eyes that experienced suprachoroidal hemorrhage during primary cataract surgery. J Cataract Refract Surg 1989;15:629–634

18. Chu TG, Cano MR, Green RL, Liggett PE, Lean JS. Massive suprachoroidal hemorrhage with central retinal apposition. A clinical and echographic study. Arch Ophthalmol 1991;109:1575–1581

19. Reynolds MG, Haimovici R, Flynn HW Jr, et al. Supra-choroidal hemorrhage: clinical features and results of secondary surgical management. Ophthalmology 1993;100:460–465

20. Scott IU, Flynn HW Jr, Schiffman J, Smiddy WE, Murray TG, Ehlies F. Visual acuity outcomes among patients with appositional suprachoroidal hemorrhage. Ophthalmology 1997;104:2039–2046

25 Strategies for Weak Zonules

David F. Chang

Weak zonules complicate every step of the cataract procedure and challenge surgeons to anticipate, recognize, and manage intraoperative zonulopathy.[1-9] If the capsular bag is successfully preserved, the surgeon must also consider and optimize long-term intraocular lens (IOL) fixation and centration in light of existing and potentially progressive zonular abnormality.[10] The most common predisposing risk factors for zonular weakness include pseudoexfoliation, prior trauma, retinopathy of prematurity, advanced age and nuclear brunescence, and prior intraocular surgery (e.g., prior vitrectomy or trabeculectomy). Less common risk factors would be conditions such as Marfan's syndrome, retinitis pigmentosa, and myotonic dystrophy.

Preoperative Signs of Zonulopathy

The presence of a traumatic mydriasis, iridodialysis, angle recession, or vitreous herniation is invariably associated with some degree of traumatic zonulopathy. Suspicion should also be high with a prior history of traumatic hyphema. Absent preoperative phacodonesis or visible zonular dialysis, however, the extent of zonular weakness is generally not known until surgery is initiated. Robert Osher's group[11] has described subtle signs of zonular weakness that include a wider iridolenticular gap (space between the iris and the anterior lens surface), a decentered nucleus, focal iridodonesis, and visibility of the peripheral lens equator upon lateral gaze.

Pseudoexfoliation syndrome is characterized by progressive zonulopathy, and the whitish deposits are found not only on the zonules but also on the posterior iris surface and pupillary margin. Therefore, smaller pupils are often associated with more advanced zonulopathy in these eyes (**Fig. 25.1a**). Likewise, a brunescent nucleus with pseudoexfoliation is frequently accompanied by weak zonules. The most worrisome sign with pseudoexfoliation, however, is an unexpectedly shallow anterior chamber despite a normal axial length; this invariably indicates diffusely weak zonules.[4,9] One should consider a retrobulbar or peribulbar anesthetic block in cases suspected of having a high risk of capsular rupture. Because of the progressive nature of the associated zonulopathy, it can be argued that cataract surgery in pseudoexfoliation eyes should be performed at the earlier end of the elective surgical window.

Capsulorrhexis

The capsulorrhexis step provides the first opportunity for surgeons to directly assess zonular integrity. If firmly anchored by the zonules, the peripheral anterior capsule is normally immobile during this step. In contrast, with weak zonular fixation, the capsule will demonstrate "pseudoelasticity" by seemingly stretching,

as the capsular flap is pulled.[12] This is not true capsular elasticity but rather due to the failure of the zonules to immobilize the peripheral lens capsule. Another sign of severe or diffuse zonular weakness is difficulty incising the anterior capsule, as though the cystotome tip was dull (**Fig. 25.1b**). If the cystotome tip depresses rather than incises the central anterior capsule, a halo-shaped light reflex may be noted. These signs represent a lack of circumferential zonular traction that should normally create a taut anterior capsule. Finally, there may be significant movement of the entire lens as the cystotome first perforates and tears the anterior capsule.

Weak zonules significantly increase the risk of a radial anterior capsular tear because of this property of pseudoelasticity. Because the zonules do not adequately immobilize the anterior capsule, the peripheral capsule moves along with the flap as it is being torn. Although a large diameter capsulorrhexis would be helpful for phaco in any challenging case, this also increases the risk of a peripheral extension if one is struggling to control the tear.

Because use of capsular retractors or a capsular tension ring (CTR) requires a continuous curvilinear capsulotomy, the overriding priority of achieving an intact capsulorrhexis dictates that one should err on the side of a smaller diameter that can be secondarily enlarged after the IOL has been implanted. If capsular pseudoelasticity is noted, one might intentionally make the capsulotomy diameter slightly smaller to improve the odds of successfully achieving a continuous curvilinear capsulotomy. Brian Little et al's[13] capsule tear-out rescue technique is particularly helpful for controlling a tear that wants to veer radially because of weak zonules and pseudoelasticity.

Hydrodissection

Upon successful completion of the capsulorrhexis, loose zonules still pose multiple problems for the phacoemulsification and cortical aspiration steps. Because of deficient capsular rotational stability and counterfixation, the nucleus is more difficult to rotate. One should always suspect significant circumferential zonular weakness if, despite proper hydrodissection technique, the nucleus does not spin easily. Finally, the epinucleus and cortex do not separate as easily from a capsular bag that is lax and loosely anchored.

Normally, we are able to rotate a hydrodissected nucleus with a single instrument because of the counterfixation provided by the capsular bag. However, to do so, the rotating instrument (e.g., hydrodissection cannula or chopper) must partially push the nucleus against the capsular bag equator to achieve the necessary rotational force and counterfixation. In fact, of all of our surgical maneuvers, I believe that rotation of either the nucleus or a three-piece IOL imparts the most force against the capsular bag. This explains why these two steps are the most likely to

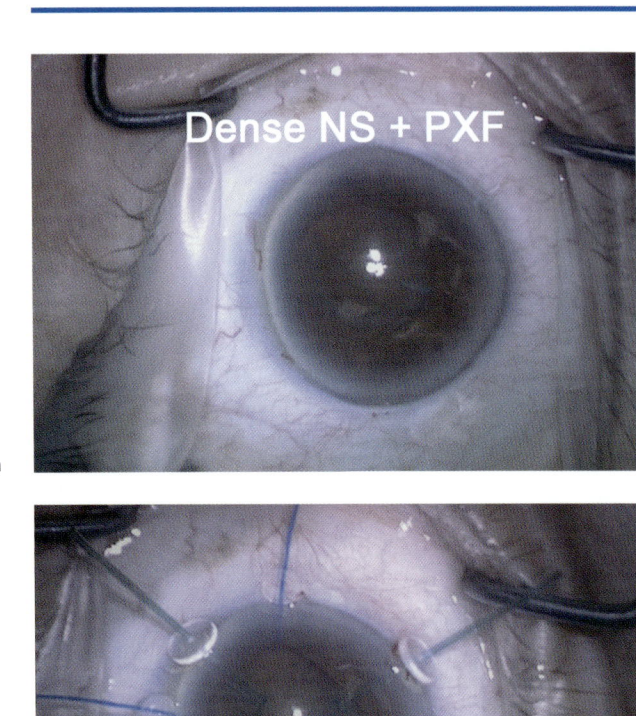

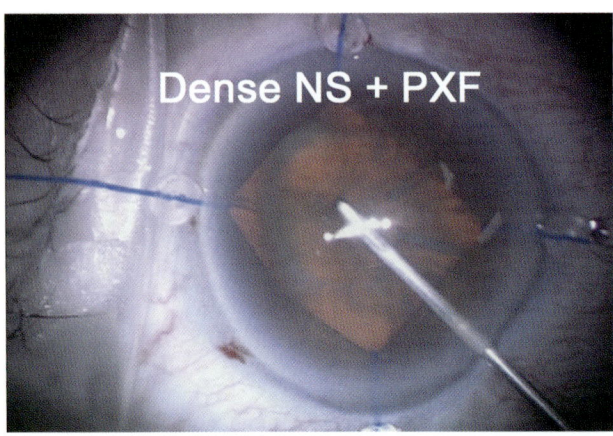

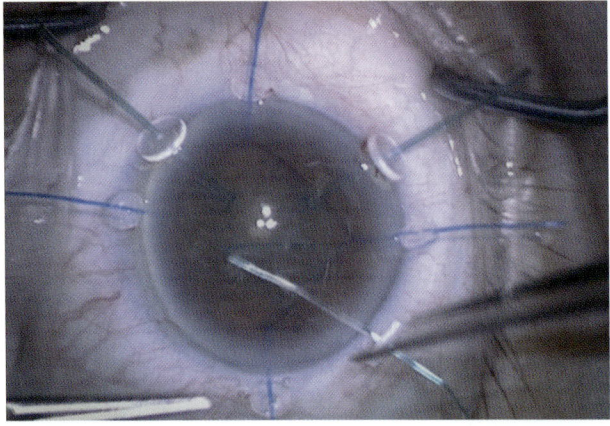

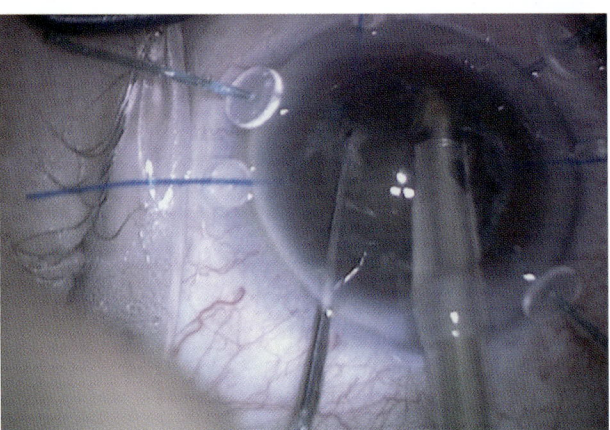

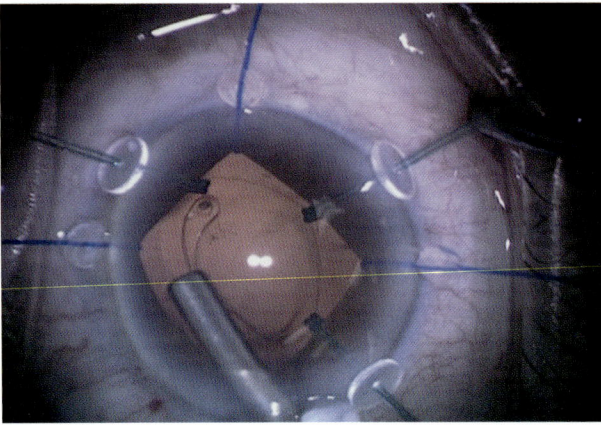

Fig. 25.1 Poorly dilated pupil in eye with pseudoexfoliation and dense nucleus (a). Following placement of iris retractors, anterior capsular striae indicate that it is difficult to puncture with the cystotome because of lax zonular tension (b). Double stranded capsule retractors (Microsurgical Technologies) are inserted around the capsulorhexis edge to support the capsular bag and equator during phaco (c). Vertical phaco chop is used to bisect the brunescent nucleus, while minimizing the zonular strain associated with sculpting (d). After cortical cleanup, a capsular tension ring is implanted while the capsule retractors are still supporting the capsular bag (e).

extend a radial anterior capsular tear into the posterior capsule. With pseudoexfoliation, overly forceful efforts to rotate the nucleus may instead shear already weakened zonules in the process. This could potentially create a large zonular dialysis or dislocate the crystalline lens even prior to insertion of the phaco tip.

One alternative is to use two instruments to bimanually rotate the nucleus. In this situation, the second instrument tip, rather than the capsular bag, becomes the counterfixating fulcrum around which to rotate the nucleus. However, when severe zonular laxity is diagnosed during the capsulotomy step and the nucleus cannot be easily rotated following hydrodissection, the safest strategy is to insert capsule retractors as described below. By fixating the capsular bag to the eye wall, capsule retractors will facilitate nuclear rotation and prevent creation of a zonular dialysis in the process.

Capsular Tension Rings

Polymethylmethacrylate (PMMA) capsular tension rings (Morcher, Stuttgart, Germany; Ophtec, Boca Raton, FL) partially compensate for a weakened zonular apparatus in several ways.[14–26] Using forceps or an injector (Geuder, Heidelberg, Germany; Ophtec), the ring can be inserted at any stage following completion of the capsulorrhexis.[27,28] If there is a focal zonular dehiscence or weakness, the ring redistributes mechanical forces, such as those of nuclear sculpting or IOL insertion, toward areas of stronger zonular support. However, if the entire circumference of zonules is uniformly weak, this benefit is negated.

A second advantage is that centrifugal equatorial pressure applied by the ring makes the flaccid capsular bag tauter. This reduces redundant capsule folds, forward trampolining of the posterior capsule, and inward collapsing of the capsular fornices toward the aspirating instrument tip. In the absence of a CTR, the stiff PMMA haptics of a three-piece foldable IOL can provide some of the same benefits during cortical aspiration. In addition, the IOL optic can block a floppy posterior capsule from vaulting toward the irrigation and aspiration (I/A) tip in the subincisional area.

The final benefit of a CTR is to counter the progressive contractile capsular forces. Postoperatively, centrifugal zonular tension normally limits capsulorrhexis diameter shrinkage as the capsular bag contracts. Therefore, severe capsulophimosis always indicates deficient zonular countertraction. Excessive or asymmetric capsular contracture can decenter the IOL and further weaken the remaining zonules. This is a likely factor in spontaneous late dislocation of the entire capsular bag and IOL in pseudoexfoliation cases.[10,29]

The CTRs have two important disadvantages to consider. Because of its larger diameter, significant compression is required to insert the ring into the capsular bag. This may stretch the capsulorrhexis and potentially shear the remaining zonules by distorting or decentering the bag. Because of this compressive force, CTRs should never be inserted in the presence of an anterior or posterior capsule tear. CTR insertion with an injector is preferable to reduce the forces exerted on the bag and zonules during insertion.[27] A second drawback to CTRs is that they may impede cortical aspiration by pinning and trapping cortex within the capsular fornix. For this reason, surgeons should consider first using capsule retractors instead of a CTR to stabilize the bag during phaco. Ideally, CTR insertion can then be delayed until after the cortex has been removed.[27] The Henderson modified CTR (FCI Ophthalmics, Pembroke, MA; Morcher) has a scalloped contour that facilitates cortical removal following placement.[30] If one area of cortex is difficult to remove because the Henderson CTR impinges on it, the ring can be rotated slightly until one of the gaps overlies the cortex.

Capsule Retractors

In addition to enlarging a small pupil, flexible iris retractors can be used to support the capsular bag in the presence of extremely loose zonules.[31–34] Merriam and Zheng[31] first described using self-retaining iris retractors through paracentesis openings to hook and fixate the capsulorrhexis. However, because the hooked ends are very short and flexible, iris retractors may tend to slip off of the anterior capsular edge during phaco and will not support the equator of the capsular bag.

Richard Mackool[35] designed the Capsular Support System (Impex Surgical, Brooklyn, NY; FCI Ophthalmics) with capsular hooks that are sufficiently elongated to support the peripheral capsular fornix and not just the capsulorrhexis edge. In this way, the retractors function as artificial zonules to stabilize the entire capsular equator and bag during phaco and cortical cleanup. Unlike a CTR, capsule retractors provide support in the anterior-posterior direction and do not trap the cortex. This is because each retractor applies only point pressure to the capsular fornix without ensnaring the cortex. The disposable nylon capsular retractors from MicroSurgical Technologies (MST; Redmond, WA) are a more recent alternative to the Mackool retractor design (**Fig. 25.1c**). They feature a double-stranded design that creates a loop at the tip, which is less likely to puncture the equatorial

capsule. One must take care, however, not to thread the CTR leading eyelet through this loop of the MST capsule retractor.

Capsule retractors can be inserted through limbal stab incisions at any surgical stage including midway through the capsulorrhexis step. By anchoring the bag to the eye wall, the additional anteroposterior support and rotational stability facilitate hydrodissection and nuclear rotation. The self-retaining capsule retractors are also strong enough to center and immobilize a capsular bag that is partially subluxated due to a severe zonular dialysis. They also restrain the peripheral anterior and equatorial capsule from being aspirated and dehisced by the phaco or I/A tip.

As a single strategy for severe zonular deficiency, capsule retractors are significantly more effective than CTRs at preventing posterior capsule rupture. Because CTRs can only redistribute instrument and mechanical forces to the remaining intact zonules, the greater the zonular defect or deficiency, the less effective a CTR can be at stabilizing the bag. However, a CTR can be used in conjunction with capsule retractors, particularly if there is a sizable zonular dialysis. If, after first inserting retractors, the unsupported equatorial regions of the capsular bag still tend to collapse inward toward the phaco tip, a CTR can be inserted to distend the equator of the bag to its proper anatomic configuration.

Although the tip of the capsule retractor is dull, it is possible for the hooks to tear the capsulorrhexis margin during surgery. A key objective is to support the capsular bag without excessive tension and stretching of the anterior capsular rim. There is a tendency to overtighten the capsular retractors because the tension is initially adjusted with a soft eye. Inserting the phaco tip with irrigation suddenly displaces the nucleus and capsular bag posteriorly, which effectively tightens the retractors further. After inserting the phaco tip, it is therefore important to momentarily assess whether the capsule retractors have become so taut that they tent the capsulorrhexis edge. If so, they should be loosened slightly so that the capsular rim does not tear during phacoemulsification. This is particularly important if the capsulorrhexis diameter is on the small side.

Nuclear Emulsification

Fragile zonules are highly prone to further damage or breakage during nuclear emulsification, and poor capsular bag stability heightens the risk of capsular rupture. Forceful sculpting or rotation of the nucleus may shear zonules in the oppositely located quadrants. Care should be taken to avoid causing excessive nuclear movement with sculpting, chopping, or rotation. Phaco chop significantly reduces the stress placed on the zonules and capsule by replacing sculpting motions with the manual forces of one instrument pushing inward against another (**Fig. 25.1d**). Because of the centrally directed instrument forces, horizontal chopping is particularly effective at avoiding nuclear tilt or displacement, and this is my preference for weak zonule cases.

The supracapsular flip technique, as popularized by David Brown,[36] prolapses and flips the endonucleus out of the capsular bag prior to emulsification. If accomplished, this prevents the capsular bag from bearing any of the phaco instrumentation forces. The ease with which this flipping maneuver can be accomplished varies depending on the size of the endonucleus relative to the capsulorrhexis diameter. Using this technique with a nucleus that is too large or a capsulorrhexis that is too small risks further zonular dehiscence. Care must also be taken to avoid endothelial trauma during the nuclear flipping maneuver (see Phaco Flip Technique, below). With chopping, one should consider bringing larger sections of nucleus out of the capsular bag where they can be sub-chopped into smaller fragments within the supracapsular space. For example, with a medium density nucleus it may be possible to lift each hemi-nucleus out of the capsular bag following the initial bisecting horizontal or vertical chop.

Throughout phaco and cortical cleanup, one should anticipate that deficient centrifugal zonular tension will result in greater posterior capsule laxity. The flaccid posterior capsule will trampoline or be drawn toward any aspirating tip as the nuclear fragments, epinucleus, and cortex are removed. Initially, the nuclear bulk will mask this situation, but one must be vigilant as increasingly more nucleus is removed to expose more of the posterior capsule. Compared with a standard 19-gauge phaco tip, a smaller-diameter, 20-gauge tip greatly reduces the risk of inadvertently aspirating the peripheral or posterior capsule. If one suspects or encounters zonular laxity, the aspiration settings can be lowered as progressively more of the nucleus is removed. To slow the pace, a lower than usual aspiration flow rate is advisable. A pre-programmed vacuum setting that usually avoids a postocclusion surge with routine cases may not be safe with a lax posterior capsule that is lacking normal centrifugal zonular tension. Therefore, one should consider decreasing the vacuum to lower than normal levels to prevent trampolining of the posterior capsule. Finally, repeatedly re-inflating the capsular bag with a dispersive ophthalmic viscosurgical device (OVD) can further restrain a flaccid posterior capsule from vaulting toward the aspirating instrument as the final fragments and epinucleus are aspirated. Guarding the phaco tip by placing the horizontal chopper tip beneath it is another strategy. These safety measures are especially important if there is no epinuclear shell remaining as the last nuclear fragment is emulsified.

Cortical Cleanup

As adherent cortex is aspirated, the usual centrifugal capsular counterfixation afforded by stronger zonules is deficient. Lacing circumferential zonular tension, a lax posterior capsule tends to cling to any epinucleus and cortex that is being aspirated; redundant capsular folds can be easily ensnared by the aspirating instrument or snagged by a capsule polisher (**Fig. 25.2**). While removing cortex, inadvertently aspirating the more pliant anterior capsule may cause a zonular dialysis. Effective hydrodissection is crucial because the more easily lens material separates from a floppy capsule, the less likely it is for the capsular folds to be aspirated.

As mentioned earlier, continually re-inflating the capsular bag with a dispersive OVD is an excellent strategy for removing cortex from a floppy bag as well. Placing both the anterior and posterior capsule on stretch prevents a pliant posterior capsule from trampolining toward the aspiration port. In this situation, cortical aspiration can be performed either with or without irrigation (dry technique). Dispersive agents are preferable to cohesive viscoelastics because they better resist aspiration. Finally, stripping the cortex tangentially rather than radially helps to distribute the tractional force across as large an area of zonules as possible.

Bimanual I/A instrumentation provides several advantages in the presence of weak zonules (**Fig. 25.3**). The ability to alternate between two aspirating ports improves access to the subincisional cortex, which can be especially challenging to remove if the capsulorrhexis diameter is small and the posterior capsule is lax. A dual-incision system also means that the aspirating port never needs to turn toward the capsular fornix. It can be kept facing the cornea and away from the posterior capsule virtually at all times. Without a constraining infusion sleeve, the surgeon is better able to reach across to the opposite equatorial quad-

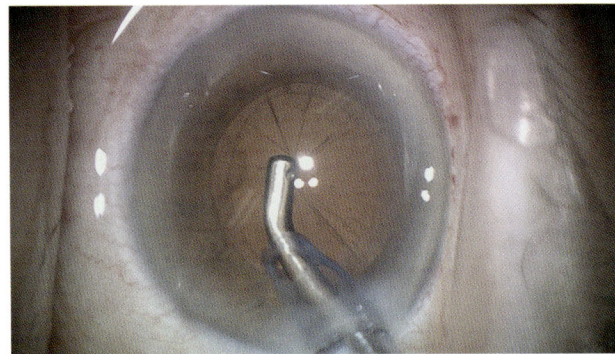

Fig. 25.2 Diffuse zonular weakness causes an excessively pliant posterior capsule due to the lack of centrifugal zonular traction. This makes inadvertent aspiration of the posterior capsule much more likely.

rants where the aspirating port can be safely buried within fluffs of cortex before vacuum builds. This prevents the tip from aspirating the pliant peripheral or posterior capsule. Finally, in the presence of a zonular dialysis, the ability to dissociate the I/A tips can minimize any misdirection of irrigating fluid through the zonular defect.

If capsule retractors are used, placing a capsular tension ring can usually be delayed until the cortex has been removed (**Fig. 25.1e**). One must be careful not to snag or tear posterior capsular folds with the leading tip of a CTR during its insertion. Fully expanding the capsular bag with viscoelastic prior to injecting the ring is critical for this reason. Brian Little's group[28] has described the fishtail method of reducing zonular stress when inserting a ring without an injector. As mentioned earlier, using an injector has the advantage of introducing the CTR into the capsular bag without excessively stretching the capsulorrhexis.[27] One can either load the ring manually with a reusable metal injector or use a preloaded, disposable plastic injector from Morcher (FCI Ophthalmics). The injector tip should be positioned as far peripherally within the bag as possible to minimize lateral displacement of the capsular bag as the ring emerges. If used, capsular retractors should be left in place to counter the lateral decentering forces of the CTR as it is injected. In fact, an additional advantage of capsular retractors is to reduce the potential for zonular damage caused during insertion of a CTR. The retractors can then be removed prior to IOL implantation.

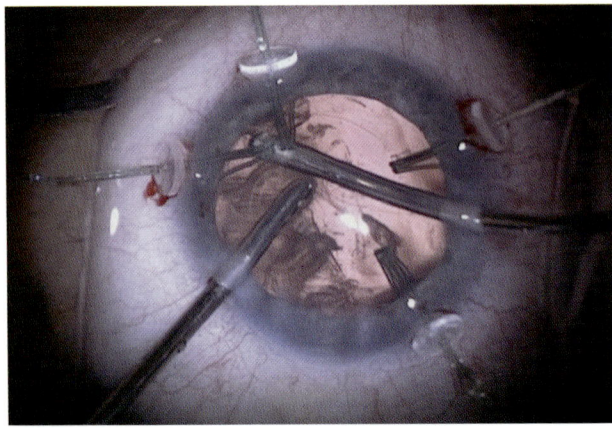

Fig. 25.3 Bimanual irrigation-aspiration instrumentation is used to remove the cortex in the presence of a lax posterior capsule. This facilitates subincisional cortical aspiration, and allows the aspirating port to face away from the posterior capsule for most of the cortical removal.

References

1. Osher RH, Cionni RJ, Gimbel HV, Crandall AS. Cataract surgery in patients with pseudoexfoliation syndrome. Eur J Implant Refract Surg 1993;5:46–50

2. Fine IH, Hoffman RS. Phacoemulsification in the presence of pseudoexfoliation: challenges and options. J Cataract Refract Surg 1997;23:160–165

3. Avramides S, Traianidis P, Sakkias G. Cataract surgery and lens implantation in eyes with exfoliation syndrome. J Cataract Refract Surg 1997;23:583–587

4. Küchle M, Viestenz A, Martus P, Händel A, Jünemann A, Naumann GO. Anterior chamber depth and complications during cataract surgery in eyes with pseudoexfoliation syndrome. Am J Ophthalmol 2000;129:281–285

5. Shingleton BJ, Heltzer J, O'Donoghue MW. Outcomes of phacoemulsification in patients with and without pseudoexfoliation syndrome. J Cataract Refract Surg 2003;29:1080–1086

6. Blecher MH, Kirk MR. Surgical strategies for the management of zonular compromise. Curr Opin Ophthalmol 2008;19:31–35 Review

7. Shingleton BJ, Crandall AS, Ahmed II. Pseudoexfoliation and the cataract surgeon: preoperative, intraoperative, and postoperative issues related to intraocular pressure, cataract, and intraocular lenses. J Cataract Refract Surg 2009;35:1101–1120

8. Belovay GW, Varma DK, Ahmed II. Cataract surgery in pseudoexfoliation syndrome. Curr Opin Ophthalmol 2010;21:25–34 Review

9. Shingleton BJ, Marvin AC, Heier JS, et al. Pseudoexfoliation: High risk factors for zonule weakness and concurrent vitrectomy during phacoemulsification. J Cataract Refract Surg 2010;36:1261–1269

10. Jehan FS, Mamalis N, Crandall AS. Spontaneous late dislocation of intraocular lens within the capsular bag in pseudoexfoliation patients. Ophthalmology 2001;108:1727–1731

11. Marques DMV, Marques FF, Osher RH. Subtle signs of zonular damage. J Cataract Refract Surg 2004;30:1295–1299

12. Chang DF. Phacoemulsification in high-risk cases. In: Wallace RB, ed. Multifocal IOLs and Refractive Cataract Surgery. Chapter 11. Thorofare, NJ: Slack; 2001

13. Little BC, Smith JH, Packer M. Little capsulorhexis tear-out rescue. J Cataract Refract Surg 2006;32:1420–1422

14. Nagamoto T, Bissen-Miyajima H. A ring to support the capsular bag after continuous curvilinear capsulorhexis. J Cataract Refract Surg 1994;20:417–420

15. Legler UFC, Witschel BM. The capsular ring: a new device for complicated cataract surgery. German J Ophthalmol 1994;3:265

16. Cionni RJ, Osher RH. Endocapsular ring approach to the subluxed cataractous lens. J Cataract Refract Surg 1995;21:245–249

17. Gimbel HV, Sun R, Heston JP. Management of zonular dialysis in phacoemulsification and IOL implantation using the capsular tension ring. Ophthalmic Surg Lasers 1997;28:273–281

18. Menace R, Findl O, Georgopoulos M, Rainer G, Vass C, Schmetterer K. The capsular tension ring: designs, applications, and techniques. J Cataract Refract Surg 2000;26:898–912

19. Bayraktar S, Altan T, Küçüksümer Y, Yılmaz ÖF. Capsular tension ring implantation after capsulorhexis in phacoemulsification of cataracts associated with pseudoexfoliation syndrome. Intraoperative complications and early postoperative findings. J Cataract Refract Surg 2001;27:1620–1628

20. Gimbel HV, Sun R. Clinical applications of capsular tension rings in cataract surgery. Ophthalmic Surg Lasers 2002;33:44–53

21. Lee D-H, Shin S-C, Joo C-K. Effect of a capsular tension ring on intraocular lens decentration and tilting after cataract surgery. J Cataract Refract Surg 2002;28:843–846

22. Jacob S, Agarwal A, Agarwal A, Agarwal S, Patel N, Lal V. Efficacy of a capsular tension ring for phacoemulsification in eyes with zonular dialysis. J Cataract Refract Surg 2003;29:315–321

23. Price FW Jr, Mackool RJ, Miller KM, Koch P, Oetting TA, Johnson AT. Interim results of the United States investigational device study of the Ophtec capsular tension ring. Ophthalmology 2005;112:460–465

24. Hasanee K, Butler M, Ahmed II. Capsular tension rings and related devices: current concepts. Curr Opin Ophthalmol 2006;17:31–41 Review

25. Hasanee K, Ahmed II. Capsular tension rings: update on endocapsular support devices. Ophthalmol Clin North Am 2006;19:507–519 Review

26. Boomer JA, Jackson DW. Anatomic evaluation of the Morcher capsular tension ring by ultrasound biomicroscopy. J Cataract Refract Surg 2006;32:846–848

27. Ahmed IIK, Cionni RJ, Kranemann C, Crandall AS. Optimal timing of capsular tension ring implantation: Miyake-Apple video analysis. J Cataract Refract Surg 2005;31:1809–1813

28. Angunawela RI, Little B. Fish-tail technique for capsular tension ring insertion. J Cataract Refract Surg 2007;33:767–769

29. Chang DF. Prevention of bag-fixated IOL dislocation in pseudoexfoliation. (letter) Ophthalmology 2002;109:1951–1952

30. Henderson BA, Kim JY. Modified capsular tension ring for cortical removal after implantation. J Cataract Refract Surg 2007;33:1688–1690

31. Merriam JC, Zheng L. Iris hooks for phacoemulsification of the subluxated lens. J Cataract Refract Surg 1997;23:1295–1297

32. Lee V, Bloom P. Microhook capsule stabilization for phacoemulsification in eyes with pseudoexfoliation-syndrome-induced lens instability. J Cataract Refract Surg 1999;25:1567–1570

33. Santoro S, Sannace C, Cascella MC, Lavermicocca N. Subluxated lens: phacoemulsification with iris hooks. J Cataract Refract Surg 2003;29:2269–2273

34. Sethi HS, Sinha A, Pal N, Saxena R. Modified flexible iris retractor to retract superior iris and support inferior capsule in eyes with iris coloboma and inferior zonular deficiency. J Cataract Refract Surg 2006;32:715–716

35. Mackool RJ. Capsule stabilization for phacoemulsification. (letter) J Cataract Refract Surg 2000;26:629

26 Capsular Tension Devices

Charles H. Weber and Robert J. Cionni

The success of cataract surgery may be uncertain when it is threatened by the presence of zonular weakness, which increases the intraoperative risk of vitreous prolapse, capsular rupture, and retained lens material, as well as the postoperative risk of intraocular lens (IOL) dislocation. Capsular tension rings (CTRs) and related endocapsular devices enable surgeons to approach zonular weakness during complex cataract surgery with improved safety and have become a well-established tool in the armamentarium of cataract surgeons.

Nagamoto and Bissen-Miyajima[1,2] as well as Hara et al[3,4] initially developed the capsular bag supporting ring independently in Japan around 1990. Although their original intent was for a device designed to maintain the circular contour of the capsular bag, they also created an effective new approach for managing zonular weakness. In 1993, Legler and Witschel[5] were the first to present the placement of an open-ringed polymethylmethacrylate (PMMA) CTR in a human eye during cataract surgery. There are now multiple variations of this simple, innovative device and its use is widespread.

Mechanics of Capsular Tension Rings

The CTR is a PMMA open-ring device with blunt-tipped eyelets at its ends. A CTR can be inserted at any point during cataract surgery following creation of a strong anterior capsulotomy created via capsulorrhexis (**Fig. 26.1a**) or femtosecond laser (**Fig. 26.2**) and can serve to support the capsular bag during surgery as well as provide long-term IOL stabilization.

The diameter of the open-ring is designed to be greater than that of the capsular bag when in its final position. The CTR creates an equally distributed centrifugal force to the equator of the bag. Thereby, the CTR recruits tension from stronger zonules to buttress areas of weak or absent zonules, stabilizing the entire complex. This distribution of support may re-center a mildly subluxed capsular bag, but it will not re-center a severely subluxed capsular bag nor will it cure a progressive zonulopathy. In these situations, a modified capsular tension ring (MCTR) or a capsular tension segment (CTS) provides a stable long-term solution through scleral fixation. A CTR decreases the prevalence of posterior capsule opacification (PCO) following cataract surgery.[6] Whether a CTR will decrease the rate capsular contraction syndrome is still being evaluated (see below).

Patient Evaluation: Indications and Contradictions

Any cause of zonular weakness or loss may be an indication for CTR placement. The most common causes of zonular insuffi-

ciency are pseudoexfoliation syndrome, trauma, previous ocular surgery (e.g., filtering surgery or vitrectomy), hypermature cataracts, and increased axial length.[7-22] Less common causes include Marfan's syndrome, homocystinuria, Weill-Marchesani syndrome, microspherophakia, retinitis pigmentosa, and intraocular neoplasms.[23-32] A full list of causes are as follows:

- Trauma, perforating, and nonperforating
  - Secondary to ocular processes ("consecutive")
    - Staphylomas, ectasias
    - Buphthalmias
    - High myopia
    - Hypermature cataract
    - Syphilis, chronic uveitis
    - Perforated corneal ulcer
    - Displacement by tumors or contracting scars
  - Unknown etiology, possibly hereditary
    - Pseudoexfoliation syndrome
- Primary hereditary systemic disease (hereditary)
  - Marfan's syndrome, inherited (autosomal dominant [AD])
  - Marfan variants (AD)
    - Congenital contractual arachnodactyly
    - Asymmetric Marfan's syndrome
  - Homocystinuria (autosomal recessive [AR])
  - Weill–Marchesani (brachymorphia–spherophakia) (AR, AD)
  - Dominant spherophakia (McGavic type) (AD)
  - Simple ectopia lentis et pupillae (AR)
  - Hyperlysinemia (AR)
  - Sulfite oxidase deficiency (AR)
- Primary hereditary systemic disease, infrequently associated with ectopia lentis
  - Aniridia with microcornea
  - Conradi's syndrome
  - Crouzon's disease
  - Dominantly inherited blepharoptosis, high myopia, and ectopia lentis
  - Ehlers–Danlos syndrome
  - Familial pseudomarfanism
  - Kniest syndrome
  - Mandibulofacial dysostosis
  - Megalophthalmos
  - Oxycephaly
  - Pfaundler syndrome
  - Pierre Robin syndrome
  - Proportional dwarfism and ectopia lentis
  - Refsum's syndrome

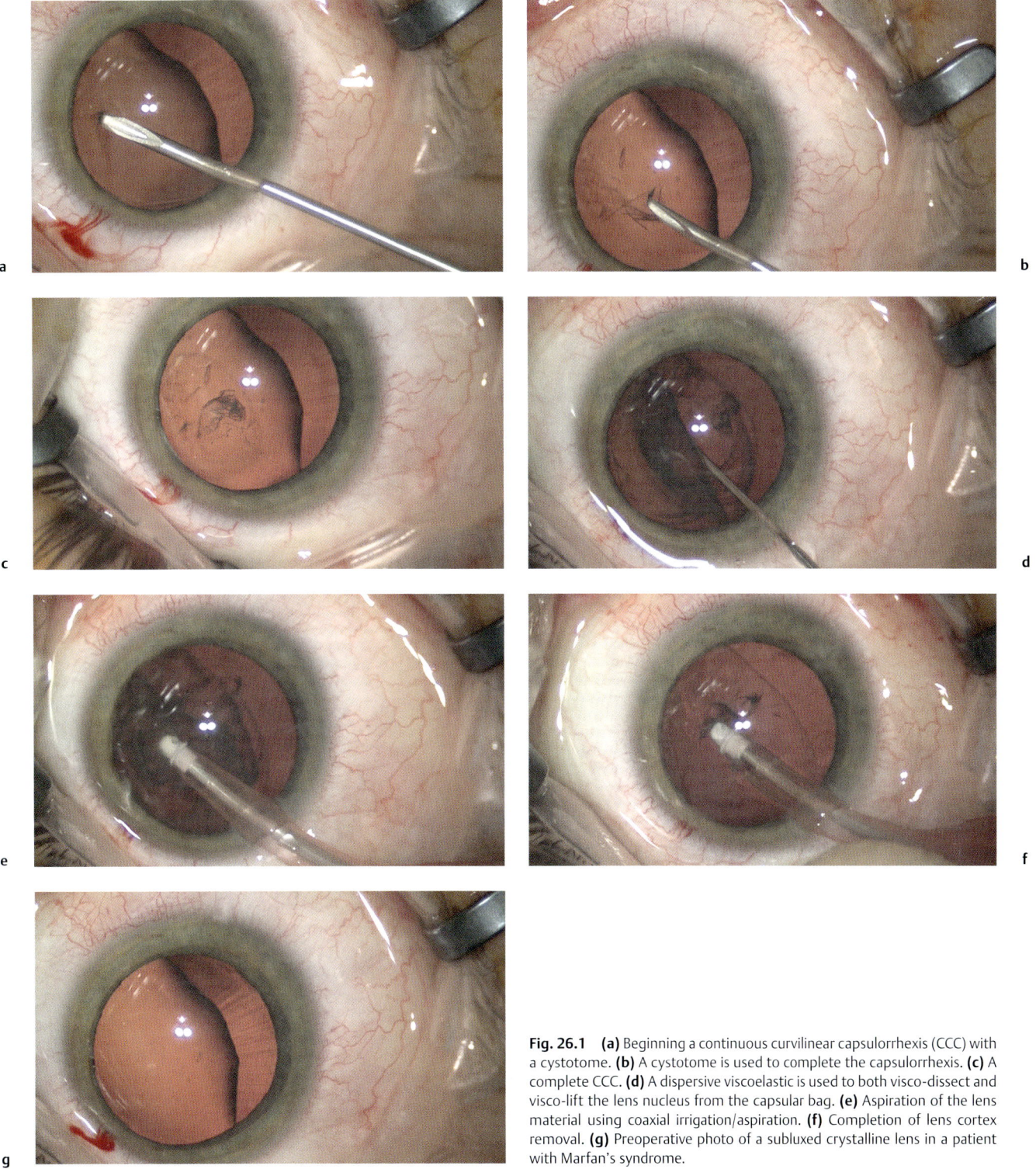

Fig. 26.1 **(a)** Beginning a continuous curvilinear capsulorrhexis (CCC) with a cystotome. **(b)** A cystotome is used to complete the capsulorrhexis. **(c)** A complete CCC. **(d)** A dispersive viscoelastic is used to both visco-dissect and visco-lift the lens nucleus from the capsular bag. **(e)** Aspiration of the lens material using coaxial irrigation/aspiration. **(f)** Completion of lens cortex removal. **(g)** Preoperative photo of a subluxed crystalline lens in a patient with Marfan's syndrome.

- Retinitis pigmentosa
- Sprengel's deformity
- Sturge-Weber syndrome
- Wildervanck syndrome

If there exists significant decentration or phacodonesis, a standard CTR is not likely to provide adequate support. When these conditions exist, a scleral fixation CTR design provides better long-term centration and stabilization.

A contraindication to the use of a CTR is an anterior or posterior capsular tear. In the setting of a noncontinuous capsular tear, the centrifugal force generated by the ring may cause tear extension and risk loss of the CTR to the posterior segment.[33] It may be possible to utilize a CTS in these cases.[13,14]

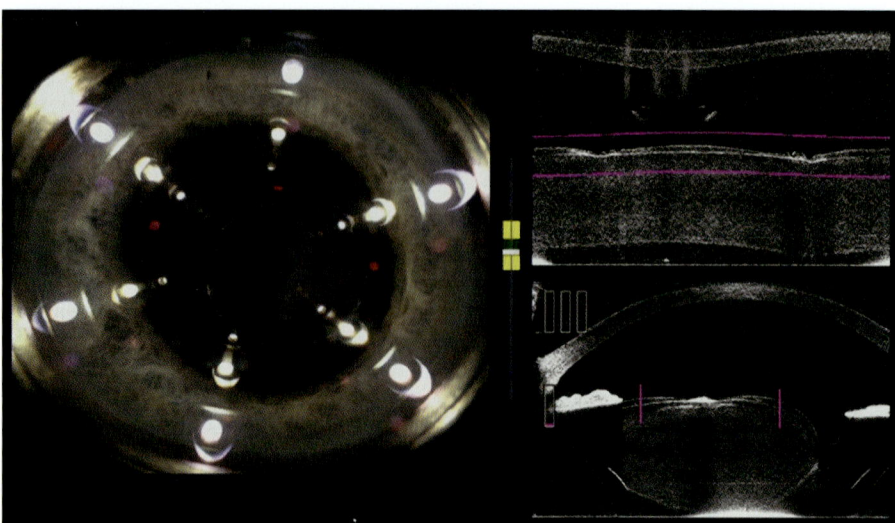

Fig. 26.2 Femtosecond laser creation of anterior capsulotomy; note the area of traumatic zonular dialysis.

Device Types

Standard Capsular Tension Ring

The general structure and mechanics of the standard CTR are discussed above. Both Morcher (Stuttgart, Germany) and Ophtec (Groningen, The Netherlands) manufacture CTRs that are approved by the United States Food and Drug Administration (FDA). The Morcher ring is currently distributed in the United States by FCI Ophthalmics (Pembroke, MA) and Alcon Laboratories, Inc. (Fort Worth, TX), and is available in three sizes: 12.3 mm (compresses to 10.0 mm), 13.0 mm (compresses to 11.0 mm), and 14.5 mm (compresses to 12.0 mm). The Ophtec ring is distributed in the United States by Abbott Medical Optics (Irvine, CA) and is available in a 13-mm ring (compresses to 11 mm) and a 12.0-mm ring (compresses to 10.0 mm). Insertion of the ring can be accomplished manually with forceps or by using an injector. All of the above rings are also available in a preloaded, single-use injector, which is our preferred method of insertion. Geuder (Heidelberg, Germany) and Ophtec make reusable injectors designed for one-handed implantation of the CTRs; Ophtec CTRs are not compatible with the Geuder injector.

A modification of the standard CTR design is the Henderson Ring,[34] which features eight equally spaced indentations spanning the circumference of the ring creating a sinusoidal shape. The indentations enable nuclear and cortical material removal while still maintaining the desired stretch of the capsular bag.

Selecting Capsular Tension Ring Size

Capsular bag dimensions dictate the size of CTR selected. *Overlap of the terminal eyelets is required for maximum circumferential support.* As shown by Vass et al[35] and others,[36] the size of the capsular bag correlates with globe axial length and corneal diameter. As such, horizontal white-to-white and axial length measurements should guide a surgeon's CTR selection. Using a larger CTR ensures overlap of the end terminals but may be more challenging to insert.

Modified Capsular Tension Ring

The modified capsular tension ring[37] was developed as a solution to profound zonular insufficiency (**Fig. 26.1g**) allowing surgeons to anchor an intact capsular bag to the scleral wall. As with the standard CTR, the MCTR utilizes a PMMA open-ring design, but, unlike the standard CTR, there are one or two fixation eyelets attached to the ring, which enable it to be sutured to the sclera (**Fig 26.3 a**). The eyelets protrude 0.25 mm forward from the ring of the CTR and sit anterior to the anterior capsule. A more recent modification designed by Boris Malyugin[38] incorporates a pigtail curve at the terminus of one end of the ring such that the fixation eyelet rests at a plane anterior to the plane of the remainder of the ring. This design enables insertion with an injector (**Figs. 26.5a,b**). An adequately sized capsulotomy (5–6.5 mm) is desired to ensure safe removal of the cataract, stable positioning of the ring, and proper interface of the hook of the MCTR eyelet with the capsulorrhexis margin (**Fig. 26.3,4,6**).[13]

Capsular Tension Segment

Similar to the MCTR, the CTS was also created for patients with extensive and/or progressive zonular loss.[13,14] The partial PMMA ring segment spans a 120-degree arc with a radius of 4.5 or 5 mm and with an anteriorly positioned fixation eyelet. Unlike the CTR and MCTR, the CTS can be utilized in cases where a discontinuous capsulorrhexis, anterior capsule tear, or a posterior capsule tear is present, as it does not generate a 360-degree expansile force. Multiple CTSs can be used when necessary. The CTS provides support in the transverse plane, and must be combined with a CTR or MCTR when circumferential support is required. The CTS may also be used for intraoperative support and removed prior to completion of the case. The CTS is available in two different radii of curvature: 4.5 mm (model 6E) and 5.0 mm (model 6D).

Choice of Device and Timing of Placement

The choice of the capsular tension device in a particular situation depends on the cause of capsular bag instability as well as surgeon comfort and preference regarding the available device options. Progressive zonular disorders (e.g., pseudoexfoliation, Marfan's syndrome) should be thought of as separate from nonprogressive zonular defects (e.g., prior trauma, iatrogenic). One must also consider the amount of zonular loss or generalized zonular instability.

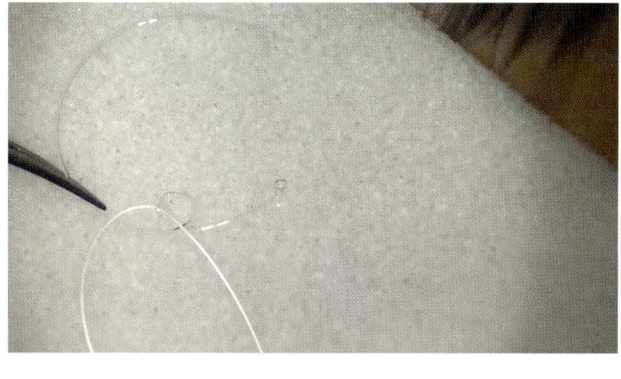

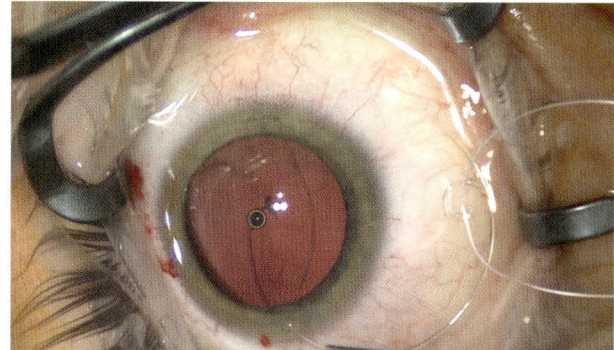

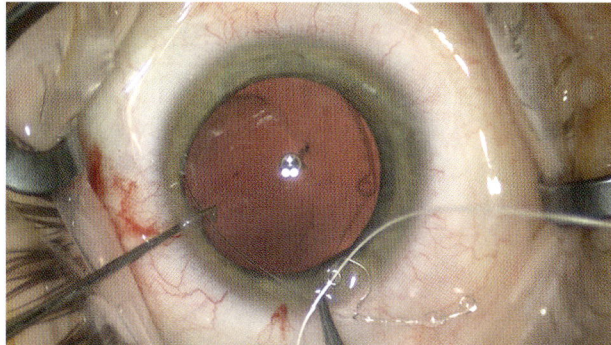

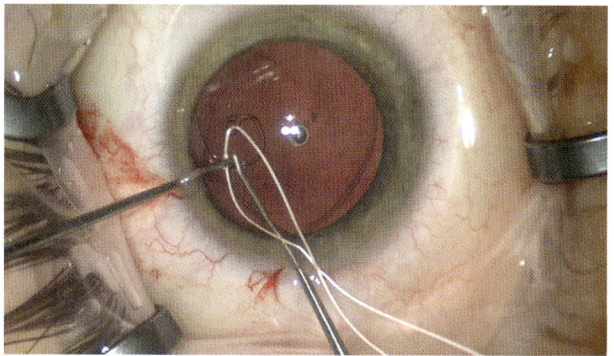

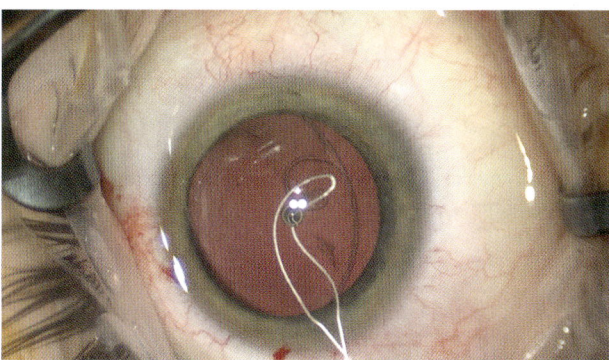

Fig. 26.3 **(a)** Passing a CV-8 expanded polytetrafluoroethylene suture through the fixation eyelet of the modified capsular tension ring (MCTR). **(b)** Manual insertion of the MCTR into the capsular bag. **(c)** Continuation of manual insertion of the MCTR, using a second instrument to guide the placement of the ring. **(d)** Continuation of manual insertion. **(e)** The MCTR within the capsular bag after dialing into position for fixation.

In cases where the remaining zonules are expected to be strong, a standard CTR may enable adequate redistribution of zonular force, compensating for an area of zonular weakness or dialysis.[7,11,12,15] More generally, CTRs are indicated in cases of mild, diffuse zonular weakness or small, localized zonular dialysis (generally less than 4 clock hour positions). In more advanced or progressive zonulopathies, a scleral-fixated MCTR or CTS paired with a CTR likely provides the best long-term solution.[13,37,39–42]

The timing of placement may also dictate the type of device used. Early ring placement provides capsular distention to prevent capsular bag collapse during phacoemulsification or cortex aspiration.[7,10] Placement of a CTR or MCTR requires the device to be dialed into position, which may require more manipulation prior to or during phacoemulsification and thus cause zonular trauma. Ahmed et al[43] demonstrated that early CTR placement leads to greater zonular stress and iatrogenic zonular trauma when compared with CTR placement after cataract and cortex removal. Early ring placement also makes cortex removal difficult. If early placement is necessary, one might consider a Henderson CTR or a CTS to provide greater ease of aspiration of cortex. In addition, a CTS can be placed relatively atraumatically on account of its smaller size, requiring less manipulation for adequate positioning. In the setting of an anterior or posterior capsular tear, which are contraindications to the use of a CTR or MCTR, a CTS

can be used due its transverse force rather than circumferential force.

Method of Insertion

As stated above, it is our preference to utilize single-use injectors with a preloaded CTR. If there is worry that the insertion of the CTR will exacerbate existing zonular damage, over-bending the ring during insertion by providing countertraction with a suture or second instrument can provide a more gentle insertion (**Fig. 26.4a–d**). When a case requires placement of an MCTR, it is our current preference to inject a preloaded Morcher-type 10 L 9 (based on the Malyugin Design) pre-loaded with suture (**Fig. 26.5a,b**). An alternative method is to insert, by hand, a standard Cionni Modified CTR. Our method for scleral fixation is a variation of an ab externo technique previously described by Slade et al[44] (**Fig. 26.3, and 26.6**). This technique uses a micro-vitreo-retinal blade to create sclerotomies and an internal limiting membrane forceps or Condon Snare (MicroSurgical Technology, Redmond, WA) to retrieve a CV-8 expanded polytetrauoroethylene (Gore-Tex, not labeled for ophthalmic use) or 9-0 polypropylene suture pre-passed through the eyelet of the MCTR (**Fig. 26.6a**). This same method of fixation is also our preference for CTS fixation.

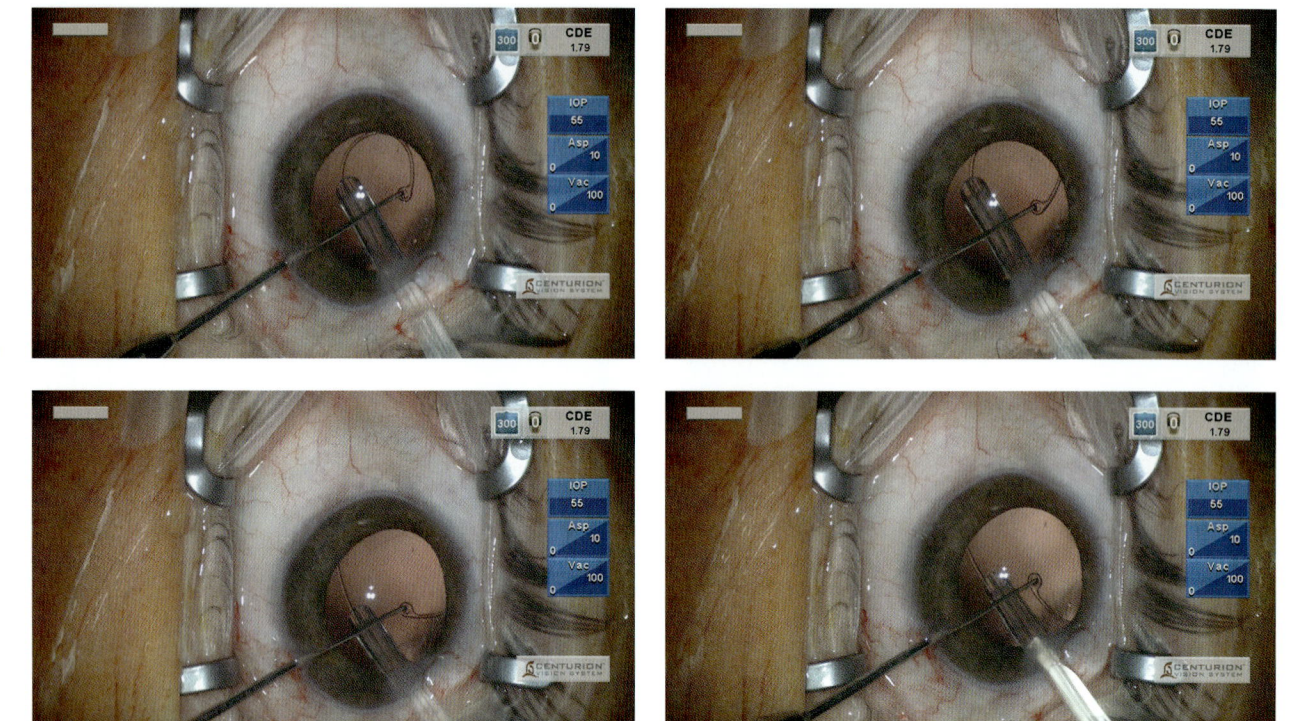

Fig. 26.4 **(a–d)** Providing countertraction with a Sinskey hook in the leading eyelet of a CTR during injection into the capsular bag to provide more uniform centrifugal force during insertion compared with standard insertion.

Intraoperative and Postoperative Capsular Stability

Early studies of capsular tension rings demonstrated their range of use, level of safety, and effectiveness.[13,18] These early studies agreed that a CTR improves capsular stability, decreases intraoperative adverse events, and maintains postoperative IOL centration in the setting of mild zonular weakness or loss.

More recent papers have also demonstrated IOL stability and centration over time after CTR placement.[16] In a small case-control series, Takimoto and colleagues[45] found no significant differences in the mean degree of IOL decentration, tilt angle, anterior capsule opening area, or refractive prediction error when comparing eyes with zonular instability requiring CTR implantation during cataract surgery to fellow eyes without zonular instability. In 2013, Wang et al[21] reported their results of a retrospective review of 84 eyes of 82 patients receiving a CTR during cataract surgery. The main indications for CTR insertion were previous trauma, pseudoexfoliation syndrome, and mature cataracts. An intraocular lens was successfully implanted in the bag in 72 eyes (85.7%) **(Fig. 26.7a,b)**. A posterior capsule tear was the most common intraoperative complication (3.6%). Postoperatively, the most common complications were a decentered intraocular lens (8.3%) and persistent corneal edema (6.0%). Overall, 61 eyes (72.6%) had better postoperative visual acuity compared with preoperative acuity, with 67 patients (79.8%) achieving vision of 20/40 or better. These recent papers demonstrate that in eyes with zonular dehiscence or weakness, a CTR can prevent marked IOL decentration, tilt, and severe anterior capsule contraction, and may lead to prevention of a refractive prediction error.

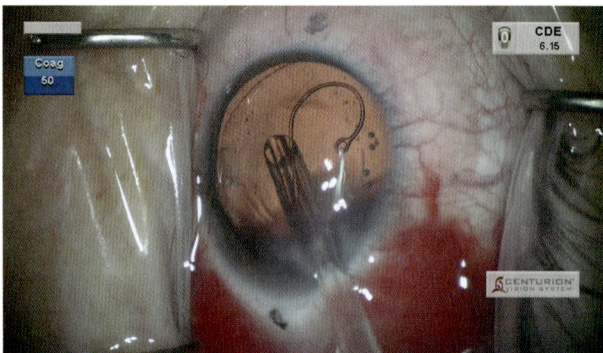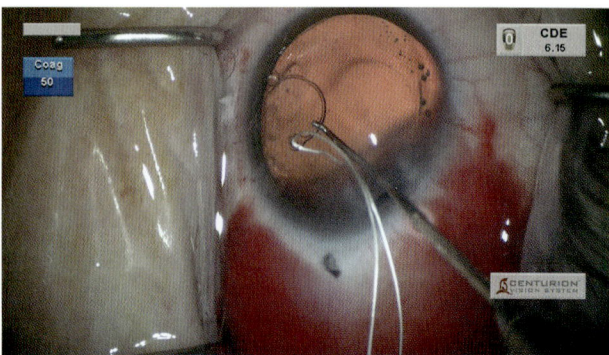

Fig. 26.5 **(a)** Injection of the Malyugin modification of the MCTR, preloaded with suture. **(b)** Positioning of the Malyugin MCTR with a Sinskey hook following injection into the capsular bag.

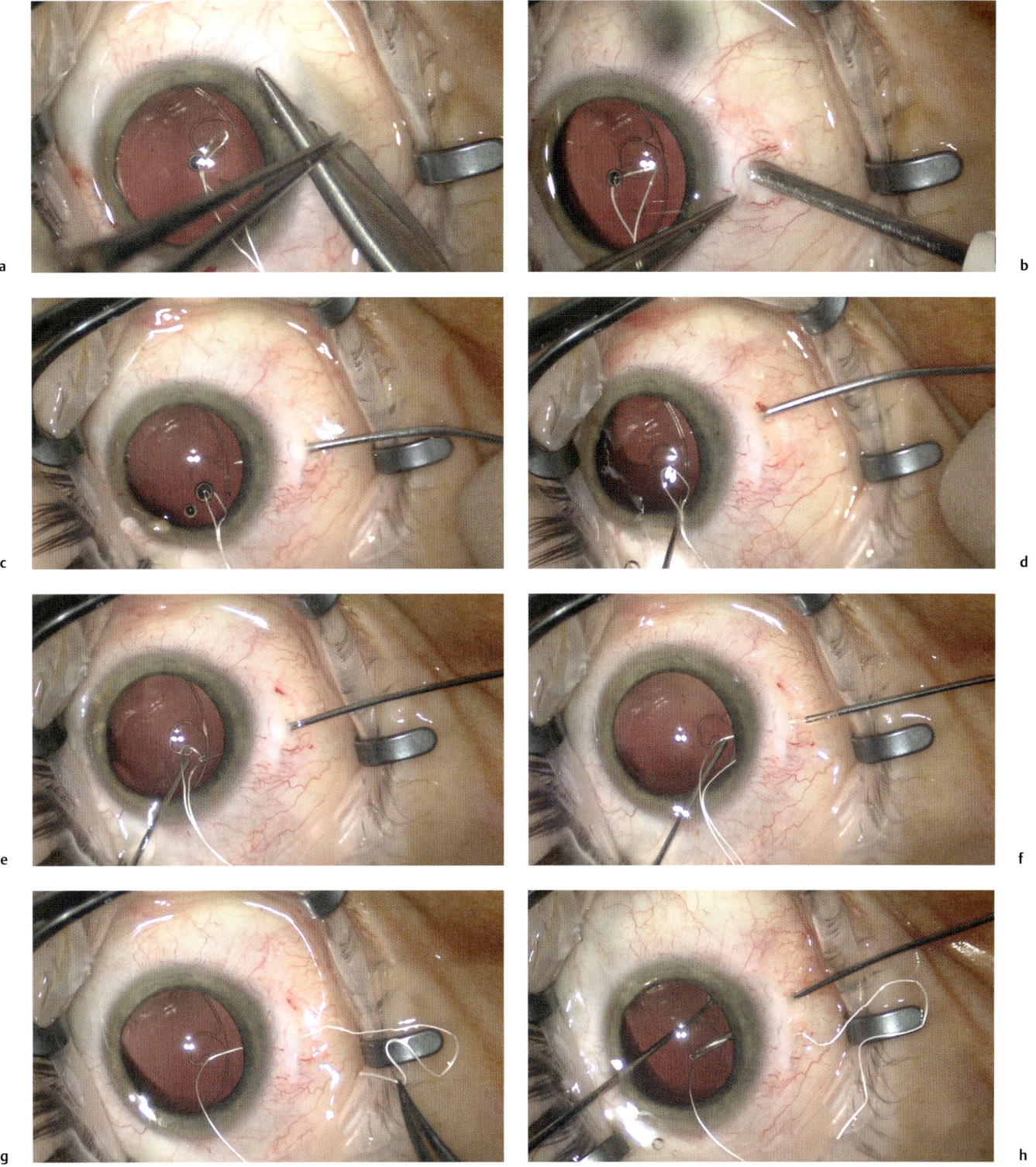

Fig. 26.6 **(a)** Creation of a localized peritomy. **(b)** Wet-field cautery to exposed episcleral blood vessels. **(c)** A 23-gauge microvitreoretinal blade is used to create a sclerotomy ~ 2 mm posterior to the limbus, with care taken to pass the tip of the blade in a plane parallel to the iris without puncturing the capsular bag. **(d)** An adjacent sclerotomy is created in a similar fashion. **(e)** The suture is retrieved using a 25-gauge internal limiting membrane forceps. **(f)** The suture is externalized. **(g)** The suture end has been fully externalized. **(h)** The other suture end is externalized in a similar fashion. (continued on page 204)

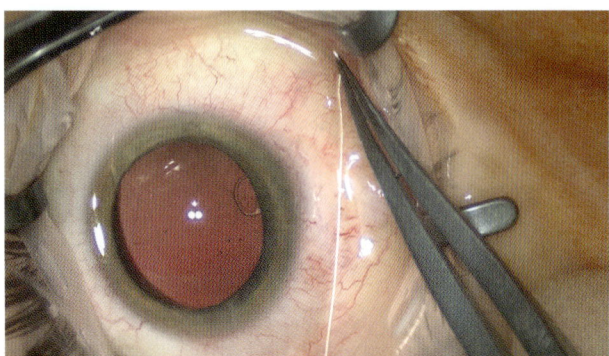

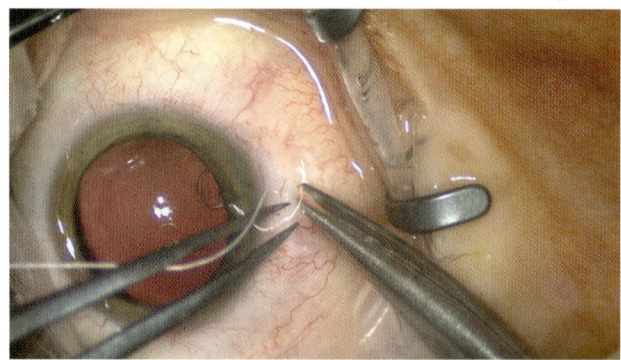

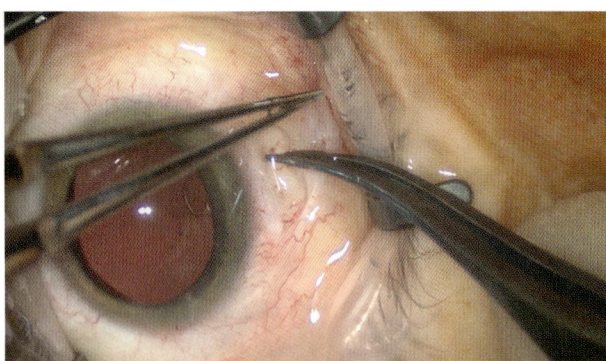

Fig. 26.6 (*continued*)   **(i)** Proper tensioning of the suture allows for centralization of the capsular bag–MCTR complex. **(j)** After locking the suture, the suture ends are trimmed. **(k)** The knot is rotated and buried within the sclerotomy. The peritomy is then closed (not pictured).

The body of evidence supporting the safety and use of CTRs in children has also continued to expand. In 2009, Das et al[29] prospectively followed 18 eyes of 15 children with subluxation of crystalline or cataractous lenses between 90 and 210 degrees after phacoemulsification, CTR, and IOL implantation. Sixteen eyes had a best corrected visual acuity (BCVA) of 20/40 or better. Nine eyes developed PCO and were managed with neodymium: yttrium-aluminum-garnet (Nd:YAG) laser posterior capsulotomy. One eye had IOL dislocation after 2 years.

Refractive Outcome

Several studies have sought to describe CTR impact on refractive outcomes.

Boomer and Jackson[46] found no statistical difference in refractive predictive errors in a small case-control series, leading them to conclude that the use of a CTR had no consistent effect on refractive outcome, and modification of IOL power calculations was unnecessary. In a separate publication,[47] they also demonstrated that following CTR placement, the CTR and IOL remained in the bag with the CTR positioned between the IOL haptics and the ciliary body.

In 2009, Rohart and Gatinel[48] found in uneventful cataract surgery that a CTR does not improve the optical quality of the pseudophakic eye. Subsequently, Schild et al[49] compared refractive outcomes in myopic eyes between phacoemulsification and IOL implantation with and without a CTR. There was no statistically significant difference in the mean absolute refractive prediction error between the CTR group and the control, but there was lower variance in the absolute refractive prediction error in the CTR group. They concluded that a CTR had no consistent effect on refractive outcomes in highly myopic eyes, although there was a tendency toward higher precision in outcomes with a CTR. As with Boomer and Jackson, their results indicated that the IOL power calculation does not have to be changed when a CTR is used.

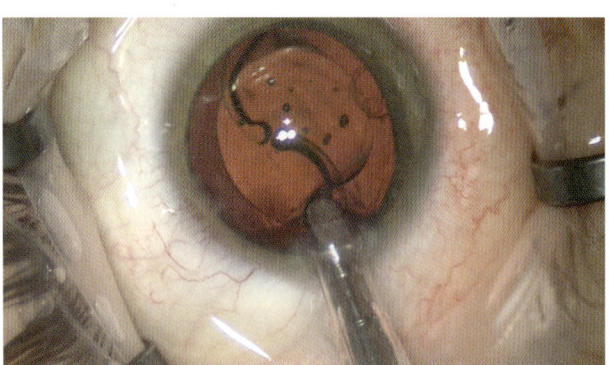

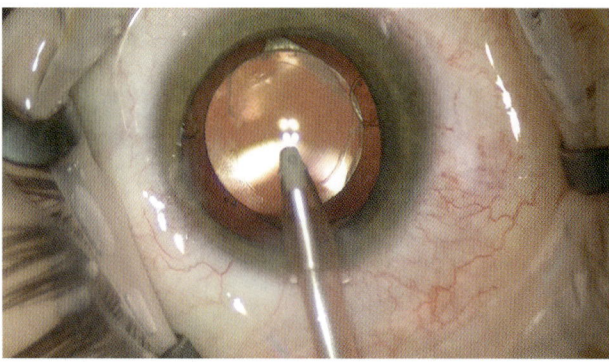

Fig. 26.7   **(a)** The intraocular lens (in this case, a single-piece acrylic diffractive multifocal IOL) is inserted into the capsular bag. **(b)** The viscoelastic is removed at the completion of the procedure.

Mastropasqua et al[50] demonstrated in a 2013 prospective, randomized trial of 60 eyes that an inclusion of a CTR implant paired with a diffractive multifocal IOL reduced the ocular wavefront error related to a reduction of third-order aberration when compared with multifocal IOL placement alone. The authors attributed this reduced wavefront error to better IOL position.

Late Spontaneous in-the-Bag IOL and CTR Dislocation

Capsular contraction syndrome (CCS) was an early reported postoperative problem despite attempted prevention with CTR placement,[24,25,51,52] and, along with pseudoexfoliation, is a leading risk factor for late spontaneous in-the-bag IOL dislocation.[53,54] More recent publications have sought to describe the conditions leading to subluxation or dislocation despite CTR use.

In a 2012 retrospective case series, Werner et al[55] described the clinical and pathological findings from cases of in-the-bag CTR and IOL subluxation or dislocation. Patients were an average age of 76 years at explantation, which was performed 6.8 years after implantation. The IOLs in these cases were of varying designs and materials. Associated ocular conditions included pseudoexfoliation (n = 17), glaucoma (n = 4), vitrectomy/retina surgery (n = 3), and trauma (n = 1). Moderate to severe degrees of Soemmering's ring formation and capsulorrhexis phimosis were observed or reported in 13 and 11 specimens, respectively. Fourteen eyes were implanted and explanted by the same surgeon, with an average interval of 7.75 years between the procedures, equating to a 0.76% rate of explantation of the CTRs implanted during the time considered.

Modified Capsular Tension Ring and Capsular Tension Segment: Recent Literature

In 2012, Vasavada et al[40] and Buttanri et al[41] published similar reports of the intraoperative performance and postoperative outcomes of MCTR implantation in eyes with subluxed crystalline lenses. The separate case series both demonstrated overall improvement in BCVA, with low rates of symptomatic decentration postoperatively. The most common complication was PCO, occurring in 34% and 50%, respectively.

In 2014, Kim et al[42] published a retrospective, observational case series of 13 consecutive pediatric patients (19 eyes) who underwent placement of in-the-bag IOL with either an MCTR or a CTS in conjunction with a conventional CTR. An MCTR was implanted in five eyes and a CTS with an unsutured capsular tension ring was implanted in 12 eyes; in two eyes, a capsular tension segment alone was placed. The mean BCVA at the final follow-up was significantly better than preoperatively, with the BCVA at final follow-up being 20/40 or better in 18 eyes (94.7%). All IOLs were well centered. Posterior capsule opacification developed in 11 eyes (57.9%), with nine eyes (47.4%) requiring Nd:YAG capsulotomy, and three eyes (15.8%) requiring pars plana vitrectomy and posterior capsulotomy.

The above studies provide additional evidence that the use of an MCTR or CTS with CTR is a safe and effective technique for visual rehabilitation in subluxed crystalline lenses in both adult and pediatric patients.

Conclusion

Zonular instability during phacoemulsification can effectively be managed intraoperatively and postoperatively using a capsular tension device. Determining the proper capsular tension device depends on the amount of zonular loss, the likelihood of progressive weakness, and capsular integrity. Skilled and knowledgeable management will reap the reward of excellent surgical results with the subsequent satisfying outcome for both patient and surgeon.

References

1. Nagamoto T, Bissen-Miyajima H. A ring to support the capsular bag after continuous curvilinear capsulorhexis. J Cataract Refract Surg 1994;20:417–420
2. Nagamoto T. Origin of the capsular tension ring. J Cataract Refract Surg 2001;27:1710–1711
3. Hara T, Hara T, Yamada Y. "Equator ring" for maintenance of the completely circular contour of the capsular bag equator after cataract removal. Ophthalmic Surg 1991;22:358–359
4. Hara T, Hara T, Sakanishi K, Yamada Y. Efficacy of equator rings in an experimental rabbit study. Arch Ophthalmol 1995;113:1060–1065
5. Legler UFC, Witschel BM, eds. The capsular ring: a new device for complicated cataract surgery. Presented at American Society of Cataract and Refractive Surgery (ASCRS) Symposium on Cataract, Intraocular Lens, and Refractive Surgery, Seattle, 1993
6. D'Eliseo D, Pastena B, Longanesi L, Grisanti F, Negrini V. Prevention of posterior capsule opacification using capsular tension ring for zonular defects in cataract surgery. Eur J Ophthalmol 2003;13:151–154
7. Gimbel HV, Sun R, Heston JP. Management of zonular dialysis in phacoemulsification and IOL implantation using the capsular tension ring. Ophthalmic Surg Lasers 1997;28:273–281
8. Lam DS, Young AL, Leung AT, Rao SK, Fan DS, Ng JS. Scleral fixation of a capsular tension ring for severe ectopia lentis. J Cataract Refract Surg 2000;26:609–612
9. Menapace R, Findl O, Georgopoulos M, Rainer G, Vass C, Schmetterer K. The capsular tension ring: designs, applications, and techniques. J Cataract Refract Surg 2000;26:898–912
10. Bayraktar S, Altan T, Küçüksümer Y, Yilmaz OF. Capsular tension ring implantation after capsulorhexis in phacoemulsification of cataracts associated with pseudoexfoliation syndrome. Intraoperative complications and early postoperative findings. J Cataract Refract Surg 2001;27:1620–1628
11. Gimbel HV, Sun R. Clinical applications of capsular tension rings in cataract surgery. Ophthalmic Surg Lasers 2002;33:44–53
12. Jacob S, Agarwal A, Agarwal A, Agarwal S, Patel N, Lal V. Efficacy of a capsular tension ring for phacoemulsification in eyes with zonular dialysis. J Cataract Refract Surg 2003;29:315–321
13. Hasanee K, Butler M, Ahmed II. Capsular tension rings and related devices: current concepts. Curr Opin Ophthalmol 2006;17:31–41
14. Hasanee K, Ahmed II. Capsular tension rings: update on endocapsular support devices. Ophthalmol Clin North Am 2006;19:507–519
15. Tribus C, Alge CS, Haritoglou C, et al. Indications and clinical outcome of capsular tension ring (CTR) implantation: A review of 9528 cataract surgeries. Clin Ophthalmol 2007;1:65–69
16. Georgopoulos GT, Papaconstantinou D, Georgalas I, Koutsandrea CN, Margetis I, Moschos MM. Management of large traumatic zonular dialysis with phacoemulsification and IOL implantation using the capsular tension ring. Acta Ophthalmol Scand 2007;85:653–657
17. Kocabora MS, Gulkilik G, Yilmazli C, Taskapili M, Kucuksahin H, Doyduk-Kocabora A. The preventive effect of capsular tension ring in phacoemulsification of senile cataracts with pseudoexfoliation. Ann Ophthalmol (Skokie) 2007;39:37–40
18. Blecher MH, Kirk MR. Surgical strategies for the management of zonular compromise. Curr Opin Ophthalmol 2008;19:31–35
19. Chee SP, Jap A. Management of traumatic severely subluxated cataracts. Am J Ophthalmol 2011;151:866–871.e1
20. Ma KT, Kim JH, Kim NR, Jang DS, Seong GJ, Kim CY. Scleral fixation of standard capsular tension ring and in-the-bag intraocular lens implantation in patients with severe lens subluxation. Ophthalmic Surg Lasers Imaging 2012;43:504–507
21. Wang BZ, Chan E, Vajpayee RB. A retrospective study of the indications and outcomes of capsular tension ring insertion during cataract surgery at a tertiary teaching hospital. Clin Ophthalmol 2013;7:567–572

22. Serna-Ojeda JC, Cordova-Cervantes J, Lopez-Salas M, et al. Management of traumatic cataract in adults at a reference center in Mexico City. Int Ophthalmol 2014

23. Groessl SA, Anderson CJ. Capsular tension ring in a patient with Weill-Marchesani syndrome. J Cataract Refract Surg 1998;24:1164–1165

24. Dietlein TS, Jacobi PC, Konen W, Krieglstein GK. Complications of endocapsular tension ring implantation in a child with Marfan's syndrome. J Cataract Refract Surg 2000;26:937–940

25. Sudhir RR, Rao SK. Capsulorhexis phimosis in retinitis pigmentosa despite capsular tension ring implantation. J Cataract Refract Surg 2001; 27:1691–1694

26. Mizuno H, Yamada J, Nishiura M, Takahashi H, Hino Y, Miyatani H. Capsular tension ring use in a patient with congenital coloboma of the lens. J Cataract Refract Surg 2004;30:503–506

27. Konradsen T, Kugelberg M, Zetterström C. Visual outcomes and complications in surgery for ectopia lentis in children. J Cataract Refract Surg 2007;33:819–824

28. Vasavada V, Vasavada VA, Hoffman RO, Spencer TS, Kumar RV, Crandall AS. Intraoperative performance and postoperative outcomes of endocapsular ring implantation in pediatric eyes. J Cataract Refract Surg 2008;34:1499–1508

29. Das P, Ram J, Brar GS, Dogra MR. Results of intraocular lens implantation with capsular tension ring in subluxated crystalline or cataractous lenses in children. Indian J Ophthalmol 2009;57:431–436

30. Guo S, Wagner R, Forbes B, Tannen B, Caputo A. Capsular tension ring in the management of occult lens zonular dehiscence in infantile glaucoma. J Pediatr Ophthalmol Strabismus 2010;47:e1–e3

31. Dikopf MS, Chow CC, Mieler WF, Tu EY. Cataract extraction outcomes and the prevalence of zonular insufficiency in retinitis pigmentosa. Am J Ophthalmol 2013;156:82–88.e2

32. Bayyoud T, Bartz-Schmidt KU, Yoeruek E. Long-term clinical results after cataract surgery with and without capsular tension ring in patients with retinitis pigmentosa: a retrospective study. BMJ Open 2013;3:3

33. Bhattacharjee H, Bhattacharjee K, Das D, Jain PK, Chakraborty D, Deka S. Management of a posteriorly dislocated endocapsular tension ring and a foldable acrylic intraocular lens. J Cataract Refract Surg 2004;30:243–246

34. Henderson BA, Kim JY. Modified capsular tension ring for cortical removal after implantation. J Cataract Refract Surg 2007;33:1688–1690

35. Vass C, Menapace R, Schmetterer K, Findl O, Rainer G, Steineck I. Prediction of pseudophakic capsular bag diameter based on biometric variables. J Cataract Refract Surg 1999;25:1376–1381

36. Dong EY, Joo CK. Predictability for proper capsular tension ring size and intraocular lens size. Korean J Ophthalmol 2001;15:22–26

37. Cionni RJ, Osher RH. Management of profound zonular dialysis or weakness with a new endocapsular ring designed for scleral fixation. J Cataract Refract Surg 1998;24:1299–1306

38. Malyugin B. Cataract surgery when capsular support is poor. Ophthamology Management. 2012;16:50–53

39. Cionni RJ, Osher RH, Marques DM, Marques FF, Snyder ME, Shapiro S. Modified capsular tension ring for patients with congenital loss of zonular support. J Cataract Refract Surg 2003;29:1668–1673

40. Vasavada AR, Praveen MR, Vasavada VA, et al. Cionni ring and in-the-bag intraocular lens implantation for subluxated lenses: a prospective case series. Am J Ophthalmol 2012;153:1144–53.e1

41. Buttanri IB, Sevim MS, Esen D, Acar BT, Serin D, Acar S. Modified capsular tension ring implantation in eyes with traumatic cataract and loss of zonular support. J Cataract Refract Surg 2012;38:431–436

42. Kim EJ, Berg JP, Weikert MP, et al. Scleral-fixated capsular tension rings and segments for ectopia lentis in children. Am J Ophthalmol 2014;158: 899–904

43. Ahmed II, Cionni RJ, Kranemann C, Crandall AS. Optimal timing of capsular tension ring implantation: Miyake-Apple video analysis. J Cataract Refract Surg 2005;31:1809–1813

44. Slade DS, Hater MA, Cionni RJ, Crandall AS. Ab externo scleral fixation of intraocular lens. J Cataract Refract Surg 2012;38:1316–1321

45. Takimoto M, Hayashi K, Hayashi H. Effect of a capsular tension ring on prevention of intraocular lens decentration and tilt and on anterior capsule contraction after cataract surgery. Jpn J Ophthalmol 2008;52:363–367

46. Boomer JA, Jackson DW. Effect of the Morcher capsular tension ring on refractive outcome. J Cataract Refract Surg 2006;32:1180–1183

47. Boomer JA, Jackson DW. Anatomic evaluation of the Morcher capsular tension ring by ultrasound biomicroscopy. J Cataract Refract Surg 2006; 32:846–848

48. Rohart C, Gatinel D. Influence of a capsular tension ring on ocular aberrations after cataract surgery: a comparative study. J Refract Surg 2009; 25(1, Suppl):S116–S121

49. Schild AM, Rosentreter A, Hellmich M, Lappas A, Dinslage S, Dietlein TS. Effect of a capsular tension ring on refractive outcomes in eyes with high myopia. J Cataract Refract Surg 2010;36:2087–2093

50. Mastropasqua R, Toto L, Vecchiarino L, Falconio G, Nicola MD, Mastropasqua A. Multifocal IOL implant with or without capsular tension ring: study of wavefront error and visual performance. Eur J Ophthalmol 2013; 23:510–517

51. Faschinger CW, Eckhardt M. Complete capsulorhexis opening occlusion despite capsular tension ring implantation. J Cataract Refract Surg 1999; 25:1013–1015

52. Waheed K, Eleftheriadis H, Liu C. Anterior capsular phimosis in eyes with a capsular tension ring. J Cataract Refract Surg 2001;27:1688–1690

53. Gimbel HV, Condon GP, Kohnen T, Olson RJ, Halkiadakis I. Late in-the-bag intraocular lens dislocation: incidence, prevention, and management. J Cataract Refract Surg 2005;31:2193–2204

54. Jakobsson G, Zetterberg M, Lundström M, Stenevi U, Grenmark R, Sundelin K. Late dislocation of in-the-bag and out-of-the bag intraocular lenses: ocular and surgical characteristics and time to lens repositioning. J Cataract Refract Surg 2010;36:1637–1644

55. Werner L, Zaugg B, Neuhann T, Burrow M, Tetz M. In-the-bag capsular tension ring and intraocular lens subluxation or dislocation: a series of 23 cases. Ophthalmology 2012;119:266–271

Section X Intraocular Lens Implantation in the Absence of Adequate Capsular Support

27 Scleral and Iris Sutured Posterior Chamber Intraocular Lenses and Intraocular Knot-Tying Techniques

Gregory S.H. Ogawa

Scleral Sutured Posterior Chamber Intraocular Lenses

The origins of transscleral sutured posterior chamber intraocular lenses (PCIOLs) date back to the 1980s,[1,2] and although it is currently performed with many different techniques, no gold-standard method has emerged. Just as several different factors affect a surgeon's choice of intraocular lens (IOL) placement in the absence of capsular support, there are also numerous factors that influence the choice of technique for transscleral IOL suturing, such as the patient's age, the availability of various suture material and needles, the patient's clinical situation, and, perhaps equally important, the surgeon's experience and level of comfort with the various techniques. We do not have high-level data from evidence-based medicine comparing different techniques, and there may be some level of inter-surgeon variation for the outcomes even with any particular technique. Despite there not being a gold-standard technique that is considered superior in all situations, transscleral sutured PCIOLs, as a category, are a useful part of the armamentarium for IOL fixation in the absence of capsule support.

Fundamental Principles

Regardless of the actual technique one uses for scleral suturing of PCIOLs, there are some core principles that may help surgeons optimize patient outcomes.

Eye Pressurization

Keeping the eye pressurized during the procedure has several advantages. It decreases the potential for intraocular bleeding associated with needle or blade passes through the sclera and ciliary body, and helps to minimize the tendency for suprachoroidal effusions or hemorrhages. A pressurized eye maintains its normal anatomic configuration, which makes it easier to properly position and secure the PCIOL. In most scleral sutured IOL situations, the lens capsule diaphragm is not intact, so an infusion source is needed to keep the eye pressurized. Most commonly that is achieved with a high-flow, self-retaining infusion cannula placed through a limbal paracentesis opening. If the procedure is done in conjunction with a retina specialist performing a pars plana vitrectomy, then the pars plana infusion cannula may be left in place for the sutured IOL portion of the procedure. The other side of the equation for maintaining pressure in the eye during surgery is to minimize fluid outflow. Perhaps the most important way to do this is to create self-sealing incisions. That principle should be applied to limbal paracentesis openings all the way up to 7-mm-wide scleral tunnel incisions

that accommodate one-piece polymethylmethacrylate (PMMA) IOLs with eyelets on the haptics. Even though various incisions may require sutures to stabilize them prior to completion of the procedure, having corneal-valve incision architecture enables outflow to be controlled during the procedure even before any sutures are placed.

Vitreous Management

Appropriate removal of vitreous from the anterior chamber and the area well behind the iris significantly decreases the chance of causing intraoperative vitreous traction with the associated risk of retinal tears and retinal detachment. There can be episodes of fluid flow out of the eye during the procedure, and because vitreous "goes with the flow" of fluid, it is desirable to keep the vitreous well away from the incisions. Much of the work in these cases occurs behind the iris, so the vitreous needs to be removed more thoroughly, and further posteriorly, than is typically done for an unplanned capsule opening during cataract surgery. It is not uncommon to remove the vitreous from the anterior third (or more) of the vitreous cavity to decrease the risk of causing vitreous traction during the surgery as needles and instruments are passed through that space. The general guideline is to keep the vitrectomy cutting tip where the surgeon can see it, but passing it a little way out of view behind the iris with the port aimed posteriorly away from the iris, in the areas where sutures will pass, may be of benefit. It is common for anterior-segment surgeons to be rather uncomfortable guiding the port of the vitrectomy probe more than a couple millimeters behind the iris. One way to improve one's comfort in working further behind the iris is to keep refocusing the microscope on the tip of the vitrectomy probe. As long as the probe is in focus, the surgeon can see anything that the probe could be getting close to, and the concern of getting too close to sensitive structures should decrease.

In a fairly well-sealed system, the vitreous goes to the port of the vitrectomy probe, regardless of where the probe enters the eye. One achieves a more posterior placement of the vitrectomy probe port immediately if the eye is entered through a pars plana incision, but the port on the probe can generally be maneuvered just as far posteriorly through a limbal paracentesis without needing to make the pars plana incisions that are less familiar to the anterior-segment surgeon. Some surgeons find it useful to inject ophthalmic intraocular triamcinolone acetonide suspension (Triesence, Alcon Laboratories, Fort Worth, TX) into the vitreous cavity to better visualize the vitreous needing to be removed. With unhurried, systematic movement of the vitrectomy probe through the desired areas, while focusing on the probe's port to be able to see vitreous entering the port, the vitreous can often be removed just about as effectively without the steroid suspension.

Suture Positioning and Management

In several types of eye surgery, the need for, and emphasis on, sutures has significantly decreased over the past couple decades. For scleral sutured IOL cases, however, positioning, tying, and managing the sutures are central parts of a successful outcome. The sutures determine the position and stability of the IOL. Having a plan for exactly how the sutures will be positioned during all parts of the procedure, and then keeping track of the sutures and consistently managing them according to the plan is necessary for the procedure to go smoothly and to achieve a satisfying outcome. The precise details of suture positioning, tying, and managing vary depending on the technique that the surgeon selects.

Peripheral Iridectomies/Reverse Pupillary Block

When a PCIOL is sutured to the sclera, it creates a relatively firm plane behind the iris with the optic of the IOL almost always being larger than the postoperative pupil. The resulting situation is a uni-chamber eye where the iris can move easily with intraocular fluid movement, but the IOL moves only minimally. The iris can be pushed back against the IOL to create either intermittent or constant from a reverse pupillary block mechanism,[3] analogous to that seen in conventional pigment dispersions syndrome. This probably results from the fluid in the anterior chamber moving posteriorly when the patient blinks. The scleral sutured PCIOL reverse pupillary block seems to be more common in individuals who have less rigid corneas, such as young people, but it can occur in anyone. If the pupil is small, the reverse pupillary block tends to cause pigment dispersion and inflammation. If the pupil is of moderate size or pharmacologically dilated, the reverse pupillary block can be significant enough to push one side of the pupil margin behind the corresponding IOL edge. Although this configuration enables fluid to flow both anteriorly and posteriorly, it usually causes notable pigment dispersion, iritis, and sometimes even iris sphincter damage from the mechanical action between the iris and the IOL. One may have the impression that this abnormal iris configuration is from a poorly positioned IOL, but unless the IOL is highly tilted, the cause is most likely to be from reverse pupillary block.

Because it is not possible to predict exactly which patients with scleral sutured PCIOLs will develop reverse pupillary block, there is merit to creating peripheral iridectomies (PIs) in all patients undergoing the procedure. The openings need to facilitate rapid flow of aqueous through the iris if all degrees of reverse pupillary block are to be avoided. This is in contradistinction to the small, low-flow peripheral iris openings created with a neodymium:yttrium-aluminum-garnet (Nd:YAG) laser to treat standard pupillary block or prevent angle closure. Experience has shown that two iridectomies ~ 0.7 mm in diameter enable adequate flow. Alternatively, a single iridectomy ~ 1.2 mm in diameter should suffice. The main advantages of the two smaller iridectomies is that there is probably less potential for unwanted optical sequelae than with a larger one, and the smaller ones are also less noticeable from a cosmetic standpoint, particularly in light-colored irides. Superior placement of the iridectomies peripheral to the optic of the IOL minimizes cosmetic side effects and does not seem to produce the dysphotopsias described in recent literature with small peripheral laser iridotomies performed in phakic patients. Because a vitrectomy is performed during most sutured PCIOL cases, a very good tool for creating iridectomies is usually already available—the vitrectomy probe (see Peripheral Iridectomy Creation with a Vitrectomy Probe, below). If a patient with a scleral sutured PCIOL who does not have a peripheral iridectomy (or who has too small of an iridectomy) develops the partial optic capture situation, then the use of dilating drops to attempt to get the pupil larger than the optic and release the partial capture configuration can help stop pigment dispersion, iris injury, and inflammation. If dilation works, then the dilation should be maintained until appropriately sized peripheral iridectomies can be created.

Transscleral Sutured Posterior Chamber Intraocular Lens Technique: Example

The following is a description of the technique with which I have two decades of experience, and for which I can provide the most insights. It is an ab-interno technique that uses small-diameter spatula needles, which have the advantage of the smaller tract that they create through vascularized tissues. Good to excellent eye pressurization is maintained throughout the procedure. IOL centration is reliably achieved using visual cues, with the second set of suture needles being passed from a paracentesis anterior to the suture location for the first haptic. (To the best of my knowledge, this maneuver is unique to the way I have been doing scleral sutured IOLs, and is something I have presented at a film festival with coauthors.[4]) Ab-interno techniques, like this one, may be a bit challenging for surgeons not accustomed to passing long, curved trans-chamber needles across the eye, but with practice, proficiency can be achieved. In the procedure description there are some general comments about instrumentation, alternate maneuvers, and tips on how to avoid problems that should broaden the usefulness of the description. At the end of the description there is an explanation of the variation I employ to allow use of expanded polytetrafluoroethylene (e-PTFE) suture (Gore-Tex, W.L. Gore & Associates, Flagstaff, AZ). After the procedure description, there is a discussion of various aspects of scleral sutured PCIOLs. After the iris-sutured IOL part of this chapter, there is a more detailed discussion of various aspects of scleral-sutured PCIOLs.

Procedure Description

Dilating drops are used prior to the procedure, but wide dilation is not as necessary as it is in cataract surgery. In fact, a pupil that is too widely dilated may be a hindrance because the iris tends to bunch up posteriorly and can get in the way of suture passes. If iris hooks are used during the removal of a dislocated IOL, then after the old IOL is removed, the surgeon may want to loosen, or remove the hooks in the areas where the sutures are to be located prior to placing a scleral sutured IOL. A retrobulbar or peribulbar block maximizes patient comfort and decreases ocular motility, but other anesthesia options are also reasonable, such as topical plus subconjunctival anesthetic injection. After placement of a lid speculum, I place superior and inferior rectus 4-0 silk bridle sutures to be able to stabilize, reposition, and even elevate the globe. The ability to elevate the globe is particularly helpful if the eye is relatively enophthalmic. Using a taper point needle on the 4-0 silk increases safety by decreasing the risk of globe penetration and bleeding. A Paufique forceps facilitates placement of bridle sutures because the size and angulation of the teeth on the tip of the forceps enable the surgeon to readily grasp the muscle tendon insertion area, rather than just grasping conjunctiva and Tenon's capsule. If a superior incision is planned, then I create a radial relaxing incision in the conjunctiva at the 10:30 clock position with a peritomy over to the 1:30 position. Next is a second radial relaxing incision in the conjunctiva at the 4 o'clock position and a peritomy carried over to the 6 o'clock position. Cautery in the exposed scleral beds is useful to help visualization of incision and suture placement. I create a half-thickness scleral groove on the superior sclera that is 7 mm wide in a "frown" configuration, with the anteriormost portion of the incision still being posterior enough to be in scleral tissue. I use a sharp, bi-bevel scleral tunneling blade to dissect anteriorly from the base of the groove in a lamellar fashion into clear cornea. To keep the dissection in a single, contiguous plane, I use wide, sweeping strokes across the entire width of the tunnel with gentle pressure at the tip of the tunneling blade to avoid deforming the tissues as the dissection proceeds. (Note: If a temporal wound is utilized, then the clock hours of the preceding and following descriptions are adjusted accordingly.)

Paracenteses at about the 10 o'clock and 2 o'clock positions are convenient locations through which to place the self-retaining infusion cannula and the vitrectomy probe. I prefer a reusable, titanium, high-flow infusion cannula (model 8–616, 20-gauge; model 8–616–1, 23-gauge; Duckworth & Kent, Baldock, UK) because it is designed with a smaller tip that facilitates entry into the paracentesis. Disposable, stainless steel cannulas, like the Lewicky infusion cannula (various manufacturers), work well, too. Infusion should be kept in the "continuous" mode throughout the procedure, with infusion only being turned off during certain times, such as prior to opening the main incision. With a gravity-feed system, a bottle height of 60 to 70 cm is usually about right during vitrectomy, but during most of the rest of the procedure, when the vitrectomy probe is not actively aspirating fluid, a bottle height about half as high is more advantageous. I usually remove the vitreous from about the anterior half of the vitreous cavity, particularly in the areas where the IOL sutures will be passed.

Incision Construction and Management

After completing the vitrectomy, the main incision is completed by opening the corneal portion of the incision in a corneal valve configuration with a sharp-tipped keratome ~ 3 mm wide. I usually use an enlargement blade next (~ 5.5 mm wide), still paying attention to the Descemet's incision line to maintain the corneal valve. I complete the enlargement to the 7-mm width using the sides of the enlargement blade. Alternatively, the sharp-tipped keratome may be used for the full wound enlargement, but in doing so, even more care and attention is needed to achieve a self-sealing incision. As the incision is enlarged, I try to maintain a corneal valve all the way to the sides of the incision for optimizing the ability of the incision to seal. In so doing, the Descemet's incision usually has a bit of a "smile" configuration, which has the mirror appearance of the "frown" configuration of the scleral groove. If the Descemet's enlargement incision tracks back to the limbus (through Schwalbe's line), then the corneal valve effect of the incision is usually lost and the incision will generally not self-seal. In this situation a significantly increased number of sutures may be required to achieve a watertight closure (**Fig. 27.1**) (see Incision Enlargement Technique, below).

I prefer using a one-piece PMMA IOL with a 7-mm optic with eyelets on the haptics (Alcon model CZ70BD) because of the rigidity it offers in spanning the distance across the front of the eye, and the presence of the eyelets. I calculate the IOL power as if it were a sulcus-placed lens, which usually achieves the desired refractive outcome. My standard suture has been a 3-inch-long double-armed 9-0 polypropylene suture with curved, long, transchamber, spatula needles (for example, Ethicon CTC-6L needles as a special order on 9-0 Prolene, D-8229; Ethicon, Somerville, NJ), which I pass through the eyelet on the lead haptic of the IOL. (This length of suture is long enough for the procedure; longer lengths have the tendency to get tangled more easily.) The suture is arranged so that one arm of the suture emerges through the top of the eyelet and the other arm comes over the top of the haptic between the optic and the eyelet (**Fig. 27.2**). Having the

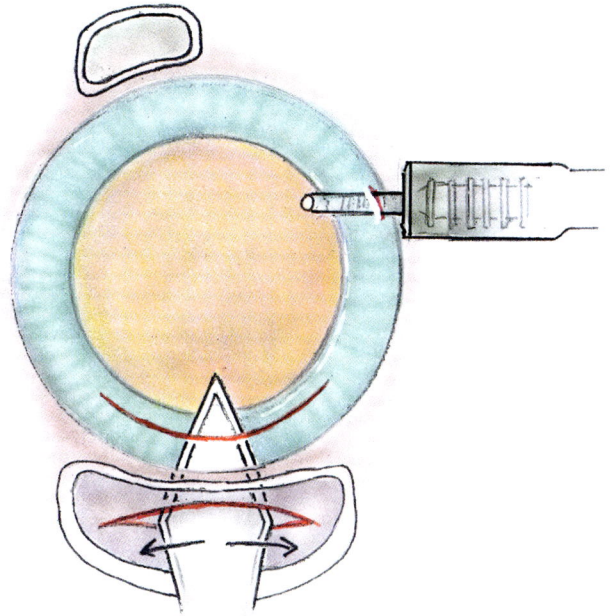

a

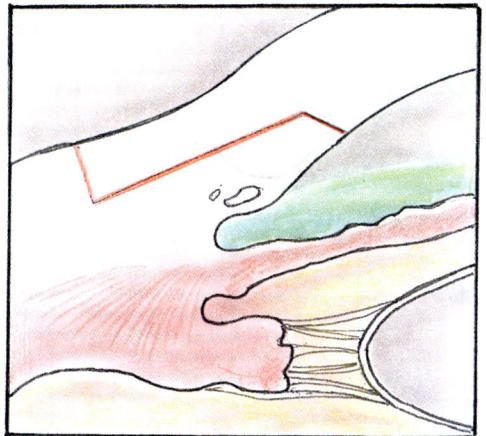

b

Fig. 27.1   (a) The keratome is slid toward each side of the initial entry through Descemet's membrane to enlarge the corneal valve portion of the incision to a full 7-mm width. Adjustments in the maneuvering of the keratome keep the proper incision line through Descemet's. Note the frown configuration of the scleral groove at the external aspect of the incision. **(b)** The cross-sectional anatomic appearance of a 7-mm-wide scleral-corneal incision.

non-eyelet suture arm come over the haptic between the eyelet and the optic decreases the risk of the suture arm inadvertently flipping over the tip of the haptic, in which case that suture arm would emerge below the haptic and have the potential to induce tilt (see Suture Configuration on Haptics and Intraocular Lens Tilt, below).

Infusion Management

During the IOL placement and IOL suturing, a relatively low infusion pressure, around 30 cm of water, helps minimize the intraocular pressure fluctuations, and decreases the risk of the iris prolapsing out through the main incision. If the iris does prolapse, then turning off the infusion for a few moments will soften the eye enough to allow gentle repositing of the iris. An additional way to help prevent iris prolapse when the main wound needs

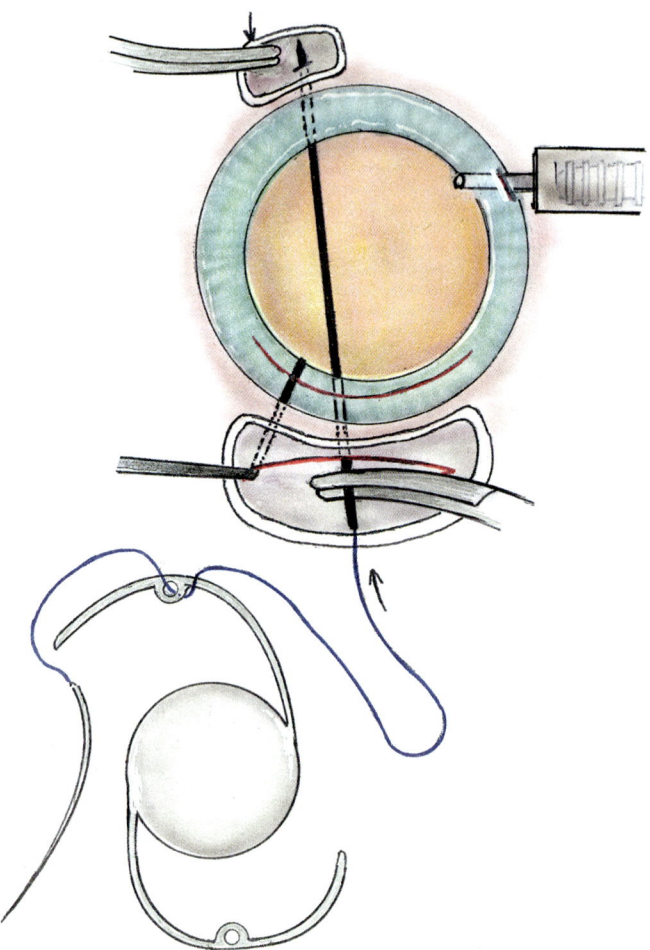

Fig. 27.2 A double-armed suture goes through the eyelet on the lead haptic of the intraocular lens (IOL) with both arms of the suture coming over the top of the haptic—one through the eyelet and the other between the eyelet and the optic. An angled tying forceps is used to depress the sclera and grasp the tip of the suture needle as it emerges from the eye. After the other end of the needle is released from the needle holder, the needle is pulled out through the sclera with the tying forceps. A cyclodialysis spatula is shown here gaping open the main incision, which is done prior to passing the needle so as to minimize the risk of catching scleral or corneal tissue; an angled tying forceps works well for this, too.

to be opened is to turn off the infusion for several seconds before opening the main wound, so that there is even less of a pressure gradient and hence minimal fluid flow out through the main incision when it is opened. Setting up the machine so that the surgeon can turn the infusion on and off with the foot pedal, as well as raise and lower the infusion bottle with the foot pedal, can facilitate the procedure. Pump-based fluidics on the machine tend to create greater flow when the eye is opened for an equivalent static pressure setting, and hence are not as user friendly for this type of surgery. If a machine with pump-based fluidics is utilized, then additional attention should be paid to turning off the infusion before opening the main incision.

First Suture Placement: Right-Hand Needle

The suture arms are physically separated on the field to keep track of which should be on the right and which should be on the left, so that they are later placed through the sclera in the correct orientation. The right-side needle is then passed through the main wound, which is slightly gaped open with an instrument, such as an angled tying forceps, to create space so that the needle tip does not catch corneal or scleral tissue inside the wound. After visualizing the needle tip in the anterior chamber, the surgeon can move the needle side to side to be sure that it has not caught any sclera or corneal tissue in the main incision. The needle tip is then passed through the pupil, under the 5 o'clock iris position and into the ciliary sulcus area. An angled tying forceps placed on the sclera near the anticipated needle exit point can be used to palpate the needle tip through the sclera and verify that

the needle tip is in the desired position. The slightly open tying forceps can be used for counterpressure on the sclera and to grasp the needle tip when it emerges from the sclera ~ 1.5 to 3.0 mm posterior to the limbus (**Fig. 27.2**). If the needle emerges in a place other than the desired location, it can be pulled back into the eye and an additional attempt can be made to place the needle in the preferred location. Once the needle shaft is about halfway through the sclera, the surgeon can pivot the needle side to side in its track through the sclera. If the iris shows corresponding motion, then this suggests that the needle pass has caught the peripheral iris, and the needle may be retracted back by gently pulling on the suture until it can be regrasped with the needle holder to make another pass without catching the iris. Reaching a location far enough behind the iris can sometimes be more challenging in large eyes due to the dimensions involved.

First Suture Placement: Left-Hand Needle

The left-hand needle is then passed through the main incision and pupil in the same manner that the right-hand needle was just passed. The needles should emerge from the sclera the same distance posterior to the limbus and ~ 1.5 mm apart from each other (**Fig. 27.3**). The needle passes may be closer to each other, ~ 1.0 mm, but when they get too close it becomes more difficult to bury the knot, and some of the four-point fixation effect becomes diminished (see Suture Configuration on Haptics and Intraocular Lens Tilt, below). The suture needle is 6 mil in diameter (0.006 inches or ~ 0.15 mm in diameter). It is less than one fifth the width of a 24-gauge microvitreoretinal (MVR) blade (0.80 mm wide),

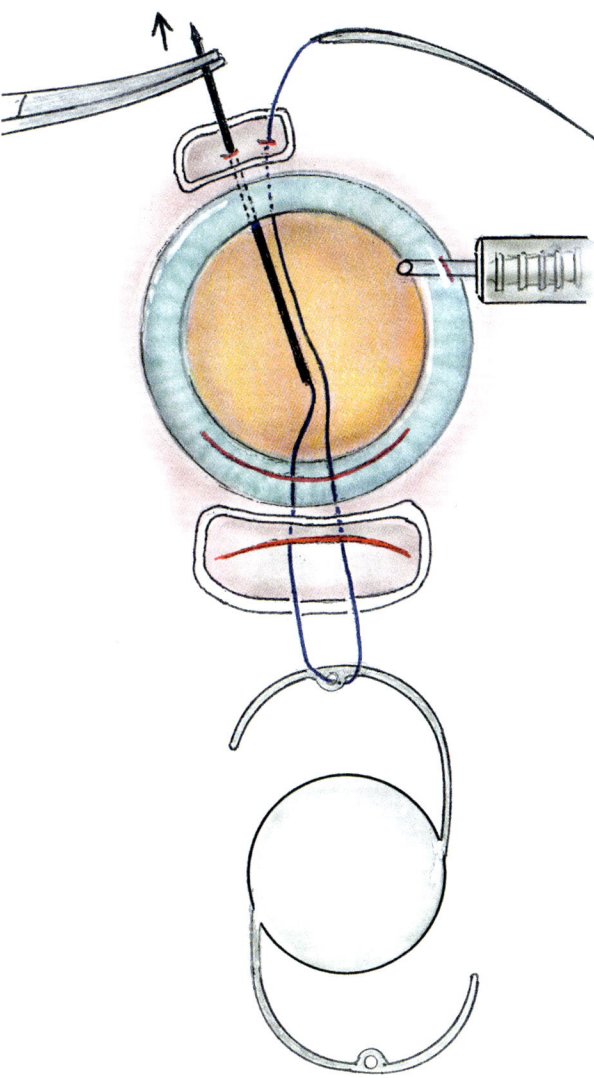

Fig. 27.3 The second suture needle for the lead haptic is brought out through the sclera adjacent to the first suture with ~ 1.5 mm of separation between them. The image shows how sutures should be oriented on the lead haptic.

so the potential for causing bleeding with transscleral passes with this needle should, theoretically, be lower than with ab-externo sclerotomies made with a 24-gauge MVR blade, and in my experience reality follows the theoretical difference. Surgeons who prefer an ab-externo approach, but still want to use 9-0 polypropylene attached to this type of suture needle often use a 27-gauge hollow-bore needle passed through the sclera from the outside of the eye. They dock the suture needle into the 27-gauge needle before it is brought out through the sclera.

Needle Position

Other locations around the eye for placement of the sutures may be selected by the surgeon if it facilitates passing the needles. That said, it is probably best to avoid the 12 o'clock and 6 o'clock positions to minimize the chance of hitting larger ciliary vessels, and also to avoid the 3 o'clock and 9 o'clock positions for the same reason, and to avoid the trunk area of the long ciliary nerves. The appropriate distance posterior to the limbus for the needle to go through the sclera in each eye is actually determined by internal anatomy, which varies from patient to patient. The needle should pass through the sclera posterior to the iris so that no peripheral anterior synechiae are created when the lens haptic is later pulled into position. The limbus is closer to the iris nasally and temporally than superiorly and inferiorly, so even in a given eye, the distance from the limbus to the appropriate place for the sutures varies depending on where around the circumference of the eye the sutures are placed. Aids for helping determine the location of the suture needle tip behind the iris before placing it through the sclera include "tickling" the back of the iris with the needle tip, mentally visualizing where the needle tip is located, and palpating the sclera.

Needle Basics

A titanium angled tying forceps is better for grasping the emerging needle because titanium instruments have better grip on stainless steel needles (due to more friction) than stainless steel instruments do. Also, using a tying forceps that is stouter than the typical fine-tying forceps helps hold the needle better and minimizes unexpected needle movement from forceps scissoring. The process of grasping and pulling the needle through the sclera is best broken down into three distinct steps: (1) Grasp the needle tip with the tying forceps, preferably with the flats of the tying forceps on the flat aspects (top and bottom) of the spatula needle. (2) Release the needle holder's grasp of the back end of the needle. (3) Pull the needle out through the sclera with the tying forceps. Although these steps seem quite intuitive while reading them, it is rather easy for a surgeon, who is focusing on the needle tip, to still hold onto the back end of the needle with the needle holder while trying to pull the tip of the needle out through the sclera with the tying forceps. The needle holder always wins, and the needle tip often pops back inside the eye, causing a setback in the flow of the surgery and often a dulled needle tip that is harder to re-pass through the sclera.

Insertion of an Intraocular Lens

After both needles have been passed, the two arms of the suture are grasped with a straight tying forceps outside the eye to pull up the suture slack as the IOL is placed in through the main incision with the angled tying forceps. The lead haptic is directed into the ciliary sulcus area where the sutures pass through the eye wall (**Fig. 27.4a**). The trailing haptic can be left in the main incision with part of the haptic just outside the eye so it is easier to later place the second suture on the trailing haptic. Having the trailing haptic in this position causes a little bit of fluid leakage out through the main incision, but the eye still remains well formed, and if the surgeon needs to raise the pressure in the eye, such as in the case of significant intraocular bleeding from the needle pass, then the haptic may be temporarily placed into the anterior chamber so that the incision can seal more completely.

Management of Needle Entrapment in the Incision

When the surgeon starts placing the IOL into the eye, it will become apparent if one of the needles caught some tissue inside the main incision because the lead haptic will stop progressing at the main incision, and the wound will deform. If this occurs, then small amounts of corneal or scleral tissue may be carefully cut with fine scissors to free the suture. If the amount of tissue is significantly greater, then the IOL may be pulled back out of the eye, and the suture may be cut in an appropriate location to enable freeing of the suture material that is caught in wound tissue. After the suture is freed, then the cut suture ends can be

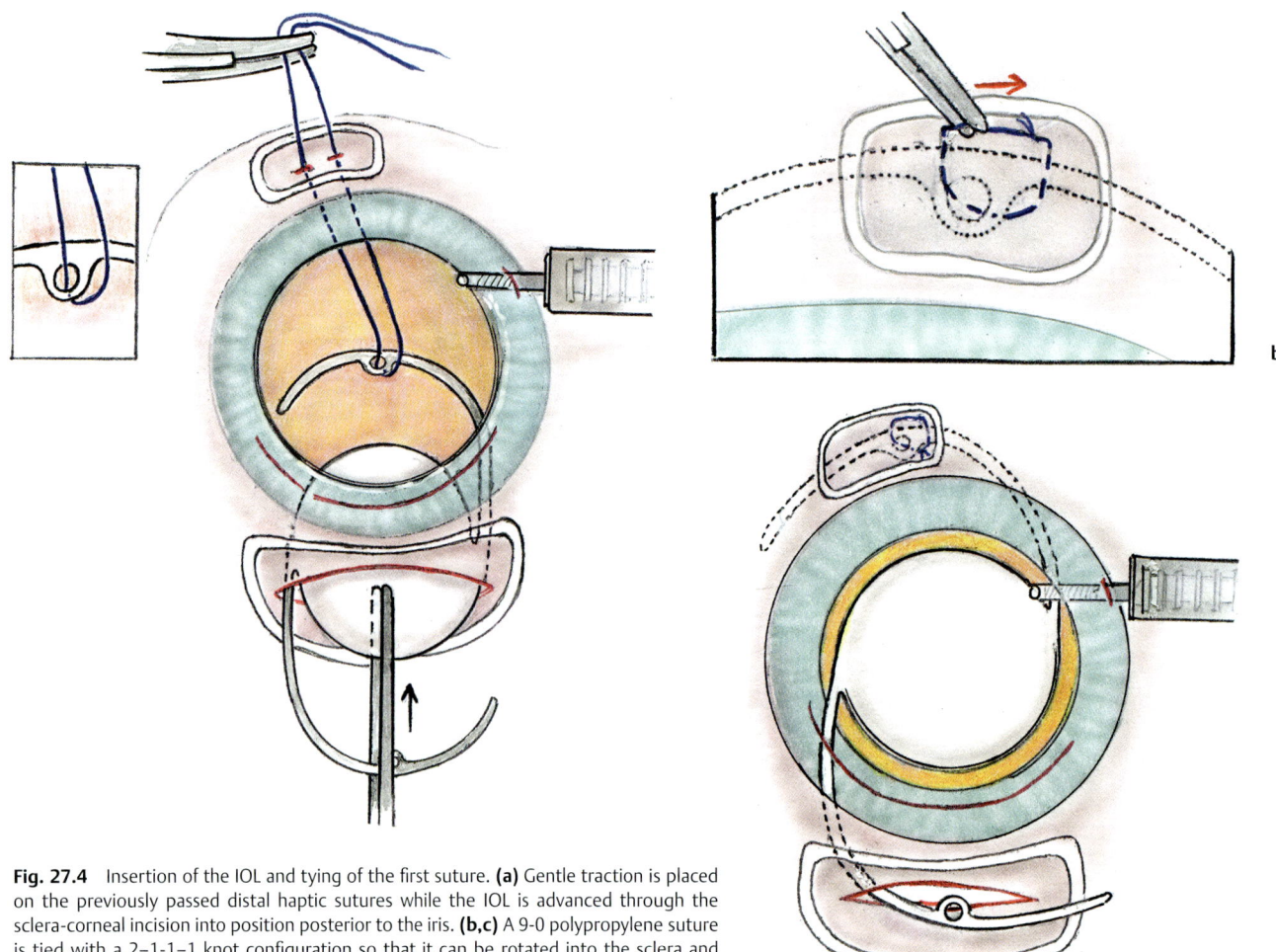

Fig. 27.4 Insertion of the IOL and tying of the first suture. **(a)** Gentle traction is placed on the previously passed distal haptic sutures while the IOL is advanced through the sclera-corneal incision into position posterior to the iris. **(b,c)** A 9-0 polypropylene suture is tied with a 2–1-1–1 knot configuration so that it can be rotated into the sclera and buried.

tied back together. This area of suture that has been retied will work fine for placing the IOL and suture in the desired location, but it should not be utilized as part of the suture that creates the final securing of the IOL to the sclera.

Once the IOL is in the eye with the lead haptic in the desired location behind the iris, the two suture arms can be carefully tied together with a 2–1-1–1 knot, being sure that each throw is laid down square and the suture arms are evenly tensioned to optimize knot configuration and strength. After the knot is tied, the arms are trimmed and the suture is rotated to bury the knot inside the eye (**Fig. 27.4b,c**) (see Suture Knot Management, below).

Second Suture Placement

To minimize the potential of sutures becoming tangled, it is not until this point in the procedure that the surgeon brings a second double-armed 9-0 polypropylene suture with curved, long, trans-chamber, spatula needles into the surgical field and passes one of the needles through the eyelet on the trailing haptic (**Fig. 27.5a**). This suture is also arranged so that that one arm of the suture emerges through the top of the eyelet and the other arm comes over the top of the haptic between the optic and the eyelet. The suture arms and needles are placed on the drapes off to their respective sides. I place an angled mini-IOL manipulator (model 6–418, Duckworth & Kent) in the eyelet on the trailing

haptic and use it to push the haptic in through the main wound, down through the pupil, while keeping the suture in the correct position on the haptic (**Fig. 27.5b**). The haptic is then released by turning the handle of the instrument obliquely away from the surgeon so that the knob rotates out of the eyelet. If the specified mini-IOL manipulator is not used, but a different instrument is going to be placed into the eyelet of the trailing haptic, then care should be taken to select an instrument that will fit into the eyelet, yet not get stuck in the eyelet (**Fig. 27.5b inset**). If such an instrument is not available, then one may choose to use forceps to place the haptic into the eye, or a different type of IOL manipulator on the outside of the haptic itself. The instrument that is used to put the trailing haptic into the eye can also be used to push the optic a little bit posteriorly to move the trailing haptic posterior to the ciliary sulcus so it is out of the way while passing the next suture needle.

I then create an additional paracentesis that is directly anterior to the location of the suture for the lead haptic—at about the 5 o'clock position. One of the needles for the trailing haptic suture is grasped a couple of millimeters from its tip with a needle holder, keeping track if it is attached to the right- or left-side suture. The needle is passed butt-end first in through the main wound, across the anterior chamber and partway out through the 5 o'clock paracentesis opening (**Fig. 27.6a**). With the butt end of the needle outside the eye at the 5 o'clock position, the surgeon is able to regrasp the needle at its back end with the needle

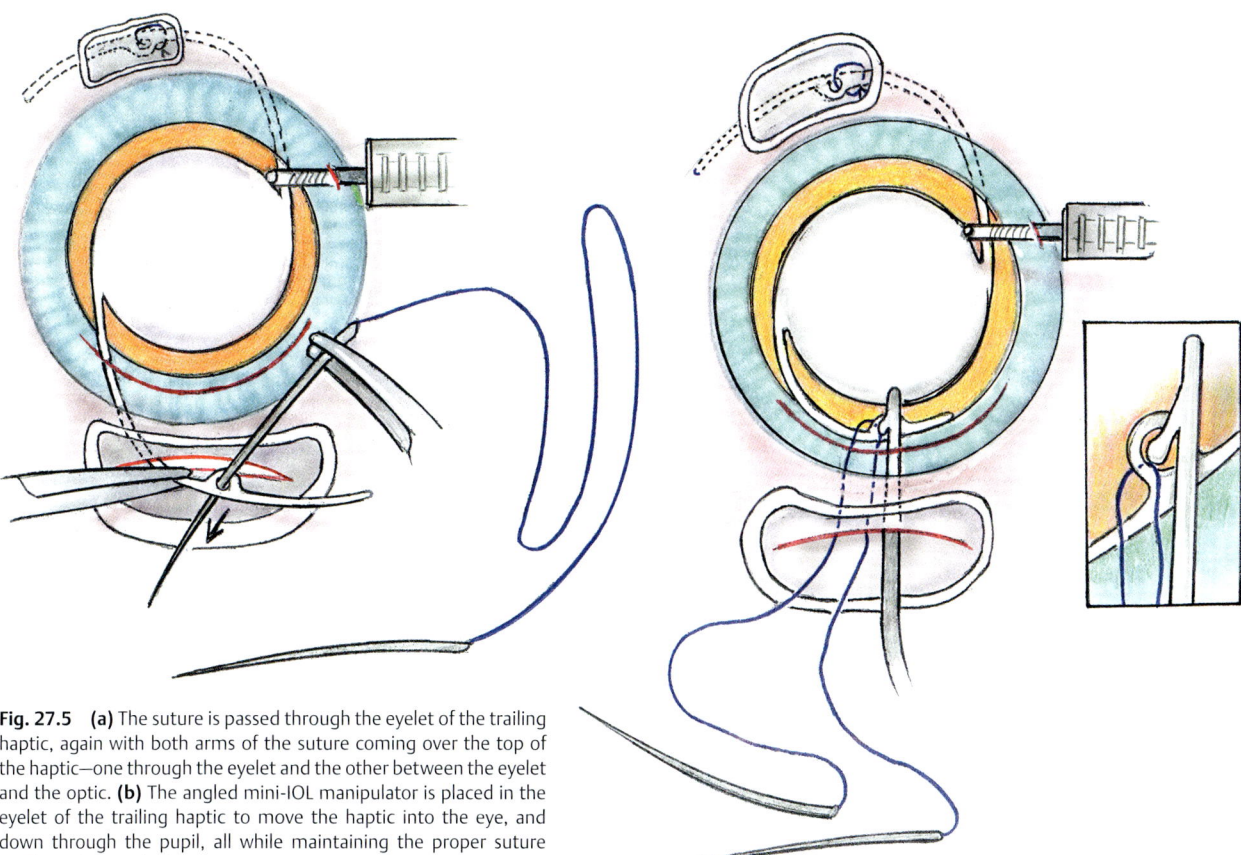

a

b

Fig. 27.5 **(a)** The suture is passed through the eyelet of the trailing haptic, again with both arms of the suture coming over the top of the haptic—one through the eyelet and the other between the eyelet and the optic. **(b)** The angled mini-IOL manipulator is placed in the eyelet of the trailing haptic to move the haptic into the eye, and down through the pupil, all while maintaining the proper suture configuration on the haptic.

holder. The needle tip can then be redirected through the pupil, under the 11 o'clock iris position and into the ciliary sulcus area (**Fig. 27.6b**). Because the needle is in a paracentesis that is directly anterior to the suture for the first haptic, the proper location for the placement of the suture for the trailing haptic can be determined by visualizing the needle as splitting the anterior segment into two equal parts before passing the needle through the sclera. For this centration method to be effective, the curved needle needs to be oriented with the plane of the needle's curve, oriented perpendicular to the plane of the iris—in other words, so that the needle appears essentially straight from the surgeons view (**Fig. 27.7**). If the surgeon desires additional help in getting the correct placement of the sutures in this or other transscleral suturing techniques, then an aid such as an inked, 180-degree marker may be used, like the type of device used to mark the axis for a toric IOL. Some surgeons place the suture through sclerotomies positioned further apart from each other, and attach the IOL to the suture using a hitch so that centration may be adjusted after the IOL sutures have been tied and the knots buried.[5] The second needle is passed in the same way, either to the left or to the right of the first needle, depending on whether it is attached to the left- or right-side suture.

The decision of whether to pass the right-side or the left-side suture first for the trailing haptic may be influenced by the position of the trailing eyelet and the sutures inside the eye. If the eyelet is to the right of the desired location for the needle pass, then it will usually pull the sutures to the right of the desired suture location. In this scenario, passing the left-side suture first minimizes the risk that it will become crossed and twisted with the right-side suture. Once the left-side suture is placed, and the

slack is taken up on the suture, then the left suture is positioned down and out of the way so the right-side suture is unlikely to cross it and create a twist. Likewise, if the eyelet is pulling the sutures to the left of the desired location for the suture placement, then passing the right-side suture first is advantageous.

Evaluation of Intraocular Lens Position and the Use of Purkinje Images

After the slack is taken up on the suture for the trailing haptic, the bridle sutures can be loosened, and the eye may be turned so it is facing directly toward the microscope. If one sees the broad reflection, or Purkinje image, off the anterior surface of the Alcon model CZ70BD IOL, when the eye is in this position and the trailing sutures are tensioned, then that is confirmation that the lens does not have significant tilt. If the reflection is not seen initially, then the eye can be rotated until the reflection is seen. Based on the direction that the eye is facing when the IOL reflection is visible, one can determine if there is a clinically significant amount of IOL tilt, or if it is insignificant. If a small amount of IOL tilt is present, it is sometimes possible to reduce the amount of tilt by either increasing, or decreasing the tension on the sutures for the trailing haptic. If the tilt is improved in this way, then the suture can be tied with either a bit more or a bit less tension to help decrease the tilt. If the amount of tilt is still unacceptable, then sometimes the IOL tilt can be reduced by using an instrument through one of the paracenteses to change the lens position, prior to tying the suture for the trailing haptic, which further secures the IOL in position. Fortunately, with the IOL suturing

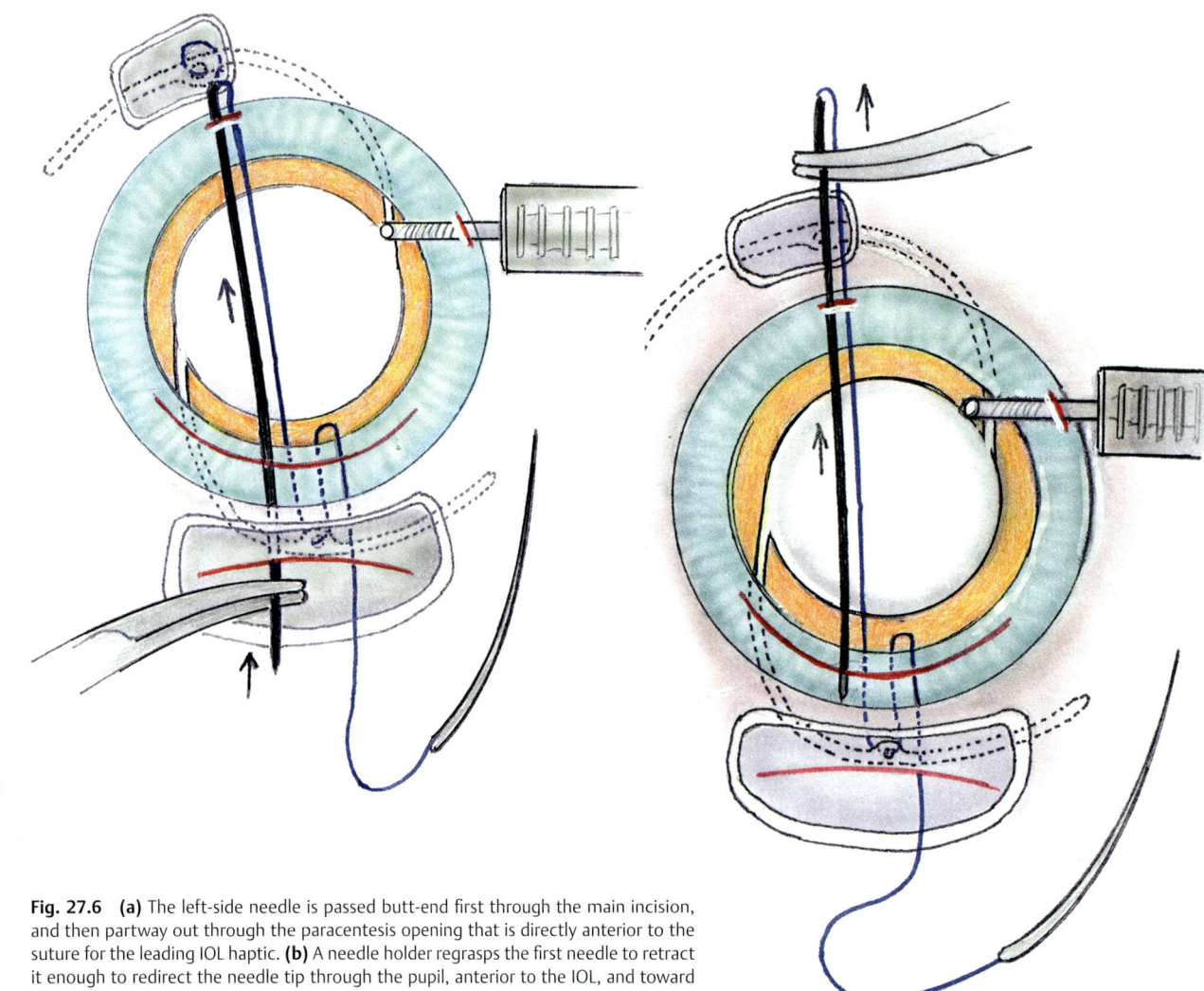

Fig. 27.6 **(a)** The left-side needle is passed butt-end first through the main incision, and then partway out through the paracentesis opening that is directly anterior to the suture for the leading IOL haptic. **(b)** A needle holder regrasps the first needle to retract it enough to redirect the needle tip through the pupil, anterior to the IOL, and toward the ciliary sulcus area 180 degrees away.

technique as described, it is rather unusual to see significant IOL tilt, so these rectifying measures are rarely needed. Once the IOL position is determined to be satisfactory, then the suture for the trailing haptic should be tied, trimmed, and the knot buried in the same fashion as was performed for the lead haptic.

An even more specific test for evaluating the IOL for lack of tilt and proper centration is if one is able to simultaneously see (1) the bright microscope light reflection off the front of the cornea positioned in the center of the cornea (first Purkinje image, P1), (2) the broad reflection off the front of the IOL (third Purkinje image, P3), and (3) the reflection off the back of the IOL (fourth Purkinje image, P4) positioned rather close to P1. P4 appears as a dimmer, inverted, and side-to-side flipped image of P1. If one aligns P1 in the center of the cornea, and P3 is visible (and centered if it is not a broad reflection), but P4 appears notably shifted off to the side, then that means the IOL does not have tilt, but that it is decentered. Retraction of the iris at the pupil margin can help one visualize the optic to determine the amount of decentration to decide if there will be IOL edge exposure issues, which might necessitate re-suturing one of the haptics. With other IOL designs and materials, some characteristics of P3 and P4 may appear different from those described **(Fig. 27.8)**. (Note: P2, off the back of the cornea, is never visible because it is directly behind P1 and much dimmer than P1.)

Incision Closure

The main incision is usually rather watertight due to its corneal valve configuration, and fairly stable with the frown configuration architecture, so three interrupted 10-0 nylon sutures are generally adequate to further stabilize the incision; more sutures should be placed as needed. When placing the 10-0 nylon sutures, care should be taken to avoid cutting the superior haptic's 9-0 polypropylene suture with the needle of the 10-0 nylon suture. If a 10-0 nylon suture needs to be placed in the area of the suture supporting the haptic, then it can be placed in a "bridge" configuration by going through the top of the scleral tunnel, then skipping over the polypropylene suture before taking a bite of sclera further posteriorly. If the 9-0 polypropylene supporting the trailing haptic is cut with the needle from the 10-0 nylon, then one can remove the 10-0 nylon sutures from the main incision before using an instrument like a cyclodialysis spatula, or a straight IOL manipulator to go through the main incision, through the pupil, and under the left side of the IOL to catch the trailing haptic, elevate it, and bring it back out through the main incision. The trailing haptic can then be re-sutured just as had already been done.

If the pupil has not spontaneously become fairly small, then injecting acetylcholine chloride (e.g., Miochol-E, Bausch & Lomb,

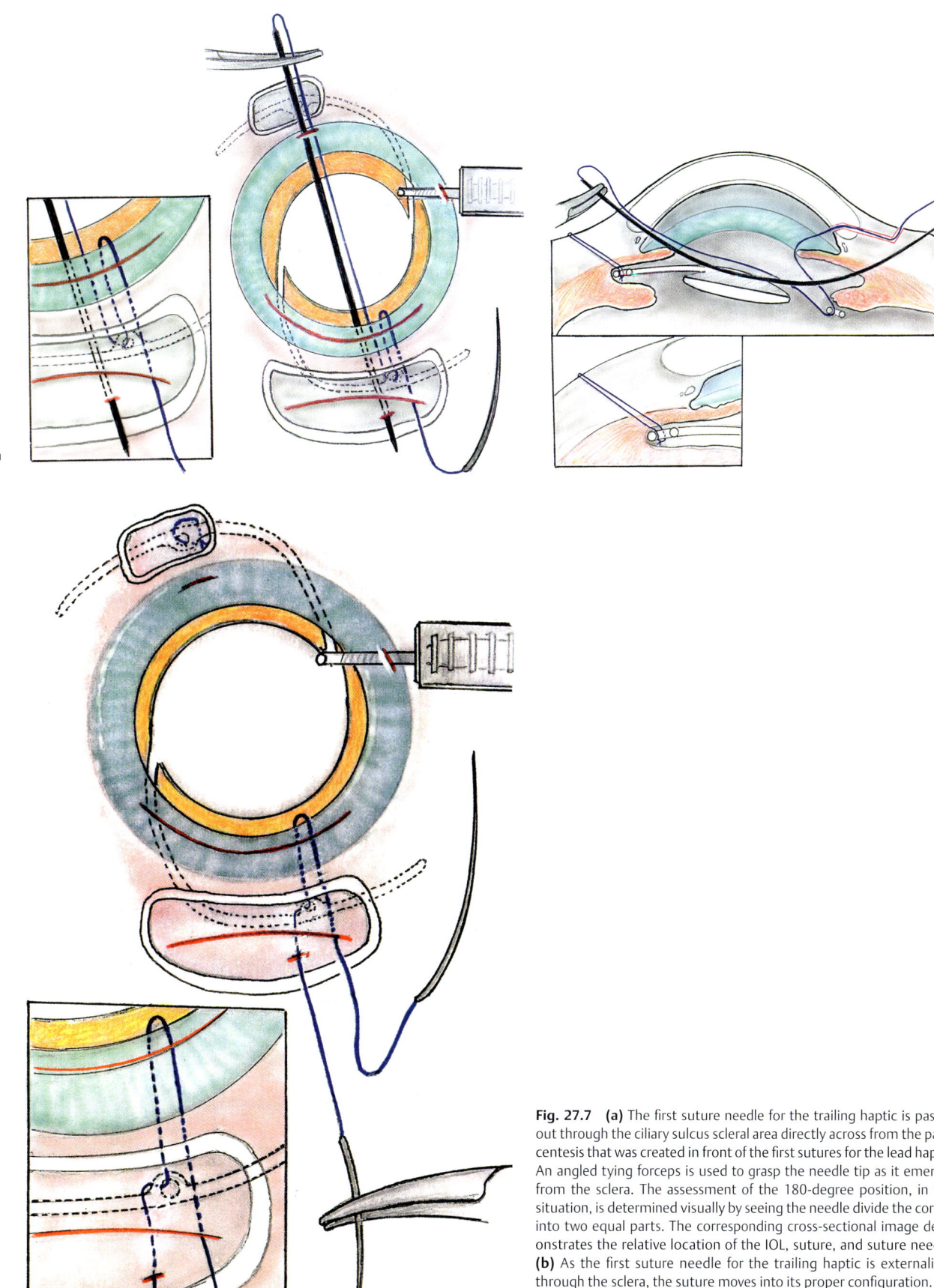

Fig. 27.7 **(a)** The first suture needle for the trailing haptic is passed out through the ciliary sulcus scleral area directly across from the paracentesis that was created in front of the first sutures for the lead haptic. An angled tying forceps is used to grasp the needle tip as it emerges from the sclera. The assessment of the 180-degree position, in this situation, is determined visually by seeing the needle divide the cornea into two equal parts. The corresponding cross-sectional image demonstrates the relative location of the IOL, suture, and suture needle. **(b)** As the first suture needle for the trailing haptic is externalized through the sclera, the suture moves into its proper configuration. Repeating the same maneuvers with the second needle for the trailing haptic completes the suture positioning prior to tying and burying the knot in the same fashion as was done for the leading haptic.

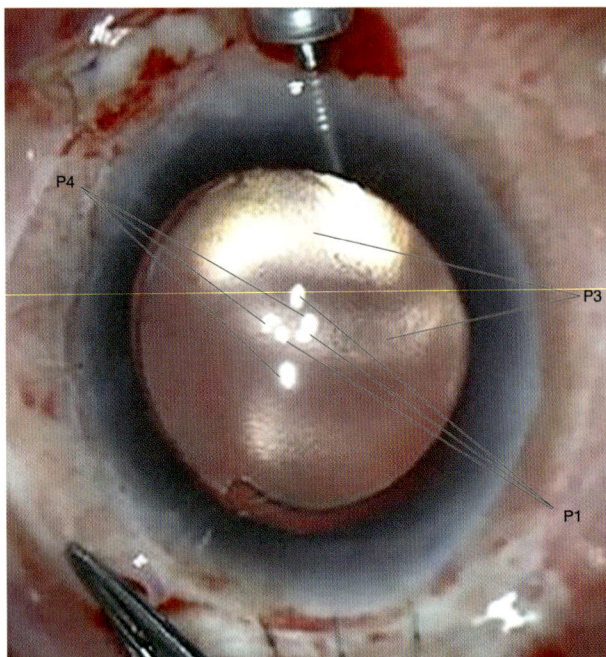

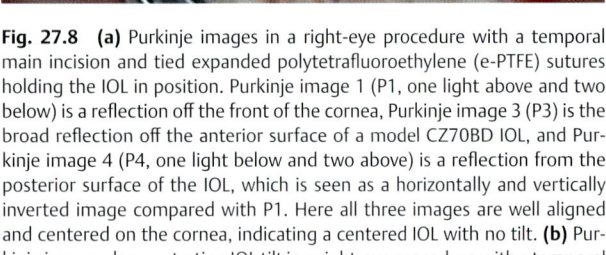

a

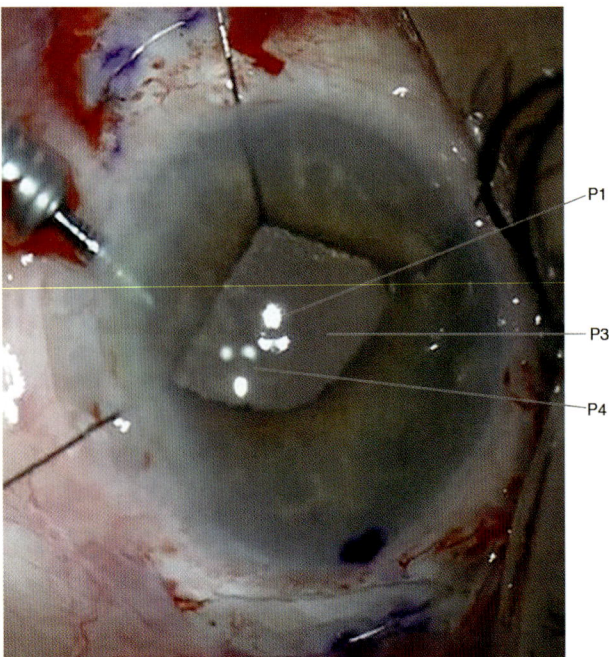

b

Fig. 27.8 **(a)** Purkinje images in a right-eye procedure with a temporal main incision and tied expanded polytetrafluoroethylene (e-PTFE) sutures holding the IOL in position. Purkinje image 1 (P1, one light above and two below) is a reflection off the front of the cornea, Purkinje image 3 (P3) is the broad reflection off the anterior surface of a model CZ70BD IOL, and Purkinje image 4 (P4, one light below and two above) is a reflection from the posterior surface of the IOL, which is seen as a horizontally and vertically inverted image compared with P1. Here all three images are well aligned and centered on the cornea, indicating a centered IOL with no tilt. **(b)** Purkinje images demonstrating IOL tilt in a right-eye procedure with a temporal

main incision and well-positioned e-PTFE sutures with buried knots. The tilt is due to residual fibrotic peripheral capsule remnants. Note that the P1 image (one light above and two below) is shifted significantly to the left (superior) of the center of the cornea in this view when the P3 image (low intensity broad light reflection from the IOL throughout the pupil area) and the P4 image (two lights above and one light below) are fairly well lined up with P1. This indicates that the IOL optic is tilted to the left in this view, which is superior. The tilt improved by adjusting the peripheral part of the haptics at the capsule remnants with an IOL manipulator.

Rochester, NY) into the anterior chamber to constrict the pupil is helpful prior to creating the superior peripheral iridectomies. If the pupil becomes relatively small prior to placing the sutured IOL, then creating the peripheral iridectomies, at that time, can decrease the iris fluctuations as fluid moves about inside the eye during insertion and suturing of the IOL (see Peripheral Iridectomy Creation with a Vitrectomy Probe, below). After creation of the peripheral iridectomies, the infusion cannula is removed. Stromal hydration may be performed, as needed, to ensure sealing of the paracentesis incisions. At this point the bridle sutures can be removed, and then the conjunctival flaps can be repositioned and held in place with 10-0 polyglactin (Vicryl, Ethicon) sutures, or another suture of the surgeon's choice. Because the conjunctival flaps cover the IOL sutures that go through the sclera, it is important that these flaps be secured so that they adequately cover, and heal in place over the IOL sutures. It is probably better to avoid cautery closure of the conjunctival flaps in these cases because the closure is not as secure as with a suture, and the cautery creates burned, dead tissue which could be a nidus for bacterial growth relatively near the transscleral sutures. I place subconjunctival injections of dexamethasone and cephazolin, with topical drops of fluoroquinolone and 5% povidone-iodine solution prior to placing some viscoelastic on the cornea and patching the eye.

Ab-Externo Variation with e-PTFE Suture Material

For certain patients, it seems appropriate to use suture made of e-PTFE in the smallest size manufactured, CV-8 (Gore-Tex)[5–7]

(see Suture Material and Suture Needles, below). Because this suture is not available on needles that can cross the anterior chamber of the eye, it is necessary to use an ab-externo technique. I perform this procedure the same way as described for the 9-0 polypropylene, with the following exceptions.

An angled 24-gauge MVR blade (0.8 mm wide) is used to create the scleral openings through which the sutures can be passed. I create the incisions for the lead haptic first, passing the blade through the sclera parallel to the iris. I choose the location to make the scleral incisions in an analogous fashion to how I place the 9-0 polypropylene sutures, by visualizing where the iris is, and trying to make the incisions an appropriate distance behind the iris. I like to pass the MVR blade centrally enough so that I can see its tip in the pupil to verify that I have made the incisions in the correct location. A sterile pen is useful to mark the round shaft of the blade just behind the cutting edges prior to each pass through sclera so that the scleral openings are easier to locate when one wants to pass coaxial forceps through the incisions. I use a cyclodialysis spatula held over the cornea so that the heel of the spatula is lined up between the sclerotomy incisions for the lead haptic and then position the tip of the spatula so that the cornea is visually bisected to see where to make the incisions for the trailing haptic sutures. I mark the 180-degree spot on the limbus with the sterile pen and then make the sclerotomies in the same fashion, just to the left and right of that mark, the same distance posterior to the limbus as the first pair of sclerotomies.

After threading a 7-cm piece of e-PTFE through the lead haptic in the same fashion as for 9-0 polypropylene technique, I pass one suture arm in through the main incision and down through the pupil with an angled tying forceps. I use a 25-gauge coaxial forceps to retrieve the suture end, usually employing a second instrument, such as an angled IOL manipulator, through a paracentesis to help move the suture into the open jaws of the forceps. A curved 25-gauge coaxial forceps facilitates suture retrieval. When reusable forceps (e.g., Snyder Grasping Forceps, DFH-0032, MicroSurgical Technology, Redmond, WA) are not available, then one can manually bend a curve into a pair of straight disposable retinal forceps using one's fingers. Adjusting the bridle sutures to rotate the eye can be very helpful during suture retrieval to work around periocular anatomy constraints. The second arm of the e-PTFE is brought through its corresponding scleral incision in the same fashion, and then the IOL is placed into the eye as is done with the 9-0 polypropylene technique. I tie the e-PTFE with a five-throw (2–1-1–1-1) knot to decrease the risk that the knot will loosen to the point of integrity loss in this slippery suture material. A 4-cm piece of e-PTFE is placed through the eyelet in the trailing haptic in the same fashion before placing the trailing haptic into the eye with the left and right suture arms left hanging out of the main incision and placed to their corresponding sides. With a second instrument pushing the optic a bit posteriorly, the 25-gauge forceps is placed through each of the scleral openings to grasp the sutures between the haptic and the iris, and then the suture ends are fed into the main incision, to minimize iris perturbation, as the sutures are extracted through the 24-gauge scleral incisions. The reason to push the IOL posteriorly is to minimize the risk that the 25-gauge forceps will enter the eye behind the haptic instead of in front of it. The knots for the trailing haptic e-PTFE are tied in the same fashion. I rotate the knots into the eye using a combination of grasping the suture with tying forceps to rotate the suture, and pushing the knot in through the sclera. I find the knob of the angled mini-IOL manipulator very helpful for pushing the knots in through the scleral incisions; the closed tip of the 25-gauge forceps, or one tip of an open tying forceps may also work.

Iris Sutured Posterior Chamber Intraocular Lenses

The practice of using the iris to support IOLs began in the late 1960s and lasted well into the 1970s during the intracapsular cataract extraction era with lenses such as the Copeland iris-plane IOL.[8] The shift from the purely iris-supported IOL to IOLs supported by the lens capsule and the iris was associated with improved visual results, as well as decreased rates of cystoid macular edema, uveitis, and other complications.[9] This shift also corresponded to the change from intracapsular to extracapsular cataract extraction techniques, so it is difficult to know how much of the difference was due to the change in IOL support versus the change in extraction technique. With that in mind, it is interesting that currently many surgeons' preferred use of iris sutured PCIOLs is in situations where the haptics are in the sulcus region or the lens capsule offers additional support to the IOL. Today, suturing a PCIOL to the iris generally involves creation of a pupillary capture of the optic of the PCIOL into the anterior chamber while the haptics remain in the posterior chamber. Sutures are passed down through the iris, under the haptic, and then back up through the iris. The sutures are tied either before or after repositing the optic back through the pupil into the posterior chamber.[10–12]

Indications and Other Considerations

Suturing a PCIOL to the posterior surface of the iris may be a desirable procedure in several situations:

1. Stabilizing or centering an IOL that was placed in the sulcus during a prior, or current cataract surgery. In this situation the IOL is already reasonably supported by the remaining lens capsule, but due to zonular defects, or the IOL overall diameter being smaller than the eye's sulcus diameter, the IOL is mobile, or decentered.

2. Primary placement of an IOL when there have been complications during cataract surgery, and there is inadequate capsule support to be able to place a sulcus-only supported IOL.

3. Secondary placement of an IOL, alone or as part of an IOL exchange, in an eye with inadequate capsule for a sulcus-only supported IOL.

Of these three scenarios, the first is probably the strongest indication for this procedure because the iris is only required to add a relatively small amount of support to the IOL, so there is less traction on the iris from the sutures, and with less iris traction there is decreased stimulus for inducing uveitis. Suturing PCIOLs to the back of the iris involves the use of long, curved transchamber type needles, which may be a bit challenging, at first, for surgeons not accustomed to using them. The procedure also involves intraocular knot tying, which may or may not be a skill with which the surgeon is already comfortable.

Intraocular Lens Selection

The IOLs for this procedure optimally have (1) rounded optic edges; (2) rounded, small-diameter haptics; and (3) an overall diameter that is large enough to offer some support to the IOL from the haptics' being able to rest in the ciliary sulcus.

If there is already an IOL in the sulcus in the eye, then that IOL should be considered as the first option, unless it has square-edged haptics or the power is considerably off from the desired power. Square-edged haptics have a notable rate of inducing uveitis, pigment dispersion, glaucoma, and hyphema when they are in the sulcus, particularly if the haptics are in contact with the iris, so these IOLs generally should be avoided when choosing a PCIOL to suture to the iris.[13,14] Once an IOL is sutured to the iris, then it effectively becomes a sulcus IOL and has close contact with the back of the iris. If the IOL in the eye is a one-piece or three-piece PMMA IOL with rounded edges and haptics, then keeping that IOL in the eye has the advantage of not needing to create an incision large enough for removing the nonfoldable IOL. It can be a little more challenging to get the optic in front of the pupil with one-piece PMMA IOLs due to the greater rigidity of the haptics, but once optic capture has been achieved and maintained, these relatively rigid haptics are easier to see and suture because they tent the iris forward better when the haptic or optic is pulled anteriorly.

If there is not an IOL in the eye, then foldable three-piece silicone optic IOLs can be a good choice because they virtually all have rounded edges on the optic and small-diameter round haptics. If there is no capsule support, and one wishes to achieve contact between the haptic and the ciliary sulcus for added support, then an IOL with a larger overall diameter is needed. Capsular bag IOLs usually have an overall diameter in the 12.5- to 13.0-mm range. In the United States, a foldable silicone IOL that has been available until 2016 with the larger, 13.5-mm overall diameter is the model AQ2010V of Staar Surgical (Monrovia, CA). In 2009, the American Society of Cataract and Refractive Surgery (ASCRS) Cataract Clinical Committee found this lens to be the most commonly selected IOL for sulcus placement,[14] suggesting that it performs well in that anatomic location. A foldable three-piece IOL with a square-edged optic (generally acrylic), and round haptics can be considered for suturing to the iris, but in a sulcus-like position the square edges of the optic have the potential to cause iris chafing with pigment dispersion, uveitis, and other problems.[15]

Procedure Description

Preoperatively, it is usually best not to use drops that dilate or constrict the pupil because too large or too small of a pupil makes it difficult to position the IOL for the creation of optic capture. Although other anesthesia options are reasonable, a retrobulbar/peribulbar block is generally a good choice for this procedure because akinesia facilitates performing the procedure, and the block provides patient comfort during the iris manipulation involved in this procedure. Superior and inferior rectus bridle sutures may be useful for elevating globes when the exposure is poor, or when the surgeon desires a more stable eye (see Procedure Description under section Transscleral Sutured Posterior Chamber Intraocular Lens Technique: Example, above, for additional bridle suture description, and see Chapter 1 for information about a peribulbar anesthetic).

Surgeon Position

The surgeon may elect to sit superiorly or temporally. Factors that influence the surgeon's seating position include (1) the best location for the main incision if an IOL needs to be put into the eye or exchanged; (2) the level of exposure of the globe, because passing long, curved, trans-chamber needles can sometimes be difficult if the brow or nose is in the way; and (3) the most comfortable position for particular maneuvers. The surgeon may change position during different parts of the procedure as needed to optimize performance of the various maneuvers.

Eye Pressurization

The optimal method for maintaining the pressure in the eye and the formation of the anterior chamber depends on whether or not there is an intact lens capsule diaphragm. If the diaphragm is intact, then an ophthalmic viscoelastic device (OVD), preferably dispersive, may be used. If the diaphragm is not intact, an anterior chamber infusion cannula can then be used with an infusion bottle to keep the eye formed and pressurized. Mydriatic agents, such as epinephrine or phenylephrine, should not be placed into the infusion bottle during these cases because it can make it difficult to achieve a solid optic capture. Any vitreous in the anterior chamber or area behind the iris should be removed with a vitrectomy probe placed through an incision matched to the size of the vitrectomy probe, usually through a limbal paracentesis. The bottle height during the IOL fixation should be high enough to keep the eye well formed, yet not so high as to create rapid fluid flow out through the paracenteses as they are opened by instruments passing through them. A bottle height of 30 to 35 cm usually achieves both of these goals. If vitrectomy needs to be performed, then the bottle height usually needs to go to almost twice this height, and a high-flow anterior chamber infusion cannula should be used (e.g., model 8–616, 20-gauge; model 8–616–1, 23-gauge; Duckworth & Kent). If one has a choice between gravity flow versus an active pump on the machine for the infusion, it is probably better to select the gravity flow option for this type of procedure because the active pump systems tend to create more flow through open incisions than is optimal.

Intraocular Lens Positioning

If the desired IOL is already in the posterior chamber, then it should be rotated so that the haptics are in the position in which the surgeon wishes to have them for placing the securing sutures

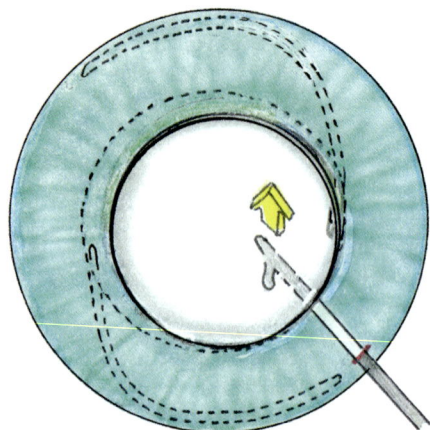

Fig. 27.9 An IOL manipulator moves the optic of the IOL anterior to the iris to begin the process of optic capture. If the IOL haptics are behind the iris, a cyclodialysis spatula or intraocular forceps may also be used.

through the iris. The optic can then be lifted up through the pupil with instruments such as a cyclodialysis spatula, various IOL manipulators, or intraocular forceps that have textured or serrated jaws. The general approach is to bring an instrument, such as a cyclodialysis spatula, in toward the optic 90 degrees away from the optic–haptic junctions, then depress the pupil edge, and slide the instrument under the optic to lift it. If the pupil is smaller than the optic, then the first instrument may need to be one with a hook or knob on it to retract the pupil edge prior to sliding the instrument under the optic (**Fig. 27.9**). In the situation of a small pupil, a second instrument may be needed on the opposite side to press the iris down under the optic. Moving the second instrument along the opposite side of the optic to progressively slide the iris under the optic may be helpful in a maneuver called "tire ironing," named after the motion of a tire iron when removing a tire from its rim. If the surgeon has appropriate coaxial intraocular forceps available to grasp the optic to elevate it, then that can sometimes facilitate the process. If the pupil is small enough, optic capture may be achieved with just these maneuvers. If the pupil is about the same size as or larger than the optic, a small amount of miotic agent can be injected into the anterior chamber to constrict the pupil to achieve optic capture after the optic has been moved anterior to the iris. Acetylcholine (e.g., Miochol-E, Bausch & Lomb) is generally the preferred agent because it causes miosis more quickly than carbachol.

Intraocular Lens Removal and Replacement

If the eye has an IOL that the surgeon wishes to replace, then the existing lens should be carefully removed through an appropriately sized incision. If the eye is already aphakic, then the IOL removal is not needed. In either of these situations, maintaining the intraocular pressure and managing vitreous is still necessary. Before placing the new lens into the eye, the surgeon should carefully assess the amount of capsule support for the lens. If there is enough lens capsule support to be able to temporarily hold an IOL in the sulcus, but not enough for permanent capsule/sulcus fixation alone, then the new IOL may be placed into the sulcus with subsequent capturing of the optic as already described for a preexisting posterior chamber IOL. If there is not any useful lens capsule support available, then the IOL should first be placed into the anterior chamber. Each of the haptics can then be placed through the pupil by a combination of flexing the haptic, retracting the iris, and tire ironing the iris in front of the haptic. The pupil needs to be relatively small to be able to capture the optic while actively repositioning the haptics behind the iris without the optic also going posterior to the iris and missing the optic capture. If an appropriate pair of serrated jaw intraocular forceps is available, the surgeon may be able to use them to grasp the optic ~ 90 degrees away from the origin of the haptics and hold it anterior to the iris while tucking the haptics behind the iris with a second instrument.

Pupillary Capture

One of the challenges of this operation is to achieve a solid pupillary capture of the IOL optic, and maintain it during the passage of sutures through the iris and under the haptics. In the situation where there is capsule support behind the IOL, losing the pupillary capture prematurely is mainly frustrating. In the case where there is no capsule support behind the iris, premature loss of the capture can mean dislocation of the IOL into the vitreous cavity— a rather undesirable event. One way to help maintain optic capture during the suturing maneuvers is to place a safety suture under the optic. This can be done by passing a 10-0 polypropylene suture on a long, curved, trans-chamber needle through the limbus, under the optic, and then back out through the limbus on the opposite side of the eye, without catching any iris tissue. The optimal orientation is for the suture pass to be ~ 90 degrees away from the optic–haptic junctions. Because the limbal plane is above the iris plane, applying a small amount of traction to each end of the suture can help elevate the optic above the iris, and keep the optic edge in front of the pupil edge while the haptics are posterior to the iris (**Fig. 27.10**). Some surgeons find the use of a suture like this to be helpful in achieving optic capture when the pupil is larger than the optic; the suture can be placed and used to elevate the optic while the miotic agent is injected. If the pupil margin does come in front of one side of the optic during the haptic suturing, then applying traction again on the

safety suture will usually elevate the optic and force the pupil margin to the desired location behind the optic (**Fig. 27.11**). If the geometry of the eye and needle are appropriate, and the haptics of the IOL are flexible enough, then the needle may actually be left in place behind the optic during the suturing of the haptics, with the ends of the needle still lodged in each side of the limbus. This not only keeps the optic anterior to the iris, but it may elevate the IOL haptics enough to make them more visible through the iris and easier to suture.

Suture Technique

Once the optic is captured and centered, sutures can be passed to secure the haptics. A long, curved, trans-chamber needle works best for the suture passes to fixate the haptics. If a fine spatula style needle is used, the needle can usually be passed directly through limbal corneal tissue. If a larger diameter tapered style needle is used, paracentesis openings need to be created in the appropriate limbal locations through which to pass the needle because this type of needle is very difficult to pass through limbal or corneal tissue. The most commonly used suture for securing the IOL haptic to the iris is 10-0 polypropylene, just as it is the most common for iris reconstruction. The 10-0 size of polypropylene seems to hold up well in this type of purely intraocular environment. Even though one might think that the additional strength of 9-0 polypropylene would be a benefit, its additional stiffness tends to cause excessive distortion of the iris during knot tying, which can lead to suboptimal results.

The surgeon should try to go down through the iris with the needle tip close to the haptic, pass the needle tip under the haptic, and then come up through the iris fairly close to the first pass down through the iris. Some surgeons find it easier to make the pass down through the iris on the concave side of the haptic's curvature because, with the haptic curving in that direction, the

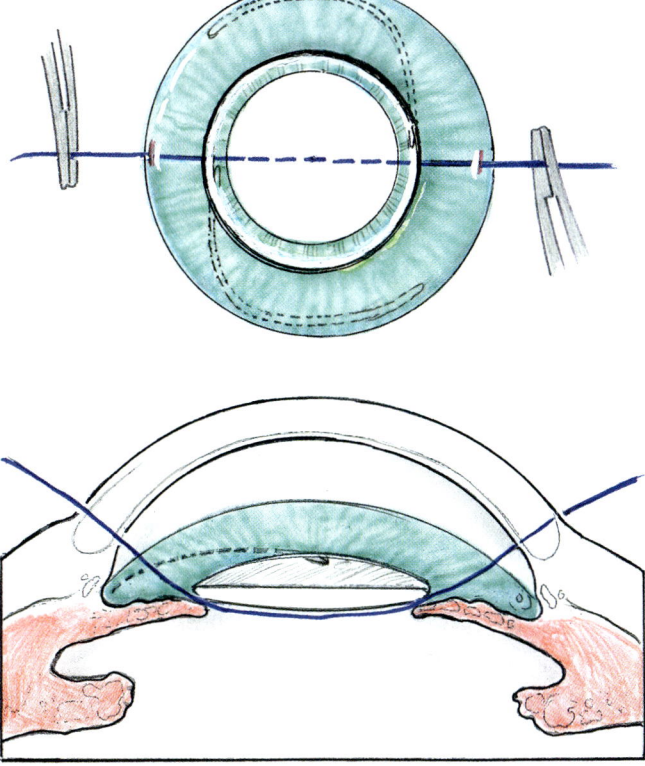

a

b

Fig. 27.10 (a,b) A 10-0 polypropylene safety suture is placed behind the optic to help keep the optic in the captured position, to make it easier to re-attain the captured position if needed, and to help prevent inadvertent posterior dislocation of the IOL if the optic capture configuration is lost.

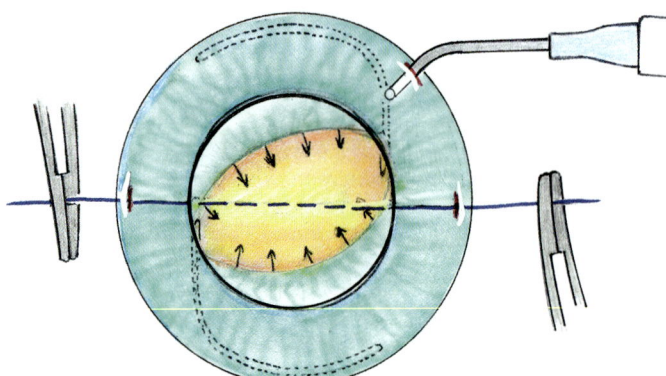

Fig. 27.11 A miotic agent is placed in the anterior chamber constricting the iris to create an IOL optic capture. The optic is displaced anteriorly to assist the pupillary miosis. The pupil takes on an oval, or cat's-eye, shape with the haptic–optic junction creating the long axis of the oval.

iris is better supported for the initial iris penetration. The direction the haptic curves is not relevant when the needle comes back up through the iris, because at that time the haptic is on the posterior side of the iris, so it is unable to provide support. Although it is possible to obtain too little iris tissue, the more common problem is incorporating too much iris tissue in the needle pass, and that causes focal bunching of the iris, with iris distortion, once the suture is tied. One may use an instrument, such as an IOL manipulator, to support the haptic through the iris or via the optic, during the passage of the needle down through the iris next to the haptic (**Fig. 27.12a**). Once the needle tip has passed under the haptic, the instrument can be shifted to push down a little on the iris to help get the needle tip up through the iris near the other side of the haptic (**Fig. 27.12b**).

After the needle tip comes up through the iris, it can be passed out through the limbus in a convenient place, or through a previously created paracentesis if a taper point needle is used. If one wishes to bring the needle out through a paracentesis, that process can be facilitated by placing a 24-gauge, plastic angiocatheter from a standard intravenous set in through the paracentesis. The needle tip can then be docked into the catheter tip before bringing them both out through the paracentesis while maintain the dock. This can also be done with steel cannulas, but the angiocatheters are soft enough that they do not dull the needle if the needle needs to be used again, and they are tapered on the outside near the tip, which makes them easier to get in through the paracentesis, while still having a generous size opening in which to dock the needle. The suture should then be left in place, with one side out through the limbal entry site and the other end out through the limbal exit site, with enough suture protruding from the eye on each side so as not to risk having the suture retract back into the eye. The needle may then be cut off of the suture. The surgeon performs the same maneuvers to pass the needle and suture through the iris, and under the second haptic.

Sometimes it can be difficult to see where the haptic is under the iris, particularly in thicker, more heavily pigmented irides. If the surgeon is having this difficulty, then using an instrument to lift the optic near the haptic can create additional tenting to highlight the location of the haptic. If that is not adequate, then moving the haptic a little bit side to side while lifting the optic can make the location of the haptic more obvious. If these maneuvers are not adequate, then the surgeon can use one instrument to lift the optic while palpating the iris with an IOL manipulator to locate the haptic, and then support the haptic through the iris while the needle is brought into position for the pass down through the iris.

The needle pass through the iris, under the haptic, and then back up through the iris should be as far into the periphery of the iris as feasible to minimize, or eliminate, an oval shape to the pupil when the procedure is complete (**Fig. 27.12a,b**). The placement of the suture through the iris delineates the part of the iris that cannot move toward the center of the pupil further than the haptic–optic junction. If the suture is placed through the iris relatively close to the pupil margin, the pupil margin will be held out near the haptic–optic junction, causing a deformed pupil. If, however, the needle pass is in the periphery of the iris, then the iris near the pupil can move more freely, which enables a round, or minimally oval, shaped pupil. There is also a theoretical advantage to placing the suture through the peripheral iris: the peripheral iris is closer to the iris root, which is the location where the iris is attached to the ciliary body. Having the suture closer to the mooring of the iris may be more effective at stabilizing the IOL and minimizing the negative sequelae associated with excessive stress on, and movement of, the iris.

At this point in the procedure, the surgeon can either tie a loose throw in each of the sutures or just keep the sutures relatively taut through the limbal pass locations, prior to repositing the IOL optic back through the pupil. If the needle was passed in and out of the limbus through paracentesis openings, then there is usually very little friction on the suture in those paracentesis openings, and greater consideration may be given to tying a loose single throw. If, however, the needles were passed directly through limbal tissue, then there is likely to be a greater amount of friction to hold the suture in place, and the surgeon may wish to reposit the optic back through the pupil without placing any throws in the suture. The main advantage of not making any throws is that it enables the iris to move more freely into a position that will minimize distortion. The main disadvantage of not

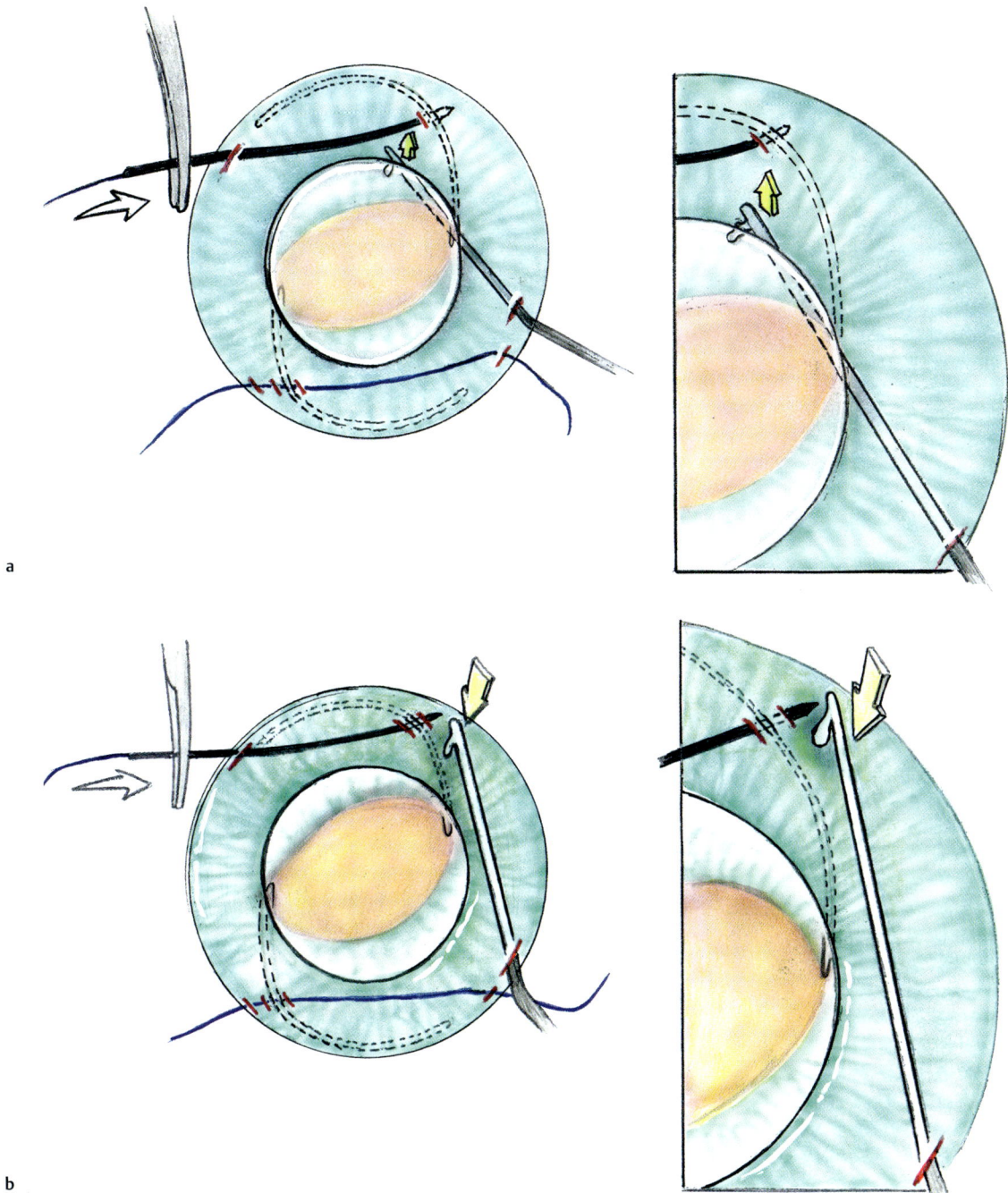

Fig. 27.12 **(a)** A long, curved trans-chamber needle going down through the peripheral iris adjacent to the IOL haptic, which is supported and elevated with an angled IOL manipulator via the optic or through the iris. The iris is constricted behind the optic demonstrating the IOL optic capture configuration. The suture is shown already in place under the other haptic. **(b)** A long, curved trans-chamber needle coming up through the peripheral iris adjacent to the haptic with an IOL manipulator pushing down on the iris as countertraction for the needle pass. The suture is shown already in place under the other haptic.

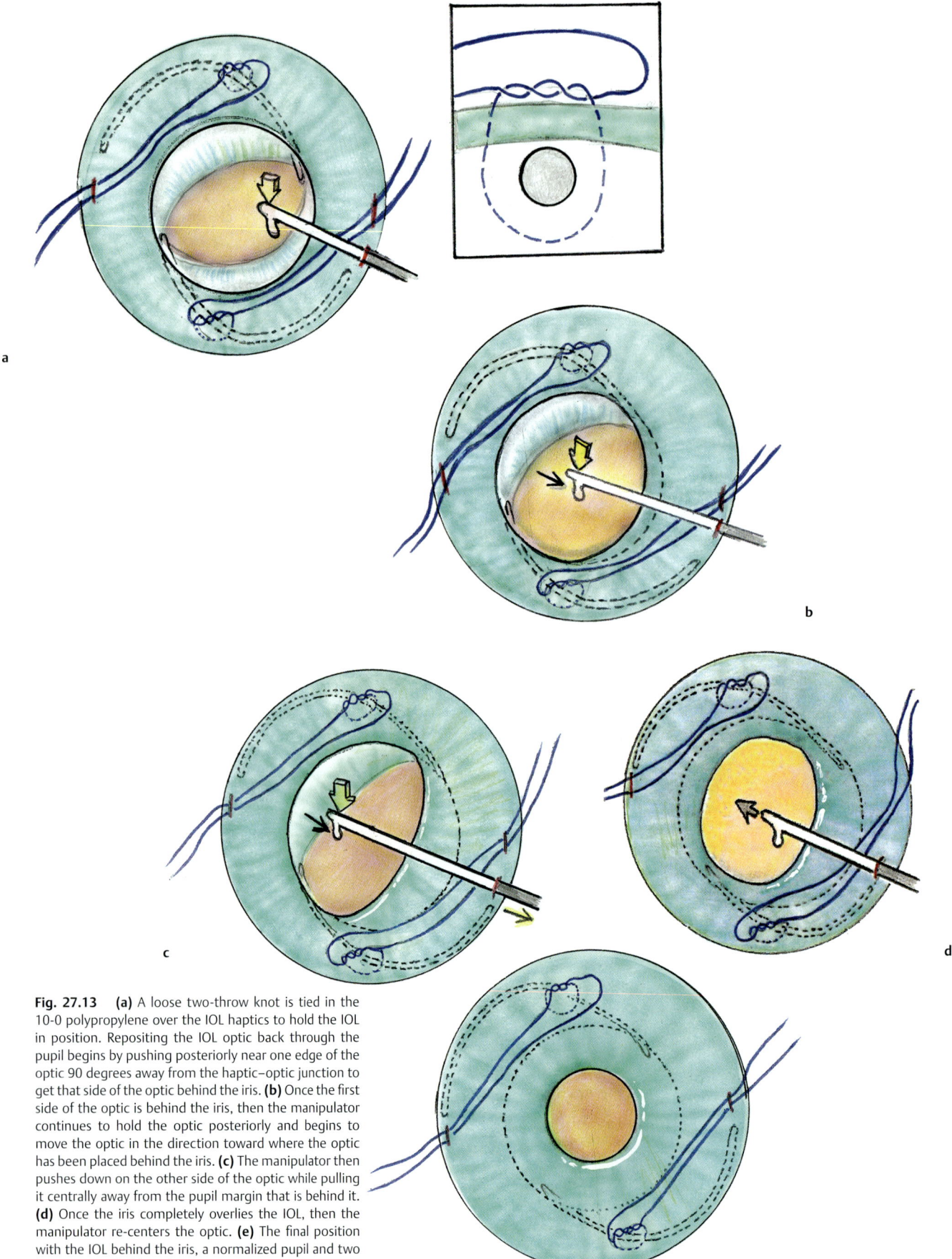

Fig. 27.13   **(a)** A loose two-throw knot is tied in the 10-0 polypropylene over the IOL haptics to hold the IOL in position. Repositing the IOL optic back through the pupil begins by pushing posteriorly near one edge of the optic 90 degrees away from the haptic–optic junction to get that side of the optic behind the iris. **(b)** Once the first side of the optic is behind the iris, then the manipulator continues to hold the optic posteriorly and begins to move the optic in the direction toward where the optic has been placed behind the iris. **(c)** The manipulator then pushes down on the other side of the optic while pulling it centrally away from the pupil margin that is behind it. **(d)** Once the iris completely overlies the IOL, then the manipulator re-centers the optic. **(e)** The final position with the IOL behind the iris, a normalized pupil and two loose sutures holding the IOL in position.

placing any throws is that there is less control of the IOL. If there is reasonable capsule support for the IOL, then the decreased control of the IOL is not of much significance. If there is no capsule support for the IOL, then the surgeon may feel more comfortable placing a single, loose throw for at least one of the haptics, prior to placing the optic back through the pupil, to decrease the risk of posterior IOL dislocation.

Repositing the IOL optic back through the pupil can usually be achieved by using an instrument through a paracentesis to push posteriorly near one edge of the optic 90 degrees away from the haptic–optic junction. Once one side of the optic is behind the pupil, and then it usually requires relatively little posterior pressure with an instrument on the other side of the optic to position the optic completely behind the iris. In situations where the iris capture of the optic is fairly tight, it can occasionally be a little more difficult to get the first side of the optic to drop behind the iris. If that is the case, then the surgeon may use the instrument on the edge of the IOL to push the optic both posteriorly and horizontally toward the middle of the pupil to reposit the first side. If this does not work, one can try pushing in the same way, plus using a cyclodialysis spatula to tire-iron the iris to the front of the optic. Retraction of the pupil margin with an instrument through a paracentesis, or an iris hook could be added in the most stubborn situations (**Fig. 27.13**).

Intraocular Lens Positioning

After placing the optic back behind the iris, the pupil will generally constrict so that it is smaller than the optic. However, having the pupil as small as possible before tightly tying the sutures minimizes the potential of pupil distortion, so injecting some additional miotic into the eye at this time may be beneficial. If the pupil still remains somewhat oval before the sutures have been tied tightly, then an instrument can be used through a paracentesis to massage that section of the iris centrally, or gently pull it centrally with an intraocular forceps. For this surgery, it is important to tighten the knots with the iris positioned in the correct location with respect to the haptics. That means that the tying techniques need to be capable of cinching the suture throws in the desired location, rather than moving the suture (and iris) to a different location (**Fig. 27.14**). A 2–1-1 knot (a knot with two wraps in the first throw, one wrap in the second throw, and one wrap in the third throw) is typically used for securing the suture around the haptic and iris. To avoid deforming the pupil or decentering the IOL, the suture ends need to be cut inside the eye without disturbing the knot or iris. These suture cuts are most easily achieved with coaxial-type intraocular scissors, which can go through a paracentesis. If coaxial scissors are not available, the cuts can be performed with fine non-coaxial scissors, like Vannas scissors, through a larger incision. Such an incision would have already been created if an IOL was inserted as part of the procedure.

Peripheral Iridotomy

Because the IOL optic is positioned very close to the iris with this type of IOL fixation, there is a noteworthy risk of pupillary block occurring as aqueous flows from behind the iris into the anterior chamber; this can be a partial or complete pupillary block. The way to prevent this adverse event is to create a peripheral iridectomy (or iridotomy). The iridectomy does not need to be large; it only needs to be big enough to stay patent and allow slow aqueous flow through it. If a vitrectomy needs to be performed for the procedure, then the vitrectomy probe may be used to create the PI (see Peripheral Iridectomy Creation with a Vitrectomy Probe, below). If not, then the PI may be created in other ways such as with intraocular scissors and forceps. The surgeon may even elect

to create a peripheral iridotomy preoperatively with an Nd:YAG laser. Although it is true that the needle passes through the iris essentially create small iridotomies, the surgeon should assess whether these are large enough to afford lasting protection against pupillary block.

Intraocular Knot Tying

There are three basic categories of knot tying that can achieve the objective of tying the suture without moving the iris and IOL haptic from the desired position:

1. The throws are formed outside the eye, and the knot is cinched with tension on the sutures outside the eye using no instruments inside the eye.
2. The throws are formed outside the eye, and the knot is cinched with tension on the sutures from both outside the eye and inside the eye using an intraocular instrument to provide tension on one of the arms as the knot is positioned prior to cinching.
3. The throws are formed inside the eye with intraocular forceps, and the knot is cinched with tension on the sutures with at least one forceps still located inside the eye to provide tension on the arms as the knot is positioned prior to cinching.

Regardless of which style or type of intraocular knot tying technique a surgeon prefers, it can be beneficial to be familiar with at least one other tying technique for when circumstances make it difficult to adequately perform one's standard tying maneuvers.

Intraocular Knot Tying with Extraocular Throws and No Instruments Inside the Eye for Knot Tightening

Siepser Sliding Knot

For the first category, the most widely known version is the Siepser sliding knot.[16,17] The fundamentals of this knot technique are that the needle needs to go through a paracentesis for at least one of the limbal passes (usually the first), the limbal needle passes need to be precisely in line with where the surgeon wants the knot to be cinched, a loop of suture is pulled out of the eye through the paracentesis opening, the wraps for each throw are performed outside the eye, and then the external ends of the suture are pulled to slide the throws inside the eye where they cinch on the iris. Because the wraps outside the eye are not intuitively familiar to surgeons, one needs to have the wrap process firmly kept in mind during surgery to complete the wraps properly. For instance, with this technique, if the wraps are not performed correctly the surgeon can pull the wrap into the eye and find that there is actually no throw to tighten down—just a twist of the suture. If the view into the eye is suboptimal, it can be difficult to see the suture to verify that the suture is oriented correctly inside the eye so that the wraps are performed on the correct portion of the suture loop. This tying technique, however, is the least complex from an instrumentation standpoint, because all that one needs to be able to form the knot are tying forceps and an instrument with which to hook a loop of suture out through the paracentesis.

As the throws are cinched with this technique, the haptic and iris move up a little out of the iris plane into the plane of the limbus, simply because that is where the sutures pass through the eye wall. Although this does create a bit of iris movement, it generally is not enough to adversely affect the outcome. The knot tying technique, as reported for iris reconstruction,[16,17] uses just

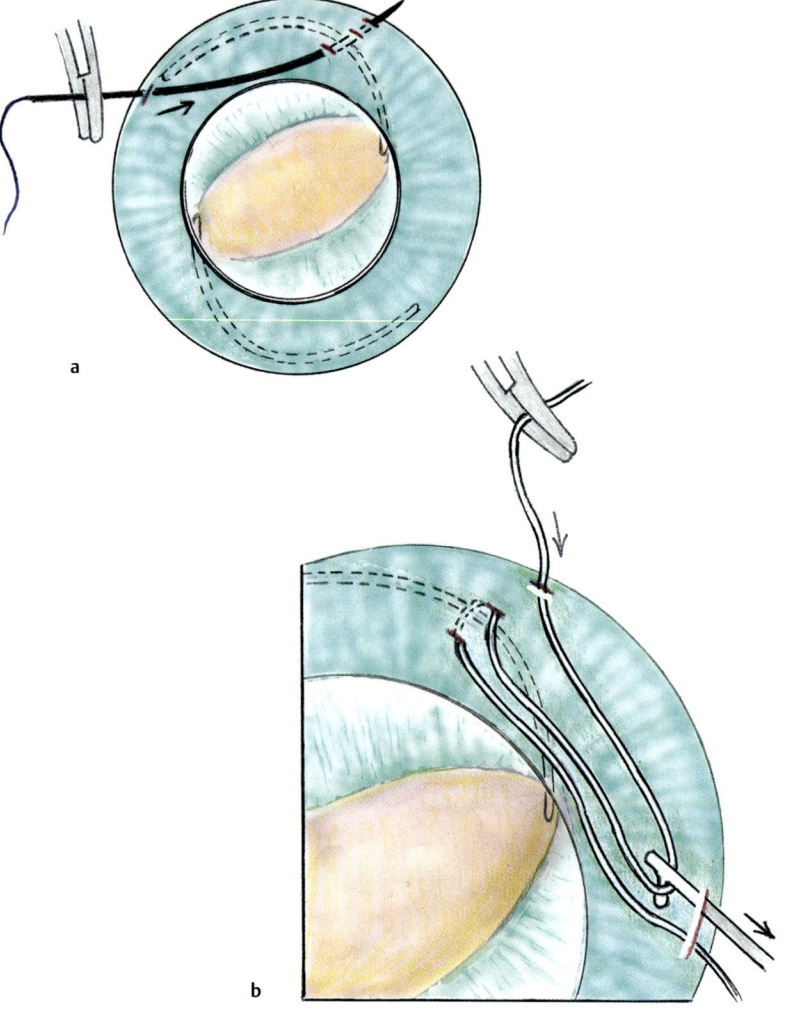

a

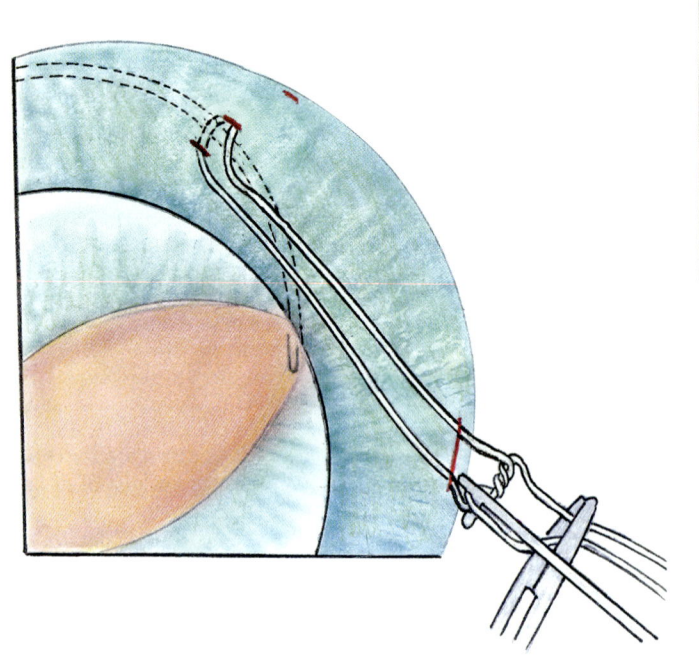

b

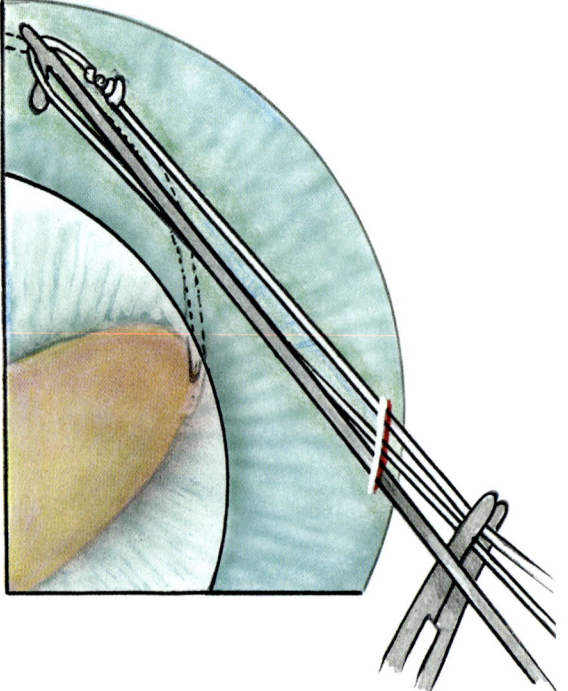

c

d

Fig. 27.14 The in-situ tying technique for suturing the IOL haptics to the iris. **(a)** After the needle and 10-0 polypropylene are passed through the limbus, through iris, under the IOL haptic, back up through iris, and out through the limbus, then one of the arms of the suture is hooked and brought out through a convenient paracentesis opening. **(b)** The second suture arm is hooked and brought out through the same paracentesis as the first suture arm after cutting the needle off the suture. **(c)** The initial throw with two wraps is formed in a conventional way with tying forceps outside the eye, and then tightened to the point where it rests at the outside of the paracentesis opening. One tying forceps is used to hold both arms of the suture while the angled mini-IOL manipulator is positioned with its knob against the longer loop of the suture, preferably on the side of the knot that will allow the throw to lie flat as it is cinched. **(d)** While both arms of the suture are held outside the eye, the knob of the mini-IOL manipulator moves past the knot location, functioning as a pulley for one of the suture arms to tighten the throw. (This throw should be left a little loose if the IOL capture has not yet been reversed. It can subsequently be cinched after the reversal of the capture and proper positioning of the iris.)

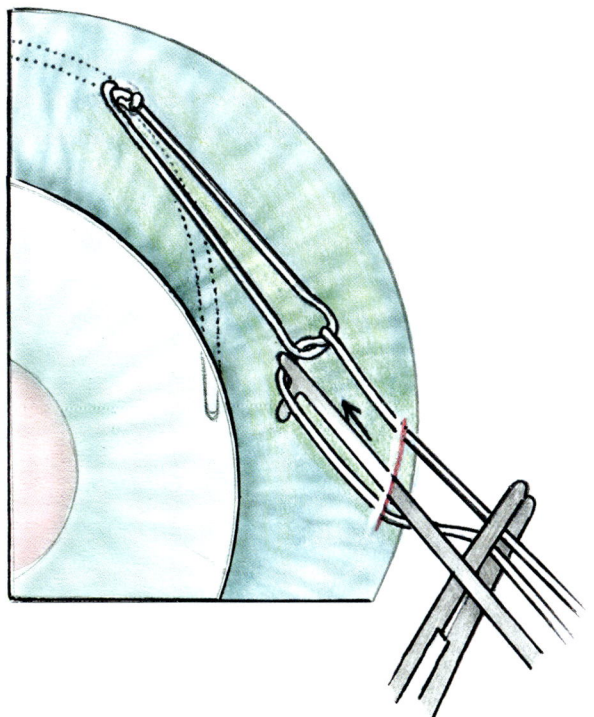

e

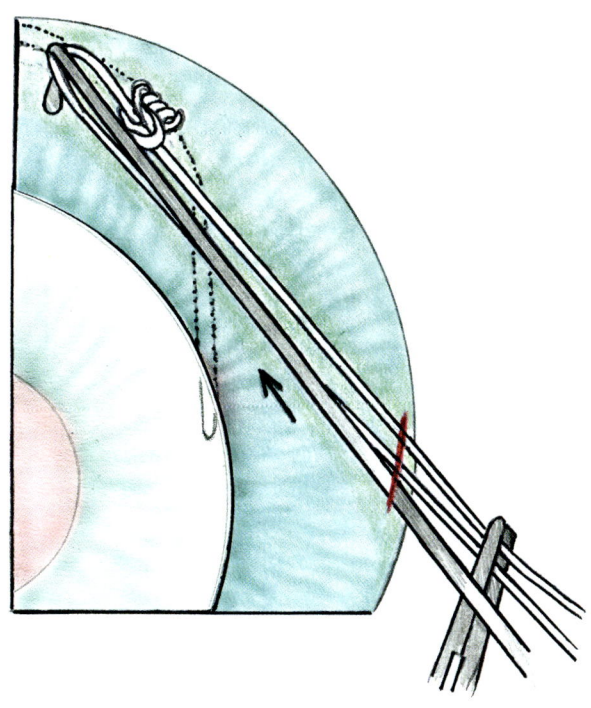

f

Fig. 27.14 (*continued*) **(e)** The second throw of the knot (a single wrap) is formed outside the eye with tying forceps, preferably in such a way that it will form a square knot configuration on the first throw, before it is tightened to the outside of the paracentesis, then pulled inside the eye and cinched in the same fashion as the first throw. **(f)** The third throw is formed outside the eye, again creating the wrap to allow a square knot formation, positioned at the paracentesis in the same way as the second throw, then taken inside the eye and cinched with the pulley action of the intraocular instrument. (Adapted from Ogawa GSH, O'Gawa GM. Single wound, in situ tying technique for iris repair. Ophthalmic Surg Lasers 1998;29:943–948.)

two throws. For adequate security in IOL suturing, it is probably prudent to place a third throw before completing the knot.

When tying a set of squared throws, the surgeon normally pulls any given arm of the suture alternatingly in one direction and then the opposite direction as the throws are cinched. With the Siepser knot, each arm of the suture is always pulled in the same direction, because each suture arm is always through its same limbal incision, which is ~ 180 degrees away from the other limbal incision. With the Siepser knot, the first and third throws are cinched with the suture arms being pulled in the opposite direction than one would normally pull to lie down and cinch a throw. Because of the flexibility of the iris, the iris usually twists to allow the throw to lie correctly when doing iris reconstruction. When tying this knot around an IOL haptic (with iris), the haptic does not twist back and forth, so the odd-numbered throws do not actually lie flat. The resulting knot is still adequately tight and strong to hold the IOL haptic to the iris. The reason for explaining this anomaly of the Siepser knot is so that those tying it will not think that they have incorrectly performed the wraps for the throw if they notice that some throws are not lying down flat as they are cinched. The schematic illustrations in **Fig. 27.15a–j** demonstrate how to perform the wraps for a 2–1–1 Siepser-style knot with the wraps performed to allow the knot to be tied so that a square knot configuration can be achieved.[17] The illustrations demonstrate the creation of the knot closing a radial iris defect for clarity and simplicity.

A further modification of this knot, known as the Condon modification, after Gary P. Condon, involves wrapping the arm of the suture loop coming from the distal side of the iris, and out the proximal paracentesis, around a tying forceps two times, with the tip of that forceps pointed toward the proximal limbus. That tying forceps is then used to grasp the arm of the suture coming from the proximal portion of the iris, and out the proximal paracentesis, before tightening the throw as described above. The second single wrap throw is formed in the same fashion except that the wrap around the forceps is conducted in the opposite direction as was performed for the first throw to enable a square knot configuration. The third single wrap throw is formed by wrapping in the same fashion, but with the direction of wrap identical to that used for the first throw. This method creates the same square knot modification of the Siepser slipping suture knot (**Fig. 27.15a–j**), but the wraps are created by moving suture around a forceps rather than moving suture around a suture. Iqbak Ike K. Ahmed posted a video demonstration on YouTube of a variant of the Condon modification. This variant wraps the suture loop coming from the distal limbus out the proximal paracentesis around the tying forceps with the forceps tip pointed toward the proximal limbus.[18] Some surgeons find it more efficient to tie the knot in this fashion, but the approach is different enough than that demonstrated in **Fig. 27.15** that one should probably understand one of the methods first before learning the other method, so as not to create undue confusion.

Intraocular Knot Tying with Extraocular Throws and One Instrument Inside the Eye for Knot Tightening

For the second category, a useful example is the single-wound in-situ tying technique.[19] For this technique, the suture needle

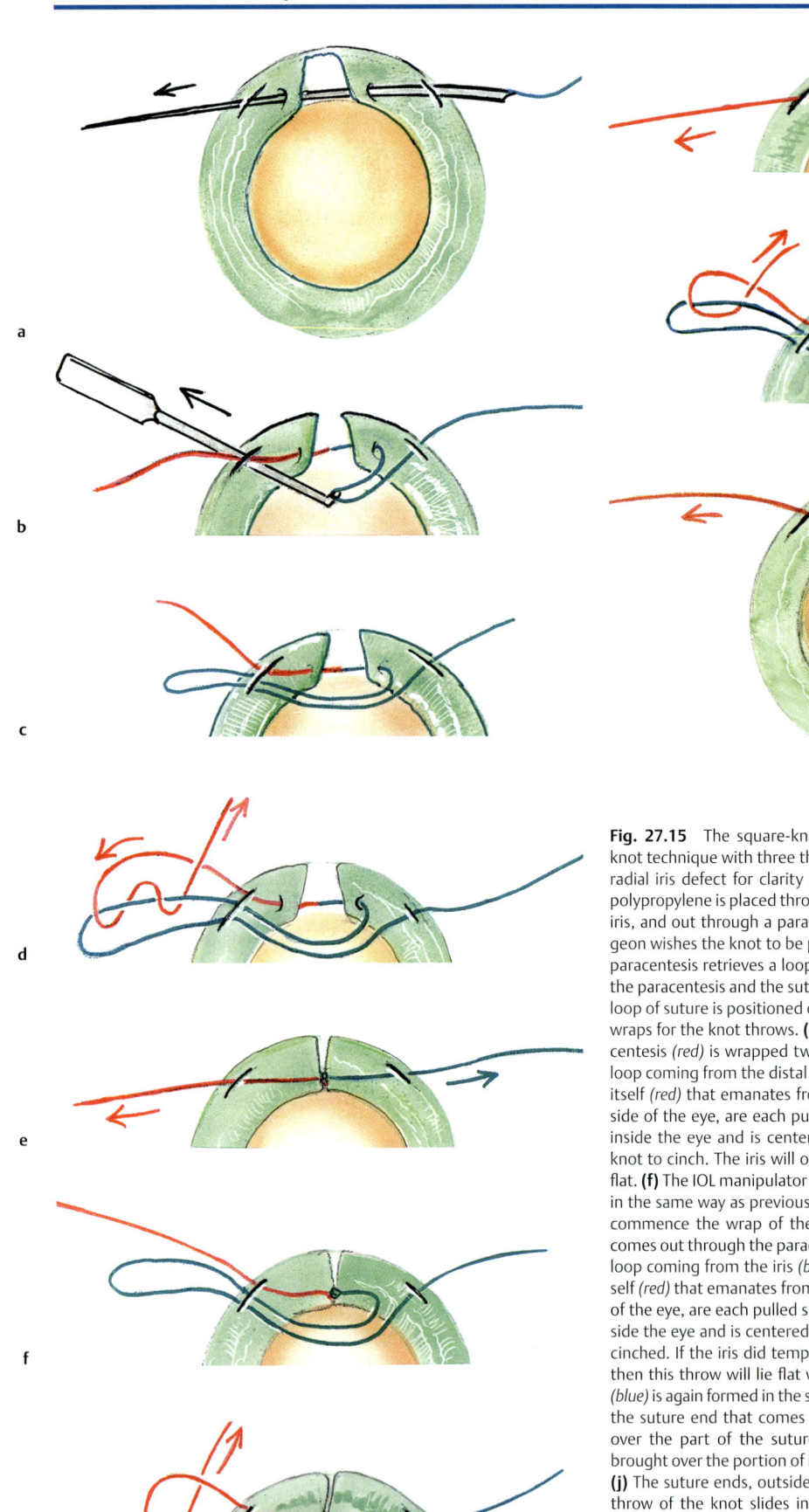

Fig. 27.15 The square-knot modification of the Siepser slipping suture knot technique with three throws (2–1-1). The knot is demonstrated with a radial iris defect for clarity and simplicity. **(a)** The suture needle on 10-0 polypropylene is placed through the limbus, through the desired portions of iris, and out through a paracentesis at a point aligned with where the surgeon wishes the knot to be positioned. **(b)** An IOL manipulator through the paracentesis retrieves a loop of suture from between the iris most distal to the paracentesis and the suture's distal passage through the limbus. **(c)** The loop of suture is positioned outside the eye in proper position for beginning wraps for the knot throws. **(d)** The suture end that is out through the paracentesis *(red)* is wrapped twice toward the eye over the part of the suture loop coming from the distal iris *(blue)*, and then brought over the portion of itself *(red)* that emanates from the paracentesis. **(e)** The suture ends, outside of the eye, are each pulled such that the first throw of the knot slides inside the eye and is centered over the iris where the surgeon wants the knot to cinch. The iris will often twist temporarily to allow the throw to lie flat. **(f)** The IOL manipulator is used again to bring a loop of suture *(blue)* out in the same way as previously described, and the suture loop is oriented to commence the wrap of the second throw. **(g)** The suture end *(red)* that comes out through the paracentesis is wrapped under the part of the suture loop coming from the iris *(blue)*, and then brought under the portion of itself *(red)* that emanates from the paracentesis. **(h)** The suture ends, outside of the eye, are each pulled such that the second throw of the knot slides inside the eye and is centered over the first throw before the second throw is cinched. If the iris did temporarily twist for the cinching of the first throw, then this throw will lie flat without the iris twisting. **(i)** The loop of suture *(blue)* is again formed in the same fashion as for the first two throws, and then the suture end that comes out through the paracentesis *(red)* is wrapped over the part of the suture loop *(blue)* coming from the iris, and then brought over the portion of itself *(red)* that emanates from the paracentesis. **(j)** The suture ends, outside of the eye, are each pulled such that the third throw of the knot slides inside the eye and is centered over the second throw before the third throw is cinched. With this throw, the iris may again twist for the throw to lie flat. (Adapted from Osher RH, Snyder ME, Cionni RJ. Modification of the Siepser slip-knot technique. J Cataract Refract Surg 2005;31:1099.)

can be passed through the limbus in any position that is convenient for achieving the desired placement of the needle and suture through the iris and under the haptic, provided a fine spatula needle is used (rather than a taper-point needle). Both ends of the suture are then brought outside the eye through a conveniently located paracentesis opening; this same paracentesis may be used for tying knots in almost any iris location, so that means the knot for both haptics can be tied through the same paracentesis. The suture arms are tied using conventional throws outside the eye, with one suture arm longer than the other to be able to keep track of which arm is the "wrapping" arm so that the throws can be created in a square knot configuration. Each throw is then brought just to the outer part of the paracentesis opening, with the slack taken out of the suture inside the eye. The suture arms are then laid down on the conjunctival surface next to each other, with one arm having a little more length between the throw and where both sutures are grasped with a tying forceps. That extra length creates a partial loop into which an instrument, such as an IOL manipulator, is placed to pull that suture arm, and the throw, inside the eye with a pulley-like effect, whereas the other ends of the suture are still held with the single tying forceps outside the eye. If the surgeon wishes, the appropriate suture arm (the arm that is coming from the part of the iris that is proximal to the paracentesis) can purposefully be formed as the longer loop to have each throw lie flat as it is cinched. The position of the IOL manipulator and the forceps holding the suture arms outside the eye are adjusted as the throw is pulled down so that the throw cinches in the desired location. The complete knot is formed using two wraps for the first throw and one wrap for the second and third throws (2–1-1). Having two wraps for the first throw gives enough friction to keep it from coming loose after it is cinched, yet still enables it to be readily pulled into the eye and tightened (a three-wrap throw can generate excessive friction, making it more difficult to tighten the throw inside the eye).

Grasping the sutures outside the eye with a single tying forceps, with one of the suture arm loops purposefully arranged to be longer, enables the surgeon to pull that arm past the location where the knot should be tied. This achieves two goals: (1) it enables the knot to be tightened with tension on the sutures to be oriented 180 degrees apart (because the IOL manipulator functions as a pulley), and (2) it keeps the knob of the IOL manipulator away from where the throws are being cinched to minimize the risk of inadvertently capturing the knob of the IOL manipulator in the throw (**Fig. 27.14**).

A variation on this technique is to use an intraocular forceps to pull one arm of the suture into the eye while holding the other arm outside of the eye with a tying forceps. The same principles are used in terms of cinching the knot in the desired location, but in this technique there is no pulley action with the intraocular instrument. If the desired knot location is close to the paracentesis through which the knot is being tied, the surgeon can grasp the suture outside the eye with the intraocular forceps and pull it inside the eye in one motion to cinch the throws. If, however, the desired location for the knot is more than halfway across the anterior chamber from the paracentesis, the suture needs to be released and regrasped inside the eye with the intraocular forceps, and sometimes more than once. Without regrasping when the knot location is on the far side of the eye from the paracentesis, the intraocular forceps will hit the cornea or anterior chamber angle before the throw is tight. Of course, if the surgeon wishes to tie the knot in this same location with this technique and not have to regrasp the suture inside the eye, then a different paracentesis closer to the desired knot location can be created.

With these single paracentesis intraocular-extraocular instrument tying techniques, the intraocular instrument can be lined up with both sutures as well as the knot location, thus

allowing the surgeon to apply force on the arms of the suture 180 degrees apart so that the knot does not shift as the throws are tightened. That said, even the small-diameter intraocular forceps shafts may be wide enough to obstruct the surgeon's view of the knot as the suture is tensioned. If the surgeon finds that the view is excessively blocked by the shaft of the intraocular forceps, but still wants to use the forceps to tighten the knot, there is the option of performing a two-paracentesis technique. This involves making the wraps of the throw outside the eye and pulling the throw into the eye through the first paracentesis, just as already described. The difference is that before the throw is cinched, the surgeon releases the suture inside the eye, and then the intraocular forceps is relocated through a different paracentesis and used to regrasp the same suture before cinching the throw. In this way the shaft of the intraocular forceps comes into the eye off-angle from the 180-degree tension line of the suture arms, enabling the surgeon to more fully view the sutures and the throw as the throw is cinched in the desired location.

Intraocular Knot Tying with Two Instruments Inside the Eye to Form the Throws and Tighten the Knot

The third category of knot tying involves cutting at least one suture end short before tying the knot with the resulting cut end of at least one arm being inside the eye. This two paracentesis technique requires a pair of intraocular forceps (see instrumentation discussion below). The sutures are tied inside the eye in the same fashion as they are normally tied outside the eye, except at least one suture end is short enough to remain inside the anterior chamber, the forceps are small, and there is a rather limited amount of space in which to create the suture wraps for each throw, just the space inside the anterior chamber. This technique provides excellent ability to cinch the throws where the surgeon desires. Because either suture arm can be pulled in either direction, it is possible to have each throw lie flat. It is most often utilized for securing haptics to the iris by surgeons who already have experience with this technique for iris repair. This type of intraocular tying is probably best demonstrated in any number of the multimedia presentations continually created for the internet and ophthalmic meetings by Ike Ahmed, MD (e.g., https://www.youtube.com/user/journey104). If this technique is used for tying haptics to the iris, it should probably be reserved for situations where (1) the IOL is already reasonably supported by remaining lens capsule, (2) the optic is solidly captured in the pupil, (3) there is a safety suture behind the optic, or (4) the first haptic has already been secured by a suture tied with a different method. The reason for this word of caution is that if the IOL is mainly supported by the sutures through the iris, and one or both cut ends of the suture are in the anterior chamber, then fluid fluctuations or gravity could create enough posterior force on the IOL to pull the cut suture end(s) posteriorly through the iris. The result could be a posteriorly dislocated IOL.

Instrumentation for Intraocular Knot Tying: The Instruments used Inside the Eye

One type of instrument that is generally used in the first two categories of intraocular knot tying (and sometimes in the third category) is something to hook sutures to bring them out of the anterior chamber through a paracentesis. A straight instrument is often most agile for this purpose because it can be rotated so that the hooking element can be positioned to most effectively retrieve the suture. Depending on the location of the paracentesis, and the surrounding anatomy, it is sometimes necessary to use an angled instrument and forgo the nimbleness of a straight instrument. The hooking element should be shaped in a way that the suture does not slide off as it is pulled to the paracentesis. This can be achieved with tip configurations of a rounded knob, a collar button, or a skeleton key, among other options. Something with a simple right angle at the tip, such as a Sinskey hook, is not configured to keep the suture from sliding off its tip, so retrieving sutures with this type of instrument can be a little more challenging and frustrating.

For the second category of knot tying that uses an instrument as a pulley inside the eye, there are several characteristics one should consider. The basic elements are an angled instrument that is small enough to go in through a paracentesis (preferably vertically), have a knob that is wider at its tip than where it is attached to the shaft of the instrument, and the knob protrude from the shaft of the instrument a short distance from the tip of the shaft. The wider the knob is at its tip, the easier it is to keep the suture arm in the desired position on the knob, but the harder it is to disengage the knob from a throw should the knob inadvertently get caught in the throw; most surgeons would find a full collar button–type instrument or a skeleton key–type instrument to be a bit broad at their tips to achieve this balance. A smaller rather than larger knob is easier to pass through the paracentesis with the loop of suture in proper position; if the knob it too large, it distorts the paracentesis and the throw, making it harder to successfully pull the suture loop into the eye. If the sides of the knob are smooth, there is less friction on the suture as it is pulled into the eye and the throw is cinched with the pulley effect from the knob. An instrument that has these characteristics and works well for the pulley-style in-situ tying technique is the angled mini-IOL manipulator (model 6–418, Duckworth & Kent). The straight version of this instrument works well for retrieving suture arms out through paracenteses.

There are a variety of different intraocular forceps that can be used for tensioning sutures inside the eye. The shaft diameters generally range in size from 20 gauge down to 25 gauge. Some have straight shafts, and others have curved shafts. The curved shafts enable the surgeon to use the forceps through paracenteses in a wider range of locations because they can be used in areas where the patient's nose or brow might make it impossible to manipulate a straight forceps in the anterior chamber. Some forceps have smooth jaws, others have micro-texturing, and still others have actual serrations to maximize the grip. For tensioning 10-0 polypropylene, smooth-jawed forceps provide adequate tension yet minimize damage to the suture. One of the forceps with smooth jaws and curved shafts, and a 23-gauge size, specifically designed for anterior segment intraocular suture tying is the Ahmed Micro-Tying Forceps (model DFH-0003, Micro-Surgical Technology).

Managing Challenges When Tying Intraocular Knots

For the Siepser style knots, the most common difficulties occur from not having the suture loop oriented correctly and from not following the prescribed wrap pattern for each throw. If the throws are not behaving as expected, the surgeon can refocus on the loop orientation and wrap configuration, and then try forming the throws again. If the surgeon is using the method where suture is wrapped around sutures, and does not tie this type of knot very frequently, it may be useful to have a copy of a schematic such as that in **Fig. 27.15** in the operating room in a place where it can be referenced during the procedure, as needed. Of the various difficulties surgeons have in tying the knot this way, it seems one of the more common problems is neglecting to thread the wrapping suture end over itself, as in the last wrap-

ping step in **Fig. 27.15d**, or under itself, as in the last wrapping step in **Fig. 27.15g**.

Using a pulley technique for the second category of knot described above, there are three principal points where difficulties may be encountered. First, the tip of the IOL manipulator may emerge inside the eye without the loop of suture on the knob. This can occur because the loop was not actually caught outside the eye to start with, or because contact between the knob and the suture was lost after the throw was pulled into the eye. In either case visualizing the location of the suture and repositioning the instrument should remedy the situation. Second, the throw does not progress across the anterior chamber in the desired fashion. This may be caused by the surgeon not having an adequate grasp of both arms of the suture with the tying forceps outside the eye, or the relative lengths of the suture arm loops spontaneously change on the first throw, so the long loop becomes the short loop. If the grasp on the sutures outside the eye has been lost, the surgeon may reestablish a grasp of both sutures to resolve the situation. If the long suture loop has become the short loop, then the surgeon may reposition the tip of the intraocular instrument on the suture arm to re-create the intended configuration, or even move the knob over to what has become the longer loop. After the first throw is cinched, this phenomenon of the long loop becoming the short loop does not occur because the prior throw has fixed the position of the suture in the iris. Third, the knob of the manipulator inadvertently gets caught in the throw that is being tightened. Although this is an infrequent occurrence, the risk of it happening is greatest when the view of the suture is suboptimal, such as with a cloudy cornea, and the knob has had to be repositioned during the tightening of the throw. If an instrument was used with a gradually tapering knob, one can use a fine-tipped second instrument in the other hand, through another paracentesis, to slide the throw off of the knob, such as a fine-tipped Sinsky hook. If a collar button or other broad-tipped knob was used for tightening the throw, the surgeon may be successful at loosening the throw with a second fine-tipped instrument, but if that does not work, the surgeon may consider using fine, intraocular scissors to cut the suture adjacent to the knob to free the instrument.

Using intraocular tying forceps for the second category of knot, the primary difficulties that may occur are (1) problems accurately regrasping the suture, (2) obstruction of the view of the throw as it is cinched, and (3) getting the forceps tip cinched into the throw. Once again, the poorer the view, the more likely it is that there will be challenges in regrasping sutures and keeping the forceps out of the cinched throw. If the forceps does get cinched in a throw, then the same maneuvers described above may be employed to free it. Depending on where the knot is being tied inside the eye, there is also the potential to hit the cornea or anterior chamber angle; avoiding this requires that the surgeon focus both on the throws being cinched and on the location of the forceps tip.

With the third category of knot, where the throws are formed intraocularly, the ability to visualize the sutures becomes even more important because all of the action occurs inside the eye. After the wraps have been created around one of the intraocular forceps, and that forceps has been used to grasp the short suture end inside the eye, it can sometimes be challenging to get the wraps off of the forceps. Using the second forceps to push the wraps off of the first forceps can make this process easier. With a poor view it can be harder to tell if the wraps have been moved off of the forceps, and the potential to cinch the forceps in the throw increases. This problem can be managed in the same ways already described, but in this situation there is also a second intraocular forceps available to help loosen the throw and free the entrapped forceps. With two forceps inside the eye, plus the throws being cinched, the surgeon needs to watch three different areas to achieve proper throw tightening, and avoid contact between the forceps and delicate intraocular structures. If the view is simply too poor for the surgeon to safely and accurately tie sutures inside the eye, there is always the fallback position of either of the other two categories of knots.

Scleral-Susured IOLs

Suture Material and Suture Needles

10-0 Polypropylene

Initially, the most commonly used material for suturing PCIOLs to the sclera was 10-0 polypropylene.[7] It is classified by suture manufacturers as a nonabsorbable suture, and years of experience with 10-0 polypropylene for suturing the iris demonstrated that it has a very long life in the intraocular environment, even though polypropylene shows signs of slow degradation in the eye.[20] The 10-0 polypropylene was available on a long curved spatula-type 6-mil-diameter needles (models CTC-6 and CTC-6L, Ethicon) and on a larger diameter tapered, curved needle with a cutting tip (CIF-4, Ethicon) that is difficult to pass through corneal and scleral tissue. Size 10-0 polypropylene was the standard suture material for scleral sutured PCIOLs until the early 2000s, when reports began surfacing that surgeons were experiencing breakage of the sutures, with subsequent IOL subluxation (dislocation) in some patients who had surgery about a decade before.[21] Although there are varying opinions, the most common belief is that the suture degrades more quickly in the scleral and subconjunctival environment,[21] compared with the purely intraocular environment. In the majority of patients with 10-0 polypropylene sutures, the IOLs did not displace, probably due to haptics healing in place,[21] but they displaced in enough patients that it created concern among surgeons, and other suture materials were sought.

9-0 Polypropylene

One of the initial responses was to shift to a larger polypropylene suture (9-0 polypropylene) to increase the longevity of suture support for the IOLs by increasing the diameter of the suture material. Size 9-0 polypropylene is 50% greater in diameter than size 10-0, so that means that the cross-sectional area of the 9-0 is 2.25 times larger than that of 10-0. In the United States, 9-0 polypropylene was made available from Ethicon on the same long, curved, trans-chamber needles (model CTC-6L, Ethicon), but as a special order (model D-8229) with a very substantial price per suture. At this time, 9-0 polypropylene is likely the standard suture for many surgeons performing scleral sutured IOL cases. As of this writing, my group practice has not experienced IOL dislocations with 9-0 polypropylene, having used it since 2003, although one surgeon at a different ophthalmology group has told me that he has seen a couple of dislocations with 9-0 polypropylene. Surgical Specialties Corp./Sharpoint (Braintree, MA) more recently started making 6-inch-long 9-0 polypropylene as a production suture with two 15-mm side cutting lancet needles that have a one eighth of a circle curvature (model J2558N). This suture is much more economical than the special-order Ethicon 9-0, with these caveats: (1) the needle has only a slight curve, (2) the needle does not go through sclera as easily, and (3) the 6-inch suture length increases the risk of suture tangling. MANI Ophthalmic (Tochigi, Japan) is reportedly developing a 9-0 polypropylene production suture, about 3 inches long, affixed, double armed, to a very sharp curved trans-chamber needle (model VI105/16-14S) that is 16 mm long (about 3 mm longer than the CTC-6L) and 0.14 mm wide, which is essentially the same diam-

eter as the CTC-6L. It is anticipated that this production suture will also be notably more economical than the Ethicon special-order option.

10-0 Polyester

Another suture used by a few surgeons is size 10-0 polyester because of the high strength of polyester and the perception that it lasts longer and does not break down as readily as polypropylene.[22] Polyester is also more resistant to crush damage from tying forceps and needle holders than polypropylene.[23] Because 10-0 polyester is only available in the United States on short needles, surgeons wishing to use it on long, curved, trans-chamber needles need to tie it to 10-0 polypropylene on long, curved, trans-chamber needles, or use it with some type of ab-externo technique.

Gore-Tex (Expanded Polytetrafluoroethylene [e-PTFE])

A third suture option that some surgeons have pursued is the use of e-PTFE in the smallest size manufactured—the CV-8 size (Gore-Tex). The CV-8 suture's mean diameter is 0.091 mm, which is essentially the same size as a United States Pharmacopeia (USP)-sized 6-0 suture, but the e-PTFE can be compressed to a smaller diameter because half of its microstructure consists of air. The needles available on the suture are short and not suitable for passing through sclera, so ab-externo techniques are employed by either docking the needles (some surgeons straighten the needles first) into hollow-bore needles or removing the needles and using forceps to externalize the suture[5,7] as described above. This suture material is highly fluorinated making it slippery, so it is advisable to use more throws than one typically uses in other suture materials to form a secure knot. The manufacturer recommends at least seven equally tensioned throws for the conventional uses of this suture,[24] but for sutured IOLs, most surgeons utilize fewer throws than that.[5,7] The manufacturer indicates that the material is very inert, and it is not subject to weakening by the action of tissue enzymes.[24]

The probable longevity and strength of this suture, resulting from its chemical composition and diameter, seem to be notable advantages. On the negative side, however, larger, separately created incisions are needed through the sclera/uvea, which adds time to the procedure and theoretically an increased potential for bleeding. If using a "needle-less" technique, specialty instrumentation, such as coaxial forceps to pull the material through the sclera, is needed. Ab-externo techniques, by nature, push the ciliary body inward away from the sclera, and in some post-trauma situations with damaged adhesion between the ciliary body and sclera, the ciliary body can actually be focally pulled away from the sclera even when using very sharp MVR blades. There is an additional, noteworthy challenge in using this suture for securing IOLs, as the manufacturer specifically states that the suture is contraindicated for ophthalmic surgery. The manufacturer's instructions for Gore-Tex suture, dated January 2012, state, "This device is contraindicated for use in ophthalmic surgery, microsurgery, and peripheral neural tissue." The instructions also offer a warning that safety and effectiveness have not been established in ophthalmic surgery.[24] Ophthalmologists frequently utilize products for off-label uses, but using contraindicated devices is a little different from simple off-label use. Communication with W.L. Gore & Associates has revealed that the manufacture does not have any data suggesting that there are safety issues with the ophthalmic or microsurgical use of the suture, but that the Food and Drug Administration (FDA) asked the company to place the contraindication in the suture instructions because

Table 27.1 The Four Controllable Variables in Descemet's Incision Widening

Variable Number	Moves the Descemet's Incision Centrally Cutting While:	Moves the Descemet's Incision Peripherally Cutting While:
1	Pushing in with the keratome	Pulling out with the keratome
2	Cutting side of keratome is tilted up	Cutting side of keratome is tilted down
3	Cutting side of keratome is angled to face centrally	Cutting side of keratome is angled to face peripherally
4	Tip of keratome is elevated up	Tip of keratome is depressed down

the suture was not studied for ophthalmic or microsurgical use.[25] All factors considered, the most compelling reason to use this suture material is in the situation where patients have a substantial life expectancy remaining after the time of surgery—a period of time that exceeds what the literature of the day indicates is the longevity of other suture materials that are not contraindicated. Because of the language in the instructions for this suture material, surgeons may wish to have and document a discussion with patients regarding the contraindication in the manufacturer's instructions as well as the reasons why the material might be recommended. If the patient elects to have this suture, the surgeon may wish to document that as well.

Intraocular Lens Options

A wide variety of IOLs have been sutured to the sclera, particularly because that is one way to secure subluxated IOLs that are already in a patient's eye. When a different IOL will be used for either secondary placement, or during IOL exchange surgery, the surgeon may choose the IOL more critically. Some surgeons suturing IOLs on a regular basis prefer an IOL with more intrinsic rigidity, and haptic configurations that are amenable to four-point fixation to minimize the potential for IOL tilt. This can be achieved with a one-piece PMMA IOL with eyelets on the haptics that help separate the suture arms where they attach to the haptics. The Alcon model CZ70BD IOL is one of the few IOLs with this configuration, plus it has a large 7-mm optic to help minimize the impact of IOL decentration. This IOL has haptics that are round and have a relatively small diameter, which probably helps minimize the potential for causing uveal irritation as well as increase the risk of the haptic healing into the ciliary sulcus.[21] Placement of a CZ70BD benefits from a well-constructed scleral tunnel incision for optimizing globe integrity and minimizing induced astigmatism (see Incision Enlargement Technique, below).

Foldable IOLs have been used by some with the goal of achieving a smaller incision size, but as noted, these generally fall short in the areas of stability, optic size, and ability to separate the suture arms on the haptic to achieve four-point fixation to prevent IOL tilt. Although the Wills Eye Hospital Retina Service (Philadelphia, PA) has published their e-PTFE scleral sutured IOL technique with the CZ70BD,[7] they have also done work using an acrylic foldable IOL [Akreos IOL, Bausch & Lomb] that has four closed loops, making it possible to achieve four-point fixation with an e-PTFE suture going through both haptic loops on each side of the IOL and then out through vitrectomy cannulas placed through the sclera, before removal of the cannulas and tying of the suture.[26] It has been well established that square-edged acrylic IOL haptics in the sulcus in nonsutured situations have a rather significant tendency to cause uveitis, pigment dispersion, and glaucoma.[15] Over time we will learn whether or not square-edged acrylic haptics sutured into the sulcus are able to avoid these problems.

Incision Enlargement Technique

Because most ophthalmic surgeons now spend very little of their time creating large incisions, it is worth focusing, for a moment, on the four controllable variables that determine the path of the incision through Descemet's membrane as a corneal valve incision is widened: (1) cutting while pushing the keratome in versus cutting while pulling it out, (2) the cutting side of the keratome being tilted up versus tilted down, (3) the cutting side of the keratome being angled in toward the center of the cornea versus angled out toward the periphery of the cornea, and (4) the tip of the keratome being elevated up toward the back of the cornea versus depressed down toward the iris. Each of these variables can be altered individually, or in concert with the others, to guide the incision enlargement along the desired path through Descemet's membrane. Variables 2 through 4 have neutral points that are roughly halfway between the extremes. If the incision is widening along the desired path, then keeping the variables close to their neutral points will generally keep the incision widening on the same path, with appropriate small adjustments being made for the fact that variable 1 does not have a neutral point. If a Descemet's incision is going acutely in an unwanted direction, then adjusting all four variables to counteract the wayward direction of the incision can rather dramatically alter the course of the incision back toward the desired direction. To utilize these maneuvers to one's advantage, the surgeon needs to focus the microscope on the Descemet's incision, with high enough magnification, to be able to see the Descemet's incision as it progresses (**Table 27.1**).

Suture Configuration on Haptics and Intraocular Lens Tilt

The configuration and orientation of the suture on an IOL haptic warrants careful preoperative and intraoperative consideration and attention to obtain the result of a stable, nontilted IOL. If an IOL tilts (deviates from the IOL's plane being parallel to the plane of the iris), then optical and mechanical problems may result.

The optical effect of a tilted IOL is a type of optical aberration called marginal oblique astigmatism that results from pantoscopic tilt—the tilting of a spherical lens such that it is no longer perpendicular to the path of the light going through it. With a positive powered lens, pantoscopic tilt induces plus-powered astigmatism, with the astigmatism axis aligned with the axis of the tilt, as well as the induction of a plus spherical component. The amount of the astigmatism is proportional to the dioptric power of the lens, and also proportional to the square of the tangent of the angle of tilt, in the theoretical model, so the greater the tilt and the greater the IOL power, the greater the aberration.[27] Marginal oblique astigmatism also contains a coma-like aberration that cannot be corrected with glasses or contact lenses, so with enough IOL tilt a patient will experience a decrease in the best corrected vision, which may be rather unsatisfactory.[28] If the tilt is great enough, a mechanical problem can result from the IOL edge chafing the iris. This may cause pigment dispersion, intraocular pressure elevation, and inflammation just as with any nonoptimal contact between an IOL and the iris. High degrees of tilt also increase the risk of partial pupillary capture of the IOL optic, even if peripheral iridectomies have been created.

Four-point fixation of some sort is generally considered to be one of the most reliable ways to achieve an IOL optic positioned parallel to the iris, and to keep the IOL from tilting postoperatively. That said, if inadequate attention is given to where and how the four-point fixation is achieved, then the lens may have an intraoperatively created tilt that remains stable postoperatively. The basic concept of four-point fixation is that there are four different points on an IOL that have their own, corresponding fixation locations in the sclera. For IOLs with two haptics, this requires a way to have suture separation on the haptic. The suture separation has been done in several ways: (1) having the suture go around a haptic perpendicular to the haptic, often through an eyelet on the haptic, so the two arms of the suture are separated by the width of the haptic[7]; (2) having the suture go through a haptic eyelet and then have both arms of the suture come out over, or under, the haptic so that the sutures are separated by part of the eyelet (as in the technique described above); (3) forming a hitch with the suture on the haptic that incorporates a spacer, such as an eyelet, to separate the two arms of the suture coming off the haptic[5]; or (4) using an IOL with four haptics.[26]

With the suture configuration in option 1, the suture arms need to either go through the sclera with one arm anterior to the other (which is usually not done due to space limitations), or with the two arms going through the sclera adjacent to each other, the same distance back from the iris, but with one of the sutures configured to tilt the IOL in one direction and the suture on the other haptic configured to tilt the IOL in the opposite direction. This is sometimes referred to as a "torque/anti-torque" suture configuration. Executed perfectly, this configuration should produce the desired result; however, this configuration is prone to two main problems. The first is that if the suture for one haptic is not tied with the same tension as the suture on the other haptic, then the tighter suture "wins" and the IOL will have a tendency to tilt in the direction dictated by the tighter suture. The second is that if the surgeon loses track and configures both sutures so they tilt the IOL in the same direction, then the torque/anti-torque balance is lost and the IOL will have a notable tendency to tilt in the direction dictated by both sutures so that, if unfettered by the iris and ciliary body, the IOL would be oriented so that light would be entering the IOL's edge rather than its optical face.

With the suture configurations in options 2, 3, and 4, it is probably best to have both of the suture arms come over the top of the haptic, rather than under the bottom of the haptic. One reason to do this is that it is easier for the surgeon to see if the suture is configured correctly before the haptic is put in its place behind the iris. Another reason is that the scleral portion (structural aspect) of the eye wall is angled such that the sclera is closer to the haptic on its anterior side and farther away from the haptic on the posterior side. With the sutures coming over the anterior portion of the haptic they can enter the sclera from a more direct angle and pull the haptic into position with minimal shifting of the haptic (anteriorly-posteriorly) as the suture is tensioned and tied.

Suture Knot Management

To complete the suturing of a transscleral fixated IOL, a knot must be tied in the suture. Knots were initially tied under scleral flaps,[2] but knots in this location have a notable tendency to erode through the sclera and overlying conjunctiva, causing complications including endophthalmitis.[29–31] At the present time scleral flaps are probably not considered an optimal way to cover the knots because of the potential for serious complications. A variety of other ways have been used to minimize the chance of knot exposure, but in considering any of these, the surgeon should carefully analyze the potential for erosion of the tissue covering the suture leading to exposure, because the downside of exposure can be so substantial.

One of the more commonly used methods for managing IOL suture knots is creating a conjunctival flap in the area of the suture pass and then rotating the knot inside the eye prior to closing the conjunctiva.[32] Getting the knot completely buried into the eye, or at least deeply into the sclera, is important to minimize the risk of the knot eroding through conjunctiva. Experience has shown that with a suture size of 9-0, there is probably essentially a zero rate of suture strand exposure through the conjictiva if the knot is buried inside the eye. The CV-8 e-PTFE (Gore-Tex) is rather soft, but it is large enough in diameter that there is likely a very small risk of suture strand exposure in patients with thin or unhealthy conjunctiva. When rotating knots through the sclera into the eye, it can be helpful to grasp the sclera with a 0.12 or Colibri forceps directly adjacent to the location where the knot is going into the sclera. During burying, one should try to minimize tying forceps pressure on the suture to lessen crush damage to the suture, because crush damage causes suture weakening. One way to minimize forceps damage to the suture is to use a separate instrument to push the knot down into the sclera at the site of one of the openings in the sclera. For openings created with just the pass of a 6-mil needle, a small-tipped Sinsky hook can be useful for this purpose. The Sinsky can even be used to help enlarge the opening through the sclera by putting the tip in the scleral opening, and then moving it in a tight, circular motion. For openings created with blades or cannulated needles, a somewhat larger instrument may be used to push the knot down into the sclera.

When creating knots, the number of wraps in a particular throw plays a bigger role in how wide it is, and hence how hard it is to bury, than the total number of throws. For instance, a 3–1–1 knot has a wider profile and is more difficult to bury than a 2–1-1-1-1 knot tied in the same suture material. In the latter case, the widest throw is a two-wrap throw, and the additional one-wrap throws create a sort of chain or tail that is only the width of a single-wrap throw, and hence does not increase the resistance to burying. Because some manipulation can be required during the burying of knots, there is the potential for the last throw of the knot to come loose or undone during the process. With this in mind, and the fact that additional throws do not widen the knot, it can be advantageous to add one more single-wrap throw to the knot when it is tied than the surgeon would feel comfortable having in the finished result with the knot buried inside the eye.

Another option for knot management that appears to avoid the risk of knot exposure is the creation of a lamellar pocket dissection posteriorly from the limbus with the knot tied inside the dissected area (see Chapter 28). This is commonly called a Hoffman pocket,[33] and neither a review of the literature nor personal communication with Dr. Richard Hoffman has yielded reports of knot erosion through the sclera and conjunctiva of these pockets when used with 9-0 polypropylene. CV-8 Gore-Tex knots are large enough that in occasional situations they may erode through the roof of a Hoffman pocket. Whether it is the preservation of scleral perfusion and innervation in the pocket area, the lack of conjunctival perturbation, or some other set of factors, at present these pockets appear to be notably more resistant to knot erosion than scleral flaps when used with sutures of the 9-0 or smaller size.

A newer variant of the procedure that avoids knots altogether is the technique of intrascleral haptic fixation (see Chapter 29). This technique generally uses fibrin glue to hold a scleral flap down over the haptic. The technique is rather enticing, but as with sutured variants, it is not free of complications, and the long-term results needed to assess sutured techniques are not yet available with intrascleral fixation techniques.[34]

Peripheral Iridectomy Creation with a Vitrectomy Probe

Peripheral iridectomies (PIs) can effectively be created with the same vitrectomy probe that was used to remove vitreous from the eye at the beginning of the procedure. The machine settings need to be adjusted considerably when creating peripheral iridectomies so that excessive amounts of iris are not inadvertently removed. For those surgeons who do not already have optimized machine settings for peripheral iridectomy creation, it may be wise to start with a very low cut rate (~ 60 cuts per minute) with a low vacuum (~ 60 mm Hg for a 20-gauge probe, and sometimes a bit higher with smaller gauge probes) and a low aspiration rate (~ 15 cc/min). If the machine has the option of irrigation and aspiration (I/A) first (foot position 2), followed by cut modality (foot position 3), this mode is good to use for peripheral iridectomies because the aspiration pulls some iris into the port before the first cut occurs. (Note that this is the opposite mode than that used while performing vitreous removal where Cut/I/A mode should be used so that the cutter starts operating before aspiration begins.) With the settings described above, it may require only two to four cuts with the vitrectomy probe face down on the anterior surface of the iris to create the PI with a 20-gauge probe. If one sees marked movement of iris tissue toward the port of the vitrectomy probe, that can be a clue that a PI of notable size may be forming, and one should stop to assess the size of the PI before continuing. If, after several cuts with the vitrectomy probe, there has been no removal of iris tissue, then one may wish to increase the vacuum in a stepwise fashion until the desired affect is achieved. As one might expect, thinner, less pigmented irides usually require less vacuum than thicker, more pigmented irides to achieve adequate iris tissue cutting during PI creation. If the surgeon creates a PI that is much larger than desired, one must assess if it will create an optical or other problem. If it seems the large size will be problematic, then a 10-0 polypropylene interrupted suture may be placed to decrease the size of the PI (**Fig. 27.14**).

Open Corneal Valve Management at the Main Incision

A 7-mm incision is relatively wide, so sometimes the corneal valve can be well formed, but it does not spontaneously close intraoperatively. If the incision is superior, a modest-sized air bubble can be placed in the anterior chamber to press the valve closed when the patient is upright. To determine if the air bubble technique will work, one can place a larger bubble intraoperatively with the patient in the standard supine position to see if the valve pushes closed and the wound stops leaking. If it seems effective, then the bubble can be made smaller prior to completing the case. (Too large of an air bubble may cause pupillary block.) Another way to close an open but well-formed corneal valve is with a corneal valve suture. This is a suture in which the needle goes full thickness straight down through the cornea central to the Descemet's incision, then comes up through the central portion of the corneal valve as the needle angles toward the anterior sclera where the needle reemerges on the ocular surface. The suture ends can be tied together outside the eye before burying the knot into the corneal tissue. Placing these sutures is actually easier with an anterior chamber filled with air because the corneal valve is pressed up into place, and it is easier to see the Descemet's incision. The corneal valve suture is particularly useful for temporal incisions because one cannot rely on a patient to position properly to close a temporal valve with an air bubble. Younger patients, who have floppier corneas, are particularly prone to having corneal valves that do not spontaneously close, or that fall open in the early postoperative period, even with smaller incisions, and especially when the incision is temporal (possibly because of the shape of the temporal limbal region, and the change in shape of the globe with blinking action). In a cooperative patient, a 10-0 nylon works well as a corneal valve suture that can easily be removed at 1 week postoperative while the patient is still on topical antibiotics. If the patient is unable to cooperate for in-office suture removal, a 10-0 polyglactin suture can be used for this purpose. However, because the suture tract is a full-thickness tract into the eye, one should probably keep the patient on topical antibiotic until the suture has completely resorbed to minimize the risk of late-onset endophthalmitis as the suture starts breaking apart about a month after it is placed.

References

1. Gess LA. Scleral fixation for intraocular lenses. J Am Intraocul Implant Soc 1983;9:453–456

2. Stark WJ, Goodman G, Goodman D, Gottsch J. Posterior chamber intraocular lens implantation in the absence of posterior capsular support. Ophthalmic Surg 1988;19:240–243

3. Higashide T, Shimizu F, Nishimura A, Sugiyama K. Anterior segment optical coherence tomography findings of reverse pupillary block after scleral-fixated sutured posterior chamber intraocular lens implantation. J Cataract Refract Surg 2009;35:1540–1547

4. Di Pascuale MA, Mootha VV, Ogawa GS. Ogawa Technique for Transsclerally Sutured PC IOL Placement. Film presented at the Film Festival of the American Society of Cataract and Refractive Surgery's Annual Symposium on Cataract, Intraocular Lens, and Refractive Surgery, San Diego, April 28 to May 2, 2007

5. Snyder ME, Perez MA. Tiltless and centration adjustable scleral-sutured posterior chamber intraocular lens. J Cataract Refract Surg 2014;40:1579–1583

6. Slade DS, Hater MA, Cionni RJ, Crandall AS. Ab externo scleral fixation of intraocular lens. J Cataract Refract Surg 2012;38:1316–1321

7. Khan MA, Gerstenblith AT, Dollin ML, Gupta OP, Spirn MJ. Scleral fixation of posterior chamber intraocular lenses using gore-tex suture with concurrent 23-gauge pars plana vitrectomy. Retina 2014;34:1477–1480

8. Jaffe NS, Duffner LR. The iris-plane (Copeland) pseudophakos. Arch Ophthalmol 1976;94:420–424

9. Jaffe NS. Results of intraocular lens implant surgery. The third Binkhorst medal lecture. Am J Ophthalmol 1978;85:13–23

10. McCannel MA. A retrievable suture idea for anterior uveal problems. Ophthalmic Surg 1976;7:98–103

11. Stutzman RD, Stark WJ. A new surgical technique for suture fixation of an acrylic IOL in the absence of capsular support. J Cataract Refract Surg 2003;29:1658–1662

12. Condon GP. Simplified small-incision peripheral iris fixation of an AcrySof intraocular lens in the absence of capsule support. J Cataract Refract Surg 2003;29:1663–1667

13. LeBoyer RM, Werner L, Snyder ME, Mamalis N, Riemann CD, Augsberger JJ. Acute haptic-induced ciliary sulcus irritation associated with single-piece AcrySof intraocular lenses. J Cataract Refract Surg 2005;31:1421–1427

14. Mamalis N. Sulcus placement of single-piece acrylic intraocular lenses. J Cataract Refract Surg 2009;35:1327–1328

15. Kirk KR, Werner L, Jaber R, Strenk S, Strenk L, Mamalis N. Pathologic assessment of complications with asymmetric or sulcus fixation of square-

edged hydrophobic acrylic intraocular lenses. Ophthalmology 2012;119: 907–913

16. Siepser SB. The closed chamber slipping suture technique for iris repair. Ann Ophthalmol 1994;26:71–72

17. Osher RH, Snyder ME, Cionni RJ. Modification of the Siepser slip-knot technique. J Cataract Refract Surg 2005;31:1098–1100

18. Ahmed IK. The Siepser Sliding Knot for Iris Repair. https://www.youtube .com/watch?v=4QipgGl1HTk. Accessed February 14, 2015.

19. Ogawa GSH, O'Gawa GM. Single wound, in situ tying technique for iris repair. Ophthalmic Surg Lasers 1998;29:943–948

20. Drews RC. Quality control, and changing indications for lens implantation. The Seventh Binkhorst Medal Lecture-1982. Ophthalmology 1983; 90:301–310

21. Price MO, Price FW Jr, Werner L, Berlie C, Mamalis N. Late dislocation of scleral-sutured posterior chamber intraocular lenses. J Cataract Refract Surg 2005;31:1320–1326

22. MacKool RJ. Intraocular lens exchange. Presented at the Cataract Surgery Telling It Like It Is symposium, Sarasota, Florida, January 18, 2014

23. Personal email communication with the medical director at Ethicon, Inc., August 21, 2014

24. Instructions for Use for. Gore-Tex suture: instructions for use. Gore Medical North America Website. http://www.goremedical.com/suture/ instructions/ Published January 2012; accessed January 4, 2015

25. Personal telephone communication on January 7, 2015 with Carrie Ortiz, product specialist at W. L. Gore & Associates, Inc.

26. Bansal AS, Khurana RN. Explanation of dislocated IOL and secondary scleral fixation. American Academy of Ophthalmology, ONE Network Website. http://one.aao.org/clinical-video/explantation-of-dislocated-iol -secondary-scleral-f Video published November 6, 2014; accessed December, 28 2014

27. Marcos S. Special circumstances: effect of IOL tilt on astigmatism. In: Hoffer KJ, ed. IOL Power. Thorofare, NJ: Slack; 2011:223–230

28. Oshika T, Kawana K, Hiraoka T, Kaji Y, Kiuchi T. Ocular higher-order wavefront aberration caused by major tilting of intraocular lens. Am J Ophthalmol 2005;140:744–746

29. Heilskov T, Joondeph BC, Olsen KR, Blankenship GW. Late endophthalmitis after transscleral fixation of a posterior chamber intraocular lens. Arch Ophthalmol 1989;107:1427

30. Schechter RJ. Suture-wick endophthalmitis with sutured posterior chamber intraocular lenses. J Cataract Refract Surg 1990;16:755–756

31. Solomon K, Gussler JR, Gussler C, Van Meter WS. Incidence and management of complications of transsclerally sutured posterior chamber lenses. J Cataract Refract Surg 1993;19:488–493

32. Lewis JS. Sulcus fixation without flaps. Ophthalmology 1993;100:1346–1350

33. Hoffman RS, Fine IH, Packer M, Rozenberg I. Scleral fixation using suture retrieval through a scleral tunnel. J Cataract Refract Surg 2006;32:1259–1263

34. Kumar DA, Agarwal A, Packiyalakshmi S, Jacob S, Agarwal A. Complications and visual outcomes after glued foldable intraocular lens implantation in eyes with inadequate capsules. J Cataract Refract Surg 2013;39: 1211–1218

28 Corneoscleral Pocket (Hoffman Pocket)

Richard S. Hoffman, Annette Chang Sims, and I. Howard Fine

Scleral fixation of intraocular lenses, adjunctive capsular support devices, and intraocular tissues has traditionally been accomplished utilizing sutures. Common to these sutured techniques is the need to rotate, cover, or bury the suture knot that is created to prevent erosion of the overlying conjunctiva and the development of subsequent endophthalmitis.[1,2] Utilization of a corneoscleral pocket for scleral fixation was originally described in 2006 and has many advantages over other techniques for suture fixation.[3]

First, there is no need for conjunctival dissection, which may sabotage the functioning of filtering blebs or the conjunctiva of future filtering blebs. Due to the elimination of conjunctival dissection and sclera cauterization, the procedure can proceed faster and result in healthier scleral tissue overlying the suture knot that is less likely to degrade with resulting suture knot exposure. In addition, patients appear to be more comfortable and the eyes are less inflamed postoperatively due to the elimination of conjunctival sutures for wound closure.

Construction of the corneoscleral pocket is fairly simple and straightforward. This chapter presents various nuances of the technique to help both the novice and the more experienced surgeon avoid some of the pitfalls that may be encountered during the simple learning curve.

Preoperative Planning

One of the common uses for the corneoscleral pocket is for scleral fixation of subluxed intraocular lens (IOL)/capsular bag complexes. During the initial examination, the patient should be placed in the supine position to ensure that the IOL is still approachable in that position. Even if the IOL appears to move posteriorly when the patient is supine, it is usually still accessible for scleral fixation. In rare instances, the IOL may appear to be accessible when the patient is upright but is completely dislocated when supine. In these instances, coordination with a retinal colleague is usually needed. As part of the preoperative evaluation, the haptics will need to be identified to plan the location of the scleral pockets for fixation. If a capsular tension ring is in place, this simplifies the surgical planning because all 360 degrees of the capsular bag fornix can be utilized as fixation sites. Any preexisting filtering blebs should be identified and avoided if possible. Large filtering blebs that may extend around the interpalpebral limbus can frequently be penetrated toward the bleb periphery by suture passes through an underlying scleral pocket without causing significant bleb leaks or failure of the bleb.

Incision and Dissection

Most surgeries are performed under a peribulbar or retrobulbar block. When two scleral pockets are needed for IOL or bag fixation, these are created 180 degrees apart. Setting a caliper to 13 mm and marking the fixation sites with gentian violet is a useful means of ensuring that the sites are not oblique to each other (**Fig. 28.1**). Creation of the scleral pockets is best done with a normal intraocular pressure; thus, an anterior chamber (AC) infusion or an AC pressurized with viscoelastic should be avoided at the onset of the pocket construction. Dissecting the pockets, and retrieving the subsequent suture passes is much more challenging when an AC infusion is in place due to the floor of the pocket being compressed against the roof of the pocket.

A 350-μm-deep grooved incision is made at the limbus just anterior to the conjunctival insertion. This can be made with a diamond or metal step blade. The limbal incision is usually 30 degrees in arc length or one clock hour. An opposing limbal groove is made 180 degrees away corresponding to the gentian violet mark on the conjunctiva. Each incision is then dissected posteriorly within the plane of the sclera. Lifting up on the posterior aspect of the grooved incision with a 0.12-mm forceps will aid in the dissection (**Fig. 28.2**). The dissection is best accomplished with a metal crescent blade, taking care to keep the blade in the plane of the sclera. Bare visualization of the blade through the overlying sclera will ensure that the dissection is not too deep.

Incision Problems

What can go wrong at this point in the procedure? First, the initial groove may not be deep enough. This usually occurs due to a timid surgeon not placing enough downward force on the step knife. Remember, it is guarded, so excessive downward force should not result in a perforation. This can be rectified by resetting the blade to a depth of 400 μm and repeating the groove depth. In regard to the pocket creation, there are two potential pitfalls. The first is cutting too deep during the posterior dissection and entering the suprachoroidal space. When this happens, there is usually a tactile sense of loss of blade resistance. Surprisingly, there is usually not significant bleeding when this happens as long as the dissection is halted before the ciliary body is incised. The pocket dissection is supposed to proceed ~ 3 to 4 mm posterior to the surgical limbus to ensure that the suture passes are within the dissected sclera. When the floor of the pocket is compromised by a dissection into the suprachoroidal space, the dissection has usually already been performed posteriorly enough so that the procedure can proceed without difficulty. The other potential pitfall is exiting the scleral pocket into the subconjunctival space during the posterior sclera dissection and effectively creating a scleral tunnel. Again, this tends to happen at the end of the dissection, and as long as the suture passes and the subsequent suture knot is covered by the overlying "bridge" of the scleral tunnel, it does not matter if there is an opening into the subconjunctival space (**Fig. 28.3**).

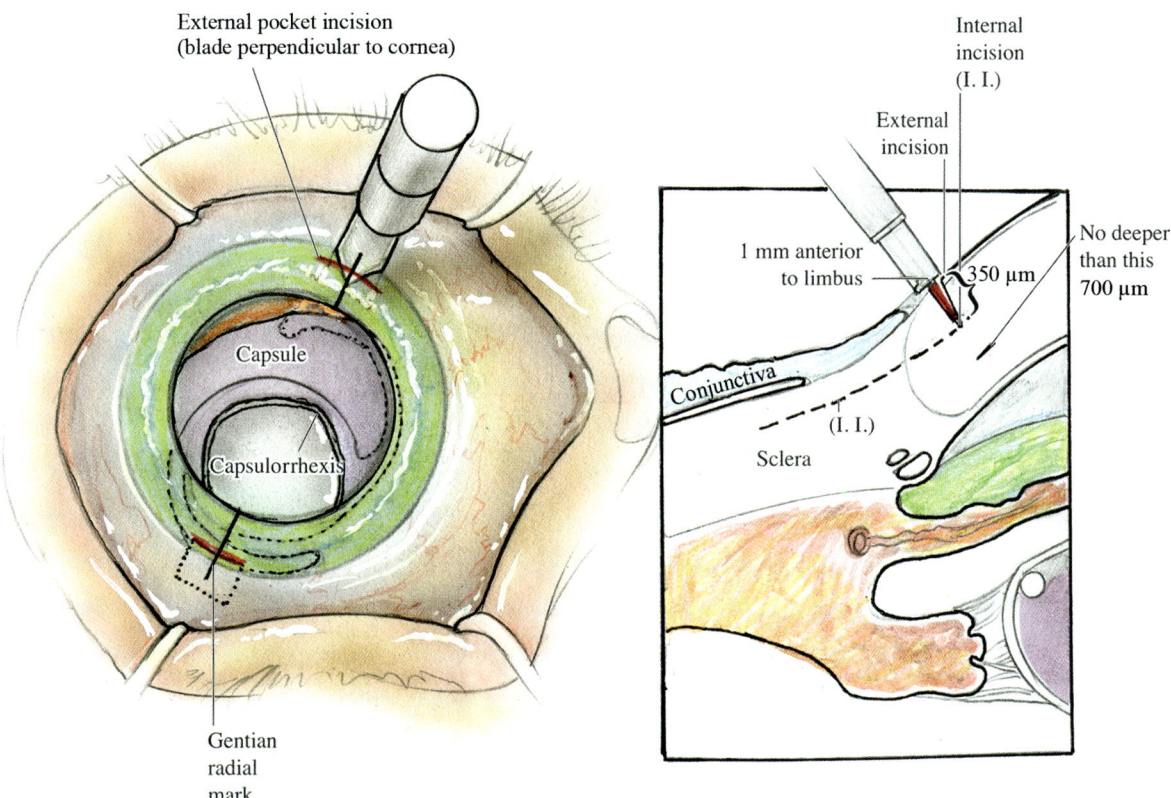

Fig. 28.1 Radial marks made with gentian violet are 180 degrees apart, marking the position of the center of the pockets. **(Inset)** A 350-μm deep grooved incision is made at the limbus just anterior to the conjunctival insertion. The limbal incision is usually 30 degrees in arc length or one clock hour.

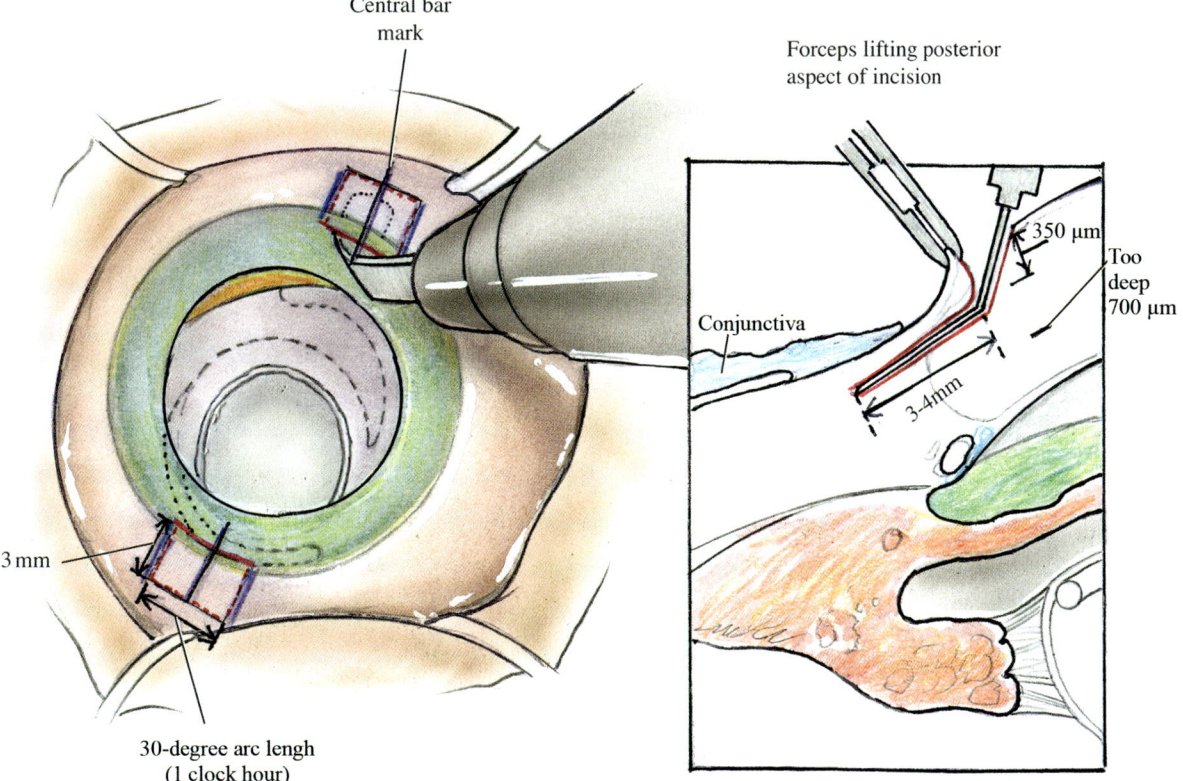

Fig. 28.2 Each incision is then dissected posteriorly within the plane of the sclera. Lifting up on the posterior aspect of the grooved incision with a 0.12-mm forceps aids in the dissection. **(Inset)** The dissection is best accomplished with a metal crescent blade, taking care to keep the blade in the plane of the sclera. Bare visualization of the blade through the overlying sclera ensures that the dissection is not too deep.

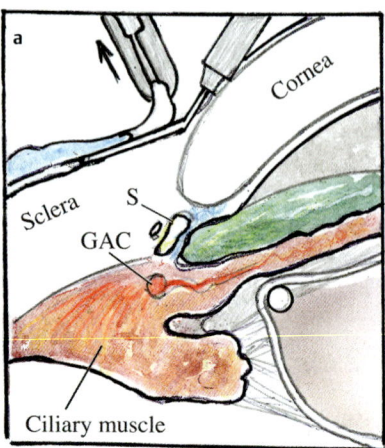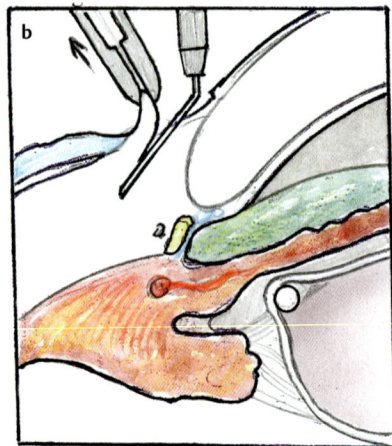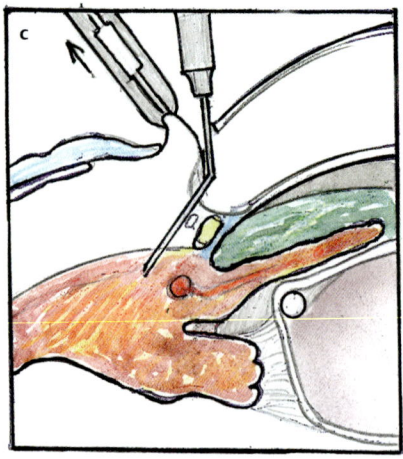

Fig. 28.3 Incision problems. **(a)** Too superficial. **(b)** Too angled. **(c)** Too deep. GAC, greater arterial circle of iris; S, canal of Schlemm.

Incision Pearls

Perhaps the most important step in this technique is to ensure that the dissection proceeds posteriorly enough so that the subsequent suture passes are within the area of the dissected sclera. Passing the sutures more posteriorly than the dissected pocket will make retrieval of the sutures through the pocket opening almost impossible. It is for this reason that it is best to dissect too far posteriorly than not far enough. Following creation of the pockets, it is also helpful for the novice surgeon to mark the lateral extent of the pockets with a radial gentian violet mark to ensure that the suture passes are not adjacent to the dissected sclera (**Fig. 28.4**). This is easily accomplished with a Sinsky hook and a gentian violet marking pad.

Following creation of the pockets, a paracentesis is then created just anterior to each of the grooved incisions, to enable a double-armed suture to pass through the paracentesis and fixate the subluxed IOL to the opposite scleral pocket. Making the paracentesis within the depth of the groove will make identification of the paracentesis opening very difficult, thus the paracentesis should be initiated anterior to the groove or adjacent to the groove in virgin cornea. These paracenteses can also be used for iris hook placement to help identify the bag equator/IOL haptics, and they can be used to remove viscoelastic at the conclusion of the procedure utilizing bimanual irrigation and aspiration (I/A) handpieces (**Fig. 28.5**).

Docking

For repair of an iridodialysis through a corneoscleral pocket, docking into a 25- or 27-gauge needle is usually not needed. Creating the paracentesis 4 clock hour positions away from the dialysis will allow the double-armed suture needles to pass through the paracentesis, through the iris root, and through the full-thickness of the globe 2 mm posterior to the surgical limbus, corresponding to the dissected scleral pocket. For secondary IOLs, capsular prosthetic devices, and subluxed IOL/capsular bag complexes, docking the suture needle into an open-bored 25- or 27-gauge hypodermic needle is the simplest approach.

Suture composition should be 9-0 Prolene or CV8 Gore-Tex for IOL and adjunctive device fixation; 10-0 Prolene should only be used for iridodialysis repair because it has been shown to degrade after 7 to 10 years when used for device fixation.[4] Passing the suture needle through the paracentesis can be one of the more frustrating steps in this procedure, and this is aggravated if

the eye is pressurized with an AC infusion due to forced closure of the paracentesis. Placing a viscoelastic cannula into the paracentesis to open the wound slightly aids in passing the suture needle into the AC (**Fig. 28.6a,b**). In addition, the needle should be moved from side to side when passed through the paracentesis to ensure that no cornea stromal fibers were incarcerated in the needle pass. Once the suture needle is in the AC, the 25- or 27-gauge hypodermic needle is then passed through the full thickness of the globe corresponding to the dissected scleral

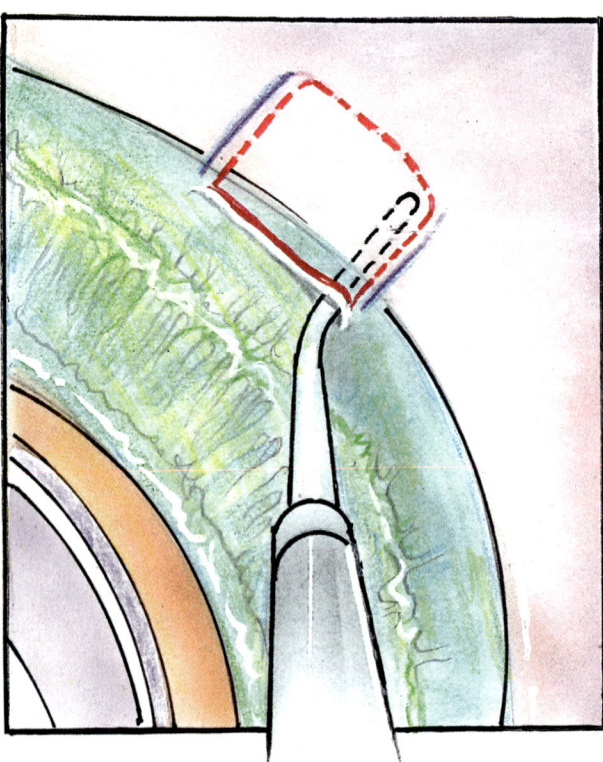

Fig. 28.4 Marking the lateral extent of the pockets with a radial gentian violet mark to ensure that the suture passes are not adjacent to the dissected sclera.

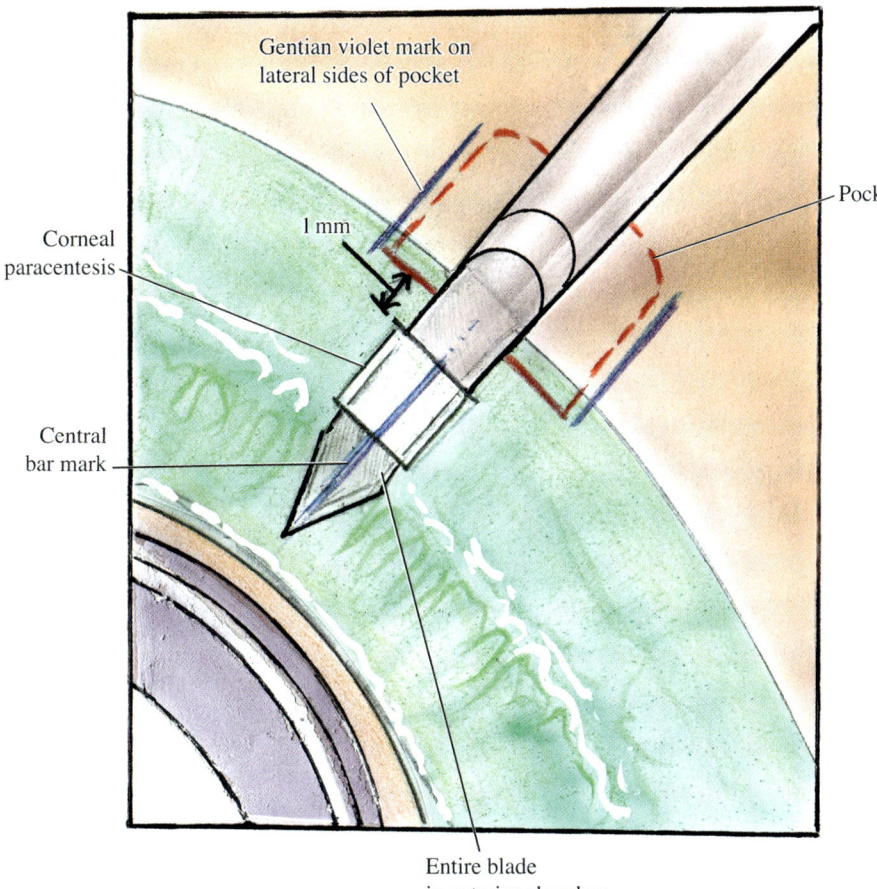

Gentian violet mark on
lateral sides of pocket

Corneal
paracentesis

1 mm

Pocket

Central
bar mark

Entire blade
in anterior chamber

Fig. 28.5 A paracentesis is initiated anterior to the pocket groove in clear cornea.

pocket, 2 to 3 mm posterior to the surgical limbus. The docking needle should be oriented somewhat parallel to the iris when initially inserted into the eye to prevent damage to the ciliary processes (**Fig. 28.6b**). The curved suture needle is then docked into the straight hypodermic needle and will lock into place due to the disparity of a curved needle inside a straight bored needle. Pulling the hypodermic needle out of the eye once the suture needle is locked will also pull the suture needle out.

When treating a subluxed IOL/capsular bag complex, passing the first suture pass through the capsular bag (behind the IOL haptic) helps support the bag so that, should the remaining zonules break, there is a point of suture support. This is then followed by passage of the second arm of the double-armed suture in front of the capsular bag so that the suture is functionally looped around the haptic (**Fig. 28.6c**). Pulling gently on these sutures helps sublux the bag away from the opposing pocket and helps with identification of the second IOL haptic. An iris hook may also be beneficial. Passage of the second set of sutures to fixate the opposite haptic is easiest if the first pass is in front of the capsular and the second pass is through the bag. The reason for this is that having the first pass through the bag tends to elevate the bag slightly and reduce the working space between the iris and the front of the capsular bag (**Fig. 28.6c**).

Intraocular Lens Tilt Prevention

A subtler nuance of this technique surrounds the avoidance of IOL tilt. Because the suture passes through the sclera are adjacent to each other and tangential to the limbus, there is the possibility of inducing some IOL tilt if the distance between the suture passes is large and if the opposing suture passes that are 180 degrees from each other are on the same side of the capsular bag. This is due to each set of sutures inducing some torque around the IOL axis in the same direction. By passing the sutures so that each set is inducing torque in opposite directions and separating the suture passes by a small amount (1 mm), the amount of torque will be reduced and IOL tilt will be eliminated.

Centration

Once the suture passes have been made, the suture needles are removed from both sets of sutures and the suture ends are retrieved through the limbal opening of the scleral pockets. This is accomplished by placing a Sinsky hook into the pocket and pulling each end out (**Fig. 28.7a**). Again, if an AC infusion is being utilized, it is easier to retrieve the sutures from the pocket if the eye is not overpressurized. Pinching the infusion briefly aids in suture externalization. Holding the first externalized suture while externalizing the second ensures that the entire suture is not pulled from the globe (**Fig. 28.7**). Each set of sutures is then tightened to center the IOL/capsular bag complex. Tying the first set with 1 to 2 mm of resulting decentration enables re-centration by tightening and tying the second set of sutures. Trimming the sutures at the knot enables the knot to slide under the protective roof of the sclera pocket. If the IOL is still slightly decentered following suture tying, the bag can usually be easily re-centered with an intraocular microincision forceps because there will be some laxity in each set of haptic sutures (**Fig. 28.8**).

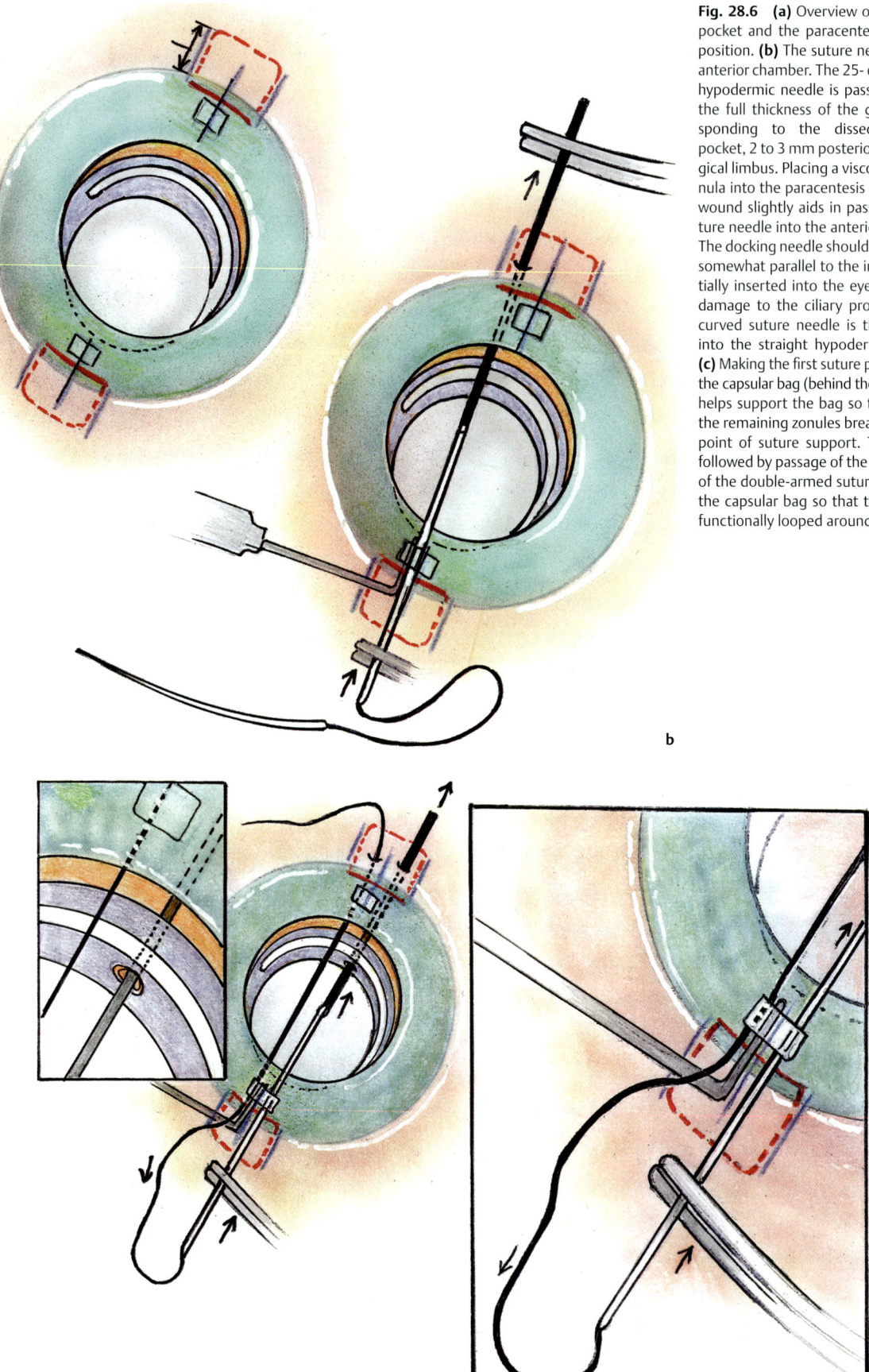

Fig. 28.6 **(a)** Overview of the scleral pocket and the paracentesis size and position. **(b)** The suture needle, in the anterior chamber. The 25- or 27-gauge hypodermic needle is passed through the full thickness of the globe corresponding to the dissected sclera pocket, 2 to 3 mm posterior to the surgical limbus. Placing a viscoelastic cannula into the paracentesis to open the wound slightly aids in passing the suture needle into the anterior chamber. The docking needle should be oriented somewhat parallel to the iris when initially inserted into the eye to prevent damage to the ciliary processes. The curved suture needle is then docked into the straight hypodermic needle. **(c)** Making the first suture pass through the capsular bag (behind the IOL haptic) helps support the bag so that, should the remaining zonules break, there is a point of suture support. This is then followed by passage of the second arm of the double-armed suture in front of the capsular bag so that the suture is functionally looped around the haptic.

a

b

c

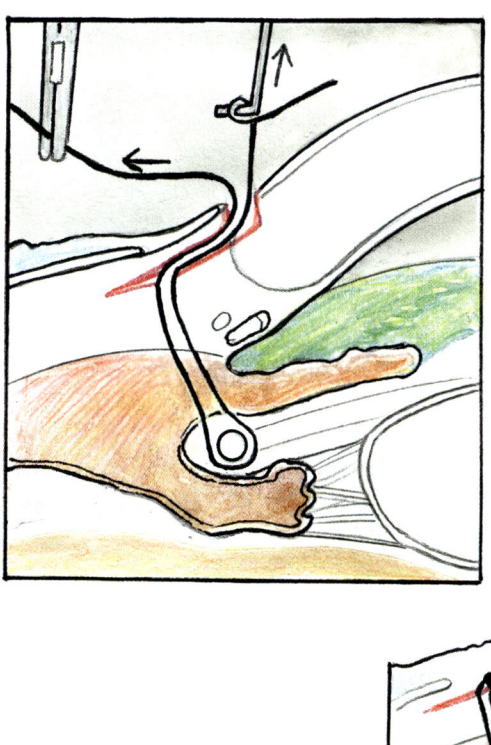

a

Fig. 28.7   (a) The suture path, after it has been pulled through the pocket, around the haptic and out of the pocket. (b) The knot in the pocket *(left)*; the knot trimmed and inside the pocket *(right)*.

b

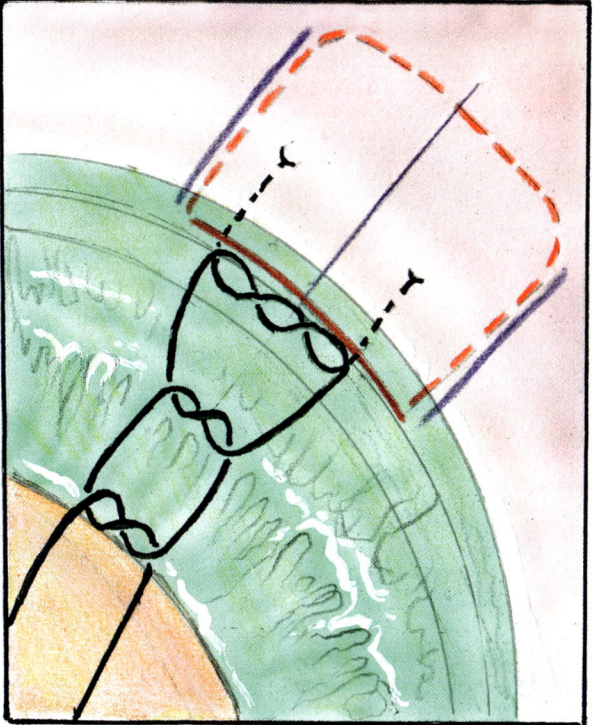

Fig. 28.8   Knot tying pattern for a secure closure in the flap.

Conclusion

Scleral fixation utilizing a corneoscleral pocket can be utilized for a variety of devices and pathologies. It has been used for secondary IOL fixation, primary subluxed IOL re-centration and stabilization, fixation of capsular bag prostheses, and iridodialysis repair. The technique is relatively simple, with a short learning curve, and it offers patients a less invasive means of sclera fixation that avoids the need for conjunctival dissection, scleral cauterization, and sutured wound closure. Each step of the procedure has various nuances that, when appreciated, can help facilitate the learning and advancement of this useful technique while reducing complications and frustration.

References

1. Heilskov T, Joondeph BC, Olsen KR, Blankenship GW. Late endophthalmitis after transscleral fixation of a posterior chamber intraocular lens. Arch Ophthalmol 1989;107:1427

2. Schechter RJ. Suture-wick endophthalmitis with sutured posterior chamber intraocular lenses. J Cataract Refract Surg 1990;16:755–756

3. Hoffman RS, Fine IH, Packer M. Scleral fixation without conjunctival dissection. J Cataract Refract Surg 2006;32:1907–1912

4. Price MO, Price FW Jr, Werner L, Berlie C, Mamalis N. Late dislocation of scleral-sutured posterior chamber intraocular lenses. J Cataract Refract Surg 2005;31:1320–1326

29 Intraocular Lens Fixation in the Absence of Support: The Glued Intraocular Lens

Amar Agarwal

Posterior capsular rent (PCR)[1,2] can occur in the early learning curve in phacoemulsification. Intraoperative dialysis or a large PCR precludes intraocular lens (IOL) implantation in the capsular bag. Implantation of an IOL in the sulcus is possible in cases of adequate anterior capsular support. The first glued posterior chamber IOL (PCIOL) implantation in an eye with a deficient capsule was performed at my eye hospital on December 14, 2007. In eyes with inadequate anterior capsular rim and deficient posterior capsule, the new technique of IOL implantation is the fibrin glue–assisted sutureless IOL implantation with scleral tuck.[3–7] The scleral tuck of a PCIOL was first performed by Gabor Scharioth from Germany (erroneously referred to as S.G. Gabor in the *Journal of Cataract and Refractive Surgery*[8]). Maggi had previously performed a sutureless scleral fixation of a special IOL.[9]

Surgical Technique

Under peribulbar anesthesia, the superior rectus is caught and clamped. Localized peritomy and wet cautery of the sclera at the desired site of exit of the IOL haptics is performed. A 23-gauge sutureless trocar infusion cannula or an anterior chamber maintainer is inserted. Two partial-thickness limbal-based scleral flaps ~ 2.5 mm by 2.5 mm are created exactly 180 degrees diagonally apart. Two straight sclerotomies with a 20- or 22-gauge needle are made ~ 1.0 mm from the limbus under the existing scleral flaps. This is followed by a 23-gauge vitrectomy via the pars plana or anterior route to remove all the vitreous traction. The 23-gauge vitrectomy probe can be passed through the sclerotomy created under the sclera flap. A clear corneal/scleral tunnel incision is then prepared for introducing the IOL. While the IOL is being introduced (**Figs. 29.1** and **29.2**), an end gripping 23- or 25-gauge micro-rhexis forceps (MicroSurgical Technology, Redmond, WA) is passed through one of the sclerotomies with the other hand. One can use any end-opening forceps such as a microrhexis forceps. The tip of the leading haptic (**Figs. 29.3** and **29.4**) is then grasped with the micro-rhexis forceps, pulled through the sclerotomy following the curve of the haptic, and externalized under the scleral flap. Similarly, the trailing haptic is also externalized through the other sclerotomy under the scleral flap. For this step, a handshake technique can be used (**Fig. 29.5**). The limbal wound is sutured with 10-0 monofilament nylon if it is a sclera tunnel incision. The tip of the haptics are then tucked inside a scleral tunnel made with 26-gauge needle. The scleral flaps are closed with fibrin glue. The anterior chamber maintainer or the infusion cannula is removed. The conjunctiva is also closed with the same fibrin glue.

Fibrin Glue

The fibrin kit we used is Reliseal (Reliance Life Sciences, Mumbai, India). Another widely used tissue glue is Tisseel (Baxter, Deerfield, IL). The fibrinogen and thrombin are first reconstituted according to the manufacturer's instructions. The commercially available fibrin glue is virus inactivated and is checked for viral antigen and antibodies with polymerase chain reaction; hence, the risk of transmission of infection is very low. But with tissue derivatives, there is always a theoretical possibility of transmission of viral infections.

Advantages

This fibrin glue–assisted sutureless PCIOL implantation technique is useful in a myriad of clinical situations in which scleral-fixated IOLs (SFIOLs) are indicated, such as luxated IOL, dislocated IOL, zonulopathy, and secondary IOL implantation.

No Need for Special Intraocular Lenses

This procedure can be performed well with rigid polymethylmethacrylate (PMMA) IOLs, three-piece PCIOLs, or IOLs with modified PMMA haptics. Therefore, there is no need to maintain an inventory of various special SFIOLs with eyelets, unlike with sutured SFIOLs. In dislocated PMMA PCIOLs, the same IOL can be repositioned, thereby reducing the need for further manipulation. Furthermore, there is no need for newer haptic designs or special instruments other than the 25-gauge forceps.

No Tilt

Because the overall diameter of the routine IOL is ~ 12 to 13 mm, with the haptic being placed in its normal curved configuration and without any traction, there is no distortion or change in shape of the IOL optic. Externalization of the greater part of the haptics along its curvature stabilizes the axial positioning of the IOL and thereby prevents any IOL tilt.[10]

Less Pseudophakodonesis

When the eye moves, it acquires kinetic energy from its muscles and attachments and the energy is dissipated to the internal fluids as it stops. Thus, pseudophakodonesis is the result of oscillations of the fluids in the anterior and posterior segments of the eye. These oscillations, initiated by movement of the eye, result

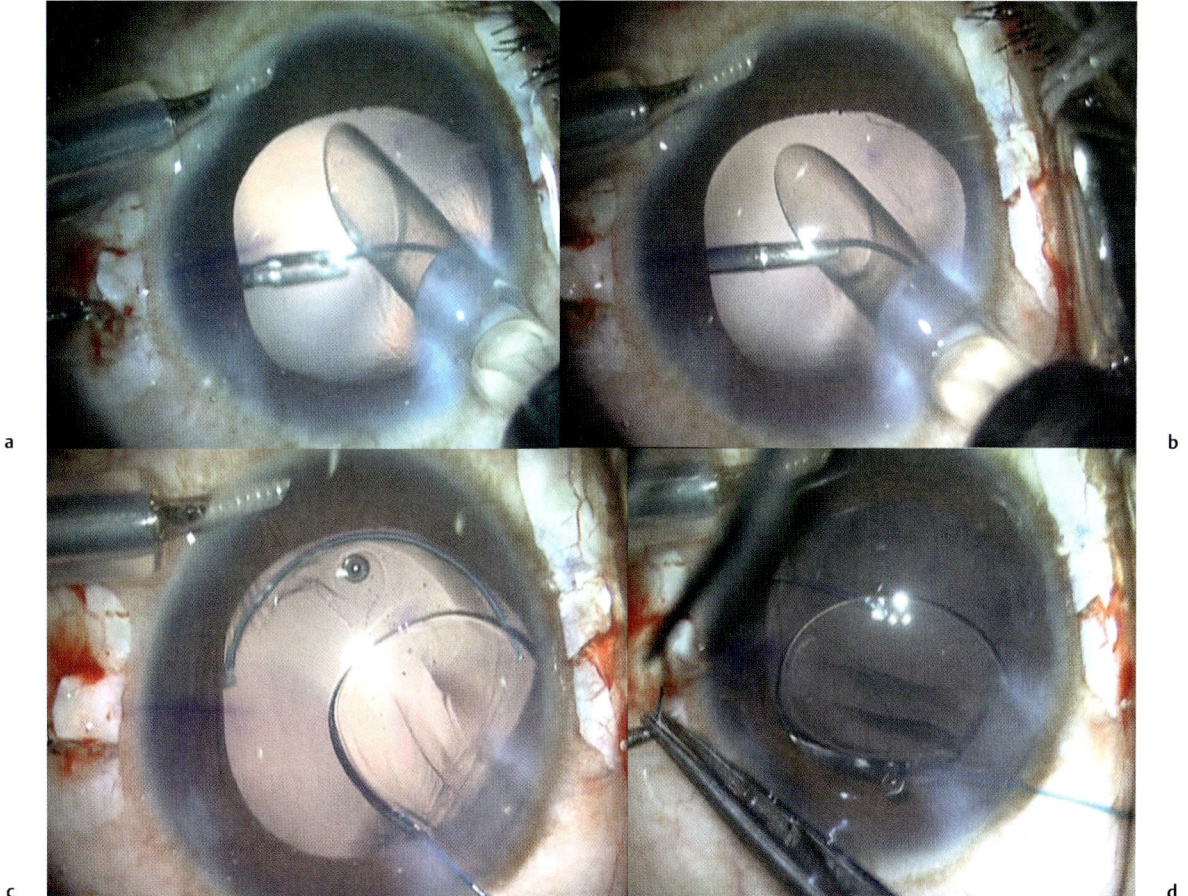

Fig. 29.1 Leading haptic externalization. **(a)** The haptic tip is slightly out of the cartridge. The glued intraocular lens (IOL) forceps is passed through the sclerotomy site. **(b)** The tip of the haptic is grasped with the glued IOL forceps. **(c)** Injection of the IOL continues. **(d)** The haptic is externalized and held by an assistant. (From Agarwal A, Jacob S, Kumar DA, et al. Handshake technique for glued intrascleral haptic fixation of a posterior chamber intraocular lens. J Cataract Refract Surg 2013;39:317–322. Reprinted with permission.)

in shearing forces on the corneal endothelium as well as vitreous motion, which leads to permanent damage. Because the IOL haptic is stuck beneath the flap, it would prevent the further movement of the haptic, thereby reducing pseudophakodonesis.[11]

Less Uveitis-Glaucoma-Hyphema Syndrome

We expect less incidence of uveitis-glaucoma-hyphema (UGH) syndrome in fibrin glue–assisted IOL implantation as compared with sutured SFIOL, because in the former the IOL is well stabilized and stuck onto the scleral bed and thus has decreased intraocular mobility, whereas in the latter there is increased possibility of IOL movement or persistent rub over the ciliary body.

No Suture-Related Complications

Visually significant complications due to late subluxation,[12] which has been known to occur in sutured SFIOLs, may also be prevented as sutures are totally avoided in this technique. Another important advantage of this technique is the prevention of suture-related complications,[13,14] such as suture erosion, suture

knot exposure, or dislocation of IOL after suture disintegration or broken suture.

Rapidity and Ease of Surgery

Passing sutures into the IOL haptic eyelets for SFIOLs, to ensure good centration before tying down the knots, and suturing scleral flaps and closing the conjunctiva take significantly less time with this procedure. The risk of retinal photic injury,[15] which is known to occur in SFIOLs, would also be reduced in our technique due to the short surgical time. Fibrin glue takes less time (Reliseal, 20 seconds; Tisseel, 3 seconds) to act in the scleral bed, and it aids in adhesion as well as hemostasis. The preparation time can also be reduced in elective procedures by preparing the glue prior to surgery, as it remains stable for up to 4 hours from the time of reconstitution. Fibrin glue has been shown to provide airtight closure, and by the time the fibrin starts degrading, surgical adhesions would have already occurred in the scleral bed. This is well shown in the follow-up anterior-segment optical coherence tomography (OCT) in which postoperative perfect scleral flap adhesion is observed.

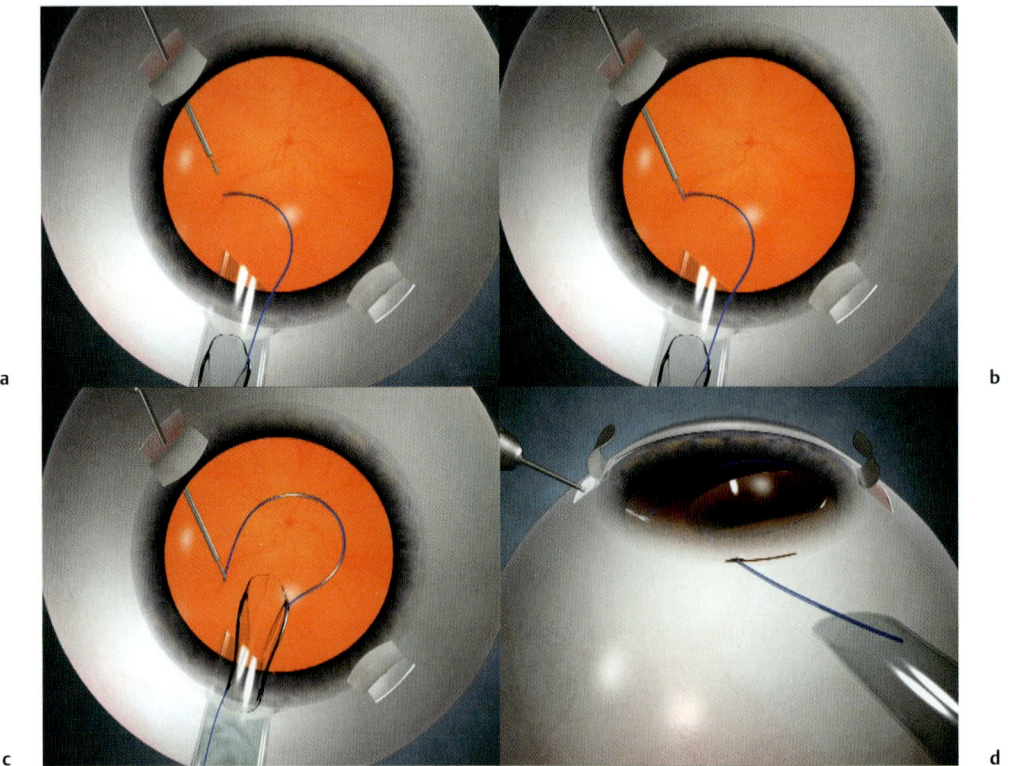

Fig. 29.2 Leading haptic externalization. **(a)** The haptic is outside the cartridge. The glued IOL forceps is ready to grasp the haptic tip. **(b)** The haptic tip is caught with the forceps. **(c)** Injection of the IOL continues until the optic unfolds inside the anterior chamber. **(d)** Haptic externalization is started. (From Agarwal A, Jacob S, Kumar DA, et al. Handshake technique for glued intrascleral haptic fixation of a posterior chamber intraocular lens. J Cataract Refract Surg 2013;39:317–322. Reprinted with permission.)

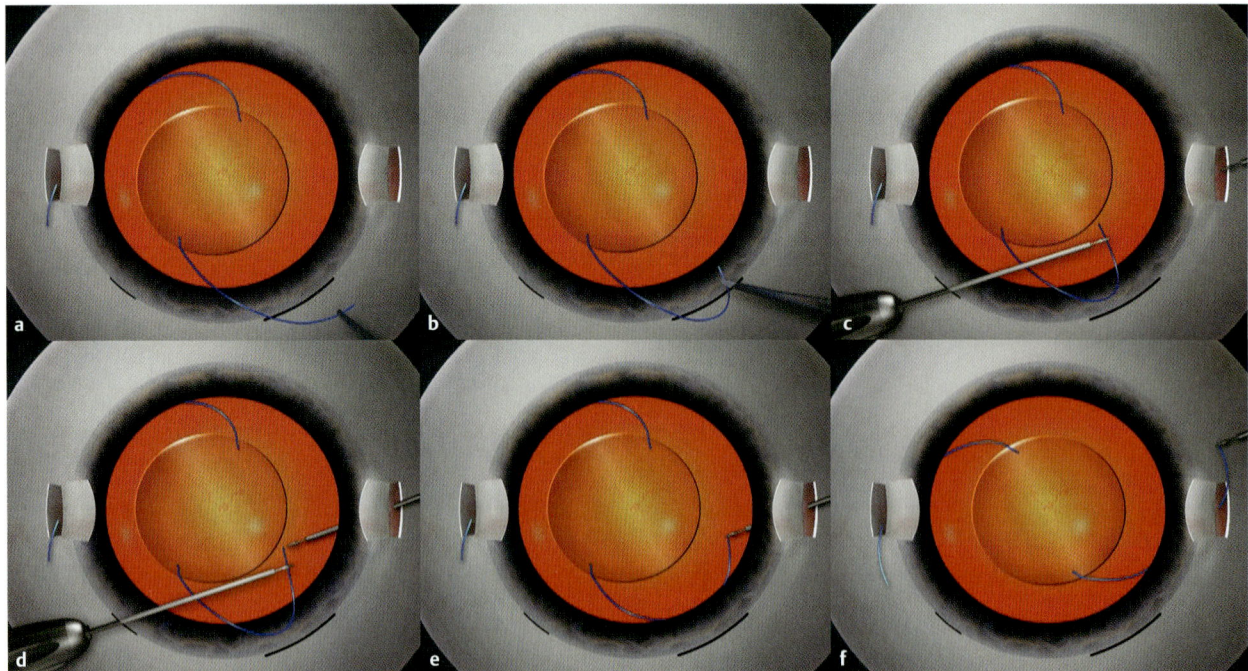

Fig. 29.3 Trailing haptic externalization. **(a)** The trailing haptic is caught with the first glued IOL forceps. **(b)** The haptic is flexed into the anterior chamber. **(c)** The haptic is transferred from the first forceps to the second forceps using the handshake technique. The second forceps is passed through the side port. **(d)** The first forceps is passed through the sclerotomy under the scleral flap. The haptic is transferred from the second forceps back to the first using the handshake technique. The haptic tip is grasped with the first forceps. **(e)** The haptic is pulled toward the sclerotomy. **(f)** The haptic is externalized. (From Agarwal A, Jacob S, Kumar DA, et al. Handshake technique for glued intrascleral haptic fixation of a posterior chamber intraocular lens. J Cataract Refract Surg 2013;39:317–322. Reprinted with permission.)

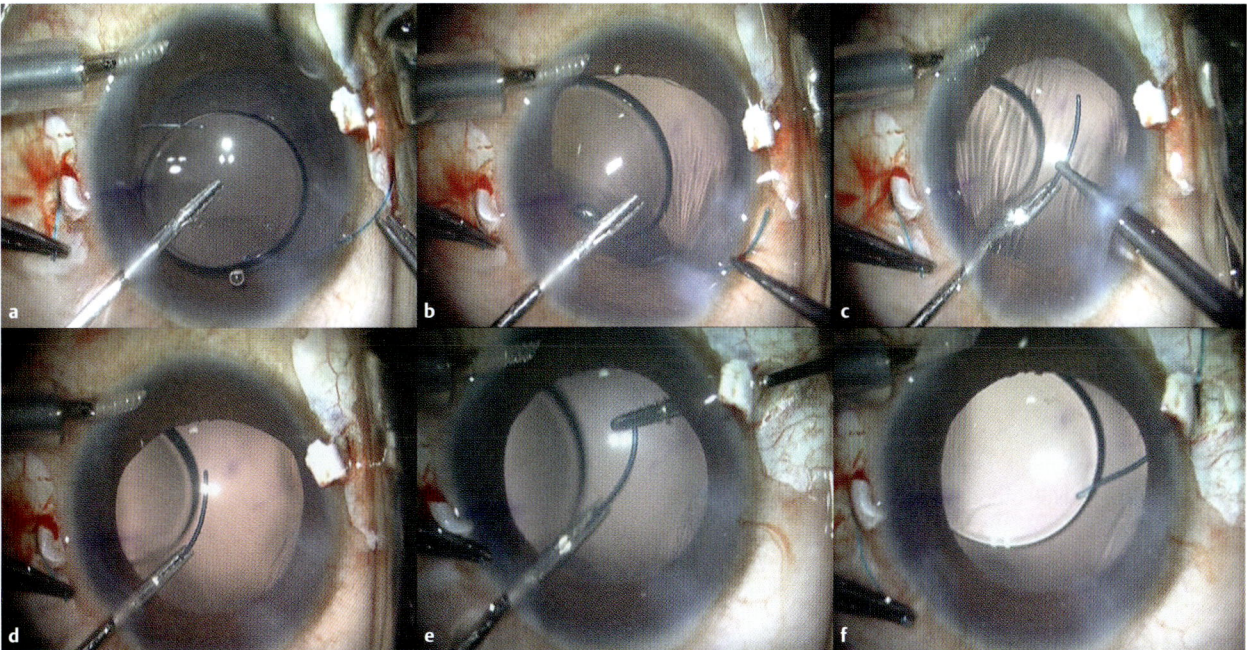

Fig. 29.4 Handshake technique for the trailing haptic. **(a)** The glued IOL forceps is passed through the side port. **(b)** The trailing haptic is grasped with a forceps and flexed to insert it into the anterior chamber. **(c)** The trailing haptic is passed into the anterior chamber and with the handshake technique, the haptic grasp is shifted from the first forceps to the second forceps. Note the dimpling on the cornea as the main incision is open due to the forceps passage. **(d)** The trailing haptic is caught with the forceps passed through the side port. Note no dimpling on the cornea as the main port incision is closed. The tip of the haptic is easily seen. **(e)** The glued IOL forceps is passed through the sclerotomy and the tip of the haptic is grasped. **(f)** The trailing haptic is externalized. (From Agarwal A, Jacob S, Kumar DA, et al. Handshake technique for glued intrascleral haptic fixation of a posterior chamber intraocular lens. J Cataract Refract Surg 2013;39:317–322. Reprinted with permission.)

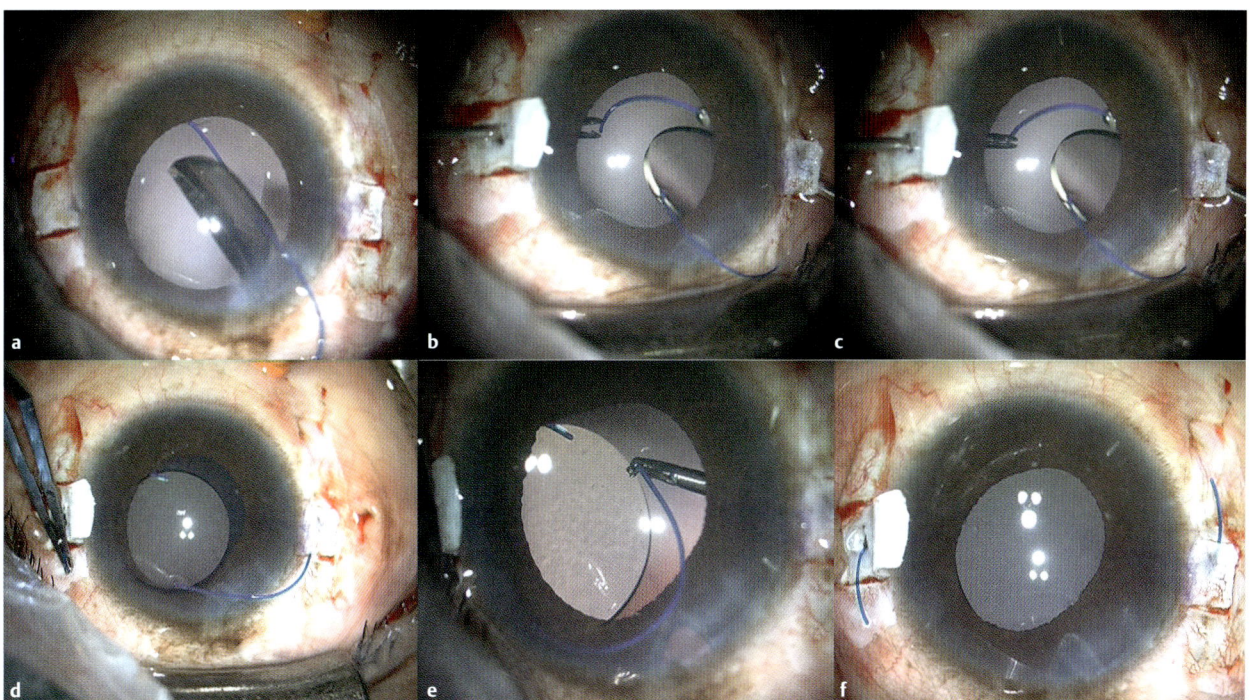

Fig. 29.5 Handshake technique to regrasp the haptic. **(a)** The foldable IOL haptic is below the iris. **(b)** The glued IOL forceps is passed through the opposite sclerotomy site while the second forceps is ready to receive the haptic. **(c)** The leading haptic is grasped with the forceps, and the haptic tip is fed into another forceps. **(d)** One haptic is externalized, and the assistant holds the haptic. **(e)** The trailing haptic is caught with the glued IOL forceps. **(f)** Both haptics are externalized under the scleral flaps. (From Agarwal A, Jacob S, Kumar DA, et al. Handshake technique for glued intrascleral haptic fixation of a posterior chamber intraocular lens. J Cataract Refract Surg 2013;39:317–322. Reprinted with permission.)

Handshake Technique for Foldable Glued Intraocular Lens

The exteriorization of the haptics is a key step in the glued IOL. Because the surgeon is maneuvering with both hands simultaneously, one hand injecting the IOL while the other grasps and exteriorizes the haptics, the surgeon needs to be familiar with the handshake technique as a means of transferring the haptic from one hand to the other. If one of the haptics is not caught or if it is released accidentally after grasping it, the situation can be easily resolved using this technique. It utilizes two glued IOL forceps, one of which holds one haptic. Depending on ease of access, the other glued IOL forceps is introduced through the opposite sclerotomy or through the side port. The first hand then transfers the haptic into the second glued IOL forceps such that the first hand now becomes free. It is essential to hold the haptic at its tip before exteriorizing it so that it does not snag on the sclerotomy while being brought out. For this reason, this handshake transfer of the haptic between the two glued IOL forceps is continued until the tip of the haptic is caught by the forceps on the side to which the haptic is to be exteriorized. This technique thus allows easy intraocular maneuvering of the entire haptic or IOL within a closed globe system.

Multifocal Glued Intraocular Lens

Multifocal IOLs enable good vision at a range of distances. Monofocal intraocular lenses, which are commonly available, provide a clear point of focus in the distance or closer, but only one focal point can be chosen. Multifocal intraocular lenses are designed to avoid the need for glasses by providing two or more points of focus. These intraocular lenses are intended to be placed in the capsular bag. Until recently, it was difficult to provide multifocality for patients who had complicated cataract surgeries and who lack normal capsules. Aphakia with deficient capsule has been a limitation for obtaining multifocality. Now multifocality is possible even in complicated cataract surgeries by the multifocal glued IOL procedure. In this multifocal IOL, implantation is done even in eyes with a large PCR and aphakias with deficient posterior capsule.

Pre-Descemet's Endothelial Keratoplasty with Glued Intraocular Lens

Pre-Descemet's endothelial keratoplasty (PDEK)[16] is the latest iteration in the set of procedures for endothelial keratoplasty; it evolved following a detailed description of the pre-Descemet's layer (PDL; also called Dua's layer) by Harminder Dua.[17] This technique enables the separation and usage of PDL, which is an additional 10-μm layer in the conventional Descemet's membrane (DM)–endothelium graft.[2] The key to the success of donor graft creation lies in the formation of a type 1 bubble, which is a central, well-circumscribed, dome-shaped bubble and typically spreads from the center to the periphery in the donor lenticule.[2]

Glued IOL[3] is a well-established form of intrascleral haptic fixation for secondary IOL procedures. The combination of PDEK with glued IOL (**Figs. 29.6, 29.7, 29.8**) serves the purpose of handling corneal endothelial dysfunction and secondary IOL fixation simultaneously.

The initial step involves successful harvesting of the donor lenticule, followed by glued IOL procedure (minus the application of glue to seal the scleral flaps), and then by recipient bed preparation and donor lenticule insertion. Application of fibrin glue to seal the scleral flaps then ensues so as to ensure that it

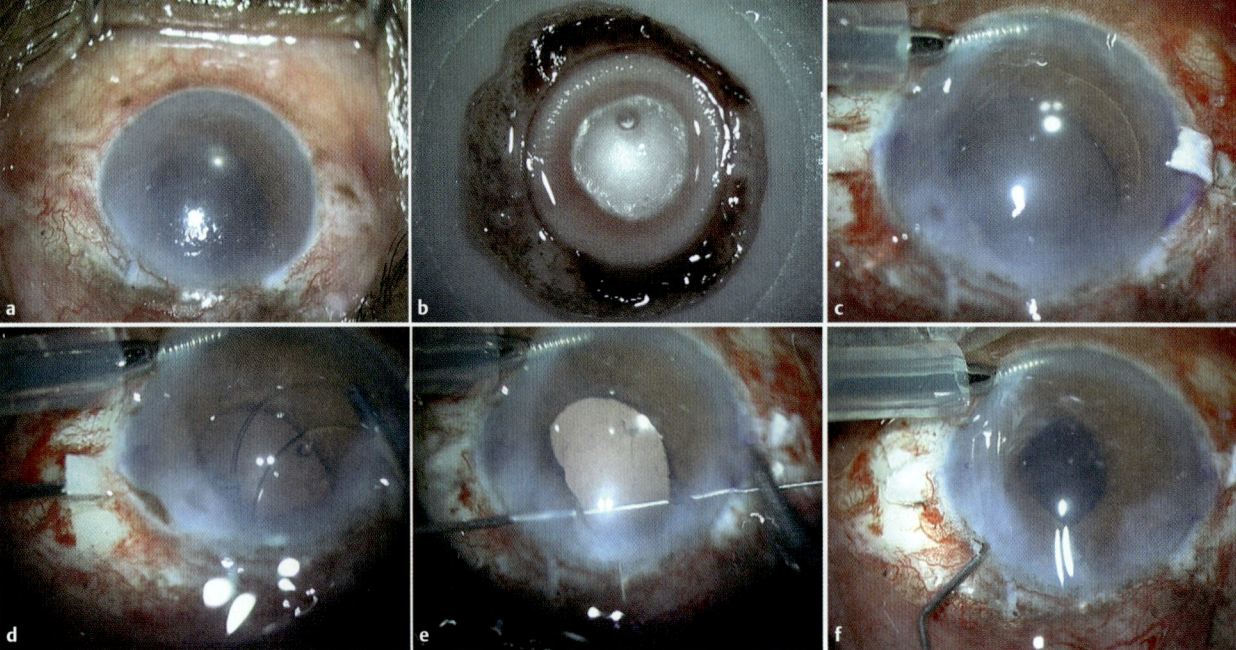

Fig. 29.6 Pre-Descemet's endothelial keratoplasty (PDEK) with a glued IOL. **(a)** Preoperative photograph of the cornea of the patient with pseudophakic bullous keratopathy. The posterior chamber IOL (PCIOL) in the anterior chamber (AC). **(b)** A type 1 big bubble (bb) between the pre-Descemet's layer (Dua's layer) and stroma is formed. Note the bb does not reach the periphery of the cornea, as there are firm adhesions between the pre-Descemet's layer and stroma in the periphery. If a bubble is created that extends to the corneoscleral limbus, it is a type 2 (pre-Descemet's) bb. This means the air has formed between the Descemet's membrane and the pre-Descemet's layer. **(c)** The AC maintainer is fixed, and the scleral flaps are created. **(d)** Glued IOL surgery is performed, and the haptics are externalized. **(e)** Pupilloplasty is performed. **(f)** Pupilloplasty is completed with glued IOL in place. The eye is now ready for PDEK surgery.

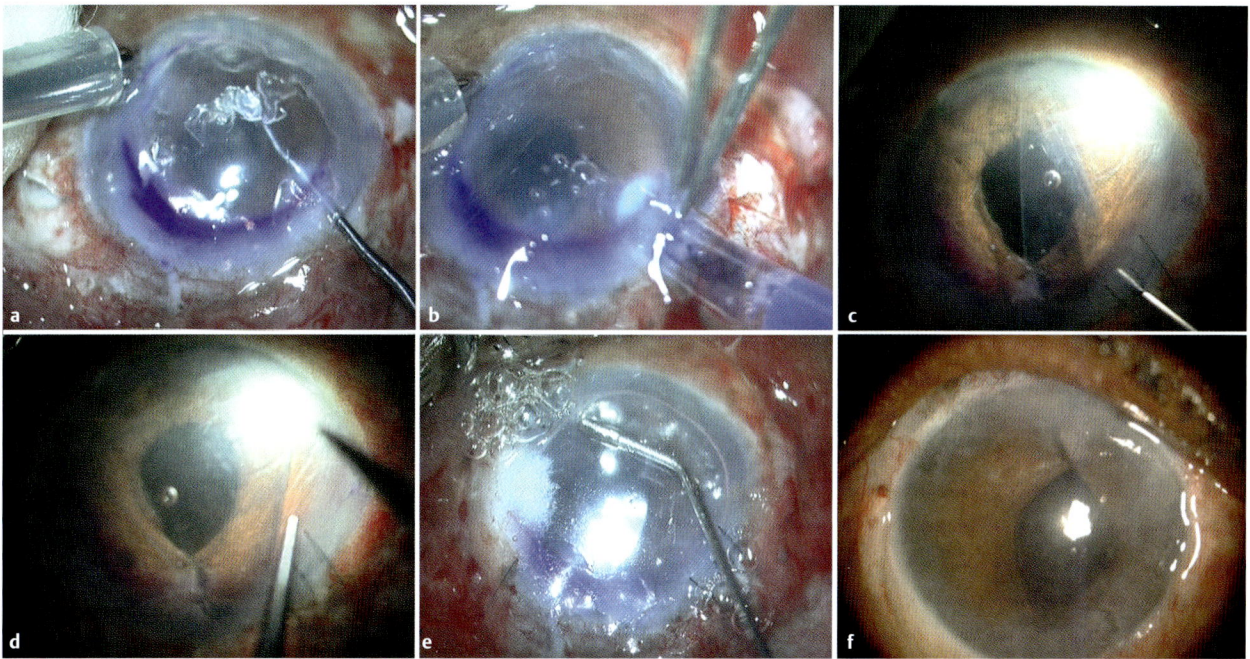

Fig. 29.7 Pre-Descemet's endothelial keratoplasty with a glued IOL. **(a)** Descematorhexis is performed. **(b)** The PDEK graft is injected into the anterior chamber with the help of the injector. **(c)** The graft is subsequently unrolled with air and fluidics. An endo-illuminator is used to help ascertain the orientation and check the unrolling of the graft (E-PDEK). **(d)** The graft is unrolled after checking that the orientation is correct. **(e)** Air is injected under the graft to appose it to the cornea. The PDEK graft is attached to the cornea with a complete air fill of the anterior chamber. Then glue is applied to the scleral flaps. **(f)** One week postoperative.

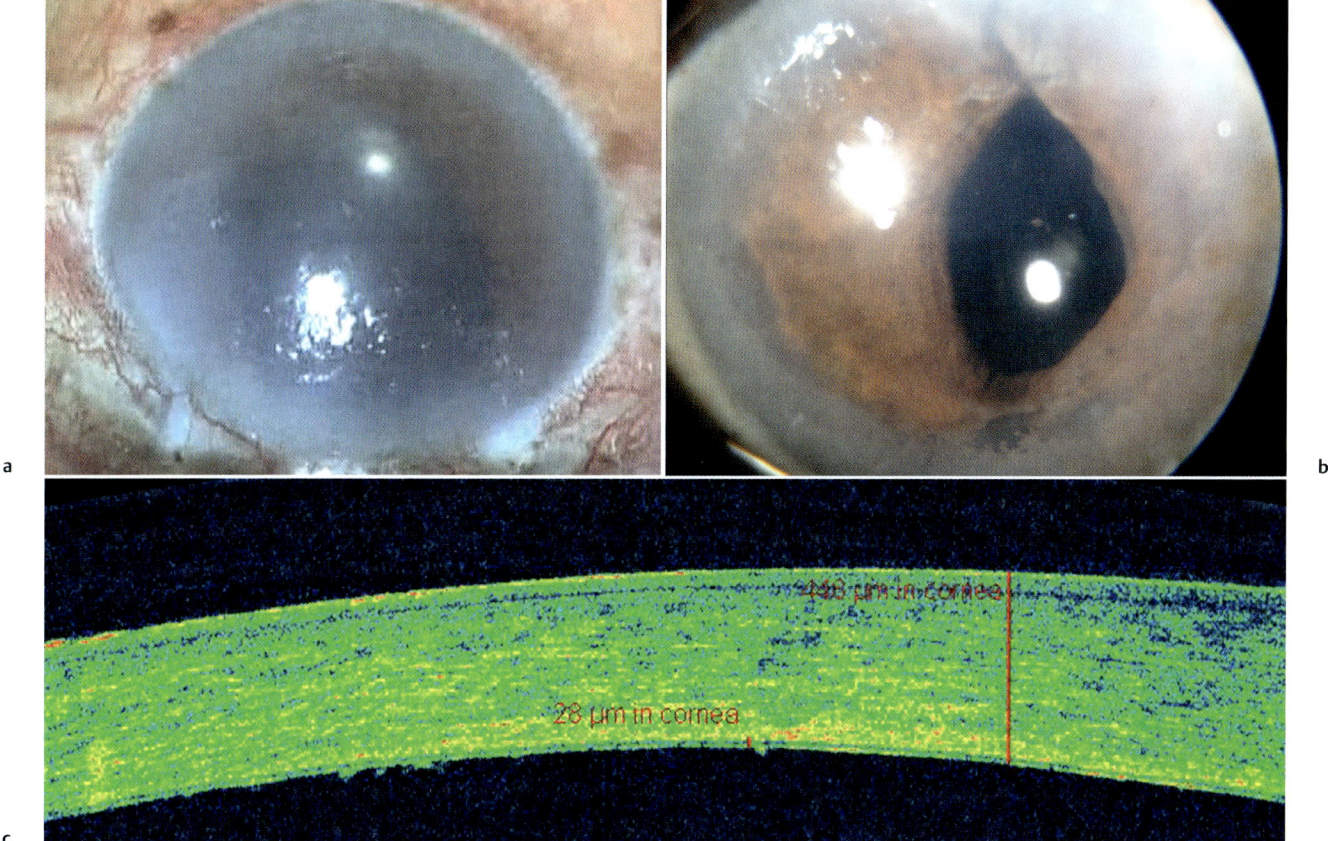

Fig. 29.8 Pre-Descemet's endothelial keratoplasty with a glued IOL. **(a)** Preoperative view of a pseudophakic bullous keratopathy with a PCIOL placed in the AC. **(b)** One month postoperative. Vision is 20/30. **(c)** Anterior-segment optical coherence tomography (OCT) showing the graft attached.

is not washed off by the fluids emanating and egressing from the eye.

Step 1: Donor Graft Preparation

The detailed method of preparation of donor graft has been previously described. Briefly, an air-filled 5-mL syringe with an attached 30-gauge needle is introduced from the corneoscleral disk with bevel up to the center of the donor lenticule with the endothelial side up. As air is injected, a type 1 bubble is formed with a distinct edge all around. A trephine of suitable diameter is used to create a mark on the endothelium. The edge of the bubble at the extreme periphery is perforated followed by the injection of trypan blue into the bubble to stain the graft, which is then cut all around the trephine mark with a corneoscleral scissors. The graft is then stored in the storage media.

Step 2: IOL Implantation by Glued IOL Method

The glued IOL technique consists of making two partial-thickness scleral flaps ~ 2.5 mm by 2.5 mm in size and 180 degrees opposite to each other. The epithelium of the recipient eye is often debrided due to epithelium decompensation, which greatly hinders the intraoperative view. An anterior chamber (AC) maintainer is introduced in the lower quadrant, and a sclerotomy wound is created with a 20-gauge needle ~ 1 mm away from the limbus beneath the scleral flaps, and the entire glued IOL surgery is performed through the tucking of the haptics in the scleral pockets. The AC maintainer is used throughout the surgery, and the use of viscoelastic is deferred, as it is important not to leave residual viscoelastic in the AC as it is thought to potentially hamper good adhesion between the donor corneal disk and the recipient corneal stroma.

Step 3: PDEK Donor Graft Insertion

The recipient cornea is marked with a trephine so as to outline the area of DM to be excised. A reverse Sinskey hook is introduced into the AC and a descematorhexis is performed corresponding to the margins of the epithelial mark. The DM is then stripped off and is removed from the AC. The donor pre-Descemet's roll is loaded onto the cartridge of a foldable IOL injector, and the spring of the injector is removed (as originally improvised by Francis Price) so as to prevent any damage to the donor graft. The donor roll is injected in to the AC, and the graft is slowly unfolded with air and fluidics, avoiding any direct contact with the graft so as to minimize the trauma. The PDEK graft rolls like a *Descemet's membrane endothelial keratoplasty* (DMEK) graft with the endothelium on the outer side, although due to the splinting effect of PDL, less rolling of tissue graft is required. After proper orientation of the graft, air is injected beneath it to facilitate proper adhesion to the posterior corneal stroma. Initial donor recipient corneal disk adherence takes about 30 minutes. Postoperatively, the patient is asked to lie flat in the recovery room for about an hour and to lie flat for the most part during the first postoperative day.

Conclusion

The glued IOL technique is an appropriate procedure for patients with defective capsules.

Sutureless 27-Gauge Double Needle Guided Intrascleral Haptic Fixation and Flanged Haptic Fixation

For an illustrated discussion of this new procedure by Jacob Soosan, see mediacenter.thieme.com

References

1. Vajpayee RB, Sharma N, Dada T, Gupta V, Kumar A, Dada VK. Management of posterior capsule tears. Surv Ophthalmol 2001;45:473–488
2. Wu MC, Bhandari A. Managing the broken capsule. Curr Opin Ophthalmol 2008;19:36–40
3. Agarwal A, Kumar DA, Jacob S, Baid C, Agarwal A, Srinivasan S. Fibrin glue-assisted sutureless posterior chamber intraocular lens implantation in eyes with deficient posterior capsules. J Cataract Refract Surg 2008;34:1433–1438
4. Prakash G, Ashokumar D, Jacob S, Kumar KS, Agarwal A, Agarwal A. Anterior segment optical coherence tomography-aided diagnosis and primary posterior chamber intraocular lens implantation with fibrin glue in traumatic phacocele with scleral perforation. J Cataract Refract Surg 2009;35:782–784
5. Prakash G, Jacob S, Ashok Kumar D, et al. Femtosecond assisted keratoplasty with fibrin glue–assisted sutureless posterior chamber lens implantation: a new triple procedure. J Cataract Refract Surg 2009;35:973–979
6. Agarwal A, Kumar DA, Prakash G, et al. Fibrin glue–assisted sutureless posterior chamber intraocular lens implantation in eyes with deficient posterior capsules. [Reply to letter] J Cataract Refract Surg 2009;35:795–796
7. Nair V, Kumar DA, Prakash G, Jacob S, Agarwal A, Agarwal A. Bilateral spontaneous in-the-bag anterior subluxation of PCIOL managed with glued IOL technique: a case report. Eye Contact Lens 2009;35:215–217
8. Gabor SGB, Pavlidis MM. Sutureless intrascleral posterior chamber intraocular lens fixation. J Cataract Refract Surg 2007;33:1851–1854
9. Maggi R, Maggi C. Sutureless scleral fixation of intraocular lenses. J Cataract Refract Surg 1997;23:1289–1294
10. Teichmann KD, Teichmann IAM. The torque and tilt gamble. J Cataract Refract Surg 1997;23:413–418
11. Jacobi KW, Jagger WS. Physical forces involved in pseudophacodonesis and iridodonesis. Albrecht Von Graefes Arch Klin Exp Ophthalmol 1981;216:49–53
12. Price MO, Price FW Jr, Werner L, Berlie C, Mamalis N. Late dislocation of scleral-sutured posterior chamber intraocular lenses. J Cataract Refract Surg 2005;31:1320–1326
13. Solomon K, Gussler JR, Gussler C, Van Meter WS. Incidence and management of complications of transsclerally sutured posterior chamber lenses. J Cataract Refract Surg 1993;19:488–493
14. Asadi R, Kheirkhah A. Long-term results of scleral fixation of posterior chamber intraocular lenses in children. Ophthalmology 2008;115:67–72
15. Lanzetta P, Menchini U, Virgili G, Crovato S, Rapizzi E. Scleral fixated intraocular lenses: an angiographic study. Retina 1998;18:515–520
16. Agarwal A, Dua HS, Narang P, et al. Pre-Descemet's endothelial keratoplasty (PDEK). Br J Ophthalmol 2014;98:1181–1185
17. Dua HS, Faraj LA, Said DG, Gray T, Lowe J. Human corneal anatomy redefined: a novel pre-Descemet's layer (Dua's layer). Ophthalmology 2013;120:1778–1785

30 The Cow-Hitch Suture Technique

Fernando González del Valle, Agustín Núñez Sánchez, Javier Celis Sánchez, Álvaro Fidalgo Broncano, Marcelino Álvarez Portela, Isabel Alonso Martínez, María José Domínguez Fernández, Francisco Javier Lara Medina, Antonio Arias Palomero, Esperanza López Mondéjar, and Ramón Lorente Moore

Late dislocation of the capsular bag–intraocular lens (IOL) complex can occur a few months to many years after surgery, usually without associated complications in the original surgery.[1–3] A slow process of progressive weakening of the zonular support, even after years of evolution, can lead to this complication. Two fundamental mechanisms contribute to the late dislocation of the capsular bag–IOL complex: age-related zonular weakness[4] and contraction of the capsular bag.[5,6] These two factors, together or individually, result in a failure of the zonular support and the subsequent displacement of the intact capsular bag containing the IOL. The anterior circular continuous capsulorrhexis, described by Neuhann,[7] could play an important role in the current incidence of this complication. Capsulorrhexis phimosis[8] might be one of the causes of the late in-the-bag IOL dislocation. Likely, the major predisposing factor for in-the-bag IOL dislocation could be pseudoexfoliation.[9–12] Furthermore, other causes might contribute to this process: retinitis pigmentosa,[12] prior vitreoretinal surgery,[13] a long axis,[12] ocular trauma,[13] and uveitis.[14]

Hanemoto et al[15,16] described the use of the cow hitch for refloating and refixating the dislocated IOL, using a needle manufactured specifically for their technique. In this chapter we describe a new technique, performing the cow hitch inside the eye, but with common microsurgical tools. Using our new surgical technique, the cow-hitch suture technique (CHST), it is possible to recuperate the dislocated late in-the-bag IOL complex.

Surgical Technique

Cow-Hitch Suture Technique for Dislocated Late in-the-Bag IOL Complex (Fig. 30.1)

For refloating the in-the-bag IOL complex, our technique of multiple globules of perfluoroctane (perfluorocarbon in the United States) is proposed,[17] with minimized risk of entrapment of the IOL between the ocular wall and the perfluoroctane. For refixating the IOL, the intraocular implementation of a cow-hitch knot is recommended, using a disposable 23- or 25-gauge microforceps

for peeling the inner limiting membrane (Revolution®, Alcon, Fort Worth, TX). It is necessary to fashion two holes in the capsular bag by the middle of each haptic, with the vitrectomy instrument. A forceps is introduced into the eye grasping a loop of 10-0 polypropylene suture using a sclerotomy in the bed of a scleral flap. Another microforceps, from the opposite 23- or 25-gauge microsclerotomy or using a corneal paracentesis, is passed through a hole made in the capsular bag by the middle of the haptic (**Fig. 30.2**). These forceps grasp the loop, and pass it to the first forceps that regrasps the loop and extracts it from the eye through the first sclerotomy under the scleral flap (**Figs. 30.3, 30.4, 30.5a**). (The handshake technique described in Chapter 29.) To complete the cow-hitch knot outside the eye, both ends of the suture must pass through the loop in the same direction (**Fig. 30.5b**). Finally, the surgeon pulls the ends of the suture, and the cow hitch goes into the eye, holding the haptic and IOL in the bag (**Fig. 30.6**). Another possible maneuver would be to pass the forceps with the loop, through the hole in the capsular bag, and then continue with the same procedure. To fix the suture on each scleral bed, both needles pass through the sclera and are tied beneath each scleral flap. One knot is made with each needle by using the corresponding suture end and a loop (**Fig. 30.7**). In that way, the capsular bag–IOL complex is sutured to the scleral wall by two cow hitches and four knots (**Figs. 30.8** and **30.9**).

We have performed the CHST in 14 cases of late in-the bag IOL complex. Preoperative vision remained unchanged or was improved after the surgery in all of the cases. Mean visual acuity prior to surgery was 0.09 ± 0.29 standard deviation (SD) Snellen and mean postoperative was 0.27 ± 0.33 SD. The average postoperative follow-up was 9.99 ± 17.55 SD months (range, 1 to 48 months). All of the late in-the-bag dislocated IOLs remained well fixated and stable throughout the postoperative period.

From these 14, 12 patients had associated predisposed ocular conditions. Six patients had a history or repaired retinal detachment by pars plana vitrectomy (42.86%). A pseudoexfoliation syndrome was present in four cases (28.6%). Other associated ocular entities were retinitis pigmentosa (one case) and ocular trauma (one case of Fuchs's heterochromic cyclitis with posttraumatic aniridia).

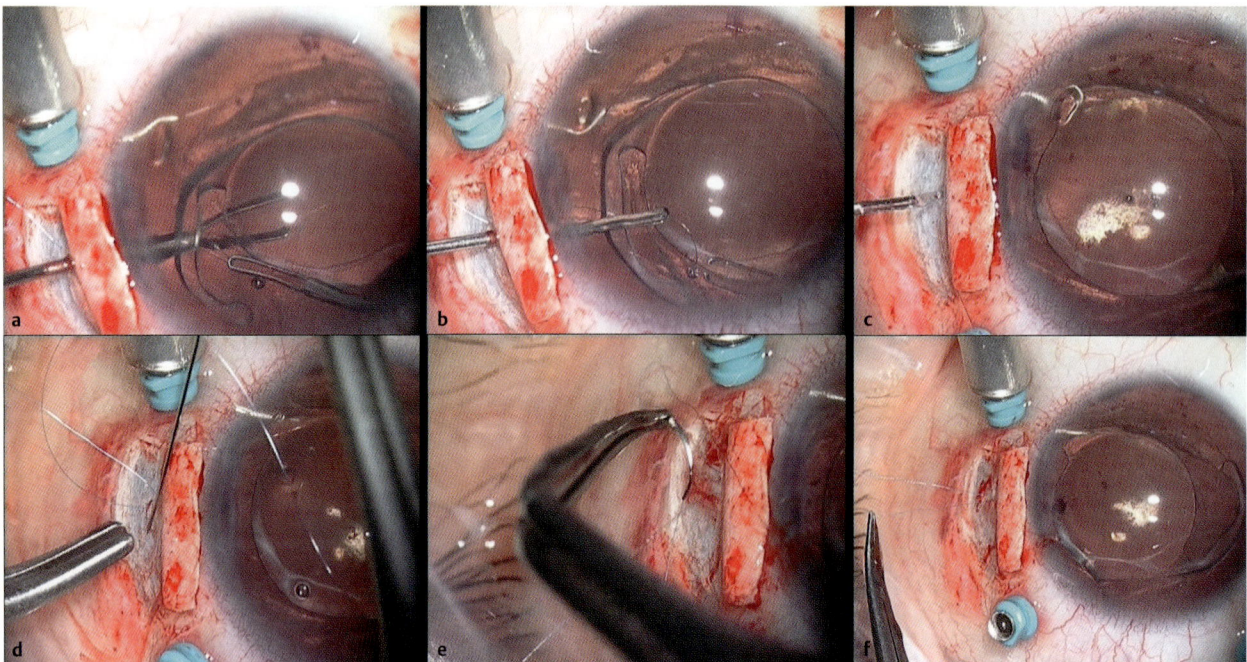

Fig. 30.1 The surgical steps of performing a cow-hitch knot are shown in this left eye of a posttraumatic aniridia with dislocated late in-the-bag intraocular lens (IOL) (one-piece AcrySof®, Alcon) complex. **(a)** The left hand introduces the loop through a hole in the capsular bag, and the right hand takes the loop. **(b,c)** The loop is pulled out by the left hand. **(d)** Once the suture is outside the eye, the polypropylene straight needle is passed through the loop. **(e)** The polypropylene curved needle is also passed through the loop in the same direction as the straight one. **(f)** Grasping the two ends of the suture, the knot passes into the eye, encompassing the haptic of the in-the-bag IOL complex.

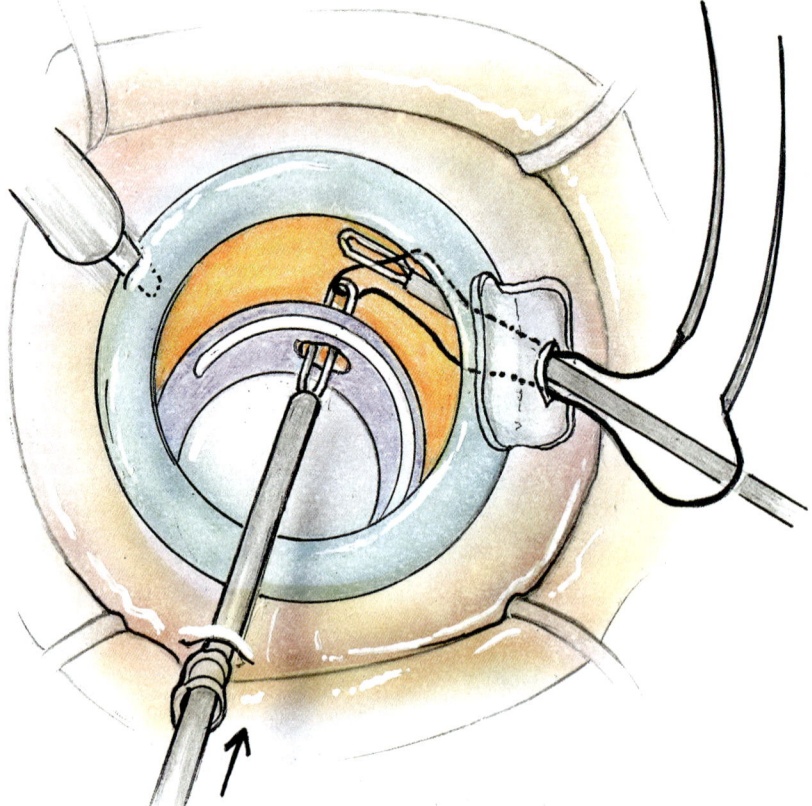

Fig. 30.2 The right hand introduces a loop into the eye with a 23- or 25-gauge inner limiting membrane (ILM) microforceps by a micro-sclerotomy in the bed of the scleral flap. The loop is passed through the hole of the capsular bag with the left hand using another ILM microforceps.

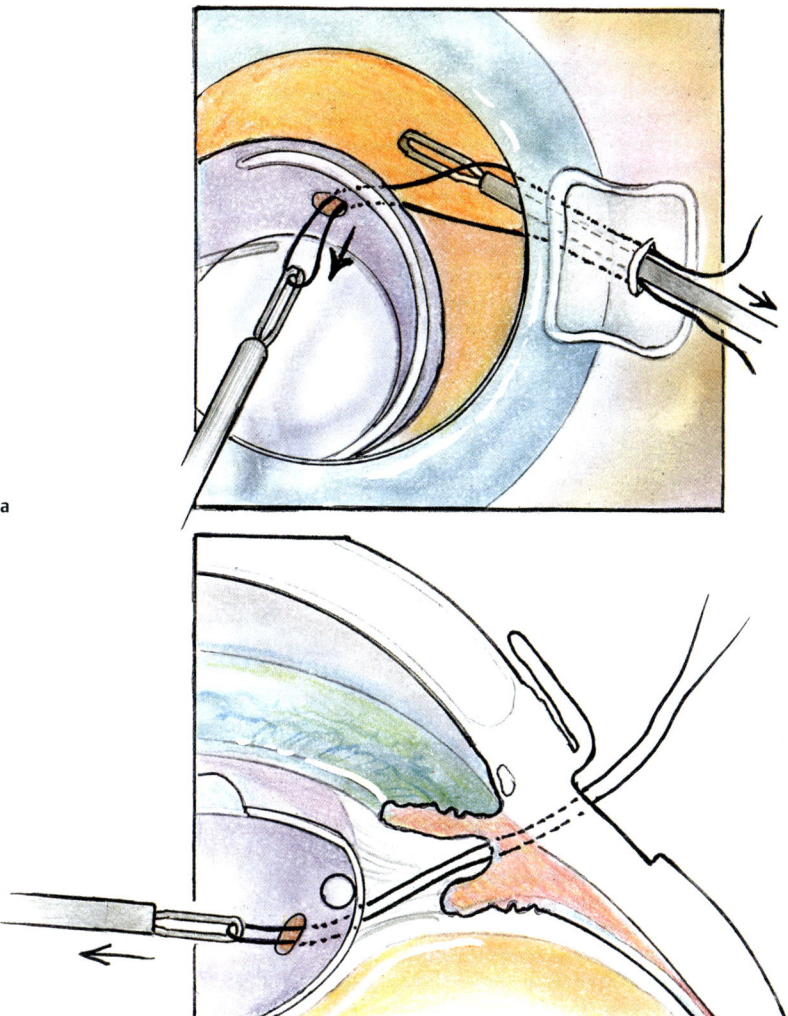

a

b

Fig. 30.3 The loop is passed from the left hand to the right hand, incorporating the haptic of the IOL.

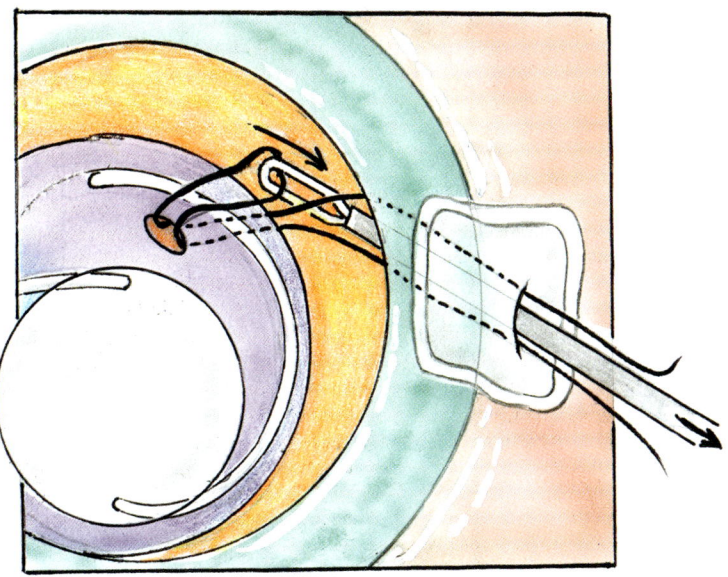

Fig. 30.4 The loop is brought out of the eye using the same micro-sclerotomy.

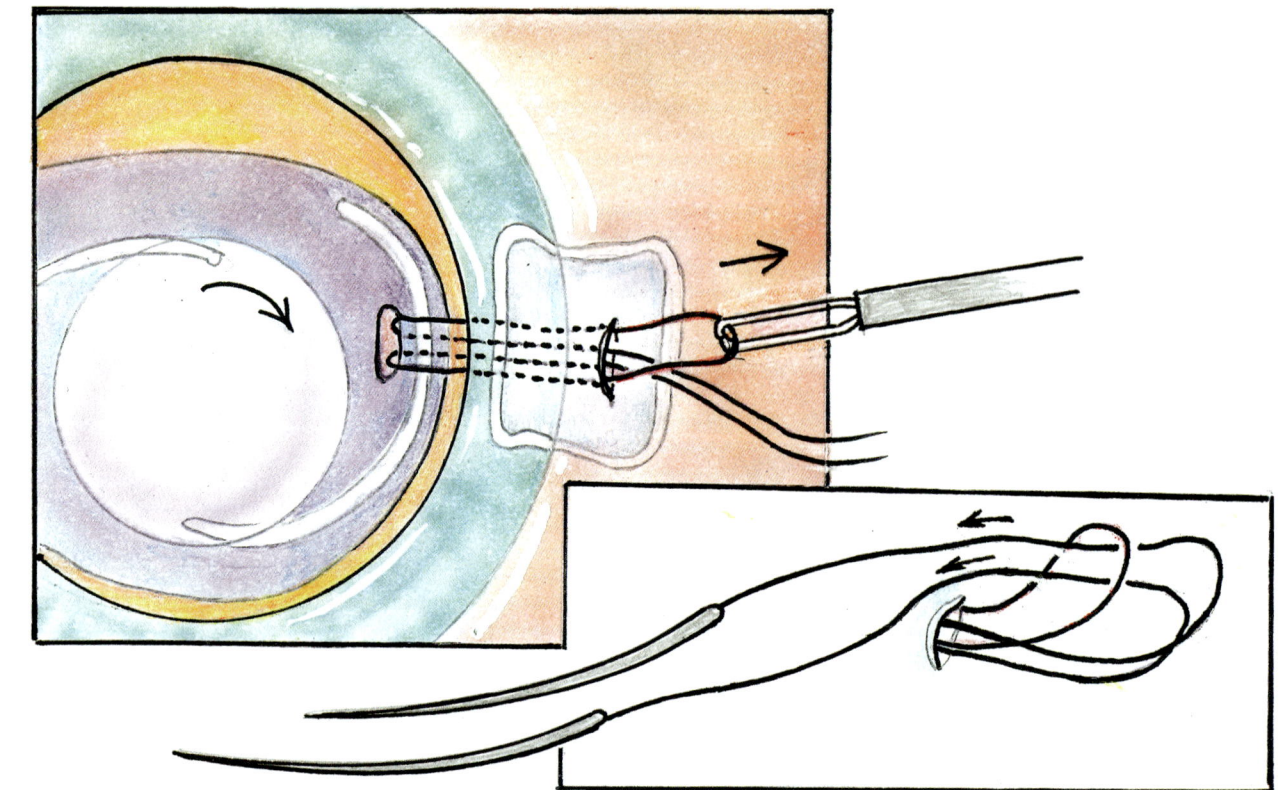

Fig. 30.5 **(a,b)** The cow-hitch knot is performed out of the eye, passing the two needles through the 10-0 polypropylene loop.

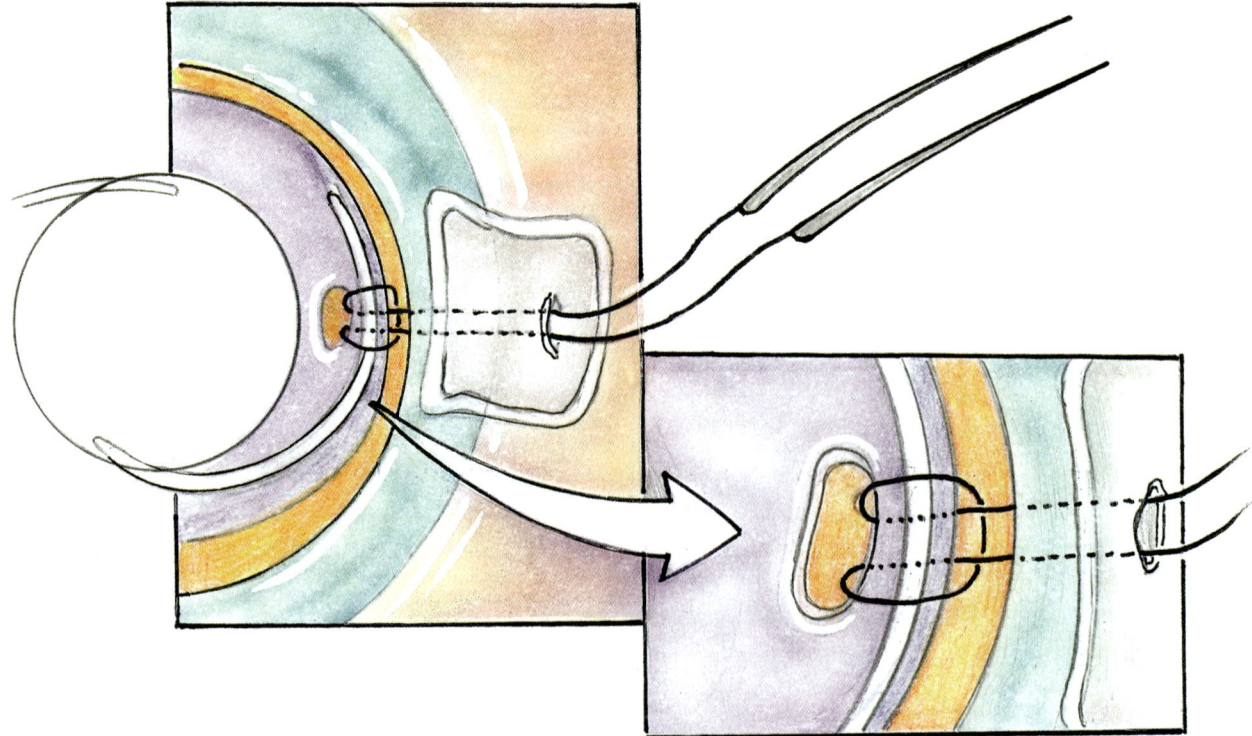

Fig. 30.6 **(a,b)** Grasping the two ends of the suture, the knot passes into the eye, securing the haptic of the in-the-bag IOL complex.

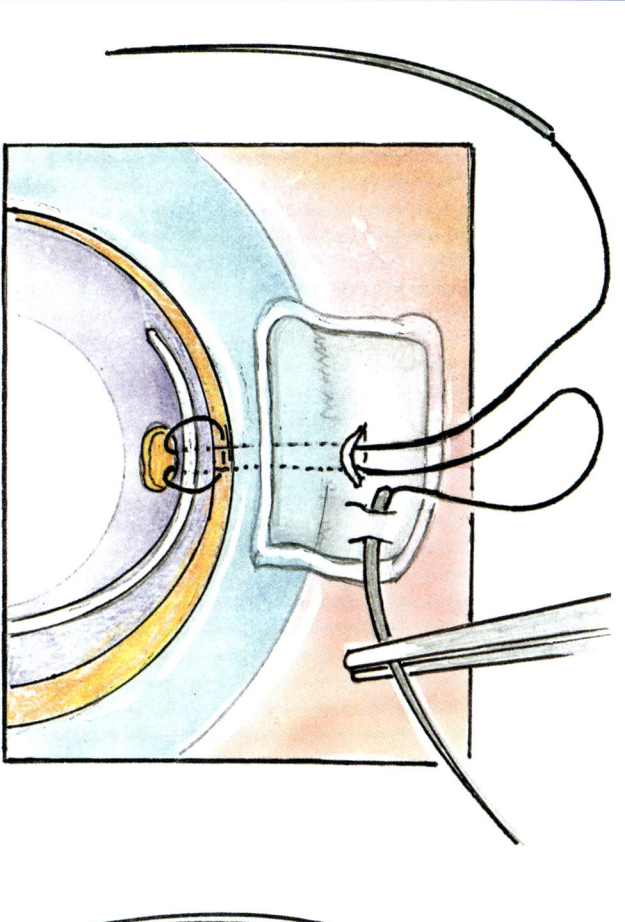

Fig. 30.7 Two ends and two needles of 10-0 polypropylene suture pass through each sclerotomy in the bed of both scleral flaps.

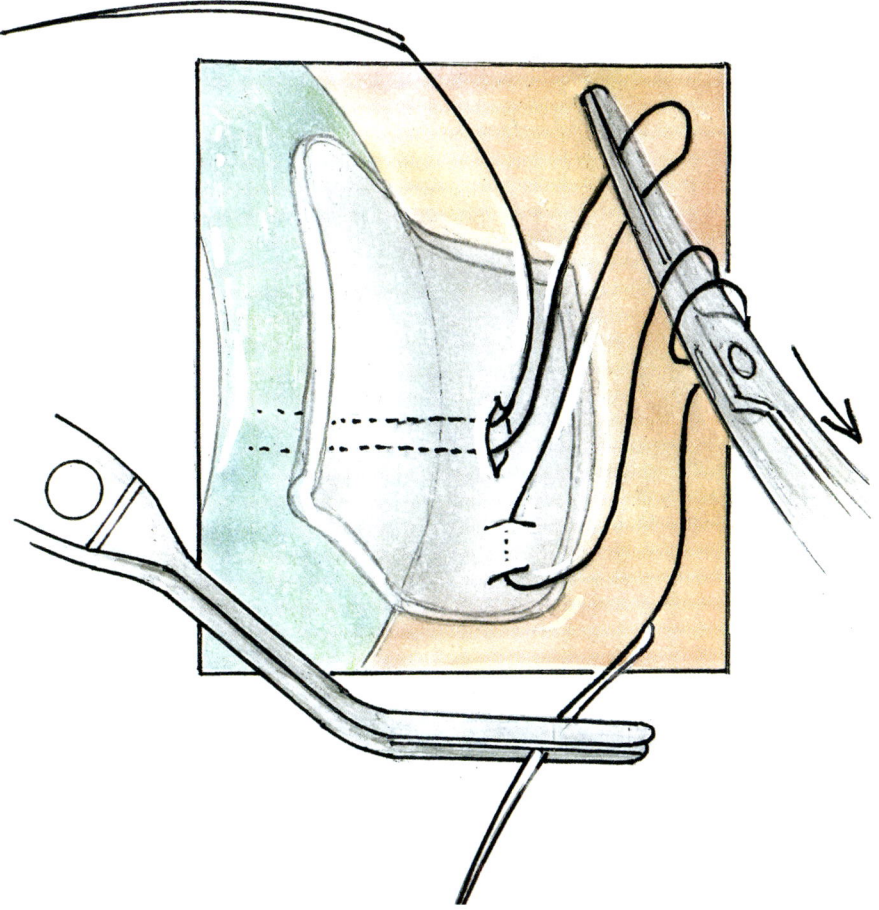

Fig. 30.8 The needle passes through the scleral bed. A knot is made with the remaining loop and the suture end, leaving the long ends to avoid late scleral erosion.

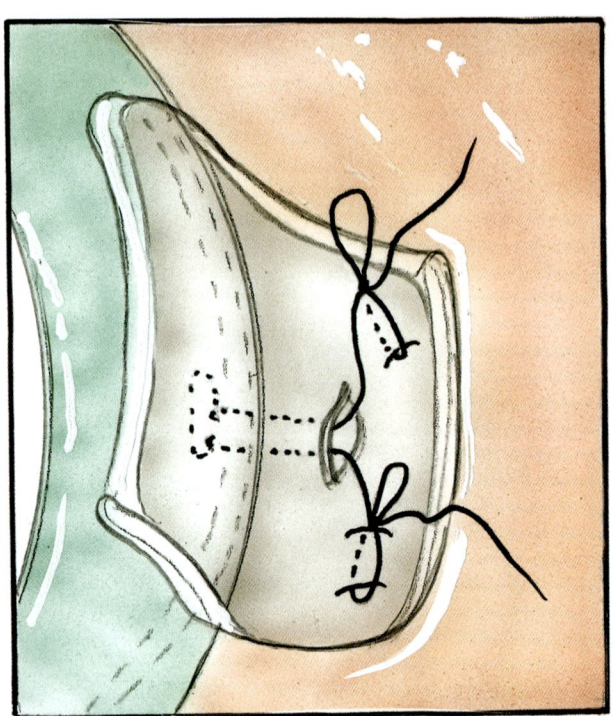

Fig. 30.9 We perform the same procedure with the second needle. Result: the capsular bag–IOL complex is sutured to the inner scleral wall by two cow hitches and four external knots.

Surgical Technique of Cow-Hitch Suture Technique for Dislocated IOL Without Capsular Bag

Greater difficulties were encountered in cases of luxation of un-encapsulated IOLs. We have used this technique in 11 eyes of 10 such patients, and it is recommended to pass each haptic into the anterior chamber to perform the cow-hitch knot there (**Fig. 30.10**). In these cases, the first haptic can be fixed with a simple knot or loop, as an alternative to the cow-hitch knot. The IOL is stabilized with the first knot in the first haptic. This is the most difficult surgical step in these cases. The loop of the polypropylene can be twisted, and then the haptic is introduced in this loop, thus performing a simple knot, like a clove-hitch knot (**Fig. 30.11**). Finally, the suture could be completed with another cow hitch.

Avoidance, Recognition, and Management of Problems

The notable problems associated with this technique are similar to those of the transsclerally sutured posterior chamber lenses, also described in this book (i.e., erosion of the polypropylene suture knots through scleral flaps, significant lens tilt/decentration

with irregular astigmatism or a secondary uveitis-glaucoma-hyphema [UGH] syndrome and vitreous hemorrhage). To avoid a late erosion of the polypropylene suture knot, we strongly recommend following the steps suggested earlier, primarily doing a deep and ample scleral flap. Also, we recommend the use of a 10-0 polypropylene, and to avoid cutting the loose ends of the suture too short, to get them flat beneath the scleral flap. To recognize a tilt in the IOL we can use a slit lamp mounted to the microscope, or we look for the correct brightness of the IOL by placing the eye centered under the microscope light. When we cannot find this reflection, we suspect that there might be a tilt of the IOL. This complication can occur if sutures are not symmetrically attached. But in our experience, when we reuse the capsular bag–IOL complex, as the IOL surface is covered by the anterior capsular bag, this could prevent a secondary UGH syndrome. Moreover, it is easier to treat this complication in these cases with CHST; we can perform another cow hitch to stabilize the late in-the-bag IOL complex. In our series, it was necessary to perform one more cow-hitch knot in one case of posttraumatic aniridia to correct the tilting of the IOL, perhaps because the iris insertion plays a role in the stability of the bag–IOL complex. We have not had a vitreous hemorrhage in our series; a pars plana infusion and the use of valved cannulas avoiding intraocular hypotension could minimize the risk of choroidal bleeding.

In our series, the main predisposing risk factor for the late-in-the bag IOL dislocation was a prior vitrectomy surgery (due to retinal detachment in all cases).

The use of 10–0 polypropylene was safe in our cases. In our 20 years of experience using this type of suture material in scleral-fixated posterior chamber IOLs, and in this new surgery (CHST), late suture lysis, suture exposure, and suture breakage have not occurred.[18] We think it is important to make a good, deep scleral flap, and to bury the suture, thus avoiding late suture problems. In fact, we think that using a heavier suture[19-22] to increase the durability of the suture, such as 9-0 polypropylene, might erode the sclera and increase the risk of endophthalmitis over the long term. Also, with this CHST, two knots are performed at each suture point, doubling the anchoring points and splitting in half the risk of late suture problems.

Other Uses for This Technique

The use of a cow-hitch knot was first utilized for IOL fixation to the ciliary sulcus in an eye without a lens capsule.[23] The use of an external cow hitch introduced into the eye with the aid of a specially designed instrument is another option for putting an end to late IOL dislocation.[16] Another similar technique has been described for the surgical treatment of the luxated IOL. This is a cow-hitch knot grasped by an intraocular microforceps in the neck of the loop and is useful for refloating and refixating the IOL within the vitreous cavity.[24] The cow-hitch knot has been suggested for transscleral fixation of IOLs.[25] Recently, a new device that enables sutureless fibrin glue–assisted transscleral fixation of the capsular bag has been described.

The total extraction of the IOL or the dislocated in the bag-IOL complex is preferred by some authors.[14] Other authors treat the aphakia by positioning an iris claw IOL.[9] Also, the use of different knots and loops for externalizing one of the haptics of the IOL can be found in the scientific literature.[27-29]

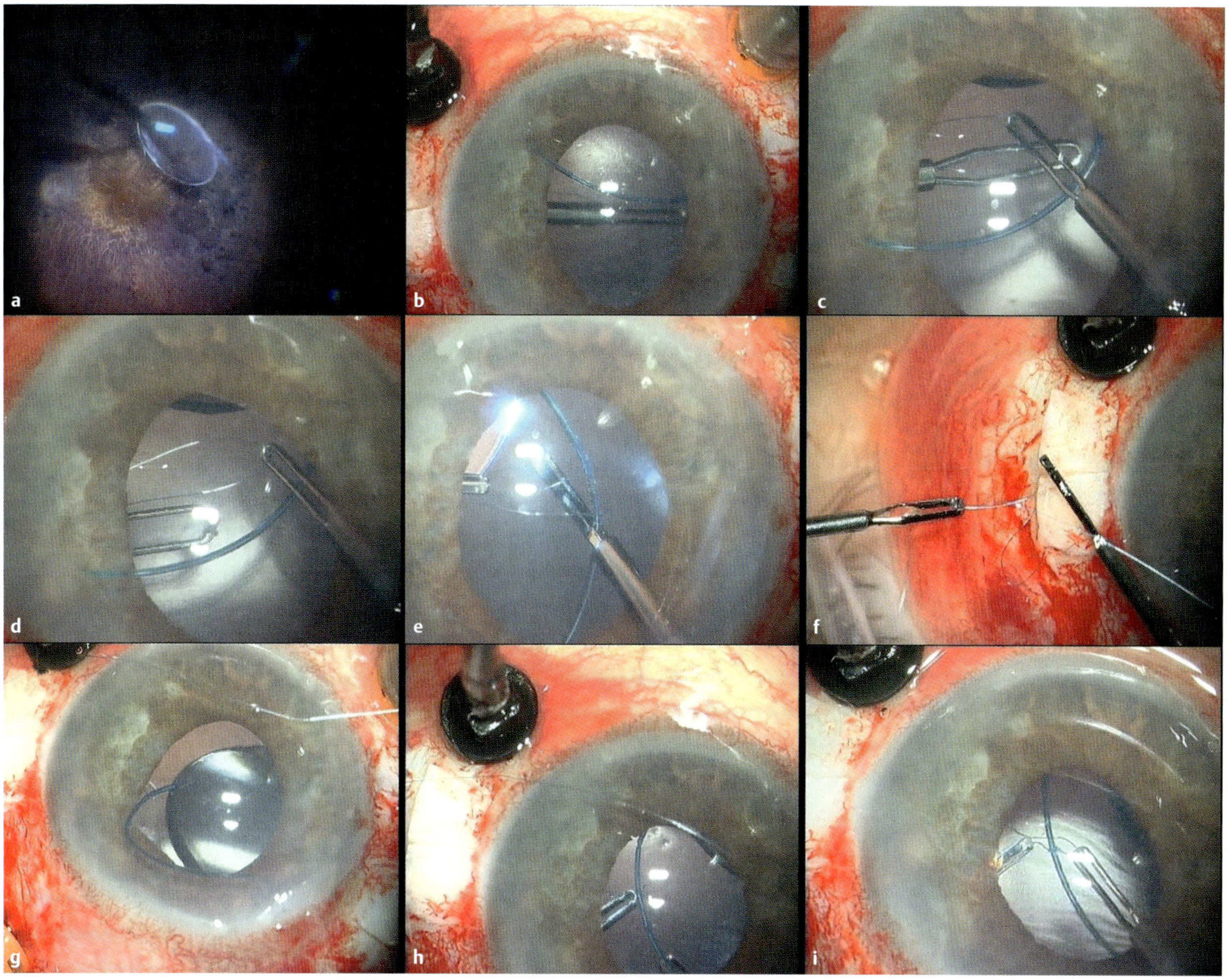

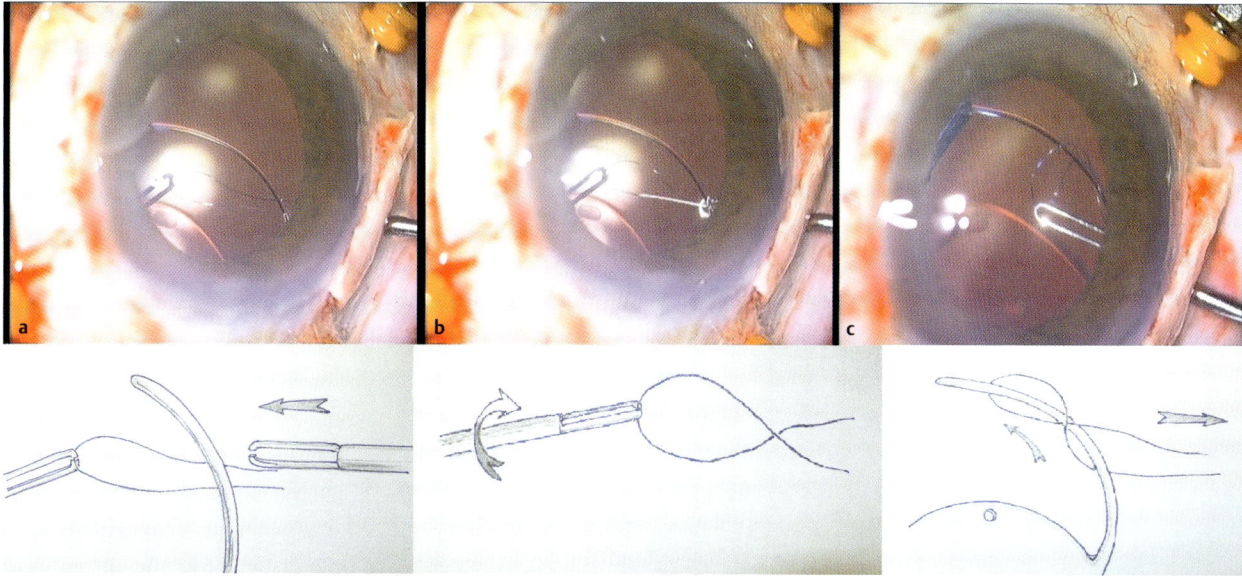

Fig. 30.10 It is possible to perform this procedure in an unencapsulated IOL (in this case a three-piece acrylic foldable Acrysof IOL). **(a)** Refloating the IOL by our technique of multiple perfluorocarbon. **(b)** The first haptic is passed to the anterior chamber. **(c–f)** The cow-hitch knot is performed in the anterior chamber, using two 23-gauge ILM microforceps. **(g-i)** The same procedure with the other haptic can be performed in the anterior chamber. In these cases, a corneal paracentesis may be of great help.

Fig. 30.11 Stabilizing one dislocated unfoldable IOL. **(a)** The loop is passed into the eye. **(b)** The second microforceps twists the loop. **(c)** The haptic passes through both created rings of the one infinite loop suture. (A variant of this type of knot, such as a clove-hitch knot, is used in Spain to secure Iberian hams to the beams where they are hung, to be dried and finally cured.)

Conclusion

This technique enables the preservation of the bag–IOL complex and suturing it to its correct anatomic site, which restores the compartmentalization of the eye. Furthermore, this technique enables the surgeon to perform a posterior capsulotomy in the same surgery. The preservation of the bag–IOL complex might avoid other complications associated with an IOL–pars plana suture, such as incorrect positioning of the IOL or secondary UGH syndrome.

References

1. Jehan FS, Mamalis N, Crandall AS. Spontaneous late dislocation of intraocular lens within the capsular bag in pseudoexfoliation patients. Ophthalmology 2001;108:1727–1731

2. Mönestam EI. Incidence of dislocation of intraocular lenses and pseudophakodonesis 10 years after cataract surgery. Ophthalmology 2009;116:2315–2320

3. Lorente R, de Rojas V. Luxación tardía del complejo saco capsular y lente intraocular. In: Lorente R, Mendicute J, ed. Cirugía del Cristalino. Madrid: Sociedad Española de Oftalmología; 2008:1751–1767

4. Assia EI, Apple DJ, Morgan RC, Legler UF, Brown SJ. The relationship between the stretching capability of the anterior capsule and zonules. Invest Ophthalmol Vis Sci 1991;32:2835–2839

5. Gimbel HV, Condon GP, Kohnen T, Olson RJ, Halkiadakis I. Late in-the-bag intraocular lens dislocation: incidence, prevention, and management. J Cataract Refract Surg 2005;31:2193–2204

6. Hayashi H, Hayashi K, Nakao F, Hayashi F. Anterior capsule contraction and intraocular lens dislocation in eyes with pseudoexfoliation syndrome. Br J Ophthalmol 1998;82:1429–1432

7. Neuhann T. [Theory and surgical technic of capsulorrhexis]. Klin Monatsbl Augenheilkd 1987;190:542–545

8. Zaugg B, Werner L, Neuhann T, et al. Clinicopathologic correlation of capsulorhexis phimosis with anterior flexing of single-piece hydrophilic acrylic intraocular lens haptics. J Cataract Refract Surg 2010;36:1605–1609

9. Lorente R, de Rojas V, Vazquez de Parga P, et al. Management of late spontaneous in-the-bag intraocular lens dislocation: Retrospective analysis of 45 cases. J Cataract Refract Surg 2010;36:1270–1282

10. Eagle RCJ Jr, Spencer WH. Lens. In: Spencer WH, ed. Ophthalmic Pathology: An Atlas and Textbook, 4th ed. Philadelphia: WB Saunders; 1996:394

11. Masket S, Osher RH. Late complications with intraocular lens dislocation after capsulorhexis in pseudoexfoliation syndrome. J Cataract Refract Surg 2002;28:1481–1484

12. Hayashi K, Hirata A, Hayashi H. Possible predisposing factors for in-the-bag and out-of-the-bag intraocular lens dislocation and outcomes of intraocular lens exchange surgery. Ophthalmology 2007;114:969–975

13. Davis D, Brubaker J, Espandar L, et al. Late in-the-bag spontaneous intraocular lens dislocation: evaluation of 86 consecutive cases. Ophthalmology 2009;116:664–670

14. Gross JG, Kokame GT, Weinberg DV; Dislocated In-The-Bag Intraocular Lens Study Group. In-the-bag intraocular lens dislocation. Am J Ophthalmol 2004;137:630–635

15. Hanemoto T, Ideta H, Kawasaki T. Dislocated intraocular lens fixation using intraocular cow-hitch knot. Am J Ophthalmol 2001;131:265–267

16. Hanemoto T, Ideta H, Kawasaki T. Luxated intraocular lens fixation using intravitreal cow hitch (girth) knot. Ophthalmology 2002;109:1118–1122

17. González del Valle F, Núñez Sánchez A, Alonso Martínez I, López Mondéjar E. Reflotamiento cristaliniano. In: Procedimientos Quirúrgicos en Oftalmología. DVD, 2005. ISBN-13: 978-84-609-9980-5

18. González del Valle F, Martínez Sanz F, Celis Sánchez J. Lentes intraoculares suturadas transescleralmente. In: Ramón Lorente, Javier Mendicute, ed. Cirugía del Cristalino. Madrid: Sociedad Española de Oftalmología; 2008. ISBN-13: 978-84-89085-36-7

19. Buckley EG. Hanging by a thread: the long-term efficacy and safety of transscleral sutured intraocular lenses in children (an American Ophthalmological Society thesis). Trans Am Ophthalmol Soc 2007;105:294–311

20. Benayoun Y, Petitpas S, Turki K, Adenis JP, Robert PY. [Sutureless scleral intraocular lens fixation: report of nine cases and literature review]. J Fr Ophtalmol 2013;36:658–668

21. McAllister AS, Hirst LW. Visual outcomes and complications of scleral-fixated posterior chamber intraocular lenses. J Cataract Refract Surg 2011;37:1263–1269

22. Lockington D, Ali NQ, Al-Taie R, Patel DV, McGhee CN. Outcomes of scleral-sutured conventional and aniridia intraocular lens implantation performed in a university hospital setting. J Cataract Refract Surg 2014;40:609–617

23. Malbrán ES, Malbrán E Jr, Negri I. Lens guide suture for transport and fixation in secondary IOL implantation after intracapsular extraction. Int Ophthalmol 1986;9:151–160

24. Nakashizuka H, Shimada H, Iwasaki Y, Matsumoto Y, Sato Y. Pars plana suture fixation for intraocular lenses dislocated into the vitreous cavity using a closed-eye cow-hitch technique. J Cataract Refract Surg 2004;30:302–306

25. Chen SX, Lee LR, Sii F, Rowley A. Modified cow-hitch suture fixation of transscleral sutured posterior chamber intraocular lenses: long-term safety and efficacy. J Cataract Refract Surg 2008;34:452–458

26. Jacob S, Agarwal A, Agarwal A, Sathish K, Prakash G, Kumar DA. Glued endocapsular hemi-ring segment for fibrin glue-assisted sutureless transscleral fixation of the capsular bag in subluxated cataracts and intraocular lenses. J Cataract Refract Surg 2012;38:193–201

27. Kokame GT, Atebara NH, Bennett MD. Modified technique of haptic externalization for scleral fixation of dislocated posterior chamber lens implants. Am J Ophthalmol 2001;131:129–131

28. Kokame GT, Yamamoto I, Mandel H. Scleral fixation of dislocated posterior chamber intraocular lenses: temporary haptic externalization through a clear corneal incision. J Cataract Refract Surg 2004;30:1049–1056

29. Chan CK, Hawkins H, Lin SG. Modified haptic externalizing technique for repositioning dislocated 1-piece acrylic posterior chamber implants. Can J Ophthalmol 2007;42:573–579

31 Intraocular Lens Exchange with an Open Posterior Capsule

Marc A. Michelson

An intraocular lens (IOL) exchange can be challenging enough with an intact capsular bag, but an IOL exchange in a eye that has undergone a previous yttrium-aluminum-garnet (YAG) laser capsulotomy presents the surgeon with a totally different set of surgical challenges. There are many circumstances, however, in which a patient may need an exchange IOL when the posterior capsule is open. This chapter discusses a step-by-step surgical technique for successful IOL removal and exchange in the face of an open posterior capsule following a YAG laser capsulotomy.

Acrylic single-piece IOLs are currently the predominant lenses of choice for cataract surgery. Multifocal lens in particular carry a risk of visual dissatisfaction in some patients.[1–3] Identifying the root cause of postoperative visual disturbance is critical before considering an IOL exchange.[4,5] However, once it is determined that an IOL exchange is necessary to improve visual function, generally the sooner the surgery is performed, the easier the lens removal will be.

In many cases, a YAG laser capsulotomy may have already been performed to help resolve the patient's vision complaints. Once a YAG laser capsulotomy has been performed, many surgeons may not attempt to remove an IOL due to the increased risk of complications. These risks may include zonular lysis from the stress induced by removing the haptic, the risk of dislocation and subluxation of the IOL or parts of the IOL into the vitreous chamber, and difficulty inserting a secondary IOL. Corneal endothelial damage with prolonged postoperative corneal edema is also a concern. In addition, a planned vitrectomy must be anticipated when removing an IOL with an open capsule.

The longer an IOL remains in the capsular bag, the greater the tendency for fibrosis of the haptics between the anterior and posterior capsule. The IOL design will also have an impact on the ease or difficulty of an IOL disinsertion from the capsular bag. If the haptics of the IOL have an expanded terminal bulb, fibrosis around the bulb may make it more difficult to extricate the lens from the capsular bag.

A successful strategy when approaching these cases must meet high expectations of an excellent vision outcome for the patient with resolution of the vision problems associated with IOL. A good technique must enable the following:

1. Small incision bimanual approach
2. Endothelial cell protection
3. Stable environment of lens disassembly and removal
4. Proper vitrectomy techniques
5. Safe removal of haptics from capsular bag
6. Secure placement of a new IOL

Step 1: The Secondary Incisions

The surgery is initiated with two 1.5-mm secondary corneal limbal incisions placed on each side of the meridian parallel to the insertion of the haptics to the optic. These incisions should be oriented perpendicular to the meridian of where the primary incision will be placed. They should be marked with a radial keratotomy (RK) marker to ensure their accurate placement.

The function of the secondary incisions is as follows:

1. Enable small-incision, closed-system bimanual surgery
2. Introduce intracameral anesthetic and viscoelastic into the anterior chamber
3. Provide access for instrumentation to open the capsule adhesions around the circumference of the optic and over the proximal optic haptic junction
4. Enable manipulation of the haptics for disengagement from the capsular bag
5. Serve as ports for small-gauge (23-gauge or smaller), high-speed bimanual vitrectomy
6. Serve to remove viscoelastic from the anterior chamber using a bimanual irrigation and aspiration (I/A) technique.

Step 2: Viscoelastic

After the two secondary incisions have been created and an intracameral anesthetic has been injected, a high molecular weight cohesive viscoelastic should be injected into the anterior chamber. A cohesive viscoelastic is essential and should not be substituted for a dispersive viscoelastic. It is important that the viscoelastic remain in the anterior chamber throughout the surgery. The viscoelastic must endure the IOL manipulation, bisection, and removal, and a vitrectomy, and as well as the insertion of the new IOL. The primary purposes of the cohesive viscoelastic are as follows:

1. Provide a stable environment for the anterior chamber during IOL manipulations
2. Tamponade any vitreous during the procedure and act as a barrier to prevent vitreous from entering the anterior chamber during the lens exchange
3. Provide a viscous environment in the anterior chamber to stabilize and prevent the IOL from dislocating into the vitreous cavity
4. Ensure that the viscoelastic is stable in the anterior chamber throughout the entire procedure

Once the lens has been bisected and the haptics amputated from the optic, components of the IOL will remain suspended and fixed within the viscoelastic and will be easily accessible for retrieval. The viscoelastic provides a stable environment for IOL disassembly and removal while both compartmentalizing and tamponading the vitreous gel. The vitreous thus becomes restricted from entering the anterior chamber by the viscoelastic while the IOL is disassembled and removed inside the anterior chamber.

Step 3: Dissect Adhesions from the Anterior Capsule and the Intraocular Lens

A small-gauge, blunt-tip spatula introduced through the secondary incision can be used to bluntly dissect the anterior capsule off of the perimeter of the IOL. Alternatively, the blunt-tip cannula can be attached to a cohesive ophthalmic viscosurgical device (OVD), and a gentle viscodissection can be performed. Dissection of the anterior capsule generally is easier if the IOL exchange is performed within 6 months of the implantation, but the anterior capsule generally can be readily dissected from an acrylic IOL optic years after the implantation. Once a separation of the anterior capsule has been achieved, the spatula can be swept 360 degrees to free the optic from the capsule. The capsule can also be dissected away from the proximal haptic–optic junction, but the distal haptic in the equatorial capsular bag should not be disturbed. As long as the distal haptics remain fibrosed in the peripheral capsule, care should be taken to avoid any stress to the zonules. Avoid any manipulation of the distal haptics at this stage of the surgery. It is important not to exert any forces that result in centripetal displacement of the distal haptic (**Fig. 31.1**).

Note that IOLs with holes at the haptic–optic junction such as the EnVista (Bausch and Lomb, Rochester, NY) may make separation of the anterior and posterior capsular adhesions more demanding.

Step 4: Displace the Optic of Intraocular Lens Anteriorly

After the IOL optic and the anterior capsule have been lysed of all adhesions from the peripheral areas of the IOL optic, the spatula is then placed under the lens optic and advanced across the posterior surface of the IOL. If using the viscodissection technique, OVD can be injected between the optic and the vitreous to elevate the optic and push the vitreous more posteriorly. The optic and the optic–haptic junction can now be displaced upward into the anterior chamber above the plane of the anterior capsule. The displacement should be enough to angle the haptics upward, exposing the optic–haptic junction above the plane of the anterior capsule while being careful not to displace the distal haptics centripetally from the equatorial the capsular bag.

Step 5: Create the Primary Incision

The primary incision should not be the first incision created, and its construction should be delayed until the IOL is ready to be removed. The incision size should be between 2.4 and 2.7 mm. The primary purposed of this incision are as follows:

1. Enable introduction of the intraocular scissors to bisect the IOL and sever the haptic optic junction
2. Remove the IOL
3. Insert the new IOL
4. Enable self-sealing during a bimanual vitrectomy

Following the anterior displacement of the acrylic IOL, the primary incision can be created. The primary incision for an IOL exchange is best placed slightly posterior to the limbus and advanced onto the cornea from the limbus. Entry into the anterior chamber should be a biplanar to create a self-sealing wound. A more posterior incision enables enlarging the wound intraoperatively, if necessary, with minimal impact on the induction of astigmatism. The ideal wound placement should be 90 degrees from the meridian of the haptic–optic junction. This provides access to disengage and remove the haptics from the capsular bag. If there is a clear corneal temporal incision present, it is recommended to avoid reopening the original incision, as irregular healing may create unpredictable astigmatism (**Fig. 31.2**).

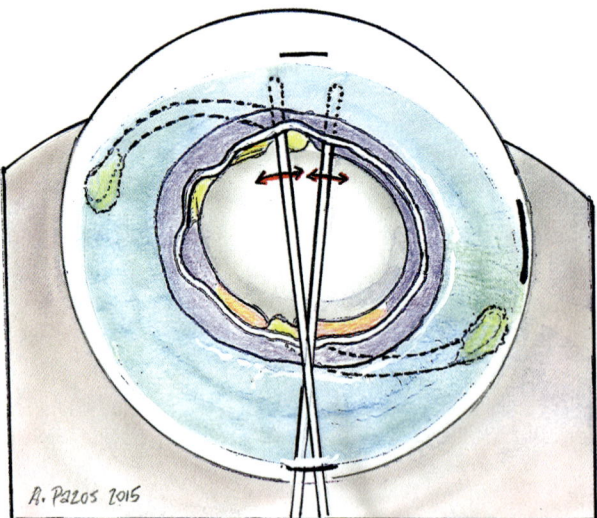

Fig. 31.1 A small-gauge, blunt-tip spatula introduced through the secondary incision can be used to bluntly dissect the anterior capsule off of the perimeter of the intraocular lens (IOL). Avoid any maneuvers that centripetally displace the distal haptic. This prevents zonular stress and zonulysis.

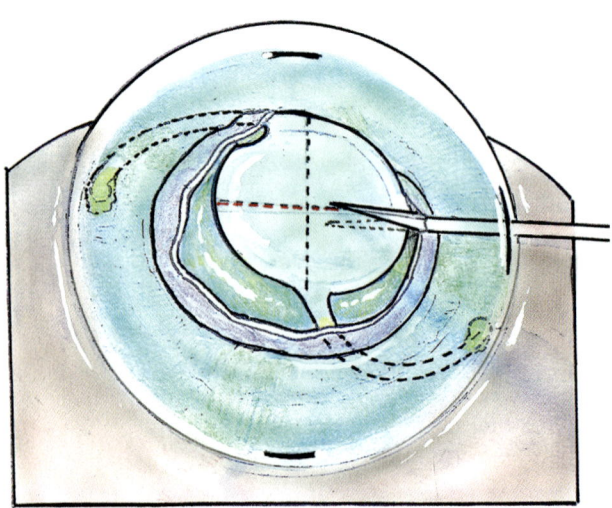

Fig. 31.2 The primary incision is created just anterior to the limbus. The optic is bisected with intraocular scissors.

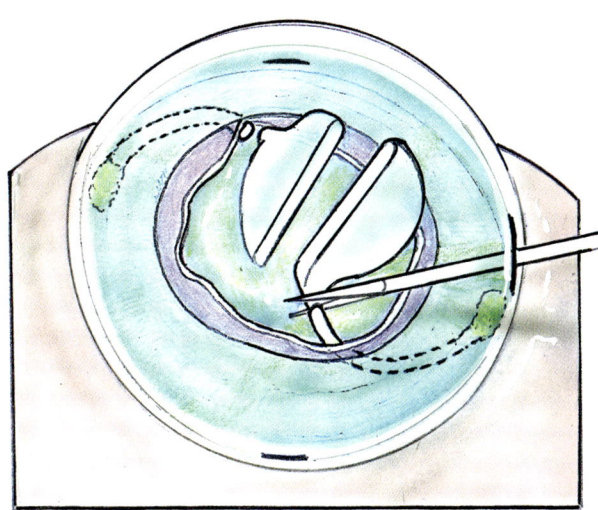

Fig. 31.3 The optic is cut in half with the intraocular scissors. After completion of the optic bisection, the scissors are then used to sever the optic–haptic junction, amputating the proximal haptic from the optic. The haptics are amputated at the optic, leaving each hemisphere of the optic suspended in the viscoelastic.

Step 6: Bisect the Optic and Amputate the Haptics

The IOL is now anteriorly displaced into the anterior chamber above the plane of the anterior capsule. The haptics have transformed from a planar position to a more acute angle, but the distal portion of the haptics remain adherent to the equatorial capsule. This in effect acts to stabilize the IOL for bisection with the intraocular scissors. The acrylic IOL is surrounded within the viscoelastic, and the vitreous is well displaced posteriorly. The intraocular scissors are introduced into the anterior chamber through the primary incision, and an intraocular forceps is inserted through a secondary incision to stabilize the IOL. The optic is then cut in half with the intraocular scissors. After completion of the optic bisection, the scissors are then used to sever the optic–haptic junction, amputating the proximal haptic from the optic (**Figs. 31.2** and **31.3**).

Step 7: Freeing the Haptics from the Capsular Bag

The distal haptic remnants can now be disengaged and removed from the capsular bag without damaging the capsule or the zonules. An intraocular forceps is now introduced into the anterior chamber and the haptic is subjected to two different maneuvers. The first is a pivoting maneuver of the distal haptic with a rocking back and forth to free the haptic from the fibrous adhesions (**Fig. 31.4a**). The second maneuver is a rotational maneuver along the axis of the haptic insertion combined with a back-and-forth rotational motion (**Fig. 31.4b**). The combination of pivoting and axis rotation of the haptic usually results in the release of the distal haptic from capsular fibrosis. If these maneuvers fail to free the haptic, the intraocular scissors can be used to trim the haptic close to the distal end of the haptic. When the haptics become free of the capsular adhesions, they are removed from the anterior chamber through the primary incision (**Fig. 31.4c**).

Anomalous Circumstances

Note that the Crystalens (Bausch and Lomb) may be more difficult to remove. First, the capsulorrhexis is larger than the optic, leading to fibrosis of the anterior and posterior capsule. Second, the Crystalens has a compound haptic. It is plate silicone topped with polyamide haptics, which are designed to closely adhere to the capsular bag equator. The polyamide haptics are considerably

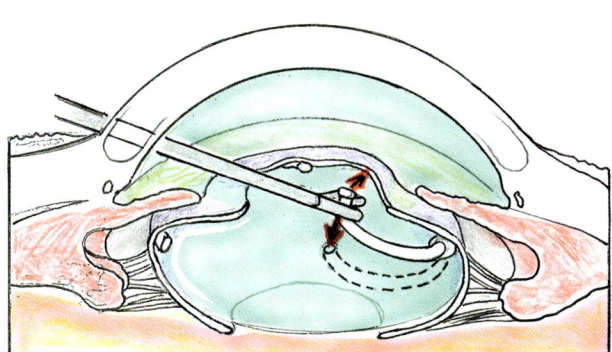

a

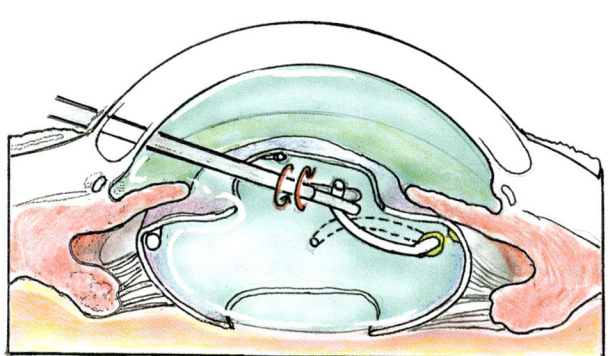

b

c

Fig. 31.4 **(a)** First, a pivoting maneuver of the distal haptic, rocking it back and forth and anteriorly and posteriorly, to free the haptic from the fibrous adhesions. **(b)** Second, a back-and-forth rotational motion is performed along the axis of the haptic insertion. **(c)** The haptic now can be disengaged from the fibrosis in the peripheral capsule without stressing the zonule. Note: the manipulation of the haptics is performed with the viscoelastic in the anterior chamber.

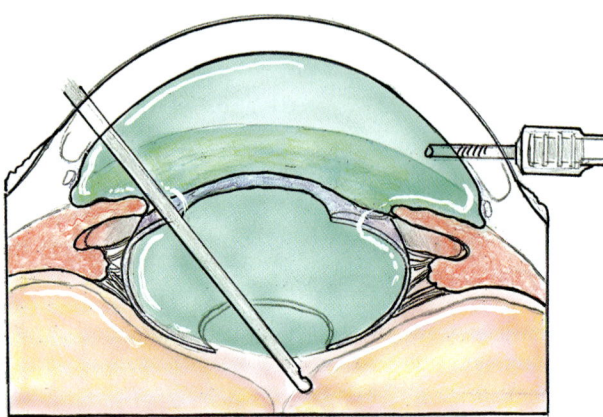

Fig. 31.5 Either a 23- or 25-gauge vitrectomy handpiece can be inserted through the side-port incision without altering the wound structure. A bimanual vitrectomy is performed with the infusion handpiece, or chamber maintainer, placed through one secondary incision and the vitrectomy handpiece placed through the other. The infusion port is placed in the anterior chamber and the vitrector is passed through the viscoelastic in the anterior chamber into the anterior vitreous.

more challenging to dissect free from the bag. It is tolerable to defer from dissecting the capsular bag or haptics rather than tear the bag. If the dissection appears unsatisfactory, it is wiser to amputate the haptics and proceed with the vitrectomy and sulcus implantation of the IOL.

Step 8: Anterior Vitrectomy

Safety and efficiency of an anterior vitrectomy has become greatly improved with advances in vitrectomy technology. When employing a either a 23- or 25-gauge vitrector with a high cutting speed with a bimanual closed system technique with constant pressure monitored infusion, the vitrectomy can be performed quickly and efficiently. Either a 23- or 25-gauge vitrectomy handpiece can be inserted through the side-port incision without altering the wound structure. A bimanual vitrectomy is performed with the infusion handpiece placed through one secondary incision and the vitrectomy handpiece placed through the other. The infusion port is placed in the anterior chamber and the vitrector is passed through the viscoelastic in the anterior chamber into the anterior vitreous. The vitrectomy can be performed while the viscoelastic remains in the anterior chamber (**Fig. 31.5**). The primary incision must either be self-sealed or sutured to enable a closed system bimanual vitrectomy to be successfully performed. Employing constant infusion pressure fluidics maintains a stable intraocular pressure, enabling the vitrectomy to be performed while minimizing or eliminating vitreous from entering the anterior chamber. Despite all precautions to prevent vitreous from advancing into the anterior chamber, the surgeon must inspect the anterior chamber to ensure that vitreous strands are not present.

Step 9: Intraocular Lens Insertion

After the vitrectomy has been completed to the surgeon's satisfaction, the eye is now ready for the new IOL to be inserted. A three-piece sulcus IOL can now be injected through the primary incision. If the volume of viscoelastic has been reduced, the amount of viscoelastic in the anterior chamber can be supplemented prior to the IOL insertion. With an adequate amount of viscoelastic in the anterior chamber, the three-piece IOL can be injected through the primary incision, allowing the distal haptic

to unfold above the iris. The trailing haptic should remain externalized at the incision site. The distal and subsequent trailing haptic can now be placed and dialed into the ciliary sulcus. Injecting the IOL into the anterior chamber and allowing the haptic to unfold over the iris will not inadvertently inject through the open posterior capsule and into the vitreous cavity the lens.

Step 10: Removal of the Viscoelastic

The IOL should now be well positioned and centered with the haptics in the ciliary sulcus over the anterior capsule. The posterior capsule is open and the anterior chamber remains filled with a viscoelastic. Despite the open posterior capsule, removal of the viscoelastic is easily performed because the IOL now becomes a physical barrier isolating the vitreous cavity from the anterior chamber. The viscoelastic can be removed from the anterior chamber with a bimanual aspiration technique. Remember, before performing a bimanual I/A, the bottle height or the infusion pressure should be lowered. If precautions are not taken to lower the infusion pressure, because the anterior chamber is filled with viscoelastic, the I/A could generate too much pressure in the anterior segment and excessively deepen the anterior chamber. This could result in a posterior dislocation of the IOL. Another approach would be to aspirate most of the viscoelastic without an irrigation cannula. The infusion cannula can be inserted into the anterior chamber to regain a stable pressure and complete the removal of any viscoelastic in the anterior chamber. No attempt should be made to remove any viscoelastic posterior to the IOL. The pupil should be round after the viscoelastic has been removed. Intracameral miotic agents may be injected to verify that there is no vitreous remaining in the anterior chamber.

The most common sources of patients' dissatisfaction with their vision following an IOL implantation that may require an IOL exchange are listed below. An open posterior capsule should not be a deterrent to a successful IOL exchange outcome. The surgeon may use the 10-step approach succinctly outlined above to successfully and confidently restore functional vision when the posterior capsule has been opened and the IOL needs to be removed. The most common reasons for IOL exchanges are as follows:

- Incorrect IOL power
- Multifocal intolerance
- Silicone oil in IOL
- IOL calcification
- Severe dysphotopsias
- Iris chafing syndrome
- Severe glistenings
- Snowflake degeneration

References

1. Cochener B, Lafuma A, Khoshnood B, et al. Comparison of outcomes with multifocal IOL: a meta-analysis. Clin Ophthalmol 2011;7:45–56
2. de Vries NE, Webers CA, Touwslager WR, et al. Dissatisfaction after implantation of multifocal intraocular lenses. J Cataract Refract Surg 2011; 37:859–865
3. Shimizu K, Ito M. Dissatisfaction after bilateral multifocal intraocular lens implantation: an electrophysiology study. J Refract Surg 2011;27:309–312
4. Santhiago MR, Netto MV, Barreto J, Gomes BA, Schaefer A, Kara-Junior N. Wavefront analysis and modulation transfer function of three multifocal intraocular lenses. Indian J Ophthalmol 2010;58:109–113
5. Toto L, Falconio G, Vecchiarino L, et al. Visual performance and biocompatibility of 2 multifocal diffractive IOLs: six-month comparative study. J Cataract Refract Surg 2007;33:1419–1425

XI Iris Reconstruction

32 Iris Defects and Complications

Kenneth J. Rosenthal

Iris defects in the context of cataract surgery may either be pre-existing or occur iatrogenically during the surgical procedure. The careful and appropriate assessment and treatment of these conditions will directly impact the success of the procedure and, indeed, make the completion of the procedure possible. Failure to address iris complications or comorbidities at the time of surgery, or in a planned sequence of surgical procedure, will cause an otherwise successful cataract extraction to fail and the patient to be dissatisfied.

Patients with iris defects present surgical challenges because the anterior segment may destabilize after cataract removal and because the implantation of a traditional intraocular lens (IOL) may result in the patient experiencing significant glare, photophobia, and polyopsia.

Furthermore, with some iris defects, such as those associated with iridocorneal endothelial syndrome, or in eyes with other comorbid conditions, such as retinal abnormalities or glaucoma, the overall success of the procedure may ultimately be compromised by the progression of the disease. These defects should be carefully assessed in determining the surgical strategy and prognosis for the patient.

It is equally important to diagnose the iris defect accurately, as its treatment will differ widely depending on its extent and on its cause. Iris repair can be accomplished by a variety of techniques and utilizing a variety of devices. In general, the repair is performed by cerclage, direct or indirect iris suture, or implantation of a prosthetic iris. Additionally, contact lenses and corneal tattooing, although infrequently performed, can be used to block unwanted excess light.

Patient Assessment

In the patient with preexisting iris defects, it is important to take a careful history. One must understand how the defect occurred, what previous treatments have been tried, and what options exist for ameliorating or repairing the condition. Of ultimate importance, however, is carefully querying the patient as to the extent of visual disability. Although larger iris defects generally have more symptoms, there are important exceptions to this paradigm, and consideration should be given to not repairing or replacing the iris tissue in patients who do not have significant symptoms.

Symptoms

Patients with iris defects may have little or no visual compromise, or may have symptoms that are so severe as to be debilitating. The most common symptoms are the following:

1. Photophobia: The aversion to light is generally extreme, so that even normal indoor lighting may be trouble-some. Patients with large iris defects are almost completely unable to tolerate outdoor sunlight without wearing dark sunglasses for protection.
2. Glare: Patients may experience starbursts, halos, or hazy vision, particularly in bright light, but even in poor lighting.
3. Decreased visual quality: Patients experience poor contrast sensitivity. This is most likely related to the transmission to the retina of higher order aberrations (particularly spherical aberration), due to light traveling through the peripheral cornea, which is unguarded by the peripheral iris. This latter is particularly important in assessing patients with congenital aniridia (discussed below). These patients frequently also suffer from foveolar hypoplasia, and accordingly their best visual potential is ~ 20/100 or less. However, despite the fact that their Snellen acuity may not significantly improve after iris prosthetic implant surgery, these patients universally note a dramatic improvement in their functional vision.
4. Cosmetic defects: Patients with iris defects may suffer from poor self-esteem, self-consciousness, and depression due to their iris color and iris configuration. Additionally, because the eyes are often the first characteristic others notice about an individual, the presence of obvious iris abnormalities may affect how patients are perceived and reacted to by others. Cosmetic improvement, particularly at the time of cataract surgery, can be helpful in improving the emotional disposition of patients suffering from externally visible iris defects, and thus the clinician should ask patients how they feel about themselves.

Function of the Iris

To appropriately repair iris defects, a clear understanding of the iris/pupil function is crucial. In addition to the obvious function of modulating light entrance through the pupil the iris has other equally important functions, particularly in the context of cataract surgery. So the repair should be designed to obliterate the pseudophakic/aphakic junction in patients with IOL implants. Other goals of treatment are as follows

1. Reduce confusional focused/unfocused images
2. Reduce peripheral asphericity and optical aberrations
3. Decrease pupil size, therefore reducing photophobia
4. Improve cosmesis

The absent or fully dilated pupil may be of a diameter in excess of 10 mm, whereas the largest IOL available in the United States is 6.5 mm in diameter (and most IOLs are 6 mm or less).

Accordingly, under these circumstances, light entering the eye presents a focused image (through the IOL) along with a super-imposed defocused image (around the edge of the IOL—aphakic). Similarly, patients with multiple iris defects may suffer from polyopsia, ghosting, poor contrast sensitivity, or reduction in visual quality. These phenomena negatively impact the patients' vision. Reducing peripheral asphericity and optical aberrations caused by light entering the peripheral cornea may reduce contrast sensitivity. Finally, the presence of iris defects, especially in light-colored eyes, may impart a significant cosmetic defect; patients may present with this defect as the sole complaint, and the risks, benefits, and advisability of repair in the absence of significant visual compromise should be given due consideration. Improvement in cosmetic appearance can be accomplished by iris repair or implantation of an iris prosthetic device.

Classification and Strategies for Repair of Iris Defects

Iris abnormalities may be assessed by their etiologies, their physical configuration, and their physiological/ophthalmic impact upon the patient.

Traumatic Etiologies

Diseases that cause iris abnormalities are summarized in **Box 32.1**. Generally, they can be divided into developmental and traumatic anomalies. The trauma can be blunt or penetrating. In such cases, the surgeon should be aware of the likely concomitance of zonular dehiscence (particularly in blunt trauma), and of lens perforation (in penetrating trauma), as well as of corneal injury. In fact, in blunt trauma with iris defects, the surgeon should be prepared to address vitreous prolapse and repair of zonular defects with capsular tension rings as they almost always occur together.

Iatrogenic conditions include surgical trauma, idiopathic postoperative mydriasis, and mydriasis related to prolonged increased intraocular pressure (IOP), both in the postoperative period and as a sequela to untreated angle closure glaucoma, as a result of IOP-related iris sphincter damage. Intraoperative snag-

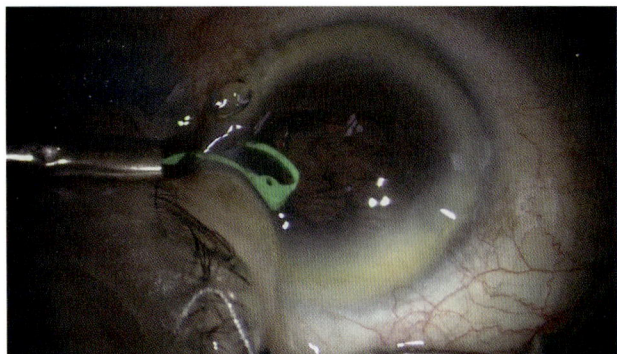

Fig. 32.1 The withdrawal of the Beaver-Visitec International (BVI; Waltham, MA) I-Ring pupil expander, resulting in snagging of the temporal iris by the insertion/removal instrument, causing a subtotal iridodialysis.

ging of the iris with instruments and devices may cause iridodialysis (**Figs. 32.1** and **32.2**).

And the preoperative use of systemic α_1-antagonists such as tamsulosin (Flomax), doxazosin (Cardura), silodosin (Rapaflo), prazosin (Minipress), alfuzosin (Uroxatral), and terazosin used in the treatment of both hypertension andbenign prostatic hypertrophy-related urinary frequency—may lead to intraoperative floppy iris syndrome (IFIS), resulting in transillumination defects, iris prolapse, and chronic mydriasis (**Fig. 32.3**). The intraoperative/preoperative management of this condition is discussed in Chapter 23. Iatrogenic traumatic aniridia has been reported in conjunction with endoscopic cyclophotocoagulation.[1]

Congenital and Developmental Etiologies

Congenital and developmental iris defects occur in a variety of conditions, including congenital aniridia, coloboma, iridocorneal endothelial syndrome, Axenfeld-Rieger syndrome, uveitis, and idiopathic postoperative mydriasis. Many patients have coexisting zonular and capsular abnormalities. In congenital aniridia, for example, the capsule may be thinned and lack elasticity, described by Robert Osher as being comparable to "wet toilet tissue." The surgeon should be prepared for this condition, and

---

Box 32.1 Causes of Iris Defects

Developmental
- Coloboma
- Iridocorneal endothelial syndrome
- Axenfeld-Rieger syndrome
- Congenital aniridia
- Ectropion uveae
- Albinism (transillumination)

Traumatic
- Surgical
  - Intraoperative floppy iris syndrome
  - Iridodialysis from instrumentation
  - Chronic elevation of intraocular pressure
- Nonsurgical
  - Percussive trauma
  - Penetrating trauma

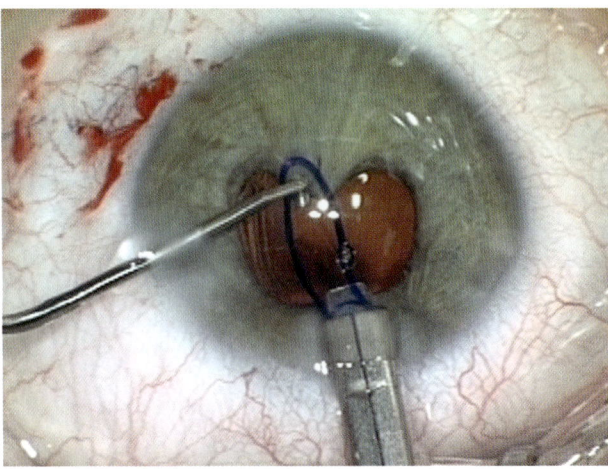

Fig. 32.2 Removal of the Malyugin pupil expansion ring, causing a snagging of the distal iris by the loop. Slow and careful removal prevents disinsertion or stretching of the iris.

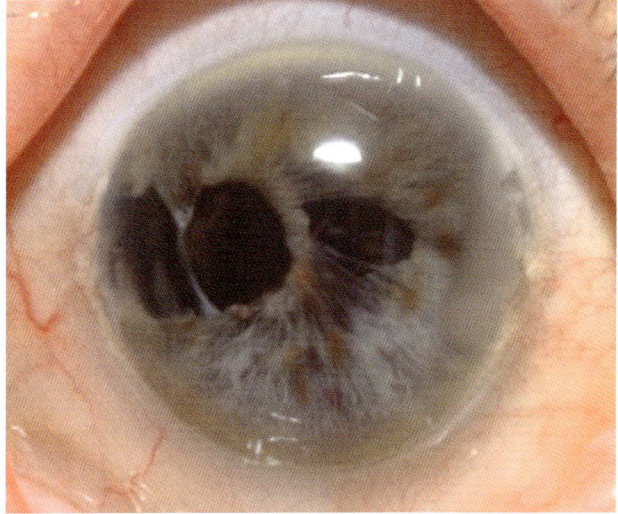

a

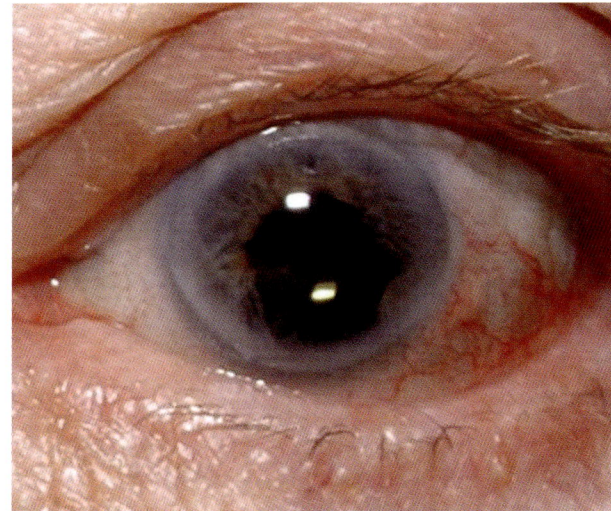

b

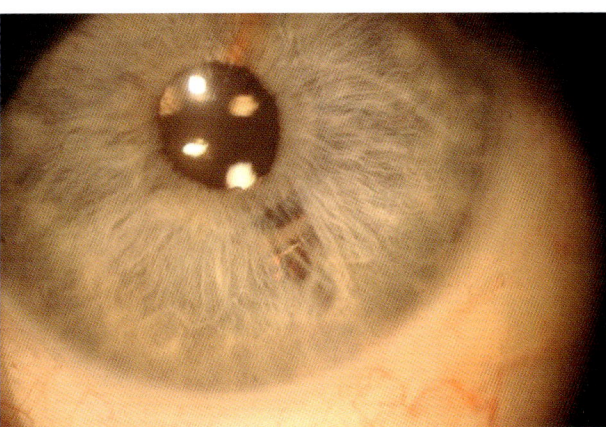

c

Fig. 32.3 **(a-c)** Various iris defects resulting from the effects of the intra-operative floppy iris syndrome (IFIS).

should modify the surgical technique to perform a well-controlled capsulotomy in these cases. In congenital aniridia in children, as in all pediatric cataracts, the capsule is universally rubbery, and a controlled rhexis can be challenging as well. Use of hyperviscous viscoelastics (e.g., Healon-5, Abbott Medical Optics, Abbott Park, IL) can aid in tamponading the capsule in both of these aniridic scenarios.

Classification of Iris Defects by Physical Types and Treatment Approach

Total or Subtotal Aniridia/Functional Aniridia

Complete functional absence of the iris occurs in patients with congenital aniridia and trauma, both surgical and penetrating. As a surgical complication, complete iridodialysis may rarely occur. Congenital and acquired ectropion uveae may also present as functional partial or full aniridia. Percussive injury may also cause complete iridodialysis. Congenital aniridia should more accurately be called "hypoplastic iris syndrome," because almost all of these patients have an iris root present, although it serves no function. Infrequently, these hypoplastic remnants can be surgically stretched toward the center of the pupil and sutured, using a cerclage or quadrantic approach (see below). However, the vast majority of such cases, both congenital and acquired, have inadequate iris tissue to provide optically useful closure, and thus care must be taken not to overstretch the iris remnants, which could cause iridodialysis or iris root hemorrhage. Most

patients with these abnormalities are likely to benefit from an iris prosthetic implant. When possible, the implant should be placed at the time of primary surgery or at the time of definitive reconstruction of trauma cases. These surgical steps can be performed sequentially. For example, in the United States it is common to perform iris implantation on a patient who has already had otherwise routine cataract surgery, because of the paucity of available devices at the time of the initial surgery. My experience is that this does not significantly impact the success of the procedure, however.

Transillumination Defects

Transillumination defects (TIDs) are not obvious in all cases. The examiner should be alerted to their possible presence by the patient's history. There is almost always diffuse transillumination in patients with ocular albinism, and the placement of an iris implant to mask this transillumination will markedly decrease photophobia and increase patients' visual potential.[2]

Transillumination defects may also occur in patients with IFIS or intraoperative iris prolapse, due to stretching of the iris tissue. TIDs have also been reported after blunt trauma, after vitrectomy, and after implantation of IOLs, usually single-piece IOLs in the sulcus,[3] or sutured to the posterior iris. We reported a case of TIDs related to in-the-bag implantation of a single piece acrylate IOL in conjunction with trabeculectomy using an EX-PRESS Glaucoma Filtration Device (Alcon Laboratories, Inc., Fort Worth, TX)[4] (**Fig. 32.4**).

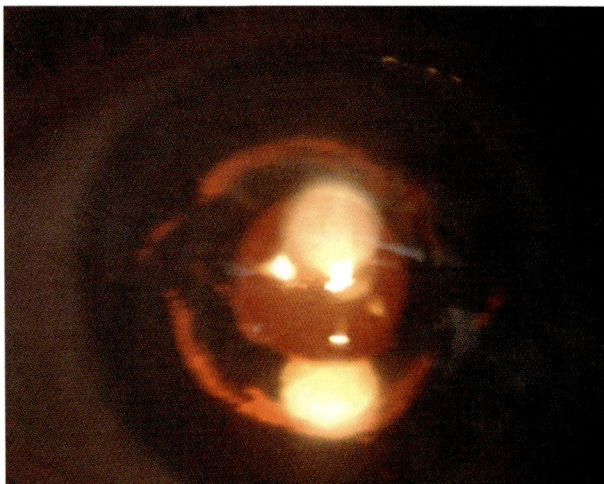

Fig. 32.4 A one-piece intraocular lens (IOL) causes extensive transillumination defects, which shadow the shape of the IOL, even though the lens was entirely within the capsular bag. Shallowing of the anterior chamber following this combined phaco-trabeculectomy may be implicated. Surprisingly, the patient was completely asymptomatic and required no further intervention.

Many TIDs are asymptomatic, particularly those covered by the upper eyelid, and they do not require treatment. However, they can be the source of poor visual quality and photophobia, especially when located within the palpebral fissure, and especially when located temporally (a common location for TIDs caused by iris prolapse). In such cases, the treatment is proportional to the extent of the defect. Smaller, well-circumscribed TIDs can be treated with a plication suture, whereas larger ones may require an iris prosthetic implant.

Polycoria

The presence of multiple pseudopupillary openings in the iris creates a "moth-eaten" appearance. This may occur in acquired disorders such as Axenfeld-Rieger syndrome or anterior embryotoxon. The first case of modular/small incision iris implantation,

which I reported in 1996, was in a patient wit Axenfeld-Rieger syndrome. This problem exists more commonly due to surgical and penetrating trauma, however, particularly with IFIS (**Fig. 32.5**). As with TIDs, the extent and location of the localized iris defect determines its treatment. Smaller areas can be treated effectively with an imbrication suture, whereas larger ones require iris implantation.

Sector Defects: Coloboma

True iris coloboma is a congenital disorder of the iris arising from failure of the embryonic optic plate to fully fuse when forming the embryonic fissure in the fifth week of gestation, resulting in a "keyhole-shaped" pupil. An iris coloboma can be associated with colobomas of the ciliary body, choroid, retina, or optic nerve. Iris colobomas are typically located in the inferonasal quadrant. They frequently affect the entire uveal tract, which therefore may include the iris, ciliary body (including the zonule), optic nerve retina, and choroid. When present only anteriorly, it creates only an iris defect with attendant photophobia and decrease visual quality. Patients with this deformity are frequently very self-conscious about their appearance, and often present for cosmetic improvement even in the absence of symptoms.

In treating such conditions as part of a cataract extraction, it is crucial to keep in mind that these patients are almost always lacking zonules in the area peripheral to the iris defect, and appropriate measures include capsular support with hooks or capsular tension ring, and placement of retentive viscoelastic overlying the area of defect, so as to prevent vitreous prolapse. This topic is discussed further in Chapters 25 and 26.

Closure of the colobomatous defect can be accomplished by the use of a Siepser knot,[5] or one of its variants,[6] if there is adequate tissue to allow it. No undue amount of tension should be placed on the iris or on the suture, as this may cause bleeding or iridodialysis; however, the iris is sufficiently elastic to allow primary closure. In iris colobomas that extend two or more clock hour positions, however, it is prudent to consider the placement of an iris prosthetic implant. This can be accomplished by using a rigid "sector" iris implant or a flexible implant in which the superior, noncolobomatous area is cut out to provide access through the superior pupil when dilated (for dilation exam and low lighting conditions) (**Fig. 32.6**).

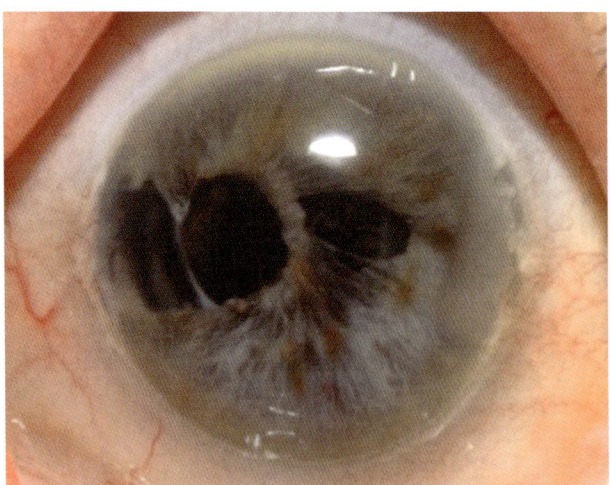

a

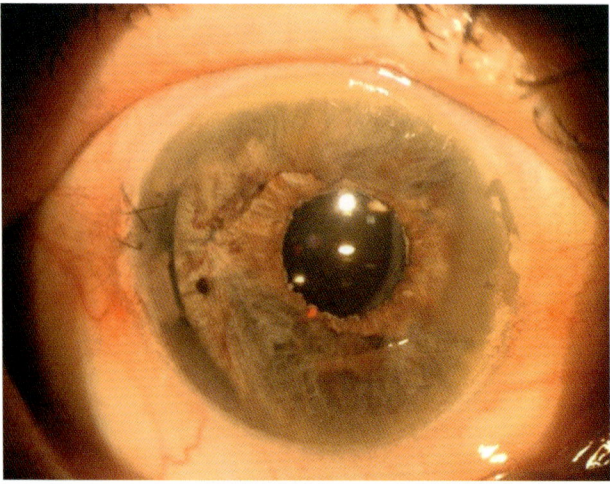

b

Fig. 32.5 Preoperative **(a)** and postoperative **(b)** appearance of a patient with polycoria secondary to presumed IFIS, with implantation of the HumanOptics CustomFlex iris prosthesis. The patient's symptoms of polyopsia and photophobia diminished markedly following this procedure.

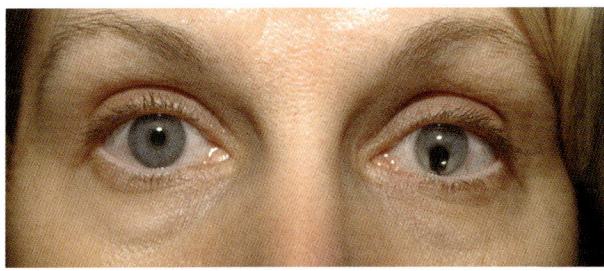

a

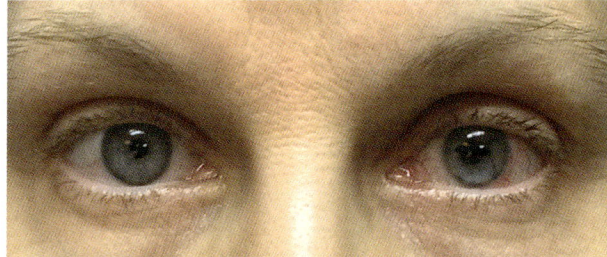

b

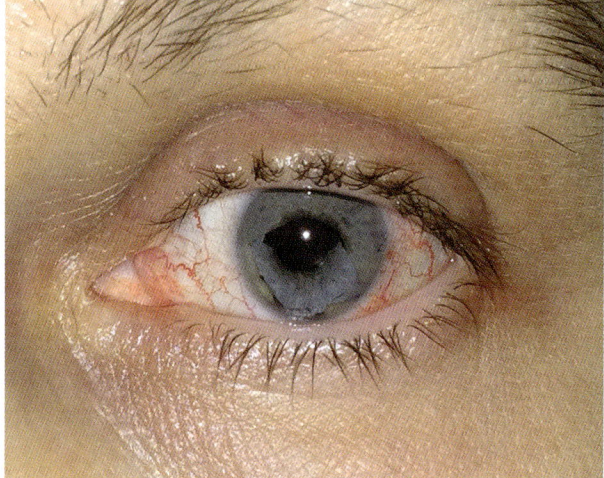

c

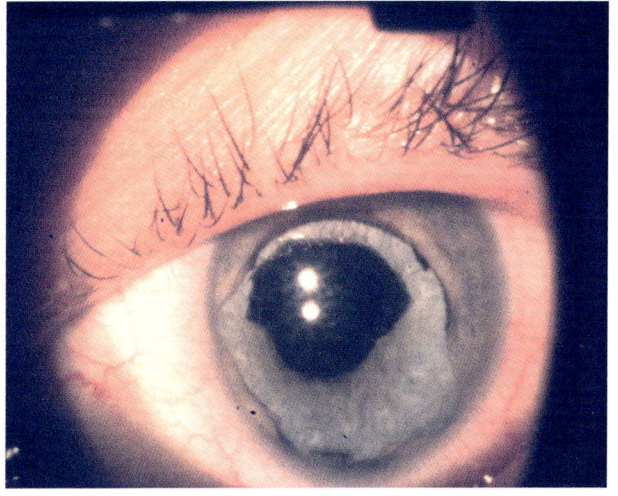

d

Fig. 32.6   Preoperative **(a)** and postoperative **(b)** appearance of a patient with coloboma of the iris and ciliary body. There was no posterior choroidal involvement. The patient had severe photophobia following cataract surgery, despite sequential opacification of the anterior capsule. The Custom- Flex artificial iris was implanted and a portion of the superior iris prosthesis was removed, to allow a full pupillary aperture on dilation. **(c,d)** Postoperative view of the Coloboma: **(c)** close-up; **(d)** dilated.

Atonic Pupil

Chronic mydriasis is generally caused by the failure of the iris sphincter, mechanical damage to the myofibrils, or stretching of the iris stroma. Common etiologies are blunt trauma (traumatic mydriasis), prolonged elevation of IOP as in acute angle closure glaucoma, in prolonged postoperative pressure spike, and inflammation. Idiopathic instances also have been known to occur.

The treatment of this condition overlaps with the strategy for congenital aniridia; however, it is much more likely that some degree of pupillary closure can be accomplished by cerclage or by quadrantic iris suture, described below. For large or chronic mydriasis, and particularly in patients with light-colored irises, where the iris stromal pigment is scant to begin with, closure, even when it can be performed, may result in inadequate pupillary closure or diffuse and visually significant TIDS. In these patients, as in all patients with inadequate iris stroma in general, an iris prosthetic device is the preferred strategy. In patients in whom there are obstacles to obtaining the iris prosthesis, or in borderline cases, due consideration should be given to a stepwise approach: repair, and then, if it fails, implantation of iris prosthesis. The patient should be aware of the relative risks and benefits of each of these approaches, particularly a patient who may be at risk for poor healing after multiple surgeries, such as a patient with poor corneal endothelial function, immune compromise, or diabetes.

Iridodialysis

Iridodialysis, in which the iris root is disinserted from the sclera, occurs most commonly due to trauma, although it may rarely occur secondary to degenerative disease. Surgically induced iridodialysis is commonly seen in conjunction with iris prolapse or with the inadvertent tethering of the iris with an instrument (**Fig. 32.7**). In such cases, prompt repair of these conditions may result in a good restoration of function.

Posterior Synechiae and Chronic Miosis

Synechiae that cause adhesion of the iris to the anterior lens capsule can present with challenges to completion of surgery. They can be addressed by viscoelevation of the normal adjacent iris combined with the use of a cyclodialysis spatula to lyse the adhesion, or by the use of a microforceps to remove a fine pupillary membrane.

Stretching of the pupil with various instruments can also be performed, but should be avoided in cases of IFIS. These techniques are covered more in detail elsewhere in this book, but it is important to keep in mind that, particularly in cases of IFIS, overzealous stretching or lysis of the pupillary ruff may result in chronic mydriasis that requires sequential surgical intervention.

Visually Detracting Iridectomies and Iridotomies

The iridectomy/iridotomy is the most commonly used surgical strategy for creation of a confluence between the posterior and anterior chambers, particularly in narrow-angle disease. Although this procedure generally is well tolerated, some patients may be sensitive to the stray light entrance through these openings, particularly when there are large areas open. These problems may

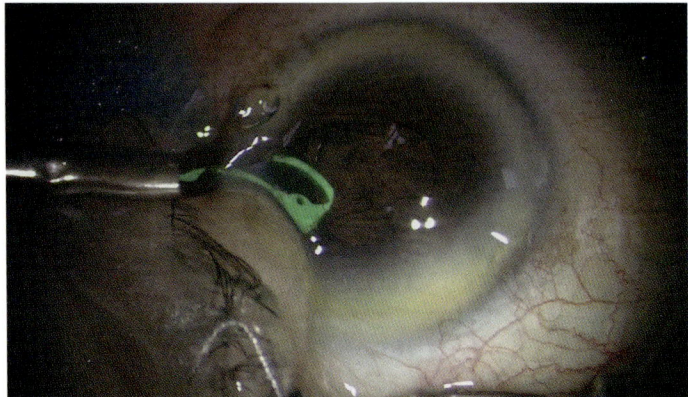
a

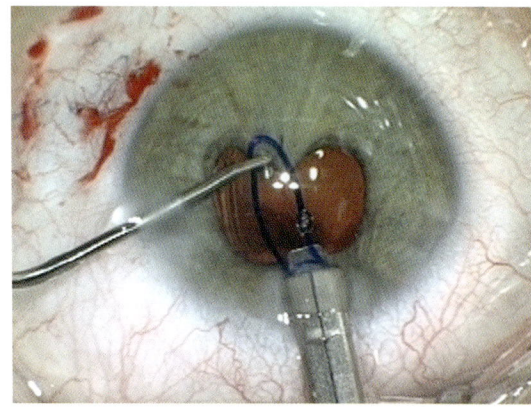
b

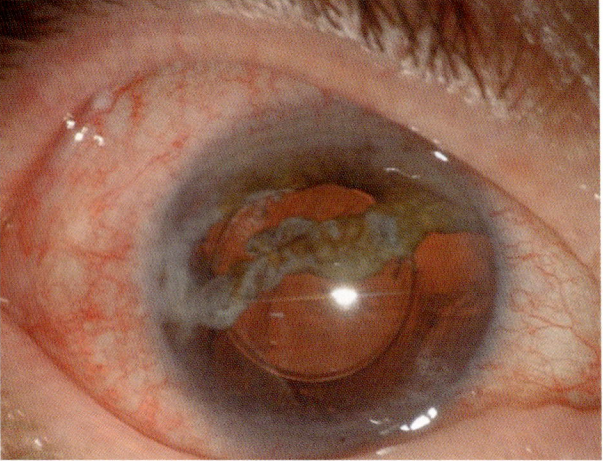
c

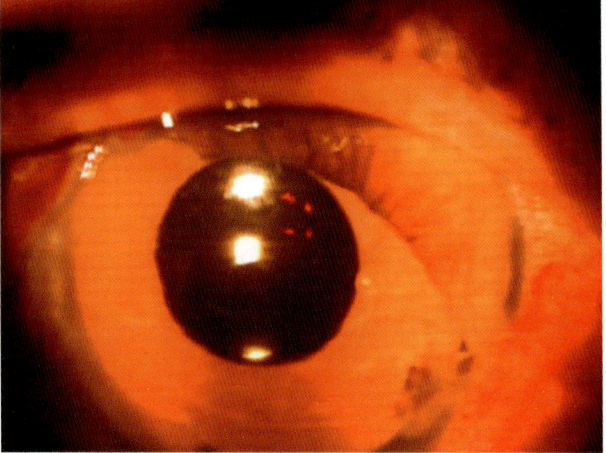
d

Fig. 32.7 **(a)** Subtotal iridodialysis caused during removal of the BVI I-Ring pupil expander. The removal instrument has snagged the proximal iris upon withdrawal. **(b)** The distal loop of a Malyugin ring is caught on the iris, causing stretch. Trauma to the iris can be avoided by careful observation of the release of the ring during removal. This patient suffered a large iridodialysis with fixed dilated curled iris tissue throughout. A fibrotic curled-up iris was excised, a partial iridodialysis repair was performed, and an Ophtec model 311 was inserted to re-form the pupil. **(c,d)** Large iridodialysis from Salz nucleus splitter: **(c)** preoperative; **(d)** postoperative.

be alleviated by partial closure of the iridotomy or by corneal tattooing overlying the iris defect.

Treatment of Iris Defects: Ocular Surface Strategies

Masking Contact Lenses

Before considering surgical intervention, due consideration may be given to prescribing nonsurgical treatments. Masking contact lenses can be offered, in which the periphery is stamped or painted with a colored material to match the color of the fellow eye, and in which an occluder layer of dark material is placed along the corneal side of the contact lens to block out the light. My experience with these contact lenses has been that they are rarely accepted by the patient because they are generally uncomfortable, and they do not provide the quality of optical correction that definitive correction can provide. The latter problem may be at least partially due to the fact that the blocking pigmentation is not in the same optical plane as the natural iris, and some light scatter is expected. Nonetheless, in patients who wish to avoid surgery, or in whom surgery is otherwise not possible, this may represent an acceptable, even if temporary, option.

Corneal Tattooing

Another, although rarely employed, method is to place permanent pigmentation in the corneal stroma. Corneal tattooing has been practiced for almost 2,000 years, first mentioned by Galen in the second century.[7] With the increasing availability of implantable iris devices, this procedure has narrow indications. It may be useful, for example, in cosmetic rehabilitation of a blind eye, or in patients who cannot have surgery or decline it. An advantage of the tatooing procedure is that it does not close a functional iris defect and may be used in treatment of stray light from iridectomies, obviating the problem of closure of a physiologically necessary ostium, which can occur with direct iris suturing. The technique requires a steep learning curve, and it yields variable results. However, some successes, particularly in improving cosmetic appearance, have been obtained.[8–14] Alio et al[9] have had success using the femtosecond laser to place the tattoo. As with contact lenses, the optical plane of the "correction" is not in the same location as the natural iris. The procedure is not reversible and may cause difficulty in performing other ophthalmic examinations, particularly fundus examination.

Capsular Fibrosis

In some cases of iris defects, the opacification of the residual anterior capsule may provide some degree of occlusion from light.

Some surgeons intentionally leave some cortical material, and do not clear the lens epithelial cells, in the hope that they will provide robust opacification. Although neither predictable nor adequate, in the absence of the availability of other techniques or expertise in their performance, this may be an acceptable form of treatment.

Treatment of Iris Defects: Surgical Approach

Because every iris defect is unique, the surgical approach must be tailored to the specific situation. Primary repair of an iris defect by means of techniques such as iris sphincterotomy, synechialysis, iris suturing, and cerclage may be adequate in some patients and should be considered before an iris prosthetic implant. However, these other forms of repair may be neither possible nor sufficient in eyes with more extensive iris defects. Overly aggressive iris suturing techniques should be avoided with these cases, because the iris tissue is almost universally abnormal and there is a risk of iatrogenic iridodialysis and hemorrhage, as well as of sequential iris atrophy in areas under tension from suturing.

Iris Defect Repair Options

Direct Iris Suture Using a Siepser Knot

The decision making and application of iris repair have been discussed above. Small areas of iris defects can be closed using either direct closure or with a Siepser knot[5] or its variants[6] (see Chapter 27). My preference is to use the direct closure for more peripheral defects, and the Siepser-type closure for more central closures. The latter does not necessitate undue pulling of the iris tissue to the periphery when tying the knot.

Direct closure entails the use of a McCannel-style suture, of 10-0 or 9-0 polypropylene on a long curved or straight needle. From the area of iris defect, the suture is passed through the near clear cornea 2 to 4 mm adjacent to the defect, passed through the iris defect on each side, and then brought out through the near clear cornea on the opposite side. A straight through (i.e., non-beveled) paracentesis is placed overlying the defect, the suture ends looped out through the paracentesis, using a Kuglen hook, and then tied, pulling the iris defect gently toward the cornea. The needle penetration can be accomplished with or without a preceding paracentesis.

The direct closure technique can also be employed in the treatment of TIDs in which the defective iris is imbricated within adjacent areas of healthy iris tissue.[15]

Iris Cerclage/Quadrantic Imbrication

Iris cerclage is performed when reduction in pupil size is desired, and where there is good iris stromal tissue with good pigmentation. The presence of TIDs, or other iris defects, especially in light-colored eyes, results in a good anatomic closure but an unhappy patient, due to persistent translucence of the remaining repaired iris, and therefore it should be avoided in favor of iris prosthetic implant surgery, when possible.

Care should be taken to avoid undue stretching of the iris tissue or tension on the sutures when performing this maneuver. Cerclage is performed by passing sutures through multiple paracenteses, using a 9-0 polypropylene suture on a long curved needle (or a comparable material), weaving the pupillary edge either through multiple individual bites (two or three per quadrant), or with a "baseball stitch" technique in which the suture weaves around the pupil with each stitch. Once passed 360 de-

grees, the suture ends are tied, either by direct closure through a straight-through paracentesis (i.e., not beveled as with traditional paracenteses) within true clear cornea, and as close to the proposed pupil size as possible, or by a Siepser or modified Siepser knot.

Quadrantic imbrication can be accomplished by placing a McCannel/Siepser suture at each quadrant, thus producing a smaller pupil in a square configuration. Four paracenteses are performed. Through each paracentesis, a 9-0 prolene suture on a long needle is passed, grasping the pupillary edge close to the entry point, approximately 1.5mm peripheral to the pupillary edge, then passed across several millimeters, and the iris is re-grasped. The needle is passed through the next paracentesis, and tied using a Siepser, or Siepser-variant technique, thus imbricating the iris. This is repeated for each quadrant, until the appropriate shape and diameter of the pupil is obtained.

Iridodialysis Repair

Small iris root dehiscences, typically less than two clock hour positions, are often asymptomatic and can be left untreated, particularly those in the area normally covered by the upper eyelid.

Repair can be accomplished by a variety of means. My favored repair technique is the make a 2- to 3-mm scleral groove beginning 2.5 mm posterior to the sclera overlying the area of dialysis. Through a paracentesis, the iris grasped with a double armed 9-0 or 10-0 polypropylene suture near its peripheral, dehisced root (some authors advocate using 8-0 Prolene).[16] Then a 25-gauge bent hypodermic needle on a 3-cc or smaller syringe is passed through the scleral groove so that it pierces the sclera at 1.5 to 2 mm posterior to the limbus and passed parallel to the iris plane into the anterior chamber. The suture needle is engaged within the 25-gauge needle, and passed out through the sclera. The second arm of the suture is passed 1 to 2 mm adjacent to this, and the sutures are tied loosely, leaving a small area of gap between the iris root and the internal scleral wall to ensure that the trabecular meshwork is not occluded. Confirmation using a gonioprism or an intraocular endoscope is helpful in cases where the placement of the suture cannot be clearly determined. For larger areas of iridodialysis, this can be repeated as many times as required, leaving some space in between the suture passes, to minimize the number of sutures required and to allow some space peripheral to the dialysis.

In moderate-sized dialyses, imbrication of the adjacent iris tissue may create an adequate closure, although a peripheral—and generally optically innocuous—space may persist.[17]

An alternative technique purposefully creates a visible space—a so-called hang-back technique to minimize the chances of trabecular occlusion.[18] A sutureless technique involves the entrapment of the iris within a sclerotomy.[19]

Iris Prosthetic Implants

The placement of a masking artificial iris implant can potentially reduce glare and improve patients' visual function. Such devices may also mask the optical aberrations prevalent in the peripheral cornea and eliminate visual competition between focused and unfocused images. Newer developments have enabled a nearly perfect cosmetic match between eyes, as well.

For eyes that have iris defects too extensive for primary surgical repair, implantable iris prosthetic devices have been developed that aid the surgeon in compensating for the deformed or imperfectly functioning iris.

Several companies produce these iris prosthetic devices. However, at the time of this writing, none is Food and Drug

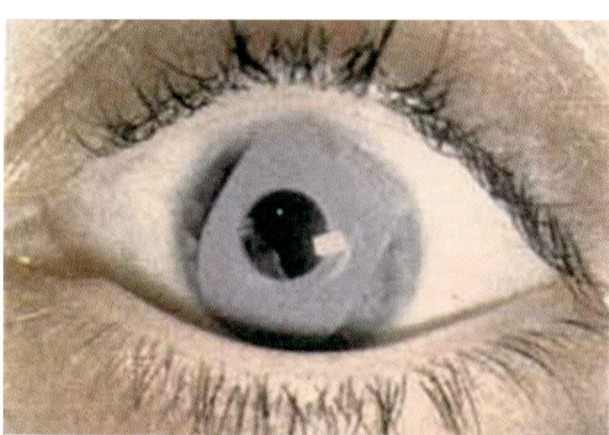

a

b

Fig. 32.8 The first iris implants invented and implanted by D. Peter Choyce failed, presumably because they were of a rigid material and were implanted in the anterior chamber angle. They all developed either corneal decompen- sation or intractable glaucoma. **(a,b)** Choyce iris implant: **(a)** preoperative; **(b)** postoperative.

Administration (FDA). There is one ongoing FDA clinical trial, for the artificial iris of HumanOptics (Erlangen, Germany). A previous FDA clinical trial for an implant manufactured by Ophtec BV (Groningen, the Netherlands), in which I participated, was halted short of FDA approval. These devices, however, are available in most of the rest of the world, and the FDA clinical trials for this device yielded excellent results overall with no reported surgical, postoperative, or optical complications caused by the device, and with no substantial difference in inflammatory response compared with that expected from traditional extracapsular surgery (the device requires an incision larger than 10 mm).

The first iris implants were developed and implanted by D. Peter Choyce[20] as iris/lens combinations, fixated in the anterior chamber angle, as early as the 1960s (**Fig. 32.8a**). However, they universally failed, due to corneal compensation or intractable glaucoma.

In 1991, Sundmacher[21] developed a polymethylmethacrylate (PMMA) IOL surrounded by an opaque black segment that serves as an artificial iris diaphragm for implantation in patients with iris defects. In patients with absent or inadequate capsular support, this lens was effective, although the black optic carrier measures up to 10 mm in diameter (and encompasses varying optic sizes), thus requiring a large incision. It is sutured to the scleral wall, through eyelets on the terminus of each haptic. Thomas Reinhard of Düsseldorf, Germany,[22] has shown that these devices provide good visual rehabilitation, although they have been associated with a greater amount of postoperative inflammation and a higher incidence of postoperative pressure elevation when compared with standard extracapsular surgery. This problem may relate to the disruption of the blood–aqueous barrier, although it should be pointed out that many of these eyes have other serious defects as well. Osher, Burke, and others have demonstrated similarly favorable results.[2,23–25]

Recently, I reported, along with Gentile et al, a technique for placement of this device without direct suture fixation, using a modified silicone oil "retention suture," in conjunction with vitrectomy and placement of silicone oil[26,27] (**Fig. 32.9**). This technique makes it possible to move or remove the iris implant (temporarily or permanently) without cutting sutures.

As with Henry Ford's Model T automobile ("Any customer can have a car painted any color that he wants so long as it is black"), the Sundmacher-designed implant is available in black only and is made of a rather brittle material that can, in some instances, fracture during or after surgical implantation. The brittle nature of the material may be related to a proprietary

alteration to the PMMA that renders the material black. Therefore, it is necessary to implant the devices gently to avoid excessive flexing or torquing, and to have spare devices available in case of breakage. The devices manufactured by Ophtec BV are available in three homogeneous standard colors (**Fig. 32.10**), and are more flexible, deriving their color from a color additive process that does not appear to reduce the elasticity of the device.

In response to the incision size limitation, in 1996, Volker Rasch of Potsdam, Germany, and I invented a series of aniridia and coloboma aperture rings (Morcher GmbH, Stuttgart, Germany), the Rasch-Rosenthal Iris Diaphragm rings, designed to be implanted in an intact capsular bag, with or without zonular instability and with a separately implanted IOL (**Fig. 32.11**).[28–31] Our devices had a 6-mm pseudo-pupil, and were designed to interface with the most popular IOL designs of 6 mm, thus

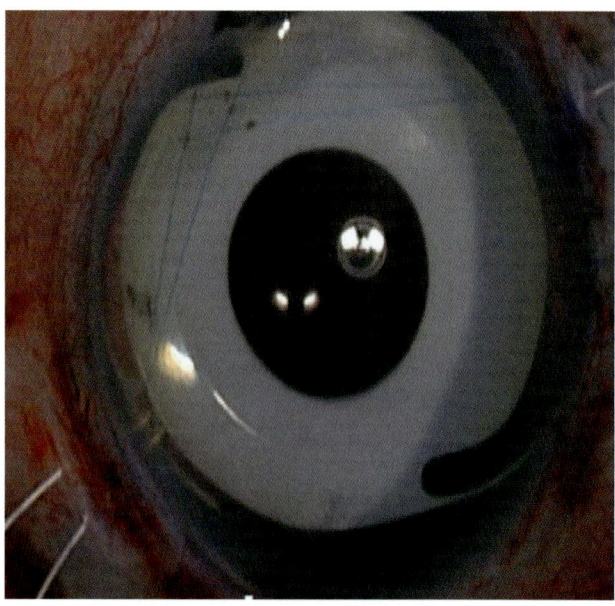

Fig. 32.9 The silicone oil tension suture crisscrosses just behind the iris root plane. In this patient with a fixed dilated pupil after vitrectomy lensectomy, an Ophtec model 311 Iris prosthesis is placed within the web of sutures. This will enable its reposition or temporary removal should further vitreoretinal surgery be required.

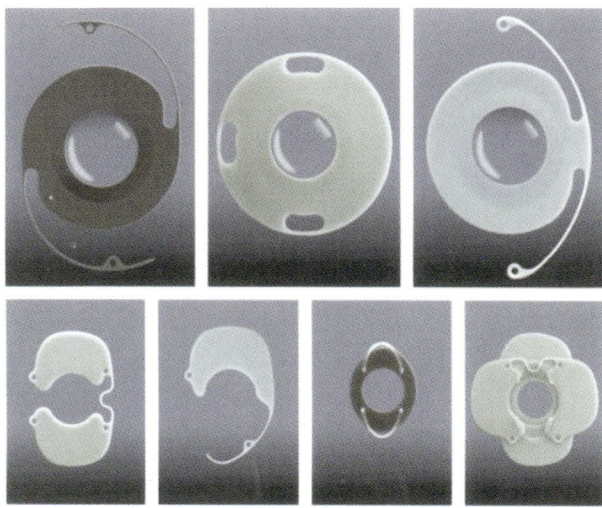

Fig. 32.10 Various models of iris prostheses are available from Ophtec. They can be implanted in the sulcus with suturing, or in the capsular bag, depending on the model.

obliterating the pseudophakic–aphakic junction. I performed the first implantation of this device (and the first iris implant of any kind in the United States) in July 1996 in a patient with Axenfeld-Rieger syndrome (**Fig. 32.11**)[28,29] in conjunction with the introduction of a sutureless phaco-trabeculectomy procedure. Since that time, Masket's group[32] has developed a similar modular iris prosthesis designed with a 4-mm pupil, thought to be more physiological in average lighting conditions.

A similar device, the Iris Prosthetic System), is manufactured by Ophtec BV but not currently available in the United States (**Fig. 32.12**).

Because these devices incorporate the properties of a capsular tension ring, they can be used to treat partial capsular instability and iris defects. Michael Snyder of Cincinnati, Ohio, had suggested that I use a 6.5-mm IOL so that an overlap between the optic and haptic occurs, thereby reducing the potential for optical problems related to the IOL's edge.

The Ophtec device is inserted similarly and in conjunction with a capsular tension ring, but it is more flexible and less prone to breakage. Both Morcher and Ophtec also produce customized devices that cover only a sector of absent iris. These implants are suitable for the management of coloboma or partial defects such

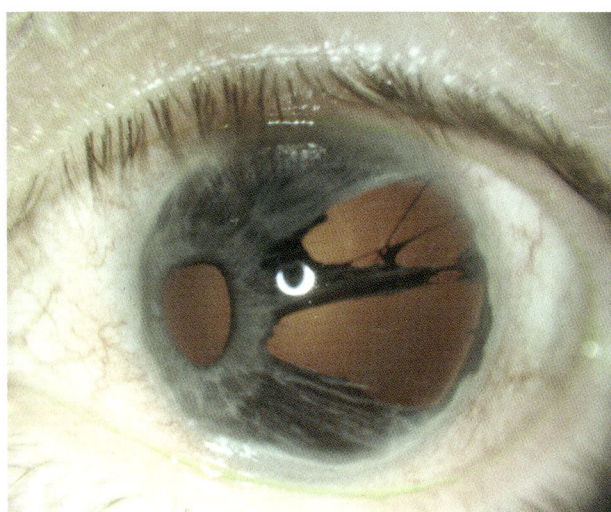

a

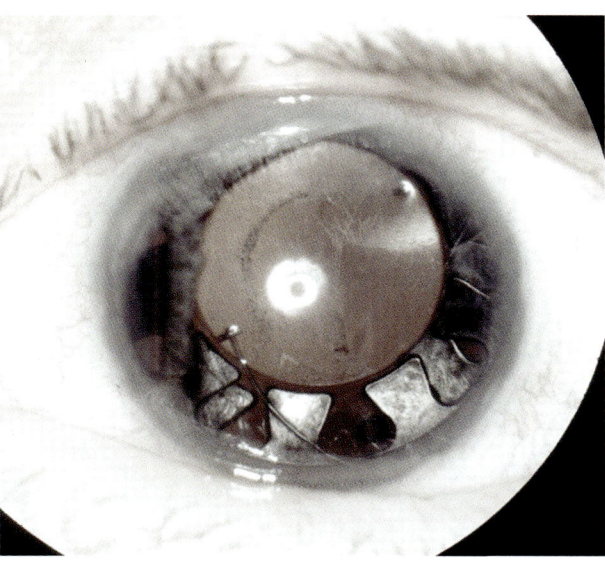

b

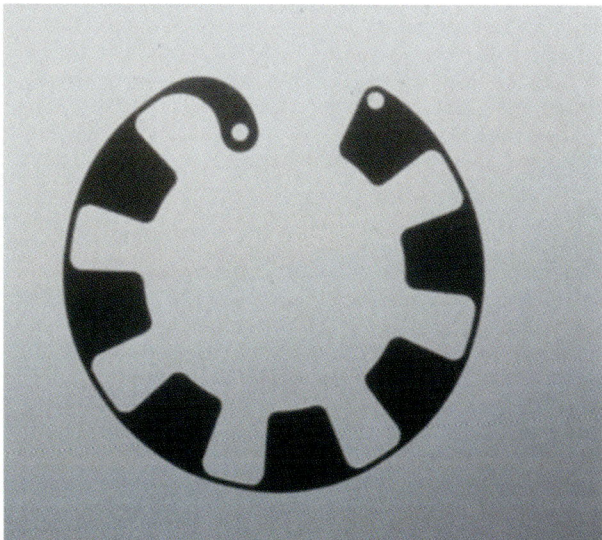

c

Fig. 32.11 The Rasch-Rosenthal iris diaphragm ring, the first small incision iris device, is implanted within the capsular bag in pairs, and dialed so that the fins interspace, forming a continuous pseudo-pupil, obliterating the pseudo-phakic/phakic. **(a,b)** Axenfeld-Rieger syndrome: **(a)** preoperative; **(b)** postoperative. **(c)** Morcher Rasch-Rosenthal iris ring.

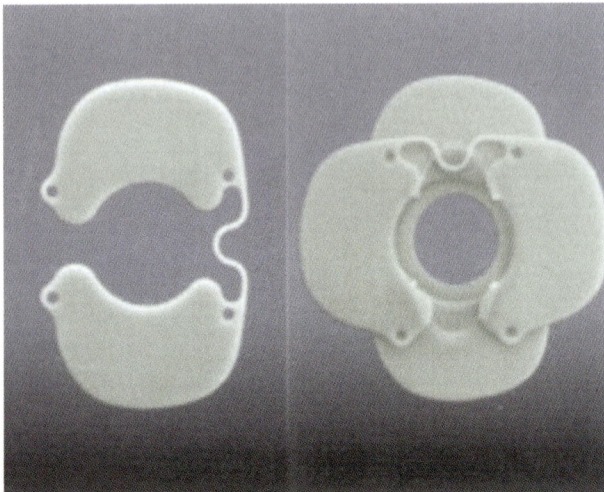

Fig. 32.12 The Ophtec Iris Prosthetic System is designed for in-the-bag implantation through a small incision.

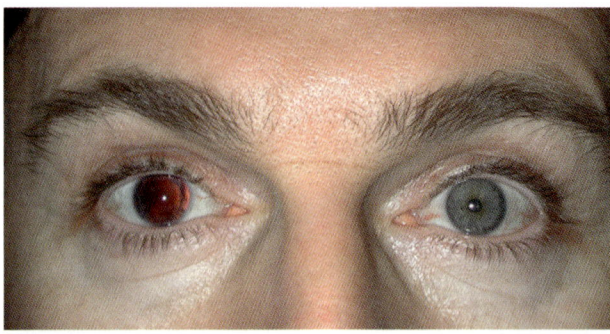

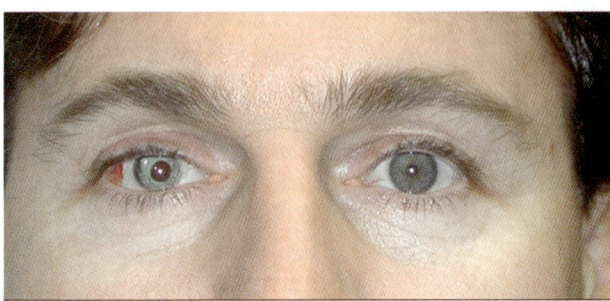

Fig. 32.13 The Ophtec model 311 is inserted: **(a)** preoperative; **(b)** postoperative.

as those seen in iris and ciliary body coloboma or in trauma (**Fig. 32.13**).

CustomFlex Artificial Iris (HumanOptics)

The CustomFlex Artificial Iris (HumanOptics AG)[29,33,34] was invented by Hans-Reinhard Koch (Bonn, Germany), and is currently being evaluated under an FDA monitor clinical trial (ClinicalTrials.gov identifier NCT01860612). It is composed of a flexible silicone disk with a 3.5-mm central pseudo-pupil aperture (**Fig. 32.14**). It is hand painted with silicone paint by matching the color texture and pattern to the properties of the fellow eye or, in cases of congenital aniridia, to those characteristics in a subject of the patient's choosing. The devices can be implanted within the capsular bag, or placed in the sulcus, with or without suture fixation. A fiber-mesh backing is available optionally to produce further structure for suture fixation (**Fig. 32.15**). The device can be trephined to the correct size, and cut so as to use a partial amount of the device. The device is flexible and can be inserted through an incision as small as 2.4 mm, through the use of an injector cartridge, making this a minimally invasive procedure, with respect to the incision, of particular importance in patients with congenital aniridia who frequently have stem cell deficiency and for whom the rigid models of iris implants were more risky. I have found that the AMO Silver Unfolder (Abbott Medical Optics) along with a cohesive viscoelastic produces the best results in insertion of the device.

Complications

Many patients, if not most, who suffer from iris abnormalities have significant comorbidities. The congenital aniridic patient, for example, frequently has concomitant limbal stem cell deficiency with its attendant corneal vascularization and pannus, as well as foveolar hypoplasia and nystagmus. Nonetheless, implantation of the iris prosthesis in such patients frequently yields better than anticipated results, presumably because the presence of the new iris causes an improvement in visual quality and enables the patient's neuroadaptive processes to progress. Be-

cause the device can be inserted through a 2.5-mm subincision, in contrast to this device's predecessors, there is minimal impact on the already deficient stem cell population in these patients (**Fig. 32.16**). However, progression of corneal vascularization and pannus can still occur. When the HumanOptics device is placed in the capsular bag, it may eventually "pea-pod" out of the bag due to capsular phimosis. We reported such a case, which stabilized and did not affect the outcome[35] (**Fig. 32.17**). In other instances, repositioning of the device was necessary.

Patients with traumatic iris defects frequently have multiple concomitant comorbidities, such as glaucoma, corneal damage, retinal detachment, and pre-retinal fibrosis. Although the iris prosthetic device is well tolerated in most of these patients, their results may be blunted by these comorbid problems.

Shifting or dislocation of the device may occur, but can almost always be repaired.

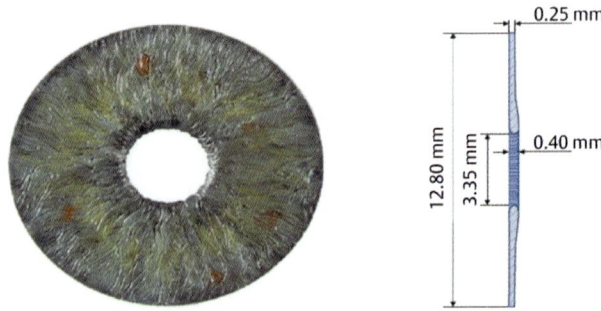

Fig. 32.14 The HumanOptics CustomFlex artificial iris is a handcrafted device on a silicone base using silicone paint, copying a photograph so that it matches either the fellow eye or an eye subject of the patient's choosing. The artisan takes into account the effect of the corneal magnification, and replicates the unique coloration and contour of the supplied photograph.

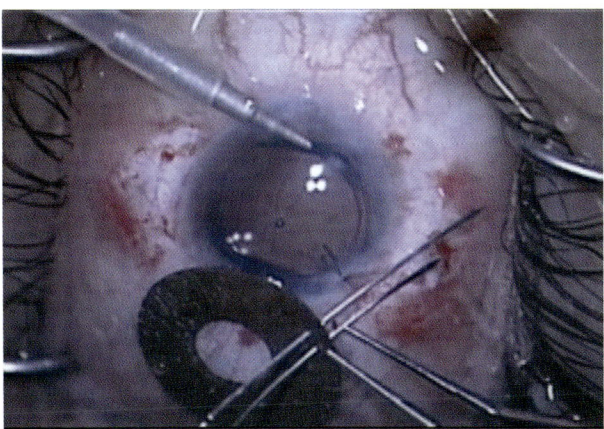

Fig. 32.15 This patient had sequelae of congenital rubella with microphthalmia, glaucoma, and hypoplastic iris. An IOL and iris prosthesis were sutured in place. The photograph shows a double-armed polypropylene suture placed through the substance of the device, which will then be fixated to the sclera. This device was produced with a fiber backing, to add support to the suture fixation.

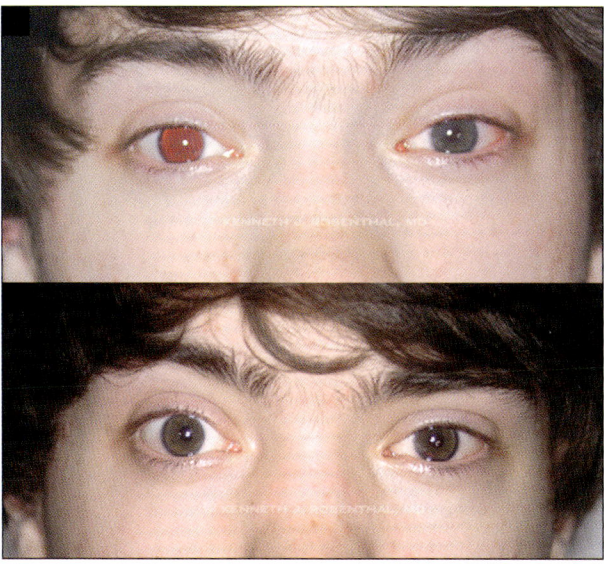

Fig. 32.16 A 17-year-old congenital aniridic, with foveolar hypoplasia, after implantation of the first eye and then fellow eye with the HumanOptics CustomFlex iris prostheses. **(a)** Preoperative: the best corrected visual acuity (BCVA) was 20/100 OU with nystagmus. **(b)** Postoperative: nystagmus is virtually absent and the BCVA is 20/30.

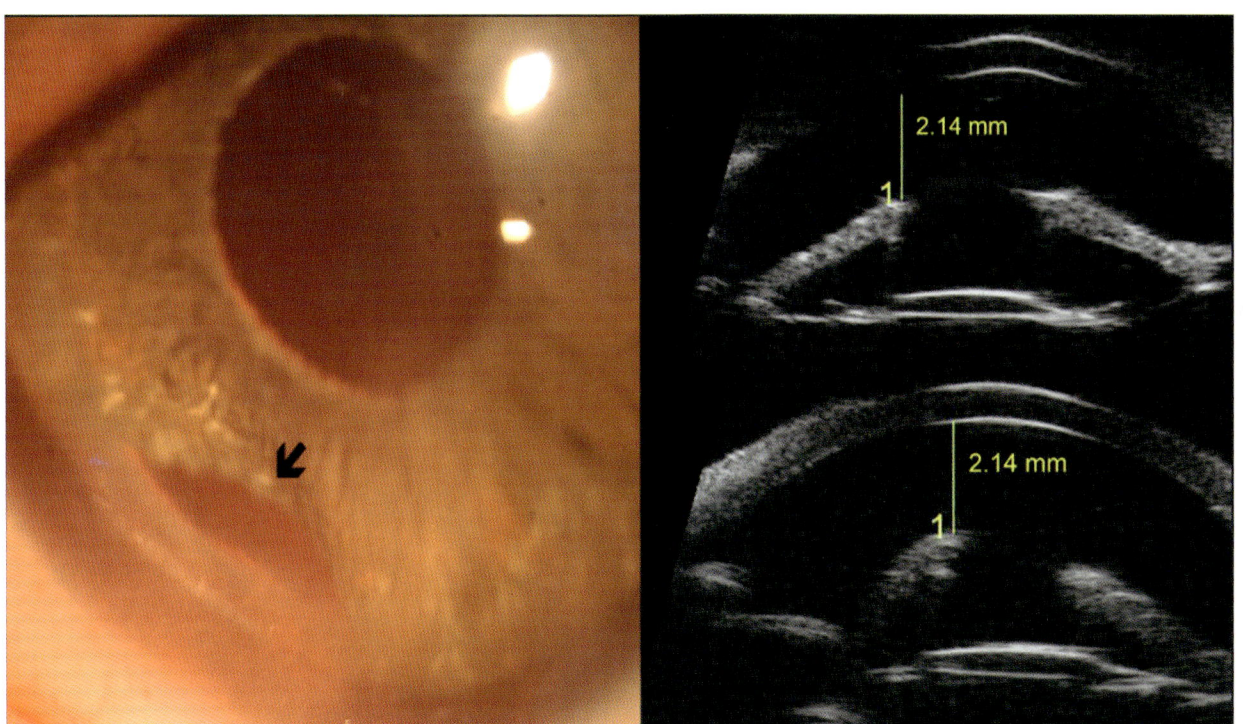

Fig. 32.17 Photograph and ultrasound biomicroscopy showing partial anterior displacement and buckling of the HumanOptics CustomFlex artificial iris. **(a)** No progression of vaulting has been noted over a three-year period. The anteior chamber depth, measured from the periphery of the pupil from the apex of the vaulted device to the corneal endothelium, is 3.29 mm. **(b)** Ultrasound biomicroscopy scan taken of the initial eye at 12 months postoperatively. Measurement of the anterior chamber depth from the periphery of the pupil at the apex of the vaulted HumanOptics CustomFlex artificial iris to the corneal endothelium was 2.23 mm and had not progressed, but rather improved, by the time of the clinical evaluation. Some investigators believe that implantation of a capsular tension ring at the time of the primary surgery may deter this problem.

The NuIris/BrightOcular Cosmetic Iris Implant

This device, made of silicone and fixated in the anterior chamber angle, has been used primarily to change eye color, although it has been used for functional iris repair as well. Although there are insufficient data as to the prevalence of complications with this device, my center and others have reported devastating ocular complications, in particular iris depigmentation, pigmentary glaucoma, end-stage and advanced glaucomatous cupping, and corneal decompensation in these individuals.[36] In some cases, explantation of the device was helpful in preventing further advancement of the disease. These devices, although not available in the United States, have been implanted extensively around the world, including a concentration of cases in the Middle East, and some American patients have traveled abroad for this surgery.

Conclusion

Iris abnormalities remain daunting obstacles to surgical success both during and after cataract surgery. Knowledge and proficiency in assessment of iris defects and their impact on the patient, and evaluation of various techniques and devices to repair these problems represent a significant step toward improving surgical outcomes.

References

1. Gayton JL. Traumatic aniridia during endoscopic laser cycloablation. J Cataract Refract Surg 1998;24:134–135

2. Karatza EC, Burk SE, Snyder ME, Osher RH. Outcomes of prosthetic iris implantation in patients with albinism. J Cataract Refract Surg 2007;33:1763–1769

3. Wintle R, Austin M. Pigment dispersion with elevated intraocular pressure after AcrySof intraocular lens implantation in the ciliary sulcus. J Cataract Refract Surg 2001;27:642–644

4. Rosenthal K, Venkateswaran N. Transillumination defects following in-the-bag single-piece intraocular lens implantation and trabeculectomy with mini-shunt. J Cataract Refract Surg 2013;39:139–141

5. Siepser SB; SB. The closed chamber slipping suture technique for iris repair. Ann Ophthalmol 1994;26:71–72

6. Schoenberg ED, Price FW Jr. Modification of Siepser sliding suture technique for iris repair and endothelial keratoplasty. J Cataract Refract Surg 2014;40:705–708

7. Pitz S, Jahn R, Frisch L, Duis A, Pfeiffer N. Corneal tattooing: an alternative treatment for disfiguring corneal scars. Br J Ophthalmol 2002;86:397–399

8. Craiu AM. [Corneal tatoo—art or science?]. Oftalmologia 2009;53:97–103

9. Alio JL, Rodriguez AE, Toffaha BT. Keratopigmentation (corneal tattooing) for the management of visual disabilities of the eye related to iris defects. Br J Ophthalmol 2011;95:1397–1401

10. Amesty MA, Alio JL, Rodriguez AE. Corneal tolerance to micronised mineral pigments for keratopigmentation. Br J Ophthalmol 2014;98:1756–1760

11. Galvis V, Tello A. Keratopigmentation: techniques and results. Br J Ophthalmol 2012;96:1270, author reply 1270–1271

12. Mannis MJ, Eghbali K, Schwab IR. Keratopigmentation: a review of corneal tattooing. Cornea 1999;18:633–637

13. Ricardo JR, Medhi J, Pineda R. Femtosecond laser-assisted keratopigmentation for the management of visual disabilities due to peripheral iridectomies. J Glaucoma 2015;24:e22–e24

14. Sirerol B, Walewska-Szafran A, Alio JL, Klonowski P, Rodriguez AE. Tolerance and biocompatibility of micronized black pigment for keratopigmentation simulated pupil reconstruction. Cornea 2011;30:344–350

15. Snyder ME, Perez MA. Iris stromal imbrication oversewing for pigment epithelial defects. Br J Ophthalmol 2015;99:5–6

16. Dağlioğlu MC, Coşkun M, Ilhan N, et al. Repair of iridodialysis using 8-0 polypropylene. Semin Ophthalmol 2014;29:159–162

17. Tsao SW, Holz HA. Iris mattress suture: a technique for sectoral iris defect repair. Br J Ophthalmol 2015;99:305–307

18. Snyder ME, Lindsell LB. Nonappositional repair of iridodialysis. J Cataract Refract Surg 2011;37:625–628

19. Richards JC, Kennedy CJ. Sutureless technique for repair of traumatic iridodialysis. Ophthalmic Surg Lasers Imaging 2006;37:508–510

20. Choyce DP. Intra-Ocular Lenses and Implants. London: H.K. Lewis; 1964:21

21. Sundmacher R, Reinhard, T, Althaus C. Black diaphragm intraocular lens in congenital aniridia. Ger J Ophthalmol 1994;3:197–220

22. Reinhard T, Engelhardt S, Sundmacher R. Black diaphragm aniridia intraocular lens for congenital aniridia: long-term follow-up. J Cataract Refract Surg 2000;26(3):375–381;

23. Burk SE, Da Mata AP, Snyder ME, Cionni RJ, Cohen JS, Osher RH. Prosthetic iris implantation for congenital, traumatic, or functional iris deficiencies. J Cataract Refract Surg 2001;27:1732–1740

24. Ozturk F, Osher RH, Osher JM. Secondary prosthetic iris implantation following traumatic total aniridia and pseudophakia. J Cataract Refract Surg 2006;32:1968–1970

25. Osher RH, Burk SE. Cataract surgery combined with implantation of an artificial iris. [In Process Citation] J Cataract Refract Surg 1999;25:1540–1547

26. Gentile R, Eliott D. Silicone oil retention sutures in aphakic eyes with iris loss. Arch Ophthalmol 2010;128:1596–1599

27. De Grande V, Rosenthal K, Reibaldi M, Gentile RC. Artificial iris-intraocular lens implantation for traumatic aniridia and aphakia assisted by silicone oil retention sutures. J Cataract Refract Surg 2012;38:2045–2048

28. Rosenthal KJ. Sutureless phacotrabeculectomy and insertion of an iris diaphragm ring in a patient with the Axenfeld-Rieger Syndrome: first reported case. Video Journal of Cataract and Refractive Surgery 1997;13

29. Rosenthal KJ. Artificial iris implants: update. Paper presented at the American Academy of Ophthalmology Annual Meeting, Anaheim, CA, November 17, 2003

30. Rosenthal K. Sutureless phacotrabeculectomy and insertion of an iris diaphragm ring in a patient with the Axenfeld-Rieger Syndrome: first reported case. Presented at the Welsh Cataract Congress, Houston, September 1996

31. Rosenthal KJ, (Osher R., ed.) The modular iris implant. Video J Viscosurg Pharmacia. 2002–2003;10

32. Olson M, Masket S, Miller K. Interim results of a compassionate-use clinical trial of Morcher iris diaphragm implantation: report 1. J Cataract Refract 2008;34:1674–1680

33. Spitzer MS, Yoeruek E, Leitritz MA, Szurman P, Bartz-Schmidt KU. A new technique for treating posttraumatic aniridia with aphakia: first results of haptic fixation of a foldable intraocular lens on a foldable and custom-tailored iris prosthesis. Arch Ophthalmol 2012;130:771–775

34. Ayliffe W, Groth SL, Sponsel WE. Small-incision insertion of artificial iris prostheses. J Cataract Refract Surg 2012;38:362–367

35. Rosenthal KJ, Venkateswaran N. Clinical and ultrasound biomicroscopic findings in a patient with anterior vaulting of a customized, flexible artificial iris. J Refract Surg 2013;29:663–664

36. Kao ARK. Surgical technique for removal of iris implants. Presented at the American Society of Cataract and Refractive Surgery, San Diego, April 2015

XII Ophthalmic Viscosurgical Devices

33 Using Ophthalmic Viscosurgical Devices to Manage Problems in Cataract Surgery

Steve A. Arshinoff and Thomas A. Berk

The developments and innovations that have occurred in the world of viscosurgery over the past 30 years have greatly enhanced our abilities and reduced our complication rates in cataract surgery. The use of ophthalmic viscosurgical devices (OVDs) in cataract surgery was first described by Balazs, Miller, and Stegmann[1] in 1979, forever revolutionizing anterior-segment surgery. Up until that point, corneal endothelial damage had been an inevitable consequence of intraocular surgery, but the unique space-creating abilities of OVDs made protection of the endothelium possible while simultaneously facilitating intraocular lens (IOL) implantation. OVDs now represent an indispensable part of even routine cataract surgery, but the diverse range of currently available OVDs and their varying chemical and physical (rheological) properties afford the skilled and knowledgeable cataract surgeon an unprecedented level of adaptability to manage virtually any intraoperative complication that may arise, as well as the ability to design techniques to facilitate management of cases previously viewed as difficult and entailing high risk.

This chapter discusses OVDs and their use in cataract surgery, with special emphasis on techniques for managing difficult cases and intraoperative complications. The chapter classifies and groups OVDs according to their rheological properties, relating each group to intraoperative strengths and weaknesses, and discusses the "soft-shell" techniques, focusing on their adaptability to different intraocular surgical situations.

The optimal use of OVDs in intraocular surgery will enhance every procedure, but there is no single preferred or universally used OVD. Understanding the rheological basis of classification of OVDs, the strengths and weakness of different groups, and how they may be combined in the most efficacious manner can provide the surgeon with an infinitely adaptable viscosurgical armamentarium.

Classification of Ophthalmic Viscosurgical Devices

Background

A viscoelastic preparation intended for intraocular use must chemically be aqueous based, isotonic, and pH balanced. The range of physical properties is governed by the molecular nature, chain length, and concentration of the rheologically active polymer constituent(s). To devise surgically useful classification criteria, the rheological parameters that best apply to OVDs in relation to their function in surgery must be identified. Currently, the two most useful laboratory-measurable OVD parameters for such a classification are (1) zero-shear viscosity (V_0), and (2) the cohesion-dispersion index (CDI).

V_0 is defined as the viscosity of the OVD at rest, or more specifically, when a shear stress equaling zero is applied to it (no turbulence). It is read off the extreme left axis of pseudoplasticity curves where shear rate is 10^{-3}, which is as near zero as is generally measured (**Fig. 33.1**). In the context of intraocular surgery, this would occur when neither phacoemulsification (phaco) nor irrigation and aspiration (I/A) are being performed. An OVD's V_0 correlates positively with both the molecular weight and concentration of its rheologically active viscoelastic component(s).

The other clinically important laboratory OVD parameter, CDI, is an objective, quantitative measure of its cohesive-dispersive behavior (physical opposites) under vacuum aspiration analogous to our use of OVDs in surgery (**Fig. 33.2**). Cohesive OVDs tend to aspirate in a bolus, as the molecules tend to entangle, are supple enough to flow around obstacles, and cohere sufficiently to avoid fragmentation when exposed to the usual vacuum aspiration forces in phaco. Dispersive OVDs tend to fragment under even mild aspiration force, and consequently a lesser volume of OVD is aspirated per unit of time when exposed to the same vacuum level compared to a cohesive OVD.

Taken together, these two parameters, V_0 and CDI, can be used to establish a classification of OVDs (**Fig. 33.3**). Long-chain ophthalmic viscoelastic molecules tend to entangle in solution, causing them to aggregate. The OVDs containing the longest chains of hyaluronic acid are therefore referred to as "higher-viscosity cohesive" and they have higher V_0 and usually higher CDI values as well. As V_0 declines below 100,000 millipascal-seconds (mPas), molecular chain entanglement becomes a far less significant factor. Consequently, these lower viscosity OVDs generally tend to be easily broken up and have lower CDI values, and are accordingly referred to as "lower-viscosity dispersives."

In the vast majority of currently marketed OVDs, the CDI correlates with the V_0 (but not in a simple linear relationship), as well as with the molecular weight and concentration of the rheologically active constituent(s) (which is hyaluronic acid in the vast majority of OVDs); thus, the degree of cohesion generally falls neatly into a classification based on only V_0. DisCoVisc (Alcon, Fort Worth, TX), however, was specifically designed with viscosity and cohesion somewhat dissociated from each other, thus giving it the V_0 of Healon (Abbott Medical Optics [AMO], Abbott Park, IL), that is, viscous-cohesive, but a CDI close to that of Viscoat (Alcon), that is, lower viscosity dispersive. Thus, the classification of OVDs had to be expanded from one- to two-dimensional in 2005, and it has been updated since.[2]

The surgical tasks for which OVDs are utilized are generally facilitated more by higher V_0. Highly viscous OVDs tend to be more cohesive (less dispersive). However, in certain situations, dispersion rather than cohesion may be desirable (e.g., to retain a thick protective layer of OVD adjacent to the corneal endothelium

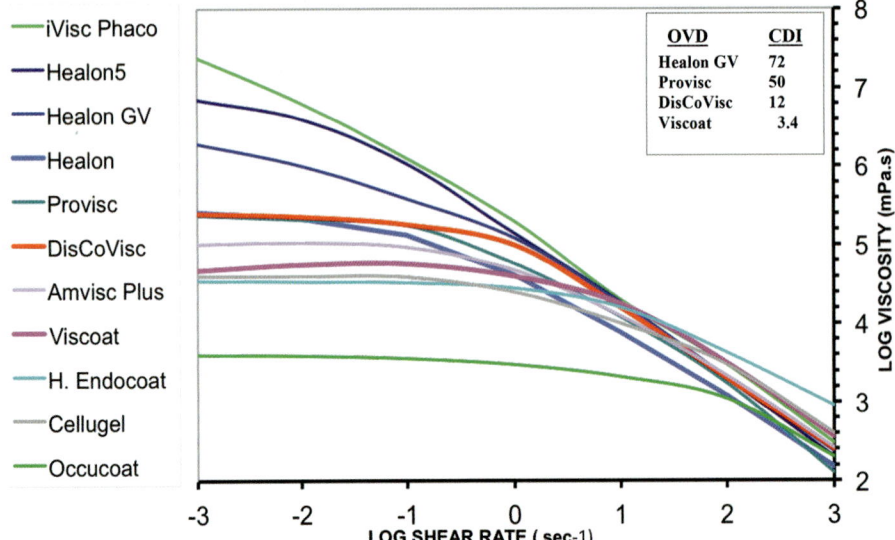

Fig. 33.1 Pseudoplasticity curves and representative cohesion-dispersion indexes (CDIs) of ophthalmic viscosurgical devices (OVDs). Graphs of log viscosity versus log shear rate are plotted for common ophthalmic viscosurgical devices sold by Alcon, Abbott Medical Optics, Bausch and Lomb, and iMed Pharma. All OVDs useful for ophthalmic surgery are pseudoplastic, which means that they exhibit low viscosity when exposed to high shear stress (right side of curve). Viscosity increases going toward the left as shear stress on the molecule decreases. iVisc phaco *(top curve)* is almost plastic in

that the graph does not level off much on the left side of the graph. The continuously rising graph indicates that iVisc phaco will have the physical properties of a solid at zero shear. All of the other OVDs exhibit flattening of their curves to the left, indicating that there is a limit to how high their viscosities become, even at low shear, thus making them pseudoplastic. The *box inset* lists the cohesion-dispersion indices of four different OVDs with the lower numbers indicating dispersive behavior, and higher numbers cohesive behavior.

to protect it from the turbulence of phaco or I/A). Consideration of this issue and the nature of the steps involved in phacoemulsification soon make it apparent that soft shell techniques (SSTs) are preferable for almost all tasks in cataract surgery, as SSTs were designed to combine the best attributes of both cohesive and dispersive OVDs, while simultaneously overcoming the drawbacks of each in different surgical situations.[3,4] SSTs have been updated to tri-soft shell techniques, permitting almost endless possibilities of partition of the anterior chamber (AC) during surgery with selective protection of chosen areas of the AC.[5] The following subsections discuss each class of OVD and highlight its strengths and weaknesses.

Higher Viscosity-Cohesive OVDs

All current OVDs in this category possess, as their active rheological agent, various concentrations and chain lengths of non–cross-linked long-chain hyaluronic acid. In addition all have zero-shear dynamic viscosities greater than 100,000 mPas. Superviscous-cohesive OVDs, a subcategory including MicroVisc Plus (Bohus BioTech, Strömstad, Sweden; iVisc Plus in Canada) and Healon GV, have zero-shear viscosities exceeding 1,000,000 mPas. Viscous-cohesive OVDs including MicroVisc (iVisc in Canada), ProVisc (Alcon), Healon, Eye Fill, Amvisc (Bausch and Lomb, Rochester, NY), Opegan Hi, Ophthalin (Hyaltech, Zeiss, Edinburgh), and others, possess zero-shear viscosities between 100,000 and 1,000,000 mPas (1 log unit less that the superviscous cohesive OVDs). Clinical trials have shown that the members of each of these subcategories share similar physical properties and behave in a similar fashion intraoperatively. However, the superviscous-cohesives appear to have an advantage over the regular viscous-cohesives in facilitating surgical maneuvers, ease of removal, and endothelial protection.

V_0 correlates well with elasticity. Highly viscous-cohesive OVDs are excellent at creating space with their viscosity, and preserving it with their elasticity. Elasticity enables the OVD to

contract and expand in the presence of the ocular pulse or externally applied force, without being expelled from the eye. These OVDs can displace and stabilize tissues in the surgical environment. Stable intraoperative intraocular pressure (i.e., the maintenance of a deep pressurized AC despite the presence of the cataract incision) is best accomplished with an elastic and viscous OVD. Only the highly viscous-cohesive and elastic OVDs are capable of neutralizing posterior positive pressure, thereby permitting "pressure-equalized cataract surgery" (below).

Areas of Strength

The higher viscosity-cohesive OVDs are best used to create space and stability where it is otherwise inadequate. A practical example of this can be recognized when surgery is performed using topical anesthesia, when the nonparalyzed extraocular muscular tone can cause shallowing of the AC. In this setting, a successful continuous curvilinear capsulorrhexis can be facilitated by using a highly viscous-cohesive OVD to pressurize the AC equal to that of the posterior pressure, thus flattening the anterior convexity of the anterior lens capsule. This neutralizes the centrifugal vector of the force generated by internal (or transmitted posterior) pressure on the anteriorly convex surface of a spheroid (the lens), encouraging the capsulorrhexis to tear toward the equator, and permits the creation of a round capsulorrhexis of the desired size and shape in the now pressure-equalized environment. A corollary of this principle pertains to the management of a rhexis that has already begun to tear toward the periphery. After injection of a superviscous-cohesive OVD into the AC (anywhere in the AC that is most convenient) to increase the pressure in the AC, thereby flattening the anterior capsule, external sources of excessive posterior pressure such as a tight lid speculum or drapes should be alleviated, and the capsulorrhexis can be rescued by gently pulling the flap centrally when it is folded over to create a shearing force at the point of tearing (**Fig. 33.4**).

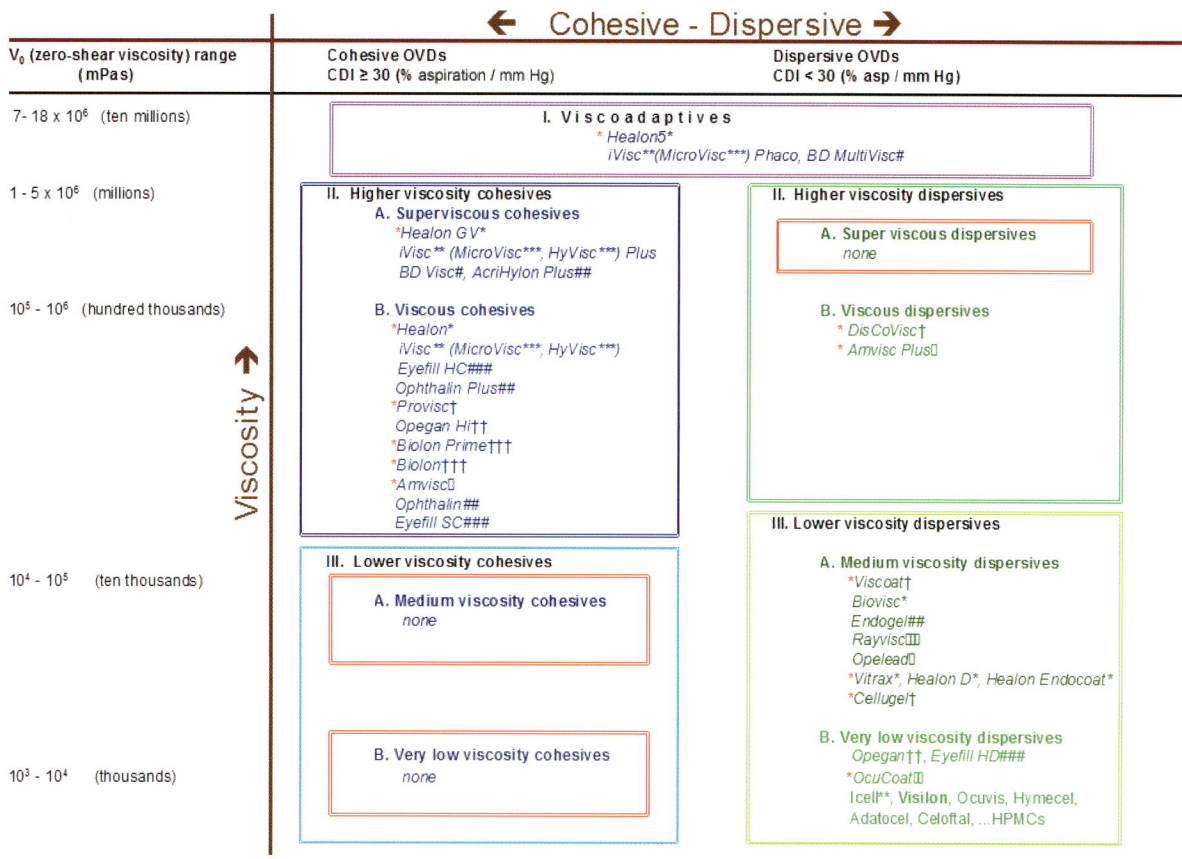

← Cohesive - Dispersive →

V₀ (zero-shear viscosity) range (mPas)	Cohesive OVDs CDI ≥ 30 (% aspiration / mm Hg)	Dispersive OVDs CDI < 30 (% asp / mm Hg)
7- 18 x 10⁶ (ten millions)	**I. Viscoadaptives** *Healon5* iVisc**(MicroVisc***) Phaco, BD MultiVisc#	
1 - 5 x 10⁶ (millions)	**II. Higher viscosity cohesives** A. Superviscous cohesives *Healon GV* iVisc** (MicroVisc***, HyVisc***) Plus BD Visc#, AcriHylon Plus##	**II. Higher viscosity dispersives** A. Super viscous dispersives none
10⁵ - 10⁶ (hundred thousands)	B. Viscous cohesives *Healon* iVisc** (MicroVisc***, HyVisc***) Eyefill HC### Ophthalin Plus## *Provisc† Opegan Hi†† *Biolon Prime††† *Biolon††† *Amvisc▯ Ophthalin## Eyefill SC###	B. Viscous dispersives *DisCoVisc† *Amvisc Plus▯
10⁴ - 10⁵ (ten thousands)	**III. Lower viscosity cohesives** A. Medium viscosity cohesives none	**III. Lower viscosity dispersives** A. Medium viscosity dispersives *Viscoat† Biovisc* Endogel## Rayvisc▯▯ Opelead▯ *Vitrax*, Healon D*, Healon Endocoat* *Cellugel†
10³ - 10⁴ (thousands)	B. Very low viscosity cohesives none	B. Very low viscosity dispersives Opegan††, Eyefill HD### *OcuCoat▯▯ Icell**, Visilon, Ocuvis, Hymecel, Adatocel, Celoftal, ...HPMCs

Viscosity ↑

Legend: * Abbott Medical Optics, ** iMed Pharma, *** Bohus Biotech, # Bectin Dickinson, ## Carl Zeiss Meditech, ### Croma Pharma, † Alcon laboratories, ▯▯Bausch & Lomb
††† Biotechnology Technology General, ▯▯▯Rayner, ▯Shisheido Co., †† Seikagaku Corporation - Santen, HPMC = hydroxypropylmethylcellulose, *Available in USA

Fig. 33.2 New classification of OVDs, 2005, modified and updated to 2015. The advent of DisCoVisc, the first OVD that claimed to be viscous-dispersive, required that the presumed correlation between zero-shear viscosity and cohesion-dispersion behavior of OVDs be abandoned, and the classification of OVDs be changed from a one- to a two-dimensional table, because viscosity and cohesion may behave reasonably independently. For rheologists, the most interesting parts of the table are the red boxes where we have no OVDs available. This encourages consideration of how OVDs with behavior of those descriptions could be helpful in surgery. If the thinking is productive, designing can begin. (Modified from Arshinoff SA, Jafari M. A new classification of ophthalmic viscosurgical devices (OVDs). J Cataract Refract Surg. 2005;31:2167–2171.)

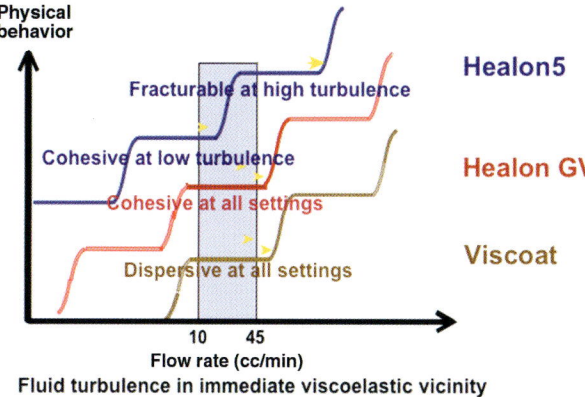

Physical behavior

Fracturable at high turbulence

Cohesive at low turbulence

Cohesive at all settings

Dispersive at all settings

Healon5

Healon GV

Viscoat

10   45
Flow rate (cc/min)
Fluid turbulence in immediate viscoelastic vicinity

Fig. 33.3 Viscoadaptive behavior of Healon5 to turbulence. Healon GV displays cohesive behavior throughout the range of aspiration flow settings (and therefore induced turbulence) commonly used in phacoemulsification surgery. Similarly, Viscoat displays dispersive behavior across this normal range of fluid turbulence encountered in phacoemulsification surgery. These two products are therefore appropriately classified as cohesive and dispersive, respectively. Healon5 was designed to have the unique property of becoming a fracturable solid at flow rates above 25 cc/mm, and therefore exhibiting typical viscous cohesive behavior at settings below 25 cc/min, and fracturable "pseudo-dispersive" behavior at flow rates above 25 cc/min. Healon5 is therefore appropriately referred to as viscoadaptive, because its rheological behavior adapts as the flow rate is increased above 25 cc/min for some parts of the phaco procedure (e.g., phacoemulsification of the lens and viscoelastic removal). It follows that to keep Healon5 in the eye during phaco, all that has to be done is to lower the flow rate to ~20 cc/min or lower.

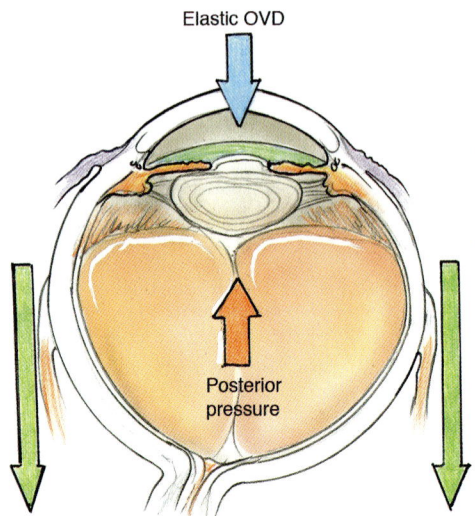

Elastic OVD

Posterior
pressure

- There is constant posterior pressure.
  -Topical or intracameral anesthesia.
  -Extraocular muscle pull.

- Anterior capsule is convex anteriorly.
  -It will always want to tear peripherally.

- Only an elastic OVD can neutralize the
  posterior pressure (HMW NaHa).

- Important for: capsulorrhexis
                  IOL implantation

Fig. 33.4 Pressure equalized cataract surgery. The concept of pressure-equalized cataract surgery is used to prevent anterior capsulorrhexis tear-outs when performing surgery on white hypermature cataracts. There is always posterior pressure due to the tension of the extraocular muscles. This is transmitted through the posterior structures of the eye to the lens, which has a convex-anterior curvature, much like a balloon. If the posterior pressure is not exceeded with anterior pressure, the tear will tend to go outward toward the equator. The use of a highly viscoelastic and cohesive OVD permits the anterior pressure on the anterior capsule to be increased until it exceeds the posterior pressure, which is noticed by the surgeon as central flattening or even concavity of the anterior capsule. Once this is done, the capsulorrhexis can be completed without centrifugal vector forces favoring extension. It will actually want to tear inward.

Other uses of higher viscosity cohesive OVDs include expanding a shallow AC in hyperopic patients, facilitating the insertion of the phaco tip where positive posterior pressure or a flaccid iris is present, stabilizing a floppy iris, enlarging a small pupil, dissecting posterior synechiae, and assisting during foldable IOL implantation by preventing the incoming lens haptic from snaring a fold in the posterior capsule and thereby tearing it.

Areas of Weakness

The high cohesion of viscous-cohesive and superviscous-cohesive OVDs results in their easy removal as a bolus by I/A at the end of the surgical procedure. However, this same desirable cohesive behavior results in these OVDs being relatively rapidly aspirated out of the AC compared to dispersive OVDs during the turbulence caused by phacoemulsification or I/A. Although an invisible, thin layer of hyaluronan bound to endothelial cell membrane specific binding sites remains behind, this may not be sufficient to protect the corneal endothelium in all cases.[6] In a similar vein, this cohesive bolus-like behavior during aspiration makes these OVDs unable to partition the AC into two adjacent fluid spaces: one zone to remain stable and to protect, and the other where the surgeon can evacuate the OVD and work in with active flow. It is impossible to use a cohesive OVD to protect and sequester a structure by coating it with OVD (e.g., protruding vitreous, frayed iris, etc.) in the AC and simultaneously work with the phaco or I/A tip in an adjacent area; the OVD and the structure that it is supposed to be protecting will be aspirated in a bolus together by the instrument.

Lower Viscosity-Dispersive OVDs

Lower viscosity-dispersives include all current OVDs with V_0 values below 100,000 mPas. Molecular chain entanglement is less prevalent in these OVDs, and so cohesion tends to be significantly weaker, resulting in dispersive behavior when exposed to the turbulence of intraocular surgery (the extreme of dispersive behavior in an aqueous solution is a grain of salt dissolving in the water). Two subgroups make up this OVD class. The first is the medium-viscosity dispersives, possessing V_0 values between 10,000 and 100,000 mPas (1 log unit less than regular viscous cohesives). They include Viscoat (Alcon), Cellugel (Alcon), Rayvisc (Rayner, Kansas City, MO), Opelead [Shisheido Co. Ltd., Tokyo], and Healon EndoCoat (AMO), to name a few. The second subclass, the very low viscosity dispersives, consists of all the unmodified

hydroxypropyl methylcelluloses, including Eyefill [Croma Pharma GMBH, Vienna (purchased by B&L 2014)], iCell (San Antonio, TX), OcuVis (Toomac Ophthalmic, Auckland, New Zealand), OcuCoat (Bausch and Lomb), Adatocel [Adatomed GMBH, Munich], Acrivisc [Acri.Tec GMBH, Henningsdorf, Germany], Visilon [Shah and Shah, Calcutta], and many others.

Areas of Strength

Surgically, the most useful properties of dispersive OVDs are their resistance to aspiration and their ability to partition spaces. Dispersive nature, negative electrical charge, and the presence of hyaluronic acid to bind to specific endothelial-binding sites are the three factors that have been demonstrated by Poyer et al[7] to improve an OVD's retention in the AC during phaco and I/A. This enables dispersives to remain adjacent to the corneal endothelial cells and protect them.

Equally important, dispersive OVDs are highly useful as surgical tools in complex situations where delicate ocular structures are exposed in the AC. It may become necessary in these settings to selectively isolate or move such a structure out of harm's way until the surgery is completed (e.g., holding back vitreous at an area of zonular disinsertion, moving aside a strand of frayed iris, plugging a small posterior capsular hole, etc.). Dispersive OVDs can accomplish these tasks by partitioning the AC into two separate fluid workspaces without the two mixing: a viscoelastic-occupied space containing the delicate structure, and a surgical zone in which phaco or I/A can be safely performed under low-flow conditions. The OVD encases the protected area in an aspiration-resistant viscoelastic shell while the surgery proceeds in an adjacent area.

Areas of Weakness

The major drawbacks of lower viscosity-dispersive OVDs is their inability to maintain or stabilize spaces as well as higher viscosity-cohesive OVDs, due to their relatively low viscosity and elasticity (e.g., to facilitate capsulorrhexis creation, as described above). In addition, lower viscosity-dispersives tend to be aspirated in small fragments during phaco and I/A, as opposed to in a bolus. This gives these OVDs their inherent resistance to aspiration, but also leads to an irregular viscoelastic-aqueous interface, which may obscure the surgeon's view of the posterior capsule during phaco. Furthermore, these OVDs tend to trap particulate matter and microbubbles generated during phaco, further impairing the surgeon's view. Finally, dispersive OVDs' aspiration resistance makes them more difficult to remove at the end of the surgical procedure. Assia et al[8] demonstrated in a controlled in vitro study that lower viscosity-dispersive OVDs such as Viscoat, Ocucoat, and Orcolon [Optical Radiation Corporation, Azusa, CA], may take more than seven times longer to remove than highly viscous-cohesive OVDs such as Healon and Healon GV. The additional manipulation and aspiration required to completely remove dispersive OVDs may actually increase the likelihood of complications such as endothelial damage or puncturing of the posterior capsule, thus offsetting the benefit derived from their use in surgery.

Viscoadaptive OVDs

As discussed above, higher viscosity-cohesive and lower viscosity-dispersive OVDs both have areas of strength and weakness. In an effort to address the weaknesses of each, the search for a single OVD that could perform satisfactorily in all aspects of cataract surgery began, and in 1998 a new class of OVDs was born with the release of Healon5, the first OVD with "viscoadaptive" properties. The method of Healon5's development is interesting because the desired rheological parameters were determined based on what was thought to be optimal for modern phacoemulsification surgery. Candidate formulations were then extensively tested, and the desired result was the creation of a highly viscous and cohesive OVD that not only possessed the best properties of Healon GV (considered to be the model of the superviscous-cohesive OVDs) but also was highly retentive in the AC throughout phacoemulsification, similar to the best dispersive OVDs. Healon5 was therefore the first OVD designed in a rheological laboratory to meet preselected rheological criteria. Another viscoadaptive OVD, iVisc Phaco (Bohus BioTech), has since been developed, but our discussion of viscoadaptives will use Healon5 as the class example because it was the first.

Viscoadaptives possess the highest V_0 values of all currently available OVDs ($\geq$ 7 million mPas). Like Healon GV and Healon, Healon5 is also very pseudoplastic; the injection of Healon5 into the AC through a 25- or 27-gauge cannula is similar, with respect to required force and feedback sensation, to that of Healon GV. The molecular weight average is 4 million daltons, the same as Healon (Healon GV is 5 million). However, its hyaluronic acid concentration is 2.3%, higher than both Healon (1.0%) and Healon GV (1.4%). It is the increased concentration at the same high molecular weight hyaluronan as Healon that enables Healon5 to display its unique characteristics. Increasing concentration increases V_0. Also increasing concentration yields more dispersive behavior (because each polymer molecular chain will occupy a smaller domain), and therefore increased retention in the AC during surgery. This is then complicated by the fact that Healon5's rheological behavior straddles the line between fluids and solids, which makes it viscoadaptive, that is, a viscous-cohesive fluid at low shear, and a pseudo-dispersive solid at higher shear rates (above 25 cc/min).

During phaco and I/A, it is the fluid turbulence that determines the character of an OVD's response; the ultrasonic energy itself has little effect at the OVD surface, which is distant from the phaco probe in molecular terms. Lower viscosity-dispersives and higher viscosity cohesives behave in dispersive and cohesive manners, respectively, across the entire range of fluid turbulence and aspiration forces typically encountered in the AC during cataract surgery (**Fig. 33.2**). Both of these OVD classes are therefore appropriately named; their surgical behavior is consistent.

"Viscoadaptives" are so named because they *adapt* their behavior in surgery to the environment that the surgeon creates around them, namely, the level of fluid turbulence. Under conditions of low turbulence, Healon5 behaves just like a viscous-cohesive fluid, whereas in increased turbulence Healon5 becomes a fracturable solid, breaking into smaller pieces and therefore mimicking the behavior of a dispersive, hence the descriptive term *pseudodispersive* (**Fig. 33.2**). Interestingly, what actually happens is that as OVDs are made ever more viscous and cohesive from Ocucoat to Viscoat to Healon to Healon GV to Healon5, they begin to approach the properties of solids and start to become brittle. This is analogous to what takes place when warm chocolate pudding is placed in the refrigerator to cool. If evaluated after increasingly longer periods of cooling, the pudding will become more and more viscous. It finally reaches a point when it appears to be almost solid, and a spoon inserted into it can easily fracture its structure and be removed with a relatively solid mound of pudding on its surface.

Like the chocolate pudding, the unique fracturability of viscoadaptives like Healon5 makes them "know" whether to display cohesive or dispersive properties based on the fluid turbulence in the immediate AC environment. Therefore, during capsulorrhexis when there is no turbulence, Healon5 acts as a superviscous-cohesive fluid, whereas during the high turbulence of phaco the viscoadaptive adopts pseudodispersive solid properties, and will come out in pieces. This quality allows the surgeon to use Healon5 to maintain space throughout surgery as if it were a viscous-cohesive OVD like Healon GV. During phaco, if low flow is used (flow rates below 20 to 25 cc/min), the Healon5 mass can be broken at the iris plane, allowing evacuation of the OVD from the capsular bag while simultaneously retaining the OVD in front of the iris in a thick layer, protecting the endothelium. Later, when removal of the Healon5 is desired, we need only turn up the flow rate and direct the irrigation ports into the mass of Healon5, fracturing it and causing the pieces to move in the fluid turbulence toward the aspiration tip (**Fig. 33.2**).

OVD Removal Techniques

The "rock 'n' roll" and "two-compartment" techniques were shown to be the most efficient ways to consistently remove OVDs at the end of surgery, prior to the advent of the ultimate soft shell technique. Healon5 is best removed using one of these three techniques. The aspiration flow rate is set at 28 to 30+ cc/min, the vacuum is set at 350 to 500 mm Hg, the bottle height is set at 70 to 100 cm above the patient's eye, and a 0.3-mm I/A tip aspiration port size is used. These settings cause sufficient turbulence to achieve easy fracturing of the Healon5 matrix. In the "rock 'n' roll" technique, the I/A tip is placed on the surface of the IOL and the foot pedal is fully depressed.[9,10] The I/A tip is now rolled back and forth across the surface of the IOL, allowing irrigation fluid to crack the Healon5 matrix with aspiration of the pieces. Simultaneously, slight posterior pressure from the I/A tip on the surface of the lens and alternately tilting the IOL ~ 45 degrees gently to the left and right mobilizes the mass of OVD posterior to it. The I/A tip is not placed behind the IOL; the IOL serves as a barrier between the I/A tip and posterior capsule, protecting it while the vacuum level is high. This part of the procedure is rapid, usually lasting less than 30 seconds, but the end point is complete removal of the OVD regardless of the time elapsed, which is usually much less than 30 seconds.

In the two-compartment technique, the IOL is placed into the capsular bag and not centered, but rather displaced remote from the incision. The I/A tip is then inserted behind the IOL into the capsular bag, and I/A is commenced with settings similar to those in the "rock 'n' roll" technique discussed above, except that the aspiration port is kept aimed toward the IOL. Once the capsular bag is evacuated, the I/A is placed in front of the IOL and is used to center the IOL, and the remainder of the OVD is aspirated. The two-compartment technique is slightly quicker than the rock 'n' roll technique but involves placing the I/A between the IOL and the posterior capsule, and so slightly increases the risk of snagging the posterior capsule.[10] Our preference is the ultimate soft shell technique, discussed below.

Soft Shell Viscosurgical Techniques

Background

The term *soft shell technique* (SST) refers to a group of viscosurgical techniques that use both dispersive and cohesive OVDs in a predetermined order and positioning method to take optimal advantage of the benefits of both OVD classes while eliminating the drawbacks of each. The SSTs are useful in all case types, but have outstanding advantages in complex surgeries. Generally, the OVDs should not mix in the eye during the period of the surgery, but rather occupy adjacent spaces within the AC. The SSTs rely on four key principles:

1. A cohesive OVD (i.e., a pressurized elastic device) in a confined space transmits pressure through adjacent fluids within the confined space. This pressurizes the entire space, transmitting the beneficial properties of cohesive OVDs throughout the entire space.
2. A dispersive OVD maintains its dispersive characteristics when subjected to moderate pressure from an adjacent cohesive fluid, thus preserving the properties of a lower viscosity dispersive OVD in the area where it is wanted.
3. Two rheologically dissimilar but transparent OVDs can be placed in adjacent spaces in the AC without significant mixing during the time period of the surgery. This utilizes, to maximum advantage, the unique properties of each, in the exact location where each is most needed. Their combined use does not blur the surgeon's view as the cohesive OVD forces the adjacent dispersive to adopt a smooth boundary, optimizing its clarity.
4. It is rheologically impossible to control the surgical environment with any single OVD as well as with a specifically placed combination of rheologically different OVDs. The more different the rheological properties of the OVDs, the greater the possibilities of creating an optimized partitioned surgical environment. This reaches the current optimal limit in tri-soft shell techniques, where three different OVDs are used together: a lower viscosity dispersive, a viscoadaptive, and an aqueous solution.[5]

The Dispersive-Cohesive Viscoelastic Soft Shell Technique (Fig. 33.5)

The first SST, the dispersive-cohesive OVD SST, was described in 1999.[3] After the paracentesis is made, through which intracameral lidocaine or lidocaine-phenylephrine solution is injected, the main phaco incision is created, through which a lower viscosity-dispersive viscoelastic is injected on the anterior lenticular surface to create a mound. It is important to note that in all soft shell techniques the OVDs are injected through the main cataract incision, not the side port, as this permits greater facility in positioning the OVD more accurately within the AC, and also in inflating the AC to the pressure desired. A higher viscosity-cohesive OVD is then injected onto the anterior capsule surface, below the dispersive mound, so that the incoming viscous-cohesive fills the center of the eye and pushes the lower viscosity-dispersive up and out, forming a smooth, even, pressurized layer

of dispersive OVD adjacent to the corneal endothelium. This protective "soft shell" of dispersive OVD, from which all soft shell techniques derived their name, will remain in place even after the cohesive OVD is aspirated out during phaco and I/A, ensuring enhanced protection of the corneal endothelium.

After phaco and I/A, but before IOL implantation, the second step of SST can be performed if IOL folding forceps are to be used.[3] This step is rarely used currently because IOL injector cartridges seal the incision as the IOL is injected, making step 2 of the SST unnecessary. However, the second, pre-IOL implantation, step of the ultimate soft shell technique (see below) is greatly advantageous in modern IOL implantation.

Several studies have experimentally validated the dispersive-cohesive OVD SST, finding less increase in postoperative central corneal thickness and less endothelial cell loss, even with dense cataracts and Fuchs's endothelial dystrophy, than with the use of a single OVD.

Ultimate Soft Shell Technique

With the advent of viscoadaptives, new SSTs became possible. The more rheologically dissimilar the properties of the two OVDs being used, the more effective the technique. Thus arose the ultimate soft shell technique (USST), extending this principle to its practical limit by pairing a viscoadaptive OVD with balanced salt solution (BSS), which has a viscosity of only 1 mPas, the same as water.[4] This dramatic rheological difference creates two adjacent but completely different physical environments within the AC. In the precapsulorrhexis step, an outer shell of viscoadaptive OVD is used to coat the corneal endothelium and block the incision, ensuring good AC pressurization. BSS, often containing a pharmacological agent (commonly trypan blue, lidocaine, phenylephrine, or a combination of lidocaine and phenylephrine), is then injected beneath it onto the lenticular surface to create a low viscosity workspace (**Fig. 33.6a–c**). The capsulorrhexis is then performed in a low viscosity aqueous environment, while the AC is highly pressurized by the blockage of the incision with the viscoadaptive OVD.

A similar soft shell arrangement is created during IOL insertion, with an outer layer of viscoadaptive OVD filling the AC entirely or partially (blocking the incisional area and extending partially into the AC) and an inner layer of BSS filling the capsular bag. The leading IOL haptic unfolds easily once it has traversed the viscoadaptive layer and enters the low viscosity BSS environment of the bag. The trailing haptic remains folded, encased in viscoadaptive near the incision. After the IOL injector is removed, the I/A device is promptly inserted into the AC, before the IOL unfolds, and when irrigation is turned on the IOL begins to fall backward into the BSS-filled capsular bag, due to increased pressure anterior to the IOL (**Fig. 33.6d–g**) Gentle nudging of the still-folded trailing haptic with the I/A tip positions the implant in the bag as aspiration is turned on to remove residual OVD. Because the IOL is inserted under an OVD shell into BSS, minimal OVD remains behind the IOL, eliminating the need to place the I/A behind the IOL, or to perform much rocking and rolling, to remove residual OVD. The two-compartment technique can be used, but it is rarely needed.[11]

Modifications to the Dispersive-Cohesive OVD SST and the USST for Special Cases

White, Intumescent, or Brunescent Cataracts (Fig. 33.7)

In cases of white or brunescent cataracts, the USST can be modified to enhance anterior capsule visualization by painting try-

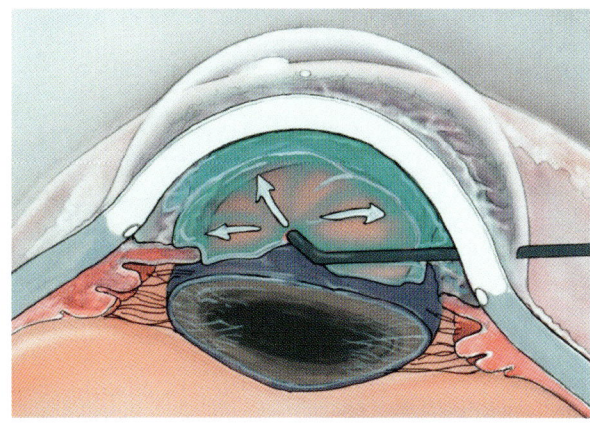
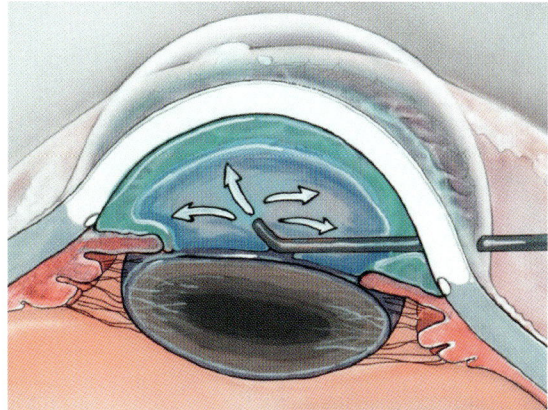
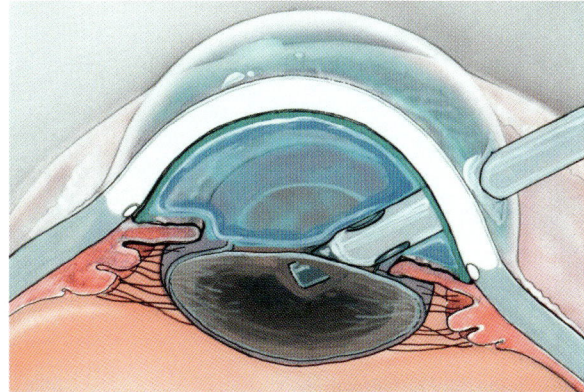
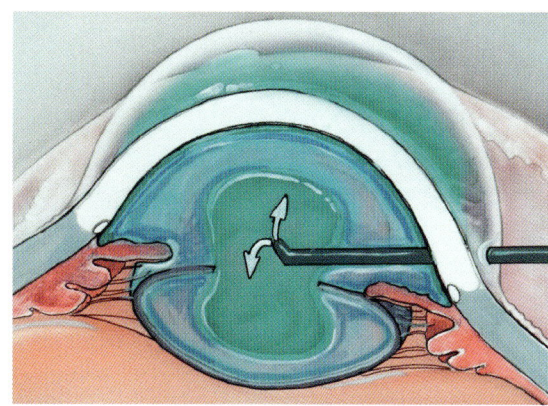
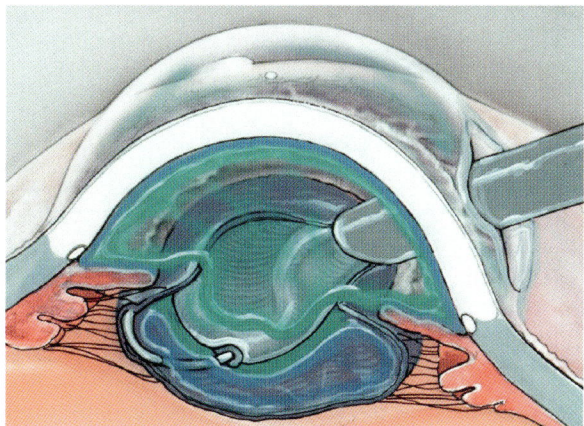

Fig. 33.5   The dispersive cohesive viscoelastic soft shell technique (SST). **(a)** The lower viscosity-dispersive OVD *(green)* is injected first to form a mound on the surface of the center of the cataractous lens. **(b)** The higher viscosity-cohesive OVD *(blue)* is injected into the posterior center of the lower viscosity-dispersive OVD, such that continued injection pushes the lower viscosity-dispersive OVD upward and outward, finally pressurizing it into a smooth layer against the corneal endothelial cells. **(c)** After performance of the capsulorrhexis, when the phaco is begun, the higher viscosity-cohesive OVD *(blue)* rapidly leaves the eye, leaving behind a layer of lower viscosity-dispersive OVD *(green)* with a smooth internal boundary, and a variable thickness, depending on how much was injected at the beginning of the procedure, adjacent to and protecting the corneal endothelial cells. This OVD layer, being dispersive in nature, thereby resisting aspiration, remains largely intact throughout the phaco and irrigation and aspiration (I/A) procedures. **(d)** After completion of removal of the nucleus and cortex, the OVDs are injected in reverse order. The higher viscosity-cohesive OVD *(blue)* is injected first to stabilize the iris, capsule, and anterior chamber (AC). The lower viscosity-dispersive OVD *(green)* is then injected into its center, placing the cannula tip approximately in the geographic center of the capsulorrhexis. **(e)** The presence of the lower viscosity-dispersive OVD *(green)* in the center of the higher viscosity-cohesive OVD mass *(blue)* allows freer movement of the incoming IOL with better stabilization of the surrounding iris and capsular bag.

pan blue into the BSS zone directly adjacent to the anterior lens surface only. This provides targeted staining of the anterior capsule with only an extremely small quantity of dye for full effect, avoiding AC clouding and reducing the potential for toxicity. The enhanced pressurization of the AC with the viscoadaptive ensures flattening of the capsule, overcoming any posterior pressure and permitting a pressure-equalized capsulorrhexis to be easily performed.

Broken Zonules or Frayed Iris Strands

In cases of broken zonules and frayed iris strands, using additional dispersive OVD to encase and isolate the damaged area is a modification of the dispersive-cohesive SST. This effect can be magnified if a viscoadaptive is substituted for the higher viscosity-cohesive partner OVD, because the rheological difference between the two OVDs is then increased (**Fig. 33.8**).

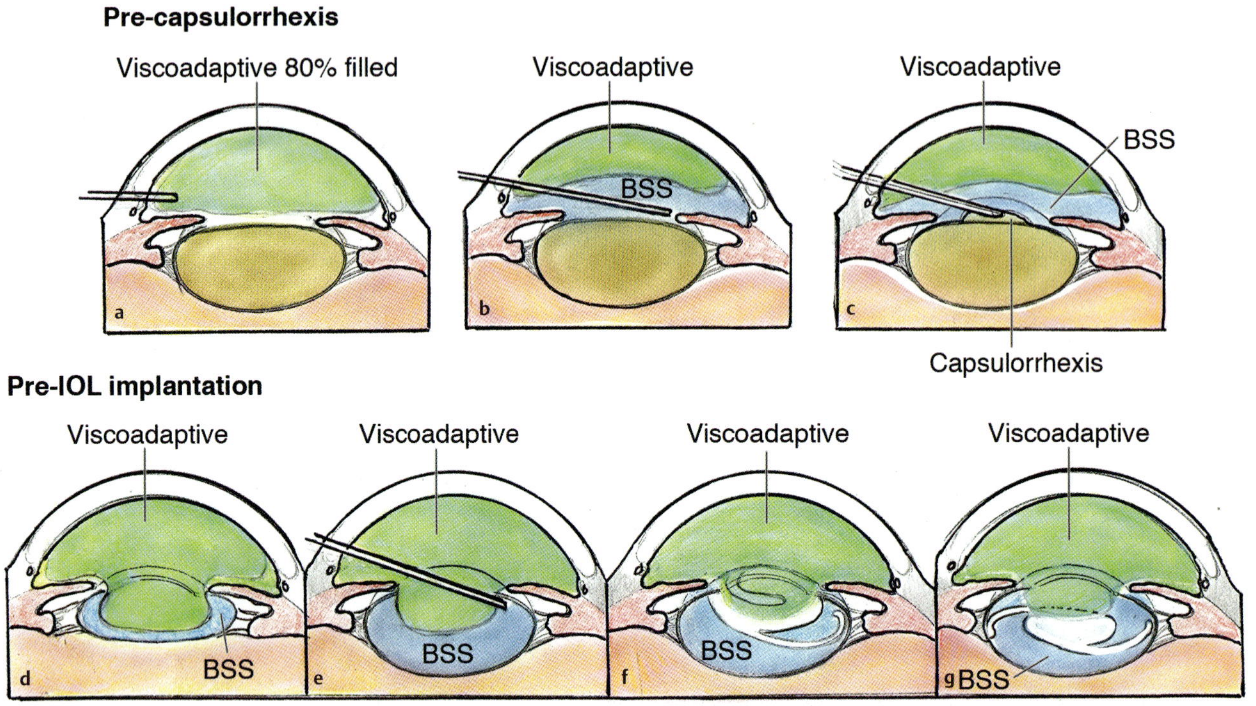

Pre-capsulorrhexis

Viscoadaptive 80% filled

Viscoadaptive

Viscoadaptive

BSS

BSS

Capsulorrhexis

a   b   c

Pre-IOL implantation

Viscoadaptive

Viscoadaptive

Viscoadaptive

Viscoadaptive

BSS   BSS   BSS   BSS

d   e   f   g

Fig. 33.6 The ultimate soft shell technique (USST). The ultimate soft shell technique is so named because it utilizes aqueous solutions, with their ultimately lowest possible viscosity, close to 1, of any aqueous solution of OVD polymers, as one of the two OVDs in the technique. This is possible because the other OVD is an extremely high viscosity viscoadaptive. The technique is performed as follows: Pre-capsulorrhexis step *(top row)*: **(a)** The viscoadaptive OVD is injected into the AC through the main phaco incision until the AC is ~ 80% filled. **(b)** A balanced salt-based solution (I prefer a mixture of lidocaine and phenylephrine) is injected through the viscoadaptive, aiming for the remote edge of the pupil. Once a small lake has been formed on the surface of the lens, the injection force is increased in a quick pulse, which forces the viscoadaptive layer upward and backward to block the incision, preventing egress of the aqueous layer below it. **(c)** The capsulorrhexis is then performed in a very low viscosity aqueous environment, while the AC is pressurized by the viscoadaptive, as if the entire AC was full of viscoadap-

tive. Pre-IOL implantation step *(bottom row)*: **(d)** Viscoadaptive is injected at the incision until the capsulorrhexis has been covered, but before the OVD significantly enters the capsular bag. **(e)** Balanced salt solution (BSS) is injected through the viscoadaptive layer into the capsular bag. This causes the bag to open and the viscoadaptive to come out of the bag, moving backward toward the incision to block it, thus pressurizing the AC and capsular bag. **(f)** The IOL is injected, preferably using a cartridge to seal the incision, through the viscoadaptive, into the BSS-filled capsular bag. The leading haptic opens quickly, as it is in a low viscosity environment, whereas the trailing haptic is surrounded by viscoadaptive, and so will open very slowly. **(g)** If the I/A is placed into the eye quickly after IOL implantation, the increase in pressure obtained by turning on the I/A causes the IOL to fall backward into the aqueous-filled capsular bag. Slight nudging of the IOL with the I/A tip ensures that it is entirely within the capsular bag. By time this is done, all of the OVD will have been cleared from the eye, as the I/A is on during this maneuver.

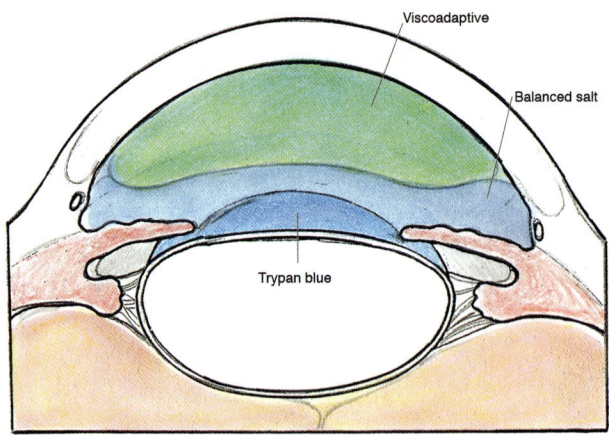

Viscoadaptive

Balanced salt

Trypan blue

Fig. 33.7 In cases of white or brunescent cataracts, the USST can be modified to enhance anterior capsule visualization by painting trypan blue directly onto the anterior capsular surface, either before or after injecting the BSS.

Tamsulosin-Induced Intraoperative Floppy Iris Syndrome

In patients taking the α_{1A}-antagonist tamsulosin (Flomax) with the resultant intraoperative floppy iris syndrome (IFIS), the dispersive-cohesive OVD SST and USST approaches are combined into a procedure referred to as the soft shell bridge (SSB).[12] After fashioning longer than usual corneal incisions to discourage iris prolapse, a peripheral low viscosity-dispersive OVD shell is created to tamponade the iris by resisting aspiration and preventing iris flutter and the propensity for prolapse commonly seen in IFIS. The pupil is dilated and the central AC stabilized with a bridge of viscoadaptive OVD. Contrary to accepted dogma, when using OVDs to stabilize the iris, it is helpful to stretch the pupil with iris hooks at this stage. Finally, a low viscosity workspace is then created adjacent to the lenticular surface with BSS or preferably a lidocaine-phenylephrine solution. Phaco is performed using low-flow parameters (vacuum 220 mm Hg, flow ~20 cc/min) within the BSS zone, sequestered underneath the viscoadaptive OVD bridge in the central region of the AC.

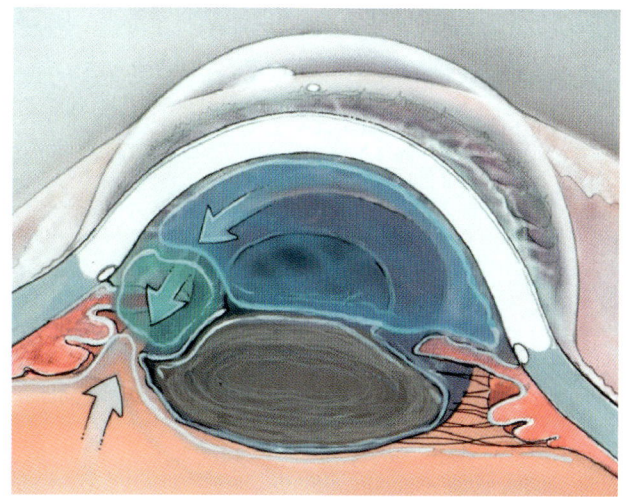

Fig. 33.8 Soft shell technique in a case of broken zonules. The dispersive OVD *(green)* is compressed by the cohesive OVD *(blue)*. This sequesters the exposed vitreous base from the turmoil of surgery. Once the OVDs are in place and the bulging vitreous has been pushed backwards behind the equator of the lens, this anatomical positioning can be assured by implantation of a capsular tension ring prior to the phaco.

The Tri-Soft Shell Technique (Fig. 33.9)

The tri-soft shell technique (TSST) was first published in 2013 in an effort to reduce surgeon confusion and unify all three SSTs (SST, USST, and SSB) and complication management scenarios into a single method from which specific applications to unusual circumstances could be simply and intuitively made.[5] It is performed by first injecting a dispersive OVD through the phaco incision to form a central mound on the surface of the anterior capsule, stopping once the AC is 20 to 25% full. Next, a viscous-cohesive OVD, or preferably a viscoadaptive OVD, to maximize the OVD rheological difference, is injected beneath the dispersive onto the anterior capsular surface. This displaces the dispersive upward against the corneal endothelium in the now familiar protective soft shell formation. Injection of the viscoadaptive should continue until the pupil stops dilating but before the eye becomes firm (~ 80% full).

Next, with the cannula aperture directed downward toward the lenticular surface, BSS or lidocaine-phenylephrine is slowly injected beneath the viscoadaptive OVD layer, creating a continuous lake of low-viscosity fluid directly on the lenticular surface. In so doing, the viscoadaptive shell is displaced upward, forming a central bridge. When viewed conceptually, what has now been created is the USST with the dispersive-cohesive SST above it. Hence the description chosen is "tri-soft shell technique."

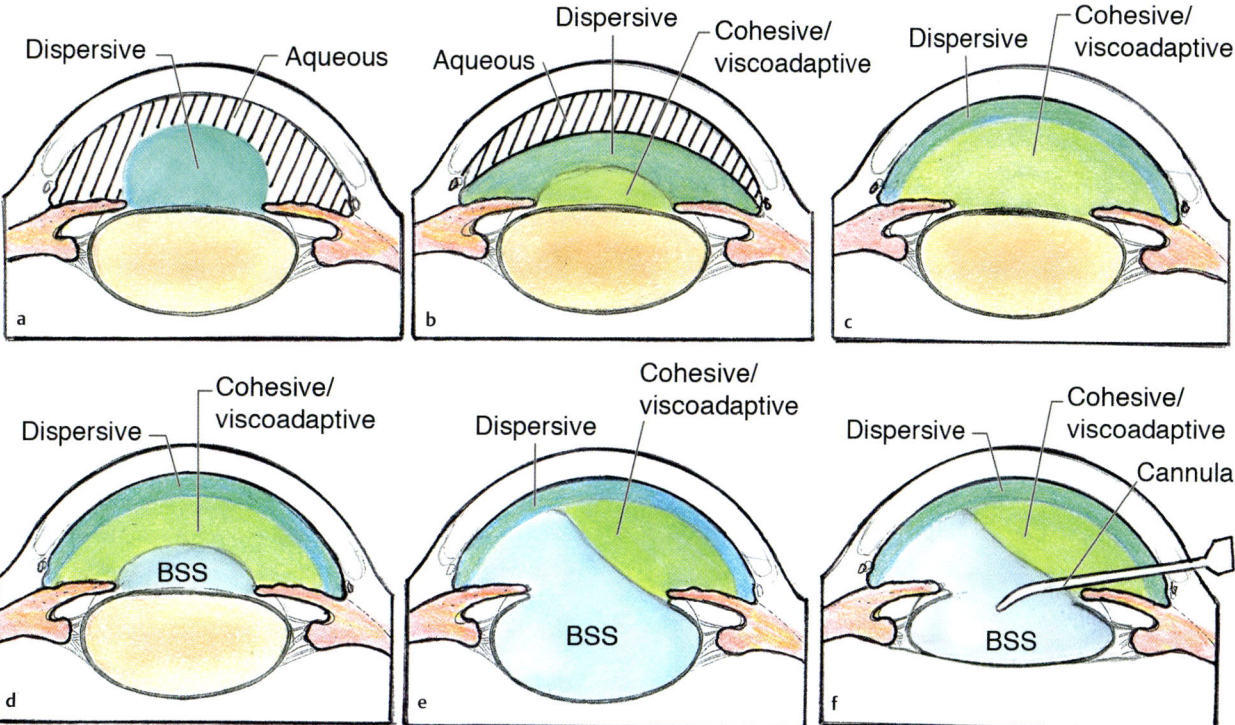

Fig. 33.9 Tri-soft shell technique. **(a)** A dispersive OVD is first injected centrally on the surface of the lens. **(b)** A viscoadaptive OVD is then injected beneath this initial shell, displacing it upward into a smooth layer coating the corneal endothelium **(c)**. **(d)** Balanced salt solution (BSS) is injected onto the anterior capsule surface, below the OVDs, creating a low-viscosity work area for capsulorrhexis. **(e)** After phacoemulsification and I/A of the lens, the viscoadaptive OVD shell is rebuilt as needed beginning at the corneal incision, with the goal of blocking the incision and creating a roof over the capsular bag to protect the corneal endothelium. **(f)** BSS is injected through the viscoadaptive OVD into the capsular gag, creating an OVD-free space in which the IOL's leading haptic can be placed and unfolded.

Pre-phaco

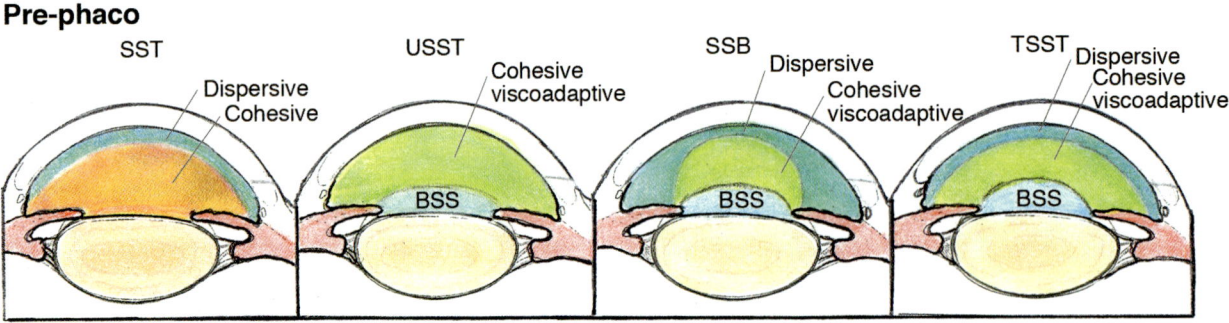

Pre IOL implantation

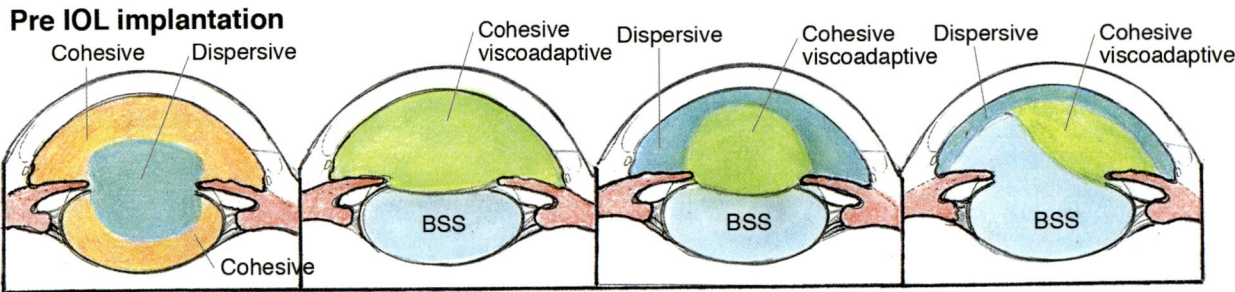

Fig. 33.10 Comparison of SSTs. For each technique, the soft shell configuration prior to the initiation of phacoemulsification and prior to IOL insertion is illustrated. The TSST is a generalization of previously described SSTs and can be easily modified to resemble each depending on the requirements of a particular surgery. SSB, soft shell bridge; SST, soft shell technique; TSST, tri-soft shell technique; USST, ultimate soft shell technique.

Once routine capsulorrhexis and hydrodissection are performed, the sequestered BSS lake actually facilitates phacoemulsification in an interesting way. Because the working space is restricted to a relatively small volume on the lenticular surface, high desired turbulence can be generated at comparatively low pump settings (e.g., 15 cc/min). This is because the ratio of flow rate to working volume is dramatically higher than if flow were higher but contained within the entire AC. Put simply, the TSST's small BSS lake makes it feel as though the pump is set at a higher setting, making it easier to draw material to the phaco tip. An intuitive analogy is using a garden hose to fill a bucket and then a swimming pool: the same flow rate in the smaller volume induces much greater turbulence. Besides making surgery more straightforward, this compartmentalized flow effectively reduces any turbulence felt by delicate endothelial cells to very low or negligible.

After routine I/A, IOL insertion can proceed as described for the USST above. As more experience is gained, viscoadaptive OVD blockade of only the incision and the area of the capsulorrhexis near the incision, pushing back the iris in the area of the incision, will be all that is necessary for IOL implantation, with the remainder of the AC and capsular bag filled with BSS injected through the viscoadaptive into the bag. The IOL is then inserted using an injector cartridge, immediately after which the I/A tip is inserted and turned on (before the IOL fully unfolds); slight posterior nudging of the trailing haptic and IOL is exerted, causing the IOL to fall backward into the BSS-filled capsular bag and open. The OVD is removed using I/A, taking only a few seconds; this is usually complete once the surgeon realizes that the IOL has fallen backward into the capsular bag. When preoperative endothelial cell counts are marginal, the surgeon may elect to leave the dispersive OVD layer in the eye by keeping the I&A tip posteriorly, avoiding exposure of the endothelium to turbulence.

While performing the TSST, careful control over the middle viscoadaptive OVD shell is of primary importance, as it plays the central role in facilitating the proposed surgery. It is responsible for four mechanical roles: (1) space creation in and (2) pressurization of the AC, (3) incisional blockade, and (4) tamponade of peripheral structures including the dispersive OVD shell, which itself tamponades iris in an IFIS case and any exposed vitreous in a zonule deficiency case. Viscoadaptives are ideal for these roles because of their extremely high V_0 values, allowing them to resist deformational stresses imposed on the eye during surgery.

The TSST is more effective and has a broader range of efficacy than older SSTs. All are shown graphically, compared with each other in **Fig. 33.10**. It can be adapted to virtually any surgical scenario, and is well suited to the most complex cataract surgeries. An example is a patient with severe Fuchs's endothelial dystrophy and IFIS, where maximal control over the operative environment is desired. The TSST is not, however, meant to be a cookie-cutter approach to cataract surgery. Clinical intuition must be exercised to guide the positioning of the different OVD layers and to choose specific OVDs in a given case. In an uncomplicated cataract, the full TSST may not be necessary; instead, for example, the dispersive OVD layer can be eliminated when only a brief phaco time is anticipated. The USST is the natural result of such omission of dispersive OVD use in the TSST, eliminating some steps and reducing cost. If a patient has severe IFIS, a little more dispersive OVD is injected, and care is taken to cover the iris well, resulting in the SSB. If there are broken zonular fibers, the dispersive OVD layer is spread to cover the area of damaged zonules and protruding vitreous. Once familiarity with the TSST is attained, simple modifications become obvious for the management of specific problems, making OVD use conceptually easier and more effective in all cases.

Conclusion

To deal effectively with the varied uses of OVDs in complicated surgery, an understanding of certain basic principles is necessary. OVDs are not all the same; the lower viscosity-dispersive, higher viscosity-cohesive, and viscoadaptive OVD classes each possess unique areas of strength, and it is through their combination in many diverse ways in the various SSTs that the anterior-segment surgeon may maximize their utility to facilitate different surgeries. In this way, OVDs can be used as powerful tools to improve surgical outcomes in complicated cases.

Disclosure

Steve A. Arshinoff has served as a consultant for most major manufacturers of OVDs globally. Thomas A. Berk has no financial conflict of interest with anything discussed herein.

References

1. Balazs EA, Miller D, Stegmann R. Viscosurgery and the use of Na-hyaluronate in intraocular lens implantation. Presented at the International Congress and First Film Festival on Intraocular Implantation, Cannes, France, 1979

2. Arshinoff SA, Jafari M. A new classification of ophthalmic viscosurgical devices (OVDs)—2005. J Cataract Refract Surg 2005;31:2167–2171

3. Arshinoff SA. Dispersive-cohesive viscoelastic soft shell technique. J Cataract Refract Surg 1999;25:167–173

4. Arshinoff SA. Using BSS with viscoadaptives in the ultimate soft-shell technique. J Cataract Refract Surg 2002;28:1509–1514

5. Arshinoff SA, Norman R. Tri-soft shell technique. J Cataract Refract Surg 2013;39:1196–1203

6. Härfstrand A, Molander N, Stenevi U, Apple D, Schenholm M, Madsen K. Evidence of hyaluronic acid and hyaluronic acid binding sites on human corneal endothelium. J Cataract Refract Surg 1992;18:265–269

7. Poyer JF, Chan KY, Arshinoff SA. New method to measure the retention of viscoelastic agents on a rabbit corneal endothelial cell line after irrigation and aspiration. J Cataract Refract Surg 1998;24:84–90

8. Assia EI, Apple DJ, Lim ES, Morgan RC, Tsai JC. Removal of viscoelastic materials after experimental cataract surgery in vitro. J Cataract Refract Surg 1992;18:3–6

9. Arshinoff S. Rock 'n' roll removal of Healon GV (video). Presented at the American Society of Cataract and Refractive Surgery Film Festival, Seattle, Washington, June 1–5, 1996

10. Arshinoff SA. Rock 'n' roll removal of Healon GV. In: Arshinoff SA, ed. Proceedings of the 7th Annual National Ophthalmic Speakers Program (Ottawa, Canada, June 1996). Medicopea; 1997:29–33

11. Tetz MR, Holzer MP. Two-compartment technique to remove ophthalmic viscosurgical devices. J Cataract Refract Surg 2000;26:641–643

12. Arshinoff SA. Modified SST-USST for tamsulosin-associated intraoperative [corrected] floppy-iris syndrome. J Cataract Refract Surg 2006;32:559–561, erratum 1076

XIII Corneal Complications

34 Corneal Problems Associated with Phacoemulsification

Mark D. Mifflin and Jason M. Feurman

Successful cataract surgery depends on a good understanding of the cornea. Optical clarity, refractive predictability, and the long-term stability and health of the cornea are necessary components for optimizing outcomes.

Anatomy of the Cornea (Fig. 34.1)

Surgical prowess is in part determined by a good foundation in anatomy. The cornea has unique structural characteristics, which are important in maintaining a clear and stable "window" for the eye. Our brief anatomy review is intended to help the surgeon achieve better outcomes and fewer corneal complications when performing cataract surgery.

The adult cornea measures 11 to 12 mm horizontally and 9 to 11 mm vertically. The thickness varies from ~ 0.5 mm in the center to 0.7 mm in the periphery.[1] It is convex and aspheric, normally steeper in the center and flatter in the periphery.[2] The anterior surface is covered by the tear film, which consists of a gradient of three layers: a superficial lipid layer, an aqueous layer, and a mucinous layer.[3] The outermost lipid layer of the tear film is produced by the meibomian glands and accessory secretory glands of the eyelid. The lacrimal gland and accessory lacrimal glands produce the aqueous layer, and the mucinous layer is produced mostly by goblet cells in the conjunctival epithelium.[2]

The central cornea consists of several layers. The most anterior layer of the cornea is stratified, squamous, nonkeratinized epithelium that is five to seven cell layers and ~ 50 μm in thickness. The deepest of these epithelial cells consist of a single layer of columnar basal cells adherent to a basement membrane via hemidesmosomes. Posterior to the epithelium is Bowman's layer, an acellular matrix of collagen fibers and proteoglycans with a smooth anterior surface, ~ 12 μm thick. The stroma, posterior to Bowman's layer, constitutes 90% of the corneal thickness, and is composed of layers of highly organized collagen fibrils embedded in a ground substance with keratocytes dispersed among these lamellae. Descemet's membrane is posterior to the stroma and is the basement membrane of the corneal endothelium. It gradually increases in thickness from ~ 3 μm at birth to ~ 10 μm in adulthood. Of note, a pre-Descemet's layer, Dua's layer, is recently purported to exist between the corneal stroma and Descemet's membrane, and may have clinical significance in lamellar keratoplasty techniques.[4] The endothelium on the posterior side of Descemet's membrane is a single cell layer ~ 5 μm thick. The endothelial cells are responsible for ion transport and maintain the cornea in a state of deturgescence. Endothelial cell density decreases with age, and it is important to protect the endothelium during surgery because human endothelial cells do not proliferate.[5]

The normal cornea is avascular, with the exception of the vascular arcade in the limbal region, which has contributions originating from both the internal carotid and external carotid arteries. The avascular cornea is supplied with glucose by diffusion from the aqueous humor and oxygen by diffusion from the tear–air interface.[2] The limbus is often the site of incisions for cataract surgery. It is ~ 1 mm wide and marks the transition between the cornea and sclera, extending from the end of Descemet's and Bowman's to the point where corneal stroma merges into sclera. Sensory nerve fibers from the ophthalmic division of the trigeminal nerve enter the limbus from the perichoroidal space and, after losing their myelin sheaths, branch into the corneal stroma, penetrating Bowman's membrane and ending as naked fibrils between epithelial cells.

Optics of the Cornea

Only the most basic concepts are discussed here. Cataract surgeons need to be concerned about two major areas when assessing the optics of the cornea. The first is opacification, which is the direct blockage of light to the more posterior structures in the eye. In addition, corneal opacities may hinder line-of-sight visualization for the surgeon, which could affect safety and efficiency during the procedure. The second type of optical problem is disruption of light rays not by direct blockage but rather by distortion of light rays due to irregularities of the optical surfaces (refraction, diffraction, scatter, decreased contrast, etc.). In many instances the disruption of light rays due to irregularity may be more clinically significant in terms of visual outcomes and certainly is a much more commonly encountered problem. In general, irregularities of the anterior refractive surface create more difficulties as compared with irregularities of the posterior corneal surface.

Helpful Hints

1. Surgeon visualization may be optimized by a variety of techniques including capsular staining and placing the main and secondary incisions strategically to facilitate performance of surgical maneuvers in areas with the best view. Indirect illumination using a light pipe is also sometimes helpful.

2. Dry eye evaluation is part of cataract surgery evaluation. At a minimum, inspection of the tear film and staining of the ocular surface are advised.

3. Perform corneal topography on all candidates for cataract surgery. A photokeratoscopic view is particularly

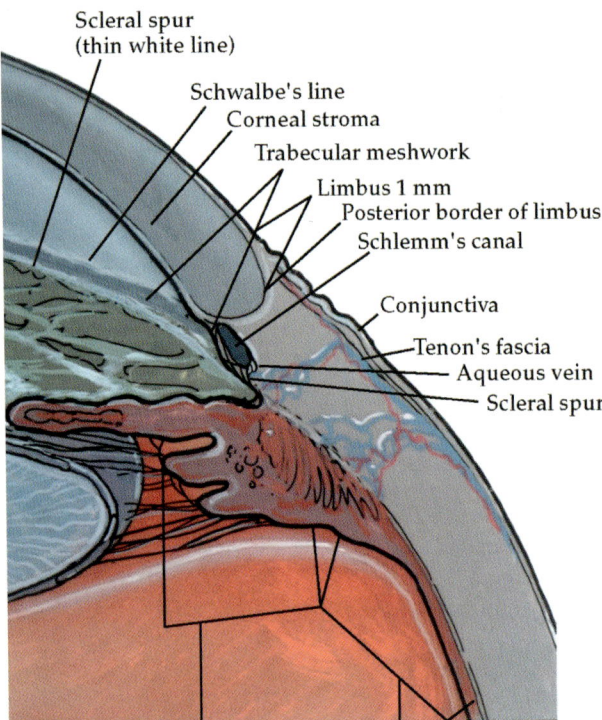

Fig. 34.1 The anatomic relationships of the cornea and limbus.

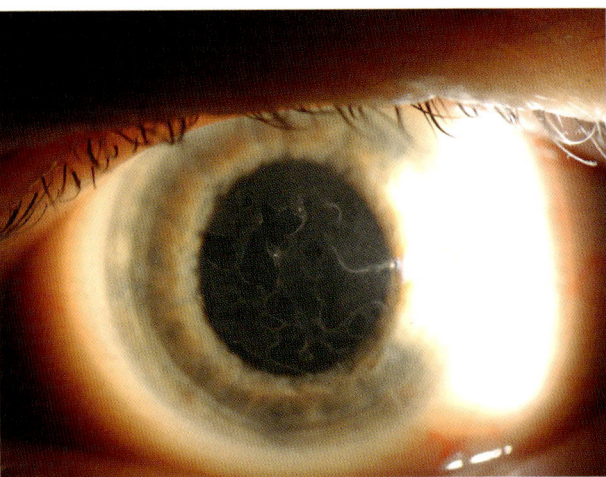

Fig. 34.2 Anterior/epithelial basement membrane dystrophy. (Courtesy of James Gilman.)

helpful and sensitive to quickly detect surface irregularities, fixation, angle kappa, and pupil size.

4. Consider corneal tomography if irregular astigmatism is detected on screening exams (topography or retinoscopy).

The Cornea and Indications for Cataract Surgery

As cataract surgery has continued to improve over the past three decades, our threshold for surgical intervention has gradually been lowered and we are more willing to operate at earlier stages of disease. The vast majority of patients seem to present in the 20/30 to 20/50 range, with significant decline in their ability to perform activities of daily living. Sometimes patients with corneal disease present at earlier stages of cataract formation, and it is imperative for the surgeon to determine the relative negative effect of the corneal pathology before performing surgery. The following subsections provide some general guidelines for managing commonly encountered conditions in cataract surgery patients.

Surface Disorders

If treatment is required to improve or optimize the ocular surface before cataract surgery, allow a minimum of 4 to 6 weeks for stabilization. Serial topography should be reproducible on two separate evaluations before the final biometry is performed.

Dry eye and blepharitis are the most common "corneal" comorbidities and must be identified, especially if "premium" (multifocal or toric intraocular lens [IOL]) cataract surgery is performed. In general, even 1–2+ punctate staining in the visual axis or tear film instability may be enough to adversely affect the biometry or the visual outcomes.

Anterior/epithelial basement membrane dystrophy (ABMD) is common and may be subtle but needs to be identified and discussed with the patient prior to surgery (**Fig. 34.2**). Severe cases will affect the biometry and the visual outcome and may require treatment (superficial keratectomy, diamond bur, photo-therapeutic keratectomy) before cataract surgery.

Pterygia may induce irregular astigmatism or in severe cases obstruct part of the visual axis. Depending on the extent, combined or separate surgery may be appropriate. In many older patients, it is very appropriate to not intervene surgically for long-standing, inactive pterygia before cataract surgery. However, if it is anticipated that pterygium surgery will be required in the future, it is advisable to perform the pterygium surgery first and allow the cornea to heal before obtaining biometry for cataract surgery.

Salzmann nodular degeneration is generally easy to recognize and more likely to be found superiorly or obliquely in a peripheral or paracentral location. Depending on proximity to the visual axis and induced astigmatism, intervention may or may not be needed prior to cataract surgery. Similar to pterygia, however, if it is clear that surgical removal will be needed in the future, this should be performed well before biometry and cataract surgery to enable the most accurate IOL calculations (**Figs. 34.3 and 34.4**).

Helpful Hints

1. Use rose bengal or lissamine green to evaluate ocular surface staining in dry-eye patients. Fluorescein is most useful for assessing tear film breakup time, which ideally should be 10 seconds or greater.[6] "Negative staining" is a useful way to detect pathology, which causes irregular elevated areas of the epithelium such as ABMD or Salzmann degeneration. Look for dark areas that stick up out of the fluorescein pool when using the cobalt blue filter at the slit lamp.

2. Corneal mapping often shows irregularity and flattening in the area of a pterygium head or Salzmann nodule. Tomography often shows thickening in these areas as well. Generalized corneal thickening may be a feature of ABMD, sometimes even in occult cases. Significant refractive shifts (usually decreased astigmatism and decreased hyperopia) may be expected when paracentral thickened lesions are removed.

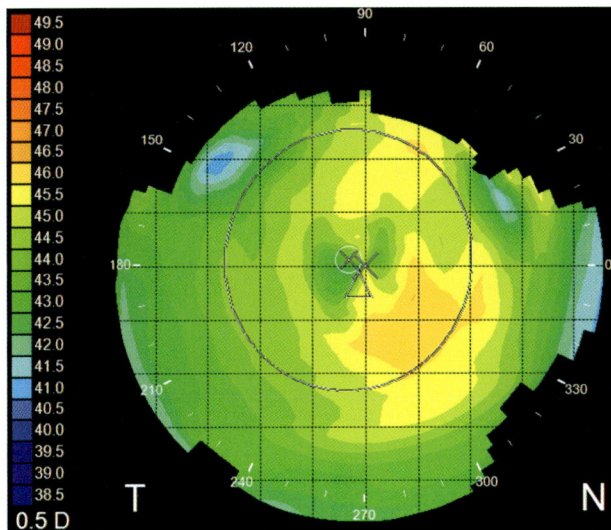

Fig. 34.3   Irregular topography due to Salzmann nodular degeneration. Note pattern of irregular flattening.

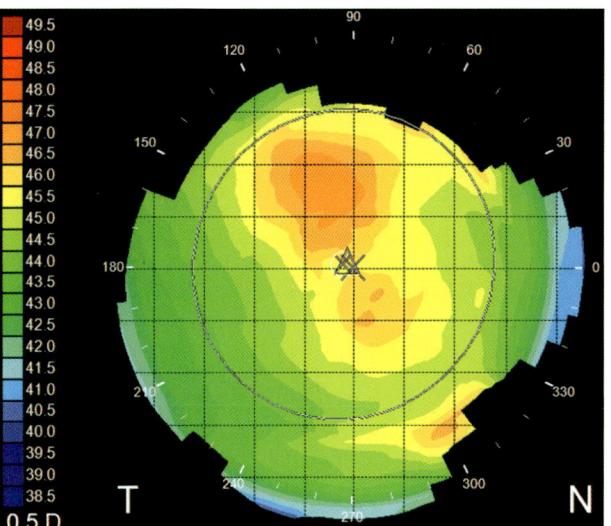

Fig. 34.4   Improved regularity of topography after superficial keratectomy for Salzmann nodules. Note overall steepening of the cornea and unmasking of the "with the rule" astigmatism.

3. Dry eye and blepharitis are often underdiagnosed and undertreated in cataract patients. Topical medications used before and after surgery may compound ocular surface disease. Avoid preserved drops when possible, and identify and treat problems preventively if possible (**Table 34.1**).

Stromal Disorders

Keratoconus is characterized by a spectrum of severity and may occasionally be diagnosed for the first time in older patients being screened for cataract surgery. This entity is typically detected using topographic and tomographic corneal mapping. The differential diagnosis includes contact lens "warpage," which may cause mild irregular astigmatism usually noted in a pattern of inferior steepening. Certainly rigid contact lenses may temporarily or permanently "mold" the cornea, and this is a point of

consideration when performing biometry for IOL calculations. Toric IOLs may be used successfully in some stable keratoconus patients after careful evaluation. The cylinder must be regular or near regular for toric IOL implantation. But toric IOLs should not be used for irregular astigmatism or in patients expecting or needing to wear rigid contact lenses after cataract surgery. Great care should be taken in performing astigmatic keratotomy or limbal relaxing incisions in patients with thin or structurally unstable corneas. Clear corneal incisions (CCIs) may be used successfully in most patients, but some surgeons prefer scleral tunnel incisions in keratoconus patients. Very careful wound design is required in the case of CCI, and suturing may be advisable for optimum safety. Patients with severe keratoconus and cataracts may need combined or sequential keratoplasty to achieve acceptable visual outcomes. This is addressed in more detail later in the chapter.

Other corneal stromal disorders that may affect outcomes in cataract surgery might include scarring, thinning, or vascular-

Table 34.1   Surface Disorders Affecting Visualization in Cataract Surgery

Pathology	Surgical Modifications
Bullous keratopathy	Trypan blue to visualize capsulorrhexis; phaco above plane of anterior capsule to protect the posterior capsule
Stromal corneal scarring secondary to advanced herpes keratitis, post-corneal ulcer, traumatic scar	Find a clear area in the cornea and perform surgery through this area
Keratoconus	Same as for bullous keratopathy, above
Severe superficial punctate keratitis (SPK) in susceptible patients especially with topical anesthesia due to exposure and epithelial toxicity	15–20 microdots dispersive ophthalmic viscosurgical device (OVD) (Viscoat is best) and a drop of balanced salt solution (BSS) until microdots coalesce, creating a clear surface
Dense arcus, if profound, may create a large band of poor visualization	Temporal approach, bimanual technique so that the eye can be rotated to enhance visualization
Band keratopathy; if able to see iris detail, okay to proceed; if unable, ethylenediaminetetraacetic acid (EDTA) scrub 6 weeks prior	All techniques noted above

ization. These conditions should be evaluated on a case-by-case basis to determine whether corneal surgery is necessary for a good outcome. Many times cataract surgery can be performed successfully by moving the incision site or performing a scleral tunnel incision.

Helpful Hint

Carefully evaluate and counsel keratoconus patients preoperatively. You will miss mild cases if you are not looking for this! Toric IOLs should be used with caution if there is a chance of rigid contact lens wear postoperatively.

Posterior Corneal Disorders

Fuchs dystrophy has a female preponderance and is more prevalent and symptomatic in the older cataract-aged patient population. The clinical hallmark is an irregular thickened posterior collagen layer of Descemet's membrane that often manifests clinically as guttae, which are excrescences associated with abnormal or missing endothelial cells **(Fig. 34.5)**.[7] It is sometimes difficult to decide whether to remove the cataract alone, perform endothelial keratoplasty (EK) alone, or perform a combined procedure. Dense, confluent guttae, anterior stromal or subepithelial scarring, or a history of marked worsening vision upon awakening ("a.m. edema") generally indicate the need for corneal surgery. Corneal pachymetry, although widely used, is a less reliable indicator for endothelial viability due to the very large range of thicknesses encountered in normal eyes. Central corneal thickness (CCT) of 620 to 650 μm or even greater should always at least prompt the cataract surgeon to consider endothelial pathology, although values well below this can be associated with marked dysfunction if the patient starts out with a lower CCT.

Prior ocular trauma or previous surgery may also be associated with significant decreases in endothelial cell density (ECD), and these patients should be addressed with similar caution.

Posterior polymorphous corneal dystrophy should be recognized and discussed but is generally low risk for causing postoperative corneal edema. This autosomal dominant disorder is bilateral but may be asymmetric. It is characterized by endothelial vesicle-like lesions, band lesions, and diffuse opacities that typically occur in the second or third decade but range in severity from asymptomatic and stable to manifesting early, severe corneal edema. These patients may have broad peripheral synechiae and advanced glaucoma.[7]

Specular microscopy is a useful tool in determining the risk of corneal decompensation following cataract surgery. ECD should be above 2,000 cells/mm² in normal adult eyes, but successful cataract surgery may be performed with levels at or below 1,000 depending on the density of the cataract and the surgical technique used.

Helpful Hints

1. Dense central guttae, stromal edema, or a history of a.m. edema are indications for EK combined with cataract surgery. Pachymetry measurements of CCT and specular microscopic measurements of ECD may also be useful.
2. In patients with known endothelial pathology where combined cornea transplant surgery is not being performed, avoid a long CCI to minimize endothelial cell loss, and use a dispersive OVD or a soft shell technique with a pocket of cohesive OVD. Consider supplemental OVD to augment endothelial protection as necessary. Minimize phacoemulsification energy and irrigation as much as possible, and manual-assisted disassembly

Fig. 34.5 Guttae in Fuchs's dystrophy.

techniques (chop, prechop, etc.) are preferred. Femtosecond laser–assisted techniques may also be helpful in selected patients.

Triple Procedures

So-called triple procedures combine keratoplasty with cataract surgery and IOL implantation. Traditionally, penetrating keratoplasty (PK) was necessary to treat significant pathology of any or all corneal layers. Recently, corneal surgery has become more specialized to target replacement of only the diseased corneal layer(s) while preserving healthy recipient layers. Deep anterior lamellar keratoplasty (DALK) and EK techniques including Descemet stripping automated endothelial keratoplasty (DSAEK) and Descemet membrane endothelial keratoplasty (DMEK) have become increasingly popular and more utilized.

Penetrating keratoplasty is still the standard for full-thickness corneal pathology. When combined with cataract surgery, regional block or general anesthesia is preferred and IOL calculations must be based on estimated postoperative corneal curvature after healing and suture removal. Depending on visualization and other factors, cataract extraction may be performed either before (usually phaco through a scleral tunnel) or during (usually manual extracapsular cataract extraction [ECCE] open sky) the actual PK. DALK preserves healthy endothelium but is technically more challenging than PK. Issues surrounding anesthesia and IOL calculations are similar to those in PK. For both PK and DALK, it is often advisable to perform cataract surgery as a subsequent surgery months to years after cornea transplant surgery to achieve the best refractive outcome. Exceptions would include a very dense cataract (limits visualization of posterior segment structures and later removal likely to damage transplant) or the desire to avoid a second surgical procedure.

Endothelial keratoplasty techniques preserve the anterior cornea, are less invasive, heal faster, and may be performed under topical anesthesia. The phaco IOL is performed first, typically through the same temporal CCI used for the EK surgery. IOL calculations are more predictable and accurate in these patients, although preoperative pathology may still contribute to uncertainty.[8] Generally, a myopic adjustment in the IOL power (–1 D for DSAEK and –0.5 D for DMEK) is advisable.

Helpful Hints

1. For combined EK/phaco IOL patients, use a cohesive OVD only to facilitate complete removal of the OVD after IOL placement and limit problems with graft adherence.

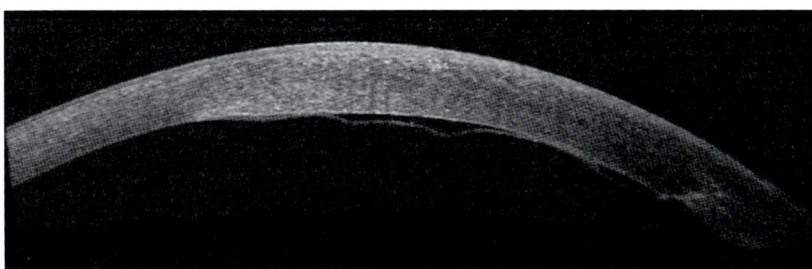

Fig. 34.6 Optical coherence tomography (OCT) of partial Descemet's detachment with overlying corneal thickening due to edema. Note the adjacent clear corneal incision.

2. A smaller capsulorrhexis diameter is preferred for most triple procedures when in-the-bag IOL placement is planned. This will limit movement of the IOL during the air/fluid/pressure shifts encountered during the transplant procedure. Three-piece foldable IOLs may provide more intraoperative stability than single-piece IOLs.

Intraocular Lens Calculations

There are several commercial devices available for biometry and IOL power calculation. In patients with known corneal pathology, especially anterior corneal pathology, caution must be used in interpreting keratometry data from these devices. Correlation with topographic and tomographic corneal mapping is advisable as are multiple measurements at different times to confirm stability before proceeding with surgery. Intraoperative real-time biometry using optical coherence tomography (OCT) imaging and wavefront analysis is an evolving technology, which may be increasingly useful in the future for these patients.

A prior history of refractive surgery poses a unique challenge when it comes to IOL selection, as standard biometry and formulas can be inaccurate. There are several published methods to address this problem, some of which require obtaining prerefractive data and others based purely on preoperative measurements. Online surgical calculators are available (www.ascrs.org) that provide data from the many proposed formulas to facilitate an informed decision. Most importantly in these patients, it is necessary to have multiple, repeatable measurements, and extensive discussion with the patient may be necessary to set appropriate expectations.

Incisions

Well-constructed and thoughtfully placed incisions are key to a successful outcome in cataract surgery. The location of the main wound should be planned carefully to minimize excessive manipulation, which can create striae that decrease visualization or create tears in Descemet's membrane **(Fig. 34.6)**. Striae are also a problem if the intracorneal portion of the incision is too long and enters the anterior chamber (AC) too anteriorly. The stress created on the stroma and endothelium may damage many endothelial cell and lead to postoperative corneal decompensation. In this situation it may be wiser to abandon the incision and create a new one that is appropriate in length and AC entry. The number of times instruments are brought in and out of the eye should be minimized in order avoid stripping Descemet's membrane and chamber depth fluctuations. A wound that is too tight puts the eye at risk for a wound burn, whereas a wound that is too loose risks leakage, chamber shallowing, and surge.

Any time it is anticipated that a wound may need to be enlarged or sutured, such as in a triple procedure, it useful to plan ahead by creating an initial perpendicular limbal groove with a guarded diamond blade. The shelved incision can then be started with the keratome at the base of this groove. The initial perpendicular groove facilitates suture passage and good wound apposition later in the case.

Prior Radial Keratotomy

In the case of prior radial keratotomy, one must avoid passing an incision through the radial scars, as this can cause gaping or leakage of the prior wound, which can add to already irregular astigmatism, increase the risk of infection, and can be difficult to suture closed. Paracentesis placement should be chosen carefully *between* radial cuts such that instruments can be comfortably passed through these with minimal torque and stress on the cornea. If radial incisions are too peripheral and close together to enable clear corneal passage with a paracentesis blade, a scleral tunnel approach can be used. Similarly, when creating a self-sealing shelved main incision, the location should be carefully chosen between radial incisions, paying close attention to how closely spaced the radial incisions are at the most anterior planned aspect of the wound. If there is any question as to whether there is sufficient space to allow for passage, a scleral tunnel incision should be made.

When astigmatism-correcting incisions are made to address corneal astigmatism during cataract surgery, proper technique will help to ensure efficacy and reproducibility. Astigmatic keratotomy or limbal relaxing incisions need to be made down to 80 to 90% depth of the cornea in order for them to achieve the desired effect. It is important to direct the guarded blade perpendicular to the plane of the cornea to ensure adequate depth. Length and optical zone can then be modified based on surgeon nomograms to accomplish appropriate astigmatic correction.

Problems Associated with Astigmatic Keratotomy

Patients are ever more demanding to be emmetropic after cataract surgery, and therefore cataract surgeons increasingly are turning to astigmatic keratotomy, as either limbal relaxing incisions or toric IOL implantation, to mitigate the postoperative astigmatic result. Of the two approaches, limbal relaxing incisions are generally quite forgiving, and with a knife blade set at 600 µm it is hard to perforate or complicate routine cataract cases. However, a large perforation can occur in exceptional cases, such as a subclinical keratoconus where the inferior cornea is thin enough. If in doubt, peripheral pachymetry will provide accurate corneal thickness. Astigmatic keratotomy with the blade set at 80% of the pachymetry will result in perforation at times. Due to the fact that such incisions are often made at the beginning of the procedure, those perforations that otherwise might be self-sealing will not hold during phacoemulsification and may even extend. Therefore, place interrupted 10-0 nylon sutures, radially or even as a mattress suture, to hold the wound together and then remove the sutures at the end of the procedure or the next day if wound integrity is adequate. It is important to remember that incisions perpendicular to the cornea do not have a lip that is self-sealing, and therefore even small perforations sometimes can persist in leaking. There is also no endothelial pump to help out; therefore, it is worth leaving the sutures in a bit longer when wound integrity is a concern. Another approach is 9-0 absorbable Vicryl sutures that will dissolve over time. With buried knots they do not cause problems. In our experience, there is little healing that will negate the effect of the astigmatic keratotomy as long as the sutures are removed within 3 weeks.

Astigmatic keratotomies that are irregular or develop significant epithelial pearls can gape, resulting in significant irregular astigmatism. They occasionally have to be cleaned out and sutured together to gain a regular corneal surface. With topical cases and unexpected eye movement, the resultant tears near the visual axis can result in enough irregular astigmatism where penetrating keratoplasty may be necessary. With appropriate attention to detail, however, all of these complications should be easily avoidable.

Toric IOLs may be helpful to correct astigmatism after prior incisional keratotomy. The authors suggest careful biometry looking for stability between morning and afternoon measurements as diurnal fluctuation of corneal shape is common after radial keratotomy (RK). Toric IOLs should only be used in patients who will not need rigid gas permeable or scleral contact lenses after cataract surgery.

Finally, femtosecond lasers are very effective in achieving precise astigmatic incisions and may be left "unopened" to titrate effect if desired.

Helpful Hints

1. Always use a sharp instrument when creating clear corneal incisions, as a dull blade can initiate a tear in Descemet's membrane.
2. Push slightly posteriorly when inserting instruments into the eye to avoid catching the anterior cut lip of Descemet's membrane.
3. Do not fight a tight wound. Have a low threshold to enlarge a wound facilitate instrument passage. Additionally, if a wound is structurally not ideal or leaking, or if placement is challenging, one can often avoid related complications by suturing the wound and creating a new one.

Corneal Complications After Cataract Surgery

The incidence of lasting corneal edema due to significant endothelial damage in phacoemulsification surgery has decreased as technology and techniques have advanced. Steps must be taken to protect and avoid the endothelium as much as possible during surgery to avoid irreversible injury, especially in susceptible patients such as those with Fuchs dystrophy. Another potential cause of edema in the early postoperative period is toxic anterior-segment syndrome (TASS). Multiple etiologies have been implicated, including intraoperative medication errors and contaminants; thus, surgical and sterilization procedures need to be investigated in depth if TASS is suspected. The edema of TASS is typically profound and diffuse, from limbus to limbus, as opposed to phaco-induced damage, which is often segmental, preferentially involving the wound and horizontal axis. TASS is also associated with elevated IOP and a nonreactive pupil, as the

toxic insult damages all sensitive anterior segment cells. The differential diagnosis includes acute endophthalmitis, which needs to be ruled out.

When pseudophakic corneal edema does occur, initial treatment with topical steroids, aqueous suppressants, and hypertonic saline solutions can alleviate symptoms in the short run. If there is minimal improvement clinically after 6 weeks, patients are unlikely to improve on their own and endothelial keratoplasty is likely necessary. If patients have demonstrated some improvement initially but are still edematous after 3 months, they are also unlikely to improve further and one can proceed with endothelial keratoplasty.

Postoperative edema due to inadvertent detachment of Descemet's membrane, if recognized early, can be managed primarily without keratoplasty. An air bubble or longer lasting gas such as SF6 can be injected into the AC under sterile conditions and the patient positioned supine to attempt reattachment. The pupil should be dilated at the time of the procedure, and if there is any concern about the potential for pupillary block, an inferior peripheral iridotomy may be performed as a preventive measure.

Corneal Refractive Surgery to Correct Residual Refractive Error

Patients' refractive expectations after cataract surgery are higher than they have ever been. Especially when patients are paying out of pocket for astigmatism and presbyopia correcting lenses, residual refractive error may need to be addressed postoperatively. One should wait at least 1 to 3 months to ensure refractive stability before proceeding with any refractive procedure. If the residual error is mostly astigmatism, corneal relaxing incisions may be the simplest and best choice to address the problem. When excimer laser corneal refractive surgery is performed postoperatively, photorefractive keratectomy (PRK) may be a better choice than laser-assisted in situ keratomileusis (LASIK). PRK is less invasive and there is less dry-eye risk. Patients who have undergone cataract surgery are already at increased risk for dry eye due to nerves severed in the creation of incisions. Dry eye can also significantly interfere with best corrected visual acuity in a patient who already has a less than ideal refractive result.

References

1. Mishima S. Corneal thickness. Surv Ophthalmol 1968;13:57–96
2. Nishida T, Saika S. Cornea and sclera: anatomy and physiology. In: Krachmer JH, Mannis MJ, Holland EJ, eds. Cornea. St. Louis: Mosby Elsevier; 2011:3–24
3. Holly FJ, Lemp MA. Tear physiology and dry eyes. Surv Ophthalmol 1977;22:69–87
4. Dua HS, Faraj LA, Said DG, Gray T, Lowe J. Human corneal anatomy redefined: a novel pre-Descemet's layer (Dua's layer). Ophthalmology 2013; 120:1778–1785
5. Laule A, Cable MK, Hoffman CE, Hanna C. Endothelial cell population changes of human cornea during life. Arch Ophthalmol 1978;96:2031–2035
6. Zeev MS, Miller DD, Latkany R. Diagnosis of dry eye disease and emerging technologies. Clin Ophthalmol 2014;8:581–590
7. Weisenthal RW, Streeten BW. Descemet's membrane and endothelial dystrophies. In: Krachmer JH, Mannis MJ, Holland EJ, eds. Cornea. St. Louis: Mosby Elsevier; 2011:845–864
8. Terry MA, Shamie N, Chen ES, et al. Endothelial keratoplasty for Fuchs' dystrophy with cataract: complications and clinical results with the new triple procedure. Ophthalmology 2009;116:631–639

35 Management of Problems with Descemet's Membrane

Randall J. Olson

The basement layer of the corneal endothelium is quite inelastic and extremely strong. It is clearly much thicker and tougher than the anterior capsule, and therefore resistant to tearing in most cases. Nonetheless, tears near the wound or the paracentesis and a significant tearing or stripping of Descemet's with large detachments are not uncommon clinical problems associated with cataract surgery (**Box 35.1**). Like so much else in medicine, prevention is the key in that, just like capsulorrhexis, small tears tend to extend into large tears![1]

To gain access to the anterior chamber (AC) for surgery with a self-sealing incision, phacoemulsification incisions, by definition, cut through Descemet's membrane. A clean cut through Descemet's membrane with a sharp instrument, be it metal or diamond, is one of the keys to avoiding further complications.

Almost all tears occur anterior to the entry wound into the AC. Tears that occur at the time of the incision or paracentesis are almost always due to an instrument or technique failure. One cause is sweeping, either anteriorly or posteriorly, as we start to enter Descemet's membrane. This is easier to do than one might imagine in our creation of a relatively long tunnel and self-sealing incision. With a sharp instrument, even with movement as we enter Descemet's, it is hard to create a tear; therefore, when a tear occurs it is most commonly created by a dull blade, be it diamond or metal. However, reused metal instruments are probably the most common cause (**Fig. 35.1**). If tears occur at the time of the incision or paracentesis, even with a sharp instrument, videotaping the technique so it can be critiqued should help in making changes in the future that obviate this problem. Even small tears are a potentially much bigger problem later.

Most anterior tears are an insertion problem created by catching the anterior Descemet's lip whenever an instrument is inserted into the eye. Due to the small size of the irrigation and aspiration (I/A) tip, it has been our experience that it is difficult to create a tear during this phase, and therefore it usually occurs when the phacoemulsification instrument or intraocular lens (IOL) is inserted into the eye. The unfortunate scenario is a small tear created at either the time of incision or with the phacoemulsification instrument insertion (**Fig. 35.2**) and then significantly extended during phaco, with the movement of the phaco tip or irrigation, or later, with IOL insertion (**Fig. 35.3**). This is also much more common with a very tight wound and difficult insertion at any time.

The following are general rules for avoiding anterior tears

1. Do not create a very tight wound! If insertion is difficult, it is much better to enlarge the wound prior to IOL insertion. An exceedingly tight wound is also a problem in regard to in inflow difficulties (pinching the sleeve), which can result in chamber depth fluctuations and phaco burns! As we torque the instrument inside the

eye, tight wounds also often result in considerable visual distortion due to wrinkling of the cornea; therefore, there is no advantage to an overly tight wound.

2. Insert the phaco instrument parallel to the wound plane. Although this may be self-evident with chambers that have collapsed, it is not uncommon to lift up the instrument to avoid the iris. We think this is a very common way that small anterior tears occur. A little viscoelastic just inside the wound, allowing room to enter the eye parallel to the incision, is one way to avoid

---

Box 35.1   Descemet's Membrane Problems

Prevention
- Use sharp instruments (diamond or new metal) to create incision and incise Descemet's membrane.

Management
- Prevent enlargement during insertion of the phaco tip and the intraocular lens (IOL).
- If the wound is tight, enlarge it.
- If the tear is on one side, enlarge the opposite side. Insert the phaco tip parallel to the wound, but do not lift the tip on insertion.
- Use viscoelastic in the wound to open it and provide room for phaco tip insertion.
- Prior to IOL insertion, enlarge the wound.

Treatment
- Make a single tear on one side of the wound less than 2 mm from the visual axis.
- Irrigate closed through the paracentesis and ignore.
- A double tear will scroll.
- Attempt irrigation; if successful, ignore.
- If unsuccessful, do viscoelastic reattachment.
- Use three full-thickness sutures.
- Leave viscoelastic; treat for potential intraocular pressure (IOP) spike with topical β-blockers and carboxy anhydrase inhibitor (CAO) (Diamox).
- Giant (or more than three quarters of Descemet's membrane detachment) is treated by a 20% sulfur hexafluoride (SSF6) bubble.

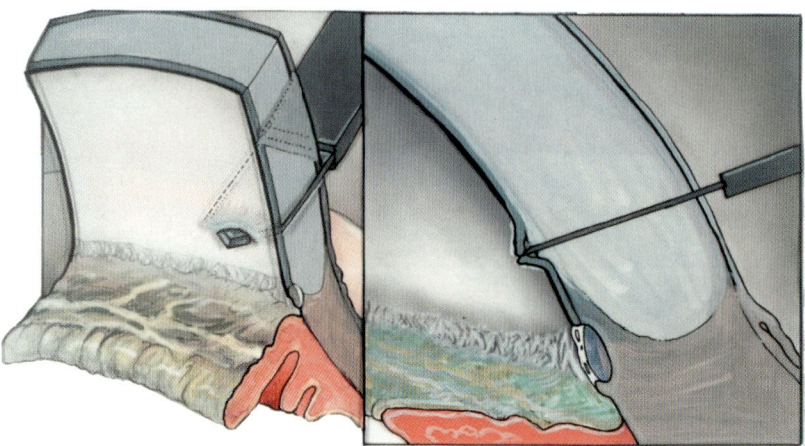

Fig. 35.1   A dull blade piercing Descemet's membrane and pushing it away from the stroma.

this problem, especially when there is a small tear that we do not want to enlarge!

3. Place posterior pressure on the wound or paracentesis. Because catching on the anterior lip is the real problem, it is our practice always to purposely push slightly posteriorly as we enter the wound to avoid putting pressure on that anterior cut edge of Descemet's.

We can often feel the resistance as we enter and engage the anterior Descemet's edge. Relieve this pressure by pushing posteriorly and actually feel Descemet's pop over the front edge of the sleeve, thereby avoiding a tear.

Remember that it is the small tear that becomes the large tear, so we need to be extra cautious if we notice a tear. I find it well worth opening the incision on the side of the wound opposite the tear to avoid additional pressure on that edge with the wound. Now is the time to be extra careful about each maneuver as we go through the wound to avoid extending this tear.

Creating a tear with IOL insertion also comes from trying to put too large a lens through too small a wound. Videotapes of insertion techniques in which surgeons seesaw their way through an extremely tight wound demonstrate that is a potential recipe for a large tear disaster. Generally, even under these circumstances, just a small tear is created, and a large tear occurring means there has already been a small one in place. All the previous rules already mentioned apply, but in particular be concerned about the overly tight wound. It only takes a second if the wound is too tight to enlarge it slightly.

What do we do when we already have a tear and therefore it is too late for prevention? At our center, we have found that most

often it is a single tear on one edge of the wound (**Fig. 35.4**), and as long as it is more than 2 mm from the visual axis, we have been able to irrigate it closed through the stab incision using balanced salt solution at the end of the procedure. It always looks fine the next day, and the endothelial pump will keep the tear attached. The only damage done under these circumstances is usually to the surgeon's ego, except for the fact that such wounds do not "self-seal" as easily, and, rarely, they also require a suture.

A double tear on both ends of the wound is fortunately harder to create but unfortunately presents a bigger problem (**Fig. 35.5**). Often one side of the tear will scroll up near the visual axis, and a single tear into the visual axis also acts in a similar way with some scrolling so that it will not easily irrigate into place. Such wounds rarely self-seal. If, however, we can irrigate the flap closed with a self-sealing wound, and it stays this way for a couple of minutes after the procedure, we still do nothing else, and it is fine the next day. Fortunately, we have not had a Descemet's tear that looks fine at the table but has been a problem the next day. However, those cases with extensive scroll detachment that will not irrigate into place require a definitive treatment on the surgical table (**Fig. 35.6**).[2]

One approach is using an ophthalmic viscosurgical device (OVD) to hold the torn area into position against the cornea (**Fig. 35.7**). Although OVD is certainly effective, it is a double-edged sword. If we are not careful, we can get the OVD between Descemet's and the stroma, and then achieving resolution on the table is exceedingly difficult.[3] Vigorous I/A to try to remove the sub-Descemet's viscoelastic can create considerable endothelial damage, and under such circumstances very gentle I/A, allowing time for the OVD to reabsorb on its own, is best. Spontaneous

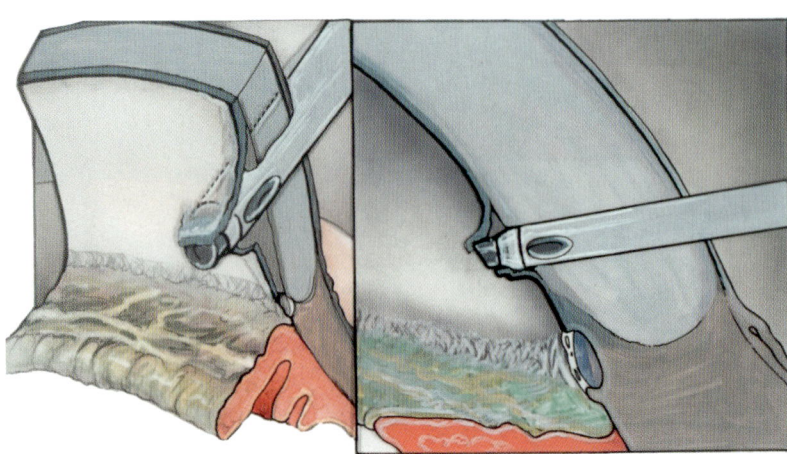

Fig. 35.2   A phaco tip catches a defect in Descemet's membrane. This can enlarge during the to-and-fro movement during phacoemulsification.

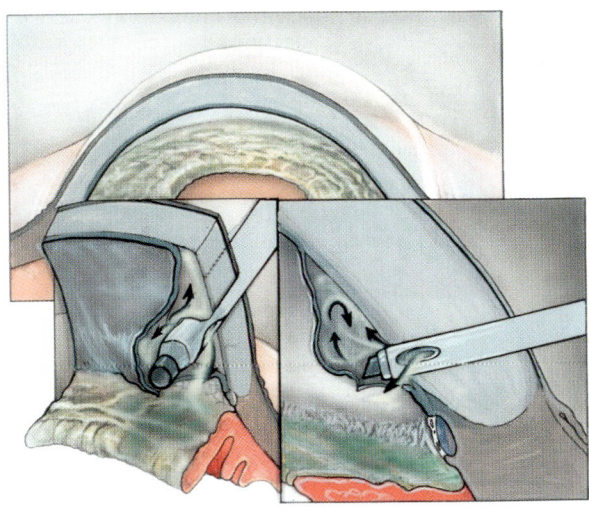

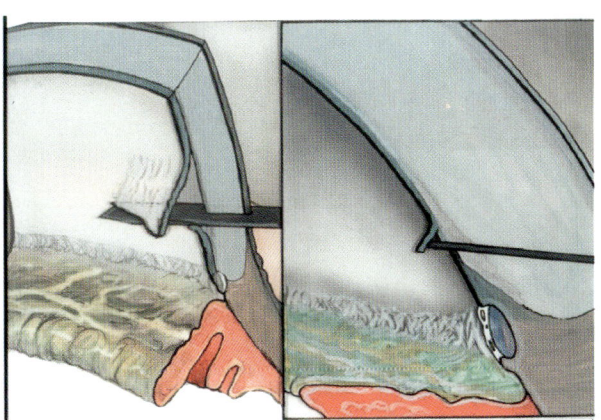

Fig. 35.4 The blade creates a single tear in Descemet's membrane.

Fig. 35.3 When irrigation is applied, irrigant flows into the cleavage plane between Descemet's membrane and the stroma. This is one scenario that may lead to a large or giant Descemet's detachment.

Fig. 35.5 The blade creates a double tear in Descemet's membrane.

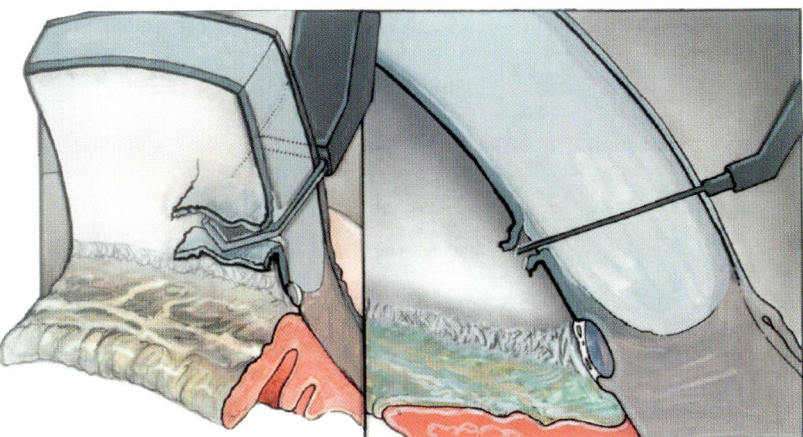

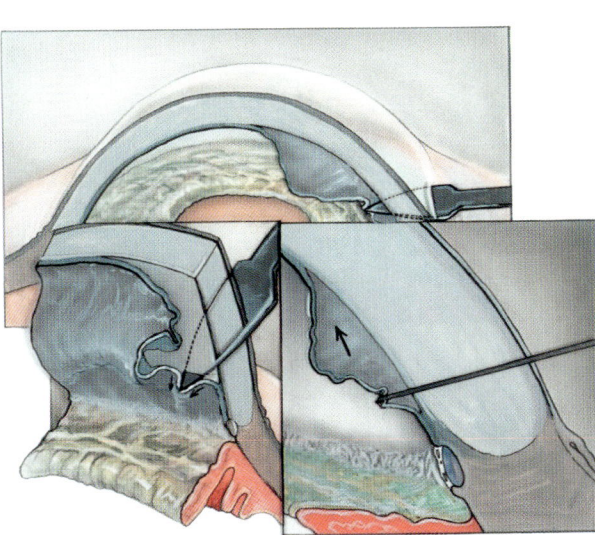

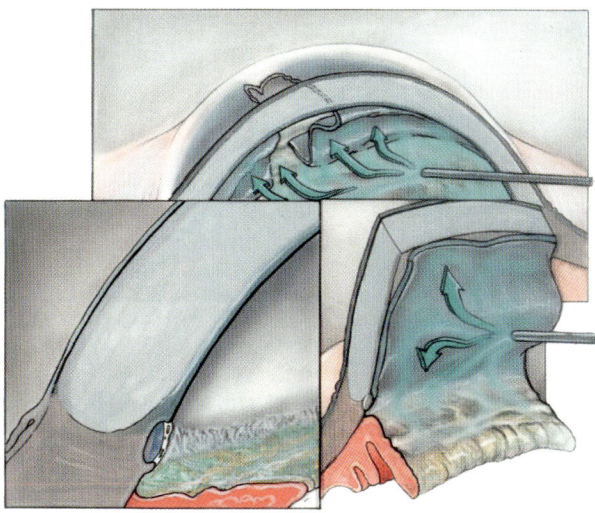

Fig. 35.7 Dispersive viscoelastic is applied to unscroll Descemet's membrane and force it into proximity with the stroma. Care must be taken to inject viscoelastic away from the tear, forcing Descemet's *against* the stroma, rather than allowing viscoelastic to insinuate itself *between* Descemet's and the stroma.

Fig. 35.6 The beginning of a giant tear. The torn Descemet's will not irrigate into place.

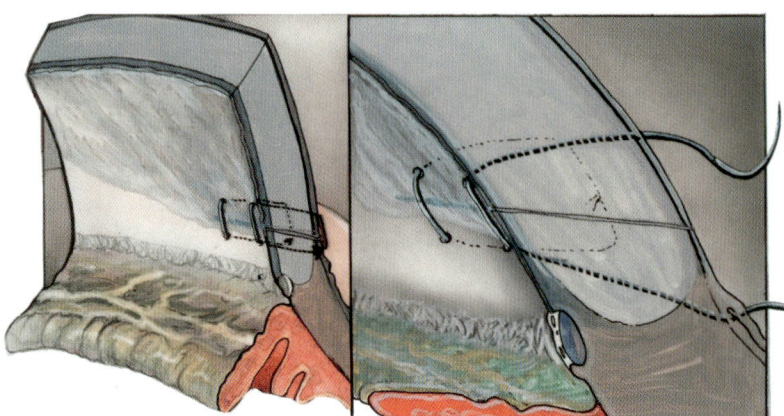

Fig. 35.8 Viscoelastic is unsuccessful. Two full-thickness sutures have been placed to hold Descemet's membrane in place.

reattachment without needing an additional surgical procedure is still common in such cases.

Ophthalmic viscosurgical device reattachment requires starting inside the scrolled Descemet's with a very small amount of OVD and slowly adding OVD to roll Descemet's back into position. Under all such circumstances, depending on the size of the tear, we place one to three full-thickness sutures to hold Descemet's in place near the wound to avoid recurrence of the scroll. We use a reverse bite on the posterior edge of the wound, and then bring the needle out of the wound. A second bite starting in the wound should be full thickness through Descemet's and the stroma (**Fig. 34.8**). One suture is often enough in combination with the viscoelastic holding things in place. Leaving a fair amount of OVD in the eye can result in significant IOP elevation, and Viscoat (Alcon, Fort Worth, TX), in our hands, has been more forgiving under these circumstances. We automatically administer topical β blockers and oral carbonic/anhydrase inhibitors to these patients until we know what the pressure is the next day. Taking these extra steps has resulted in no long-term problems with Descemet's detachment in our practice.

Air could also be used in place of viscoelastic, and it has the advantage that it can be removed if it is incorrectly placed. Longer-lasting gases have also been used to hold Descemet's in place and avoid the sutures. The head position is critical, which is not easy for all patients, and all of the gases, including air,[4] are endothelial toxic to some degree. We still find reattachment with a few full-thickness sutures the best approach when Descemet's does not stay in place by irrigation alone.

Complete Descemet's Detachment

Fortunately, we have not had the inauspicious situation where the entire, or almost the entire, Descemet's membrane detaches during a surgical procedure. We have had an experience in corneal transplantation where Descemet's membrane was so loosely attached that it was left in the AC inadvertently. However, rarely a large or complete Descemet's detachment may uncommonly occur, and it seems to be an exceedingly unusual patient variation. This condition is very easy to recognize, with Descemet's ballooning into the AC and visualization becoming difficult shortly thereafter (**Fig. 35.9a**). I have heard accounts of an unsuspecting surgeon seeing this membrane, assuming it is an edge of the capsule, and pulling an entire Descemet's out of the eye.

A total detachment often happens early in the procedure. However, it can start as a small separation and extend during the procedure. Sutures alone are a very difficult way to handle such a profound detachment, and air often does not last long enough to

hold Descemet's in place before reattachment occurs. The intracameral injection of 20% sulfur hexafluoride (SF6) gas filling the AC approximately half full, with expansion occurring later, is often a better way to make sure there is contact long enough for the normal pumping mechanism of the endothelium to resolve this problem.[5,6] The injection is performed by filling a tuberculin (TB) syringe with 20% SF6 and injecting with a 30 gauge needle through a de novo injection site. Be sure to pass the needle through or under the detached Descemet's membrane (**Fig. 35.9b**).[7,8]

If SF6 is not immediately available, we use air to fill the AC.[1] On the first postoperative day, examination reveals if this initial treatment is adequate. If it is not, severe corneal edema and the floating Descemet's membrane, or a space between Descemet's and stroma, would be apparent. We then use 20% SF6. In the operating room, as a sterile procedure, we inject a half AC volume bubble with a 27-gauge needle on a 3-cc syringe. The needle is passed directly into the AC without a paracentesis to prevent escape of the gas. If necessary, prior to gas injection, a small amount of OVD can be injected adjacent to the AC needle entry site to act as a cork preventing egress of the SF6 gas. The patient must be examined the next day, as the SF6 gas bubble will increase dramatically in size and may cause severe elevation of IOP. It will also, however, push Descemet's against the stroma, so that the endothelial pump may become active and generate a pressure gradient holding Descemet's in place. If the IOP is too high, a small amount of gas can be released through a paracentesis. However, only a sufficient amount of gas to lower the IOP should be released so that enough remains to continue to put pressure on Descemet's. Daily observation and gas release on an as-needed basis should be performed for 1 week. The SF6 gas will then resorb.[10,11]

A large Descemet's detachment is a most uncommon problem, but one that is vital to recognize. If it occurs early, continuing with irrigation under these circumstances could result in an even greater trauma. Therefore, upon early recognition, the cataract procedure should be aborted. If this is impossible, a dry cataract removal should be done under OVD with as little I/A forces as possible.

We should keep in mind that if there is a large Descemet's detachment and it does not appear to be repairable, after a short period of observation a *Descemet's membrane endothelial keratoplasty* (DMEK) or Descemet's stripping automated endothelial keratoplasty (DSAEK) can be performed. This will undoubtedly solve the problem and salvage excellent postoperative visual acuity.

Many smaller detachments are not noticed until the first postoperative day. Small scroll tears that are not near the visual axis usually can be handled conservatively and will resolve on their own. Even with large tears we wait at least 1 week to see if

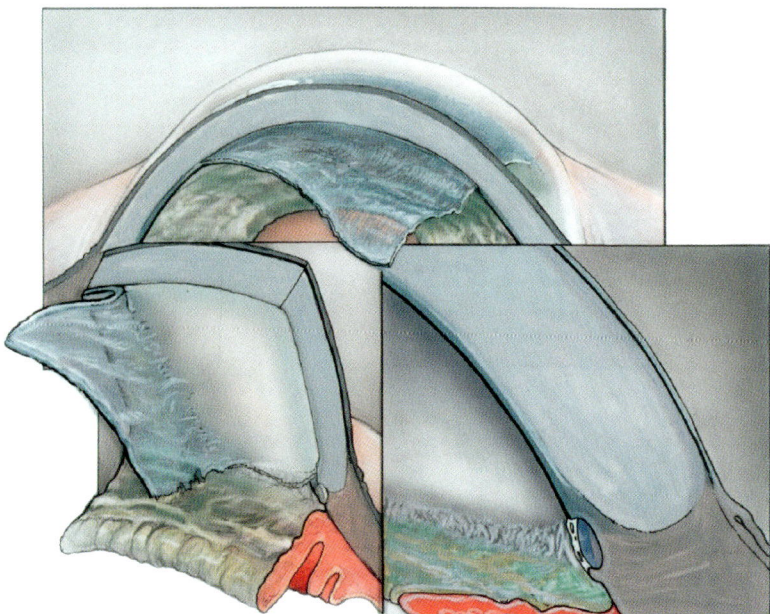

Fig. 35.9 **(a)** A giant tear. Descemet's membrane billows in the anterior chamber, and the cornea becomes hazy due to the loss of the barrier effect of Descemet's and subsequent corneal hydration. **(b)** Sulfur hexafluoride (SF6) gas is placed in the anterior chamber, half filling it. The gas bubble will expand and push Descemet's in proximity to the stroma.

a

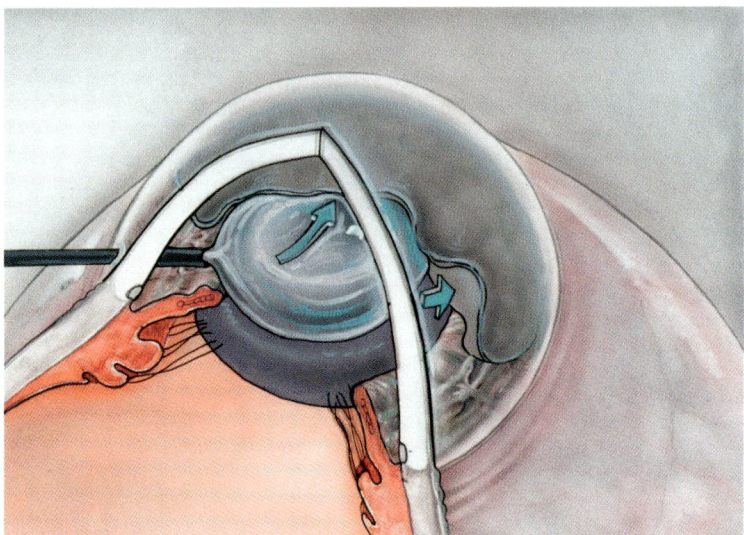

b

they are resolving, as many will spontaneously move back into position. Generally, by 2 weeks if there is no resolution, it is easy to unscroll them using either air or a viscoelastic with a few strategically placed full-thickness sutures through a stab incision. We see no reason to put the patient through any more agony to take care of this problem. An ounce of prevention is worth a pound of cure in how we handle small tears. We must fix them on the operating table if they are significant!

References

1. Zeiter HJ, Zeiter JT. Descemet's membrane separation during five hundred forty-four intraocular lens implantations. 1975–1982. J Am Intraocul Implant Soc 1983;9:36–39

2. Assia EI, Levkovich-Vebin H, Blumenthal M. Management of Descemet's membrane detachment. J Cataract Refract Surg 1995;21:714–717

3. Ostberg A, Tornqvist G. Management of detachment of Descemet's membrane caused by injection of hyaluronic acid. Ophthalmic Surg 1989;20:885–886

4. Olson RJ. Air and the corneal endothelium: a cat in vivo study. Arch Ophthalmol 1980;98:1283–1284

5. Kremer I, Stiebel H, Yassur Y, Weinberger D. Sulfur hexafluoride injection for Descemet's membrane detachment in cataract surgery. [see comments] J Cataract Refract Surg 1997;23:1449–1453

6. Gault JA, Raber IM. Repair of Descemet's membrane detachment with intracameral injection of 20% sulfur hexafluoride gas. Cornea 1996;15:483–489

7. Macsai M. Total detachment of Descemet's membrane after small-incision cataract extraction. Am J Ophthalmol 1992;114:355–366

8. Amaral CE, Palay DA. Technique for repair of Descemet membrane detachment. Am J Ophthalmol 1999;127:88–90

9. Sparks GM. Descemetopexy surgical reattachment of stripped Descemet's Membrane. Arch Ophthalmol 1967;78(1):31–34

10. Marcon AS, Rapuano CJ, Jones MR, Laibson PR, Cohen EJ. Descemet's membrane detachment after cataract surgery: management and outcome. Ophthalmology 2002;109:2325–2330

11. Mahmood MA, Teichmann KD, Tomey KF, Al-Rashed D. Detachment of Descemet's membrane. J Cataract Refract Surg 1998;24:827–823

36 Ultrasound-Induced Thermal Incision Contracture

Randall J. Olson

An incision burn is a complication that is infrequent but can be devastating. I have seen video examples of severe wound burns that happened within three seconds of the introduction of ultrasound, and yet resulted in such profound scarring that, even with a partial transplant in the area of the burn, vision did not return to 20/20 even a year after the surgery. Because we generally look at the phacoemulsification tip during surgery, our first indication of an incision burn are the corneal folds from the thermal contraction that have made their way into the central cornea, obscure our view, and make us realize we have a major problem on our hands (**Fig. 36.1**).

Studying the Problem

Our in vitro work over the years points to a temperature of 60°C at the incision site as the level at which a second or two is enough for a wound burn to start to form. It is important to understand that this is not really a burn or an oxidative change as such, but rather is what happens to collagen once it reaches ~ 60°C; there is a contracture of the collagen, which has been used in the past to contract the cone in keratoconus prior to keratoplasty. This contracture starts as a focal change and extends, if the heat source is maintained, to the point of substantial blurring of the central cornea as well as induction of huge amounts of astigmatism. One case referred to me had over 20 diopters of induced irregular astigmatism! So clearly it is important to understand this process and strive to do all we can to avoid it.

I first became very interested in this problem when claims were being made about different thermal properties of phaco machines that simply did not make sense. What was claimed did not follow the laws of thermodynamics, and so I became curious about understanding the thermal properties of phacoemulsification instruments. Everyone agreed that wound burns were due to ultrasound-induced heat change in the incision. With an ultrasound needle having a peak velocity of about 50 miles per hour, even though the length it travels is very short, friction is generated very rapidly. To demonstrate, lightly squeeze a vibrating phaco needle between your fingertips to realize how fast it can get hot.

Our first major publication on this subject showed that the percentage of power was not a constant that you could use to compare one machine to another[1] (**Fig. 36.1**). Looking at the three common machines available at the time, and performing the experiment in saline solution (some earlier work had even been done in air, which made no sense at all), we found that Legacy (Alcon, Fort Worth, TX) at 100% power produced the same heat that Sovereign (Abbott Medical Optics [AMO], Abbott Park, IL) did at 43% power and Millennium (Bausch and Lomb, Rochester, NY) did at 36% power. Therefore, any comparisons without understanding this difference made very little sense.

Additional work demonstrated that the machines also behaved quite differently when there was a load in place[2] (**Table 36.1**). Just going from air to water dramatically changes the load; however, we further used weight on the sleeve, thereby creating increased friction on the tip, just as a tight incision would do, or in trying to phacoemulsify a hard nuclear fragment, and here the clear outlier was Legacy, which had an eightfold increase in its overall heat production over that of Sovereign and Millennium. In fact, with a load, the total heat generated by Legacy exceeded at the same power setting what Sovereign and Millennium created. Thus, it became clear that a stroke-protected machine such as Legacy acts like a cruise control in a car such that if you set it for 50 miles per hour, you will have very little energy needed to go downhill and a lot of energy to go uphill. In contrast, Millennium and Sovereign and most machines today are more like a gas pedal—you push the pedal a certain distance down and then the energy created is the same so you would race downhill and then go more slowly uphill. We surmised that this potentially was a wound burn risk for Legacy, because the surge in power would occur without any movement of the foot peddle and would occur at the riskiest time—when there was a lot of friction on the phaco needle or a hard nuclear fragment was being removed, often associated with occlusion of flow through the needle tip.

All of this early work also showed that the riskiest step we take is when we block fluid flow through the tip and engage long runs of ultrasound, such as when we have impaled and are removing a nuclear fragment. Heat buildup to near 60°C was not possible without blocking flow, but we could rapidly meet and exceed this temperature with the loss of the cooling effect of fluid flow. So we surmised that long runs of ultrasound with a hard nuclear fragment that also blocks the flow of fluid is the main cause of incision burns.

More recently, we have seen entirely new ultrasound modalities in the marketplace where the needle tip subtends an arc (OZil [Alcon] or torsional phaco) or an ellipse (Ellips [AMO] or transversal phaco). Claims were made that these types of tip action essentially prevented the risk of wound burn, and all studies to date show a dramatic decrease in frictional heat generation. So is that the end of the story and the end of wound burns?

Looking at this in more detail, we measured the heat generated, especially looking at metal stress heat generated from the wagging motion of the tip[3] (**Table 36.2**). We were able to document that there was heat generated in the direction of the tip motion, and then compared it to the same amount of power with the same machine with continuous as well as micropulsed (6 ms on and 12 ms off) longitudinal ultrasound. We found, as did others, that continuous longitudinal ultrasound created three times or more heat than torsional, but micropulsed ultrasound created less heat, being on only a third of the time when compared with continuous longitudinal ultrasound. Repeating this experiment

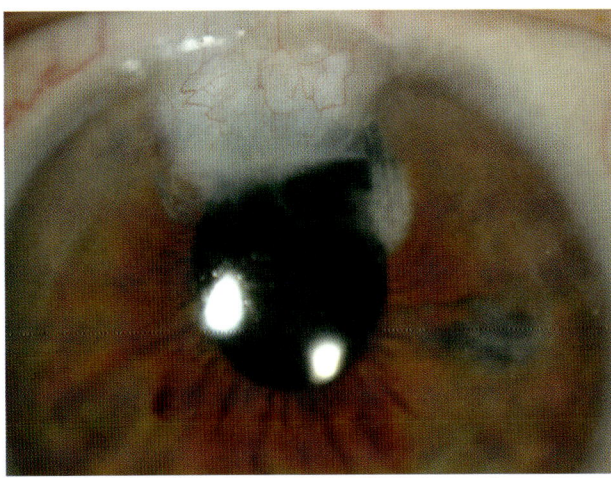

Fig. 36.1   A wound burn a year after the procedure. (Courtesy of Jorge Alio, Professor and Chairman of Ophthalmology, Universidad Miguel Hernandez, Alicante, Spain.)

Table 36.1   Temperature Increase (in Centigrade) at 1 Minute Per 20% Increment of Power Increase (40% Divided by 2, 60% by 3) for Four Phacoemulsification Machines with 20 mL/min of Free Flow (n = 25 for Each Category)

Machines	Unweighted	Weighted	Ratio of Weighted/ Unweighted
Millennium	5.67 ± 0.51	6.80 ± 0.80	1.20[b]
Sovereign	4.59 ± 0.70	5.65 ± 0.72	1.23[b]
Infiniti	2.79 ± 0.62	3.96 ± 0.31[a]	1.42[c]
Legacy	1.99 ± 0.49	4.27 ± 0.76[a]	2.15[c]

Source: Sovereign and Legacy data from Brinton JP, Adams W, Kumar R, Olson RJ. Comparison of thermal features associated with 2 phacoemulsification machines. J Cataract Refract Surg 2006;32:288–293.
[a]p = 0.06.
[b]p = 0.34.
[c]p = 0.0016.
Note: $p < 0.0001$ for all unweighted versus weighted comparisons. The weight used was 200 g.

Table 36.2   Thermal Comparison of Infiniti OZil and Signature Ellips: Comparative Ratios of Temperature Increases

Category	Position (Degrees)	Ultrasound Setting	Aspiration	Ratios
OZil/Ellips	0	Continuous	Unblocked	1.57
OZil/Ellips	90	Continuous	Unblocked	1.53
OZil/Ellips	180	Continuous	Unblocked	1.55
OZil/Ellips	270	Continuous	Unblocked	1.50
OZil/Ellips	0	Continuous	Blocked	2.49
OZil/Ellips	90	Continuous	Blocked	2.33
Ellips/Signature	0	Cont/Micropulse	Unblocked	0.87
Ellips/Signature	90	Cont/Micropulse	Unblocked	0.83
Ellips/Signature	0	Cont/Micropulse	Blocked	0.56
Ellips/Signature	90	Cont/Micropulse	Blocked	0.56
OZil/Signature	0	Cont/Micropulse	Unblocked	1.36
OZil/Signature	90	Cont/Micropulse	Unblocked	1.26
OZil/Signature	0	Cont/Micropulse	Blocked	1.39
OZil/Signature	90	Cont/Micropulse	Blocked	1.31
Signature/OZil	0	Continuous	Unblocked	2.57
Signature/Ellips	0	Continuous	Unblocked	4.03

Source: Schmutz JS, Olson RJ. Thermal comparison of Infiniti OZil and Signature Ellips phacoemulsification systems. Am J Ophthalmol 2010;149:762–7.e1. Reprinted by permission.
Note: Micropulse is 6 milliseconds on/12 milliseconds off. All results are $p < 0.0001$.

with fluid flow blocked showed that torsional heat could rise to levels where wound burns were possible. Clearly, therefore, blockage is a key concern, and even though the horizontal motion associated with torsional creates about one third the heat of continuous longitudinal ultrasound, if it were used consistently at a very high power, and longitudinal ultrasound were used at a much lower power setting, which we felt was the more likely clinical scenario, then there may not be any wound burn protection with torsional ultrasound as it was currently being used.

Another key element had to be the efficiency with which we are using ultrasound energy. Some surgical approaches use mainly mechanical energy in which no heat is produced and very little ultrasound energy is used. We suggested that such approaches should be protective of wound burn. Furthermore, we have had a chance to study in some detail just what makes a phaco machine more efficient in the cataract removal process.[4,5] From this particular combination of work, we have been able to discover many variables in association with efficiency—all of which suggests that how the machines operate, the parameters chosen, and the cataract surgical approach are all potentially important factors in wound burn creation.

Another important clinical consideration gleaned from studies using thermography of the incision site during surgery showed that temperatures close to the "cliff" of wound burn (60°C) are not uncommon, and there is no clinical clue that we are nearing the cliff. So we are blindfolded and wandering near a cliff that we can only appreciate once we are actually falling off (a wound burn occurs). Using this cliff analogy and without any simple means of removing this blindfold, it only makes sense to do all we can to stay as far from this cliff as possible. We can't fall off a cliff if we never get close!

An additional important finding had to do with the role of viscoelastics in the creation of wound burns. Videos have documented that such burns can happen in a matter of seconds after applying ultrasound! A possible explanation is that the viscoelastic could block fluid flow through the needle, but the rapidity with which these wound burns have occurred simply cannot be explained by just fluid blockage. This was a mystery that had to be unraveled. So we studied different viscoelastics in an artificial chamber and compared them to the heat generated with saline solution with flow through the needle blocked.[6] Incredibly, we found that all viscoelastics were variably exothermic when ultrasound is applied when compared with saline solution. These heat generation ratios when compared with that of saline were on the low side, with Healon GV (AMO) 2.4 to 7.1 times that of Viscoat (Alcon) **(Table 36.3)**. This would mean that when you combine both this exothermic factor with the loss of fluid flow, you could reach wound burn temperatures in a matter of a couple of seconds, which is exactly what we have seen clinically. So clearly, viscoelastics would also appear to be a potential major risk for incision burn creation.

All of this work was theoretical and did not pinpoint the actual clinical factors related to, or the incidence of, wound burn. We had too many potential variables to ever discern the clinical basis of wound burns in prospective clinical studies, and with no clue as to the incidence, it would be impossible to power such a study. So we felt our best next step was a clinical survey. Surveys looking at absolute numbers of cases is always problematic, as they are based on a guess as to the number of cases; however, we were confident that surgeons would not forget a wound burn that they had in their clinical practice, so we felt that comparative ratios would be valid. Our first survey **(Table 36.4)** reported on 75 wound burns from a projected total of 75,000 surgeries, for an incidence of 1 in 1,000.[7] We were able to determine that the vast majority of them (53) occurred during fragment removal, which supports exactly what we felt was the riskiest moment,

Table 36.3 Table Comparison of Heat Buildup for Different Viscoelastics During Ultrasound as a Ratio Where Heat Buildup for Balanced Salt Solution Is Given a Value of 1.0

Ophthalmic Viscosurgical Device	Power	Legacy Ratio	Sovereign Ratio
Viscoat	20%	1.90	7.14[a]
	40%	3.53	6.30[a]
Healon5	20%	2.97	3.86[b]
	40%	3.25	5.20[a]
Provisc	20%	1.71	4.00[c]
	40%	2.25	3.87[d]
Vitrax	20%	2.31[e]	2.88
	40%	2.25	3.72[b]
Healon GV	20%	1.57[f]	2.26
	40%	2.11	2.38[b]
Healon	20%	1.52	1.98
	40%	1.64	3.56
Amvisc Plus	20%	1.51	1.70[g]
	40%	1.95	2.77

Source: Floyd M, Valentine J, Coombs J, Olson RJ. Effect of incisional friction and ophthalmic viscosurgical devices on the heat generation of ultrasound during cataract surgery. J Cataract Refract Surg 2006; 32:1222–1226. Reprinted by permission.
[a]20-second comparison.
[b]40-second comparison.
[c]50-second comparison.
[d]30-second comparison.
[e]$p = 0.004$.
[f]$p = 0.008$.
[g]$p = 0.002$.
Note: Except where specified, comparisons are with 60-second data and p-values less than 0.0001 when comparing Legacy and Sovereign.

and that is when the port of the needle is occluded and there is no cooling going on inside of the needle.

We were also able to determine that there was a significant difference in incidence among the Sovereign, Millennium, and Legacy machines commonly used at that time, with a 0.12% incidence with Legacy, 0.056% with Sovereign, and 0.038% with Millennium ($p = 0.014$). Obviously, there were many other factors we know we had to look at before we could say the machines created a differential risk.

We also were able to show that a surgeon's approach was very protective, with the chop technique decreasing the overall incidence in comparison with the divide-and-conquer technique or the Carousel technique by four- to fivefold. This certainly supported our hypothesis that approaches relying more on mechanical forces were protective. Looking at the type of ultrasound used, and remember this was before either torsional or transversal ultrasound was available, we found that micropulsed longitudinal ultrasound was protective in comparison with burst, pulse,

Table 36.4 Survey Response Rates and Phacoemulsification Wound Burn Rates as Reported by Surgical Approach, Phacoemulsification Unit, and Usual Settings

	Surgeries	Wound Burns	Wound Burn Rate (per 1,000)
Surgical approach:			
Divide and conquer	41,125	53	1.29
Carousel	10,057	12	1.19
Horizontal chop	11,359	7	0.62
Vertical chop	11,554	3	0.26
Other	2,487	0	0
1 versus 3 ($p = 0.003$),[a] 2 versus 3 ($p = 0.009$)[b]			
Phaco unit:			
Legacy	46,416	54	1.16
Millennium	5,140	2	0.39
Sovereign	20,885	11	0.56
Other	4,141	8	1.93
1 versus 2 ($p = 0.014$)[c]			
Unit setting:			
Continuous	23,899	42	1.76
Pulse	8,685	12	1.38
Burst	18,588	16	0.86
White Star	19,260	5	0.26
1 versus 3 ($p = 0.013$),[d] 1 versus 4 ($p < 0.0001$),[e] 2 versus 4 ($p = 0.0004$),[f] 3 versus 4 ($p = 0.013$)[g]			

Source: Bradley MJ, Olson RJ. A survey about phacoemulsification incision thermal contraction incidence and causal relationships. Am J Ophthalmol 2006;141:222–224. Reprinted by permission.
[a]Divide and conquer versus vertical chop,
[b]Carousel versus vertical chop.
[c]Legacy versus sovereign.
[d]Cont versus pulse.
[e]Cont versus white star.
[f]Pulse versus white star.
[g]Burst versus white star.

or continuous longitudinal ultrasound and in a highly significant fashion. Although a multivariate analysis did not show anything independently significant, micropulsed longitudinal ultrasound and vertical chop came out as the two most likely factors to protect against would burn.

Hating to leave so many questions unanswered, the decision was made to undertake a much larger study that would be Web based in both the United States and Canada. We felt that we needed to expand the number of incision burns by a factor of at least five, and therefore we decided we ought to look at a million surgical cases to see if we could better understand this problem. Fortunately, we were able to get 910 surgeons to report on 419 incision burns in 963,543 surgeries. This study **(Table 36.5)** for

the first time gave us a detailed understanding of not only the incidence but also the risk.[8] The first survey was conducted in 2005, and the most recent survey was conducted in 2009 at a time when torsional ultrasound was commonly used.

Determining the Significant Factors

We now had enough power to complete a thorough multivariate analysis. We found that the most significant independent factor correlated with wound burn was surgical volume ($p < 0.0001$). This was an inverse relationship, meaning that the busier the surgeon, the less likely there was going to be an incision burn. Although the study itself could not look at this specific issue in

Table 36.5 Multivariate Analyses: Adjusted Rates and 95% Confidence Intervals

Variable	Adjusted Rate	Lower CL	Upper CL
Machine/power setting			
Legacy continuous	0.354	0.151	0.828
Signature hyperpulse	0.333	0.074	1.505
Millennium continuous	0.198	0.052	0.753
Infiniti continuous	0.196	0.077	0.499
Millennium pulse	0.191	0.065	0.563
Infiniti OZil longitudinal	0.185	0.097	0.354
Legacy burst	0.150	0.037	0.617
Sovereign hyperpulse	0.149	0.068	0.325
Millennium burst	0.112	0.011	1.131
Legacy OZil	0.106	0.033	0.345
Infiniti OZil	0.105	0.053	0.209
Infiniti burst	0.101	0.028	0.366
Legacy pulse	0.083	0.022	0.316
Infiniti pulse	0.082	0.021	0.318
Legacy OZil longitudinal	0.082	0.033	0.201
Millennium hyperpulse	0.043	0.003	0.696
Ophthalmic viscosurgical device			
Healon 5	1.349	0.338	5.382
Ocucoat	0.275	0.068	1.119
Duovisc/Viscoat	0.197	0.112	0.345
Provisc	0.172	0.076	0.391
Discovisc	0.114	0.046	0.285
Amvisc Plus	0.102	0.040	0.260
Amvisc	0.051	0.012	0.216
Healon GV	0.046	0.009	0.240
Healon	0.042	0.010	0.171
Approach			
Divide and conquer	0.326	0.198	0.537
Carousel	0.315	0.109	0.915
Stop and chop	0.216	0.121	0.386
Vertical chop	0.102	0.049	0.212
Phaco flip	0.082	0.028	0.245
Horizontal chop	0.067	0.023	0.189
Prechop	0.063	0.008	0.516

Table 36.5   (*Continued*)

Variable	Adjusted Rate	Lower CL	Upper CL
Incision size			
2.40 mm or less	0.140	0.069	0.285
2.41 mm or greater	0.129	0.073	0.228
Region			
Canada	0.181	0.081	0.404
Southeast US	0.141	0.070	0.284
West US	0.120	0.063	0.225
Northeast US	0.106	0.055	0.205

Abbreviation: CL, confidence level.
Source: Sorensen T, Chan CC, Bradley M, Braga-Mele R, Olson RJ. Ultrasound-induced corneal incision contracture survey in the United States and Canada. J Cataract Refract Surg 2012;38:227–233. Reprinted by permission.
Note: Shown are adjusted rates of reported incision contracture for each indicated factor in a multivariate analysis of 618 surgeons. This analysis included machine/setting combination, ophthalmic viscosurgical device, approach, incision size, and region as predictor variables. Surgery volume ($F = 36.25$, $p < 0.001$), approach ($F = 4.8$, $p < 0.001$), and viscoelastic ($F = 2.8$, $p = 0.004$) but not machine/power setting combination ($F = 1.3$, $p = 0.20$), region ($F = 1.0$, $p = 0.40$) or incision size ($F = 0.1$, $p = 0.75$) were independent predictors of reported incision contracture. Each doubling of surgery volume was independently associated with a 45% (95% confidence interval 38% to 55%) reduction in the incidence of reported thermal incision contracture. After adjusting for each factor listed in the table, the incidence of reported incision contracture varied significantly among the surgeons ($p < 0.001$).

any greater detail, it is apparent that those who do a lot of surgeries learn to be efficient, and efficient use of ultrasound makes it less likely that prolonged use of ultrasound will be the result. There is no reason why all surgeons cannot take the same approach; clearly, the important point here is to understand that wound burn risk is associated with the use of ultrasound and that we should be as parsimonious as possible wit its use, especially with long runs with the phaco tip blocked.

The second significant independent factor was the surgical approaches utilized, which confirmed not only our earlier work, as well as our smaller survey, but also provided greater detail. So when looking at burn rates adjusted for other significant factors, we found that the divide-and-conquer technique had an incidence of ~ 0.33 per 1,000 cases, the Carousel technique had an incidence of 0.32, and the stop-and-chop technique somewhere right in the middle with an adjusted rate of 0.22, whereas the different chopping approaches all gave us a rate of between 0.06 to 0.1 wound burns per thousand. This was high statistically significant ($p = 0.0001$) and clearly supports that fact that the more mechanical force we use during surgery, the less likely wound burn is to occur. In fact, I submit that if one is very careful using mechanical forces in the chop technique that I call ultrasound-assisted phacoaspiration, then incision burn is essentially impossible as long as we avoid our third significant independent factor.

The third significant independent factor was the use of viscoelastics. Indeed, very early onset wound burn, which can happen in a matter of seconds, correlates completely with using ultrasound within an anterior chamber full of viscoelastic. Our findings here correlated extremely well with the two factors we thought were important with viscoelastic-induced wound burns: the ability of the viscoelastic to block any fluid flow through the bore of the needle, and its exothermic effect. We found Healon 5 was the worst offender, which had a burn rate of 1.35 per 1,000

surgeries, compared with Healon, which had an incidence of 0.04 per 1,000. This is a huge range of incision burn incidence, with other viscoelastics falling somewhere in between. The critical point to remember in regard to viscoelastic-associated wound burn that it is 100% preventable. All it takes is a few seconds to create a wound burn and just 10 to 15 seconds to prevent one! Take this time to aspirate all viscoelastic over the dome of the lens so that phacoemulsification occurs in a pool of balanced salt solution free from any viscoelastic. This is a simple habit to form and a habit that can absolutely prevent a severe burn right at the start of the procedure.

Interestingly, when everything is adjusted for, we did not find a statistically significant difference between any of the machines or in any ultrasound modulation. Although Legacy again seemed to be an outlier on the high side, even after adjusting for surgical volume, the difference was not significant in a multivariate analysis. This was also the case in regard to ultrasound modulation. We found that neither micropulsed nor torsional ultrasound was protective. Anyone, therefore, who feels that there is essentially a free ride from wound burn risk with torsional or transversal ultrasound may be in for a rude awakening. All studies to date show that torsional ultrasound decreases frictional heat generation when compared with continuous longitudinal ultrasound, but it is often used at 80 to 100% power and often for long stretches, because there is little chatter, so the risk of wound burn, as documented in this large survey, is not decreased. It is true that continuous longitudinal ultrasound-adjusted wound burn risk was the highest by a fair margin, but this difference was not quite statistically significant in our multivariate analysis, and therefore not a factor that we could say was critical in the creation of incision burns.

To recap, we know that the risk is always greatest when ultrasound is used no matter what the modality and, therefore, our approach should be to use mechanical forces as much as possible. We also know the risk is greatest when we have a fragment blocking the tip so that fluid cannot flow through the needle to cool it down. This is a particularly important time, with very hard fragments, not to have long runs of ultrasound and to strive to take similar steps as secondary mechanical forces break up the fragment rather than just using ultrasound. The third key factor is the very important one, as ultrasound in an anterior chamber full of viscoelastic can create a very rapid and devastating incision burn in a matter of seconds. Our conclusions are that attention to all three of these issues would make the overall incidence of incision burn extremely low, and, personally, I think wound burn can be completely prevented with a little attention to the details outlined.

But what happens if you already have an incision burn? It is important to recognize it as early as possible. I have seen incision burns so small that all they did was induce some astigmatism and they were easily closed with sutures, which astigmatism tended to relax, or could be corrected with a relaxing incision. More severe incision burns can be almost impossible to close with sutures, and the amount of astigmatism induced is such that trying to close it by sutures alone is not going to lead to a very good outcome. I have found making a 600-μm-deep relaxing incision in the cornea just ahead of the burn often enables the tissue to more easily close with much less induction of irregular cylinder. Remember, the problem is collagen contracture, which is the same as loss of tissue in the incision area. I have also been able to take a partial-thickness scleral flap posteriorly and flip it over to fill in the space, rather than try to close it primarily. This both decreases a lot of the induced astigmatism and makes for an easier closure. Suturing this partial-thickness flap is relatively straightforward, and if eye bank tissue is available, it also can be used to help close the incision.

The astigmatism often has to be addressed, and so it is worth waiting 3 or 4 months for it to stabilize. I have seen cases of tremendous induced astigmatism finally relax to something much more reasonable. Relaxing incisions are surprisingly powerful in that the contracture right at the incision is largely eliminated thereby. I have also had some cases where a small patch graft had to be placed in the incisional area to make up for this loss of tissue and relax the induced irregular cylinder. The key detail is to make sure you have a watertight closure at the end of the procedure. If the incision is badly contracted and gaping, I would close it and move to a totally new site to complete the procedure.

Conclusion

It is clear that by using mechanical forces as well as using ultrasound very parsimoniously and never using ultrasound in an anterior chamber full of viscoelastic, that the incidence of this problem can be extremely small and possibly completely prevented. We know that in the United States and Canada, at least as of 2009, the incidence is 1 in 2,000 surgeries, but quite variable depending on one's approach and whether ultrasound is used inside of viscoelastic in particular. With our most important finding showing that efficient surgery is protective, it is clear that all of this taken together should make wound burn an extremely uncommon problem today. Sadly, reliance on ultrasound variations does not appear to be protective as they are actually used in clinical practice and, therefore, the other approaches described here are more important.

References

1. Brinton JP, Adams W, Kumar R, Olson RJ. Comparison of thermal features associated with 2 phacoemulsification machines. J Cataract Refract Surg 2006;32:288–293

2. Floyd MS, Valentine JR, Olson RJ. Fluidics and heat generation of Alcon Infiniti and Legacy, Bausch & Lomb Millennium, and advanced medical optics sovereign phacoemulsification systems. Am J Ophthalmol 2006; 142:387–392

3. Schmutz JS, Olson RJ. Thermal comparison of Infiniti OZil and Signature Ellips phacoemulsification systems. Am J Ophthalmol 2010;149:762–767.e1

4. Oakey ZB, Jensen JD, Zaugg BE, Radmall BR, Pettey JH, Olson RJ. Porcine lens nuclei as a model for comparison of 3 ultrasound modalities regarding efficiency and chatter. J Cataract Refract Surg 2013;39:1248–1253

5. DeMill DL, Zaugg BE, Pettey JH, et al. Objective comparison of 4 nonlongitudinal ultrasound modalities regarding efficiency and chatter. J Cataract Refract Surg 2012;38:1065–1071

6. Floyd M, Valentine J, Coombs J, Olson RJ. Effect of incisional friction and ophthalmic viscosurgical devices on the heat generation of ultrasound during cataract surgery. J Cataract Refract Surg 2006;32:1222–1226

7. Bradley MJ, Olson RJ. A survey about phacoemulsification incision thermal contraction incidence and causal relationships. Am J Ophthalmol 2006;141:222–224

8. Sorensen T, Chan CC, Bradley M, Braga-Mele R, Olson RJ. Ultrasound-induced corneal incision contracture survey in the United States and Canada. J Cataract Refract Surg 2012;38:227–233

XIV Machine Management in Complicated Cases

37 Understanding the Phaco Machine

Barry S. Seibel and William J. Fishkind

Modern phaco machine technology upgrades the phaco hand-piece to the role of our most diverse and elegant handheld instrument. It can be used to prevent tears in the capsule during phaco, and it can be reprogrammed to minimize further damage if the capsule should rupture.

Overview

The patient will have the best visual result when the phaco energy delivered to the anterior segment is minimized. Additionally, phaco energy should be directed into the nucleus. This avoids injury to iris blood vessels, trabecular meshwork, and endothelium. Finally, skillful emulsification leads to shorter overall surgical time. Therefore, a lower amount of irrigation fluid passes through the anterior segment.

Normally, all phaco procedures have two phases: first, creation of fragments, which requires sculpting or chopping; second, the removal of the fragments in a controlled approach. Occlusion is mandatory to move fragments to the iris plane. Fragment removal is assisted by partial to complete occlusion phaco.

All phaco techniques are preceded by capsulorrhexis, cortical cleaving hydrodissection, and removal of the anterior cortex and epinucleus to expose the endonucleus.

Complications related to the phaco machine can generally be grouped into two categories. First, the inappropriate use of machine parameters may result in direct tissue damage through such mechanisms as chamber collapse, corneal wound burn, iris incarceration, and capsule rupture. Second, failure to optimally adjust machine parameters so as to facilitate efficient surgery will result in the surgeon having to compensate by more frequent and exaggerated manual maneuvers that can increase the possibility of tissue damage. Although some surgical complications are inevitable by-products of preexisting anatomy, many can be avoided by judiciously examining the relationship of the machine technology and the fundamentals of the microsurgical techniques to modern phaco surgical methods. Many aspects of the machine technology's contribution to surgical complications can be understood by first simplifying the role that the machine plays in a routine case. That role is to create and maintain a fluidic circuit that starts at the elevated irrigating bottle, passes through the eye and then the phaco pump, before draining into a collection chamber.

If a cataract has a soft, gel-like density, then the nuclear material can propagate along the fluidic circuit as the phaco needle's aspiration port is placed against the nucleus, aspirating it. As the nuclear density increases, the pump must create more vacuum to deform the nuclear material sufficiently for aspiration. If the nucleus has still greater, crystalline-type density, then an appropriate amount of ultrasound must be titrated so that the material can be emulsified sufficiently to enable pump vacuum and flow to deform it into and through the phaco needle and aspiration line. The ultrasonic vibrating phaco needle tends to push material away from it with traditional longitudinal non-torsional ultrasound.

During sculpting, the nucleus is held in place by the capsule and zonules, but during fragment emulsification, fluidic parameters of vacuum, flow, and bottle height must be adjusted to counteract the ultrasonic repulsion so as to aspirate the nuclear material into the phaco needle.

The anterior chamber (AC) must be maintained during all phases of cataract surgery; its fluid pressure, therefore, must be greater than the ambient atmospheric pressure. Any vacuum created in the fluidic circuit by the pump is optimally located between the aspiration port and the pump; any vacuum (pressure lower than atmospheric pressure) in the eye portion of the fluidic circuit would result in a chamber collapse, leading in turn to potential damage to the capsule, zonules, and corneal endothelium. One of the main determinants of intraocular pressure (IOP) is the height of the irrigating bottle, which yields an IOP of 11 mm Hg (above ambient atmospheric pressure) for every 15 cm (6 inches) of elevation above the eye. This relationship is accurate for hydrostatic pressures in pedal position 1. In pedal positions 2 and 3, the IOP decreases (but remains greater than atmospheric pressure) with induced flow in proportion to the commanded pump strength, as well as the degree of aspiration port occlusion.

New modifications in the Centurion (Alcon, Fort Worth, TX) have "active fluidics" where the surgeon sets the target IOP during surgery and software in the unit maintains that IOP throughout the surgery, thus enhancing AC stability. The Stellaris (Bausch and Lomb, Rochester, NY) has surgeon-controlled pressurized infusion to maintain AC stability during phaco.

Chamber collapse may potentially occur if the surgeon uses a standard bottle height for most cases but neglects to appropriately raise it if the flow rate is subsequently increased to enhance followability. The converse is also true. For example, a surgeon may lower the bottle height to achieve a lower IOP for such conditions as weak zonules or a posterior capsule tear, but chamber instability will result if the flow rate is not correspondingly adjusted to a lower setting that is appropriate for the lower bottle height. Once again, bottle height must be titrated not only for hydrostatic pressures in pedal position 1 but also hydrodynamically to a given pump strength for positions 2 and 3. Needless to say, the highest elevation of the bottle will be inadequate if the irrigating fluid is completely depleted; operating room staff vigilance is required in this area for longer procedures. The potential for this problem is increased if the surgeon has the room lights dimmed partly or completely during cataract surgery. In those machines with pressurized infusion, it is obvious that the infusion rate must be adjusted to balance the aspiration rate.

Pump Types

To create a vacuum, a pump of some type is necessary. Classically, pumps have fallen into two categories. The flow pump, the best example being a peristaltic pump, enables the surgeon to directly program both flow and vacuum parameters. The vacuum pump, for example the Venturi pump, enables direct surgeon control over vacuum only. The amount of flow is dependent on the vacuum setting and cannot be set by the surgeon. Recently, pumps have evolved such that flow pumps are so responsive that they can be programmed to respond as if they were vacuum pumps. Additionally vacuum pumps can be manipulated to act as if they were flow pumps. These modern pumps are therefore considered as "hybrid pumps."

Irrespective of pump selection, flow, measured in cubic centimeters per minute (cc/min), is the force that brings material toward the phaco tip. In general, the higher the flow, the faster events will occur within the AC. Vacuum setting, measured in millimeters of mercury (mm Hg), will hold material on the phaco tip, once occlusion has occurred.

Fluidic Problems: Flow Management

The flow rate (cc/min), being an important factor in determining IOP, can be increased directly on a flow pump by increasing the commanded flow rate or indirectly on a vacuum pump by increasing the commanded vacuum; in both cases, the actual flow rate is dependent on the degree of aspiration port occlusion. The actual flow rate is also affected by the fluidic circuit's resistance, which is in turn determined by the internal diameters of the phaco needle as well as the fluidic tubing (especially the aspiration line). In addition, flow rate is affected proportionately by bottle height, but only when using a vacuum pump. One potential arrangement that may lead to complications is using a vacuum-priority pump for a high-vacuum technique. A high commanded vacuum setting produces a high flow rate with the unoccluded phaco tip. The surgeon may compensate for this with an elevated bottle height to maintain adequate IOP in the face of the high flow rate. However, the higher bottle height produces an even higher flow rate, with the aspiration port unoccluded, which not only diminishes the effectiveness of increasing the IOP but also produces potentially dangerously fast intraocular currents that can uncontrollably attract and incarcerate unwanted material such as iris and capsule.

The induced flow rate from a high commanded vacuum can be limited to a safer level by the use of a high-resistance phaco needle with a small internal diameter, such as a flare tip needle. In addition, the surgeon should titrate the amount of commanded vacuum during phaco with linear pedal control according to the clinical application and the status of the aspiration port. Appropriately high vacuum may be used safely when the aspiration port is occluded, for example, when gripping a hemi-nucleus in preparation for chopping. However, when anticipating an occlusion break at the end of a chop, the surgeon should linearly titrate vacuum to a lower, safer, and more appropriate level.

Aspiration Line Obstruction

Another potential area of complication related to IOP maintenance and flow concerns is the presence of an obstruction between the aspiration port and the pump. Although kinked aspiration line tubing can produce this effect, it is most often caused by the localized accumulation of nuclear emulsate, clogging the aspiration line, especially when sculpting dense, mature cataracts. This type of obstruction does not occur regularly, but

it can significantly impair the effectiveness of the phaco machine by limiting the pump's ability to transfer its force (either via flow or vacuum) past the obstruction to the phaco tip where it is needed. The surgeon can recognize this problem when free (e.g., chopped) nuclear fragments fail to be effectively drawn to the phaco tip when in pedal position 2 and using a flow setting that usually is effective in this situation. Similarly, an aspiration line obstruction is suspected when faced with insufficient grip of an occluding nuclear fragment when using a vacuum setting that usually achieves a good grip. An aspiration line clog is also a strong possibility when observing intraocular flocculence ("lens milk" or "phaco dust") during sculpting, indicating the inability for pump-induced flow to effectively clear the AC of the ultrasonically induced emulsate.

Any of these scenarios must prompt the surgeon to interrupt the surgery so that the problem can be isolated and rectified. Verification of a clog is achieved by placing a test chamber over the visibly unobstructed phaco needle and engaging pedal position 2 while observing inadequate or absent activity in the irrigating bottle's drip chamber. The accumulation of emulsate can sometimes be visualized in the aspiration line, often at the junction of the aspiration tubing/handpiece junction, or at the aspiration tubing/cartridge connection; in these cases, digital massage of the tubing at this area often breaks up the obstruction. Sometimes, very high commanded flow and vacuum along with high ultrasound will free a nonvisualized obstruction; remember to perform this maneuver extraocularly with a test chamber over the phaco needle. If the clog is within the handpiece, forcibly irrigating it with a balanced salt solution (BSS) syringe is usually an adequate solution.

The greatest danger of an aspiration line obstruction is the surgeon's failure to recognize the situation and rectify it. The most benign outcome of such a failure is the impairment of the machine's effectiveness in producing the desired intraoperative flow and vacuum. However, a greater danger occurs if, as a result of the subsequently impaired followability and grip, the surgeon chases after nuclear fragments into the periphery of the AC rather than maintaining the phaco needle in a safer, more central position and having the machine fluidics attract fragments to and into the aspiration port. With the needle in a peripheral position, an aspiration line obstruction might spontaneously clear, inducing a surge that can incarcerate and damage the juxtaposed iris or capsule. Furthermore, if the obstruction does not clear spontaneously, the probability of a corneal wound burn becomes progressively greater as more ultrasound energy is engaged without sufficient cooling flow.

Vacuum Settings

The appropriate setting of the machine's vacuum parameter, measured in millimeters of mercury (mm Hg), is another key element in avoiding complications. As discussed previously, adjusting the commanded vacuum on a vacuum priority pump (e.g., Venturi) proportionately adjusts the flow rate when the phaco tip's aspiration port is not occluded. But when the phaco tip is occluded, adjusting the commanded vacuum (vacuum priority pump) or the vacuum limit preset (flow priority pump) proportionately adjusts the grip and deformational force that is applied to the material that is occluding the aspiration port. The amount of grip for a given amount of pump vacuum is proportional to the surface area of the phaco needle's aspiration port; the surgeon, therefore, should anticipate the need for increasing the vacuum from the usual levels when changing to either a smaller gauge or less beveled phaco needle. As with any parameter, the vacuum should be adjusted appropriately for a given surgical function; a higher adjustment would needlessly compromise the operation's safety margin.

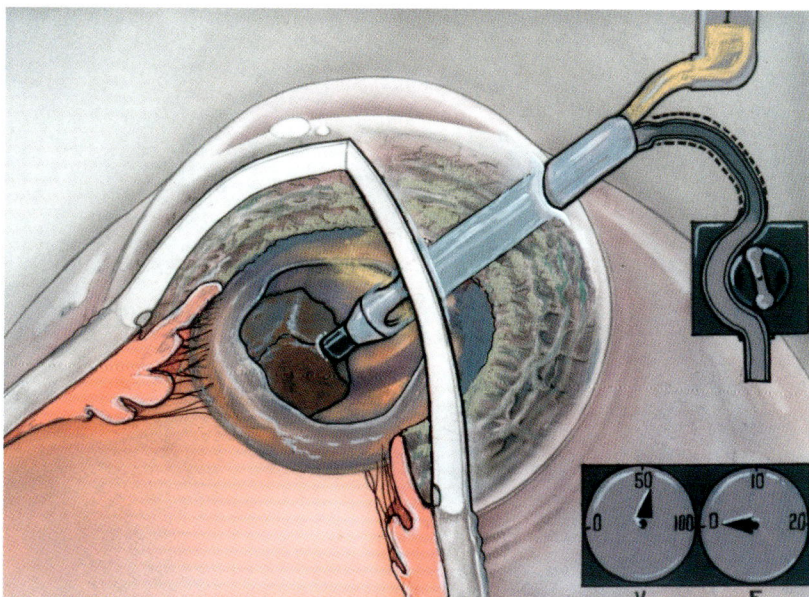

Fig. 37.1 Immediately preocclusion. The nuclear fragment is almost occluded on the phaco tip. There is no flow. Vacuum will rise to the preset limit. The aspiration tubing begins to collapse.

For example, a high vacuum level of 350 mm Hg might be required during a chop maneuver to grip and pull the engaged hemi-nucleus centrally so as to facilitate the peripheral placement of the chopping instrument. However, once the hemi-nucleus is mechanically fixated between the chopper and the phaco tip, high vacuum is no longer required. Indeed, it can subsequently become a liability if maintained beyond the completion of the chop, with breaking of the vacuum seal between the phaco tip and the nucleus. When using a vacuum pump, the high induced flow from the high vacuum level with an unoccluded tip can produce shallowing or collapse of the AC. Therefore, after higher vacuum has been applied when needed with complete aspiration port occlusion, the vacuum level should then be lowered in anticipation of using pedal position 2 or 3 along with partial or complete unocclusion of the aspiration port.

Partial Occlusion Phaco

To better identify the concept of partial occlusion we must analyze the events surrounding occlusion. It is important to understand that partial occlusion phaco occurs during fragment removal.

When removing a fragment, the fragment is pulled toward the phaco tip by the flow of fluid drawn into the phaco needle. When it reaches the phaco tip, it occludes the needle orifice and vacuum holds it in place. At this moment the flow stops and the vacuum rises to its preset maximum limit when using a flow pump, or equilibrates with the commanded vacuum on a vacuum pump. This is occlusion (**Figs. 37.1** and **37.2**). It represents a specific moment in time. During occlusion, the vacuum rises, the aspiration line tubing constricts, and the fragment is held

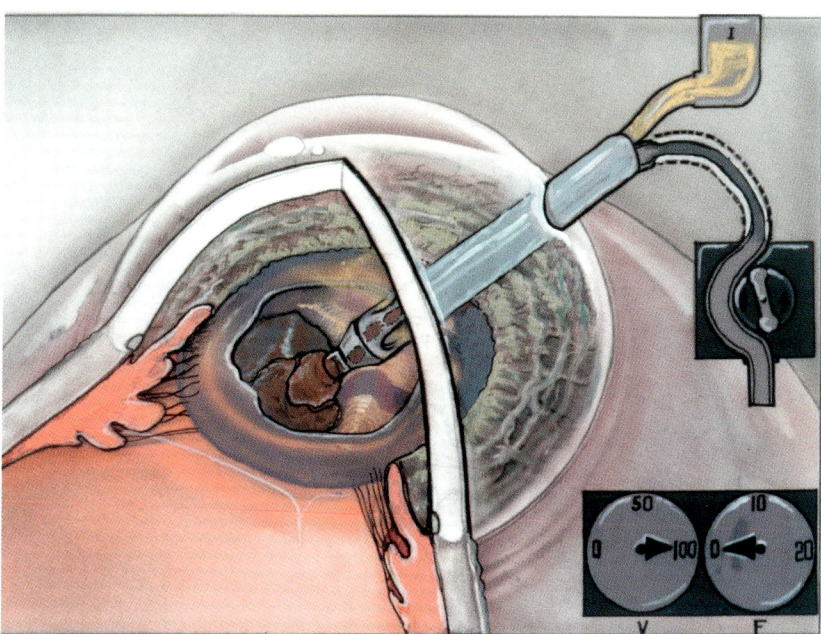

Fig. 37.2 Occlusion. The fragment is firmly held to the phaco tip. Vacuum increases to the preset maximum. The tubing collapses. There is inflow but no outflow. The chamber is deep. (Occlusion is just about to break, as evidenced by the presence of nuclear fragments at the phaco tip.)

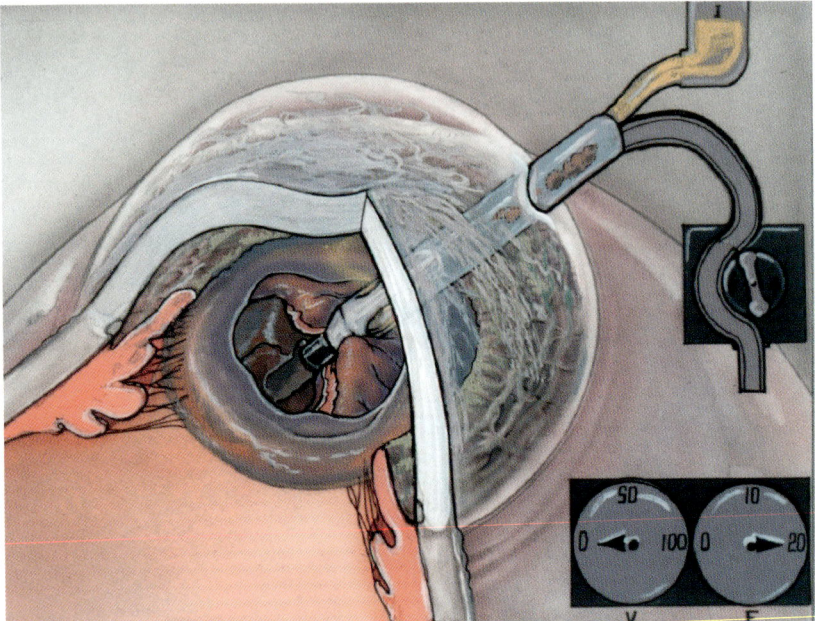

Fig. 37.3 Postocclusion. After the application of phaco power, the fragment is emulsified and the vacuum immediately falls to 0. Flow immediately rises to the preset maximum. This enables the high vacuum and expanding aspiration tubing to pull fluid out of the anterior chamber (AC) more rapidly than it can be replaced by infusion. The rapid loss of AC volume causes the posterior capsule to move anteriorly and the cornea to collapse. The posterior capsule is "snapped," or stretched, around the nuclear fragment, resulting in a tear.

more and more firmly to the phaco tip. When the surgeon activates phaco energy, the emulsification of the fragment instantaneously permits flow to begin (**Fig. 37.3**). The flow volume increases to its preset maximum exceptionally rapidly based on pump speed and due to expansion of the vacuum tubing. The inflow of the fragment particulates and fluid into the phaco needle momentarily exceeds the inflow from the irrigation line, and the AC shallows. This abrupt forceful flow of fluid, beyond the steady-state flow with an unoccluded aspiration port, is defined as surge, and results in simultaneous anterior movement of the posterior capsule as well as collapse of the cornea. The event may be violent enough to tear the capsule by itself, tear a preexistent tear of the AC at the equator, or tear around a sharp edge of partially emulsified hard nucleus. It also can be aspirated into the phaco tip and breached (**Fig. 37.4**).

If we deem that the moment of occlusion symbolizes a specific instant in time, we can partition the emulsification of fragments into three divisions: preocclusion, occlusion, and postocclusion. Obviously, surge is undesirable. However classically we have performed phaco by using occlusion to hold fragments and postocclusion to emulsify them. Thus we unconsciously inhabited the world of unwelcome surge!

Partial occlusion phaco is the method by which we break the cycle of occlusion and surge! During fragment emulsification, if the fragment is brought close to the phaco tip orifice, but never completely occludes it, there is never full occlusion. Thus, a distinct new term, *partial occlusion,* describes the monumental change. If there is no occlusion there cannot be surge (**Table 37.1**).

The fragment emulsification occurs in the interval between preocclusion and occlusion. Therefore, if we never have occlusion

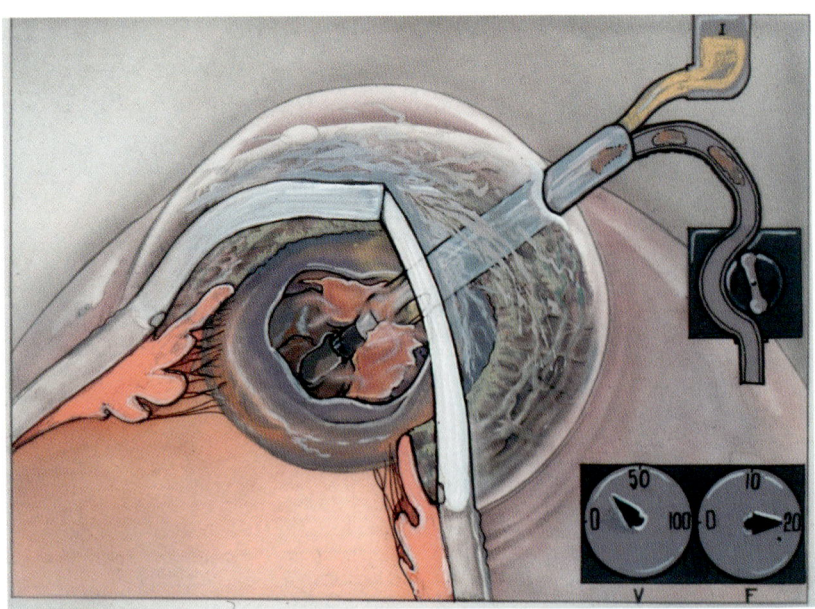

Fig. 37.4 Late postocclusion. If the surge is violent, the posterior capsular tear may enlarge and the vitreous face may rupture. Vacuum moderately increases as vitreous is aspirated. Eventually, inflow equilibrates with outflow and the AC will stabilize.

Table 37.1 Stages of Partial Occlusion Phaco

Preocclusion $\Longrightarrow$	Occlusion $\Rightarrow$	Postocclusion
	↑	↑
	Partial Occlusion	Surge

during sculpting due to low vacuum settings, and we never have occlusion during fragment removal due to partial occlusion, the surgeon never has to encounter the unnerving occlusion/surge event. The incidence of torn posterior capsules and unplanned vitrectomy lessen. Patients experience superior surgery and outcomes.

Partial occlusion occurs when the fragment is in close proximity to, but not occluding, the phaco tip (**Fig. 37.5**). If no occlusion occurs, there will be no surge. The question then becomes, How do we shift the equation to the preocclusion side? The answer resides in the understanding of the elements of phaco energy.

Phaco Energy

There are three types of phacoemulsification energy in evidence at the phaco tip: jackhammer energy, low-frequency cavitation energy, and high-frequency cavitation energy.

Jackhammer energy is created by the mechanical striking of the phaco needle against cataractous material. It is a powerful force.

Low-frequency cavitational energy is created by the vibration of the phaco tip. It has a relatively long wavelength and penetrates into tissues a great distance from the phaco tip. The manufacturer of the machine determines the frequency. This energy creates both transient and sustained cavitational energy.

High-frequency cavitation occurs during fragment emulsification and facilitates removal of the fragment. This energy also discharges from the phaco tip, injuring surrounding tissues.

Transient Cavitation

When there is adequate fuel (in this case aqueous fluid/BSS) at the phaco tip, and it is energized, the backward movement of the tip pulls dissolved gases out of solution and creates micro-bubbles. The forward movement of the tip compresses the bubbles repeatedly until they implode. The implosion causes a shock wave of 75,000 pounds per square inch, which discharges from the tip in the direction of the bevel of the needle. The equivalent process occurs along the needle barrel and at any point of change in diameter of the needle. Therefore, cavitation is enhanced at the narrowing of the shaft of a flared tip, the angulation of the Kelman tip, or at the needle hub. Transient cavitation is short-lived, lasting only 2 to 4 ms as fuel is rapidly depleted.

Sustained Cavitation

After 2 to 4 ms, when fuel is depleted, the needle continues to vibrate, but bubbles just vibrate without imploding. This is useless and wasted energy.

Modifications of Phaco Power

Two modifications of phaco energy release are instrumental in shifting the procedure away from occlusion phaco and in the direction of partial occlusion phaco: micro-pulse energy production and partial occlusion phaco mechanics.

Micro-Pulse Energy Production

Micro-pulse (hyper-pulse) phaco can be delivered by one of the three machines that are most available in the United States that have this modification; it is called by different names. However, in all cases, changes in machine software and handpiece piezo-electric crystal inertia enable exceedingly short bursts of phaco energy coupled with exceedingly short periods of aspiration only. The duration of energized times, as well as aspiration only time, are independently adjustable. The result of this important modification is to maximize the use of transient cavitation associated

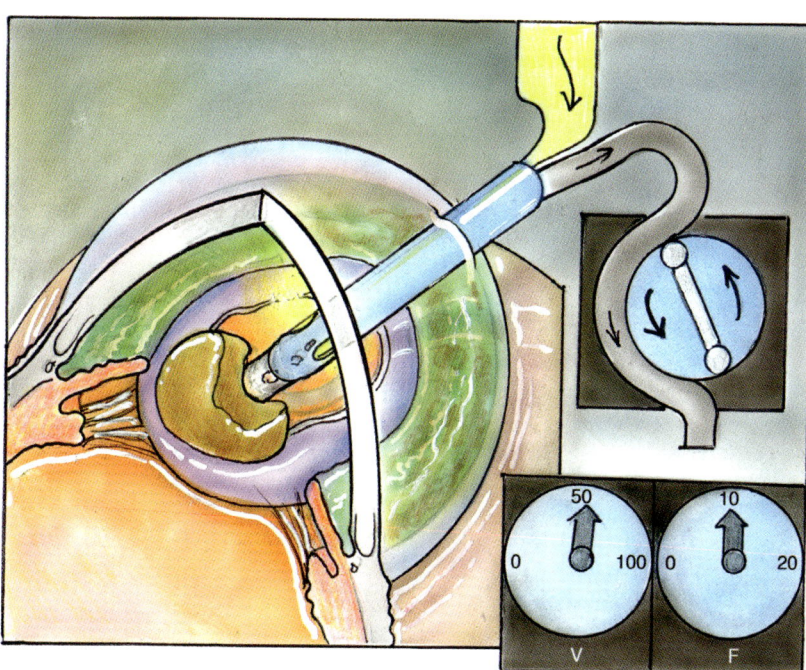

Fig. 37.5 The fragment is extraordinarily close to the tip but never entirely occludes it. There are various amounts of vacuum and flow. Therefore, the emulsification is performed preocclusion or with partial occlusion.

with jackhammer mechanical energy. The power bursts are so short that all the cavitational energy generated is powerful transient cavitation. The needle vibration stops before fuel is burned and stabilized cavitation begins.

There are three important consequences of microburst energy generation[2–8]:

1. Energy misuse, produced by periods of stabilized energy expenditure with its worthless injury to endothelium, iris blood aqueous barrier, and trabecular meshwork, is curtailed.
2. There is a dramatic decrease in heat production and energy delivery without any loss of phaco efficiency.
3. The micro-pulse phaco initiates partial occlusion phaco.

Partial Occlusion Phaco Mechanics

In this scenario, the fragment is drawn toward the phaco tip orifice by fluid flow. It almost occludes the tip when micro-pulse phaco is energized. The fragment is emulsified by the short powerful bursts of transient cavitational energy, in harmony with the jackhammer effect. This combined energy drives the fragment away from the phaco tip. However, 4 ms later, energy production pauses, aspiration brings the fragment back toward the orifice, and just as it is about to occlude the tip, energy is again resumed, and on and on the cycle repeats. The fragment is extraordinarily close to the tip but never entirely occludes it. Thus, micro-pulse phaco is the generator of partial occlusion phaco (**Fig. 37.5**).

The philosophy of the Bausch and Lomb Stellaris is to employ micro-pulse coupled with a lower frequency cavitation generator. The lower the frequency, the larger the cavitation bubble produced. In fact, the cavitation bubble at 28.5 KHz is 73 µm, whereas that of 40 KHz is 52 µm, for a difference of 71%. The larger bubble, upon implosion in a micro-pulse environment, must give off more powerful cavitational energy. The partial occlusion is enhanced both by removing larger chunks of the fragment and by not requiring as close proximity of the fragment to the tip for emulsification, as with smaller bubble formation.

Nonlongitudinal Phaco

The discussion above has referenced the movement of the phaco needle in a longitudinal, or forward and backward movement. An innovation in design enables the tip to move in nonlongitudinal directions. The importance of this change to nonlongitudinal power is the augmentation of the shaving characteristic of the phaco needle. Longitudinal power cores material so that cavitational energy can emulsify it. Nonlongitudinal energy shaves fragments of cataractous material, further enhancing partial occlusion phaco while additionally improving followability (**Fig. 37.6**).[9–11] Two manufactures have adopted this style of power generation.

Alcon Laboratories (Fort Worth, Texas) has created OZil torsional power generation. By utilizing an angled Kelman phaco tip driven with an oscillatory movement, a zone of cavitational energy is created around the angled tip. The torsional needle movement enhances the jackhammer effect, which predominantly shaves and removes fragments. Cavitational energy does not play much of a role. However, the shaved fragments are often larger than the cored fragments created by longitudinal phaco. In an effort to further emulsify the shaved fragments, Alcon has developed Intelligent Phaco (IP). This software creates an occlusion threshold that is surgeon selected. When it is reached, longitudinal movement of the needle replaces the torsional movement. This instantly produces cavitational energy through-

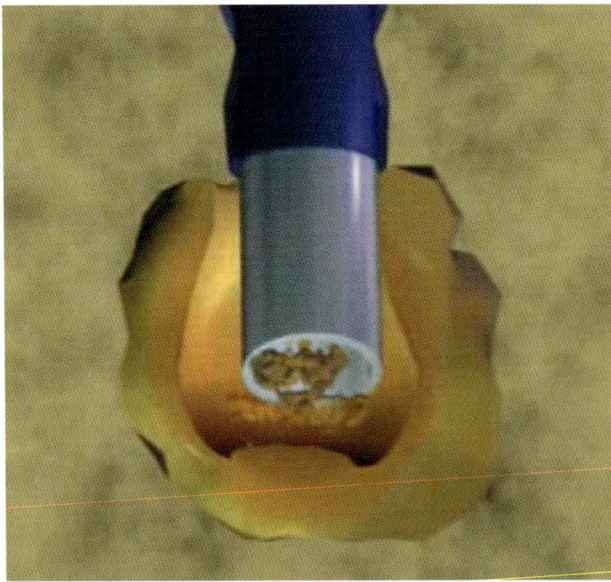

Fig. 37.6 Nonlongitudinal shaving of material with a lateral movement. The material is then aspirated. (Courtesy of Abbott Medical Optics.)

out the needle barrel and at the hub. Thus, trapped fragments are emulsified, clearing the needle, allowing vacuum to decline, and beginning torsional movement once again.

Abbott Medical Optics (AMO; Orange County, CA) has chosen a different approach. It uses a standard tip driven in an elliptical motion. The needle path resembles the shell of an egg. This modification also shaves cataractous fragments but is less prone to clogging, as it emits a high level of cavitational energy.

Nonlongitudinal phaco, like micro-pulse phaco, gives rise to partial occlusion phaco. Therefore, when using nonlongitudinal phaco it is not necessary to use micro-pulse phaco. Nonlongitudinal phaco effectively shaves material, reducing overall time of phaco energy release. It is so efficient at generating partial occlusion phaco that it seems to the surgeon that fragments hug the phaco tip and are effortlessly removed in a quiet and stable AC.

Aspiration Solutions to Surge

The use of micro-pulse and nonlongitudinal phaco to promote preocclusion phaco is accompanied by fluidic management. Manufacturers have developed software modifications to recognize occlusion and instantaneously slow the pump or decrease vacuum. This smart-pump technology can be combined with low-compliance tubing to additionally minimize surge.[12] Finally, phaco tips can be designed as flow restrictors; 21-gauge needles and flare-tip designs effectively decrease an outflow to decrease the surge.[13,14]

Aspiration Problems

In Paul Koch's stop-and-chop method, an appropriately titrated vacuum level enables the surgeon to firmly grip an engaged hemi-nucleus so as to displace it centrally prior to chopping; this maneuver enables the chopper to be more easily engaged at the hemi-nuclear periphery while minimizing danger to the anterior and peripheral capsule. If the phaco tip pulls out of the hemi-nucleus instead of pulling it centrally, the surgeon may perhaps suspect that the vacuum parameter was insufficient. However, this ineffective grasp might have been caused by a vacuum level that was, in fact, too high for the given nuclear density, such that

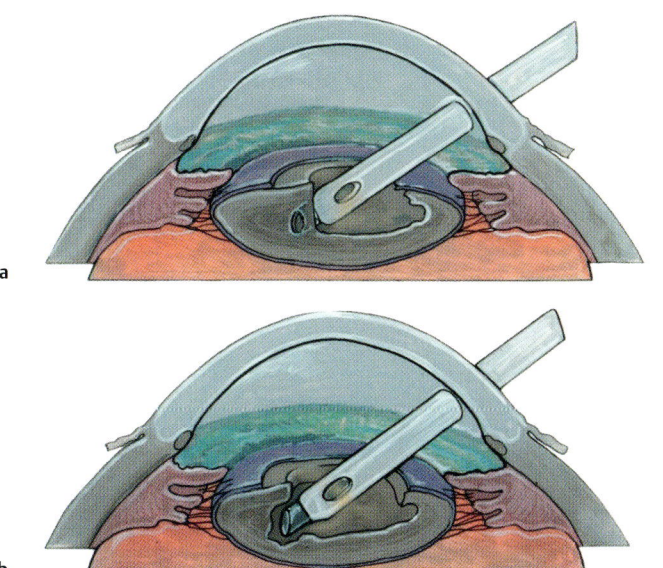

Fig. 37.7   (a) Excessive vacuum in relation to nucleus density leads to removal of excess nuclear material contiguous with the tip. This disrupts the vacuum seal. **(b)** There is resultant poor holding power.

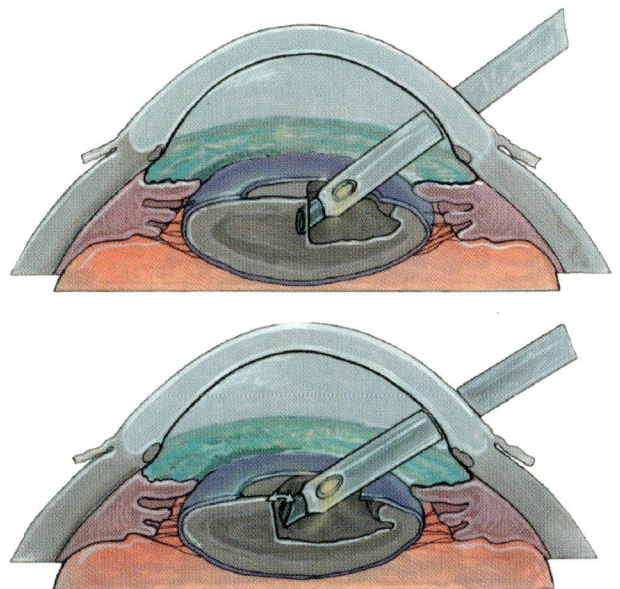

Fig. 37.8   (a) Correct approach. The phaco tip is held at the appropriate angle to match the tip angle to the fragment. This enhances occlusion and holding power. **(b)** Incorrect approach. The phaco tip at the wrong angle does not occlude well, thus diminishing the holding power or creating the need for excessive phaco energy to bury the tip.

the nuclear material just around the tip was abruptly aspirated (**Fig. 37.7**). Without a relatively snug fit around the phaco tip to give a good vacuum seal, it is impossible to effectively transmit the machine's gripping force, regardless of whether a flow pump or a vacuum pump is used. A similar disruption of material just around the tip might have been caused by the excessive use of ultrasound when embedding the tip. Only mild ultrasound should be used at this point to ensure a tight vacuum seal, and it should always be discontinued as soon as the tip is buried to an adequate depth of 1 to 1.5 mm. Maintaining ultrasound beyond this point not only can preclude a good vacuum seal, as just described, but also will further preclude an effective grip of a hemi-nucleus by allowing the needle to vibrate free when pulled rather than pulling the hemi-nucleus with it.

With regard to the importance of a good vacuum seal, as discussed above, the concept of the phaco needle bevel must be examined relative to its ease of occludibility. A good occlusion is obtained when the aspiration port is buried a sufficient amount over its entire surface. If part of the aspiration port is only shallowly embedded in the nucleus, the vacuum seal can easily be broken with only modest physical manipulation of the phaco (**Fig. 37.8**). The surgeon might mistakenly think that more vacuum parameter is needed when in fact the needle bevel and the surface to be occluded simply needed to be adjusted so that they are parallel to each other to achieve an effective vacuum seal. It can be seen that both a 0-degree tip and a 45-degree tip can achieve either a good or a poor occlusion based on this relationship (**Fig. 37.9a,b**). It is only necessary to turn the beveled tip bevel down to maximize the capability for occlusion (**Fig. 37.9c**). If bevel-down sculpting is to be performed, it is undesirable to have occlusion near the equator. Therefore, low or zero vacuum should be programmed. This will prevent an inopportune occlusion. Thus, it is vital to first optimize the surgical technique to facilitate the most efficient utilization of the phaco machine so as to avoid setting unnecessarily high parameters that compromise intraoperative safety.

Ultrasonic Problems

In addition to the ultrasonic and fluidic modulation discussed above, ultrasound power must also be modulated correctly so as to avoid complications. Ultrasonic problems typically fall into three categories. First, failure to utilize adequate ultrasound power can produce zonular and capsular stress and even rupture

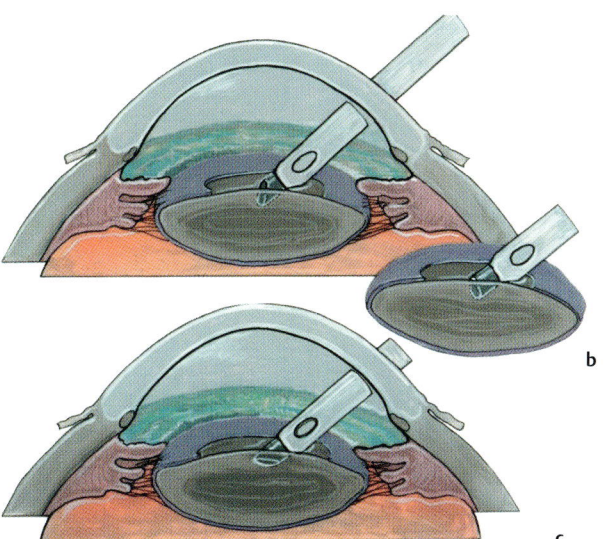

Fig. 37.9   (a) Incorrect approach. The bevel-up 45-degree phaco tip is not completely embedded in the nucleus. There is no occlusion and therefore no holding power. **(b)** Incorrect approach. The 0-degree phaco tip is not adequately occluded. Holding power is poor. **(c)** Correct approach. Performed correctly, the 45-degree bevel-down phaco tip is easily occluded with nuclear material. Holding power is excellent.

during sculpting. Ultrasound should be titrated along with the linear speed of the sculpting pass as well as the amount of the tip engaged so as to enable effective carving through the nucleus without pushing it. Second, the use of too high a power setting when inadvertent material such as iris is incarcerated can generally be avoided by the effective use of mechanical force (cracking and especially chopping) to segment the nucleus to minimize the need for sculpting, which typically involves the highest power settings and closest proximity of the tip and capsule or iris. The surgeon then uses effective titration of fluidic parameters (flow and vacuum) so as to attract and aspirate these segments, minimizing the need to move the phaco tip toward the periphery of the AC to chase after the segments. Furthermore, ultrasonic aspiration of fragments is more efficient than sculpting because the full tip occlusion enables vacuum to augment ultrasonic action; therefore, lower power levels are used with correspondingly lower risk of damage to inadvertently incarcerated tissue. During emulsification of fragments, flow and vacuum are titrated to the level of applied ultrasound, which is itself titrated to the nuclear density. Preferably, fluidics and ultrasound are titrated simultaneously in a linear fashion for the most effective and efficient control. Third, there is a potential for thermal injury at the incision because of frictional energy from the rapidly vibrating phaco needle. Surgical technique is particularly relevant in avoiding corneal wound burns. For example, one should avoid maintaining high ultrasound power for long, continuous intervals. Furthermore, avoiding handpiece positions that result in lifting or extreme angulations at this location can prevent unnecessary wound pressure. Therefore, a temporal incision that is not too long will provide a better outcome.

Control of Heat Generation

Fluidic parameters can influence heat production by affecting the flow rate; less heat is produced to the extent that more AC fluid exchange and more fluid flow around the needle shaft provides cooling. Recall that aspiration line fluid becomes more viscous as viscoelastic and dense nuclear emulsate are aspirated, and that flow is consequently diminished, especially with vacuum pumps; machine parameters should be adjusted accordingly, especially when sculpting. One should avoid maintaining high ultrasound power while the aspiration port is occluded and thereby prohibits any cooling flow. This can occur at the initia-

tion of phaco when the AC is filled with any ophthalmic viscosurgical device (OVD) but has been shown to be most likely to occur after the initial entry into an AC filled with Healon 5 (AMO). To avoid heat production, apply a short period of aspiration only while moving the phaco tip to remove some of the OVD prior to applying power. This enables aspiration to be reestablished before power is utilized.

Chopping maneuvers require the aspiration port to be fully occluded to effectively build vacuum and gripping power, but this can be accomplished by a brief application of moderate ultrasound to embed the tip followed quickly by a return to pedal position 2 to titrate vacuum appropriately without any further ultrasound until the chop is completed (**Fig. 37.8a, 37.9c**). Furthermore, occlusion methods of fragment removal do not necessarily produce excessive heat even though ultrasound power is applied from short to moderate periods. The reason is twofold: first, only moderate levels of ultrasound are required because of the greater efficiency of occlusion methods; second, full occlusion is rapidly and intermittently interspersed with moments of flow that facilitate cooling as well as removal of emulsified material.

Different needle designs have been developed to decrease the likelihood of wound burns as the silicone sleeve is pressed against the vibrating needle by the surgical incision. Graham Barrett designed the MicroFlow needle to incorporate longitudinal grooves along the outer shaft, which continue to channel cooling irrigation fluid even when the silicone sleeve is compressed against the outer needle surface. The Surgical Design (Armonk, NY) silicone sleeve applies this principle in reverse, with the sleeve itself having the grooves that maintain irrigation flow even with compression against the needle. Richard Mackool developed the MicroSeal needle (as well as the similarly designed Mackool System needle), which maintains flow via a rigid polyimide (plastic) sleeve between the needle and the compressed sleeve; the polyimide additionally provides heat insulation via its own material properties.

With regard to avoiding wound burns, surgical technique is important not only relative to handpiece manipulation as mentioned previously, but also with regard to correct handling of nuclear segments when attempting ultrasonic aspiration. For example, the phaco tip in **Fig. 37.10a** has impaled a nuclear fragment, boring almost completely through it. Maintaining pedal position 3 in this case invites disaster because of the aspiration flow tending to draw unwanted material like iris or capsule into the port. Furthermore, without complete occlusion of the aspira-

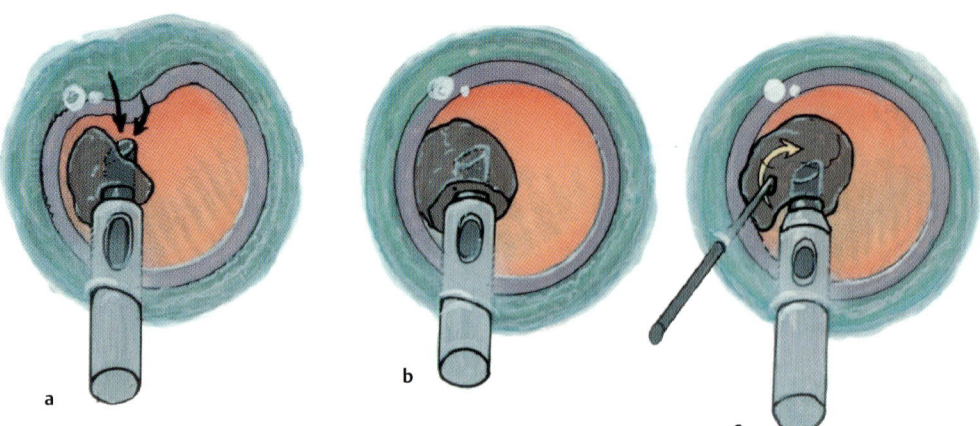

Fig. 37.10 **(a)** The phaco tip has bored through the fragment. As the tip emerges from the distal aspect of the fragment, a surge occurs. The now exposed tip, during the postocclusion surge, may aspirate the iris or the capsular bag. The *arrows* indicate the aspiration flow. **(b)** The fragment is immobile on the phaco tip. Further emulsification is impossible. The sleeve prevents fragment rotation. A wound burn is a possible result. **(c)** A second instrument is utilized to push the fragment to a new position to assist its emulsification.

tion port, vacuum cannot aid in aspirating the fragment; similarly, the flow does not help to aspirate the fragment because fluid is drawn into the tip prior to affecting the fragment. Recall that because of the axial orientation of ultrasound needle vibration, continuation of position 3 will not accomplish any further emulsification of the fragment; the needle will simply vibrate back and forth along the axis of the hole it has bored. In **Fig. 37.10b**, the phaco needle cannot progress any further through the fragment because of the physical obstruction from the silicone irrigation sleeve. The corrective action in this case is to back off to foot pedal position 1 to maintain the AC; then use a second instrument through the side-port incision to push the fragment off of the phaco tip and then reengage to emulsify the fragment, manipulating and feeding the fragment to the tip with the second instrument as necessary (**Fig. 37.10c**). Note how the segment's sharp tip was ultrasonically removed prior to emulsification to prevent it from spinning into the capsule or cornea.

Engaging fragments in a tangential fashion enables efficient emulsification as both flow and vacuum continue to feed new material into the phaco tip as the previously engaged portion is emulsified and aspirated in an efficient occlusion mode of operation. Note the nontangential fragment engagement (**Fig. 37.11a,b**) in which the phaco needle has bored into part of the fragment; maintaining position 3 with a dense nuclear sclerotic fragment would not produce any further emulsification because the silicone sleeve prevents vacuum from drawing the fragment any further into the needle. Furthermore, because the aspiration port is completely occluded, maintaining position 3 causes potentially dangerous heat buildup from incisional friction caused by the vibrating ultrasonic needle in the absence of a cooling flow current. Fragments engaged in this fashion should be removed by refluxing or with a second instrument so that they can be reengaged for emulsification (**Fig. 37.11c,d**). Larger fragments generally require more manipulation by a second instrument to maintain optimum tangential positioning; therefore, chopping methods, because smaller nuclear fragments are generated, are typically more efficient than quadranting techniques.

In all cases heat production decreases when selecting micropulse or nonlongitudinal phaco modulations.

Specific Phaco Techniques: Machine Settings and Modifications for Management of Complicated Scenarios

Divide-and-Conquer Phaco

Sculpting

To concentrate cavitational energy into the nucleus, a 0-degree tip, or a 15- or 30-degree tip turned bevel down, should be utilized. Low vacuum (depending on the manufacturer's recommendation) and moderate flow are mandatory for bevel down phaco. This prevents occlusion. Occlusion, at best, causes excessive movement of the nucleus during sculpting. At worst, occlusion occurring near the equator, or deep within the nucleus, may capture the nucleus, adherent cortex, the capsule, and vitreous. This is the origin of tears in the equatorial or posterior bag early in the phaco procedure. Alternatively, sculpting can be performed bevel up with panel power so that there is no ramp-up of power, which can push the nucleus ahead of the time during the low-power phase of the linear foot pedal.

Once the groove is judged to be adequately deep (about three phaco tip diameters deep), the bevel of the tip should be rotated to the bevel-up position and vacuum can be increased. This improves visibility and prevents the risk of phaco through the posterior nucleus and posterior capsule. Sculpting is assisted by the use of panel controlled continuous phaco. This is because the nucleus is held in place by the capsular bag. Therefore, pressure against the nucleus enables the jackhammer effect to take over and emulsify a groove.

If micro-pulse phaco is used for sculpting, duty cycles with longer power on than off should be selected. This enables phaco to proceed with clean emulsification and avoids pushing the nucleus ahead of the phaco tip, potentially damaging zonules.

When the initial groove is judged adequate, the nucleus is rotated 90 degrees and another groove is created. Next, a 180-degree rotation provides access for creation of the final groove.

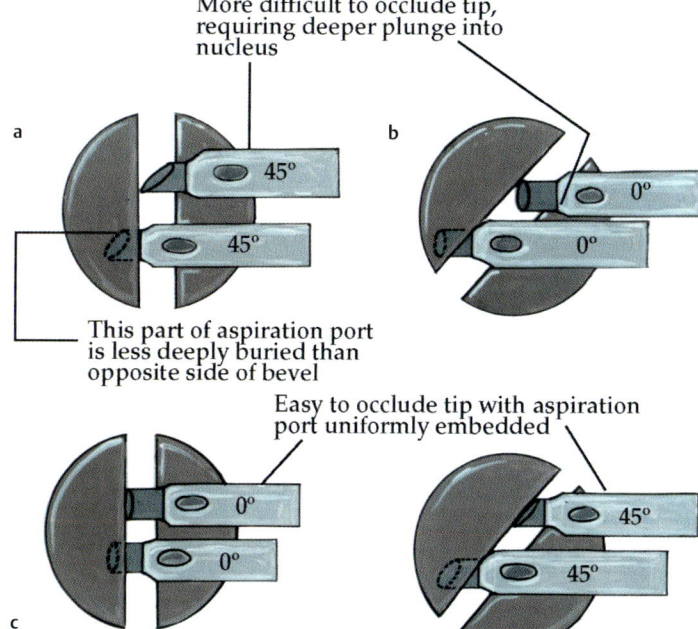

Fig. 37.11 **(a,b)** The fragment is not aligned with the phaco tip. Occlusion is difficult. If emulsification is successful, the tip will eventually be stuck within the fragment with the sleeve precluding further efficient emulsification. **(c,d)** The fragment has been maneuvered such that the fragment angle matches the tip angle. This facilitates occlusion and promotes efficient emulsification of the fragment.

Quadrant and Fragment Removal

The grooves are expanded, cracking a fragment, which is then mobilized to the level of the iris. The tip selected, as noted above, is retained. Vacuum and flow are increased to reasonable limits governed by the machine being used. The limiting factor to these levels is the development of surge. Therefore, micro-pulse phaco or nonlongitudinal phaco is best used at this stage. The bevel of the tip is turned toward the quadrant or fragment. Low pulsed or burst power is applied at a level high enough to emulsify the fragment without driving it away from the phaco tip.

Epinucleus and Cortex Removal

If cortical cleaving hydrodissection has been performed, the endonucleus is removed first, as noted above. The result is a shell of epinucleus and cortex. For removal of epinucleus and cortex, the vacuum is decreased while flow is maintained. This enables grasping of the epinucleus just deep to the anterior capsule. The low vacuum helps the tip hold the epinucleus on the phaco tip, without breaking off chunks. High vacuum results in breaking off pieces of epinucleus and cortex, making it more difficult to remove. With the fluid parameters balanced, the epinucleus/cortex scrolls around the equator and can be pulled to the level of the iris. There, low power pulsed or hyper-pulse phaco is employed for emulsification.

Stop-and-Chop Phaco[15]

Groove creation is performed as noted above (see Divide-and-Conquer Phaco). Once a single deep groove is adequate, vacuum and flow are increased to improve the holding capability of the phaco tip. The nucleus is rotated 90 degrees, and the phaco tip is driven into the mass of one hemi-nucleus using pulsed linear phaco. The sleeve should be 1.5 mm from the base of the bevel of the phaco tip to create adequate exposed needle length for sufficient holding power. Excessive phaco energy application is to be avoided, as this will cause nucleus immediately adjacent to the tip to be emulsified. The gap thus created in the vicinity of the tip is responsible for interfering with the seal around the tip and, therefore, the capability of vacuum to hold the nucleus. The nucleus will then pop off the phaco tip, making chopping more difficult. With a good seal, the hemi-nucleus can be drawn toward the incision and the chopper can be inserted at the endonucleus–epinucleus junction (**Fig. 37.12**). The chopper is then drawn down and left, while the phaco tip is pushed up and right. This results in chopping of the hemi-nucleus.

After the first chop, a second similar chop is performed so that the hemi-nucleus is divided into three pieces. One of the pie-shaped pieces of nucleus thus created is elevated to the iris plane (occlusion is utilized to move fragments) and removed with low-power hyper-pulsed phaco or nonlongitudinal phaco, as discussed above (see Divide-and-Conquer Phaco). Each fragment and the remaining hemi-nucleus are removed in turn. Epinucleus and cortex removal are also performed as noted above.

Phaco Chop[16]

Phaco chop requires no sculpting. Therefore, the procedure is initiated with high vacuum and flow and linear pulsed or micro-pulse phaco power. Nonlongitudinal phaco does not work well for the actual chopping, as the shaving movement of the phaco tip prevents an adequate vacuum seal to assist chopping and fragment mobilization. For a 0-degree tip, especially when emulsifying a hard nucleus, a small trough may be required to create adequate room for the phaco tip to push deep into the nucleus.

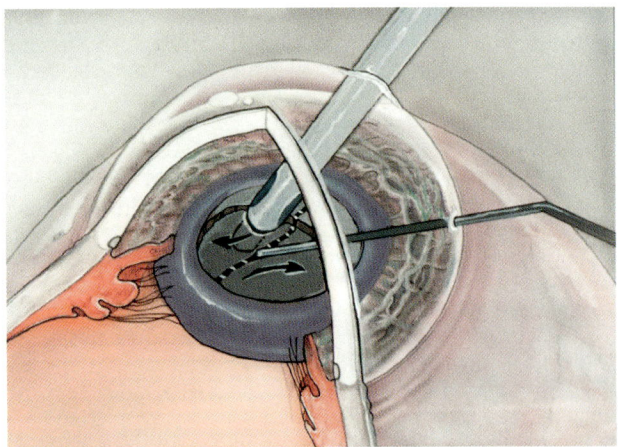

Fig. 37.12 Excessive vacuum in relation to nucleus density leads to removal of excess nuclear material contiguous with the tip. This disrupts the vacuum seal. There is resultant poor holding power.

For a 15- or a 30-degree tip, the tip should be rotated bevel down to engage the nucleus. The phaco tip should be encased within the endonucleus with the minimal amount of power necessary. All chopping procedures require 1 mm of exposed phaco tip to create adequate holding power for chopping. If the phaco tip is inserted into the nucleus with excess power, the adjacent nucleus will be emulsified, creating a poor seal between the nucleus and the tip. This makes it impossible to remove fragments, as the tip will just "let go" of the nuclear material. Additionally, the bevel should be turned toward the fragment to create a seal between the tip and the fragment, enabling vacuum to build and create holding power.

Horizontal Chop

A few bursts or pulses of phaco energy enables the tip to be encased within the nucleus. It then can be drawn toward the incision to provide the chopper access to the endonucleus–epinucleus junction. The chopping instrument is passed over the nucleus and under the anterior capsule into this junction. It may be helpful to rotate the chopper to horizontal as it passes below the anterior capsule. If the nucleus comes off the phaco tip, excessive power has produced a space around the tip, impeding vacuum-holding power as noted above. Pulling the chopper down and left and pushing the phaco tip up and right generates the first chop. Minimal rotation of the nucleus enables creation of the second chop. The first pie-shaped piece of nucleus is mobilized with high vacuum and elevated to the iris plane. There it is emulsified with low linear hyper-pulse or nonlongitudinal power, high vacuum, and moderate flow.

Vertical Chop

Once the phaco tip is embedded within the nucleus as previously described, a sharp chopper (Nichamin, Katina Products, Denville, NJ) is pushed down into the mass of the nucleus at the same time that the phaco tip is elevated. The chopper is then drawn down and left and the phaco tip is moved up and right. This creates a cleavage plane in the nucleus. With a second chop, the fragment created is mobilized to the iris plane and removed as noted above. When the nucleus is noted to be hard, the process of rotation and vertical chopping is repeated until the entire nucleus is chopped. Usually, at this point, the nucleus loses its rigidity, enabling the segments to be mobilized without difficulty.

Micro-Incisional Phaco

The development of micro-pulse and nonlongitudinal phaco ("cold phaco") has led to the performance of phaco through increasingly small incisions with tighter irrigation sleeves, no irrigation sleeves, and decreased inflow.

Bimanual Micro-Incisional Phaco

Two incisions are created 90 degrees apart. Their size is dependent on the instrumentation: 20-gauge instruments require 1.4-mm incisions, whereas 21-gauge instruments require 1.2-mm incisions. There is no irrigating sleeve on the phaco tip. The instrumentation for this procedure is important, and the relationship between the instrument and incision size is essential. If the wound is too tight, it is difficult to manipulate the instruments. If the wound is too large, excessive outflow permits chamber shallowing with an unstable anterior segment. The instruments can be moved forward and backward through the incisions without creating corneal distortion. If the instruments are angled in the incision, corneal distortion makes the procedure appreciably more difficult. The irrigating chopper should be parallel to the iris and above it. The inflow current thus created tends to wash fragments toward the unsleeved phaco tip. The small incisions cause less disruption of the blood–aqueous barrier, and are more stable and secure. Presently a new incision is created for intraocular lens (IOL) implantation. In the future, with insertion of an IOL through the 1.4-mm incision, there should be less disruption of ocular integrity, immediate return to full activities, and less risk of postoperative wound complications.

Micro-Incisional Coaxial Phaco

A thin-walled, flared, 21-gauge phaco tip and thinner irrigation sleeve is available for the Infinity (Alcon) machines and now permit phaco though a 2.2-mm incision. Bausch and Lomb has designed a coaxial phaco tip for a 1.8-mm incision. Despite the smaller incision, inflow is adequate to maintain a deep AC due to the forced infusion systems. The procedure is no more difficult than when performed through a 2.4-mm, or larger, incision. Alcon also manufactures a one-piece acrylic IOL and injector, which is capable of implanting the IOL through the 2.2-mm unenlarged incision and Bausch and Lomb IOL is implanted through a 1.8-mm incision.

Irrigation and Aspiration

Similar to phaco, AC stability during irrigation and aspiration (I/A) is due to an equilibrium of inflow and outflow. Employing a soft sleeve around the I/A tip can minimize wound outflow. Combined with a small incision (1.8 to 2.4 mm), a deep and stable AC will result. Generally, a 0.3-mm I/A tip is used. With this orifice, a vacuum of 500 mm Hg and flow of 20 cc/min can tease cortex from the capsular fornices. Linear vacuum enables the cortex to be grasped under the anterior capsule with low vacuum and drawn into the center of the pupil at the iris plane. There, in the safety of a deep AC, vacuum can be increased and the cortex aspirated.

Bimanual I/A is also a viable procedure. A 21-gauge irrigating cannula provides inflow through one paracentesis while an unsleeved 21-gauge aspiration cannula is used through the opposite paracentesis. The instruments can be easily switched making removal of stubborn cortex considerably easier.

Machine Settings

Every machine, by virtue of its pump dynamics, software, tubing, foot pedal, venting, and tuning, has distinctive settings. The manufacturer's surgical representative can help the surgeon fine-tune the settings.

Capsular Tears

The capsule can tear at any time during phaco surgery. If the capsule tears before phaco is initiated, the likely causes are the following:

1. Extension of an anterior capsulorrhexis tear centripetally around the equator into the posterior capsule
2. Hydrodissection, with or without capsular block, "blowing out" the anterior capsule or posterior capsule
3. Preexistent posterior capsule pathology such as a posterior polar cataract or a vitrectomy in which the posterior capsule sustained damage from the vitrector

If the capsule tears during phaco procedure, the likely causes are the following:

1. Aspirating the capsule either at the equator or posteriorly and energizing phaco energy, resulting in an immediate tear at the site of occlusion. The likelihood of rupture of the vitreous face is high.
2. Attempting to phacoemulsify a mature cataract through too small a capsulorrhexis, causing a tear in the anterior capsule extending into the posterior capsule. The vitreous face may remain intact.
3. Aspirating the posterior capsule during a surge. The likelihood of rupture of the vitreous face is high.

If the capsule tears during I/A, the likely causes are the following:

1. Aspirating the capsule instead of cortex, pulling and tearing it
2. Aspirating the capsule instead of cortex and having a sharp bur in the aspiration orifice tear it
3. Aspirating cortex and continuing to aspirate the attached capsule until it tears
4. Aspirating OVD and, secondary to surge, aspirating and tearing the posterior capsule

Although there are many variations on the above themes, they represent a distillation of the problems, and enable us to distinguish the scenarios required for successful outcome. The following universal principles affect the outcome in all cases of torn capsule:

1. Attempt to maintain a small wound and a closed chamber.
2. Attempt to prevent enlargement of the tear.
3. If the capsule is intact, attempt to preserve the integrity of the anterior capsule and capsulorrhexis to provide support for a sulcus fixated or a bag-fixated IOL.
4. Attempt to avoid rupture of the vitreous face.
5. Never withdraw the phaco tip in the presence of a torn capsule without first filling the AC with OVD. Without OVD, the forceful shallowing of the AC will likely produce extension of the tear and in all probability rupture of the vitreous face.
6. Prevent loss of the nucleus into the vitreous.
7. Have unpreserved triamcinolone acetonide injectable suspension, 40 mg/mL (Triesence, Alcon) available.

8. Have a vitrectomy kit containing the vitrector, tubing, irrigating cannulas, needle holder, and suture available.

Management of a Tear in the Anterior Capsule Without a Tear in the Posterior Capsule

Once a tear of the anterior capsule is recognized, it is imperative to maintain a stable AC. Pressure posteriorly, for example, from the phaco tip pushing posteriorly while attempting to chop the nucleus, or pressure anteriorly from removing the phaco tip and allowing the vitreous to move anteriorly, is adequate stimulus to tear the capsule through the equator and into the posterior capsule.

Therefore, the anticipated approach is to maintain a stable AC. Actual machine settings are dependent on the machine, the grade of the cataract, the surgical technique, and the surgeon. Certain generalizations however, hold true.

Techniques for a Hard or Moderate Cataract

Chop

Confirm that there is 1.5 mm of exposed phaco tip. This is important, as it establishes that there is sufficient holding force for chopping maneuvers. If there is not enough exposed tip, simply slide the sleeve back a bit more. Switch to panel control for faster impaling of the nucleus, or, if desired, use linear power until the tip is completely embedded, up to the sleeve, in the nucleus. Turn the power to 50% or more. Use longitudinal power (i.e., not OZil or Elliptical). Increase vacuum slightly (our setting is 340 mm Hg). Increase the flow slightly (our setting is 30 cc/min unoccluded, increasing to 38 cc/min with occlusion to improve holding ability), and lower the irrigating bottle 20 cm (our setting is 70 cm). These changes cause the tip to energize at 50% power immediately on entering foot pedal position 3. The increased flow and vacuum enable the tip to pass into the central nucleus without posterior pressure. The decreased inflow also decreases posterior pressure. The avoidance of OZil or Elliptical power affects the nonlongitudinal movement of the phaco tip. This brings about a tight fit between the tip and the nucleus for improved holding power. This is required for either vertical or horizontal chopping. With the tip firmly embedded in the nucleus, in foot pedal position 2 so that vacuum holds the nucleus firmly on the phaco tip, the phaco tip can slightly lift the nucleus and vertical chopping can be accomplished within the confines of the capsular bag, without pressure on the posterior capsule. The nucleus is rotated, and this process is repeated until the entire nucleus is chopped into small pieces and nuclear rigidity is disrupted. Then, the phaco machine is set to linear power, with, if available, micro-pulse or nonlongitudinal power. The power is decreased to 30%, and vacuum and flow are set to appropriate levels to prevent surge. The bottle remains in position. Each fragment of nucleus is then elevated to the central pupil at the plane of the anterior capsule, where it is emulsified.

Prior to removing the phaco tip, OVD is utilized to fill the AC. This prevents positive posterior pressure from moving the vitreous anteriorly, consequently enlarging the tear. It also prevents

the initial infusion surge from the I/A tip from pushing the posterior capsule and vitreous posteriorly and enlarging the tear.

Assuming the posterior capsule has remained, intact the cortex is removed with I/A. The cortical removal is begun opposite from the anterior capsular rent. As the location of the rent is approached, the cortex is engaged with low linear aspiration; then, as aspiration is increased, the cortex is pulled toward the rent, in an attempt to prevent enlargement. Venturi pump technology makes the aspiration control more precise in this situation.

Alternatively, a dispersive OVD can be used to fill the capsular fornices and then can be aspirated, revealing the cortex below it and enabling cortex removal in a more expanded capsular bag environment.

After IOL insertion, remaining OVD is removed with moderate linear vacuum and a lowered irrigation bottle. An even more gentle solution to remove the OVD is to do so in aliquots by aspirating a few tenths of a cubic centimeter in a 3-cc syringe with a 25-gauge cannula and then replacing the volume with BSS. This procedure is repeated until most of the OVD is removed.

Alternatively, bimanual I/A provides a nicely controlled environment for both the cortical cleanup and removal of the OVD. The larger fluid fluxes seen with coaxial I/A are avoided with this technique.

Divide and Conquer

Confirm that there is 1.5 mm of exposed phaco tip. This is important, as it establishes that there is sufficient groove depth for grooving maneuvers. If the is not enough exposed tip, simply slide the sleeve back a bit more. Switch to panel control for faster sculpting at adequate power to emulsify the nucleus, or use linear power for slower titrated energy application. Use nonlongitudinal continuous power (i.e., OZil or Elliptical) if available. Decrease vacuum significantly so that there is no tendency for the phaco tip to grab and pull the nucleus during grooving. Keep flow at the usual setting. It is important to have adequate inflow to cool the phaco tip. Lower the irrigating bottle 20 cm. In panel control, the immediate power prevents the phaco tip from pushing the nucleus ahead of it and posteriorly potentially further tearing the torn anterior capsule. The nonlongitudinal power assists in cutting the groove. The decreased inflow from the lower infusion bottle diminishes the posterior pressure. Create the groove with minimal posterior pressure, shaving and deepening the groove gradually, dependent on the consistency of the nucleus. When groove depth is judged sufficient, gently rotate the nucleus 180 degrees in the plane of the capsular bag and complete the groove. For stop and chop, rotate the nucleus 90 degrees and proceed as above for chopping with the new machine settings. If continuing to divide and conquer, rotate the nucleus 45 degrees and create another groove. Once all eight grooves are complete, they can be separated with minimal force and distance. The pie-shaped fragments thus produced are then emulsified at the plane of the anterior capsule in the mid-pupil with the settings as noted for chopping techniques.

Viscoat Sandwich

Another alternative to the above scenarios is to create a "Viscoat sandwich." Because there is already a tear in the anterior capsule, it is straightforward to mobilize the entire cataract into the

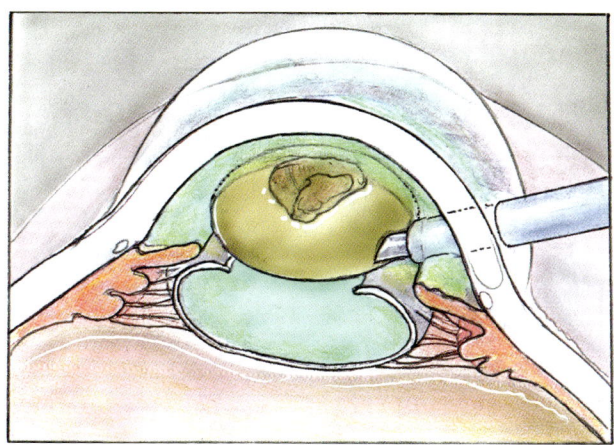

Fig. 37.13 The "Viscoat sandwich." The nucleus is elevated above the plane of the anterior capsule and isolated with dispersive ophthalmic viscosurgical device (OVD) above and below it. It is therefore emulsified within the stabilizing OVD.

AC (**Fig. 37.13**). This is accomplished by injecting a dispersive OVD behind the cataract while simultaneously elevating the cataract into the AC. More OVD is placed over the nucleus to suspend it in the AC and protect the endothelium. The nucleus is then emulsified in the AC, employing whatever technique is preferred. Obviously, this prevents any posterior pressure on the capsule, minimizing the risk of tear extension.

It is important to have the nucleus immediately adjacent to the phaco tip when power is energized. The high power, moderate vacuum, low flow, and low infusion bottle settings assist in pulling the nucleus into the phaco tip while maintaining a stable AC. In machines where torsional or elliptical nonlongitudinal and micro-pulse power settings are available, they should be utilized.

Capsular Tears During Phaco

As soon as the capsule tears during phaco, the normal fluid dynamics of the anterior segment are disturbed. The open capsule enables inflow fluid to flow through the rent, into the vitreous. As a result the irrigation inflow from the phaco sleeve will tend to push fragments away from the tip. This dynamic is so enhanced that it is difficult for aspiration forces to overcome it. In addition, hydration of the vitreous and turbulence bring vitreous into the AC, where it is easily aspirated by the large-bore phaco tip. This occludes the needle orifice, making aspiration of the nucleus even more difficult. It may appear that the nucleus will not come up to the phaco tip, or even be pushed away from it.[8]

To prevent this, the infusion bottle must be lowered significantly (~ 70 cm). The aspiration flow rate and vacuum should also be lowered. If possible, dispersive OVD can be used to push vitreous posteriorly and provide a barrier between the vitreous and the phaco tip. It also serves to elevate nuclear material above the plane of the anterior capsule, where it can be emulsified. The AC can even be filled with OVD as described by Chang and Packard[17] in the "Viscoat trap" technique.

If there is already too much vitreous in the AC for the use of OVD, limited vitrectomy may be necessary to remove vitreous, which will otherwise prevent aspiration of the nucleus. Excessive vitrectomy should be avoided at this stage as it may possibly allow nucleus, or pieces of nucleus, to fall into the vitreous. OVD then can be used as a barrier, as described above. The phaco tip should be placed adjacent to the nuclear fragment before aspiration is engaged. The second instrument should be utilized to hold the fragment against the phaco tip, ensuring that it will be aspirated rather than vitreous. Only then can aspiration overcome inflow and enable emulsification of the remaining nucleus. If the nucleus begins to fall posteriorly, it must be secured with OVD and a Sheets' glide technique as described by Michelson[18] (**Fig. 37.14**) or a Kelman[19] posterior assisted levitation (PAL) technique (**Fig. 37.15**) can be employed. Finally, Kumar and Agarwal's group[20] described using a three-piece foldable IOL as a scaffold to create a pseudophakic posterior capsule. The IOL is injected below the nucleus and over the posterior capsule to permit emulsification of the residual nuclear material above the IOL. This is particularly beneficial if there is residual posterior capsule.

Once the nucleus is removed the cortex should next be removed. This can be done efficiently with a vitrector, if available; it enables aspiration without cutting. Set for aspiration in foot pedal position 2 and cutting in foot pedal position 3 (I/A–Cut setting), the cortex can be aspirated without cutting, and vitrectomy, with cutting, can be performed intermittently as is necessary. Bimanual I/A would be the next best option for cortex removal. The absence of an irritating sleeve and the separation of irrigation from aspiration prevent the irrigation fluid flow from pushing cortex away from the aspirating tip. The last choice is obviously coaxial I/A. Again it is advantageous to use a lowered infusion bottle, low aspiration flow rate (20 cc/min), and linear vacuum (300–500 maximum mm Hg). The aspiration orifice should be placed close to the cortex to aspirate it preferentially over OVD and vitreous. Once cortex is engaged, the vacuum is progressively increased until aspiration is complete.

A thorough vitrectomy should be performed once all cortex is removed. Vitrectomy should also be performed intermittently, whenever vitreous prevents either emulsification of nucleus or aspiration of cortex. In this case the cutting mode of the vitrector should be engaged before the aspiration mode so as not to create vitreous traction. This is the Cut–I/A setting. Therefore, cutting is engaged in foot pedal position 2 and aspiration in foot pedal position 3. New vitrectomy instruments cut at high rates. The cutting rate should be set as high as possible on older machines, usually 350 to 550 cuts per minute. On newer machines, cutting rates of 1,500 cuts per minute actually enable sculpting of the vitreous and decrease the volume of vitreous removal. Vacuum of 100 to 125 mm Hg and aspiration flow of 20 cc/min are appropriate settings for vitrectomy. These parameters may be modified in different machines and with different pumps.

Irrigation is provided by a 21-gauge cannula placed through the paracentesis. If a small paracentesis is initially created, it must be enlarged for cannula passage. Similarly, the vitrectomy instrument should be placed through a new paracentesis and appropriately sized.

Alternatively, pars plana vitrectomy can be performed (see Chapters 19 and 20). Conversion to extracapsular cataract extraction is another alternative (see Chapter 19). Unpreserved triamcinolone acetonide injectable suspension, 40 mg/mL (Triesence,

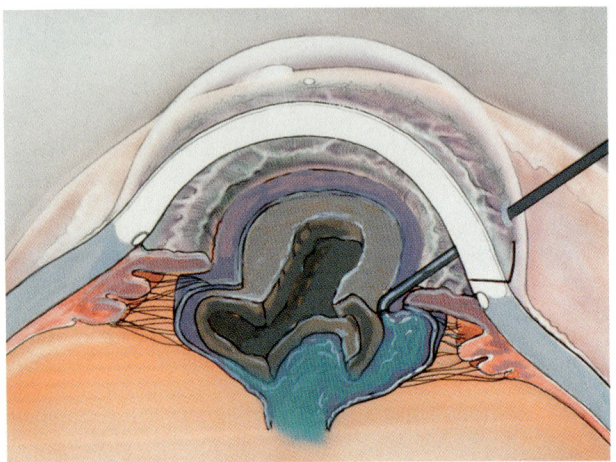

a

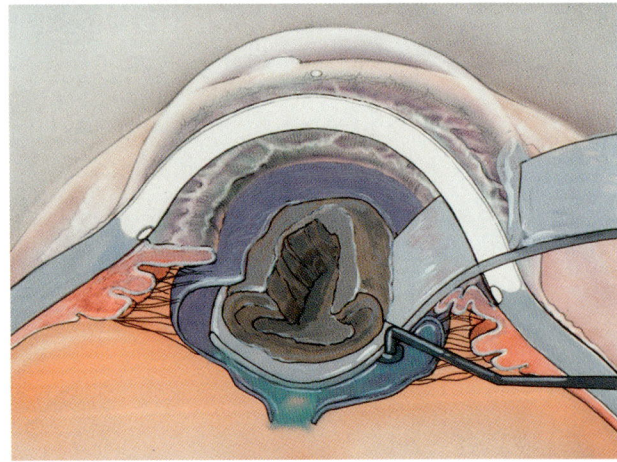

b

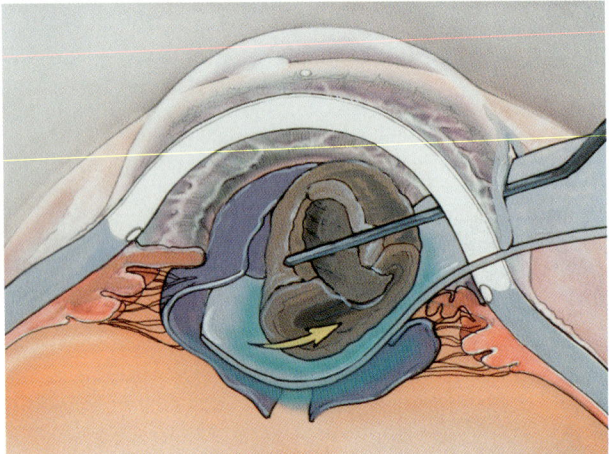

c

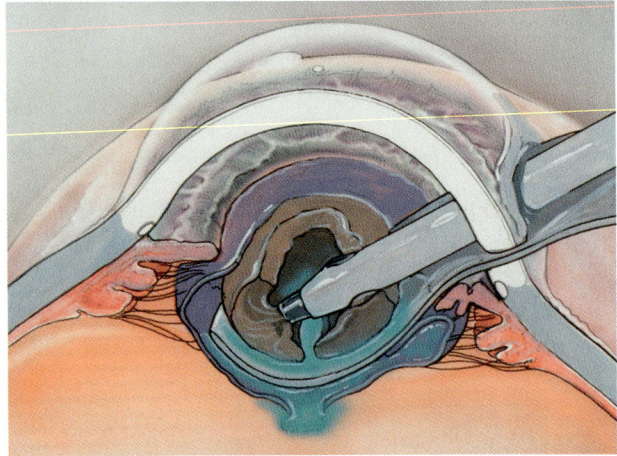

d

Fig. 37.14 **(a)** Dispersive viscoelastic is placed below the lens fragment to make space for the Sheets' glide. **(b)** The Sheets' glide is placed below the lens fragment. A second instrument is used to guide it into position. **(c)** Using the glide as support, a Sinskey or Kuglen hook is used to maneuver the lens fragment out of the incision. No external pressure is used. **(d)** Phaco is performed over the glide. The glide prevents lens fragments from falling into the vitreous as well as restraining anterior movement of vitreous.

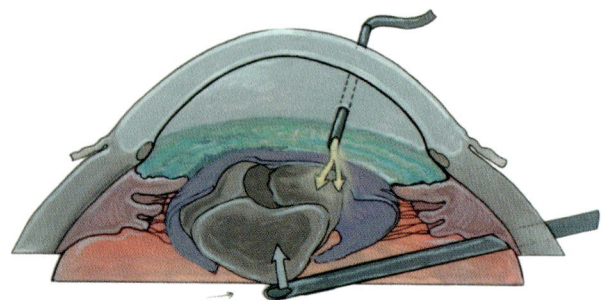

Fig. 37.15 A single sclerotomy through the pars plana 3.0 mm posterior to the limbus has many advantages. Infusion is performed through the limbus. A vitrectomy performed in this manner pulls vitreous out of the AC and does not enlarge the capsular defect. If lens fragments threaten to fall posteriorly, the vitrector or another instrument passed through the pars plana enables the surgeon to apply a posterior force to prolapse the fragments into the AC.

Alcon) is a superb adjunct to vitrectomy. It can be diluted one part Triesence to four parts BSS. Injected into the AC is reveals residual vitreous and importantly vitreous strands incarcerated in the various incisions.

Conclusion

When challenged by a critical crisis, such as the torn capsule, a carefully designed surgical plan is an enormous advantage. Understanding the principles of the fluid dynamics in the altered anterior segment may well avert a major complication. Possessing the instruments to perform vitrectomy, and the awareness of the machine settings that will enhance the effectiveness of the instruments, can salvage the visual outcome for the patient.

Booker T. Washington said, "Excellence is to do a common thing in an uncommon way." It is our legacy as cataract surgeons to relentlessly strive for excellence.

References

1. Schafer ME. Cavitation generation and cavitational effects in phacoemulsification (abstract 329). Presented at the American Society of Cataract and Refractive Surgery Symposium, San Francisco, April 12–16, 2003

2. Soscia W, Howard JG, Olson RJ. Bimanual phacoemulsification through 2 stab incisions. A wound-temperature study. J Cataract Refract Surg 2002;28:1039–1043

3. Soscia W, Howard JG, Olson RJ. Microphacoemulsification with White-Star. A wound-temperature study. J Cataract Refract Surg 2002;28:1044–1046

4. Donnenfeld ED, Olson RJ, Solomon R, et al. Efficacy and wound-temperature gradient of WhiteStar phacoemulsification through a 1.2 mm incision. J Cataract Refract Surg 2003;29:1097–1100

5. Osher RH, Injev VP. Thermal study of bare tips with various system parameters and incision sizes. J Cataract Refract Surg 2006;32:867–872

6. Fishkind W, Bakewell B, Donnenfeld ED, Rose AD, Watkins LA, Olson RJ. Comparative clinical trial of ultrasound phacoemulsification with and without the WhiteStar system. J Cataract Refract Surg 2006;32:45–49

7. Braga-Mele R. Thermal effect of microburst and hyperpulse settings during sleeveless bimanual phacoemulsification with advanced power modulations. J Cataract Refract Surg 2006;32:639–642

8. Chang DF. Phaco chop: mastering techniques, optimizing technology, and avoiding complications. In: Chang DF, ed. Strategies for Managing Posterior Capsular Rupture. Thorofare, NJ: Slack; 2004:212–217

9. Liu Y, Zeng M, Liu X, et al. Torsional mode versus conventional ultrasound mode phacoemulsification: randomized comparative clinical study. J Cataract Refract Surg 2007;33:287–292

10. Rekas M, Montés-Micó R, Krix-Jachym K, Kluś A, Stankiewicz A, Ferrer-Blasco T. Comparison of torsional and longitudinal modes using phacoemulsification parameters. J Cataract Refract Surg 2009;35:1719–1724

11. Vasavada AR, Raj SM, Patel U, Vasavada V, Vasavada V. Comparison of torsional and microburst longitudinal phacoemulsification: a prospective, randomized, masked clinical trial. Ophthalmic Surg Lasers Imaging 2010;41:109–114

12. Georgescu D, Kuo AF, Kinard KI, Olson RJ. A fluidics comparison of Alcon Infiniti, Bausch & Lomb Stellaris, and Advanced Medical Optics Signature phacoemulsification machines. Am J Ophthalmol 2008;145:1014–1017

13. McNeill JI. Flared phacoemulsification tips to decrease ultrasound time and energy in cataract surgery. J Cataract Refract Surg 2001;27:1433–1436

14. Davison JA. Performance comparison of the Alcon Legacy 20000 straight and flared 0.9 mm Aspiration Bypass System tips. J Cataract Refract Surg 1999;25:1386–1391

15. Koch P. "Stop and Chop" [film]. American Society of Cataract and Refractive Surgery Film Festival Award Winner, 1993

16. Chang DF, ed. Bimanual Microincision Chopping in Phaco Chop and Advanced Phaco Techniques: Strategies for Complicated Cataracts, 2nd ed. Thorofare, NJ: Slack; 2013:77–83

17. Chang DF, Packard RB. Posterior assisted levitation for nucleus retrieval using Viscoat after posterior capsule rupture. J Cataract Refract Surg 2003;29:1860–1865

18. Michelson MA. Use of a Sheets' Glide as a pseudoposterior capsule in phacoemulsification complicated by posterior capsule rupture. Eur J Implant Surg 1993;570–572.

19. Kelman C. New PAL method may save difficult cataract cases. Ophthalmology Times 1994;19:51

20. Kumar DA, Agarwal A, Prakash G, Jacob S, Agarwal A, Sivagnanam S. IOL scaffold technique for posterior capsule rupture. J Refract Surg 2012;28:314–315

Further Reading

Phaco chop and advanced phaco techniques. In: Chang DF, ed. Strategies for Complicated Cataracts, 2nd ed. Thorofare, NJ: Slack; 2013: sections 1 and 2

Phacodynamics: Mastering the Tools and Techniques of Phacoemulsification Surgery, 4th ed. Thorofare, NJ: Slack; 2004

The phaco machine: the physical principles guiding its operation. In: Steinert RF, ed. Cataract Surgery, 3rd ed. Philadelphia: Saunders Elsevier; 2010:75–92

XV   Intraocular Lenses and Complications

38 Aspheric Intraocular Lenses

Uday Devgan

Photographers have known for many years that the key to great images is the optical properties of the lenses used in the cameras, almost all of which are aspheric. We have adopted the same concept in ophthalmology, with the introduction of precisely made intraocular lenses (IOLs) with aspheric optics.

Using an aspheric lens, particularly at large pupil sizes (or large camera apertures) ensures that all light rays entering the lens, both in the center and in the periphery, are focused at the same point or plane (**Fig. 38.1**). This gives a better image quality in terms of both sharpness as well as contrast (**Fig. 38.2**).

The traditional lenses are spherical because they have the same, constant curvature on the optic. In essence, they can be thought of as being carved out of a sphere of glass. This spherical lens has a higher power in the periphery than in the center, thereby inducing positive spherical aberration (SA).

An aspheric lens with zero SA has a variable curvature but produces a lens with an even power from center to edge. It can be more technically challenging to make, but it produces better optical quality. An aspheric lens can also be designed to have a negative degree of SA wherein the power of the lens is higher in the center than it is in the periphery (**Fig. 38.3**).

Incorporating aspheric IOLs in cataract surgery can help to restore a better quality of vision to our patients. Although the most important optical function of an IOL is correcting the lower order aberrations, such as sphere and cylinder, the ability to modulate the SA of the eye can lead to further improvements in vision.

Lower Order Versus Higher Order Aberrations

Lens power calculations depend on accurate biometry of the corneal power and axial length, but also on the ability to predict the effective lens position of the IOL after surgery. This last factor ends up being the source of much of the variance in refractive outcomes in our cataract surgery patients. Ideally, we would like to address the spherical component of the refraction, the astigmatism, as well as the SA with cataract surgery and the IOL implanted.

Optical aberrations, as best explained by the Zernike polynomials, can be divided into lower order aberrations and higher order aberrations. Patient satisfaction and visual outcomes are very well associated with achieving precise results in correcting these lower order aberrations, such as myopia, hyperopia, and astigmatism. In most eyes, it is far more important to accurately address the lower order aberrations than to focus on SA, which is just one of the many higher order aberrations. Higher order aberrations are more important in eyes with larger pupils. At a pupil size of 3 mm or below, SA plays only a minor role in image quality.[1]

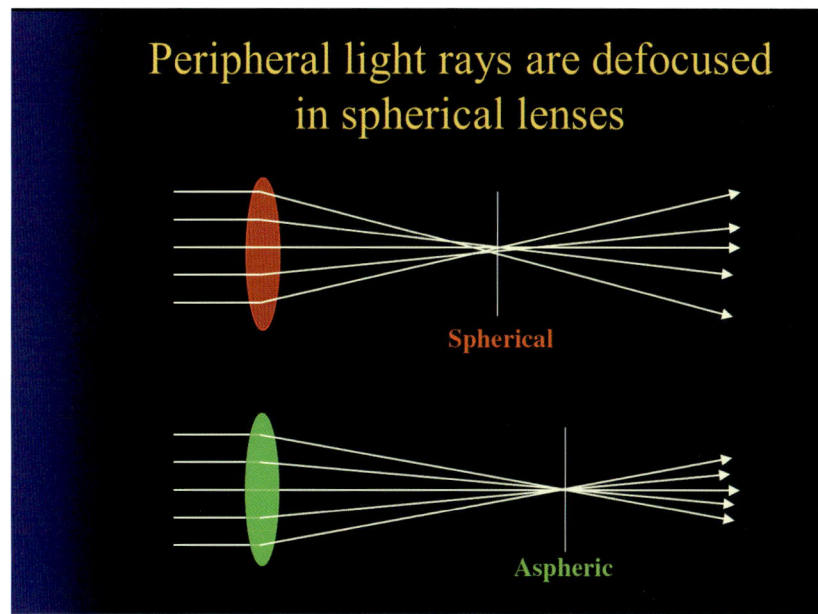

Fig. 38.1 In a spherical lens, the rays in the periphery of the lens focus differently than the rays in the center of the lens, thereby producing spherical aberration (SA) and degrading image quality. The aspheric lens enables all rays from the center to the periphery to focus at the same point.

329

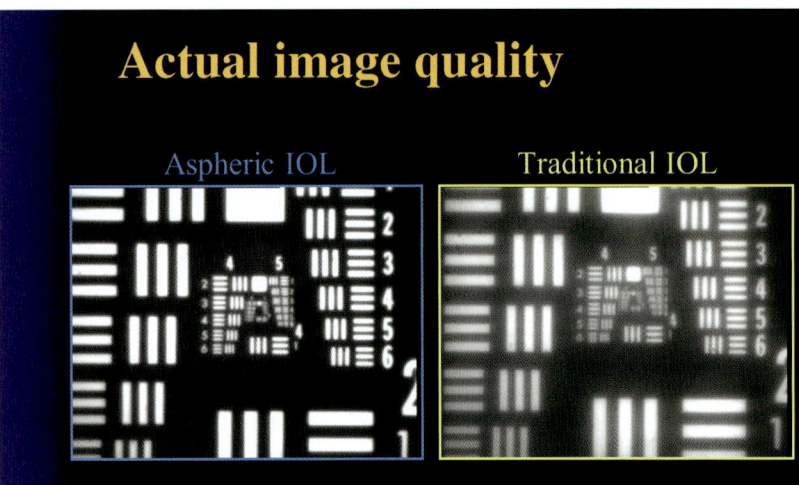

Fig. 38.2   Image quality taken through an intraocular lens (IOL) with aspheric optics and traditional optics showing the difference in image quality.

Addressing Spherical Aberration

Studies done by Li Wang and Douglas Koch's group[2,3] demonstrate that when we look at the average of the various corneal aberrations in a sample of normal eyes, the only one that has a nonzero mean is SA. The average cornea has a small degree of positive SA, which the young crystalline lens typically neutralizes because it has a small degree of negative SA. This produces an eye with a total of zero SA. As we age, the lens changes toward a less negative SA and the eye as a whole develops a small degree of positive SA. This may be helpful because it may increase the depth of field as the eye becomes presbyopic and loses accommodation.

In selecting an IOL for the eye, we have a choice of lenses with negative SA, such as the AcrySof line (Alcon, Fort Worth, TX) and the Tecnis line (Abbott Medical Optics [AMO], Abbott Park, IL), or those with zero SA, such as the EnVista, Akreos, SofPort, and Crystalens lines (Bausch and Lomb, Rochester, NY) (**Fig. 38.4**). In eyes in which we want to maximize the depth of field, there may be a benefit to the zero SA IOLs. In eyes in which we want to prioritize image quality at a specific focal point, the negative SA IOLs would be selected.

Of particular importance is to remember that in order for a negative SA IOL to address the positive SA of the cornea, the IOL must be very well centered in the visual axis. Decentration of negative SA IOLs can induce other higher order aberrations such as coma, whereas zero SA IOLs are relatively immune to mild decentration and do not induce coma.[4] Because the center of the visual axis is slightly nasally displaced when compared with the center of the capsular bag, it is helpful to orient the IOL in the vertical axis, with the haptics at the 12 and 6 o'clock positions, so that the axis can be nudged nasally to achieve optimal centration.

We know that lenticular SA changes as the eye ages. By age 60, most eyes have excessive positive SA, which degrades the quality of vision. The beauty of an aspheric IOL is that it can

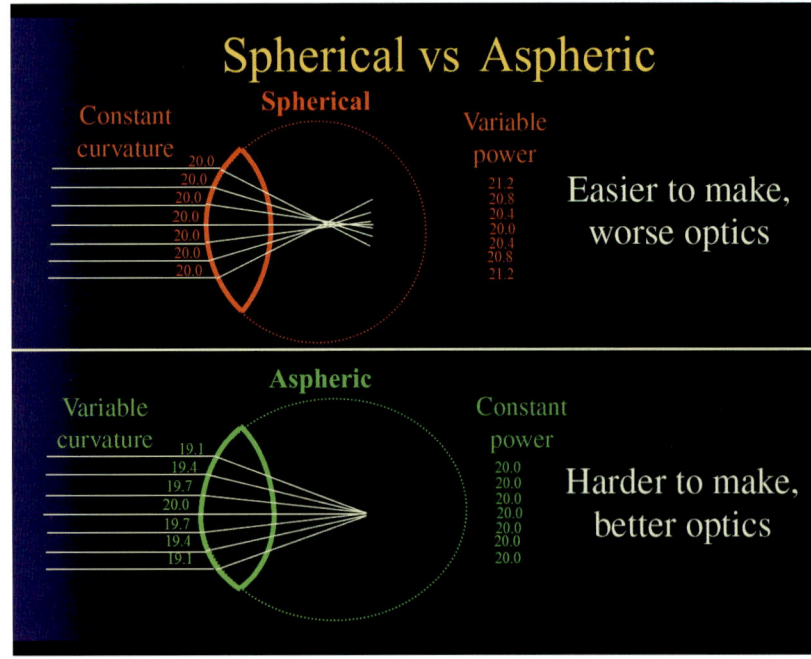

Fig. 38.3   Spherical versus aspheric lenses comparing curvature and power.

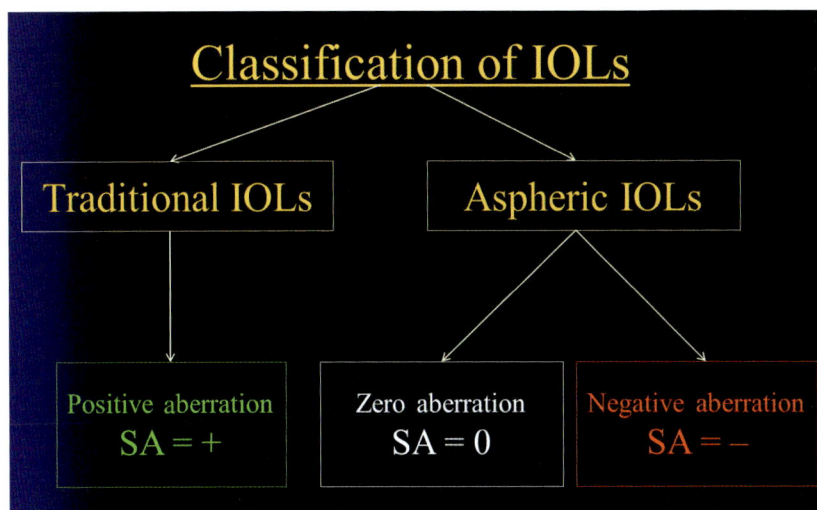

Fig. 38.4 Intraocular lenses are classified as either traditional, with a positive SA, or aspheric, with either zero or a negative SA.

restore the sharper image quality of the young eye. By addressing the SA, in addition to the lower order error, we can offer the patient improved contrast sensitivity and better visual performance in suboptimal lighting (**Fig. 38.5**).

With the variety of lens choices we now have, it is the surgeon's responsibility to tailor the lens choice to best suit the patients' eye anatomy, lifestyle, and needs and desires for their vision (**Fig. 38.6**). My decision tree has evolved to a very simple one that favors an aspheric IOL of one type or another in almost every case.

The acrylic Alcon AcrySof and AMO Tecnis IOLs offer a significant degree of negative SA. For most patients, this brings the total SA of the eye closest to the 20-year-old level of zero. This lens is also great for patients with prior myopic refractive surgery who probably have a significant level of induced positive SA. It is the lens I choose when I want the absolute sharpest vision, especially at night (**Fig. 38.7**).

The Bausch and Lomb silicone SofPort AO and acrylic Akreos AO IOLs have zero SA. They keep SA neutral and are relatively immune to centration issues. I choose a zero-SA lens if the patient has a highly aberrated cornea, perhaps from previous refractive surgery, or if there are loose zonules, a broken capsule, prior trauma, or anything else that leads me to expect trouble with lens centration (**Fig. 38.8**).

The only situation in which I implant a traditional spherical IOL is the occasional patient with a history of a large degree of hyperopic laser-assisted in situ keratomileusis (LASIK). These eyes often have too much negative SA, so the positive SA induced by a traditional lens balances out their aberrations.

Aspheric Intraocular Lens Selection in Special Cases

In eyes with prior keratorefractive surgery such as LASIK or photorefractive keratectomy (PRK), the laser ablation can alter the SA of the cornea. Typically, myopic ablations induce more positive SA in the cornea, whereas hyperopic treatments lessen the

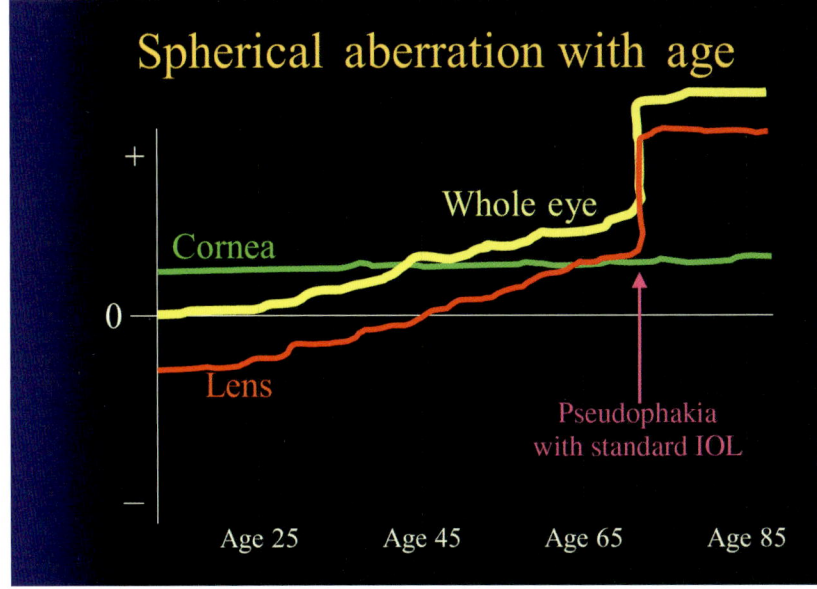

Fig. 38.5 Throughout life the cornea has a small degree of positive SA that is relatively constant. The lens, however, changes from negative SA to zero and then to positive SA with age.

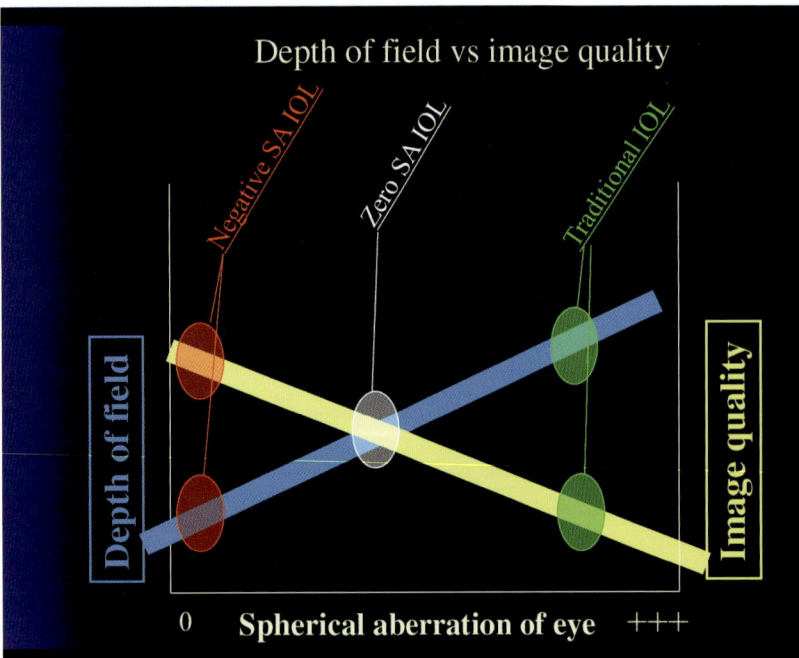

Fig. 38.6 Graph showing the relationship of SA, image quality, and depth of field.

corneal SA. Most of the excimer laser systems that we have used in the past decade have been optimized to minimize the SA changes, so extreme changes to corneal SA are now unusual. Using a negative SA IOL can help improve vision quality in eyes with prior myopic treatments. In eyes with prior hyperopic treatments, the zero SA IOL is usually the best choice, though in some cases a traditional IOL with positive SA may be useful (**Fig. 38.9**).

Prior myopic LASIK tends to induce positive corneal SA, so an aspheric monofocal IOL with negative SA is a good choice to return the eye to an overall status of no SA. The IOL with the highest ability to balance out a cornea after myopic LASIK is the AMO Tecnis, which comes in both a one-piece acrylic design (model ZCB00) as well as a three-piece acrylic design (model ZA9003). The Alcon Acrysof model SN60WF is a one-piece acrylic design that has less ability to balance out the SA of a post-LASIK cornea, but offers a yellow tint should that be desirable.

Eyes with complex aberrations, such as post–radial keratotomy (RK) eyes, may benefit from IOLs that induce zero SAs. These IOLs do not help to offset any corneal SA, but they also do not induce any aberrations. When there is a significant degree of corneal irregularity, a zero SA IOL such as the Bausch and Lomb

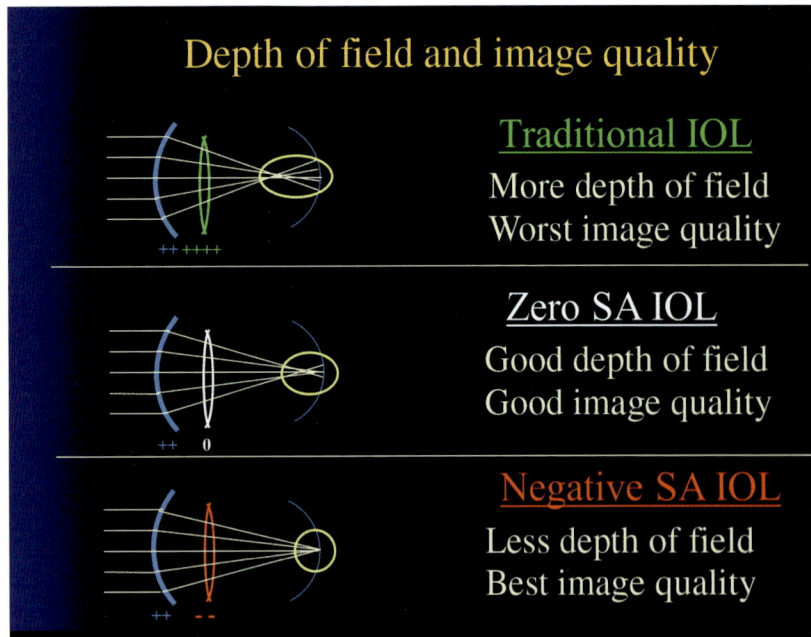

Fig. 38.7 Ray-tracing diagram showing the cornea and the various IOLs available with regard to depth of field and image quality.

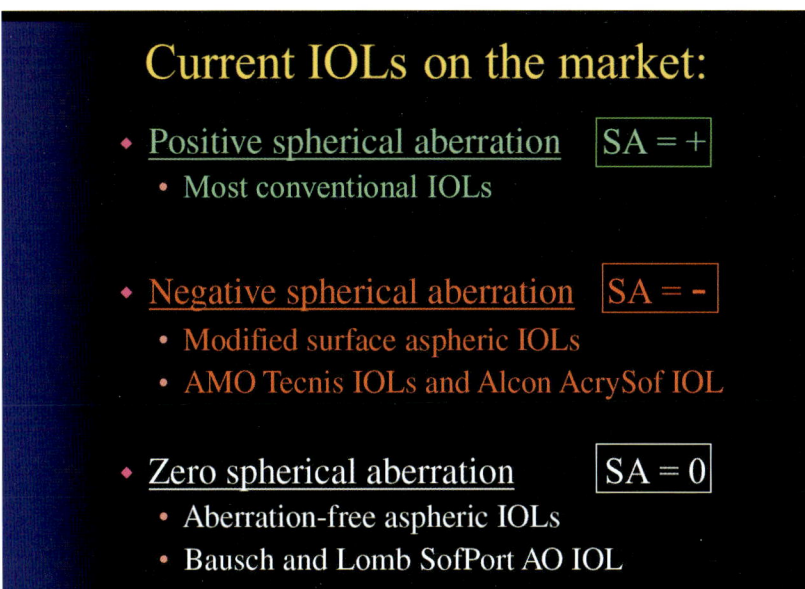

Fig. 38.8   Ray-tracing diagram showing the cornea and the various IOLs available with regard to SA.

SofPort AO silicone three-piece IOL, the Bausch and Lomb Akreos AO one-piece acrylic IOL, or the Collamer and Silicone aspheric IOLs (Staar, Monrovia, CA) are good choices.

Some eyes have preexisting corneal aberrations or anomalies such as scars, irregular astigmatism, corneal dystrophies, or decentered ablations. Using a zero SA IOL in these eyes does no harm in terms of higher order aberrations, whereas a negative SA IOL may confound the existing aberrations and degrade image quality.

Leaving the eye with the existing mild positive SA of the cornea by implanting a zero SA IOL may provide an improvement in depth of field. There are many other factors that influence depth of field as well, such as pupil size, other aberrations, and even ambient lighting. Modulating the SA of the eye with aspheric

IOLs can help to provide better vision outcomes for our patients in both routine and special cases. Surgeons should have access to both zero SA and negative SA IOLs to tailor the lens to each patient's situation (**Fig. 38.10**).

In the future, I think an aspheric design is something we will all take for granted, the way that we now expect nearly all lenses to have ultraviolet blocking and squared edges to prevent posterior capsule opacification (PCO). For the vast majority of patients, all of the above aspheric IOLs outperform traditional IOLs when it comes to image quality and contrast sensitivity, and all are appropriate choices. Aspheric IOLs now account for 95% of the monofocal lenses that I implant in my own practice, and I anticipate that other practices will soon notice similar trends.

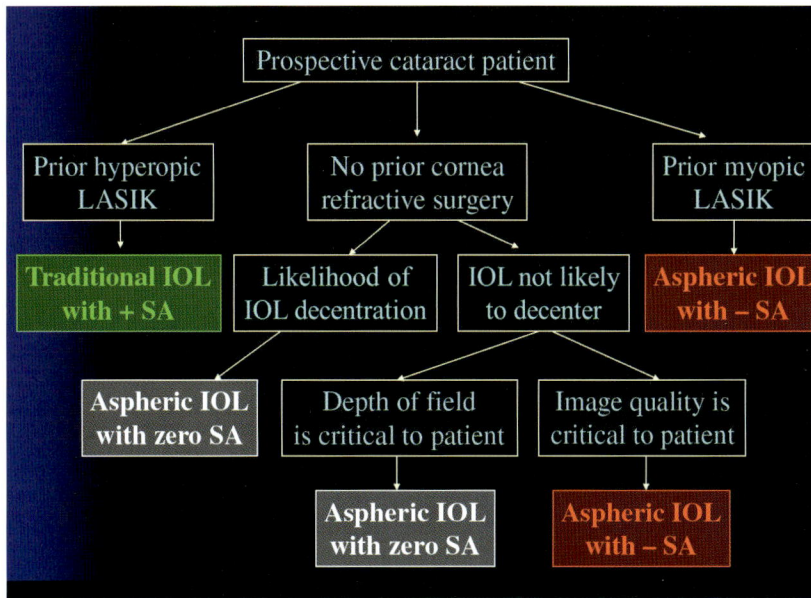

Fig. 38.9   Decision tree for IOL selection.

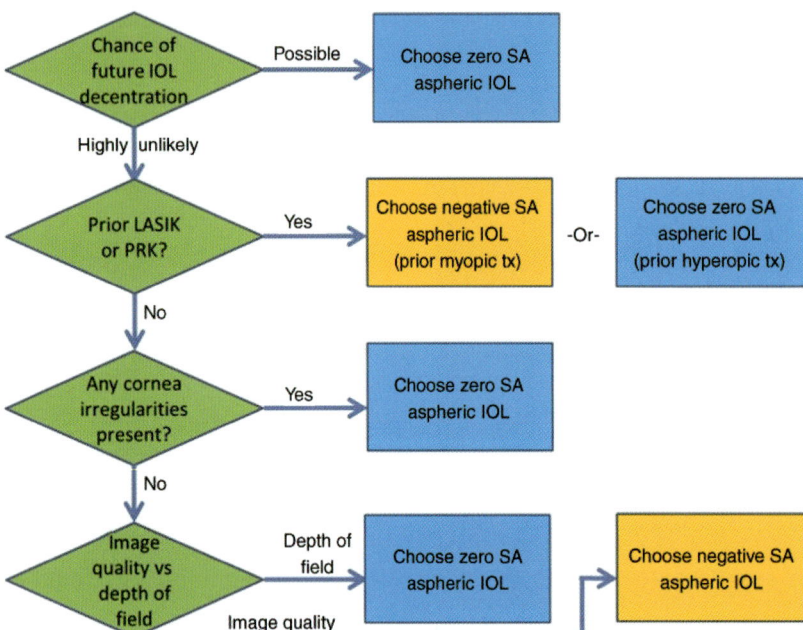

Fig. 38.10 Algorithm for selection of the most appropriate aspheric IOL. tx, treatment.

Financial Disclosure

Uday Devgan is a consultant/speaker for Alcon and Bausch and Lomb, and formerly for AMO.

References

1. Wang L, Santaella RM, Booth M, Koch DD. Higher-order aberrations from the internal optics of the eye. J Cataract Refract Surg 2005;31:1512–1519

2. Yeu E, Wang L, Koch DD. The effect of corneal wavefront aberrations on corneal pseudoaccommodation. Am J Ophthalmol 2012;153:972–981.e2

3. Koch DD, Wang L. Custom optimization of intraocular lens asphericity. Trans Am Ophthalmol Soc 2007;105:36–41, discussion 41–42

4. Wang L, Koch DD. Effect of decentration of wavefront-corrected intraocular lenses on the higher-order aberrations of the eye. Arch Ophthalmol 2005;123:1226–1230

39 Intraocular Lens Implantation

Harry B. Grabow and William J. Fishkind

Intraocular lens (IOL) implantation, whether phakic or aphakic, entails complications that can occur before, during, or long after implantation. They can result in damage to the eye, the IOL, or both. Surgeons and manufacturers alike, in an effort to minimize the incidence and severity of IOL-related complications, have been studying implantation techniques and IOL behavior since the late 1970s. The method of insertion of an IOL into the eye, and the IOL design, material, and location are all associated with potential complications.

The effect of the location of an IOL inside the eye has been under continuous scrutiny. IOLs have been fixated in the anterior chamber (AC) angle, the anterior iris stroma, the pupil, the posterior chamber (ciliary sulcus), the lens capsular bag, and the pars plana. IOL materials have proliferated since the first polymethylmethacrylate (PMMA) IOL was implanted by Harold Ridley[1] in 1949. Brought on by the success of small-incision phacoemulsification in the 1970s,[2] rigid PMMA lenses have been supplanted by foldable lenses of silicone, polyhydroxyethylmethacrylate (poly-HEMA), acrylic, and biologic collagen.[3] Each material behaves differently from the others during and after implantation.

The introduction of any physical object through an incision into the eye can result in damage to the intraocular structures (**Box 39.1**). If an IOL is forced through an incision that is too small, the incision might enlarge by tearing or stretching, with the possible result of an unstable and leaking wound, requiring suturing to prevent leakage. Wound leakage is thought to be one cause of postoperative infectious endophthalmitis.

In an attempt to pass the insertion device through the tight incision, excessive posterior angulation may cause inadvertent iridodialysis, with associated hyphema, or a torn posterior capsule. This is especially possible if substantial force is used to push the insertion device through the tight incision. The release of the cartridge into the AC can be so forceful that the cartridge passes though the posterior capsule. Similarly, an insertion forceps, or cartridge angled too anteriorly, might cause stripping of Descemet's membrane. The improper wound and chamber dynamics thus created could result in iris prolapse, chamber collapse, corneal endothelial damage, and subsequent postoperative corneal edema.

Improper attention during implantation may traumatize the capsule, resulting in zonulodialysis, tearing of the anterior capsule, tearing of the posterior capsule, and rupture of the anterior hyaloid face, increasing the incidence of postoperative cystoid macular edema (CME) and retinal detachment.

With proper attention paid to wound size and construction, chamber maintenance, ophthalmic viscosurgical device (OVD), and careful intraocular manipulation, the incidence of traumatic IOL implantation can be greatly minimized.

Just as the ocular tissues may be damaged during IOL implantation, so may the IOL itself (**Box 39.2**). Damage to an IOL ranges from minor optic surface damage from implant forceps or injectors causing scratches, or scuffing of acrylic or silicone IOLs, to major optic fracture or transection. IOL haptics may also be deformed or fractured.

Three-piece foldable IOLs may sustain damage to the haptics during implantation. When an insertion cartridge or forceps is used, the leading or trailing haptic may be caught by the folder and crimped. A bend in the haptic can be gently straightened and the IOL implanted. To do this, withdraw the damaged haptic

---

Box 39.1 Operative Ocular Complications of IOL Implantation

- Unstable wound/leakage
- Stripped Descemet's membrane
- Corneal endothelial trauma
- Iris prolapse
- Iridodialysis
- Hyphema
- Zonulodialysis
- Torn anterior capsule
- Torn posterior capsule
- Rupture anterior hyaloid

Box 39.2 Operative IOL Complications

- Haptic deformation
- Haptic fracture
- Haptic avulsion
- Optic excoriation
- Optic deformation
- Optic fracture
- Asymmetric bag/sulcus implantation
- Reversed-optic implantation*
- Off-axis implantation**
- Posterior IOL dislocation

*Angled haptics, toric, and multifocal IOLs.
**Toric IOL.

Box 39.3 Complications of IOL Injectors

Problem	Cause	Management
Torn leading or trailing haptic	Crimped trailing haptic; torn IOL	Careful observance of placement guide
	Improper placement in cartridge	Careful observance of placement guide
	Aggressive injector speed	Inject more slowly
	Inadequate viscoelastic	Use Adequate OVD
Plunger damage	Aggressive injector speed	Inject more slowly
	Improper placement in cartridge	Careful observance of placement guide
		Watch plunger as it contacts posterior IOL; avoid contact with haptic
		Use preloaded IOL
	Too long dwell time	Do not load IOL into cartridge more than 5 minutes before intended insertion.

through the wound and utilize two instruments to straighten the bend. Then dial the IOL into position. If the haptic fractures or is broken during the straightening process, it must be removed and the IOL replaced.

Infrequently, when injecting three-piece lenses, if the lens is not positioned properly in the cartridge, the leading or trailing haptic may be torn off during implantation. This IOL also must be removed and replaced. Additionally, improper plunger positioning may crimp the leading or trailing haptic. This can usually be straightened, but if severe, or broken, the IOL must be removed and replaced. Overriding plungers can damage the optic. Minor scratches can be left alone, but if in doubt about the severity of a scratch or scuff, remove the IOL and replace it with an undamaged one. It is far more difficult to go back later if the patient complains of dysphotopsia. Let your conscience be your guide on this issue.

One-piece IOLs have problems with the haptics or optics similar to three-piece IOLs. However, the haptic–optic junction is more robust, so haptic avulsion is more rare and haptic crimping does not occur. The surface of the one-piece acrylics, depending on the manufacturer, may be more prone to scuffing

Silicone three-piece IOLs that are left in the barrel of the injector too long can often stick to the plastic cartridge and tear

during insertion. Therefore, it is important not to load the IOL into the cartridge more than 5 minutes prior to insertion, and not to start the IOL down the barrel until the actual time of intended insertion (**Box 39.3**). Plate haptic silicone 6.0-mm optic lenses were originally designed to go through cartridges large enough for 4.0-mm scleral incisions. However, they are now going through cartridges tapered to fit through sub–3.0-mm clear-corneal incisions. Subsequent compression and occasional piston override can result in either haptic or optic fracture. If the fracture has completely transected the trailing plate haptic, destabilizing the optic centration, the IOL must be removed and replaced (**Fig. 39.1**). However, if the fracture involved avulsion of only a corner of a plate or is only partially through a haptic, the lens may be left in situ, as the centration of the IOL will not be affected (**Fig. 39.2**). The general rule regarding optic tears is as follows: A partial fracture of an optic that does not involve the central 3 to 4 mm of the "optical zone" may be left in place; if the tear enters the visual axis, the possibility of dysphotopsias is significant and the IOL should be removed and replaced.

In these cases with small tears, rotation of the peripheral optic fracture to the 12 o'clock position enables the upper eyelid to cover the peripheral optic aberration. In addition, capsulor-

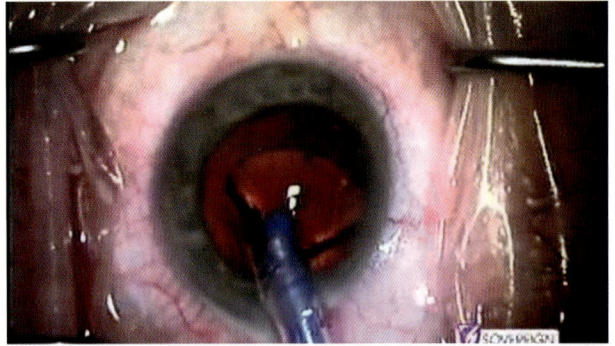

Fig. 39.1 A tear during insertion caused by the intraocular lens (IOL) catching on the edge of the injector. (Courtesy of William J. Fishkind, MD.)

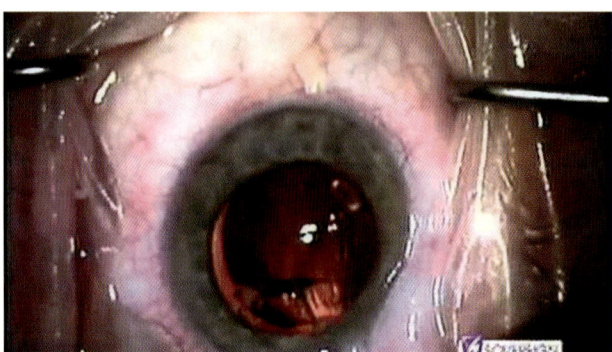

Fig. 39.2 The tear of the optic is extensive. This IOL must be removed and replaced. (Courtesy of William J. Fishkind, MD.)

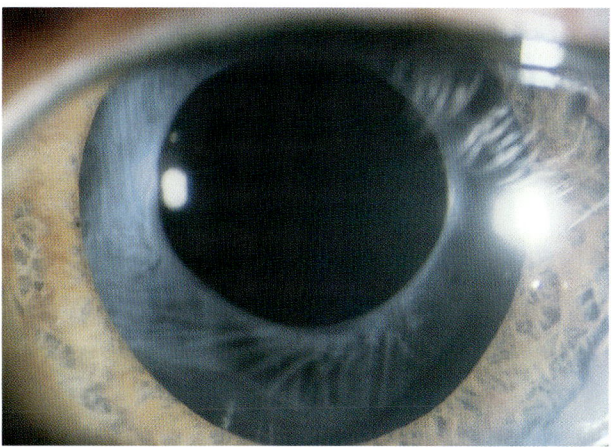

Fig. 39.3 Anterior capsular fibrosis over a plate-haptic silicone IOL.

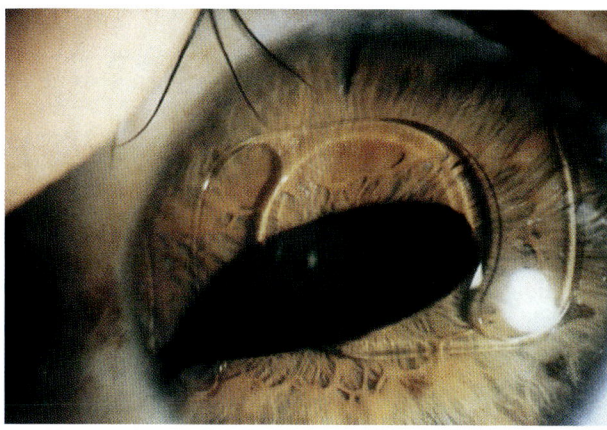

Fig. 39.4 Progressive postoperative pupillary ovalization with a polymethylmethacrylate (PMMA) anterior chamber (AC) IOL. (Courtesy of J. Alio.)

rhexis contraction and fibrosis may cover the area (**Fig. 39.3**), as well as the pupil itself.

Phakic Intraocular Lens

Errors of implantation may also occur without damage to the IOL. Although AC IOL implantation is now rarely performed during cataract surgery, it is currently used, although usually not a first choice, for the phakic correction of ametropia. As the pupil is often intentionally miotic for AC implantation, damage to the iris may occur. Iridodialysis with hyphema can occur both on the proximal side, due to dragging of the subincisional iris while moving the leading haptic toward the pupil, and on the distal side, when attempting to force the trailing haptic of an oversized IOL into the proximal angle. Tucking of the distal iris causes an acute ovaling of the pupil (**Fig. 39.4**). Excessive manipulation of an AC IOL may result in chamber collapse with IOL contact with the corneal endothelium.

The implantable Collamer lens (ICL; Staar Surgical, Monrovia, CA) is an extremely soft and friable Collamer material. It must be loaded carefully and injected slowly. If the lens is damaged in any way, it should be removed and replaced. Lens length and vault are difficult to determine and are directly related to postoperative complications. A full discussion of the ICL is beyond the scope of this chapter.

Phakic and aphakic iris-supported IOL implantation is also currently available in Europe. The Worst-Fechner "lobster-claw" IOL[4] (Artisan, Ophtec, Groningen, the Netherlands) is enclaved onto the anterior iris stroma, unlike their first-generation predecessors, such as the Binkhorst iris-clip IOL, the Worst two-loop medallion IOL, the Copeland Maltese cross IOL, the Fyodorov Sputnik IOL, and others, which were pupil-supported. The enclavation process of these newer version iris-supported IOLs, in the event of phakic implantation, can result in pressure damage to the lens in back with subsequent development of cataract, or to endothelial damage in both phakic and aphakic implantation if care is not taken to suture or secure the wound before enclavation to prevent viscoelastic escape and chamber collapse (assuming that proper stabilization of the IOL was maintained).

Posterior Chamber Intraocular Lens

Implantation of the posterior chamber (PC) presumes the presence of an intact or mostly intact zonulocapsular apparatus. The zonule may be complete or incomplete. The capsule may be intact or partially collapsed from sectoral zonulodialysis or torn anteriorly or posteriorly. Just as an AC IOL can tuck the peripheral anterior iris stroma, so can a PC IOL tuck the peripheral posterior iris pigmented layer. The haptic, in this case, may push the iris forward at that location, causing sectoral angle closure and peripheral anterior synechiae formation. Chronic chafing of the pigmented layer can result in a transillumination defect and pigment dispersion syndrome. Vigorous implantation of haptics into the ciliary sulcus can result in traumatic zonulodialysis and inadvertent posterior loop location on the pars plana.[5,6] Implantation in the PC in the absence of capsular support requires suturing of loops to the sclera.[7,8] Avoiding damage to the ciliary sulcus structures by the blind passage of a needle behind the iris can be facilitated by passing a hollow needle ab externo to guide the intraocular suture needle out through the proper anatomic location[9–11] (see Chapters 27 to 31).

Implantation of the capsular bag entails potential complications. Unintentional asymmetric bag/sulcus implantation, with one haptic in the capsular bag and one in the ciliary sulcus, may occur, particularly in cases of large capsulorrhexis openings where the continuous curvilinear capsulorrhexis (CCC) is larger than the diameter of the optic, in cases of small pupils with impaired visualization of haptic placement, or in cases of anterior radial tears.[12,13] This may be recognized by inspection at the time of implantation or may not be recognized until a postoperative dilated slit-lamp examination. Careful IOL rotation before removal of the OVD can verify the haptic position in the capsular bag. Early repositioning of the optic into the capsular bag may be performed in the operating room. However, if not recognized until later, when capsular fibrosis has caused decentration or anterior subluxation of the IOL, then loop-haptic and plate-haptic IOLs must be treated differently.

A three-piece rounded optic loop-haptic IOL may simply be dialed out of the fibrosed capsular bag into the ciliary sulcus, provided that significant loop deformity has not occurred. This is usually possible with a three-piece foldable lens with extruded PMMA haptics.

A one-piece IOL with a square edge cannot be placed in the ciliary sulcus (**Fig. 39.5**). The square edge and lack of angulation will invariably cause recurrent iris chafe, with subsequent pigmentary dispersion and glaucoma, and iris atrophy. Therefore, the capsular bag must be viscodissected and opened and the IOL repositioned into the capsular bag. Viscodissection of the capsular bag can be performed years after the original surgery and is more successful when the anterior capsulotomy is smaller than

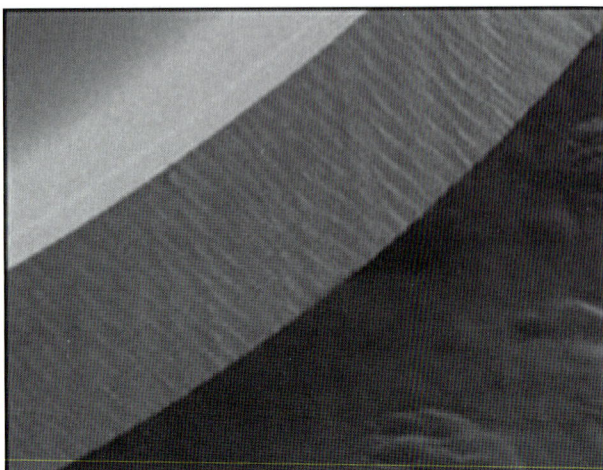

Fig. 39.5 Square edge of the Abbott Medical Optics (AMO) Tecnis one-piece IOL. (Courtesy of AMO.)

the IOL optic, preventing fibrosis of the anterior capsule to the posterior capsule. To do this, OVD should be gently injected through the opening in the bag created at the haptic–optic junction. If successful, the capsule will distend, enabling gentle viscoseparation of the anterior from the posterior capsule. The plane of separation is then performed for 360 degrees. The IOL can then be dialed out of the capsular bag and inspected. It then can be repositioned with both haptics within the capsular bag, or, if the haptics are significantly distorted, replaced. If it is impossible to separate the anterior capsule from the posterior capsule due to capsular fibrosis, further attempts should be curtailed rather than risk tearing the capsular bag or disinserting the zonule. The IOL can nevertheless be dialed out of the bag, but the new IOL must be placed in the ciliary sulcus.

Three-piece IOLs with polypropylene haptics cannot be repositioned, as the haptic has no memory and the permanent deformation of the haptic will interfere with stable IOL positioning. They must be removed and replaced or sutured into the ciliary sulcus.

A plate haptic IOL, measuring less than 11.2 mm in overall length, is too short for sulcus fixation. It must be either repositioned into the capsular bag, after reopening with OVD, or, if that is not possible, removed and replaced with a three-piece, rounded optic edge, PMMA loop-haptic IOL in the sulcus.

A second implantation error is that of implanting an IOL upside down, the front side in back, or anteroposteriorly reversed. A foldable IOL can easily unfold upside down if the insertion process is too fast and not properly controlled. Upside-down implantation of the IOL would be of potential refractive significance in the case of an IOL with angled haptics and specific optic edge configurations. Additionally, with an aspheric IOL or toric and multifocal IOLs, where the IOL power is on the posterior surface of the optic, postoperative refractive errors may occur and may be significant. Three-piece IOLs with polypropylene or extruded PMMA haptics, and a non-aspheric design, have no significant memory. Therefore, after a short time they flatten in the capsular bag, inducing little change in the calculated postoperative power. In the case of a spherical monofocal IOL, even with angulated haptics, the IOL may be left in place with usually no more than 0.25 diopter of induced postoperative myopia. However, the silicone plate–haptic toric IOLs (Staar models AA4203T and AA4203TL) and the acrylic single-piece haptic multifocal IOLs (Tecnis models ZMB, ZKB, ZLB, Abbott Medical Optics [AMO], Abbott Park, IL), with their added corrections intended for the

posterior IOL surface after implantation, lose their intended effects when implanted reversed (**Fig. 39.6**).

Because it has been estimated that there may be a distance of as much as 8.0 mm from the corneal endothelium to the posterior capsule when fully distended with a dispersive viscoelastic, it is usually possible to turn over a 6.0-mm optic IOL inside the eye. Refolding an IOL inside the eye with two instruments has also been demonstrated, but is usually unnecessary.[14] Otherwise, but also rarely necessary, the incision may be extended, and the inverted IOL may be removed and reimplanted right side up. The choice of corrective maneuver depends on the surgeon's judgment and experience.

Off-axis implantation relates specifically to toric IOLs. It would be unlikely for a toric IOL to be inadvertently implanted at the incorrect axis. However, it is a simple matter to rotate a plate-haptic silicone IOL to its correct axis at the time of implantation with an instrument through the 1.0-mm side-port incision.

Decentered IOL implantation is important for implantation of all aspheric IOLs and especially multifocal IOLs. Small amounts of decentration may lead to dysphotopsias as well as decreased near or far visual acuity. Toric and aspheric IOL decentration may result in a diminished quality of vision. It is prudent to mark the center of the visual axis, on the cornea, in the preoperative area. Despite parallax, this mark is effective in determining centration

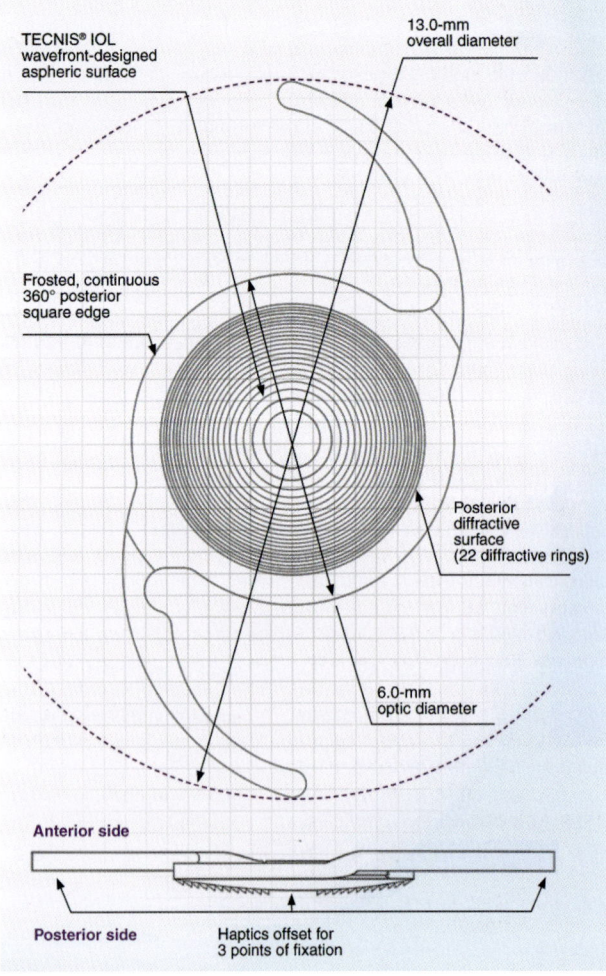

Fig. 39.6 Technical drawing of the AMO Tecnis Multifocal with the IOL power on the posterior surface. (Courtesy of AMO.)

in the presence of the dilated pupil. Femtosecond laser–assisted cataract surgery (FLACS) is also helpful, as IOL centration on the precise capsulorrhexis ensures IOL centration.

If using a femtosecond laser, the capsulorrhexis can be centered over the visual axis, rather than the anatomic axis. If the IOL is then centered in the capsulorrhexis, it will automatically be centered on the visual axis.

Additionally, complete removal of OVD behind the IOL promotes better adhesion of the IOL to the capsular bag, minimizing the risk of decentration in the immediate postoperative period. Use of cohesive OVD for IOL implantation assists in OVD removal. Finally, leaving the eye soft, that is, at an intraocular pressure (IOP) of 10 to 15 mm Hg also promotes IOL–capsular bag contact.

Posterior IOL dislocation into the vitreous at the time of primary implantation is also a rare occurrence. There is a particular propensity for this to occur during unfolding of a three-piece silicone IOL for sulcus implantation in the presence of a large rent in the posterior capsule, particularly after vitrectomy has already been performed. Silicone IOLs have considerable potential energy when folded in an injector. As the IOL is delivered, it can unfold explosively, catching and tearing the posterior or equatorial capsular bag.

Posterior IOL dislocation into the vitreous can also occur during routine foldable IOL implantation in the presence of an intact capsule, when the act of insertion or unfolding causes the capsule to tear, allowing the IOL to fall into syneretic vitreous. Tears in the posterior capsule during unfolding usually occur when the unfolding leading haptic catches a fold in the posterior capsule. This can be avoided by the use of adequate OVD to deeply fill the capsular bag to prevent the folds that can capture the unfolding haptic. With slow, controlled implantation, and manipulation of the injector, the tendency for the leading haptic to unfold in the wrong direction can be detected, and redirected, before implantation is completed. This will avert this complication.

For the novice surgeon, maintaining orientation of the unfolding IOL in the AC ensures proper IOL orientation. The unfolding leading haptic should point to the left. If it points right, up or down, it is easy to rotate the injector 180 degrees so that the haptic points to the left. Additionally if the haptic is unfolding superiorly or inferiorly, it is a simple process to slow down, and rotate the injector to ensure that the haptic is in the horizontal plane.

Postoperative Intraocular Lens Complications

Postoperative IOL-related complications are usually associated with either malfunction or malposition of an IOL. Malfunction includes either unwanted optical images, such as dysphotopsias, glare, halos, or edge reflections, as seen with square-edged acrylic IOL designs, as well as with concentric multifocal designs, or incorrect or undesirable IOL power, resulting in unwanted anisometropia with secondary ametropia. Heavy glistening formation is included in this category; however, glistenings have not been categorically associated with dysphotopsia.

Intraocular lens malpositions are traditionally classified into these categories:

1. Decentration
2. Subluxation
3. Dislocation

With the advent of capsular-fixated single-piece acrylic and plate-haptic toric IOLs, a fourth category, rotation, can occur, which is especially significant with toric IOLs.

Anterior Chamber Intraocular Lens Malposition

In the AC, decentration may occur when the AC IOL is improperly sized. An AC IOL that is too short will decenter and be unstable. The haptic may repeatedly traumatize the corneal endothelium with subsequent endothelial damage. An unstable AC IOL may also rotate until a haptic migrates through the peripheral iridectomy, resulting in optic decentration and complaints of monocular diplopia. If an AC IOL is to be utilized, a peripheral iridectomy is mandatory to prevent pupillary block glaucoma. The iridectomy, however, should not be placed at the iris root, but rather in the mid-stroma. Should the IOL rotate, the mid-stromal position of the iridotomy will prevent entrapment and migration of the IOL haptic.

An AC IOL that is too long may push the peripheral iris posteriorly, ovaling the pupil and causing chronic inflammation and secondary glaucoma—the uveitis-glaucoma-hyphema (UGH) syndrome. Iris-enclaved IOLs may become un-enclaved.[15] The loosely fixated IOL may then become decentered with visual symptoms. In addition, endothelial damage may occur.

Posterior Chamber Intraocular Lens Malposition

Decentration of a PC IOL in the ciliary sulcus may also occur if the IOL's overall size is too small for the diameter of the ciliary sulcus. If there is partial absence of the zonule (often unrecognized), a haptic may migrate posteriorly, resulting in decentration of the IOL optic; however, this form of decentration may be more accurately described as a subluxation.

Decentration of an IOL fixated in the capsular bag may be caused by the IOL size, by the IOL haptic material, or by the postoperative behavior of residual lens epithelial cells. In the case of fixed-size IOLs whose haptics do not expand to fill the capsular space, such as plate-haptic designs, the overall diameter of the IOL may be shorter than the diameter of the capsule, resulting in decentration along the short or long axis of the IOL. This is particularly likely to occur in the presence of a large anterior CCC or an anterior capsular rent. One haptic may dislocate anteriorly, out of the bag into the ciliary sulcus, or may actually dislocate through the dilated pupil into the AC, resulting in pupillary optic capture (**Fig. 39.7**). Finally, the optic of a loop-haptic PC IOL

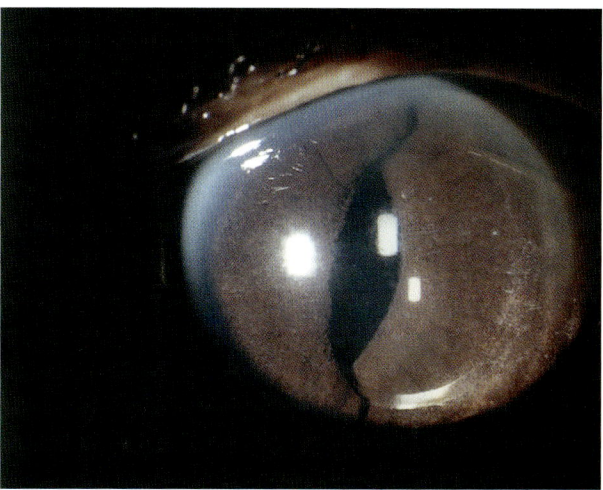

Fig. 39.7 Anterior plate haptic dislocation with pupillary optic capture: one day postoperative.

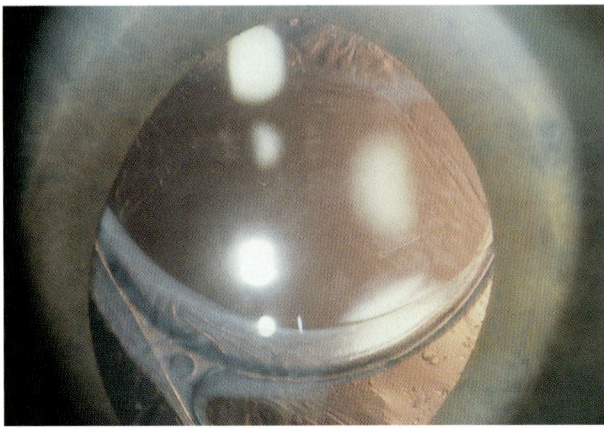

Fig. 39.8 Superior haptic decentration due to superior haptic anterior dislocation with resultant asymmetric bag–sulcus fixation.

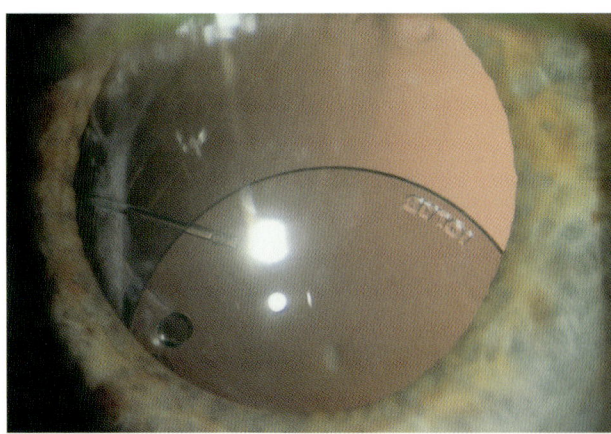

Fig. 39.9 Postoperative subluxation of loop-haptic posterior chamber (PC) IOL due to unstable posterior capsule.

placed into the ciliary sulcus or capsular bag may be captured by the pupil and may cause pupillary block.[16] Flexible loop haptics made of material with poor elastic memory, such as polypropylene, may decenter under the contractile influence of metaplastic capsular fibrosis. The same fibrotic forces may also force a loop to dislocate anteriorly out of the capsule. Such asymmetric "bag–sulcus" fixation often results in optic decentration (**Fig. 39.8**). If an unrecognized equatorial capsular tear occurred at the time of original surgery, late subluxation or total posterior dislocation may occur, both being the result of capsular fibrotic activity (**Fig. 39.9**). Both loop-haptic[17] and plate-haptic IOLs are subject to such occurrence (**Fig. 39.10**). If adequate adhesion has developed between the anterior and posterior capsules around the remaining encapsulated loop-haptic or through the fenestration of a plate-haptic (**Figs. 39.11** and **39.12**), then total posterior dislocation into the vitreous (**Fig. 39.13**) may not occur.

Management of Intraocular Lenses

Complications

The first decision to be made intraoperatively, when an IOL complication is observed, is whether or not to change the intended surgical procedure. If an IOL problem has been determined to have the potential to threaten positional stability or proper optical performance, then surgical correction is indicated. Similarly, postoperatively, if an IOL is determined to be the cause of pathophysiology or suboptimal optical performance, then secondary surgical intervention may be likewise indicated.[18]

Whether primarily or secondarily, the action taken usually falls into one of the three R's: repositioning, removal, and replacement.

Intraocular Lens Repositioning (See Chapters 25 to 31)

Intraocular lens repositioning presumes that the desired IOL was implanted but that it is not in the desired anatomic position. A repositioning procedure may move an IOL without changing its

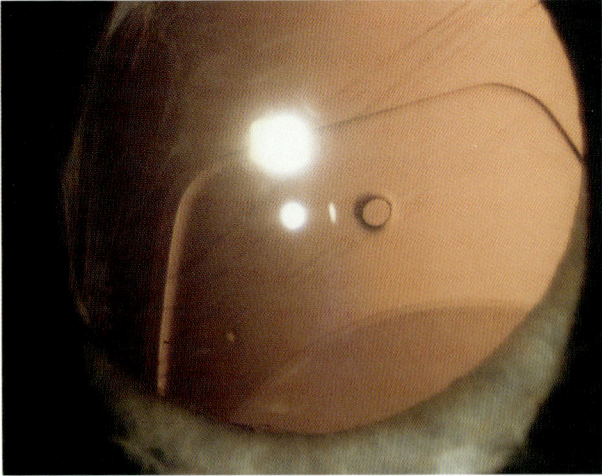

Fig. 39.10 Postoperative subluxation of small-fenestration plate-haptic PC IOL.

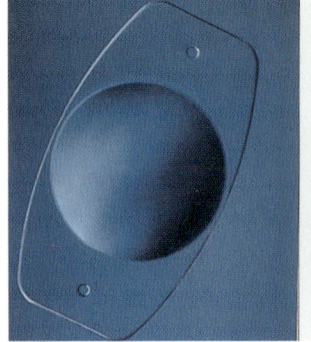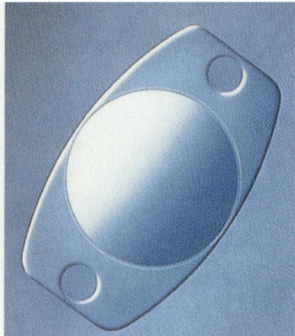

Fig. 39.11 Older, small-fenestration and newer, large-fenestration plate-haptic IOL designs.

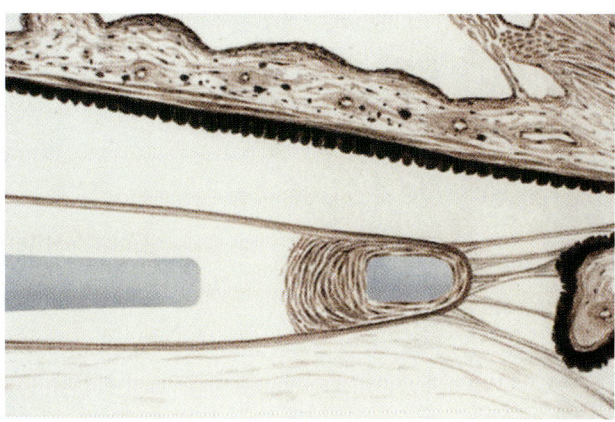

Fig. 39.12 Artist's enhancement of capsular fibrosis through large-fenestration plate haptic.

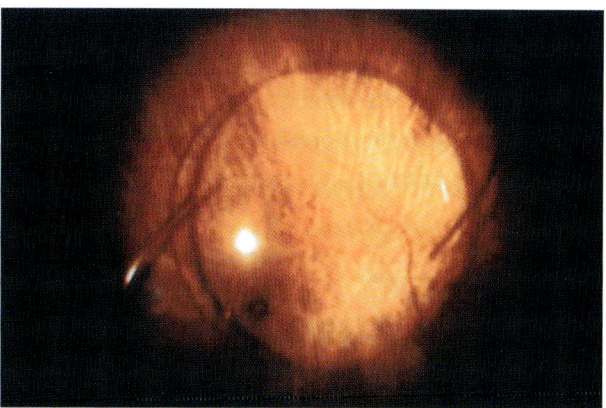

Fig. 39.13 Total posterior dislocation of a loop-haptic PC.

location, such as rotating a toric IOL within the capsular bag or rotating an AC IOL to retrieve a haptic that has migrated through an iridectomy, or to release an incarcerated peripheral iris to circularize an oval pupil. An asymmetric IOL position, such as the bag–sulcus location, with one haptic in the bag and one in the sulcus, with optic decentration, is a common cause of IOL repositioning. The surgeon then has the choice either to replace the sulcus haptic back into the bag or to place the bag haptic into the sulcus. Similarly, an optic or a haptic of a PC IOL may be partially or totally through the pupil, with "optic capture" necessitating haptic repositioning. All of these maneuvers can be performed under topical anesthesia through a 1-mm paracentesis incision, with appropriate viscoelastic, at the slit lamp, or in the operating room, depending on patient compliance.

There is another circumstance that may indicate surgical IOL repositioning, and that is total posterior dislocation. A lens that has gone through a large opening in the posterior capsule may be repositioned into the ciliary sulcus. This requires pars plana vitrectomy. If there is adequate anterior capsule remaining and the IOL is of appropriate size, the IOL may be placed into the sulcus without sutures.[19,20] Some cases may necessitate polypropylene suture fixation of one or both haptics to the posterior surface of the iris[21] or to the sclera.[22–25]

In the absence of adequate capsular support, elevation of the IOL to the ciliary sulcus, externalizing and gluing the haptics, has become a noteworthy alternative.

Intraocular Lens Removal

Intraocular lens removal without replacement is an extremely rare event. It is sometimes performed in eyes in which the IOL itself is thought to be the cause of chronic uveitis, chronic endophthalmitis, recurrent spontaneous hyphema, pigmentary glaucoma, or progressive corneal endothelial cell loss—even though there is no malposition or refractive dysfunction of the IOL. In these instances, an IOL may be removed and not replaced, almost as a diagnostic or therapeutic trial, to see if the chronic pathology will be corrected. Once the underlying problem is ascertained, a secondary IOL implantation in the sulcus can then be performed.

Vitreoretinal surgeons also occasionally perform IOL removal. This might occur if, at the time of posterior vitrectomy or scleral buckle, a well-tolerated IOL loses its proper support or loses its transparency due to chemical adhesion, such as silicone oil adhering to a silicone IOL. In these cases, if the appropriate corrective measure is not undertaken at the time of the posterior segment procedure, the eye will be left, intentionally, temporarily aphakic, with reimplantation to be undertaken later by a cataract surgeon.

Technique

The method of IOL removal depends on the type and location of the IOL being removed. The incision size required for IOL removal depends on the IOL optic material. PMMA IOLs require incisions large enough to accommodate the rigid optic to be removed; this usually means 5 to 6 mm. An incision of this length can affect the corneal curvature. Therefore, its location, whether scleral or corneal, superior or temporal, may be preselected by the surgeon to achieve the desired astigmatic effect. Sclerocorneal frown incisions minimize induced astigmatism if the IOL must be removed. Some AC IOLs (especially those with closed loops) may have formed peripheral anterior synechiae, "fibrotic cocoons," around the haptics in the angle. The attempt at manual extraction may then be met with resistance. Excessive traction may result in iridodialysis and hyphema. In these cases, haptic amputation with scissors enables atraumatic optic removal; the haptics then may be either left in or removed by dialing them out of their fibrotic tunnels.

Removal of PMMA PC IOLs that are in the ciliary sulcus must be done carefully by dialing the haptics until they are free of any adhesions. Similarly, loop haptics encapsulated in the capsular bag may also be fixed by equatorial fibrosis. Attempt at IOL removal from the capsular bag may then be met with resistance, and continued traction may result in either a capsular tear or, more likely, zonulodialysis. Therefore, if resistance is encountered, after OVD separation of the anterior and posterior capsules, haptic amputation may then be performed and the optic removed. The replacement PC IOL may still be implanted into the capsular bag or into the sulcus.

Foldable lenses may be removed "flat," unfolded, and in one piece, through 3- to 5-mm incisions,[26] if the intention is to use that incision length to alter the astigmatism. However, these IOLs are more easily removed through astigmatically neutral 3-mm incisions by bisecting the IOL. Several optic cutting instruments have recently been designed for this purpose: the Utrata snare (Rhein, St. Petersburg, FL) the Chang/Packer IOL cutter (MicroSurgical Technologies [MST], Redmond, WA; **Fig. 39.14**), the Osher IOL scissors (Bausch and Lomb Storz, Rochester, NY) and the Mackool IOL cutter (MSI Precision, Phoenixville, PA).

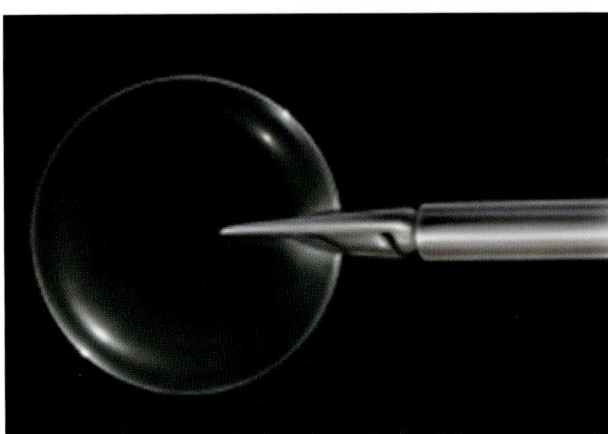

Fig. 39.14 Osher IOL scissors (Bausch and Lomb Storz) and the Mackool IOL cutter.

All foldable IOLs can be bisected safely with one of these instruments. To perform this maneuver, the AC is partially filled with cohesive OVD. The OVD is then used to dissect the anterior capsule from the IOL by placing gentle downward pressure on the IOL and slipping the cannula under the anterior capsule. The OVD is gently used to viscodissect the capsule from the IOL for 360 degrees. Once the IOL is free of the capsule, it can be elevated by injection of OVD below it. This pushes the PC backward away from the IOL and provides support to dial the IOL out of the posterior capsule into the AC. The IOLs need not be completely transected; a cut that is at least 50% across the optic enables the two halves of the optic to separate as one half is being withdrawn through the 3-mm incision. The trailing hemioptic is either completely severed at the incision or remains attached and follows the leading hemioptic out of the eye.[27]

Bisecting single-piece acrylics and three-piece acrylics or silicone IOLs is the least traumatic method of removal. Once in the AC, the IOL is stabilized with an intraocular forceps placed through a paracentesis and cut with the IOL cutter. Each half is then removed.

Removing a plate-haptic silicone IOL may be accomplished in one piece, without sectioning, through a 4-mm incision; firm purchase on the leading haptic with forceps is necessary. However, bisection along the long axis may be achieved by bisecting the proximal haptic and hemioptic first, and then rotating the IOL 180 degrees for bisection of the second haptic and hemioptic. Each half may then be removed through a 3-mm incision with the forceps.

Intraocular Lens Replacement

Intraoperative

Replacing an IOL may be indicated at the time of primary IOL implantation or as a secondary procedure. Removing and replacing an IOL at the time of primary implantation may be indicated if it becomes immediately apparent that the incorrect IOL type or power had been inadvertently implanted—usually an IOL for a different patient or a mistake in IOL selection from the consignment. A second indication for immediate replacement is a damaged IOL, such as a fractured haptic that did not permit proper centration or a fractured optic that would interfere with proper visual function. In each of these cases, the damaged IOL may be removed and replaced by an intact IOL of the same power and

design. However, if the primary IOL was a plate-haptic design and a tear in the posterior capsule occurred after implantation, the primary plate-haptic IOL must be removed and replaced with a loop-haptic IOL with the loops now being placed into the ciliary sulcus.

Postoperative

There are many indications for secondary IOL replacement (**Box 39.4**). Whether primary or secondary, IOL replacement is, by definition, always a two-stage procedure: removal of the primary IOL followed by implantation of the secondary IOL. Depending on the anatomy of the eye following IOL removal, replacement implantation may be back into the capsule, into the ciliary sulcus, or into the AC. If the capsule is intact, this is the preferred location for reimplantation. If the posterior capsule was torn in the process of IOL removal, but the anterior capsulorrhexis is still intact, a PC IOL may be placed into the ciliary sulcus or with the haptics in the sulcus and the optic captured through the anterior capsulorrhexis.

Similar secondary bag/sulcus implantation may be performed if a posterior capsular opening was previously created by a neodymium:yttrium-aluminum-garnet (Nd:YAG) laser; if the posterior capsular opening is completely stabilized by marginal fibrosis, the IOL may be placed completely into the bag. Additionally, if a small posterior tear occurred during primary IOL explantation, this may be converted to a posterior CCC (see Chapter 6). The capsule, now stabilized, may be implanted with the secondary PC IOL. If, upon removal of the primary IOL from the capsular bag, partial zonulodialysis occurred but the capsule remained intact, a capsule tension ring may be implanted into the capsular equator to support the remaining zonule prior to IOL implantation.

The secondary loop-haptic IOL can then be implanted into the intact capsular bag, orienting the loop axis in the meridian of the zonulodialysis. The combination of the ring and the loop haptic at the meridian of zonulodialysis helps to provide resistance to post operative capsular fibrotic contraction in that meridian, which, if it occurred, could lead to further "unzipping" of the zonule.

In the event that both the anterior and posterior capsules have lost all integrity or the capsule has become completely dia-

---

Box 39.4 Causes of IOL Repositioning, Removal, or Replacement

- Primary operative complications
- Undesirable optical phenomena
- Damaged (dysfunctional)
- IOL Incorrect power
- Rotation (toric IOL)
- Decentration
- Subluxation
- Dislocation
- Corneal edema/bullous keratopathy
- Iritis/uveitis-glaucoma-hyphema (UGH) syndrome
- Secondary glaucoma
- Cystoid macular edema Infectious
- Endophthalmitis
- Removal to facilitate vitreoretinal surgery

lyzed, the surgeon has three remaining choices for secondary IOL implantation (see Chapters 27 to 31):

1. A sutured/glued PC IOL
2. An iris-sutured three-piece PC IOL
3. An AC IOL[28] with a peripheral iridotomy performed with a scissor, vitrectomy instrument, or YAG.

Conclusion

Problems during IOL implantation are reported regularly. Many of these problems can be avoided by careful implantation and appropriate IOL positioning. Many can be managed by surgeon observation of IOL damage with removal and replacement. In those circumstances when IOL decentration or subluxation occurs late, appropriately planned surgery with multiple options should provide for a satisfactory outcome.

References

1. Ridley H. Intra-ocular acrylic lenses after cataract extraction. Lancet 1952;1:118–121

2. Kelman CD. Phaco-emulsification and aspiration. A new technique of cataract removal. A preliminary report. Am J Ophthalmol 1967;64:23–35

3. Leaming DV. Practice styles and preferences of ASCRS members—1998 survey. J Cataract Refract Surg 1999;25:851–859

4. Fechner PU, van der Heijde GL, Worst JGF. The correction of myopia by lens implantation into phakic eyes. Am J Ophthalmol 1989;107:659–663

5. Foster JA, Lam S, Joondeph BC, Sugar J. Suprachoroidal dislocation of a posterior chamber intraocular lens. Am J Ophthalmol 1990;109:731–732

6. Sandramouli S, Kumar A, Rao V, Khosla A. Subconjunctival dislocation of posterior chamber intraocular lens. Ophthalmic Surg 1993;24:770–771

7. Behndig A, Otto M. Scleral suturing of intraocular lenses. J Cataract Refract Surg 1997;23:1454–1456

8. Stark WJ, Goodman G, Goodman D, Gottsch J. Posterior chamber intraocular lens implantation in the absence of posterior capsular support. Ophthalmic Surg 1988;19:240–243

9. Chakrabarti A, Gandhi RK, Chakrabarti M. Ab externo 4-point scleral fixation of posterior chamber intraocular lenses. J Cataract Refract Surg 1999;25:420–426

10. Helal M, el Sayyad F, Elsherif Z, el-Maghraby A, Dabees M. Transscleral fixation of posterior chamber intraocular lenses in the absence of capsular support. J Cataract Refract Surg 1996;22:347–351

11. Epley KD, Levine ES, Katz HR. A simplified technique for stable transscleral suture fixation of posterior chamber intraocular lenses. Ophthalmic Surg Lasers 1999;30:398–402

12. Wasserman D, Apple DJ, Castaneda VE, Tsai JC, Morgan RC, Assia EI. Anterior capsular tears and loop fixation of posterior chamber intraocular lenses. Ophthalmology 1991;98:425–431

13. Assia EI, Legler UFC, Merrill C, et al. Clinicopathologic study of the effect of radial tears and loop fixation on intraocular lens decentration. Ophthalmology 1993;100:153–158

14. Burrill A, Morrill KA. Two ways to make foldable IOL explantation easier. Rev Ophthalmol 1998;87–95.

15. Risco JM, Cameron JA. Dislocation of a phakic intraocular lens. Am J Ophthalmol 1994;118:666–667

16. Nagamoto S, Kohzuka T, Nagamoto T. Pupillary block after pupillary capture of an Acrysof intraocular lens. J Cataract Refract Surg 1998;24:1271–1274

17. Tognetto D, Agolini G, Ravalico G. Spontaneous dislocation into the vitreous of a poly (methylmethacrylate) disc lens 9 years after surgery. J Cataract Refract Surg 1999;25:289–292

18. Carlson AN, Stewart WC, Tso PC. Intraocular lens complications requiring removal or exchange. Surv Ophthalmol 1998;42:417–440

19. Schneiderman TE, Johnson MW, Smiddy WE, Flynn HW Jr, Bennett SR, Cantrill HL. Surgical management of posteriorly dislocated silicone plate haptic intraocular lenses. Am J Ophthalmol 1997;123:629–635

20. Smiddy WE. Modification of scleral suture fixation technique for dislocated posterior chamber intraocu- lar lens implants. Arch Ophthalmol 1998;116:1116–1117

21. Panton RW, Sulewski ME, Parker JS, Panton PJ, Stark WJ. Surgical management of subluxed posterior-chamber intraocular lenses. Arch Ophthalmol 1993;111:919–926

22. Shakin EP, Carty JB Jr. Clinical management of posterior chamber intraocular lens implants dislocated in the vitreous cavity. Ophthalmic Surg Lasers 1995;26:529–534

23. Woldoff HS, Newman B. Management of dislocated posterior chamber intraocular lens. Ann Ophthalmol 1997;29:293–295

24. Seo M-S, Yoon K-C, Yang K-J, Park Y-G. A new technique for repositioning a posteriorly dislocated intraocular lens. Ophthalmic Surg Lasers 1998;29:147–150

25. Akduman L. Transscleral fixation of a dislocated silicone plate haptic intraocular lens via the pars plana. Ophthalmic Surg Lasers 1998;29:519–521

26. Rao SK, Sharma T, Parikh S, Madhavan HN, Padmanabhan P. Explantation of silicone plate haptic intraocular lenses. Ophthalmic Surg Lasers 1999;30:575–578

27. Batlan SJ, Dodick JM. Explantation of a foldable silicone intraocular lens. Am J Ophthalmol 1996;122:270–272

28. Mittra RA, Connor TB, Han DP, Koenig SB, Mieler WF, Pulido JS. Removal of dislocated intraocular lenses using pars plana vitrectomy with placement of an open-loop, flexible anterior chamber lens. Ophthalmology 1998;105:1011–1014

40 Angle-Supported Intraocular Lenses

Manus C. Kraff

On November 29, 1949, Sir Harold Ridley implanted the first intraocular lens (IOL) in London, England. In the following years, the first early adapting surgeons and researchers tried to determine the best place in the eye optically to implant, and the best place to support, the IOL. Ridley implanted the first lens in the posterior chamber (PC) (**Fig. 40.1**).[1,2]

Angle-supported, iris-supported, and later the reemergent PC lenses appeared. The angle was a logical area for support because it simplified the surgical procedure.

Dannheim, Strompelli, Barraquer, and Choyce developed the first angle-supported lenses. The Dannheim, Strompelli, and Barraquer lenses were either poorly designed or poorly manufactured, or of inappropriate material, and they all failed shortly after implantation, requiring explantation in almost all cases (**Fig. 40.2**).

Peter Choyce working in the United Kingdom persisted through the 1950s, 1960s, and 1970s in developing eight iterations of his angle-supported (anterior chamber [AC]) lens. The United States Food and Drug Administration (FDA) officially approved the Mark VIII (Rayner, Kansas City, MO) in 1981 (**Fig. 40.3**).

The manufacturing of IOLs began in the United States in the mid-1970s. The initial lenses were poorly manufactured copies of the European Choyce Mark VIII lens, with rough edges and warpage, and complications soon arose, including uveitis, glaucoma, and uveitis-glaucoma-hyphema (UGH) syndrome. The manufacturing techniques improved in the next phase of development (the late 1970s and early 1980s). In an effort to improve the design, tubular haptics were employed. With these new lenses, complications took slightly longer to develop but also included UGH syndrome, because of cocooning of the tubular elements in the angle, producing inflammation.

It was Charles Kelman who observed that properly manufactured Choyce lens lacked the UGH complication and determined that a plate haptic in the angle, as Choyce had originally designed it, eliminated the risk of UGH. Kelman, whose primary interest was always the small incision, developed flexible haptics with triangular and quadripedal angle support in the mid-1980s to accommodate these lenses. The Kelman quadripod flexible lens design is still the angle-supported lens implanted today. These lenses are called "new-design" IOLs, even though they are almost 30 years old, and they are still the gold standard (**Figs. 40.4, 40.5, 40.6**).[3,4]

Indications for the Use of Angle-Supported Lenses

The current indications for angle-supported (AS) IOLs are as follows:

1. Primary implantation
   a. Rupture of the posterior capsule during cataract surgery with insufficient capsular support for a PC IOL
   b. Inadequate capsular support, and the surgeon chooses to use a far less traumatic procedure in the eye than suturing it
2. Secondary implantation
   a. After a current or previous intracapsular cataract extraction
   b. As an alternative to sutured, glued, or iris-supported PC IOLs.
   c. After removal of a subluxated PC IOL with insufficient capsular support remaining

Suturing of a PC IOL, currently being performed when inadequate capsular support exists for the implantation of a PC IOL, may be a traumatic and lengthy process. Unless the surgeon has performed this procedure many times, suturing the lens may subject the eye to avoidable trauma. An angle-supported lens may be a better choice for both the patient and the surgeon, especially in elderly patients, for the following reasons:

1. An AS IOL is technically more straightforward to implant.
2. Less surgical time is required for the procedure.
3. The implantation of an AS IOL is less traumatic to the eye than is suturing of a PC IOL.

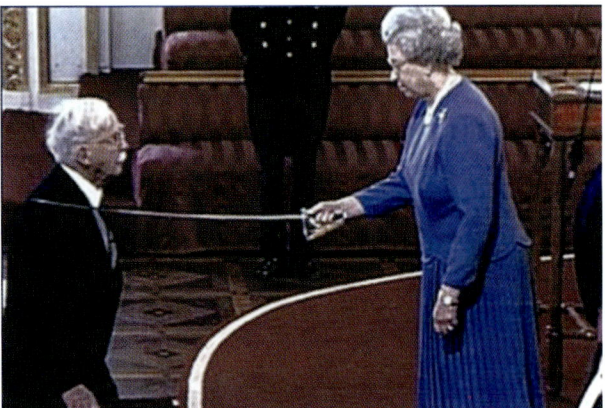

Fig. 40.1 Queen Elizabeth Knighting Sir Harold Ridley in London, March 2000. (From Steinert RF, ed. Cataract Surgery, 3rd ed. Philadelphia: Saunders, Elsevier; 2010.)

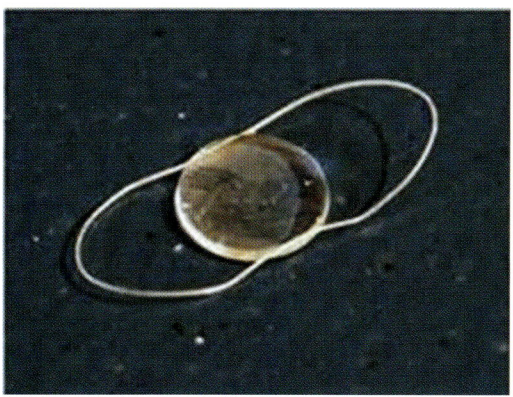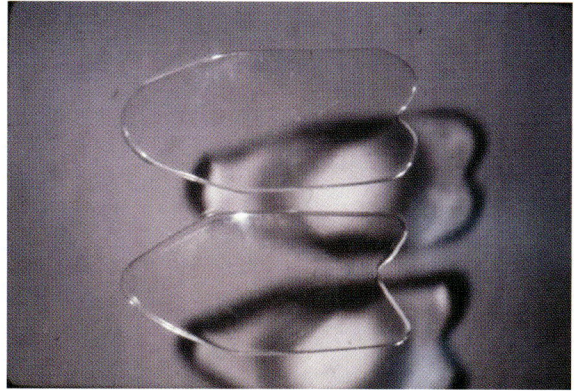

Fig. 40.2 **(a)** Dannheim intraocular lens (IOL) for the anterior chamber (AC): closed loop IOL design. **(b)** Strampelli plate IOL. (From Steinert RF, ed. Cataract Surgery, 3rd ed. Philadelphia: Saunders, Elsevier; 2010.)

4. If it becomes necessary, the AS lens is easier to remove than a sutured PC IOL.
5. An AS lens is in contact with the anterior surface of the iris. This cell layer is derived from mesodermal tissue. This is in contrast to a sutured PC IOL that is in contact with the iris pigment layer. This layer is derived from neural ectoderm, which causes intensified intraocular inflammation and cystoid macular edema in the postsurgical period. Additionally, there is the possibility of

a greater incidence of late hemorrhaging into the AC and PC.
6. In a review of my own data from more than 1,500 AS IOLs over a 25-year period, the results are superior to those with sutured PC IOLs.

Sizing

Sizing of these lenses is determined by measuring the white-to-white corneal diameter under the microscope with a caliper. A 12-mm white to white calls for a 12-mm AS IOL, and similarly for other size measurements. But this is changing with the anterior segment imaging devices such as the Visante optical coherence tomography (OCT; Carl Zeiss Meditec, Jena, Germany), the Oculus Pentacam (Arlington, WA), and the Artemis VHF digital ultrasound scanner (ArcScan, Morrison, CO).

Insertion Technique

The AS lens is inserted through a 6-mm limbal incision, usually temporally, on top of a Sheets' glide. The AC should be filled with an ophthalmic viscosurgical device (OVD) until the iris is flat. It is best not to overfill the AC, making the iris concave and making the insertion more difficult. Once the IOL is positioned, each haptic on the three-point fixation IOL, and the single leading and trailing haptic on the four-point fixation IOL, should be withdrawn slightly from the angle with an inverted Sinsky hook. This step, and the observation of a round pupil, will verify that there is no iris capture. If the pupil is oval, there is likely peripheral iris capture, and it must be released.

Peripheral Iridectomy

At least one surgical peripheral iridectomy (PI) is required to prevent postoperative papillary block. This must be done even if a vitrectomy has been performed. The PI should not be in the iris periphery, as the IOL may rotate until one loop passes through the peripheral PI and causes damage to the ciliary body. The PI, therefore, should be more central and should be adequately constructed, confirming that the posterior pigment epithelium has been excised. The procedure is as follows:

1. An intraocular forceps is utilized to grasp the peripheral iris and excise it with an intraocular scissor.

Fig. 40.3 Peter Choyce, MD. (From Steinert RF, ed. Cataract Surgery, 3rd ed. Philadelphia: Saunders, Elsevier; 2010.)

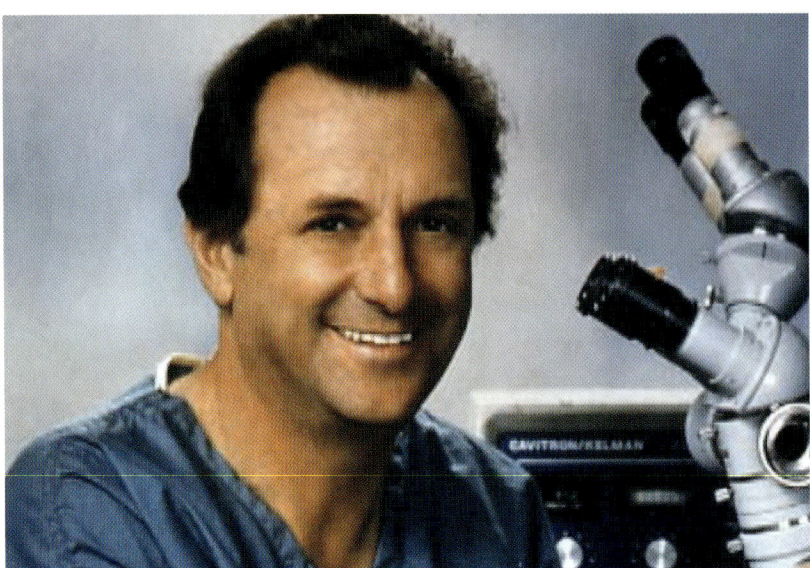

Fig. 40.4 Charles D. Kelman, MD. (From Steinert RF, ed. Cataract Surgery, 3rd ed. Philadelphia: Saunders, Elsevier; 2010.)

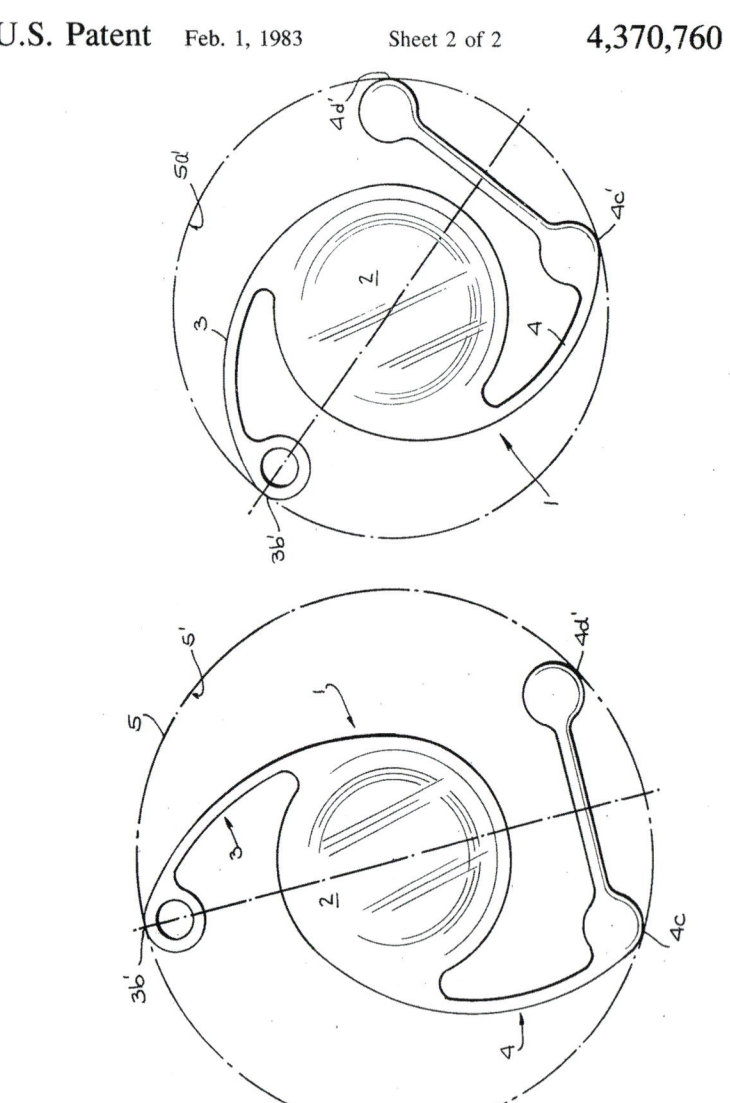

U.S. Patent Feb. 1, 1983 Sheet 2 of 2 **4,370,760**

Fig. 40.5 Patent on the Kelman AC IOL used by Cilco, Abbott Medical Optics (AMO), Hyer-Schulte, and Precision Cosmet. (From Steinert RF, ed. Cataract Surgery, 3rd ed. Philadelphia: Saunders, Elsevier; 2010.)

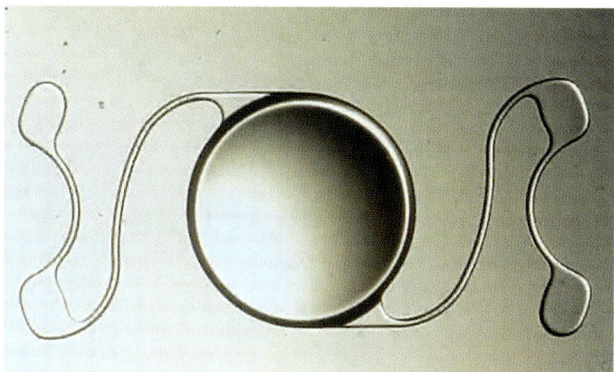

Fig. 40.6   A single-piece AC IOL from the Kelman patent manufactured by Cilco as the Multiflex II. (From Steinert RF, ed. Cataract Surgery, 3rd ed. Philadelphia: Saunders, Elsevier; 2010.)

2. A vitrector is the perfect device to cut a small PI. Alternatively, this is accomplished by a small limbal incision superior to the temporal wound with pressure on the posterior lip. If the iris does not prolapse spontaneously, one may extract it with a fine-tooth forceps and perform the iridectomy.
3. Another approach is to make two small PIs with the yttrium-aluminum-garnet (YAG) laser immediately after the surgery, before corneal edema becomes a barrier to the laser pulses.
4. The incision is closed with two or three interrupted 10-0 nylon sutures. The absence of wound leak must be verified.

Flexible Haptic Intraocular Lenses in the Anterior Chamber

The surgeon should never implant a PC lens in the AC. Past experience has established that AC IOLs must be slightly flexible and have flat footplates at the periphery of the haptics, not the highly flexible tubular haptics found in PC IOLs that will promote cocooning.

Posterior chamber IOLs, therefore, will produce the same complications that occurred in the era of the poorly designed AC lens, that is, cocooning of the haptics in the angle, which caused the formation of synechiae around the haptics. The result of this is inflammation-uveitis, cystoid macular edema, UGH, and progressive corneal endothelial cell loss with potential corneal decompensation[5] **(Fig. 40.7)**. These problems inevitably require late lens removal. The synechiae make removal of the haptics from the chamber angle almost impossible without hemorrhage and damage to the iris root.[6,7]

The Future of Angle-Supported Intraocular Lenses

Although the implantation of AS IOLs in cataract surgery is a rare event, in the future AS IOLs may well be used for the correction of phakic refractive errors. Currently, American and European companies are conducting ongoing clinical trials of AS phakic IOLs.

Implanting these lenses will be straightforward. The procedure will be reversible so that the IOL may be explanted easily, if

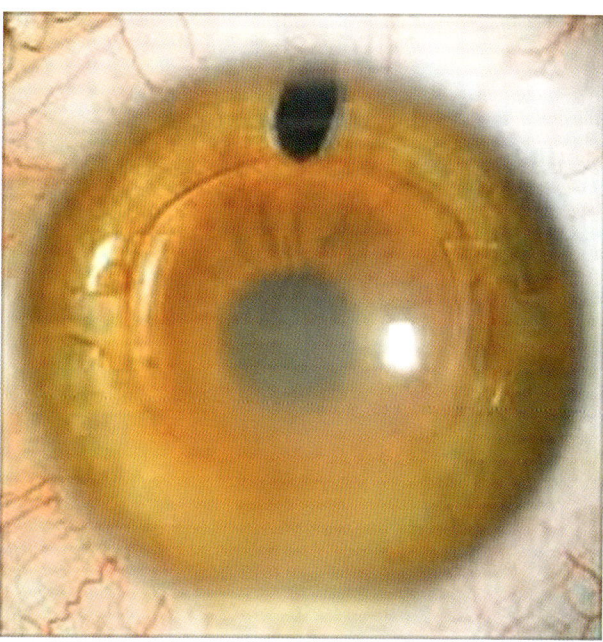

Fig. 40.7   End result of uveitis-glaucoma-hyphema (UGH) with the AC IOL and corneal decompensation. (From Steinert RF, ed. Cataract Surgery, 3rd ed. Philadelphia: Saunders, Elsevier; 2010.)

necessary. The lenses will fold into a cartridge and be injected into the AC through a precise small wound that is astigmatically neutral. There will be a very low degree of cataract formation. The lens will not rotate within the AC. Finally, these IOLs will have superior design features compared with the currently available AS IOLs. All European and Asian studies have shown that lenticular correction of refractive errors produces optical superiority to corneal procedures in refractive surgery. Vision return is immediate, producing high patient satisfaction.

Conclusion

Although seldom used, in unusual circumstances an AC angle-supported IOL may be the least traumatic or demanding IOL to utilize. Surgeons should be familiar with them and with the techniques required to ensure successful outcomes.

References

1. Ridley H. Intra-ocular acrylic lenses. Trans Ophthalmol Soc U K 1951;71: 617–621
2. Ridley H. Intra-ocular acrylic lenses after cataract extraction. Lancet 1952;1:118–121
3. Hoffer KJ. The evolution of the intraocular lens. In: Steinert RF, ed. Cataract Surgery, 3rd ed. Philadelphia: Saunders, Elsevier; 2010:419–437
4. Lindstrom RL. Peripheral iridectomy lenses. In: Steinert RF, ed. Cataract Surgery, 3rd ed. Philadelphia: Saunders, Elsevier; 2010:439–447
5. Ellingson FT. The uveitis-glaucoma-hyphema syndrome associated with the Mark VIII anterior chamber lens implant. J Am Intraocul Implant Soc 1978;4:50–53
6. Keates RH, Ehrlich DR. "Lenses of chance" complications of anterior chamber implants. Ophthalmology 1978;85:408–414
7. Osher RH, Cionni RJ, et al. Surgical repositioning and explantation of the intraocular lens. In: Steinert RF, ed. Cataract Surgery, 3rd ed. Philadelphia: Saunders, Elsevier; 2010:570–571

41 Understanding and Managing the Dysphotopsias

Samuel Masket and Nicole R. Fram

The dysphotopsias, both positive dysphotopsia (PD) and negative dysphotopsia (ND), represent subjective undesired optical phenomena that are associated with otherwise uncomplicated cataract and lens implant surgery. They are unanticipated photic consequences that are, at least in part, related to intraocular lens (IOL) design and, to some extent, surgical methods. No significant physical or demographic characteristics have been attributed to symptomatic patients. PD is typically described by patients as light streaks, arcs of light, central light flashes, and starbursts; these observations are induced by external light sources. PD is to be distinguished from entoptic light flashes resulting from vitreoretinal traction. In contrast, ND is observed by the patient as a temporal dark shadow much like the effect of wearing "horse blinders." The etiology and symptomatology may be somewhat different between the two conditions, although there can be some crossover and both conditions can coexist in the same patient, as described by Davison.[1] Indeed temporal light "flickering" is commonly associated with ND. Adding to the clinician's frustration with evaluating these conditions is that there are no objective tests to qualify or quantify symptoms; we rely solely on patient-reported outcomes (PROs). Furthermore, there are no "absolutes" with the dysphotopsias; although most cases can be codified, some are atypical in symptoms, causes, and cures.

Olson's group[2] has reported that dysphotopsia represents the chief cause of dissatisfaction following routine cataract surgery. In fact, the term *dysphotopsia* was coined in a publication from Olson's department. In that report, 49% of patients had a degree of dysphotopsia, either ND or PD, at some time following surgery. Additionally, Bournas et al[3] reported that 19.5% of patients complained of dysphotopsia at 1 day after surgery. Specific to ND, Osher[4] reported a 15.2% incidence at 1 day postoperatively, which was reduced to 3.2% at 1 year postoperatively.

Given that the volume of cataract surgery in the United States is 3 million eyes annually, somewhere between 30,000 and 100,000 new cases of chronic dysphotopsia occur each year. As mentioned, evaluating the patient with dysphotopsia is very difficult. However, in the optical laboratory setting, one can use ray-tracing analysis and reflectometry of IOL materials, surfaces, shapes, and edge designs.

Dysphotopic complaints should also be distinguished from Purkinje images, which are a series of reflections from the corneal and lens surfaces. The accentuated third Purkinje images may be associated with lens implants and represent purely a cosmetic blemish, as they are not associated with functional vision deficits. Additionally, patients may notice a Maddox rod effect (with point sources of light) from striae in the posterior capsule; this undesired optical phenomenon is not specific to the intraocular lens and may be managed by laser capsulotomy, as necessary.

Traditionally, the nonsequential ray tracing from Zemax (Kirkland, WA) has been used to analyze optical pathways, surfaces and edges; Franchini et al[5] found good laboratory evidence

that the square edge of IOLs is associated with the production of halos, rings, and arcs of light. In fact, edge-induced positive dysphotopsia was first reported by one of us (S.M.) and coworkers[6] in 1993 with regard to the truncated squared edge of ovoid IOLs. At that time, prior to wide acceptance and distribution of foldable IOLs, oval polymethylmethacrylate (PMMA) IOLs were in wide use as a means to reduce incision size. The vast majority of implanted IOLs were made of PMMA and typically had round or thin (knife) edges. Oval lens implants were created by truncating the parallel edges of the optic, reducing one dimension from 6 to 5 mm, and hereby allowing implantation through a smaller incision. However, an optical effect of truncating the edge was creation of a flat surface that induced internal reflection from oblique illumination. This effect was investigated by reflectometry and ray tracing in the 1993 publication.[6] A clinical example of internal light reflection is provided in **Fig. 41.1**, in which the oblique slit-lamp beam strikes the surface of a square-edged acrylic IOL, and the edge becomes highly luminescent. Given the above, we remain concerned about the recent reintroduction of ovoid IOLs. However, the square-edge design reduces posterior capsule opacification (PCO) by inhibiting migration of equatorial lens epithelial cells (LECs) along the posterior capsule. This aspect of the square edge was established by the work of Nishi et al.[7] As a result, the (posterior) square edge has been maintained as a feature of most IOLs to limit PCO. The trade-off, however, can be induction of positive dysphotopsia.

Other facets of IOL design may induce PD. According to the work Erie et al,[8] positive dysphotopsia may be caused by internal reflection from the posterior surface of the front of the IOL. In keeping with their theory, the occurrence of PD is more likely with IOLs that have relatively flat surfaces associated with a high index of refraction optic material.

The ophthalmic industry has responded to PD in several ways:

1. Modifying the square edge of the IOL by reducing its thickness and by rounding the anterior edge
2. Leaving the edge unpolished or frosted; one wonders, however, how this modification reduces *internal* light reflection
3. Moving more of the IOL optical power to the anterior rather than posterior surface of the optic

Other opportunities to reduce PD might include using materials with a lower index of refraction or reduced surface reflectivity. The latter property has not been addressed by the manufacturing sector and may be an important consideration with both ND and PD.

Negative dysphotopsia is perhaps a less well understood phenomenon. As mentioned, it is typically manifest as a temporal dark crescent, similar to wearing "horse blinders," which may be very disconcerting and annoying to the patient. Temporal "shim-

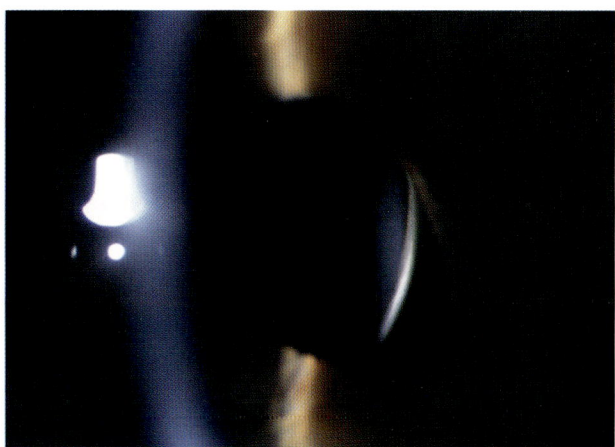

Fig. 41.1 Oblique slit-lamp view of an acrylic square-edged intraocular lens (IOL). The angulated light beam induces enhanced illumination of the edge due to internal reflection.

mering" or "smudging" of vision may also be present, suggesting an occurrence of both ND and PD in the same eye. Interestingly, although PD symptoms may be improved with pharmacological pupil constriction, the opposite is true of ND symptoms, which almost invariably improve with pupil dilation.

The etiology of ND remains a topic of debate, and there are a few theories about its origin. Osher[4] suggests that edema surrounding a temporal corneal incision could be responsible for the high early incidence of ND. But the fact that ND has been reported with superiorly oriented cataract incisions makes that theory less likely. Furthermore, the corneal cataract incision is seemingly not a likely source, as ND has never been reported with radial or arcuate keratotomies, nor has it been reported with penetrating keratoplasty or laser-assisted in situ keratomileusis (LASIK) flaps. But it is well recognized that ND symptoms improve over time, suggesting that neuro-adaptation reduces the severity and incidence of ND over time.

Another theory about the etiology of ND is offered by Holladay et al.[9] Their premise is that ND represents a penumbra primarily associated with IOL edge design but is also related to posterior chamber depth and the index of refraction of the IOL material. However, their theory cannot explain the clinical phenomena that we reported.[10] Corroborating our suggestions is the study from Burke and Benjamin,[11] in which five patients with ND and a variety of "in-the-bag" IOLs were relieved of their symptoms when the IOLs were exchanged for sulcus-placed AcrySof IOLs (Alcon Labs, Fort Worth, TX). Interestingly, that particular IOL has been impugned as causal for ND when placed in the capsule bag.

Our experience, in agreement with other reports in the literature, strongly suggests that the final common path for ND is the presence of the IOL within the confines of the capsule bag, irrespective of lens material or design.[12] Frustrating for both surgeon and patient is the fact that ND seemingly only occurs with what we consider to be "perfect" surgery with a well-centered IOL with the edge fully covered by the anterior capsulotomy. Interestingly, and in concurrence, ND has not been associated with anterior chamber IOLs or sulcus-fixated IOLs. Furthermore, Vámosi et al[13] first reported that ND symptoms could only be relieved surgically by elevating the IOL from the capsule bag to the sulcus; when the bag-placed IOL was exchanged for an IOL of different material and design, ND symptoms persisted. We have had a similar experience. In one of our reported cases, the patient was highly symptomatic with a square-edged acrylic IOL in the cap-

sule bag. At surgery the acrylic IOL was exchanged for a round-edged silicone IOL placed in the capsule bag; symptoms persisted without change. However, when that same IOL was brought anterior to the capsule bag in a subsequent surgery, the ND symptoms fully abated. We also have reported that placing a piggyback IOL atop the existing implant may relieve or improve symptoms in roughly 75% of patients. We particularly noted improvement (in 13 of 14 eyes) in ND symptoms when the previously implanted optic edge was elevated above the anterior capsulotomy, leaving the haptics in the capsule bag. This orientation is referred to as reverse (or anterior) optic capture (ROC). We have also employed ROC with universal success (11 eyes) for second eyes of patients who were significantly bothered by ND in the previously operated eye; however, one cannot be certain that the second eyes would be equally symptomatic.

In our investigation we employed ultrasound biomicroscopy (UBM) to evaluate the relationship of posterior chamber depth and ND.[10] Interestingly, and in distinction to the Holladay et al[9] report, we did not find that increased posterior chamber depth was associated with ND. Two cases are illustrative: In one case the patient complained of ND following surgery with a single-piece acrylic IOL. A second surgeon exchanged the offending lens for a round-edged silicone IOL and added a capsule tension ring as diffuse zonulopathy was noted. The patient's symptoms were unchanged and he was referred to one of us (S.M.) for evaluation and management. UBM testing revealed exaggerated posterior chamber depth. At a subsequent surgery the bag/IOL/capsular tension ring (CTR) complex was suture fixated to the iris, significantly collapsing the posterior chamber depth; however, the ND symptoms persisted unchanged. In another patient with severe ND, the UBM demonstrated a remarkably shallow posterior chamber in accord with high hyperopia preoperatively and the need for a +30 D IOL implant.

The above observations have led us to believe that the optical interaction between the anterior capsulotomy and anterior surface of the IOL is a potential contributing factor for ND or even a causative factor. Toward that end, certain features of the IOL might enhance the risk of ND, among them a high index of refraction and high surface reflectivity. It is interesting to note two reports in the literature indicating relief of ND symptoms in some patients after neodymium:yttrium-aluminum-garnet (Nd:YAG)[14,15] laser anterior capsulectomy over the nasal aspect of the IOL.[14,15] Although not uniformly successful, this finding seems to corroborate the concept that the anterior capsule/IOL interface may be causal of ND. This finding also speaks against progressive anterior capsule opacification as responsible for reduction of ND symptoms with time. Moreover, given no movement of the IOL after anterior laser capsulotomy, it is not likely that the "penumbra" has been shifted away from visible retina. All these considerations point to an optical relationship between the anterior capsulotomy and anterior surface of the IOL as contributing to ND. Nevertheless, the etiology of ND remains unsettled and is likely multifactorial.

Unlike PD, to date there has been no significant response from the manufacturing sector regarding an IOL design specific for reducing the incidence of ND. However, there have been unsubstantiated reports that a given oval IOL precludes ND. Presently, there are no meaningful studies to address the issue. Moreover, the concern regarding PD with oval IOLs, as discussed above, remains problematic.

Recently, however, one of us (S.M.) has been granted a United States patent for an IOL that is specifically designed to prevent ND **(Fig. 41.2)**. The design concept was based on the effect of reverse (anterior) optic capture in reducing ND. As such, an anteriorly placed peripheral groove is featured to accept the anterior capsulotomy. In this fashion a lip of the optic overrides the anterior capsule. This facet of the design should prevent ND.

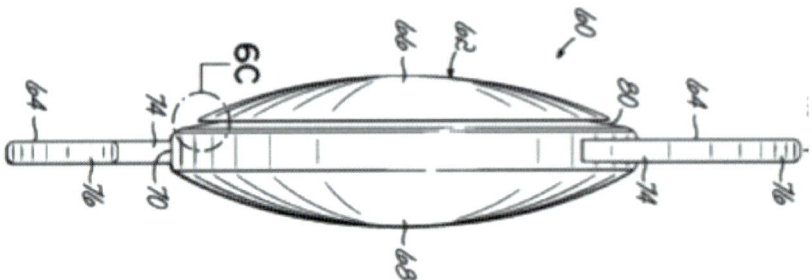

Fig. 41.2 Artist's drawing of the IOL design from the United States patent. 6C indicates the groove designed to capture the anterior capsulotomy.

Other aspects of the IOL concept would enable any preferred haptic or optic design, be it toric, multifocal, or another design.

In accord with the design, Morcher (Stuttgart, Germany) created an IOL that achieved CE marking in 2013, and a small number of patients have been implanted with the device in a preliminary clinical trail (**Fig. 41.3**). Burkhard Dick and Tim Schultz, employing a femtosecond laser for the anterior capsulotomy, performed the surgery (**Figs. 41.4** and **41.5**). Oliver Findl in Vienna, using an image-guided manual anterior capsulorrhexis, has performed subsequent cases. To date, all patients in both settings have been free from ND.

Interestingly, the bag-in-the-lens design of Tassignon et al,[16] which features an equatorial groove to receive anterior and posterior capsule leaflets, is seemingly unassociated with ND. In an unpublished investigation, 30 patients were examined (Bostanci Ceran, personal communication, 2011), and none were noted to have ND complaints at any time following surgery. This seemingly adds credence to the concept that ND is prevented if the anterior portion of the optic overlies the anterior capsule edge. Earlier, Nishi and Sakka[17] designed a grooved IOL to act as a "plug" in the anterior capsule for capsule bag refilling of an accommodative polymer. Nevertheless, no IOL of their design has come to clinical use.

Clearly, the dysphotopsias represent a sizable source of dissatisfaction for patients following uncomplicated cataract surgery. The incidence and significance should not be overlooked. We remain hopeful that new IOL design concepts and surgical methods will prove valuable toward that end.

Management strategies for dysphotopsia vary with patient symptoms and the type of IOL in situ. Helping the patient with PD requires careful and sensitive patient counseling as an initial phase. The patient can be reassured that the optical phenomenon is typically associated only with anatomically "perfect" surgery and that the surgery was uncomplicated. The patient may take solace from the fact that symptoms often dissipate over the first few months. The next line of treatment is the use of topical agents that reduce pupil diameter. Brimonidine 0.15% or pilocarpine 0.5 to 1.0% may reduce symptoms, in particular during the evening. The patient needs to be made aware of the side effects of the medication(s).

Should PD symptoms persist beyond 6 months and topical agents prove ineffective, IOL exchange can be considered. For pure PD, a "bag-to-bag" exchange can be successful if the new IOL is of different design and material and the posterior capsule is intact. An IOL with a low surface reflectivity, low index of refraction, and absence of a square edge would be ideal. We have had a high degree of success with placing model AQ 2010V, CQ 2015A, or CC 4204 (all from Staar Surgical, Monrovia CA) in the capsule bag. However, if capsule bag placement is not possible for any reason, we prefer model AQ 2010V for sulcus placement as it has a round edge, 13.5-mm haptics, and a 6.3-mm optic. When placing a secondary posterior chamber IOL in the ciliary sulcus, unless employing optic capture, we generally suture the loops of the IOL to the iris to prevent movement and possible decentration.

In contrast, patients suffering from ND cannot benefit from miotic therapy, as it generally worsens symptoms; although ND may improve with pupil dilation, the associated glare makes intentional pharmacological dilation an inappropriate strategy. Surgical options can benefit the majority of patients. However, we generally request that patients wait 6 months from the initial procedure before considering reoperation. We have come to recognize that final pathway to alleviating ND is to place the IOL

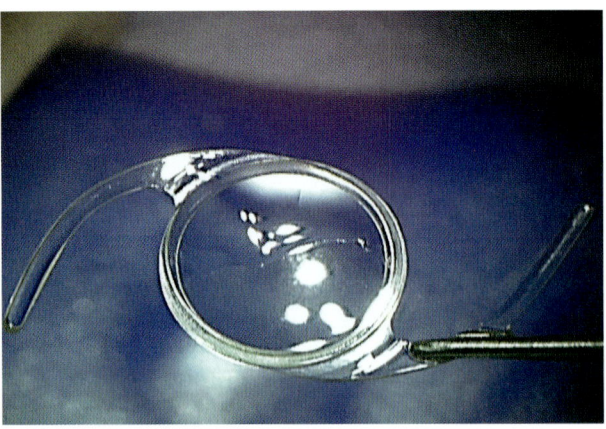

Fig. 41.3 Overview of the Masket™ (Morcher, Stuttgart Germany) negative dysphotopsia (ND) IOL.

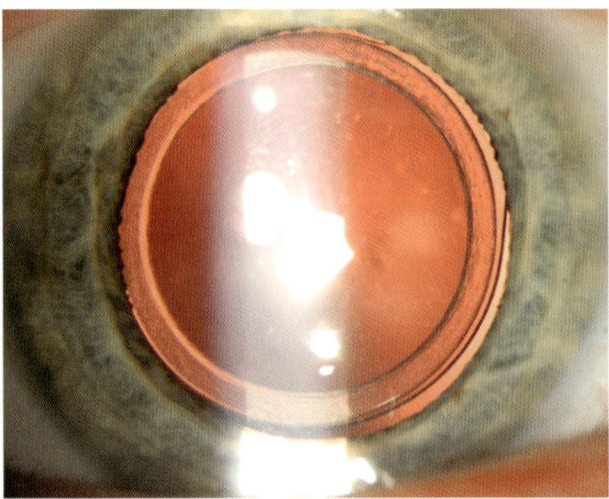

Fig. 41.4 Postoperative appearance of patient with the Masket ND IOL. (Courtesy of Samuel Masket.)

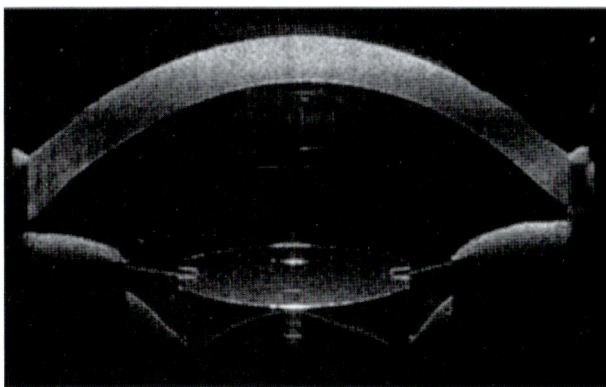

Fig. 41.5 Intraoperative optical coherence tomography (OCT) of the Masket ND IOL demonstrates the groove in the optic holding the anterior capsulotomy. (Courtesy of Samuel Masket.)

optic (in part or in whole) anterior to the anterior capsulotomy. This may be achieved by elevating the optic alone while leaving the supporting haptics in the capsule bag (referred to as reverse or anterior optic capture). However, should the anterior capsulotomy not allow this maneuver by virtue of size, centration, or condition, the existing IOL may brought anteriorly from the capsule bag into the ciliary sulcus. Alternatively, the existing IOL may be exchanged for a sulcus-placed implant lens as necessary. IOL options for exchange would be similar to those mentioned for PD (see above); however, many if not all IOLs that can be safely placed in the sulcus may be employed for anterior (reverse) optic capture.

Patients complaining of both ND and PD are generally benefited by IOL exchange for the aforementioned IOLs and anterior optic capture or sulcus placement.

Although we currently employ the above management methods, alternative strategies for ND include use of a secondary piggy-back IOL[18] and Nd:YAG laser anterior capsulectomy or relaxing incisions.[14,15] Not presently available in the United States, the Sulcoflex (Rayner, East Sussex, UK) "add on" sulcus-fixated IOL has been used with success in Europe for management of ametropia and dysphotopsia. Nevertheless, there are concerns associated with the use of "add on" IOLs with regard to iris chafe and decentration over the long term. We have not opted for laser management of the anterior capsule, as it removes the possibility of anterior optic capture. Finally, one might consider a strategy of generating an anterior capsulorrhexis deliberately larger than the optic to prevent overlap of the capsulotomy. However, this concept induces baring of the optic edge with an increased likelihood for positive dysphotopsia.

In conclusion, both PD and ND create the potential for dissatisfaction after otherwise uncomplicated cataract surgery. Given high expectations by patients, particularly those who pay premiums for advanced lens implant technology and femtosecond laser augmentation, these enigmatic conditions require further attention from both the profession and the manufacturing sector.

References

1. Davison JA. Positive and negative dysphotopsia in patients with acrylic intraocular lenses. J Cataract Refract Surg 2000;26:1346–1355

2. Tester R, Pace NL, Samore M, Olson RJ. Dysphotopsia in phakic and pseudophakic patients: incidence and relation to intraocular lens type (2). J Cataract Refract Surg 2000;26:810–816

3. Bournas P, Drazinos S, Kanellas D, Arvanitis M, Vaikoussis E. Dysphotopsia after cataract surgery: comparison of four different intraocular lenses. Ophthalmologica 2007;221:378–383

4. Osher RH. Negative dysphotopsia: long-term study and possible explanation for transient symptoms. J Cataract Refract Surg 2008;34:1699–1707

5. Franchini A, Gallarati BZ, Vaccari E. Computerized analysis of the effects of intraocular lens edge design on the quality of vision in pseudophakic patients. J Cataract Refract Surg 2003;29:342–347

6. Masket S, Geraghty E, Crandall AS, et al. Undesired light images associated with ovoid intraocular lenses. J Cataract Refract Surg 1993;19:690–694

7. Nishi O, Nishi K, Wickström K. Preventing lens epithelial cell migration using intraocular lenses with sharp rectangular edges. J Cataract Refract Surg 2000;26:1543–1549

8. Erie JC, Bandhauer MH, McLaren JW. Analysis of postoperative glare and intraocular lens design. J Cataract Refract Surg 2001;27:614–621

9. Holladay JT, Zhao H, Reisin CR. Negative dysphotopsia: the enigmatic penumbra. J Cataract Refract Surg 2012;38:1251–1265

10. Masket S, Fram NR. Pseudophakic negative dysphotopsia: Surgical management and new theory of etiology. J Cataract Refract Surg 2011;37:1199–1207

11. Burke TR, Benjamin L. Sulcus-fixated intraocular lens implantation for the management of negative dysphotopsia. J Cataract Refract Surg 2014;40:1469–1472

12. Trattler WB, Whitsett JC, Simone PA. Negative dysphotopsia after intraocular lens implantation irrespective of design and material. J Cataract Refract Surg 2005;31:841–845

13. Vámosi P, Csákány B, Németh J. Intraocular lens exchange in patients with negative dysphotopsia symptoms. J Cataract Refract Surg 2010;36:418–424

14. Folden DV. Neodymium:YAG laser anterior capsulectomy: surgical option in the management of negative dysphotopsia. J Cataract Refract Surg 2013;39:1110–1115

15. Cooke DL, Kasko S, Platt LO. Resolution of negative dysphotopsia after laser anterior capsulotomy. J Cataract Refract Surg 2013;39:1107–1109

16. Tassignon MJ, De Groot V, Vrensen GF. Bag-in-the-lens implantation of intraocular lenses. J Cataract Refract Surg 2002;28:1182–1188

17. Nishi O, Sakka Y. Anterior capsule-supported intraocular lens. A new lens for small-incision surgery and for sealing the capsular opening. Graefes Arch Clin Exp Ophthalmol 1990;228:582–588

18. Ernest PH. Severe photic phenomenon. J Cataract Refract Surg 2006;32:685–686

42 Pathology of Complicated Phacoemulsification

Liliana Werner

The Intermountain Ocular Research Center at the John A. Moran Eye Center, University of Utah (Salt Lake City, UT), codirected by Nick Mamalis and myself, is a laboratory specializing in the evaluation of ocular implantable biodevices, particularly intraocular lenses (IOLs), for cataract surgery. Pathological analyses and experiments involving pseudophakic human eyes obtained postmortem, as well as IOLs explanted because of various problems, have proved to be very useful in the understanding of different complications of cataract surgery procedures with IOL implantation. This chapter discusses the pathological aspects of the phacoemulsification procedure with IOL implantation as well as the postoperative complications, based on the most recent work of our laboratory using pseudophakic human eyes and explanted IOLs. These complications may necessitate secondary procedures for lens explantation or repositioning.

In-the-Bag Intraocular Lens Subluxation/Dislocation

Multiple conditions may play a role in contributing to inherent zonular weakness and instability. The most commonly correlated conditions include pseudoexfoliation (PXF) syndrome, previous vitreoretinal surgery, trauma, and myopia. Additional causes include connective tissue disorders (Marfan's syndrome, Ehlers-Danlos syndrome, homocystinuria, Weill-Marchesani syndrome) and retinitis pigmentosa.[1-3] PXF is a condition in which abnormal extracellular matrix and basement membrane structural and metabolic proteins are deposited into virtually all structures within the anterior chamber (**Fig. 42.1**). These accumulations mechanically weaken the zonular lamella and impair zonular anchoring to the epithelial basement membrane at both its origin and insertion. Because zonules are mainly composed of elastic fibers, and because patients with PXF exhibit an increase in elastolysis, the disease likely also enzymatically weakens the zonules.[4]

We have been receiving an increasing number of specimens in our laboratory from cases of in-the-bag IOL subluxation/dislocation.[5-7] The findings of 86 consecutive cases sent for pathological analysis were described in 2009.[6] Two of the specimens were submitted before 2003, and all others between 2006 and 2008. The mean time from surgery to spontaneous IOL dislocation was 8.5 years. Associated conditions included PXF (50%), prior vitreoretinal surgery (19%), history of trauma (6%), uveitis (2%), and none/unknown (23%). None of the specimens contained an accompanying capsular tension ring (CTR), which indirectly suggests the efficacy of this device in preventing this complication (**Fig. 42.2a**).[6]

In a follow-up study, 23 specimens corresponding to explanted subluxated/dislocated capsular bags containing a CTR and an IOL were evaluated (**Fig. 42.2b**).[7] Explantation was performed 81.5 ± 32.2 months after implantation. Available information on associated ocular conditions included PXF (N = 17), glaucoma (N = 4), vitrectomy/retina surgery (N = 3), and trauma (N = 1). Excessive contraction of the capsular bag with capsulorrhexis phimosis was observed in 11 specimens: one with an associated history of vitrectomy, seven with an associated history of PXF, and three with an associated history of glaucoma (**Fig. 42.3**). Explantation was performed 72.1 ± 41.3 months after implantation (~ 6 years) in eyes with capsulorrhexis phimosis.[7] It is not surprising that the mean explantation time was shorter in the series of 23 specimens containing a CTR (6.8 or 6 years, without or with capsulorrhexis phimosis, respectively),[7] in comparison with the series of 86 specimens without a CTR (8.5 years),[6] considering that CTRs are usually implanted when zonular weakness is observed before or during surgery. Stress to the zonules during CTR insertion can also not be ruled out.[3]

It is noteworthy that histopathological assessment completed in selected specimens showed material consistent with PXF, although there was no history or clinical signs of this condition.[7] We hypothesized that the prevalence of PXF in our subluxation/dislocation series may be higher than the rate based on clinical history and clinical examination. Therefore, we undertook a study involving a retrospective case series with complete histopathological examination of 40 explanted subluxated/dislocated capsular bags containing an IOL, or a CTR and an IOL.[8] Excessive contraction of the capsular bag with capsulorrhexis phimosis was observed in 24 specimens; 26 specimens had histopathological evidence of PXF, whereas only 13 had a clinical history/evidence of PXF. Therefore, PXF may be implicated in a larger proportion of late in-the-bag IOL subluxations/dislocations than previously thought due to significant clinical underdiagnosis. This may impart a need to consider new factors during the pre- and postoperative cataract surgery assessments and follow-up. It is also noteworthy that different IOL materials and designs were represented in the above-mentioned studies performed in our laboratory, with no apparent preference. Also, the amount of Soemmering's ring (SR) formation within the capsular bags varied from mild to severe.[5-8]

Sulcus Intraocular Lenses and Pigmentary Dispersion

One-piece and three-piece hydrophobic acrylic AcrySof lenses (Alcon, Fort Worth, TX) have a square optic edge on the anterior and posterior optic surfaces. The finishing of the square edges of these lenses was modified to give the side walls an unpolished or "textured" appearance, which was found to improve postoperative glare phenomena.[9] This feature was extended along the length of the optic and haptics in the one-piece lenses. Because of the flexibility and thickness/bulk of its haptics, the square optic and haptic edges, and the unpolished side walls, implantation of the one-piece AcrySof lens in the sulcus is not recom-

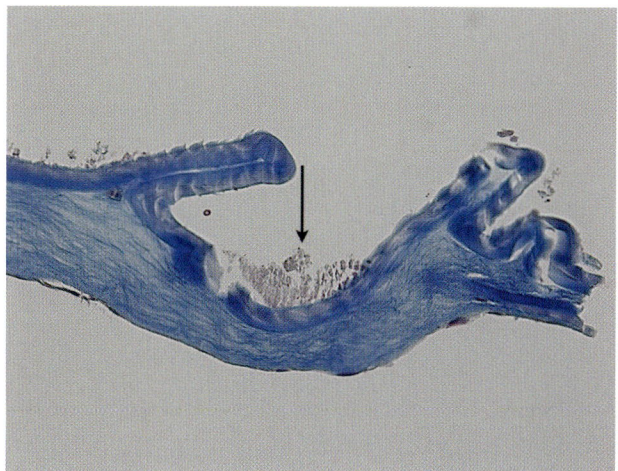

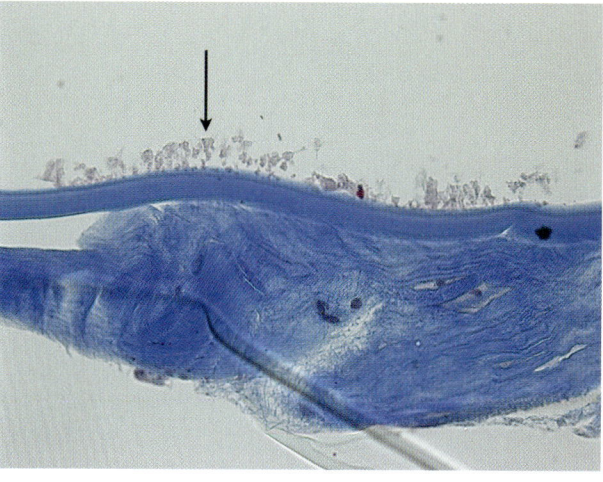

Fig. 42.1   Histopathological sections of capsular bags from in-the-bag subluxation/luxation cases (Masson's trichrome stain). The *arrows* show the pseudoexfoliation material on the anterior capsules. There are significant amounts of fibrotic material attached to the inner surface of the anterior capsules, with contraction and folds. **(a,b)** Original magnification ×400.

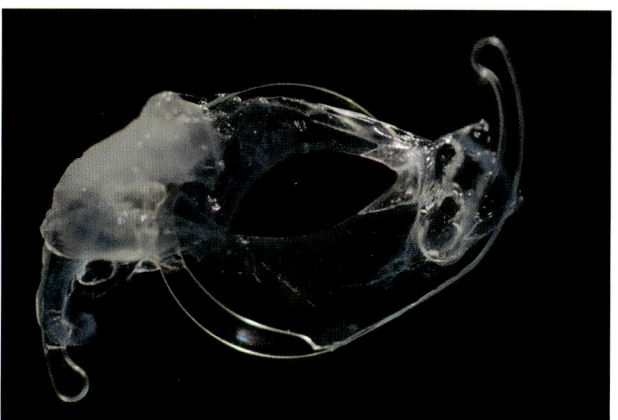

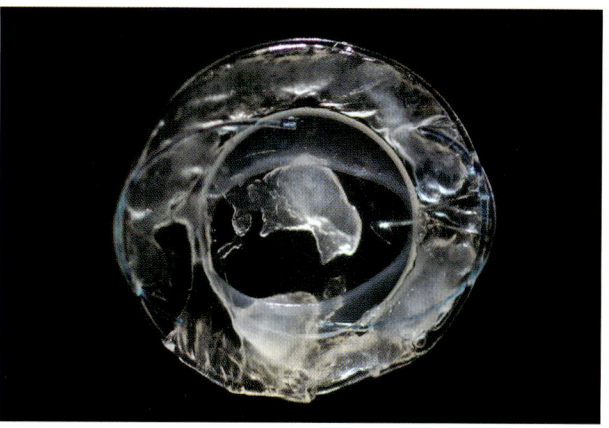

Fig. 42.2   Gross photographs of in-the-bag subluxation/luxation cases. **(a)** In-the-bag luxation of a one-piece hydrophobic acrylic lens. There is capsulorrhexis phimosis and mild Soemmering's ring formation. **(b)** In-the-bag luxation of a three-piece hydrophobic acrylic lens with a capsular tension ring (CTR). There is significant fibrosis of the rhexis edge and moderate Soemmering's ring formation.

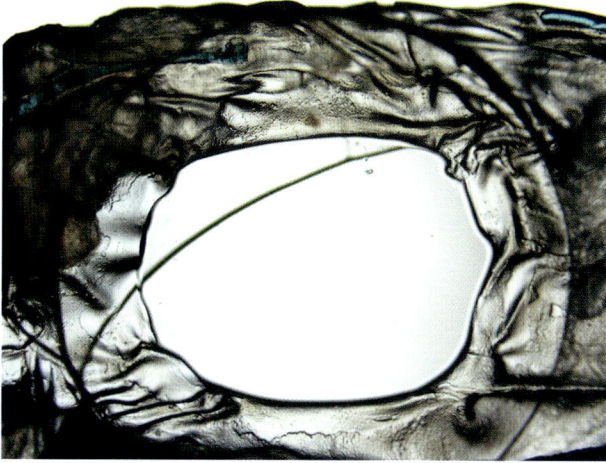

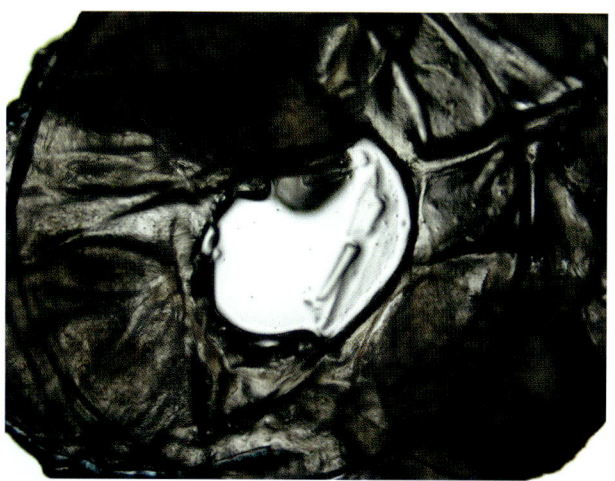

Fig. 42.3   Light photomicrographs from in-the-bag subluxation/luxation cases (three-piece hydrophobic acrylic lenses). There are different degrees of capsulorrhexis phimosis, capsular contraction, and capsular folds. **(a)** Without a CTR. **(b)** With a CTR.

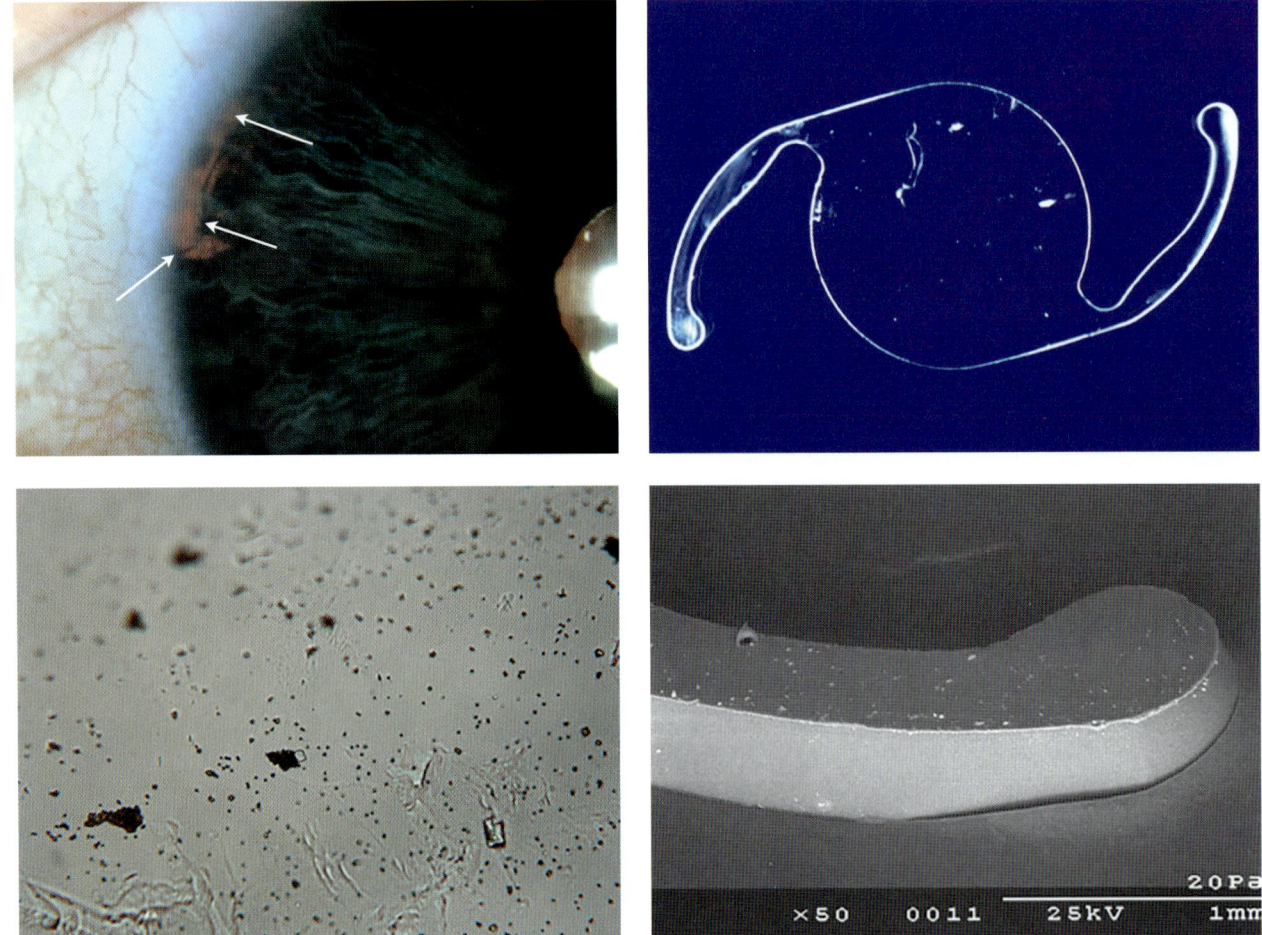

Fig. 42.4 A case of asymmetric (bag-sulcus) fixation of a one-piece hydrophobic acrylic lens. **(a)** Clinical photograph showing the loop in the sulcus through a transillumination defect *(arrows)*. **(b)** Gross photograph of the explanted lens. **(c)** Light photomicrograph of the lens showing pigmentary dispersion (×200). **(d)** Scanning electron photomicrograph showing the thick loop with rough edges. (From LeBoyer RM, Werner L, Snyder ME, et al. Acute haptic-induced ciliary sulcus irritation associated with single-piece AcrySof intraocular lenses. J Cataract Refract Surg 2005;31:1421–1427. Reprinted by permission.)

mended, and this design is not indicated for sulcus fixation, according to the directions-for-use labeling. Furthermore, the haptics of the one-piece lens are planar and therefore do not vault the optic posteriorly from the iris. The overall lens diameter is up to 13.0 mm, which is too short for many eyes; if the haptics do not fully extend because of their low compressive force, the IOL will be prone to decentration in the ciliary sulcus of larger eyes.[10] A study from our laboratory reported on three one-piece lenses that were explanted because of pigmentary dispersion syndrome related to the presence of their haptics in the ciliary sulcus **(Fig. 42.4)**.[11] These cases revealed the presence of significant amounts of iris pigment on the anterior surface of the lens (optics and haptics). Other similar cases of pigmentary dispersion with this lens have been described in the literature, which were generally managed with explantation/exchange of the lens, or by surgical repositioning within the capsular bag.[10]

In a retrospective study, Chang et al[10] described the findings in 30 eyes with sulcus-fixated one-piece lenses (29 of those were one-piece AcrySof; one was a Rayner [Kansas City, MO] model 570C hydrophilic acrylic design). Posterior capsule rupture and IOL decentration were observed in approximately two thirds of the eyes. No IOL was suture fixated to the iris or sclera. Approximately one third of the patients were taking at least one intraocular pressure (IOP)-lowering medication. The most common

complications were pigment dispersion and iris transillumination defects, followed by IOL edge symptoms and elevated IOP. Intraocular hemorrhage and cystoid macular edema were relatively infrequent. The authors hypothesized that the latter may have been underreported because of the retrospective nature of the data collection.

Similar complications have also been reported with three-piece AcrySof lenses, in a piggyback configuration or standard sulcus fixation.[12–16] In piggyback implantation, fixation of the anterior lens in the sulcus has been recommended to prevent interlenticular opacification. However, a previous publication from our laboratory described a case of pigmentary dispersion syndrome resulting from secondary piggyback implantation of a low power three-piece hydrophobic acrylic, square-edged IOL in the ciliary sulcus (AcrySof IOL model MA60MA; +5 D).[12] Chang and Lim,[13] as well as Iwase and Tanaka,[14] have also described cases of pigmentary dispersion syndrome with the same three-piece hydrophobic acrylic lens implanted in a piggyback configuration.

Wintle and Austin[15] reported a case of pigmentary dispersion syndrome 1 month following implantation of a three-piece hydrophobic acrylic lens (AcrySof IOL model MA60BM, 6.0 mm optic, 13.0 mm overall length) placed electively in the ciliary sulcus following a posterior capsule tear. A similar case was also described by Almond et al.[16] Other studies did not show excessive interaction between these three-piece, sulcus-fixated lenses and the posterior iris surface.[17,18]

We performed a donor eye study in our laboratory that provided pathological evidence of complications related to out-of-the-bag fixation of one- or three-piece hydrophobic acrylic IOLs with anterior and posterior square optic edges.[19] Eighteen eyes with the targeted lenses exhibited asymmetric or sulcus IOL fixation (6 one-piece, and 12 three-piece IOLs). These eyes underwent complete histopathological evaluation and were compared with the contralateral eyes with symmetric in-the-bag IOL implantation. The pathological findings were IOL decentration and tilt, pigmentary dispersion within the anterior segment and on the IOL surface, iris transillumination defects, iris changes including vacuolization/disruption/loss of the pigmented layer, iris thinning, and iris atrophy, as well as synechiae and loop erosion in the case of three-piece lenses. Findings were more significant in comparison with the control contralateral eyes and were particularly evident in relation to the sulcus-fixated haptic in the case of one-piece lenses (**Fig. 42.5**). The majority of the eyes with three-piece lenses in the above-mentioned study showed signs of complicated surgery; therefore, all pathological findings in those cases could not be strictly attributed to the out-of-the-bag fixation of the IOL. To further understand these findings, we compared the pathological findings from 13 eyes with three-piece hydrophobic acrylic IOLs with anterior and posterior square optic edges to those from 14 eyes with three-piece lenses with anterior round edges (13 silicone lenses, and one hydrophobic acrylic lens) (**Fig. 42.6**). All lenses had sulcus fixation or asymmetric fixation.[20] In both groups, more significant defects were especially evident in relation to the side of the IOL fixated in the sulcus (in asymmetric fixation cases). Gross/macroscopic decentration, tilt, pigment dispersion, and iris transillumination defects were statistically similar in both groups, and to a great extent could have been related to the complicated surgery itself. However, the most striking findings in this second study came from the analyses of the histopathological sections of the eyes. The severity of the iris changes was more prominent in relation to three-piece lenses with square anterior optic edges. Also, all eyes with these lenses had pigmentary dispersion within the trabecular meshwork, in comparison to only one eye in the group of lenses with round anterior edges. This indicates continuous trauma to the posterior surface of the iris, likely related to rubbing by the square optic edge.[20] Our pathological findings, therefore, appear to confirm that IOLs with round anterior edges are more suitable for sulcus fixation.

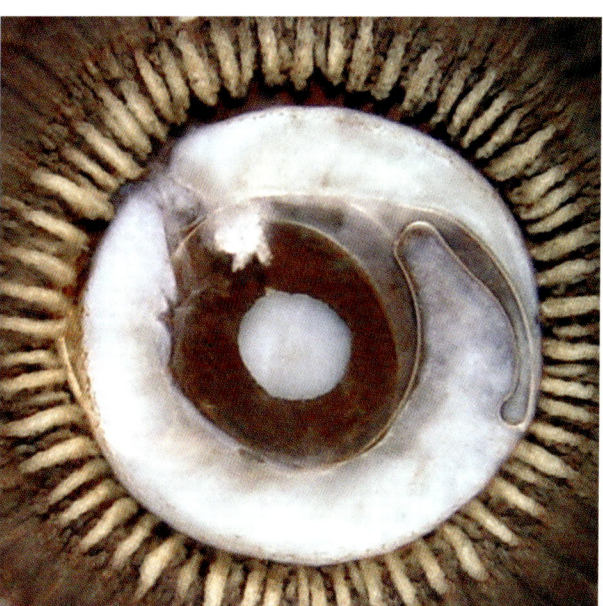

a

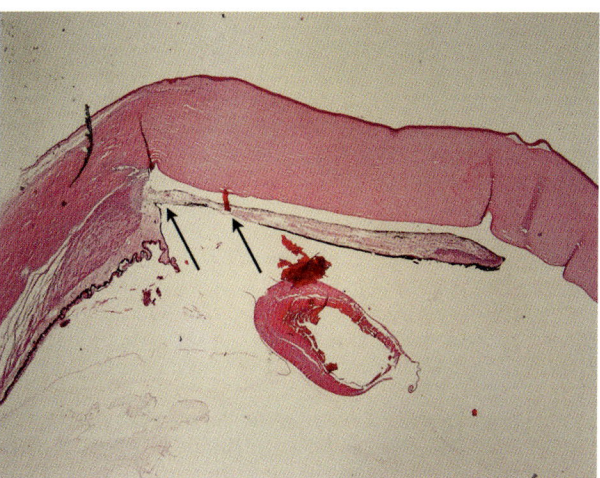

b

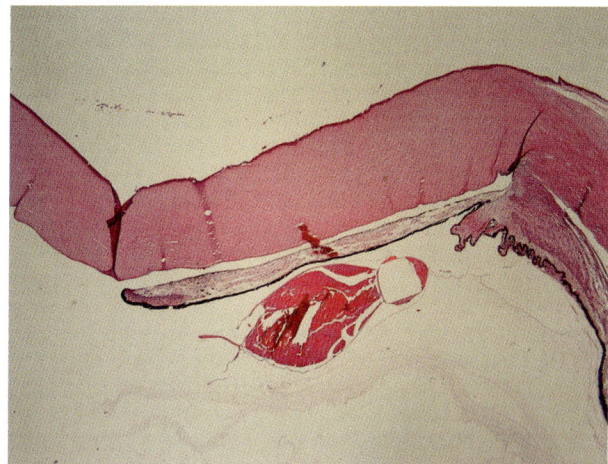

c

Fig. 42.5 A pseudophakic human eye obtained postmortem with asymmetric (bag-sulcus) fixation of a one-piece hydrophobic acrylic lens. **(a)** Gross photograph from the Miyake-Apple view. **(b)** The haptic on the left was in the sulcus, which caused disruption of the iris pigmented layer in regions close to the iris root and midperiphery *(arrows)*. **(c)** The haptic on the right was in the bag. The iris pigmented layer on this side does not exhibit any major disruption. **(b,c)** Hematoxylin & eosin stain; original magnification ×20. (From Kirk KR, Werner L, Jaber R, et al. Pathological assessment of complications with asymmetric or sulcus fixation of square-edged hydrophobic acrylic intraocular lenses. Ophthalmology 2012;119:907–913. Reprinted with permission.)

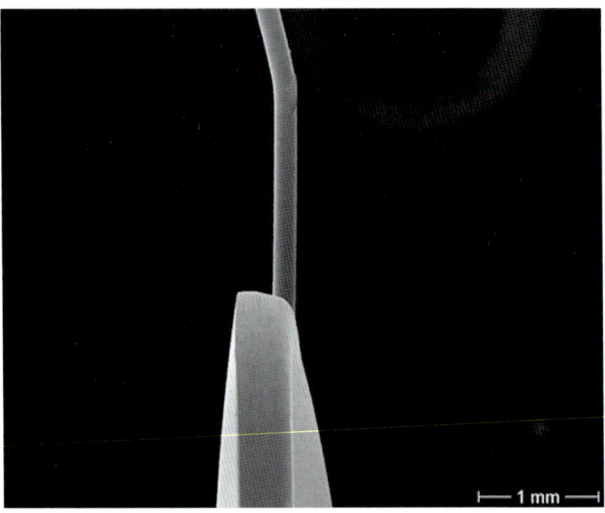

Fig. 42.6 Scanning electron photomicrographs showing the edges of three-piece hydrophobic acrylic lenses. The anterior surface is shown on the right side of each photo. **(a)** Square anterior optic edge and unpolished side wall. **(b)** Round anterior optic edge and smooth side wall.

Intraocular Lens Opacification

The majority of IOLs explanted in the United States because of optic opacification and sent to our laboratory for analyses are calcified hydrophilic acrylic lenses. We also still receive a relatively significant number of calcified silicone lenses as well as polymethylmethacrylate (PMMA) lenses with snowflake degeneration.[21,22]

Calcification of Hydrophilic Acrylic and Silicone Intraocular Lenses

Postoperative optic opacification of modern hydrophilic acrylic IOL designs has been a significant complication since 1999, leading to IOL explantation. Different studies using histopathological, histochemical, electron microscopic, as well as elemental or molecular surface analytic techniques demonstrated that the opacification was related to calcium/phosphate precipitation on or within the lenses. The four major designs manufactured in the United States that had this problem were the Hydroview (Bausch and Lomb, Rochester, NY), the MemoryLens (Ciba Vision, Duluth, GA), the SC60B-OUV (Medical Developmental Research, Clearwater, FL), and the Aqua-Sense (Ophthalmic Innovations International, Claremont, CA). Although in many cases it was difficult to determine the time that the optic opacification was first observed, the lenses that had the problem were on average explanted during the second year postimplantation. The opacification was not associated with anterior segment inflammatory reaction, and the neodymium:yttrium-aluminum-garnet (Nd:YAG) laser was ineffective in removing the calcified deposits from the lenses.[21,22]

Dystrophic calcification of hydrophilic acrylic lenses appears to be a multifactorial problem, and factors related to IOL manufacture, IOL packaging, surgical techniques and adjuvants, as well as patient metabolic conditions, among others, may be implicated. As the exact combination of factors and sequence of events ultimately leading to calcification of the lenses is still unknown, continuous research on this complication is warranted. This requires a multidisciplinary approach, which is further complicated by the fact that detailed manufacturing procedures are considered proprietary information, and some IOL designs are distributed in different countries with different commercial names.[21,22] In the meantime, surgeons must be able to recognize this condition during clinical examination, to avoid performance of unnecessary procedures, such as Nd:YAG laser posterior capsulotomy (after a misdiagnosis of posterior capsule opacification), or vitrectomy (after a misdiagnosis of some form of vitreous opacity). We have described eight cases in which calcification of the implanted MemoryLens IOLs was not recognized, resulting in unnecessary procedures and repeated interventions, ultimately leading to complications such as retinal detachment and endophthalmitis.[23] Explantation/exchange of the opacified/calcified IOL is to date the only possible treatment.

There have also been sporadic reports of postoperative IOL calcification involving different hydrophilic acrylic lens designs manufactured in Europe.[21,24] They have mostly been related to complicated cases, with significant postoperative inflammation, multiple surgical procedures, and intraocular use of adjuvants such as tissue plasminogen activator (for severe fibrinous reaction), silicone oil, air, or gas. The onset of signs and symptoms may occur much earlier than in the cases of dystrophic calcification mentioned above, and the pattern of calcium deposition may vary. In cases following different surgical procedures involving use of air or gas inside the eye (e.g., Descemet stripping endothelial keratoplasty), the pattern of calcification appears to be more superficial, on or close to the anterior surface of the lens, and confined to the pupillary/capsulorrhexis area **(Fig. 42.7a)**.[24] Further research is also warranted to understand the local factors involved in this relatively well-demarcated pattern of IOL calcification.

Calcified deposits leading to significant opacification requiring explantation were observed on the surface of silicone IOLs in eyes with asteroid hyalosis.[21,25,26] The composition of asteroid bodies was found to be similar to that of hydroxyapatite (calcium and phosphate). Whitish deposits appear on the posterior optic surface of the lenses only in the late postoperative period. In some cases, the deposits were noted before Nd:YAG laser capsulotomy was performed. Fast reaccumulation of the deposits on the posterior surface of the lenses was described after the procedure. More recently, we reported on 16 new cases involving eight designs of silicone lenses manufactured from five different silicone material.[26] It is unclear why there are so few reported cases of opacification despite the numerous silicone IOLs that have probably been implanted in patients with asteroid hyalosis since their introduction to the market in the 1980s. In light of

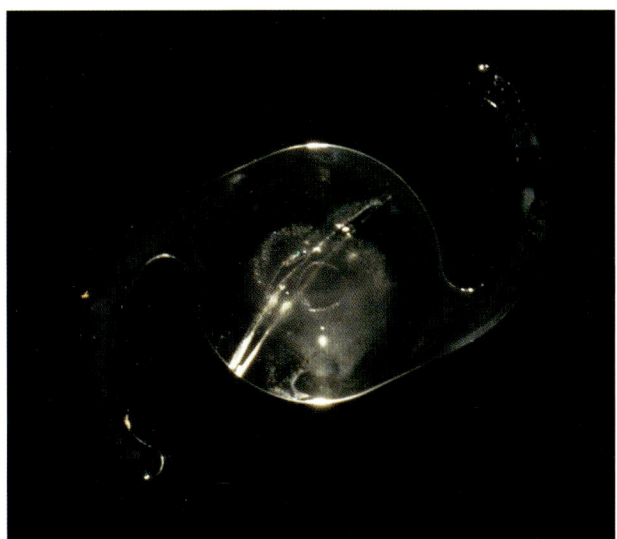

a

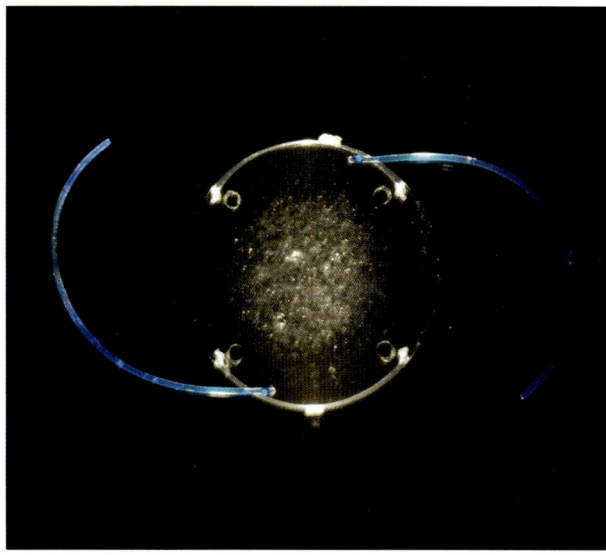

b

Fig. 42.7 Intraocular lenses explanted because of postoperative optic opacification. **(a)** Single-piece hydrophilic acrylic lens explanted because of localized calcification after Descemet's stripping automated endothelial keratoplasty (DSAEK). **(b)** A three-piece polymethylmethacrylate (PMMA) lens explanted because of snowflake degeneration.

the increasing number of opacified silicone lenses in these eyes, involving a variety of IOL designs, surgeons should consider our findings when selecting or recommending an IOL.

Snowflake Degeneration of Polymethylmethacrylate Intraocular Lenses

Snowflake degeneration entails a slowly progressive opacification of PMMA lenses, occurring sometimes 10 years or longer after implantation.[21,27] It has been observed in three-piece PMMA lenses implanted between the early 1980s and the mid-1990s, which were generally manufactured by injection molding (**Fig. 42.7b**). It has been hypothesized that this degeneration is a result of long-term ultraviolet (UV) light exposure. The explanted lenses had spherical lesions, which were interpreted as foci of degenerated PMMA material clustered in the central zone and midperipheral portion of the optic. This led to the hypothesis that the central optic was exposed to UV light over an extended period, whereas the peripheral optic may be protected by the iris. Therefore, snowflake lesions are generally not observed in the optic periphery, they generally involve the anterior third of the optic substance, and they do not disappear when the lens is in the dry state. Although the snowflake lesions are dry, it has been observed that an unusual amount of water is collected within the affected optic area upon hydration of explanted PMMA lenses with this condition, leading to more significant optic opacification. Therefore, the clinical significance of snowflake degeneration may depend on the amount of water collected within the IOL optic.[27]

Glistenings and Nano-Glistenings

Two hydration-related phenomena have been described in the literature in IOLs made of different materials, particularly in hydrophobic acrylic lenses: glistenings, and surface light scattering.[28] Ophthalmologists should be aware of these findings, which generally do not prompt IOL explantation. Glistenings are fluid-filled microvacuoles (1 to 20 µm in diameter) that form within the IOL optic when the lens is in an aqueous environment (**Fig. 42.8a**). Although they are largely described in association with hydrophobic acrylic IOLs, they can actually be observed with different IOL materials, including PMMA. The majority of peer-reviewed articles on glistenings available in the literature describe them in relation to the AcrySof material. Literature regarding glistening formation with other hydrophobic acrylic lenses is relatively scarce. There are differences in wettability or water content of different hydrophobic acrylic lenses as a function of temperature changes, which may account for different tendencies for glistening formation among these lenses, besides possible influences of the manufacturing technique.[28]

Although it is difficult to compare different clinical studies due to differences in patient population and grading system used, among others, the majority of them show an increase in the incidence or severity of glistenings up to 3 years postoperatively.[28] One study following 12 eyes implanted with AcrySof lenses for 5 years demonstrated stabilization of the degree of glistenings between 3 and 5 years, as indicated by light scattering within the IOL optic using Scheimpflug photography.[29] It is therefore reasonable to hypothesize that the incidence and degree of glistenings may increase until the IOL is completely hydrated and all available voids within the polymer network are visible as glistenings, under the influence of temperature fluctuations. Further long-term, prospective clinical studies are necessary to confirm this hypothesis. In terms of clinical impact, the majority of clinical studies show no influence on visual acuity, and there are few reports of a possible influence on contrast sensitivity, under specific test conditions. Review of the available literature and database mechanisms, such as Food and Drug Administration (FDA) reporting, revealed that explantation due to glistenings has been rarely reported, although underreporting of such cases remains a possibility. However, in the majority of these cases it has also been challenging to establish a direct relationship between the degree of glistenings and the patient symptoms leading to explantation.[28]

Surface light scattering is a "whitening" appearance of the lens surface when the light is directed at the IOL at an angle of incidence of 30 degrees or greater during slit-lamp examination

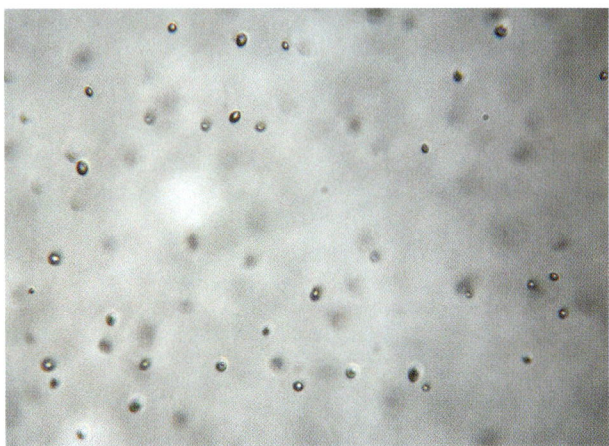

a

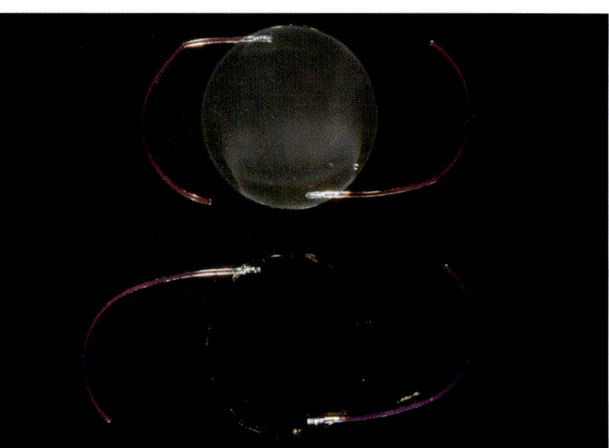

b

Fig. 42.8   Glistenings and nano-glistenings. **(a)** Light photomicrograph of a three-piece hydrophobic acrylic lens with glistenings inside the optic substance (×400). **(b)** Gross photograph (dark-field image with a 90-degree off-axis illumination) of a three-piece hydrophobic acrylic lens removed from a cadaver eye *(top)* with corresponding control lens *(bottom)*. Both lenses are immersed in solution. The cadaver eye-removed lens exhibits an overall optic haziness in comparison with the control, which is related to light scattering due to subsurface nano-glistenings.

or during image capture at an angle of 45 degrees at Scheimpflug photography.[28,30,31] Studies analyzing explanted lenses in dry and hydrated states as well as analyses under cryo-focused ion beam scanning electron microscopy (SEM) showed that scattering was predominantly caused by phase separation of water (from aqueous humor) as subsurface nano-glistenings. Surface light scattering/nano-glistenings have also been particularly studied and described in IOLs made of the AcrySof material (Alcon) **(Fig. 42.8b)**.[28]

Ogura et al[30] analyzed the optical performance of cadaver-eye explanted AcrySof lenses with significant surface light scattering, as well as clinical explants removed at least 8.5 years after implantation. The authors did not find any effect on image resolution or on modulation transfer function values of the lenses. Although light transmittance was slightly decreased, the magnitude appeared to be inconsequential for optical performance. In a study performed in our laboratory, 49 single-piece AcrySof IOLs were obtained from human cadaver eyes (36 with blue light filter), and power/model matched to unused control IOLs.[31] Although surface light scattering of cadaver-eye removed lenses was significantly higher than that of controls and appeared to increase with time, no effect was observed on the light transmittance of single-piece hydrophobic acrylic lenses with or without blue light filter. Finally, clinical studies attempted to correlate surface light scattering with clinical complaints or effects on visual function, but to date no specific correlation was found.[28]

Conclusion

Complications occurring after phacoemulsification with IOL implantation, such as in-the-bag IOL subluxation/dislocation, pigmentary dispersion, and IOL optic opacification in general, prompt performance of secondary procedures for IOL explantation/exchange or IOL repositioning. Although a significant finding during slit-lamp examination, the occurrence of glistenings and nano-glistenings in hydrophobic acrylic lenses generally does not require explantation, as their precise association with a decrease in the visual function remains to be established. Pathological and laboratory analyses of the above-mentioned complications and findings are helpful in gaining a better understanding of the underlined conditions, as well as in the selection of the best clinical/surgical approach in each case.

References

1. Gimbel HV, Condon GP, Kohnen T, Olson RJ, Halkiadakis I. Late in-the-bag intraocular lens dislocation: incidence, prevention, and management. J Cataract Refract Surg 2005;31:2193–2204

2. Hayashi K, Hirata A, Hayashi H. Possible predisposing factors for in-the-bag and out-of-the-bag intraocular lens dislocation and outcomes of intraocular lens exchange surgery. Ophthalmology 2007;114:969–975

3. Lorente R, de Rojas V, Vazquez de Parga P, et al. Management of late spontaneous in-the-bag intraocular lens dislocation: Retrospective analysis of 45 cases. J Cataract Refract Surg 2010;36:1270–1282

4. Naumann GO, Schlötzer-Schrehardt U, Küchle M. Pseudoexfoliation syndrome for the comprehensive ophthalmologist. Intraocular and systemic manifestations. Ophthalmology 1998;105:951–968

5. Jehan FS, Mamalis N, Crandall AS. Spontaneous late dislocation of intraocular lens within the capsular bag in pseudoexfoliation patients. Ophthalmology 2001;108:1727–1731

6. Davis D, Brubaker J, Espandar L, et al. Late in-the-bag spontaneous intraocular lens dislocation: evaluation of 86 consecutive cases. Ophthalmology 2009;116:664–670

7. Werner L, Zaugg B, Neuhann T, Burrow M, Tetz M. In-the-bag capsular tension ring and intraocular lens subluxation or dislocation: a series of 23 cases. Ophthalmology 2012;119:266–271

8. Liu E, Cole S, Werner L, Hengerer F, Mamalis N, Kohnen T. Pathological evidence of pseudoexfoliation in cases of in-the-bag intraocular lens subluxation/dislocation. J Cataract Refract Surg 2015;41:929–935

9. Meacock WR, Spalton DJ, Khan S. The effect of texturing the intraocular lens edge on postoperative glare symptoms: a randomized, prospective, double-masked study. Arch Ophthalmol 2002;120:1294–1298

10. Chang DF, Masket S, Miller KM, et al; ASCRS Cataract Clinical Committee. Complications of sulcus placement of single-piece acrylic intraocular lenses: recommendations for backup IOL implantation following posterior capsule rupture. J Cataract Refract Surg 2009;35:1445–1458

11. LeBoyer RM, Werner L, Snyder ME, Mamalis N, Riemann CD, Augsberger JJ. Acute haptic-induced ciliary sulcus irritation associated with single-piece AcrySof intraocular lenses. J Cataract Refract Surg 2005;31:1421–1427

12. Chang WH, Werner L, Fry LL, Johnson JT, Kamae K, Mamalis N. Pigmentary dispersion syndrome with a secondary piggyback 3-piece hydrophobic acrylic lens. Case report with clinicopathological correlation. J Cataract Refract Surg 2007;33:1106–1109

13. Chang SHL, Lim G. Secondary pigmentary glaucoma associated with piggyback intraocular lens implantation. J Cataract Refract Surg 2004;30:2219–2222

14. Iwase T, Tanaka N. Elevated intraocular pressure in secondary piggyback intraocular lens implantation. J Cataract Refract Surg 2005;31:1821–1823

15. Wintle R, Austin M. Pigment dispersion with elevated intraocular pressure after AcrySof intraocular lens implantation in the ciliary sulcus. J Cataract Refract Surg 2001;27:642–644

16. Almond MC, Wu MC, Chen PP. Pigment dispersion and chronic intraocular pressure elevation after sulcus placement of 3-piece acrylic intraocular lens. J Cataract Refract Surg 2009;35:2164–2166

17. Brazitikos PD, Balidis MO, Tranos P, et al. Sulcus implantation of a 3-piece, 6.0 mm optic, hydrophobic foldable acrylic intraocular lens in phacoemulsification complicated by posterior capsule rupture. J Cataract Refract Surg 2002;28:1618–1622

18. Mackool RJ. Pigmentary dispersion syndrome. J Cataract Refract Surg 2001;27:1341–1342 (letter)

19. Kirk KR, Werner L, Jaber R, Strenk S, Strenk L, Mamalis N. Pathologic assessment of complications with asymmetric or sulcus fixation of square-edged hydrophobic acrylic intraocular lenses. Ophthalmology 2012;119:907–913

20. Ollerton A, Werner L, Strenk S, et al. Pathologic comparison of asymmetric or sulcus fixation of 3-piece intraocular lenses with square versus round anterior optic edges. Ophthalmology 2013;120:1580–1587

21. Werner L. Causes of intraocular lens opacification or discoloration. J Cataract Refract Surg 2007;33:713–726 (Review)

22. Werner L. Calcification of hydrophilic acrylic intraocular lenses. Am J Ophthalmol 2008;146:341–343 (Editorial)

23. Haymore J, Zaidman G, Werner L, et al. Misdiagnosis of hydrophilic acrylic intraocular lens optic opacification: report of 8 cases with the MemoryLens. Ophthalmology 2007;114:1689–1695

24. Werner L, Wilbanks G, Nieuwendaal CP, et al. Localized opacification of hydrophilic acrylic intraocular lenses after procedures using intracameral injection of air or gas. J Cataract Refract Surg 2014; In press

25. Foot L, Werner L, Gills JP, et al. Surface calcification of silicone plate intraocular lenses in patients with asteroid hyalosis. Am J Ophthalmol 2004; 137:979–987

26. Stringham J, Werner L, Monson B, Theodosis R, Mamalis N. Calcification of different designs of silicone intraocular lenses in eyes with asteroid hyalosis. Ophthalmology 2010;117:1486–1492

27. Dahle N, Werner L, Fry L, Mamalis N. Localized, central optic snowflake degeneration of a PMMA intraocular lens: clinical report with pathological correlation. Arch Ophthalmol 2006;124:1350–1353

28. Werner L. Glistenings and surface light scattering in intraocular lenses. J Cataract Refract Surg 2010;36:1398–1420 (Review)

29. Yoshida S, Fujikake F, Matsushima H, Obara Y, Rin S. Induction of glistening and visual function of eyes with acrylic intraocular lenses inserted. IOL&RS. 2000;14:289–292 (Japanese)

30. Ogura Y, Ong MD, Akinay A, Carson DR, Pei R, Karakelle M. Optical performance of hydrophobic acrylic intraocular lenses with surface light scattering. J Cataract Refract Surg 2014;40:104–113

31. Werner L, Morris C, Liu E, et al. Light transmittance of 1-piece hydrophobic acrylic intraocular lenses with surface light scattering removed from cadaver eyes. J Cataract Refract Surg 2014;40:114–120

XVI Premium Intraocular Lenses and Their Management

43 Management of Astigmatism with Peripheral Corneal Relaxing Incisions and Toric Intraocular Lenses

Jonathan B. Rubenstein

The goal of modern cataract surgery has been evolving over the past few years aided by significant improvements in intraocular lens (IOL) implant technology as well as advancements in preoperative and intraoperative surgical technology. Today, the majority of patients desire postoperative emmetropia, and the preoperative consideration of this goal has become an essential aspect of cataract surgery. With the advent of IOLs that correct astigmatism and presbyopia, in addition to the incisional methods of managing astigmatism, the tools necessary to fulfill patient expectations are now available. This chapter reviews two of the methods to achieve refractive neutrality—toric IOLs and peripheral corneal relaxing incisions (PCRIs; also referred to as limbal relaxing incisions [LRIs])—and discusses the preoperative, intraoperative, and postoperative considerations.

Preoperative Assessment

The first step in the management of astigmatism is to perform a thorough preoperative ophthalmologic examination. A stable tear film, normal ocular surface, corneal epithelium, and basement membrane are critical in obtaining precise measurements. The amount of astigmatism, the location of the axis of cylinder, and the refractive status of the other eye should be determined during the examination, and the patient's age is another factor to take into consideration. For patients to achieve spectacle independence, cataract surgeons should aim to treat preoperative corneal astigmatism > 0.50 diopters.

There are multiple methods of measuring preoperative astigmatism, and advances in technology continue to provide addi-

tional techniques. It is important to measure both the astigmatic axis and the astigmatic power. Every evaluation should begin with a manifest refraction, which takes into account both the corneal and lenticular astigmatism. Because lenticular astigmatism is eliminated with removal of the cataractous lens, only the measured corneal astigmatism should be corrected. The corneal astigmatism can be measured with manual keratometry, automated keratometry, Placido-based corneal topography, Pentacam Scheimpflug elevation mapping (Oculus, Optikgeräte, Arlington, WA), Galilei Dual Scheimpflug analysis (Ziemer, Port, Switzerland; Alton, IL), partial coherence interferometry, and optical low-coherence reflectometry.

A recent study compared manual keratometer, partial coherence interferometry, Pentacam, and auto keratometry and demonstrated that all methods were equally satisfactory in measuring preoperative corneal astigmatism.[1] More advanced technology utilizing corneal elevation mapping, such as the Oculus Pentacam and Ziemer Galilei, evaluate both the anterior and posterior corneal surfaces. Recent studies have shown the importance of posterior corneal astigmatism in overall corneal toricity, and a nomogram has been developed at Baylor University (Houston, TX), which takes this into consideration (**Fig. 43.1**).[2] In our experience, the best assessment of corneal astigmatic power comes from careful manual keratometry plus IOL Master interferometry (Carl Zeiss Meditec, Jena, Germany) or Lenstar reflectometry (Haag-Streit, Mason, OH), and the best assessment of astigmatic axis location comes from IOL Master interferometry or Lenstar reflectometry combined with qualitative guidance from corneal topography and corneal elevation mapping.

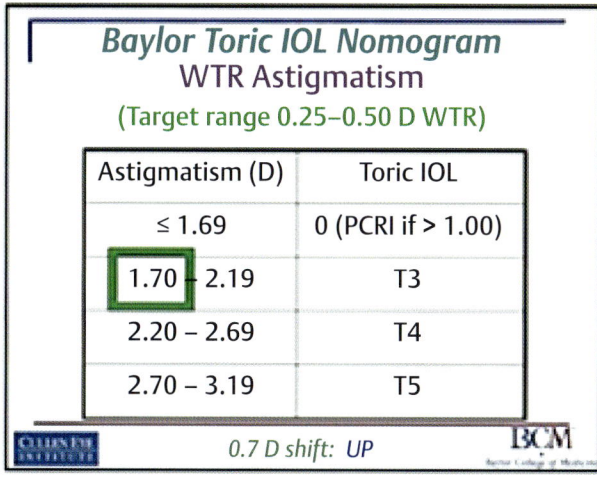

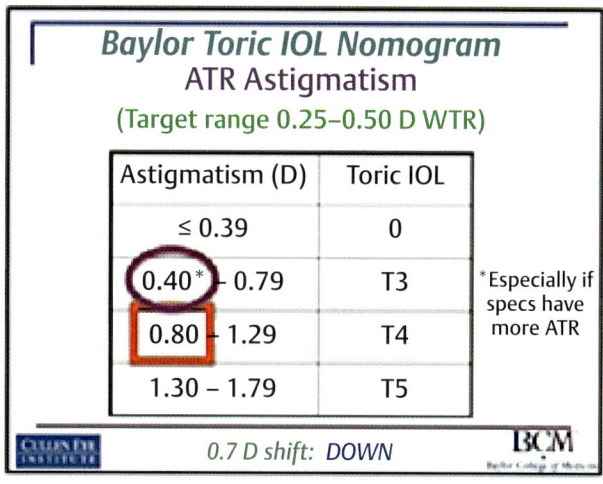

Fig. 43.1 Baylor toric nomogram, with the rule (WTR) and against the rule (ATR), takes into account posterior corneal astigmatism.

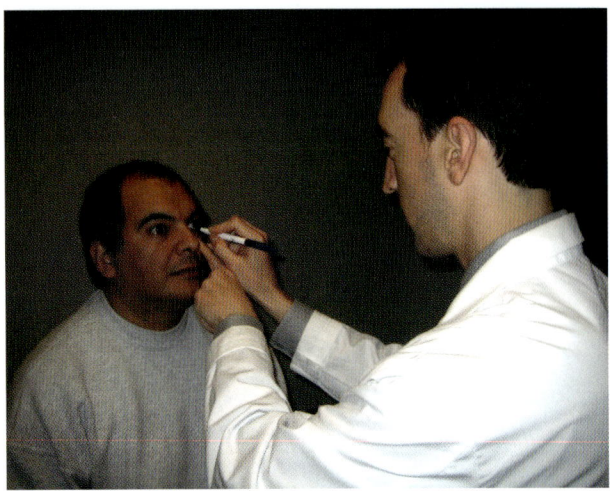
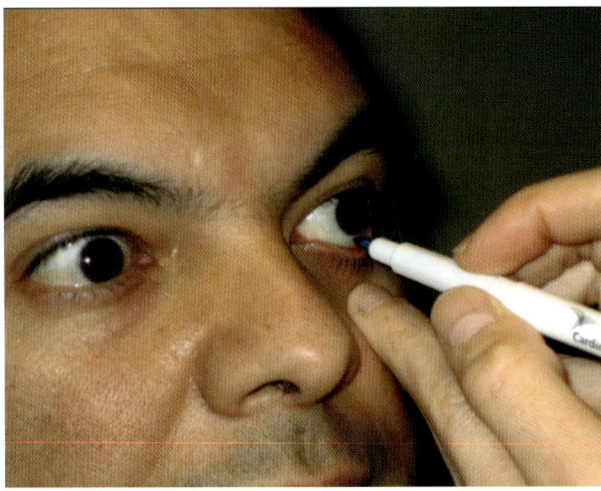

a   b

Fig. 43.2 **(a)** Preoperative patient is seated fixating at a distance. **(b)** The steep corneal axis is marked with gentian violet.

Intraoperative Marking

Prior to the patient's arriving in the operating room, the eye must be marked to correctly place the PCRIs or toric IOL on axis. The surgeon manually marks the 6 o'clock and/or 3 and 9 o'clock positions on the cornea while the patient is sitting up and looking straight ahead with both eyes open to avoid cyclotorsion (**Fig. 43.2**). Then, in the operating room, a marked fixation ring, astigmatic ruler, or arcuate axis marker is centered and oriented on the previously marked 6, 3, or 9 o'clock positions to identify and mark the steep corneal axis.[3] Precise axis marking and alignment is critical for effective reduction of astigmatism. For toric IOLs, 1 degree of misalignment is equivalent to a 3.3% decrease in astigmatic correction. When a toric IOL rotates 30 degrees, there is no astigmatic correction induced, and when rotation is greater than 30 degrees there is an induction of increased astigmatism.[4] Newer

methods have been developed to further increase the accuracy of astigmatic axis marking. These techniques involve preoperative digital imaging that captures keratometry values and iris, limbal, and conjunctival vessel patterns, and uses these landmarks to map the steep axis of astigmatism. One example of this is the VERION™ system (Alcon, Fort Worth, TX) that links preoperative diagnostic imaging data to the operative procedure to orient the positive axis of astigmatism without the use of manual markers. A reference unit in the office captures images and data such as keratometry and limbus and pupil location and transfers this data to the VERION digital marker in the operating room via a USB key (**Fig. 43.3**). Real-time eye registration and tracking is generated in the surgeon's microscope view and on a flat screen monitor to provide intraoperative astigmatic guidance for the surgeon. Callisto (Zeiss) has a similar intraoperative guidance system, as does the Cassini Truevision 3D system (Leica Microsystems, Buffalo Grove, IL).

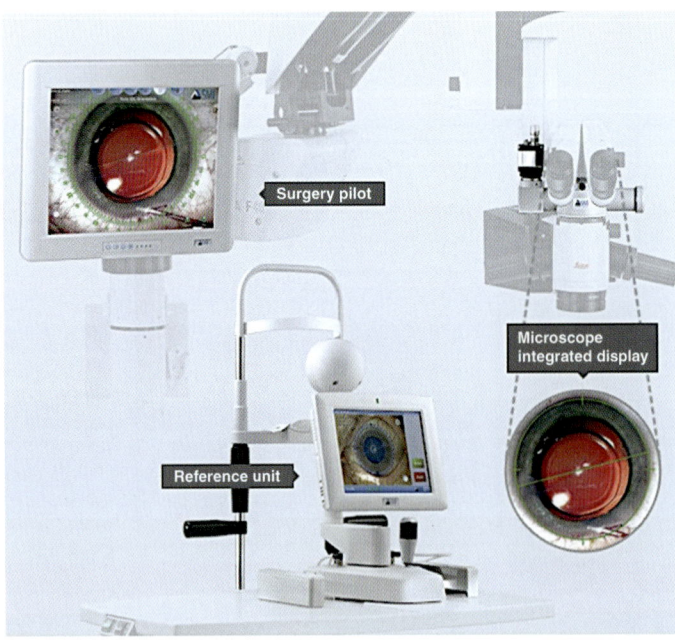

Fig. 43.3 VERION™ system (Alcon).

Choosing the Appropriate Surgical Correction

Peripheral corneal relaxing incisions continue to be a viable method of intraoperative astigmatic correction even with advances in toric IOL technology. The procedure is cost-effective and can correct one to three diopters of corneal astigmatism. The advent of femtosecond laser technology has provided another platform for utilizing intraoperative corneal relaxing incisions. PCRIs can also be used in conjunction with toric IOLs to correct larger amounts of astigmatism than corrected by toric lens implants alone. The correction of astigmatism with multifocal and accommodating IOLs has traditionally been accomplished with the addition of PCRI incisions, with toric presbyopic IOLs only recently becoming available in the United States. However, the addition of PCRIs can still be helpful to correct high amounts of astigmatism in patients with astigmatic presbyopia correcting lenses. In addition, patients who have low degrees of astigmatism of +0.75 to +1.00 D do well with PCRIs instead of toric IOLs, as there is a risk of overcorrection with even the lowest powered lenses. Lastly, intraoperative PCRIs can be used to correct astigmatism when a lack of zonular or capsular integrity precludes the use of a toric IOL.

Most cataract surgeons are more comfortable correcting astigmatism with a toric IOL versus corneal relaxing incisions. The techniques for the use of a toric IOL is not significantly different from that used for conventional one-piece foldable lens implant. The first toric lens was a plate haptic one-piece silicone Staar toric IOL (Staar Surgical, Monrovia, CA) that was approved by the Food and Drug Administration (FDA) in 1998 **(Fig. 43.4a)**. Wide adaptation of this IOL was hindered because its toric position was not always stable, and the lens was found to occasionally rotate off the axis.[5] In 2005, the one-piece acrylic AcrySof toric IOL (Alcon) was approved by the FDA and was noted to have excellent rotational stability, with less than 4 degrees of rotation at 1 year[6] **(Fig. 43.4b)**. More recently, Abbott Medical Optics (AMO, Santa Ana, CA) has released its Tecnis toric IOL **(Fig. 43.4c)**. This acrylic IOL also shows excellent rotational stability. Bausch and Lomb (Rochester, NY) has introduced the Trulign toric IOL. This lens is based on the same platform as the Crystalens (Bausch and Lomb) accommodating lens implant. Currently, in the United States, toric IOLs can correct 1.00 to 4.11 D of corneal astigmatism. It is important to note that toric IOLs cannot correct irregular astigmatism and higher order aberrations. Also, they should not be used in patients with zonular instability, lack of capsular integrity, or significant pupil irregularity, and should never be implanted in the ciliary sulcus. Furthermore, caution should be taken in patients with very high axial myopia with a large capsular bag because of a higher risk of postoperative lens rotation.

There are situations in which patients have greater than 4.5 D of astigmatism, and the use of PCRIs in addition to a toric IOL should be considered because this enables correction of up to 7 diopters of corneal astigmatism. Gills et al[7] found that implanting a toric IOL in combination with PCRIs allowed for the

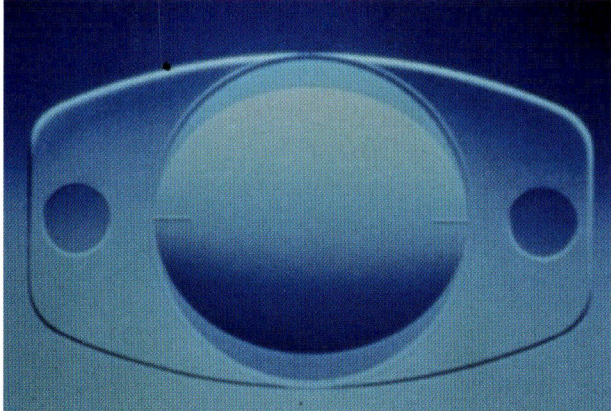

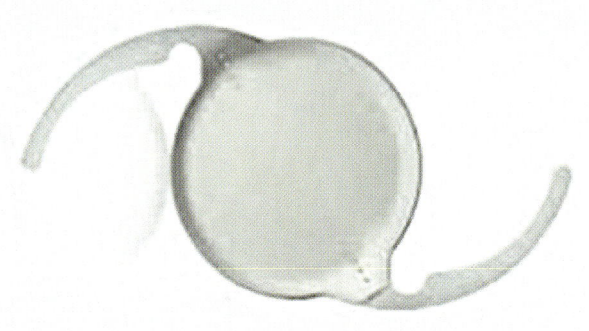

Fig. 43.4 **(a)** The Staar toric intraocular lens (IOL) is the first FDA-approved toric IOL. It has a silicone plate haptic design. As with all plate lenses, it should not be implanted in a compromised capsular bag. It is available in two models with different lengths. Model AA4203-TF (10.8 mm in length) comes in spherical powers of 24.0 to 28.5 D. Model AA4203-TL (11.2 mm) comes in spherical powers of 9.5 to 23.5 D. This lens comes in two cylindri-cal corrective powers: +2.0 D is intended for patients having 1.5 to 2.25 D of preexisting corneal cylinder, whereas the 3.5 D toric IOL is intended for patients having greater than 2.25 D of preexisting corneal astigmatism. The axis of toric power is marked with two hash marks at the optic periphery. (Courtesy of the Staar Surgical Company, Monrovia, CA.) **(b)** AcrySof Toric IOL. **(c)** AMO Tecnis Toric IOL.

correction of high astigmatism while avoiding the induction of corneal irregularities.

Technique

Limbal Relaxing Incisions

There are multiple PCRI and toric IOL nomograms available in the literature as well as on the Internet. Widely used PCRI nomograms include those by Doug Koch and Skip Nichamin (**Figs. 43.5** and **43.6**). Online nomograms are available from Alcon, AMO, and PalmScan AP2000 (Micro Medical Devices, Calabasas, CA). These nomograms take into account the amount of astigmatism, the patient's age, and the location of the steep axis. The online software available at LRIcalculator.com enables the physician to choose between the DONO (Donnenfeld) and the NAPA (Nichamin age and pachymetry adjusted) nomograms depending on physician preference. Surgeons should try multiple nomograms, record their postoperative results, and then modify the chosen nomogram to fit their surgical technique. It is thought that nomograms that plan incisions based on degrees of arc are more accurate than those based on millimeters of arc.[8] The number of incisions can be single or double, depending on the amount of astigmatism that needs correction. In addition, the incision should be tailored to correspond with the astigmatic "bow tie" that is seen on corneal topography. For example, in asymmetric astigmatism, the longer PCRI should be in the larger arm of the bow tie and the shorter incision in the smaller arm.

The PCRI incisions are created at the beginning of cataract surgery on the steep corneal axis in the peripheral clear cornea using a preset 550- to 600-µm double-cutting diamond knife (**Fig. 43.7**). Some nomograms require a pachymetry-adjusted blade thickness using intraoperative assessment of the corneal thickness at the site of the incisions. With the introduction of femto-second laser–assisted cataract surgery, PCRIs can be placed very precisely using the laser at the beginning of the procedure just after the capsulorrhexis and lens softening. These incisions can be opened at the time of surgery, or the incisions can be opened postoperatively to enable adequate astigmatism correction.[9]

There are currently four femtosecond laser platforms available in the United States to treat astigmatism at the time of cataract surgery. The incision axis location, peripheral location, depth, and length can be planned preoperatively, and this information can then be programmed into the laser's computer program. The incisions are created in a posterior to anterior direction and can be programmed to either break through the epithelium or remain intra-stromal. Nomograms for femto incisions are currently being created with preliminary nomograms available from Skip Nichamin and Julian Stevens.

To avoid intraoperative complications, it is recommended that the PCRIs be performed prior to beginning cataract surgery. In addition, it is important to avoid intersecting the corneal incisions; for example, if an PCRI incision is coincident with the temporal clear corneal cataract incision, which occurs with against-the-rule astigmatism, the PCRI should be limited to the length of the cataract incision (for example, 2.4 mm) and only lengthened after the IOL is placed. If the PCRI incision is near the paracentesis incision, as occurs in with-the-rule astigmatism, the paracentesis should be made peripheral to the PCRI to avoid intersecting incisions. Once the PCRI incision is made, intraoperative assessment of the effectiveness of the PCRIs can be assessed using intraoperative wavefront aberrometry. This information can be used to titrate the length of the incision.[10] After the PCRI incisions are created, the phacoemulsification cataract surgery proceeds in a routine fashion. The spherical power of the lens implant does not need to be altered if PCRIs are used secondary to corneal coupling, which entails no net change in overall corneal power.[11]

Cataract WTR Astigmatism (steep meridian at 090)*			
Preoperative astigmatism	Age	Number	Length
0.75–1.00 D	< 65	2 or 1	45° = 4.5 mm 60° = 6.0 mm (if asymmetric)
	> 65	1	45° = 4.5 mm
1.01–1.75 D	< 65	2	60° = 6.0 mm
	> 65	2 or 1	50° = 5.0 mm 60° = 6.0 mm (if asymmetric)
> 1.75 D	< 65	2	80° = 8.0 mm
	> 65	2	60–70° = 6.0–7.0 mm
*Combined w/3.0 mm corneal temporal wound (150°–30° OD, 0°–30° OS).			
Cataract ATR/Oblique Astigmatism (steep meridian at 180)*			
Preoperative astigmatism	Age	Number	Length
1.00–1.25 D**	—	1	35–40° = 3.5–4.0 mm
	—	2	30° = 3.0 mm
1.26–2.00 D**	—	1	45° = 4.5 mm
	—	2	40° = 4.0 mm
> 2.00 D	—	2	45° = 4.5 mm
*Combined w/3.0 mm corneal temporal wound (150°–30° OD, 0°–30° OS).			

Fig. 43.5 Koch limbal relaxing incision (LRI) nomogram. From Wang L, Misra M, and Koch DD. Peripheral corneal relaxing incisions combined with cataract surgery. J Cataract Refract Surg 2003;29:712–722.

♦Astigmatic status = "with-the-rule": (steep axis 45°–145°):
Intraoperative keratoscopy determines exact incision location

Incision design = *"neutral" temporal clear corneal along with the following peripheral arcuate incisions:*

Preoperative cylinder		30–40 yo	41–50 yo	51–60 yo	61–70 yo	71–80 yo	81–90 yo	> 90
+1.00 → +1.50	Paired limbal arcs on steep axis	50°	45°	40°	35°	30°		
+1.75 → +2.25	Paired limbal arcs on steep axis	60°	55°	50°	45°	40°	35°	30°
+2.50 → +3.00	Paired limbal arcs on steep axis	70°	65°	60°	55°	50°	45°	40°
+3.25 → +3.75	Paired limbal arcs on steep axis	80°	75°	70°	65°	60°	55°	45°
						Degrees of arc to be incised		

a

Nomogram
for
clear corneal phaco surgery

Louis D. "Skip" Nichamin, M.D.
Laurel Eye Clinic, Brookville, PA

♦ Astigmatic status = "spherical": (+0.75 × 90 ◄──► +0.50 × 180)

Incision design = *"neutral" temporal clear corneal incision*
(3.5 mm or less, single plane, just anterior to vascular arcade)

♦ Astigmatic status = "against-the-rule": steep axis 0–30°/150–180°):
Intraoperative keratoscopy determines exact incision location

Preoperative cylinder		30–40 yo	41–50 yo	51–60 yo	61–70 yo	71–80 yo	81–90 yo	> 90
+0.75 → +1.25	Nasal limbal arc only						35°	
	*Paired limbal arcs on steep axis	55°	50°	45°	40°	35°		
+1.50 → +2.00	*Paired limbal arcs on steep axis	70°	65°	60°	55°	45°	40°	35°
+2.25 → +2.75	*Paired limbal arcs on steep axis	90°	80°	70°	60°	50°	45°	40°
+3.00 → +3.75	*Paired limbal arcs on steep axis	↓ o.z. to 8 mm 90°	↓ o.z. to 9 mm 90°	85°	70°	60°	50°	45°
					Degrees of arc to be incised			

*The temporal incision is made by first creating a two-plane, grooved phaco incision (600-μm depth),
which is then extended to the appropriate arc length at the conclusion of surgery.

b

Fig. 43.6 (a,b) Nichamin LRI nomogram.

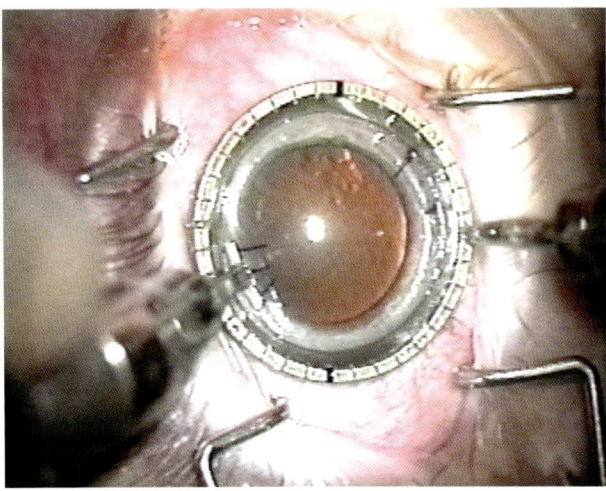

Fig. 43.7 Surgical image of PCRI.

Table 43.1 AcrySof Toric IOL Models T3 to T9 (**Fig. 43.4b**)

Model	Cylinder Power (D) at IOL Plane	Cylinder Power (D) at Corneal Plane
SN6AT3	1.50	1.03
SN6AT4	2.25	1.55
SN6AT5	3.00	2.06
SN6AT6	3.75	2.57
SN6AT7	4.50	3.08
SN6AT8	5.25	3.60
SN6AT9	6.00	4.11

Toric Intraocular Lenses

Toric IOL calculators are available online and are specific to the toric IOL that is being placed. Examples are the online calculator for the Alcon AcrySof toric IOL (acrysoftoric.com), for the AMO Technis toric IOL (tecnistoriccalconline.com), and for the Bausch and Lomb Trulign toric IOL (truligntoric.com). Recently, Warren Hill has promoted the Barrett toric calculator as the most accurate for both toric positioning and power. Its formula takes into account the variable effective lens position, the IOL power, and the posterior cornea. The formula is available on the American Society of Cataract and Refractive Surgery (ASCRS) Web site. When using this formula, Hill makes a point of recommending that, for best results, use a less sensitive centroid surgically induced astigmatism (SIA) value, such as 0.12 D for a 2.4-mm clear corneal incision[12] (see Chapter 43).

Prior to surgery, the patient's information is inputted into the calculator, including patient name, right or left eye, keratometry data, IOL spherical power calculated using the surgeon's preferred method, surgically induced cylinder, and axis of incision location. The calculator then determines the correct toric IOL model, optimal axis orientation in the capsular bag, and expected residual astigmatism. Recent studies have shown that posterior corneal curvature should be taken into consideration and the toric power adjusted accordingly.[2]

In patients who have with-the-rule astigmatism, the toric power should be decreased by 0.50 to 0.60 D, and in patients who have against-the-rule astigmatism, the toric power should be increased by 0.20 to 0.30 D[2] (**Tables 43.1** and **43.2**). Ideally,

surgeons should review the outcomes of their previous cases, comparing the preoperative keratometric measurements with the postoperative readings.

It is important to bring the toric IOL calculator results to the operating room and place the printout in a location that is easily visible to the surgeon. This eliminates confusion regarding the location of the steep axis and the desired location of the toric IOL. A fine-tipped marking pen should be used to mark the steep axis after the limbus is thoroughly dried to create the thinnest possible discreet mark. In addition, the introduction of the astigmatic guidance systems, such as the VERION system, can be particularly useful to help correctly identify the steep axis, control for intraoperative cyclotorsion, and enable proper IOL placement. After the IOL is placed, intraoperative aberrometry systems such as the ORA™ (Optiwave Refractive Analysis) system with VerifEye™ (Alcon) can facilitate verification of the refractive effect of the lens implant and adjustment of the IOL axis to minimize astigmatism.

When using toric IOLs, cataract surgery is performed in the routine fashion with a standard capsulorrhexis, hydrodissection, and phacoemulsification; however, it is crucial to place the cataract incision at the precisely marked location. The incision can be made superior or temporal depending on surgeon preference, and this is taken into account with the preoperative planning in the online toric calculator. An ideal capsulorrhexis size is 5 to 5.5 mm to allow for overlap of the toric IOL optic, which ensures toric stability. If the integrity of the capsulorrhexis is compromised, a single-piece toric IOL cannot be used and instead a three-piece monofocal IOL is placed in the sulcus and optic captured, instead of a one-piece toric IOL. The astigmatism, in the presence of a ruptured capsule and nonastigmatic IOL, can be treated at the end of the procedure, when the eye is normally pressurized,

Table 43.2 Tecnis Toric One-Piece IOLs, IOL Center (**Fig. 43.4c**)

IOL Model	Cylinder Power		Correction Ranges Based on Combined Corneal Astigmatism (Preoperative Kcyl + Surgically Induced Astigmatism) Kcyl = Corneal Cylinder
	IOL Plane	Corneal Plane	
ZCT150	1.50	1.03	0.75–1.50 D
ZCT225	2.25	1.55	1.50–2.00 D
ZCT300	3.00	2.06	2.00–2.75 D
ZCT400	4.00	2.74	2.75–3.62 D

with an PCRI. After the removal of the nucleus and cortex, a cohesive viscoelastic is used to fill the capsular bag, and the IOL is inserted. As the lens begins to unfold, it is important to achieve gross alignment of the lens with the lens ~ 10 degrees counterclockwise to the final position. As the viscoelastic is removed, stabilize the lens with a soft-tipped irrigation and aspiration (I/A) handpiece or with a second instrument to avoid lens rotation. Residual viscoelastic, especially behind the lens, can cause the lens to rotate postoperatively and must be diligently removed. Utilizing a cohesive ophthalmic viscosurgical device (OVD), such as Healon GV (AMO), makes complete elimination of OVD considerably easier and ensures that all OVD behind the bag is eliminated. After complete removal of the viscoelastic and stromal hydration of the wounds, it is important to ensure that the lens is centered on the pupil and that the IOL is rotated until the toric hash marks are perfectly aligned with the marking of the steep axis at the limbus. When the anterior chamber is replenished with balanced salt solution (BSS), the final IOP should be between 10 and 15 mm Hg so that the eye is soft. This promotes more contact of the IOL and the posterior capsule, helping to reduce the risk of IOL rotation. At this time, if using intraoperative aberrometry, the toric alignment can be adjusted accordingly to the overlay-axis markings.

Peripheral Corneal Relaxing Incisions and Toric Intraocular Lenses

There are certain clinical scenarios in which the amount of astigmatism cannot be corrected simply with a toric IOL or a PCRI alone. For example, when the amount of corneal astigmatism is > 4.11 D, a combination of a toric IOL and PCRIs should be considered. For these patients, the preoperative calculations are performed using the online toric calculator, and the residual amount of astigmatism is entered into the PCRI calculator. The PCRIs should be completed prior to the cataract surgery, taking into account the placement of the cataract incisions. This combination method can potentially correct eyes with high astigmatism > 5.00 D without causing corneal irregularities.[7]

Postoperative Results and Complications

Limbal Relaxing Incisions

With proper and meticulous technique, the desired astigmatic correction is excellent, with most patients having less than +0.50 D of astigmatism.[13] However, results can vary depending on the surgeon's technique, preoperative planning, and patient healing factors. The most important cause of undercorrection is poor surgical technique causing inadequate incision depth. Attention to the proper blade depth and knife angle can minimize this undercorrection.

Complications

Complications include overcorrection, undercorrection, perforation, wound leak, and infection. It is better to achieve an undercorrection than an overcorrection, as the creation of astigmatism with a flipped axis can be disconcerting to the patient.[11] Overcorrections should be corrected postoperatively with excimer laser refractive surgery rather than the use of additional PCRIs, as the addition of further incisions can weaken and destabilize the cornea. In contrast, undercorrection can be managed with either extension of the PCRI or with excimer laser refractive surgery.

Perforations can occur when the cornea is abnormally thin in the area of the relaxing incision secondary to scarring or dellen formation, which emphasizes the importance of careful preoperative examination of the peripheral cornea and accurate preoperative corneal pachymetry. Some surgeons advocate intraoperative pachymetry to help avoid perforations. Perforations can also occur if the diamond knife is not set at the expected depth due to a malfunction of the knife or a loosening of the blade in its epoxy. Lastly, leaking incisions can occur when the phaco incision is coincident with the PCRI, and the phaco incision becomes stretched during the course of the procedure. Crossing the paracentesis with a PCRI can also produce wound leaks. Perforations leading to a significant wound leak should be addressed intraoperatively with the placement of corneal sutures. These can be removed 1 to 4 weeks postoperatively depending on their effect in the induction of astigmatism. Postoperative wound leaks can also be addressed with the placement of bandage contact lenses. To decrease the risk of infection, patients should be placed on postoperative topical antibiotics.

Toric Intraocular Lenses

In toric IOL patients, the desired postoperative correction is excellent, with most patients having less than +0.75 D of astigmatism.[14] However, results can vary depending on preoperative planning, intraoperative toric IOL alignment, and postoperative IOL rotation.

Complications

Complications include overcorrection or undercorrection of corneal astigmatism, improper lens orientation, lens rotation or tilt, and lens power miscalculations. Intraoperatively, if the toric IOL rotates off the desired axis, the intracapsular bag can be reinflated with viscoelastic and the IOL can be repositioned in a clockwise fashion to achieve final alignment. Once the lens is on axis at the end of surgery, it does not generally rotate postoperatively. However, if a patient has a significant postoperative astigmatic refractive error, the eye should be dilated and the position of the IOL examined. Careful attention should be paid to the exact position of the IOL axis. Assessment of the postoperative axis can be made at the slit lamp with the aid of smart phone applications such as I-Handy level and Axis Assistant to assess the exact IOL alignment. In addition, online Web sites such as astigmatismfix.com and smart phone applications such as Eye Vectors are available to aid in appropriate postoperative management and possible realignment of the toric IOL.

Realigning and repositioning a toric IOL postoperatively requires a return to the operating room. This can be done easily within the first 2 weeks, as the capsular bag has not formed a bioadhesive bond with the posterior capsule. The eye is entered through the same wounds, a dispersive viscoelastic is inserted to protect the cornea, the anterior capsule is lifted off the IOL with a needle or a viscoelastic cannula, a cohesive viscoelastic is inserted into the intracapsular bag, and the lens is rotated clockwise to prevent tearing of the posterior capsular bag.[15] Care should be taken to fully release the terminal bulbs at the end of the IOL haptics before rotating. The use of intraoperative guidance with wavefront aberrometry such as the ORA is very useful in ensuring proper IOL alignment and minimizing postoperative astigmatic refractive error. In general, the newer generation acrylic one-piece IOLs have improved rotational stability and have yielded excellent results in patients who desire spectacle independence.

If the IOL rotated a second time after repositioning it, is necessary to consider reverse optic fixation to hold the IOL in position. In this situation, once the IOL is mobilized in an OVD-supported anterior chamber, it is positioned at the selected axis. The optic is then elevated above the anterior capsule and captured, anterior to the anterior capsule, with the haptics in the capsular bag. This secures the IOL at the desired axis and prevent rotation.[16]

Conclusion

Today's cataract surgeons have excellent options for the correction of astigmatism with PCRIs and toric IOLs. The further advent of newer IOL designs, femtosecond corneal incisions, preoperative astigmatic guidance systems, and postoperative aberrometry will help to advance the accuracy of astigmatic management and provide even better outcomes for our patients.

References

1. Chang M, Kang SY, Kim HM. Which keratometer is most reliable for correcting astigmatism with toric intraocular lenses? Korean J Ophthalmol 2012;26:10–14

2. Koch DD, Jenkins RB, Weikert MP, Yeu E, Wang L. Correcting astigmatism with toric intraocular lenses: effect of posterior corneal astigmatism. J Cataract Refract Surg 2013;39:1803–1809

3. Ouchi M, Kinoshita S. Prospective randomized trial of limbal relaxing incisions combined with microincision cataract surgery. J Refract Surg 2010;26:594–599

4. Shimizu K, Misawa A, Suzuki Y. Toric intraocular lenses: correcting astigmatism while controlling axis shift. J Cataract Refract Surg 1994;20:523–526

5. Till JS, Yoder PR Jr, Wilcox TK, Spielman JL. Toric intraocular lens implantation: 100 consecutive cases. J Cataract Refract Surg 2002;28:295–301

6. Holland E, Lane S, Horn JD, Ernest P, Arleo R, Miller KM. The AcrySof toric intraocular lens in subjects with cataracts and corneal astigmatism: a randomized, subject-masked, parallel-group, 1-year study. Ophthalmology 2010;117:2104–2111

7. Gills Jp, Van der Karr M, Cherchio M. Combined toric intraocular lens implantation and relaxing incisions to reduce high preexisting astigmatism. J Cataract Refract Surg 2002;28:1585–1588

8. Cristóbal JA, del Buey MA, Ascaso FJ, Lanchares E, Calvo B, Doblaré M. Effect of limbal relaxing incisions during phacoemulsification surgery based on nomogram review and numerical simulation. Cornea 2009;28:1042–1049

9. Cleary C, Tang M, Ahmed H, Fox M, Huang D. Beveled femtosecond laser astigmatic keratotomy for the treatment of high astigmatism post-penetrating keratoplasty. Cornea 2012

10. Packer M. Effect of intraoperative aberrometry on the rate of postoperative enhancement: retrospective study. J Cataract Refract Surg 2010;36:747–755

11. Nichamin LD. Astigmatism control. Ophthalmol Clin North Am 2006;19:485–493

12. Hill WE. American Academy of Ophthalmology (AAO) Skills Transfer Course: Advanced Refractive Cataract Surgery and Anterior Segment Reconstruction, course number LEC 110. Using Toric IOLs: What You Need to Know. AAO, Las Vegas, November 15, 2015

13. Ganekal S, Dorairaj S, Jhanji V. Limbal relaxing incisions during phacoemulsification: 6-month results. J Cataract Refract Surg 2011;37:2081–2082

14. Hoffmann PC, Auel S, Hütz WW. Results of higher power toric intraocular lens implantation. J Cataract Refract Surg 2011;37:1411–1418

15. Chang DF. Repositioning technique and rate for toric intraocular lenses. J Cataract Refract Surg 2009;35:1315–1316

16. Gimbel HV, Amritanand A. Suture refixation and recentration of a subluxated capsular tension ring-capsular bag-intraocular lens complex. J Cataract Refract Surg 2013;39:1798–1802

44 Avoiding Unexpected Outcomes with Toric Intraocular Lenses

Graham D. Barrett

Our ability to provide excellent unaided acuity after cataract surgery improved dramatically with the introduction of toric intraocular lenses (IOLs). Nevertheless, despite accurate keratometry, precise alignment, and complex calculations, the refractive outcome after toric IOL implantation is not always predictable. Choosing the correct toric IOL for patients is challenging, as we have to consider the magnitude and axis of the toric cylinder required. To avoid unexpected astigmatic outcomes, we need to consider which devices should be used to measure the cornea, how to interpret the measurements, what methods to use to predict the required cylinder, and what techniques to use to accurately align the toric IOL axis.

Devices Used to Measure the Cornea

The first practical device able to measure the corneal curvature accurately was developed by Louis Emile Javal in the late 19th century. The optics were described initially by Helmholtz and even earlier by Ramsden. Essentially if the size of an object reflected in the cornea is known and the image size can be measured, the radius of curvature of the anterior cornea can be accurately determined.

Today we have many different devices capable of measuring the corneal curvature. These include manual keratometers, optical biometers, and topographers based on placido videokeratography or Scheimpflug imaging devices.

Interpreting Measurements from Multiple Devices

The challenge we face is that different devices can provide different measurements for the same patient. The best way to understand the utility of multiple devices is to embrace the concept of primary and secondary instruments introduced by Warren Hill,[1] who used the analogy of a pilot selecting an altitude indicator to determine his orientation but due to the critical nature of the activity always considers secondary instruments to confirm or validate the primary instrument. Predicting residual astigmatism for a specific patient is critical to the outcome, and so we should use these same principles.

My personal practice is to use three different devices: an optical biometer, a topographer, and a manual keratometer. I rely on the optical biometer as my primary instrument for the magnitude and axis of astigmatism but use the Javal type kerometer (Gm 300; CSO, Milan, Italy) and Pentacam (Oculus, Optikgeräte, Arlington, WA) to confirm the Lenstar (Haag-Streit, Mason, OH) or IOL Master (Carl Zeiss Meditec, Jena, Germany) measurement.

If they do not correspond, then the correct measurement is located somewhere within the triangle of agreement. It is feasible to combine the results of different devices mathematically, and I have been able to demonstrate that the mean or median of the measurements from multiple devices does improve the prediction of residual astigmatism compared with a single device. The one scenario in which I do consider the cylinder in the patient's spectacle correction is when all devices provide different values.

Methods to Predict the Required Cylinder

The predicted residual astigmatism (predRA) is the sum of the predicted corneal vector of the toric IOL cylinder plus the corneal astigmatism obtained from our keratometer and method of prediction.

The predRA is in error when it differs from the actual refraction. This can be expressed as a median value or the percentage of cases with an error of predRA less than 0.5 D. Even more informative, however, is the centroid value, which is the mean or median vector value reflecting both the axis as well as the magnitude of the error.

Louis Émile Javal, the noted 19th century ophthalmologist, acknowledged that he could not account for total ocular astigmatism by simply measuring the power of the anterior cornea. This phenomenon is known as Javal's rule and is thought to be due to the posterior cornea contributing on average 0.5 D against the rule astigmatism.

Doug Koch, in his Innovators Lecture in 2012, noted that posterior corneal astigmatism increased with increasing amounts of with-the-rule (WTR) astigmatism but showed no relationship with against-the-rule (ATR) astigmatism measured from the anterior corneal surface. Ignoring the posterior cornea results in an overcorrection of ~ 0.5 D in patients with WTR astigmatism and an undercorrection of ~ 0.3 D in patients presenting with ATR astigmatism. Commonly used methods to account for the contribution of the posterior cornea include a nomogram introduced by Doug Koch and Li Wang or actually measuring the posterior corneal radius with a Scheimpflug device such as the Pentacam or Galilei instruments (Ziemer, Port, Switzerland; Alton, IL).[2–4]

There are several different calculators available. The Alcon (Fort Worth, TX) calculator uses a fixed ratio in calculating the corneal vector of the cylinder power of the toric IOL. This can be adjusted for the posterior cornea using the Baylor nomogram. The Holladay Calculator (Holladay Consulting, Bellaire, TX) uses the effective lens position (ELP) to calculate the corneal vector of the toric IOL and can be adjusted by the Baylor nomogram or direct measurements of the posterior cornea. The alternative is to go online to the Asia-Pacific Association of Cataract and

Refractive Surgeon (APACRS) or American Society of Cataract and Refractive Surgery (ASCRS) Web sites and use the Barrett Toric Calculator that I developed, which is also available on the Lenstar.

The Barrett Toric Calculator uses the Universal II formula to predict the required spherical equivalent IOL power. The calculator derives the posterior corneal curvature based on a theoretical model proposed to explain the behavior of the posterior cornea. The toric IOL cylinder power required to correct the corneal astigmatism, including the posterior corneal astigmatism, is calculated from the predicted effective lens position using vector math for each eye. In a study conducted at the Ein-Tal Eye Center (Tel Aviv, Israel), the most accurate prediction of residual astigmatism was achieved with the Barrett Toric Calculator in combination with the Lenstar.

In a subsequent study that I performed with Adi Abulafia in Perth, Australia, we analyzed the outcome in 54 eyes that had a toric IOL implanted. We compared the results using preoperative versus postoperative keratometry K value, the intended versus the actual axis of alignment, and different calculators to identify the relative contribution of each of these factors to the errors in predicted residual astigmatism.

The results of the study demonstrate that errors in estimating surgically induced astigmatism (SIA) adversely impact the predictably of toric outcomes, and utilizing the centroid value for SIA offers significant improvement. Similarly eliminating errors in axis alignment offers further improvement but the impact is less.

The most important benefit, however, that can be obtained in improving toric outcomes is to use an improved calculator.

A double angle plot of the x and y values for each vector demonstrates that the Alcon and Holladay calculators result in significant unintended ATR astigmatism. Adjusting the measured K's with the Baylor nomogram improved the percentage of cases with an error in predRA within 0.5 D to 50%, as did utilizing the Pentacam 4.5 mm *equivalent K-reading* (EKR) value. Both these modifications, however, proved to be less accurate than the Barrett Toric Calculator, with which 70.4% of cases had an error in predRA within 0.5 D and these differences were statistically significant (**Fig. 44.1**).

Techniques to Accurately Align the Toric IOL Axis

An error in alignment of 1 degree reduces the effective correction of a toric IOL by an estimated 3%. Although clinically the impact of misalignment appears to be less than not taking into account factors such a posterior corneal astigmatism there are several techniques that can be considered to improve alignment.

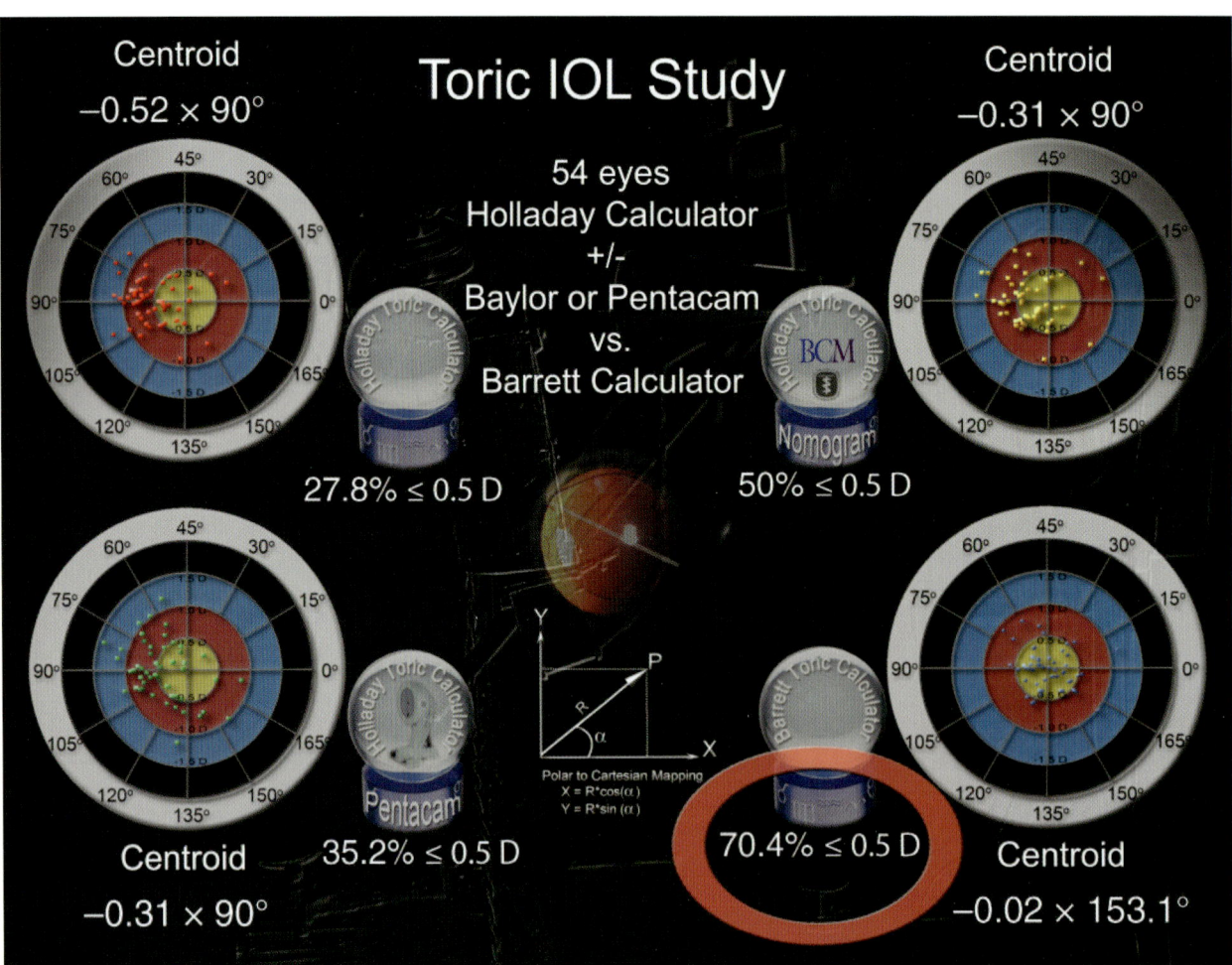

Fig. 44.1 Toric Intraocular Lens (IOL) Study Summary of the Holladay Calculator ± Baylor or Pentacam versus Barrett Calculator.

First I dry the limbus with a spear to prevent smearing and mark the limbus at what I perceive to be 180 degrees. I then use my ToriCAM App to align the red reference axis indicator with the limbal marks and press the camera button to capture an image. The images are stored in the ToriCAM in the photo album of your iPhone, along with a record of the reference axis, patient name, and date and time of the image. I then set the desired Toric axis on my marker and offset the reference axis accordingly. A custom toric marker specifically for the ToriCAM App is available, which enables the surgeon to set the reference axis as indicated by the app independently from the toric axis recommended by the toric calculator. Applying the inked marker then provides accurate marks with which the toric IOL is aligned after inserting the IOL. My personal preference is to maintain the posterior pressure on the IOL with a coaxial irrigation and aspiration (I/A) cannula while removing the viscoelastic. I do not find it necessary to go behind the IOL to remove the viscoelastic, but many surgeons do so, particularly with bimanual I/A, and then position the IOL correctly while maintaining fluid infusion.

I analyzed the difference in axis indicated by the ToriCAM App from the intended reference axis in 45 consecutive eyes and found a mean error of 3.5 degrees, indicating that overall simply eyeballing the horizontal axis is reasonably accurate, but for patients with errors up to 7 degrees using the app would certainly improve the refractive outcome.

Avoiding unexpected outcomes with toric IOLs is as important as selecting the appropriate spherical IOL power. Understanding the source of potential errors during measurement, prediction, and alignment with careful attention to each step in the process can minimize the likelihood of an unexpected astigmatic result.

References

1. Hill WE. American Academy of Ophthalmology (AAO) Skills Transfer Course: Advanced Refractive Cataract Surgery and Anterior Segment Reconstruction, course number LEC 110. Using Toric IOLs: What You Need to Know. AAO, Las Vegas, November 15, 2015

2. Koch DD, Ali SF, Weikert MP, Shirayama M, Jenkins R, Wang L. Contribution of posterior corneal astigmatism to total corneal astigmatism. J Cataract Refract Surg 2012;38:2080–2087

3. Zhang L, Sy ME, Mai H, Yu F, Hamilton DR. Effect of posterior corneal astigmatism on refractive outcomes after toric intraocular lens implantation. J Cataract Refract Surg 2015;41:84–89

4. Wang L, Shirayama M, Ma XJ, Kohnen T, Koch DD. Optimizing intraocular lens power calculations in eyes with axial lengths above 25.0 mm. J Cataract Refract Surg 2011;37:2018–2027

5. Adi Abulafia, Douglas D. Koch, Li Wang, Warren E. Hill, Ehud I. Assia, Maria Franchina, Graham D. Barrett. J Cataract Refract Surg 2016;42:663–671.

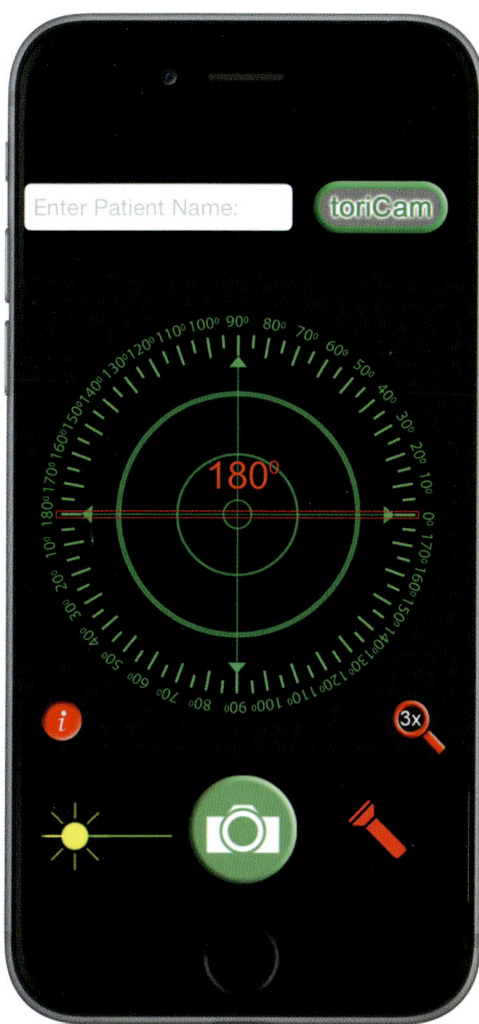

Fig. 44.2   Illustration of the ToriCAM System.

Today we have sophisticated systems to help minimize errors in alignment of the toric IOL on the required axis. These include intraoperative determination of the axis with wavefront devices or image-guided systems.

Personally I use the ToriCAM System I have developed, which is simple to use but very accurate (**Fig. 44.2**).

45 Crystalens/Trulign Intraocular Lenses

Mitchell A. Jackson

We are fortunate to have several options in presbyopia-correcting intraocular lenses (IOLs) to offer our cataract patients. These fundamentally different lens designs give us an opportunity to tailor the implant to each patient's needs and lifestyle, especially as we pursue the ideal of an emmetropic outcome. But being able to recommend the best choice for each patient also requires a thorough knowledge of the strengths and weaknesses of these lens technologies so that we can manage patients' expectations appropriately. Having had extensive experience with both multifocal and accommodating lens designs, I have found that the latter design provides the range and quality of vision that more of my patients hope to achieve following surgery, with fewer of the complaints commonly associated with multifocal IOLs. Since the United States Food and Drug Administration's (FDA) approval of the Crystalens (Bausch and Lomb, Rochester, NY) in 2003, many changes have occurred to the original model AT-45 platform including the introduction of the toric version known as Trulign (Bausch and Lomb). This chapter reviews the FDA approvals for both Crystalens and Trulign, the Centers for Medicare and Medicaid Services (CMS) ruling on presbyopia-correcting IOLs, the design evolution of the Crystalens, patients' preoperative expectations with this technology, intraoperative and postoperative tips to optimize visual outcomes, and management of adverse events or complications, including yttrium-aluminum-garnet (YAG) laser approaches to treat and prevent Z syndrome/capsular contraction syndrome.

Food and Drug Administration Approval of Crystalens/Trulign

There is only one FDA-approved accommodating IOL available to U.S. surgeons (as of September 2015)—the Crystalens family of IOLs including the most current Crystalens Advanced Optics (AO) and the Trulign Toric (**Figs. 45.1** and **45.2**). The Crystalens models AT50AO and AT52AO were approved in the United States in 2009, whereas the Trulign Toric was FDA-approved in 2013. Unlike multifocal IOL designs, the Crystalens lens platform is aspheric and aberration-free and has uniform center-to-edge power,[1,2] producing a more natural range of vision through physical accommodation in the eye (forward movement),[3] and typically requires less neuroadaptation than multifocals. The optic design also enables the lens to use 100% of available light regardless of pupil size or lens centration for enhanced contrast sensitivity.[4]

Robert Ang's[4] prospective randomized subject-masked 6-month study, as presented at the European Society of Cataract and Refractive Surgeons (ESCRS) 2011 meeting compared the contrast sensitivity among three FDA-approved lenses: the Crystalens AT50AO, the Acrysof ReStor 3.0 (Alco, Fort Worth, TX), and the Tecnis ZMB00 (Abbott Medical Optics, Abbott Park, IL). The Crystalens AT50AO demonstrated statistically significant improved binocular mesopic contrast sensitivity without glare compared with the two multifocal IOLs at both 1.5 cycles/degree and 3.0 cycles/degree spatial frequencies. In binocular low-contrast uncorrected distance visual acuity (UDVA),[4] Crystalens was statistically better than Tecnis ZMB00 (+4.00 add); in binocular cumulative low- and high-contrast uncorrected intermediate visual acuity (UIVA), Crystalens statistically outperformed both multifocals. As for binocular cumulative low- and high-contrast uncorrected near visual acuity (UNVA), Crystalens was statistically similar to both multifocal designs. Because the Crystalens is an aspheric aberration-free optic design, it avoids any of the light-splitting disturbances seen with multifocal designs described above. The newer FDA-approved low add Acrysof Restor 2.5 and Tecnis ZKB00 and ZLB00 (+2.75 and +3.25, respectively) multifocal designs have improved contrast and glare complaints in low light conditions such as night driving compared with its predecessor designs but still have not reached mesopic contrast sensitivity levels seen with the Crystalens AO and Trulign platforms (**Fig. 45.3**).

One of the key clinical advantages of the Crystalens AO (AT50 and AT52) platform is its long-term refractive stability as published

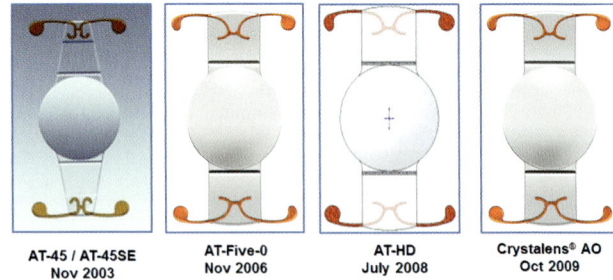

Fig. 45.1 Crystalens family of intraocular lenses (IOLs). (Courtesy of Bausch and Lomb.)

AT-45 / AT-45SE
Nov 2003

AT-Five-0
Nov 2006

AT-HD
July 2008

Crystalens® AO
Oct 2009

Built on an Innovative Platform

Fig. 45.2 Food and Drug Administration (FDA) approval dates for Crystalens/Trulign. (Courtesy of Bausch and Lomb.)

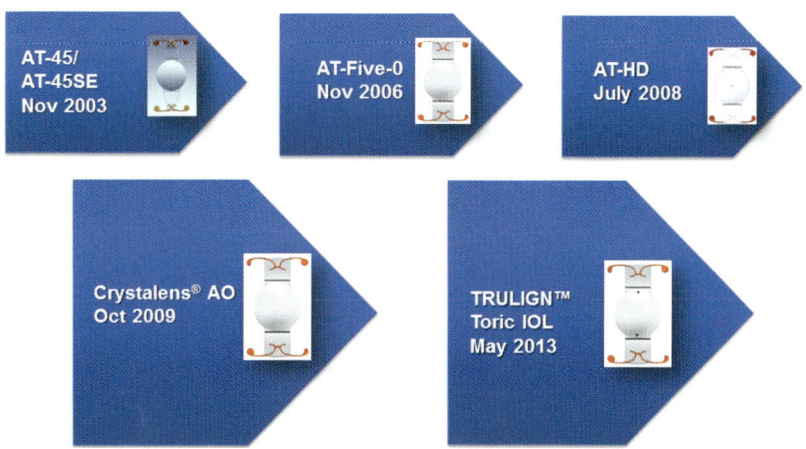

in 2011[5] and continues to date in 2015. Colvard[5] found that binocular UDVA was sustained over 7 years such that 96% of the 24 patients seen this far out retained 20/40 or better UDVA and 75% retained 20/20 or better. Binocular UIVA was also sustained and even improved from year 1 out to 7 years, such that 100% of the 24 patients saw 20/40 or better and 83% saw 20/20 or better.

Both the Crystalens AT50AO and Crystalens AT52AO IOLs have a central prolate anterior and posterior aspheric aberration-free 5.0-mm BioSil silicone elastomer optic body with index of refraction of 1.43 (35°C), an equiconvex shape, a 360-degree square edge to reduce posterior capsular opacification (PCO), rectangular hinged haptics to increase forward translation, a plate haptic diameter of 10.5 mm, and round-to-the-right asymmetric polyimide loops ("knobs"), the latter designed to prevent inadvertent upside down implantation intraoperatively (**Figs.**

45.1 and **45.4**). The overall diameter of the Crystalens AT50 AO and Trulign Toric BL1UT is 11.5 mm, and the Crystalens AT52AO is 12.0 mm in length, the latter designed to be placed in eyes with axial lengths > 25 mm and maintain improved effective lens position (ELP) per FDA labeling. The FDA-approved IOL powers for the Crystalens AT50 AO range from +17 to +33 D (in 0.5-D increments) and +18 to +22 D (in 0.25-D increments) and for the Crystalens AT52AO range from +4 to +9 D (in 1.0-D increments) and +10 to +24 D (in 0.5-D increments) (**Fig. 45.2**). **Table 45.1** summarizes the Crystalens platforms approved since 2003; the Crystalens models AT50AO and AT52AO are the most commonly used designs as of 2015.[6]

The FDA-approved model BL1UT Trulign Toric IOL has a central anterior aspheric axis mark just inside the haptic junction and a posterior aspheric toric aberration-free 5.0-mm BioSil optic

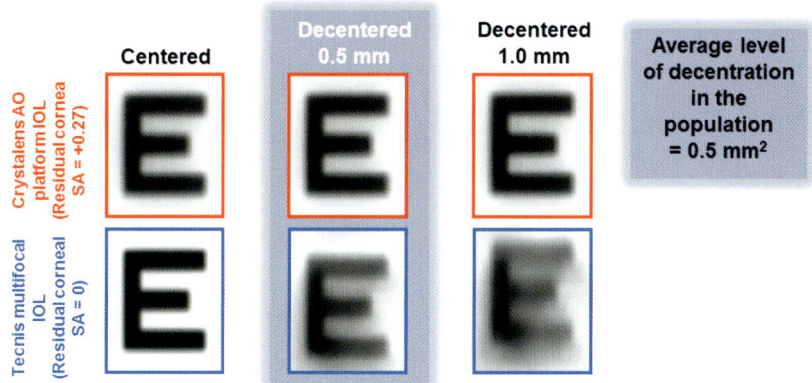

20/20 Letter E, 4-mm Pupil.

Fig. 45.3 Due to the aspheric aberration-free optic of Crystalens, there is significantly decreased aberration with IOL decentration.[1]

Crystalens AT50AO & AT52AO

Trulign BL1UT

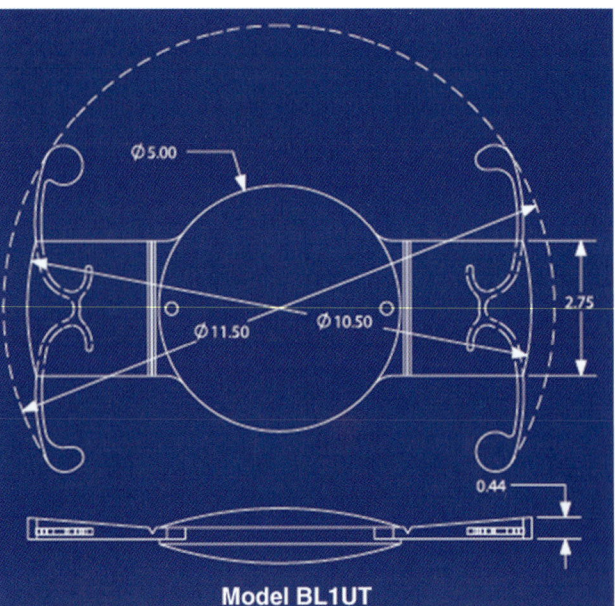

Fig. 45.4 Crystalens models AT50AO and AT52AO and Trulign model BL1UT: design elements.

body, with index of refraction of 1.43 (35°C), an equiconvex shape, a 360-degree square edge, rectangular hinged haptics with a plate haptic diameter of 10.5 mm, and round-to-the-right polyimide loops similar to those in the Crystalens AO designs (**Figs. 45.2** and **45.4**). The BL1UT comes in three FDA-approved IOL labeled cylindrical powers of 1.25, 2.00, and 2.75 D that correlate to a corneal cylindrical correction of 0.83, 1.33, and 1.83 D, respectively. The FDA-approved powers for all three cylindrical designs are +4 to +10 D spherical equivalent (SE) (in 1.0-D increments) and +10.5 to +33 D SE (in 0.5-D increments).

The original FDA labeling for each of the two platforms (Crystalens and Trulign) enables near, intermediate, and distance vision without spectacles. The Crystalens is intended for primary implantation in the capsular bag of the eye for the visual correction of aphakia secondary to the removal of a cataractous lens in adult patients with and without presbyopia. The Crystalens provides approximately 1 D of monocular accommodation, which enables near, intermediate, and distance vision without spectacles.[7] The Trulign Toric posterior chamber IOL is intended for primary implantation in the capsular bag of the eye for the visual correction of aphakia and postoperative refractive astigmatism secondary to removal of a cataractous lens in adult patients with or without presbyopia who desire reduction of residual refractive cylinder with increased spectacle independence and improved uncorrected near, intermediate, and distance vision. The original FDA pivotal clinical trial based on the Crystalens model AT-45 paved the way for all future platforms. In this trial prior to 2003 approval, 497 eyes of 324 patients had the AT-45 platform implanted, with a range of axial lengths of 21.0 to 26.6 mm and dioptric power range between 16.5 and 27.5 D. The clinical results were obtained using an A constant of 119.0, the SRK/T formula, and immersion biometry or interferometry and manual keratometry. In 124 bilaterally implanted patients, the proportion

of patients achieving uncorrected visual acuities of 20/32 (J2) or better at 1 year was 97.6% at distance, 100% at intermediate (80 cm), and 93.5% at near (40 cm). In 74 bilaterally implanted patients who were within ±0.5 D of plano in each eye, the proportion of patients achieving uncorrected visual acuities of 20/32 (J2) or better at 1 year was 100% at distance, 100% at intermediate (80 cm), and 97.3% at near (40 cm).

The pivotal clinical trial in the United States of the Trulign Toric IOL was conducted on 229 eyes of 229 patients, of which 227 eyes had it implanted. The dioptic power range was 16.0 to 27.0 D with cylindrical powers at the lens plane of 1.25, 2.00, and 2.75 D for the AT50T/AT52T. The Crystalens Accommodating IOL models AT50SE/AT52SE (nontoric optic) were used as the control IOLs. To facilitate toric IOL selection and axis placement, a proprietary Toric Calculator was used to determine the appropriate Trulign Toric IOL model and axis of placement for each eye (**Fig. 45.5**). The Trulign Toric IOL Calculator was used to calculate the predicted postoperative corneal astigmatism using preoperative keratometry, phaco/insertion incision location, and predicted magnitude of surgically induced astigmatism (SIA) inputs entered by the physician. The calculator accounted for SIA, incision location, and the patient's preoperative corneal astigmatism, and determined the toric IOL cylinder power needed and placement orientation to best correct the patient's predicted postoperative corneal astigmatism. In the trial, all cataract incisions were placed on the preoperative keratometric steep axis and a fixed SIA value of 0.50 D was used in the Trulign Toric IOL Calculator for all study subjects. The results achieved by 227 patients followed postoperatively for 6 months provide data to support the conclusion that eyes implanted with a Trulign Toric IOL following cataract extraction achieved visual correction of aphakia and astigmatism. The data also support a percent reduction in absolute cylinder, cylinder correction accuracy, rotational

Table 45.1 Crystalens and Trulign Intraocular Lenses: Power

Model	Crystalens AT-45	Crystalens AT50SE	Crystalens AT52SE	Crystalens HD500	Crystalens HD520	Crystalens AT50AO	Crystalens AT52AO	Trulign Toric BL1UT
Complete power range	10.0–27.0 D	4.0–33.0 D		10.0–33.0 D		4.0–33.0 D		10.0–33.0 D
Power	10.0–27.0 D in 0.5-D increments	17.0–26.75 D in 0.25-D increments; 27.0–33.0 D in 0.5-D increments	4.0–9.0 D in 1-D increments; 10.0–16.0 D in 0.5-D increments; 16.25–16.75 D in 0.25-D increments	17.0–18.0 D in 0.5-D increments; 18.0–22.75 D in 0.25-D increments; 23.0–33.0 D in 0.5-D increments	10.0–16.5 D in 0.5-D increments	17.0–33.0 D in 0.5-D increments; 18.0–22.0 D in 0.25-D increments	4.0–9.0 D in 1-D increments; 10.0–24.0 D in 0.5-D increments	10.0–33.0 D in 0.5-D increments; cylinder powers (corneal plane): 1.25, 2.00, 2.75 D
Length	11.5 mm	11.5 mm (17.0–33.0 D)	12.0 mm (4.0–16.75 D)	11.5 mm (17.0–33.0 D)	12.0 mm (10.0–16.5 D)	11.5 mm (17.0–33.0 D)	12.0 mm (4.0–24.0 D)	11.5 mm
Optic size	4.5 mm	5.0 mm	5.0 mm	5.0 mm	5.0 mm	5.0 mm	5.0 mm	5.0 mm
Shape	Biconvex	Biconvex	Biconvex	Biconvex	Biconvex	Biconvex	Biconvex	Aspheric (ant.)/toric (post.)

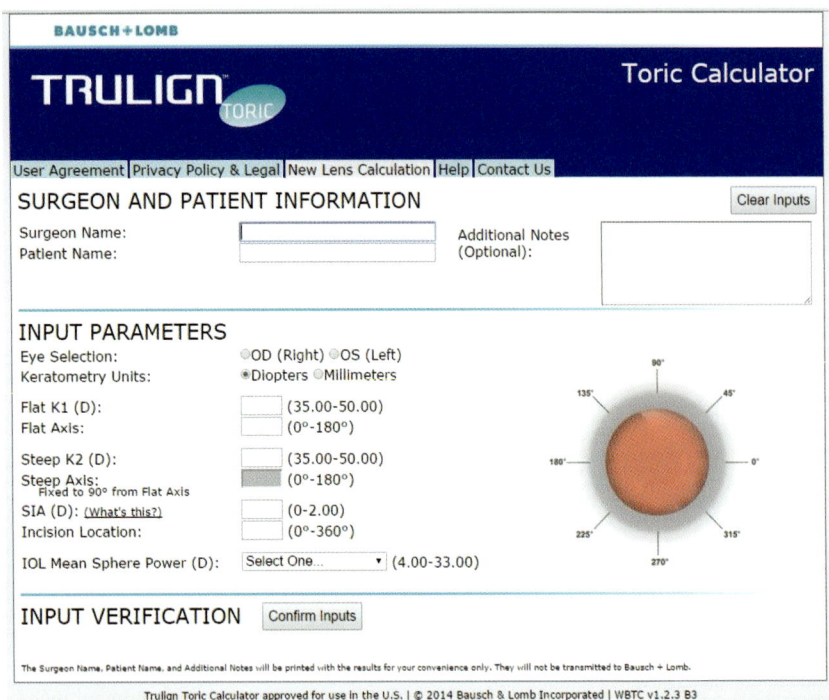

Fig. 45.5 Trulign Toric Calculator. (Courtesy of Bausch and Lomb.)

stability of the lens, and improvement of UDVA following implantation of Trulign Toric IOL (**Figs. 45.6, 45.7, 45.8, 45.9**). All three toric powers implanted cumulatively had a 78.4% cylinder correction accuracy within 0.5 D of intended target compared with 45.1% in the control group, and 95.5% were within 1.00 D of the intended target compared with 72.1% in the control group (**Fig. 45.6**).

The data in **Fig. 45.8** show quantitatively that the Trulign Toric IOL provides a range of vision from distance to intermediate, and at 6 months 97.8% of patients achieved at least 20/40 in both UDVA and UIVA, the latter measured at 32 inches. Rotational stability is vital in terms of final visual outcome with a toric IOL and even as little as a 4-degree misalignment or a cyclotorsion effect can cause a loss of 14% of the cylindrical correction effect,

Cylinder correction accuracy. Results at 4 to 6 months.

	Control IOL	Toric IOL 1.25 D	2.00 D	2.75 D	All Toric
Within 0.50 D of intended, %	44.1	79.7	79.5	71.4	**78.4**
Within 1.00 D of intended, %	72.1	96.0	92.3	100.0	**95.5**

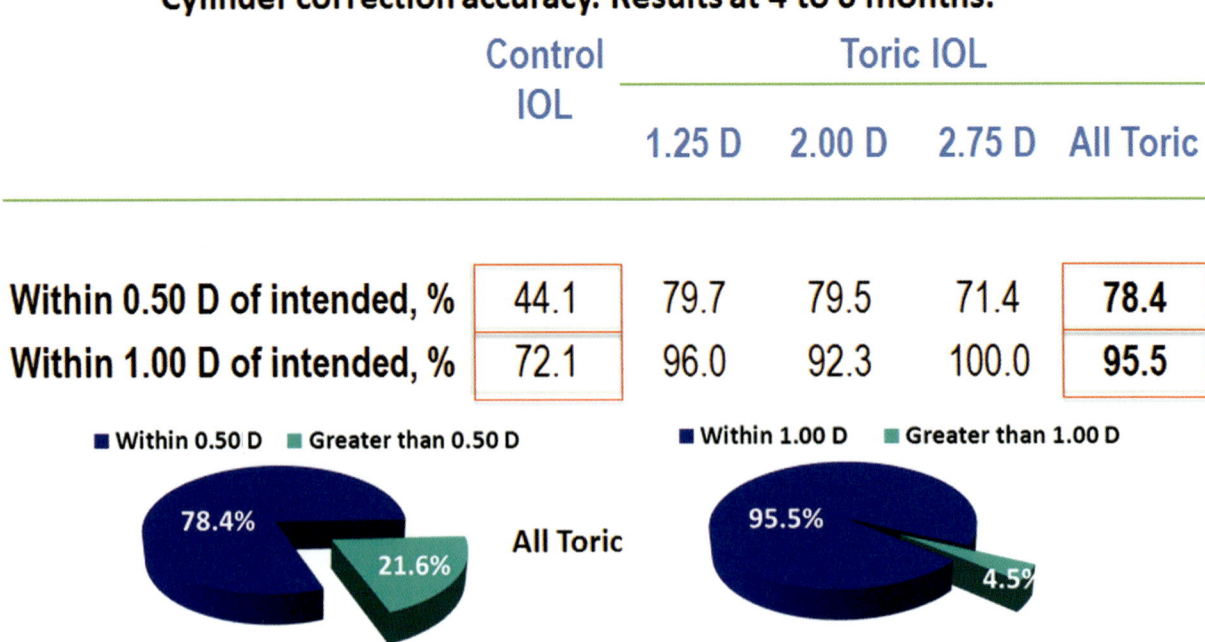

Fig. 45.6 Cylinder correction at 4 to 6 months. (Data from Bausch and Lomb's study 650.)

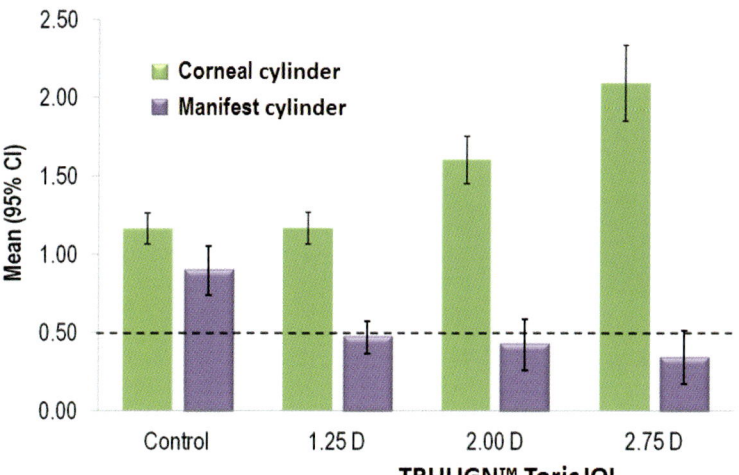

Fig. 45.7   Cylinder correction at 4 to 6 months, continued.

correlating to an approximate 3.3% decrease in cylinder correction per degree of rotation (**Fig. 45.10**). Looking at all toric cohorts at 4 to 6 months postoperatively, the mean rotation was less than 2 degrees, and 96.1% of all eyes had 5 degrees or less of rotation (**Fig. 45.10**). When comparing the pivotal trial data for Trulign Toric compared with the other two FDA-approved toric IOLs, Trulign achieved 96.1% rotational stability less than 5 degrees, whereas the Acrysof IQ monofocal toric achieved only 81.1% rotational stability less than 5 degrees, and the Tecnis monofocal toric achieved only 94.0% less than 5 degrees (**Fig. 45.11**). By far, the Trulign Toric definitely did not any show any noninferiority compared with its two toric IOL predecessors on the U.S. market.

Centers for Medicare and Medicaid Services Ruling on Presbyopia-Correcting IOL Implants

When the first-generation Crystalens AT-45 was approved by the FDA in 2003, there were no existing rules in the insurance process for patients to gain access to this technology. Initially, patients had to pay in full for all levels of service surrounding cataract surgery and placement of this first-of-a-kind presbyopia-correcting IOL in the United States. Payment was strictly a self-pay model, and included the professional fee, the facility fee, and the anesthesia fees, totaling $10,000 to $15,000 per eye depending on the location and facility involved. Not until May 3, 2005,

	Uncorrected Distance VA*	Uncorrected Intermediate VA*
≥ 20/25	72.4%	86.6%
≥ 20/32	86.6%	94.1%
≥ 20/40	97.8%	97.8%

*TRULIGN Toric IOL effectiveness cohort. Results at 4 to 6 months.

Fig. 45.8   Distance and intermediate visual acuity of 20/40 or better at 6 months. (Data from Bausch and Lomb's study 650.)

did CMS approve Ruling 05–01, which allowed patients to pay above and beyond as an out-of-pocket expense for cataract surgery with a presbyopia-correcting IOL in addition to what their insurance plan would cover for routine cataract surgery.[8] The rule specifically states that the beneficiary is responsible for the payment of facility charges for resources required for fitting and vision acuity testing of a presbyopia-correcting IOL that exceeds the facility charges for resources furnished for a conventional IOL following cataract surgery. The beneficiary is also responsible for payment of the charges for physician services that exceeds the physician charge for insertion of a conventional IOL following cataract surgery. This CMS ruling paved the way for all presbyopia-correcting IOLs, and as a result really expanded

Absolute rotation results at 4 to 6 months

	1.25 D	2.00 D	2.75 D	All Toric
≤ 5.00°, %	93.1	100	100	**96.1**
≤ 10.00°, %	98.6	100	100	**99.2**

- Mean IOL rotation < 2°
- **96.1% exhibited IOL rotational stability of ≤ 5°**

Fig. 45.9   Rotational Stability at 6 months. (Data from Bausch and Lomb's study 650.)

- 4°: ↓ 14%
- 10°: ↓ 34%
- 30°: No Δ
  - Axis shifts!
- If > 30°,
  ↑ astigmatism!

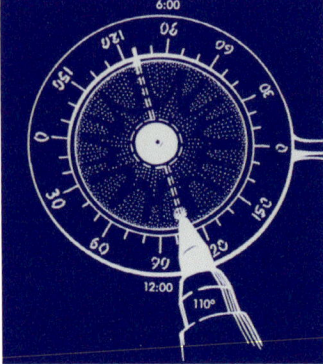

Fig. 45.10 Effects of misalignment/cyclotorsion.

the patient population that could potentially qualify for this technology.

Preoperative Patient Selection and Surgical Optimization

The largest group of patients who have readily purchased the presbyopia-correcting IOL option has historically been the baby boomers, which account for 78 million people in the United States born between 1946 and 1964.[9] In this baby boomer generation, 90% use computers, at least 66% text-message on their cell phones, and 72% plan to work after retirement age. The most important source of independence is the ability to maintain a driver's license to drive, and 82% of seniors drive on a daily basis.[10,11] Despite this vast group of potential presbyopia-correcting IOL candidates, patient selection is the key to optimal outcomes postoperatively. Patients should have the potential for good visual acuity in each eye postoperatively, have an understanding that corneal astigmatism must be corrected, have minimal ocular surface disease,[12] and have realistic expectations that in certain circumstances spectacles for near vision may be needed such as in restaurants with dim illumination and for the tiny print on medicine bottles.

The most important part of the preoperative process to achieve a successful outcome with either the Crystalens or Trulign platform is conducting a full range of comprehensive diagnostic testing. Corneal topography is performed to assess the preoperative magnitude and axis of corneal astigmatism, to rule out irregular astigmatism from keratoconus, pellucid marginal degeneration, or epithelial basement membrane disease (which could prevent future postoperative enhancement options if needed), and to measure posterior corneal astigmatism effect[13,14] to avoid over- or undercorrection of astigmatism if applicable. Optical coherence tomography (OCT) imaging of the macula to rule out epiretinal membrane and other macular pathology, which could prevent good visual outcome postoperatively, is critical as well. Past studies have found that a high angle kappa can have a negative impact on the final visual outcome in multifocal IOL technology, and measurement of the angle kappa preoperatively can help determine if a patient should have Crystalens/Trulign versus multifocal IOL technology.[15] Recently, light scattering has become an excellent means to differentiate corneal from lenticular pathology, and objective scatter index (OSI) scores have been highly correlated to the Lens Opacities Classification System III (LOCSIII)-accepted cataract grading scale.[16] Using OSI for tear film stability along with other point-of-care diagnostic ocular surface tests such as tear osmolarity, *matrix-metalloproteinase-9* (MMP-9) assay analysis (InflammaDry, Rapid Pathogen Screening, Sarasota, FL), and LipiView (TearScience, Morrisville, NC) with dynamic meibomian imaging (DMI) facilitates the need for ocular surface disease optimization prior to cataract surgery.[17]

The Prospective Health Assessment of Cataract Patients Ocular Surface (PHACO) study was paramount in demonstrating preoperatively that 87% of patients being worked up for cataract surgery are asymptomatic for dry eye but on exam 63% demonstrated a tear breakup time (TBUT) of under 5 seconds, and 77% had positive corneal staining, of which 50% was central in location.[12] Not only can a poor ocular surface have impact on vision quality postoperatively, it can have impact on keratometry and topography readings such that a wrong IOL power or cylinder axis treatment could occur. Proper ocular surface management preoperatively is paramount for achieving precise outcomes postoperatively. Lastly, proper IOL power calculation is essential for achieving the intended refractive target postoperatively. Adjustment for high axial length in axial myopia[18] and adjustment for post-refractive surgery using fourth-generation formulas, such as the Shammas and Haigis L formulas,[19-21] is critical to avoid hyperopic surprises in patients undergoing Crystalens/Trulign surgery. After performing the correct preoperative IOL calculations, the Crystalens/Trulign platforms perform best with a targeted blended vision ranging from plano to –0.25 D sphere in the distance eye and –0.25 D sphere to –0.50 D sphere in the near eye (**Fig. 45.12**). The Trulign Toric Calculator (**Fig. 45.5**) displays the array of visual outcomes based on the target selected

	Trulign® Toric IOL	AcrySof® IQ Toric (Monofocal Toric)	Tecnis® Toric IOL (Monofocal Toric)
Astigmatism correction	Yes	Yes	Yes
Intermediate -≥20/32	94.1%	NA	NA
Uncorrected distance visual acuity: eyes ≥20/40	97.8%	93.8%	97.0%
Rotational stability <5	96.1%	81.1%	94.0%

Fig. 45.11 Comparison of rotational stability.

Monocular Vision Chart				
Distance	**Intermediate**	**Near**	**Target Spherical Equivalent**	
20/60	20/20	J1+	−1.25	
20/50	20/20	J1+	−1.00	
20/40	20/20	J1+	−0.75	
20/30	20/20	J1	−0.50	Near eye
20/25	20/20	J2+	−0.25	Near and distance eye
20/20	20/20	J3	0.00	Distance eye
20/15–20	20/20	J3	+0.25	
20/20–30	20/25	J5	+0.50	

Note: If the results are different from the intended DVA or NVA, measure the patient's actual refraction.

Fig. 45.12 Target and outcome chart. DVA, distance visual acuity; NVA, near visual acuity.

preoperatively, with the dominant eye typically the distance eye and the nondominant eye typically the near eye. When planning surgery with the Trulign Toric, it is important to utilize the Trulign calculator to adjust for vector analysis from the main incision location, the SIA, and preoperative corneal astigmatism. Surgeon should know their own SIA (ideally for both the right and left eye), and this can easily be calculated at Web sites such as Warren Hill's www.sia-calculator.com.

Intraoperative Pearls and Optimization Techniques

With the recent approval of several femtosecond lasers for cataract surgery, tailoring the eye to meet the needs of the selected IOL preoperatively has improved immensely. Variance of capsulotomy size, reduced phacoemulsification times, reduced corneal endothelial trauma, and enhanced astigmatism management have brought cataract surgery to a level that meets the demands of premium IOLs such as the Crystalens and Trulign Toric. Specific intraoperative techniques critical to a successful Crystalens/Trulign Toric outcome first involves creating a symmetrical capsulorrhexis, preferably larger than the 5.0-mm optic size. With the utilization of the femtosecond laser to create near-perfect capsulotomies, there still remains debate as to what the exact capsulotomy/capsulorrhexis size should be; nevertheless, the capsulotomy should be large enough to allow free movement of the lens at the optic–hinge junction. Regarding the correction of astigmatism intraoperatively, the effectiveness of the Trulign Toric in reducing the visual effect of preoperative corneal astigmatism of less than 1.33 D has not been established per FDA labeling. In the lower levels of astigmatism management under 1.50 D of corneal cylinder, manual or femtosecond laser astigmatic incisions have a long history of being successful and less affected by the regression effect of wound healing and pose an excellent alternative when the Trulign Toric cannot be used or if the Crystalens 50AO/52AO is the IOL of choice. Higher levels of astigmatism can be managed with the Trulign Toric up to a level of ~ 2.00 D of corneal cylinder. If higher levels are needed, a combination of corneal astigmatic incisions with a Trulign Toric can be considered, or just proceeding with a monofocal toric approved for higher ranges of corneal astigmatism may offer the best option.

The Crystalens or Trulign Toric should never be placed into the capsular bag in the event of zonular compromise or a disrupted posterior capsule at the time of cataract surgery. Meticulous cortical cleanup and careful attention to polishing the anterior and posterior capsule is very important to minimize capsular contraction and PCO. The Crystalsert® IOL Delivery System (Bausch and Lomb) requires a 2.85-mm opening through the main incision for injection of either the Crystalens or Trulign Toric platforms. Use of a cohesive viscoelastic is recommended for lubrication in the injector, and it is important to verify that the IOL is right side up, determined by the round knob on the loop of the leading haptic being on the right ("round to the right"). Prevention of wound leak is important because if the IOL moves even slightly forward postoperatively, this will change the ELP and usually cause an unwanted myopic shift. Likewise, over-inflation of the capsular bag with balanced salt solution (BSS) at the end of the procedure could produce a hyperopic surprise postoperatively. Methods to prevent wound leak range from corneal suturing to the Wong hydration maneuver to using tissue glues such as the FDA approved ReSure sealant (Ocular Therapeutix, Bedford, MA).[22–24] Use of intraoperative aberrometry can be helpful in aphakic power selection for both the Crystalens and Trulign Toric, especially in eyes that have undergone prior refractive surgery. Pseudophakic axis verification with intraoperative aberrometry can also be helpful in the final positioning of the Trulign Toric as well. The use of a capsular tension ring (CTR) in the presence of the Crystalens and Trulign Toric has been controversial, but it has been reported anecdotally to reduce the risk of capsular contraction syndrome in patients with higher axial length. When deciding to place a CTR with either of the two platforms, it is recommended to place the CTR first into the capsular bag followed by injection the Crystalens or Trulign Toric. Placement of the CTR after IOL placement could cause IOL tilt or malposition.

Postoperative Pearls and Optimization

Postoperatively, several factors still are in play when trying to achieve the perfect outcome with Crystalens or Trulign Toric. Measuring and demonstrating UDVA, UIVA, and UNVA[25] OU for all three levels of vision is the best simulated way to show patients their final outcome in terms of visual function (patients typically function with both eyes being used together in real life). Measuring manifest refraction for each eye is important from the surgeon's perspective to determine, first, if the intended target was achieved, and second, if any induced astigmatism is developing as a consequence of capsular contraction syndrome. Maintenance of an optimized ocular surface is probably the most important factor in stabilizing vision and avoiding fluctuation in vision. A very low threshold should be maintained for deciding when to treat the ocular surface postoperatively. Some studies have suggested the use of prolonged topical steroids or nonsteroidal anti-inflammatory drug (NSAID) eyedrops to prevent capsular contraction syndrome and to prevent the development of cystoid macular edema (CME).[26] A refractive enhancement can be performed on a patient postoperatively if the patient demonstrates stable refraction, stable corneal topography, lack of macular pathology such as CME, and lack of capsular contraction syndrome. The decision to place corneal astigmatic incisions versus laser vision correction (photorefractive keratectomy [PRK], laser-assisted in situ keratomileusis [LASIK]) depends on the corneal topography appearance and refraction being treated.

When performing corneal astigmatic incisions, corneal coupling must be accounted for to avoid hyperopic surprises or myopic undercorrections. A YAG laser capsulotomy should be considered as well prior to performing refractive enhancements, as the effective lens position could shift post–YAG capsulotomy, thus altering the refraction to be treated by the intended enhancement method. Once the ideal intended refractive target is achieved, the ocular surface is optimized, and all other pathology is ruled out, patient satisfaction with the outcome can still, unfortunately, be poor. Word-finding puzzle books (originally created by Eyeonics, now part of Bausch and Lomb) have six levels of decreasing fonts so patients can help increase their accommodative function and neuroadaptation. The use of apps on cell phones and tablets, such as the Glasses Off App, can help patients self-motivate their near visual activity postoperatively. In the exam lane, keeping a pair of –2.50 D spherical glasses ("purple frame pair") and demonstrating to an unhappy patient what their uncorrected near visual acuity would have been with a monofocal IOL helps put in perspective how successfully the Crystalens or Trulign Toric is actually performing.

Capsular Contraction

The most cumbersome adverse event postoperatively with the Crystalens and Trulign Toric IOL platforms is capsular contraction.[27] Capsular contraction has a variety of etiologies, including lens capsule epithelial cell metaplasia, fibronectin, laminin, and inflammatory mediators or other unknown factors yet discovered. The primary mechanism of action is a decrease in capsular bag diameter, and it can present in many different scenarios. Anterior capsular contraction syndrome (ACCS) results in loss of accommodative amplitude and a hyperopic shift (**Fig. 45.13**) Posterior capsular contraction syndrome (PCCS) results in lens tilt, causing a myopic shift without induced astigmatism (**Fig. 45.14**) or in a Z-pattern causing a myopic shift frequently with induced astigmatism (**Figs. 45.15** and **45.16**). Equatorial capsular contraction syndrome (ECCS) in not usually a problem seen with Crystalens or Trulign Toric IOLs.

When treating PCO without capsular contraction, a central round posterior capsulotomy is recommended without extending the capsulotomy beyond the edge of the optic to prevent inadvertent vitreous prolapse into the anterior chamber. When treating ACCS, besides a central YAG posterior capsulotomy, described above, additional YAG pulses should be delivered 90 degrees away from the hinge–optic junctions (**Figs. 45.17** and **45.18**).[28,29] When treating PCCS with lens tilt alone, a central YAG capsulotomy should be performed with additional YAG pulses placed just outside the hinge–optic junction in the posterior capsule in the area of the vaulted hinge (**Fig. 45.19**).[28,29] When

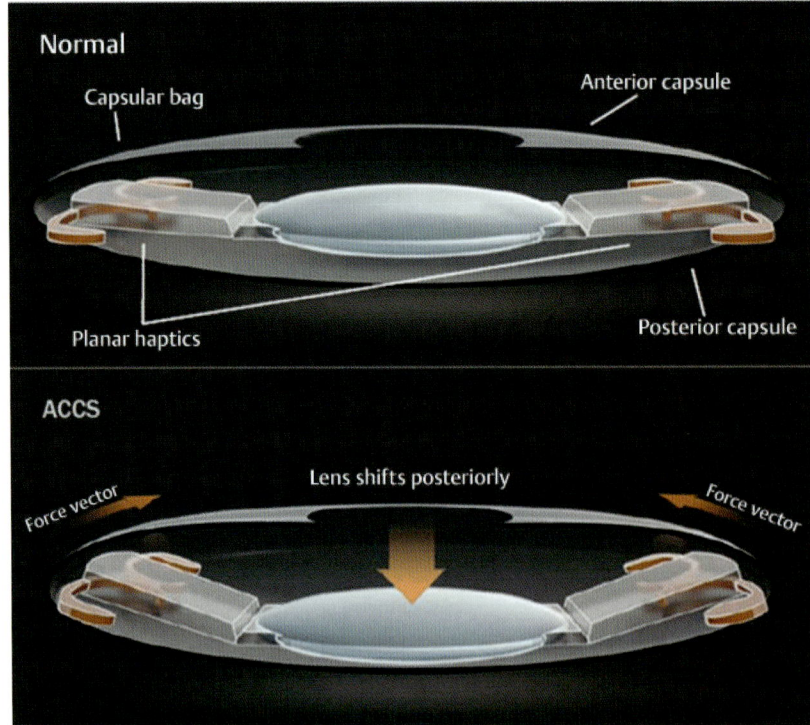

Fig. 45.13 Intraocular lens configuration of a normal lens position and an anterior capsular contraction syndrome (ACCS).

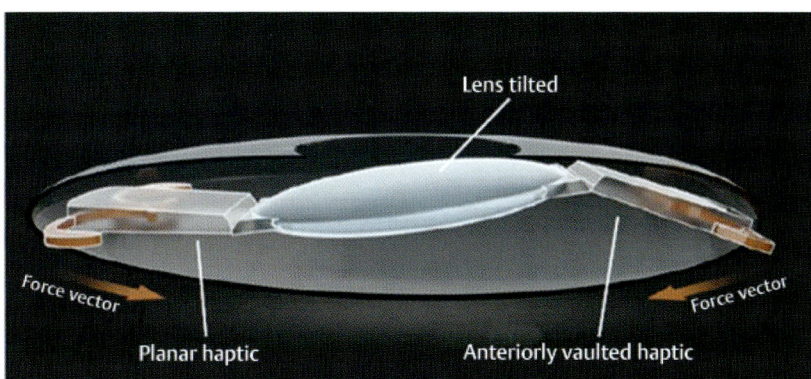

Fig. 45.14   Intraocular lens configuration of posterior capsular contraction syndrome (PCCS) with lens tilt.

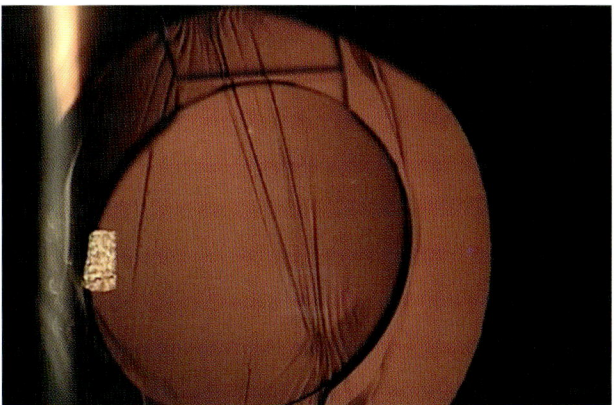

Fig. 45.15   Slit-lamp photo of PCCS with Z syndrome.

PCCS occurs as a Z-pattern, a central YAG round capsulotomy is performed along with additional YAG pulses in the posterior capsule behind both the anteriorly vaulted and posteriorly vaulted haptics (**Fig. 45.20**).[28,29] YAG laser selective capsulotomy as described can successfully resolve all capsular contraction syndromes successfully if diagnosed early enough. It is very important to see Crystalens or Trulign Toric patients at 1 month, 3 months, 6 months, 9 months, and 12 months until the YAG laser capsulotomy is performed to avoid any of the capsular contraction syndromes aforementioned. Although there have been trends of earlier capsular contraction post–femtosecond laser cataract surgery, there has not been enough evidence to prove a statistical correlation. But no matter whether manual phacoemulsification is performed with or without femtosecond laser assistance, close monitoring of capsular contraction is warranted to avoid a poor vision outcome.

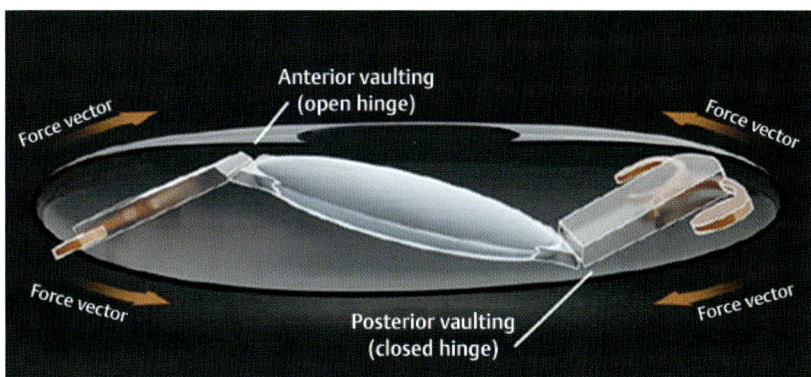

Fig. 45.16   Configuration of PCCS with Z syndrome.

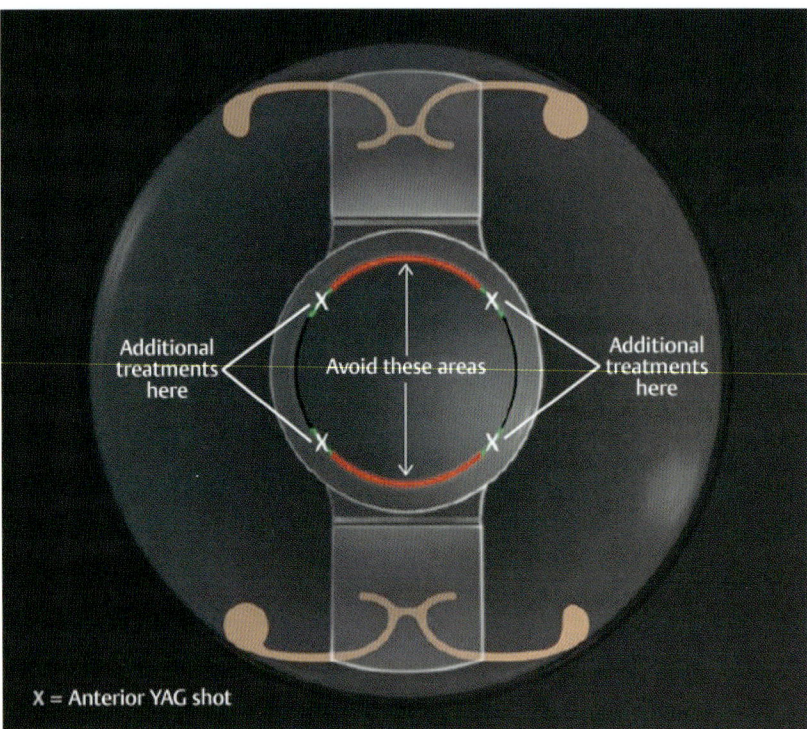

Fig. 45.17 Anterior capsular contraction syndrome: YAG treatment pattern.

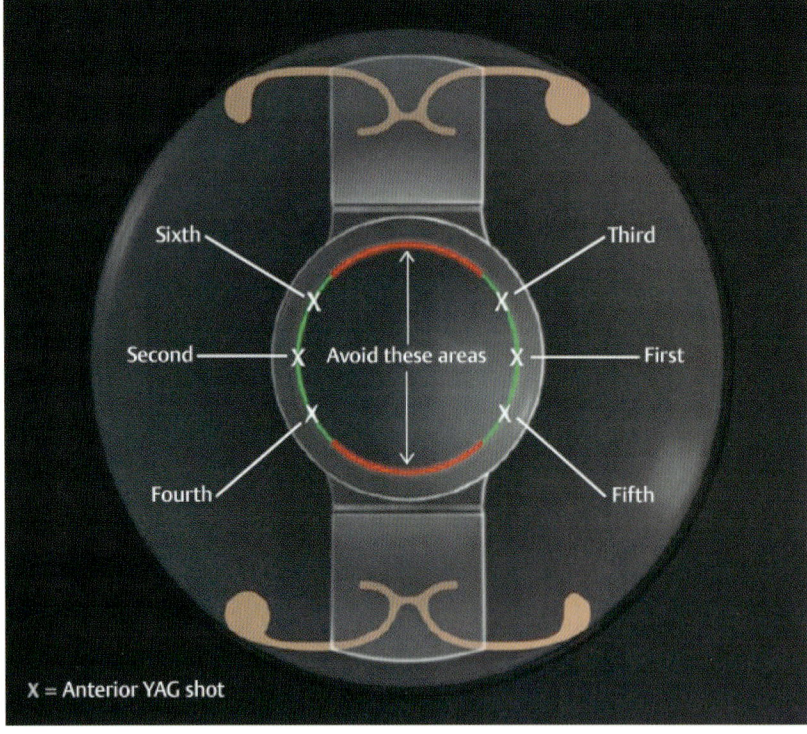

Fig. 45.18 Anterior capsular contraction syndrome: YAG treatment pattern.

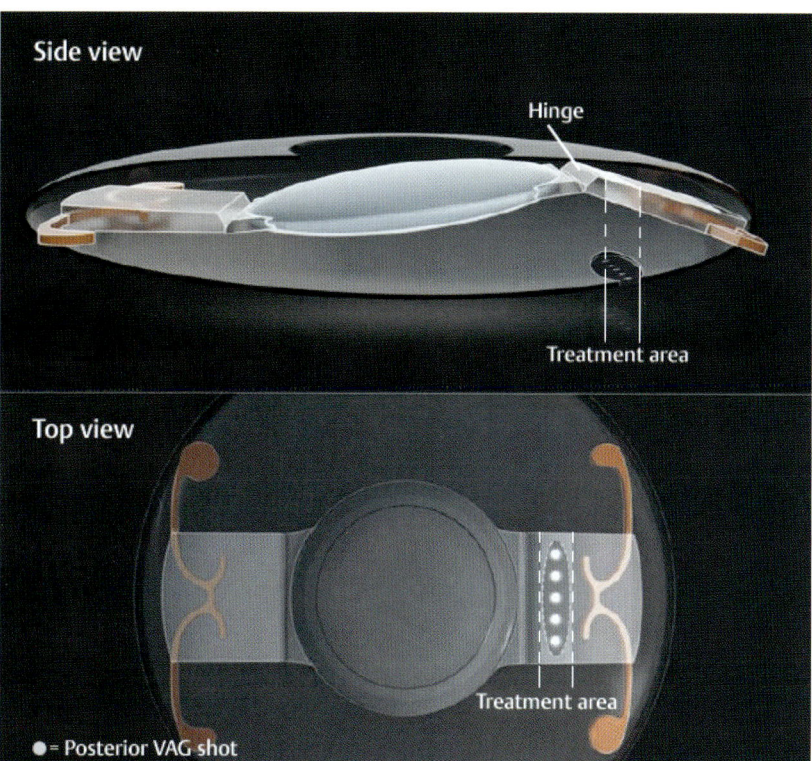

Fig. 45.19 Posterior capsular contraction syndrome with lens tilt: YAG pulses placed just outside the hinge–optic junction in the posterior capsule in the area of the vaulted hinge.

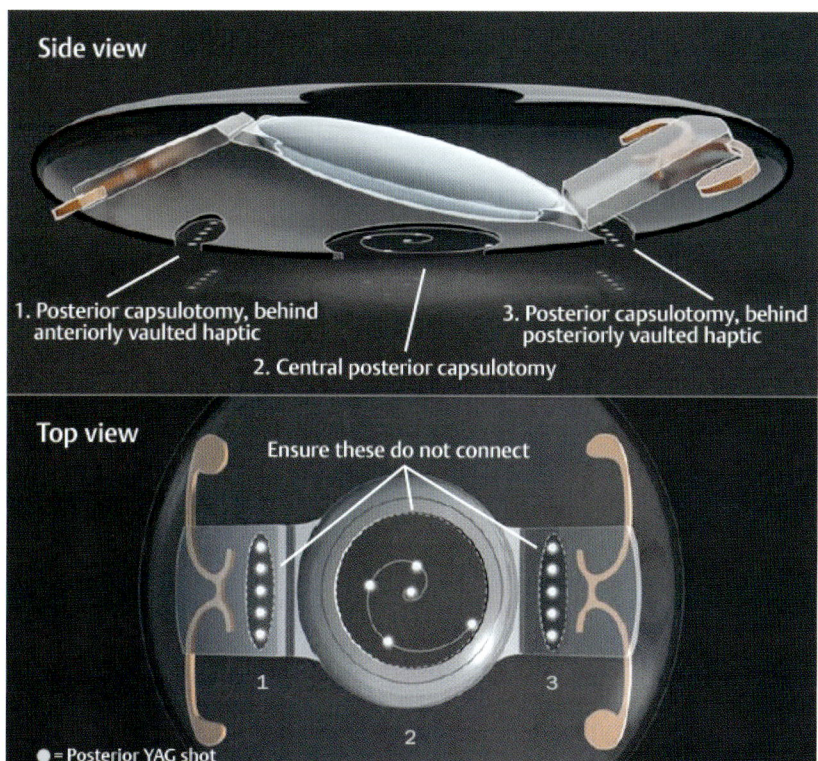

Fig. 45.20 Posterior capsular contraction syndrome with Z-syndrome treatment: central YAG round capsulotomy and additional YAG pulses in the posterior capsule behind both the anteriorly vaulted and posteriorly vaulted haptics.

Conclusion

Surgeons are faced with many obstacles today in trying to achieve near perfection with the Crystalens or Trulign Toric IOL platforms. This chapter has reviewed some of the critical components to achieving the best possible outcome with these advanced IOLs: preoperatively, setting proper patient expectations and performing proper advanced diagnostics and optimizing the ocular surface; intraoperatively, paying meticulous attention to IOL placement and preventing wound leaks and appropriate astigmatism management; and postoperatively, continuing to manage patient expectations, avoiding capsular contraction syndrome, and making proper enhancement decisions if needed. In the end, the CMS ruling created in 2005 has led to a new generation of happy baby boomers achieving visual freedom after cataract surgery with the Crystalens or Trulign Toric IOL implants.

References

1. Altmann GE, Nichamin LD, Lane SS, Pepose JS. Optical performance of 3 intraocular lens designs in the presence of decentration. J Cataract Refract Surg 2005;31:574–585

2. Schaeffel F. Binocular lens tilt and decentration measurements in healthy subjects with phakic eyes. Invest Ophthalmol Vis Sci 2008;49:2216–2222

3. Pepose J. The longevity revolution. Ophthalmol Manage. 2011;(suppl):3–7

4. Ang R. Comparison of 3 presbyopia-correcting IOLs used in cataract surgery. Presented at the 29th Congress of the European Society of Cataract and Refractive Surgeons (ESCRS), Vienna, September 17–21, 2011

5. Colvard DM. Long-term stability of accommodative IOLs. Ophthalmol Management. 2011;(suppl):13–15

6. Bausch and Lomb, unpublished data

7. Cumming JS, Slade SG, Chayet A; AT-45 Study Group. Clinical evaluation of the model AT-45 silicone accommodating intraocular lens: results of feasibility and the initial phase of a Food and Drug Administration clinical trial. Ophthalmology 2001;108:2005–2009, discussion 2010

8. Centers for Medicare and Medicaid Services (CMS). Ruling 05–01. Determining payment for insertion of presbyopia-correcting IOLs. May 3, 2005

9. Hurley T. Baby boomer statistics. Love to Know website. http//www.seniorslovetoknow.com/Baby_Boomer_Statistics

10. Bulic BS. Boomers—yes, boomers—spend the most on tech. Ad Age Digital website. 2010

11. Webb D. Del Webb Baby Boomer Survey. 2010

12. Trattler W, Goldberg D, Reilly C. Incidence of concomitant cataract and dry eye prospective health assessment of cataract patients. Presented at the World Cornea Congress, Boston, April 8, 2010

13. Koch DD, Ali SF, Weikert MP, Shirayama M, Jenkins R, Wang L. Contribution of posterior corneal astigmatism to total corneal astigmatism. J Cataract Refract Surg 2012;38:2080–2087

14. Koch DD, Jenkins RB, Weikert MP, Yeu E, Wang L. Correcting astigmatism with toric intraocular lenses: effect of posterior corneal astigmatism. J Cataract Refract Surg 2013;39:1803–1809

15. Tyson F, Jackson M, Solomon J. Combining multimodal wavefront examination and digital refraction to create a rapid and accurate approach (XFraction) for a total visual system assessment for intraocular lens selection. US Ophthalmic Review 2013;6:110–117

16. Artal P, Benito A, Pérez GM, et al. An objective scatter index based on double-pass retinal images of a point source to classify cataracts. PLoS ONE 2011;6:e16823

17. Jackson M. A systematic approach to dry eye using LipiFlow treatment. US Ophthalmic Review 2014;7:104–108

18. Wang L, Shirayama M, Ma XJ, Kohnen T, Koch DD. Optimizing intraocular lens power calculations in eyes with axial lengths above 25.0 mm. J Cataract Refract Surg 2011;37:2018–2027

19. Aramberri J. Intraocular lens power calculation after corneal refractive surgery: double-K method. J Cataract Refract Surg 2003;29:2063–2068

20. Masket S, Masket SE. Simple regression formula for intraocular lens power adjustment in eyes requiring cataract surgery after excimer laser photoablation. J Cataract Refract Surg 2006;32:430–434

21. Davison JA. Capsule contraction syndrome. J Cataract Refract Surg 1993; 19:582–589

22. Wong RW, Kokame GT, Mahmoud TH, Mieler WF, Tornambe PE, McDonald HR. Complications associated with clear corneal cataract wounds during vitrectomy. Retina 2010;30:850–855

23. Mifflin MD, Kinard K. Prospective comparison of clear corneal incisions for cataract surgery: stromal pocket hydration versus conventional hydration. Presented at the American Society of Cataract and Refractive Surgery (ASCRS), San Francisco, April 4, 2009

24. Wong M. Securing clear corneal incisions. Cataract Refract Surg Today 2003;March:25–27

25. Kohnen T. New abbreviations for visual acuity values. J Cataract Refract Surg 2009;35:1145

26. Mukai K, Matsushima H, Gotoh N, et al. Efficacy of ophthalmic nonsteroidal antiinflammatory drugs in suppressing anterior capsule contraction and secondary posterior capsule opacification. J Cataract Refract Surg 2009;35:1614–1618

27. Davison JA. Capsule contraction syndrome. J Cataract Refract Surg 1993; 19:582–589

28. Wang YL, Wang ZZ, Zhao L, et al. Finite element analysis of neodymium: yttrium-aluminum-garnet incisions for the prevention of anterior capsule contraction syndrome. Chin Med J (Engl) 2013;126:692–696

29. Deokule SP, Mukherjee SS, Chew CK. Neodymium:YAG laser anterior capsulotomy for capsular contraction syndrome. Ophthalmic Surg Lasers Imaging 2006;37:99–105

46 Diffractive Multifocal Intraocular Lenses

Quentin B. Allen

The ultimate goal of visual rehabilitation in cataract surgery has always been to restore the best level of visual acuity, across a natural range of focal distances, much like the normal pre-presbyopic human eye. Utilizing the optical property of diffraction and interference to separate light rays into two distinct focal lengths enables an individual to perceive both near and distant images simultaneously, depending on the target of regard. Newer aspheric diffractive multifocal intraocular lenses (IOLs) provide high-quality images at both distance and near foci, and improved near vision quality compared with refractive multifocal lenses.[1]

Multifocal Intraocular Lenses

There are two types of multifocal diffractive IOLs currently available in the US in different models and iterations. First, the aspheric Restor (Alcon, Fort Worth, TX) is a biconvex apodized diffractive acrylic lens with an embedded blue-filtering cromophore. This lens is available in a single-piece IOL design in 3 different add powers, 4.0 D, 3.0 D, and 2.5 D (models SN6AD3, SN6AD1, and SV25T0). It is also available in a 3 piece design suitable for sulcus fixation with either a 4.0 D or 3.0 D add power (MA60 D3, MA60D1). All of the Restor lenses have a central anterior surface diffractive , ringed, multifocal optic encompassing the central portion of the IOL. The central diffractive optic measures 3.6 mm in the Restor 4.0 and 3.0 add, while the 2.5 D lens model has a central diffractive optic measuring 3.4 mm. The peripheral portion of all of the Restor lenses is devoted to distance focus. This lens design is intended to reduce glare and halo under mesopic and scotopic conditions when the pupil is potentially larger. At small pupil sizes, the lens provides an equal distribution of light rays for both near and distant foci. However, at a 5mm pupil size, 84% of light rays entering the Restor lens are distributed to distance focus, due to the peripheral refractive zone of the lens. The 2.5 D model has other modifications to enhance distance vision quality, including a larger central ring which is 100% distance-dominant (0.94 mm vs 0.84 mm), as opposed to 60% distance focus in the Restor 3.0 D lens. The 4.0 D and 3.0 D Restor lenses have –0.10 of negative asphericity, while the 2.5 D version and –0.20 um of negative asphericity. (All of this information is Alcon, data on file)

Second, the Tecnis multifocal (Abbott Medical Optics, Abbott Park, IL) is also available in 3 different add powers, a 4.0 D, 3.25 D, and 2.75D single-piece IOL design (ZMB00, ZLB00, ZKB00). It too is available in a 3-piece design suitable for sulcus fixation, with a 4.0 D add power (ZMA00). All of the Tecnis multifocal lenses add –0.27 um of negative asphericity to the optical system of the eye. The Tecnis multifocal lens is designed to be pupil-independent, with a 50/50 light split at all pupil sizes, due to the full-optic diffractive design. Three multifocal diffractive IOL types are available in the United States. First, the Tecnis Multifocal (model ZMB00, Abbott Medical Optics, Abbott Park, IL) is a one-piece acrylic, pupil-independent full optic diffractive lens with a +4.00 add power (**Fig. 46.1**).

Second, the aspheric Restor (Alcon, Fort Worth, TX) multi-focal lens is a biconvex one-piece acrylic, apodized diffractive multifocal lens with an embedded blue-filtering chromophore (**Fig. 46.2**). This lens is available in the United States in two add powers, 3.0 D and 4.0 D (models SN6AD1 and SN6AD3). In other parts of the world a 2.5 D add power is available as well. The lens has a central anterior surface diffractive, ringed multifocal optic encompassing the central 3.6 mm of the lens, whereas the peripheral 2.4 mm of the remaining optic is a full distance refractive portion. This design is intended to reduce glare and halo under mesopic and scotopic conditions when the pupil is dilated. The aspheric Restor lens corrects –0.10 µm of spherical aberration.

Third, the Restor lens is also available in a three-piece format (models MA60D1 and MA60D3) that may be sulcus fixated.

Patient Selection

Before discussing surgical options with the patient, the patient exam may be used as a time-saving screening tool to eliminate lens choice options based on patient anatomy and comorbidities. Performing a corneal topography and macula optical coherence tomography (OCT) in the cataract evaluation helps to effectively tailor the discussion of IOL options and reduce the need to discuss options for which the patient is not a candidate. A multifocal lens should not be implanted if there is evidence of significant ocular pathology. The splitting of light rays into near and distant foci in a diffractive multifocal optic causes 18% of light rays to be lost to high orders. The inherent reduction of contrast sensitivity associated with a multifocal lens may further compromise any preexisting contrast loss related to macular dysfunction.[2] This may include epiretinal membrane and any other macular degenerative process. Optic nerve disease may also produce impaired contrast sensitivity. Therefore, in any patient with documented optic nerve dysfunction or visual field loss, caution with multi-focal lens implantation is warranted.[3]

Corneal topography is helpful in identifying preexisting corneal astigmatism. If a corneal topography is available at the time of surgical evaluation, discussion may then be further tailored to include the need for concomitant astigmatic correction, or to eliminate a multifocal IOL option if there is corneal pathology. Significant corneal irregular astigmatism is a contraindication to the use of a multifocal IOL, as poor vision quality may result from preexisting high-order aberrations (HOAs) and the combined impact of reduced contrast sensitivity.[4] Treatable forms of irregular astigmatism such as pterygium or anterior basement membrane dystrophy should be identified and addressed prior to obtaining biometric measurements. If a patient elects to

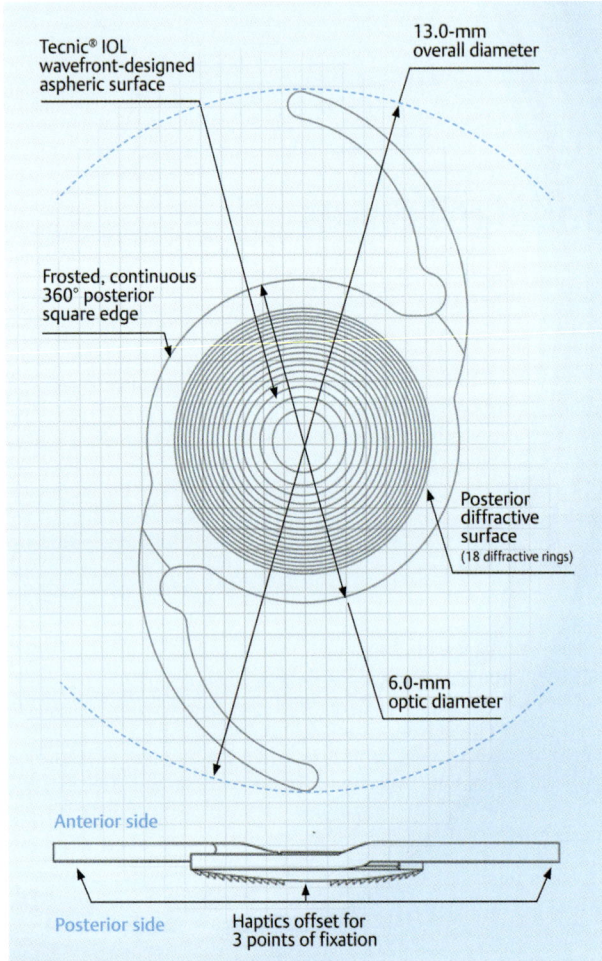

Fig. 46.1 Tecnis multifocal lens, model ZMB00. The lens has a prolate anterior surface with –0.27 μm of asphericity and a back-surface diffractive ringed multifocal surface. This lens provides a 50/50 split for distant and near foci for pupil sizes greater than 1.00 mm. The central 1.00 mm of the lens is distance focus only. This lens is also available in a three-piece platform that may be used for sulcus placement. (Courtesy of Abbott Medical Optics.)

undergo pterygium excision or superficial keratectomy due to preexisting corneal disease, then several months of corneal stabilization should be allowed prior to obtaining corneal measurements for cataract surgery. If repeat corneal topography or wavefront aberrometry shows an acceptable improvement in corneal regularity, a multifocal IOL may be considered. Ideal candidates for multifocal IOLs should have minimal amounts of corneal irregularity or HOA. There are few studies regarding acceptable parameters for irregular astigmatism or HOAs to guide candidacy for multifocal IOLs. However, patients with coma measuring greater than 0.32 μm implanted with multifocal IOLs have been demonstrated to have increased dysphotopsia.[5]

Corneal topography may also help identify patients with underlying aqueous tear deficiency that may impact corneal regularity and visual quality.[6] If significant dry eye is identified, a regimen of artificial tears or punctal occlusion should be considered as well. Use of topical cyclosporine or lifetegrast may be considered as well. If corneal irregularity is noted due to dry eye, it is often necessary to treat the dry eye aggressively for 1 to 2 weeks prior to obtaining biometric measurements.

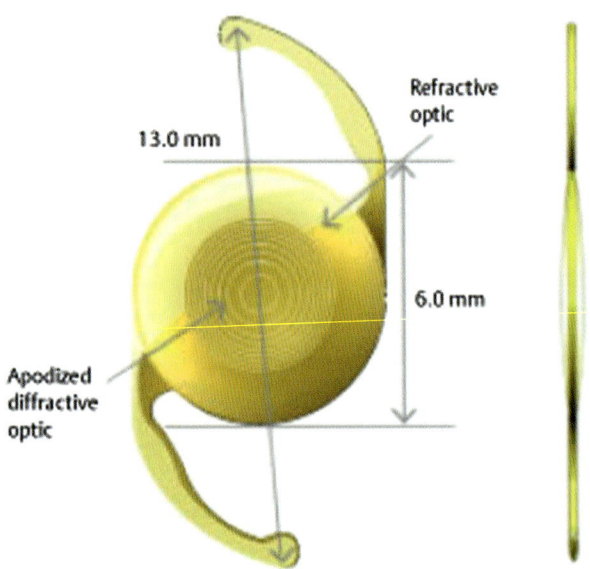

Fig. 46.2 Alcon model SN6AD1 Restor apodized diffractive multifocal intraocular lens (IOL). (Courtesy of Alcon.)

Pupil Size

Pupil size may be an important variable to consider in terms of candidacy for a multifocal lens. The Tecnis multifocal lens is pupil independent, providing a 50/50 split of light rays focused for distance and near across all pupil sizes from 1.0 mm and larger. This lens provides excellent near and distance acuity even in patients with large or irregular pupils. The Restor lens is pupil dependent, due to its central diffractive optic being 3.6 mm in diameter. Therefore, in patients with a mesopic pupil measuring significantly larger than 3.6 mm, near function of this lens may be compromised. Conversely, the shift in function from a diffractive to a refractive optic when the pupil is larger than 3.6 mm may reduce photic phenomena with nighttime driving.[7] Careful measurement of mesopic pupil size as a part of preoperative testing may help identify which multifocal lens is appropriate for each patient's unique anatomy and functional needs. Certain medication, such as antidepressants, may cause pupillary dilation due to anticholinergic properties. This should be a consideration in preoperative planning, as large pupil size may contribute to glare and dysphotopsia symptoms.[8] Conversely, in patients with poorly dilating small pupils, where mechanical pupil enlargement or a Malyugin ring may be required, a non–pupil-dependent lens may be favorable to achieve effective near vision, as pupil size and function may be permanently altered.

Other Preoperative Considerations

Advances in corneal imaging now make identification of abnormal corneas much simpler. Parameters such as HOA may be evaluated as well. Wavefront analyzers such as the iTrace (Tracey Technologies, Houston, TX) and the optical path difference (OPD)-Scan III (Marco, Jacksonville, FL) enable the evaluation of other information such as angle kappa, spherical aberration, and HOA. These indices may be predictors of patient satisfaction, and also help to guide the choice of appropriate IOL[9] (**Fig. 46.3**).

Patients with prior refractive surgery may be suboptimal candidates due to corneal irregularity and HOA. However, some

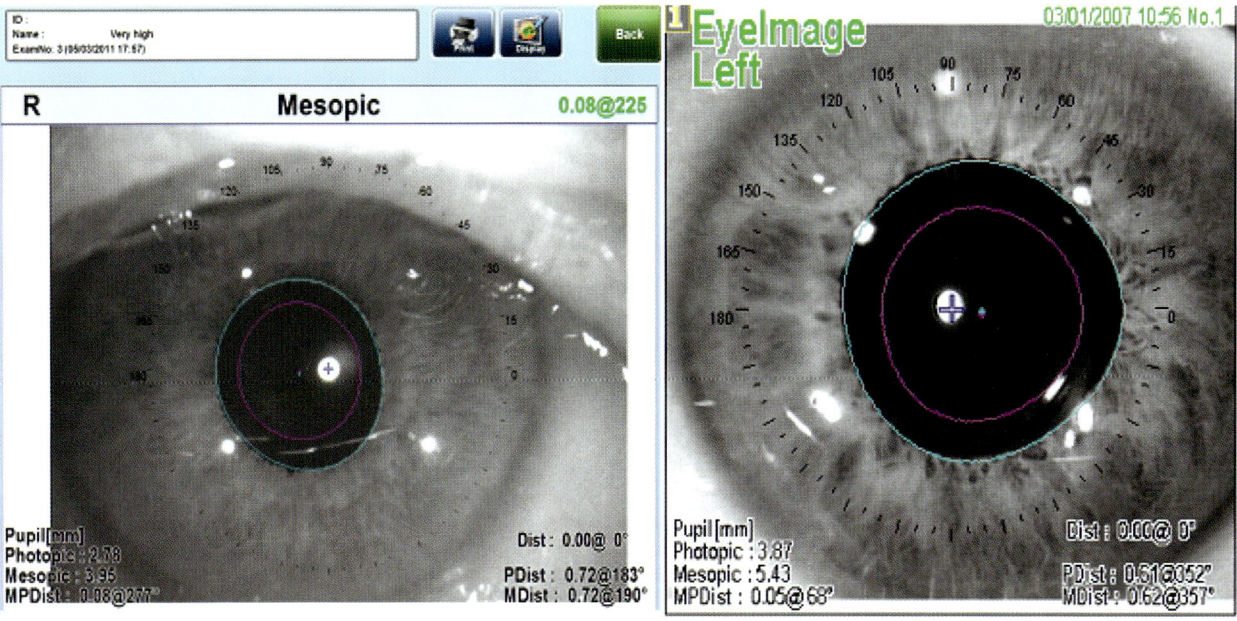

Fig. 46.3 Nidek optical path difference (OPD) III. Images show high angle kappa and large mesopic pupil size. Large angle kappa may be a relative contraindication to multifocal IOL usage. (Courtesy of Mitchell Jackson, MD.)

studies have demonstrated that diffractive multifocal IOLs may be implanted successfully in post-refractive patients.[10] The regularity of the post-refractive cornea and measured HOA should be a strong consideration in these cases, and additional discussion with the patient regarding vision quality is advisable. Use of intraoperative aberrometry to refine IOL selection may be helpful in prior myopic refractive surgery patients.[11]

Patients with prior myopic refractive surgery typically have high positive spherical aberration (oblate cornea), whereas those with prior hyperopic refractive surgery more typically have negative spherical aberration (prolate cornea). Spherical aberration matching with the most appropriate lens based on preexisting spherical aberration may help to normalize postoperative spherical aberration. Highly aberrant corneas typically have some degree of induced multifocality and reduction in contrast sensitivity. Placement of a multifocal lens in this clinical scenario is more likely to adversely impact visual quality.

Preoperative Counseling

Utilizing presbyopia-correcting lenses enables us to offer patients more options for visual rehabilitation after cataract surgery. Every lens option or vision system such as monovision has some inherent compromise: accommodating lenses may not provide a uniformly satisfactory degree of near acuity, whereas multifocal lenses reduce contrast sensitivity and are associated with increased risk of photic phenomena. Therefore, it is incumbent upon the surgeon to educate the patient so that an informed decision can be reached, while considering all options. There are numerous video education platforms available, including Eyemaginations™ (Baltimore, MD) and even iPad based apps for patient education including SightSelector™ (Patient Education Concepts, Houston, TX). It is helpful to have patients watch one of these educational videos prior to meeting with the surgeon or surgical counselor so that the concepts of accommodation, lens removal, and multifocality can be clearly grasped. If patients do not fully understand the absolute loss of accommodation typically experienced with a monofocal lens, they are more likely to be

disappointed with their lack of near vision postoperatively. Also, patients are correspondingly less likely to consider a presbyopia-correcting lens if the loss of accommodation with standard cataract surgery is not clearly understood.

Specific examples of tasks that could require glasses postoperatively may be helpful to explain the anticipated range of visual function with a monofocal lens, such as needing glasses for seeing the dashboard instrument panel in a car, or needing glasses for computer use. Most cataract patients anticipate the need for reading glasses, but are less aware of the need for glasses for intermediate tasks after cataract surgery. Explaining that even seeing the food on one's dinner plate may be less clear than one would anticipate, due to the profound accommodation loss with a monofocal lens, may be helpful.

During preoperative counseling, it is also important to determine patient lifestyle, hobbies, reading needs, and personality type. To successfully implant multifocal lenses and reduce patient dissatisfaction and risk of lens exchange, a full and thorough discussion of the potential for aberrant light phenomena (glare and haloes) is warranted. Occupational night drivers may not be ideal candidates. The process of neuroadaptation, and allowing 3 to 6 months for reduction in glare and halo phenomena, should be explained. It is also extremely important to demonstrate and discuss the typical focal distance of the lens being considered. For a Tecnis Multifocal or Restor with +4 add, the optimal reading distance is 33 cm, with a fairly rigid depth of focus in front or behind this zone. For the Restor +3 lens, the optimal near focus is 43.5 cm, with a larger depth of focus. With lower add power, intermediate acuity is logically improved, as illustrated by the binocular defocus curve of the lower add power lens, measuring 20/25 compared with 20/40 with the +4 add[12] (**Fig. 46.4**).

An additional consideration is the amount of intermediate-range work that the patient does on a regular basis. Multifocal lenses with lower powers are designed to better optimize intermediate-range vision. The highest add power (+4) multifocal lenses lead to more patient complaints in this regard, although over time the intermediate vision can improve with neuroadap-

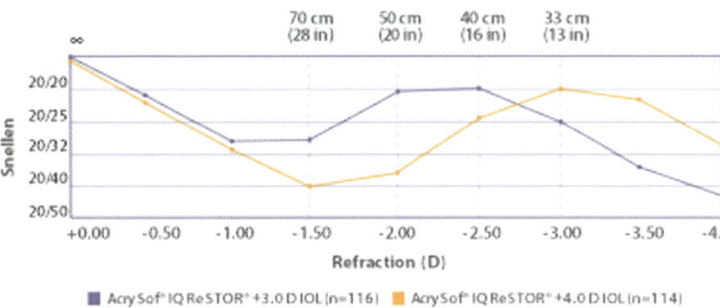

Fig. 46.4 A plano refractive target is ideal; a +4 D add lens plano to +0.25 is targeted to avoid a myopic outcome that would shorten the focal distance to an unacceptable near point. For a 2.5 to +3 D add lens, a plano to –0.25 result is optimal to maintain good near acuity.

tation. Even so, +1.00 reading glasses are often required to optimize intermediate vision in patients implanted with a +4 add multifocal. Lower power multifocal lenses such as the ZKB00 or Restor +2.5 add lens may provide increased intermediate acuity. However, these low add multifocal lenses do not provide the amount of near correction to reliably provide consistent unaided near acuity for most reading tasks. If a low-add multifocal lens is implanted in the first eye, sometimes it may be desirable to implant a higher power MFIOL in the second eye to optimize patient needs. Other products available outside the United States such as the FineVision trifocal IOL (PhysIOL, Liège, Belgium) seek to address this shortcoming of multifocal IOLs with more than two optimal focal distances.

Each cataract patient has unique vision needs and lifestyle considerations. It is important to ask each patient, "If you had to wear glasses after cataract surgery, would you rather wear them for reading or for the computer?" It is equally important to ask, "Would you be willing to have glare and haloes at night while driving, if you could have good reading vision without glasses?" These two questions help to identify good multifocal lens candidates. The final factor here is patient personality. The Dell questionnaire attempts to elucidate this factor by asking patients to rate their personality type from easygoing to very particular, or type A, on a scale of 1 to 10. One can also query patients whether the people who know them well would describe them as "picky" or "particular." The classic type-A personality type is often manifested in engineers. Scientists, math professors, and any person who is a meticulous, keen observer may also be type A. This personality type, in my experience, is best served by monofocal or accommodating lens technology. If patients describe themselves as easygoing, with realistic expectations, and they have a strong desire for spectacle independence, they would benefit from a full discussion of the advantages and disadvantages of multifocal lenses.

Low add multifocal counseling, in particular the Restor 2.5, is similar to preoperative counseling for accommodative lenses. The low-add Restor lens provides excellent distance and intermediate vision, with minimal night-time photic phenomena. Patients should be advised that low power readers will be necessary for reading. The ZKB00 lens also has been reported to have less glare and halo than the higher add Tecnis multifocals, however, as it is still a full diffractive multifocal, it may theoretically have a tendency towards more nightime photic phenomena.

Surgical Planning

Careful preoperative measurements are paramount in achieving tight refractive outcomes in cataract surgery. Uncorrected refractive error in multifocal lens patients may lead to unacceptable vision quality and photic phenomena. A plano refractive target is ideal; a +4 D add lens plano to +0.25 is targeted to avoid a myopic outcome that would shorten the focal distance to an

unacceptable near point. For a +3 D add lens, a plano to –0.25 result is optimal to maintain good near acuity. For low add multifocal lenses, targeting -0.25 for the first eye may prevent an indavertent hyperopic overcorrection, which would significantly reduce the already lessened near vision with these lens models. It is preferred in this setting to employ the most accurate method of obtaining axial length, optical biometry, using either partial coherence interferometry (Zeiss IOL master™, Carl Zeiss Meditec, Jena, Germany) or low coherence reflectometry (Lenstar™, Alcon). The IOL master has demonstrated the capability of obtaining reproducible measurements to within 20 μm, five times better than ultrasound biometry.[13] The Lenstar has also been shown to provide this degree of accuracy and is considered to be biometrically equivalent.[14,15] Additionally, the Lenstar provides lens thickness measurements, which are required for newer lens power calculation formulas such as the Holladay 2 and Olsen formula.[16] Outcomes should be analyzed and lens optimization performed to continue to "fine-tune" refractive results.

Astigmatism Control

Control of preexisting corneal astigmatism is extremely important in achieving excellent refractive outcomes and high levels of patient satisfaction. Corneal approaches to correction of regular astigmatism can be very successful in reducing or eliminating moderate amounts of astigmatism. The effect of corneal arcuate incisions is lessened in younger patients, and regression may be more of an issue in younger patients as well. Manual or femtosecond corneal arcuate incisions are both effective modalities. If manual incisions are employed, it is critical to use a nomogram that considers corneal pachymetry, such as the Nichamin Age and Pachymetry Adjusted (NAPA) nomogram (Beaver-Visitec International, Waltham, MA). There is tremendous variability in corneal thickness, and a standard 600-μm depth peripheral corneal relaxing incision will undercorrect patients with thick corneas, and overcorrect or even perforate in patients with thinner corneas. Ultrasonic pachymetry measurements may be taken preoperatively over the peripheral cornea in the areas to be incised. Alternatively, 9-mm optical zone measurements may be used from Scheimpflug measurements (Pentacam, Oculus, Arlington, WA). The Mastel PhDII adjustable depth diamond blade (Mastel Precision Surgical Instruments, Rapid City, SD) is an excellent instrument for manual corneal arcuate incisions. Femtosecond laser corneal arcuate incisions are typically set to a true 85% of corneal thickness in the area of the arcuate incision. Many nomograms are available for femtosecond arcuate incisions.

Given the effect of age on response to corneal correction of astigmatism, a reasonable rule of thumb is that patients 60 to 70 years of age can achieve 1.5 diopters of correction with either manual limbal relaxing incisions (LRIs) or femtosecond LRI. For patients over 70 years of age, multifocal IOL and concomitant manual or femtosecond corneal arcuate incisions may typically be expected to correct up to 2.0 diopters of corneal astigmatism. When a patient under 60 years of age with high astigmatism is encountered and a multifocal IOL is appropriate, preplanned sequential laser vision correction is advised. Patients with high astigmatism should be counseled that the risk of needing a laser vision correction enhancement is always higher than average. Smaller optical zones may be used to increase the range of astigmatic correction, but laser-assisted in situ keratomileusis (LASIK) may be more precarious through previous corneal arcuate incisions if an enhancement is required. Aggressive astigmatic keratotomy may also be associated with induction of HOA.[17] Residual corneal astigmatism may be corrected with photorefractive keratectomy (PRK) or LASIK in a second procedure after refractive stabilization, typically 2 to 3 months postoperatively.

Another option for patients with high astigmatism is to correct the corneal astigmatism via a lenticular approach using an accommodating toric IOL (Trulign, Bausch and Lomb, Rochester, NY), or use conventional monofocal toric lenses in a monovision strategy. There are toric multifocal lenses available outside of the United States that address this need as well.

Intraoperative Pearls

Cataract surgery with implantation of a multifocal lens requires meticulous attention to detail, technique, and prevention of intraoperative complications. Topical anesthesia with monitored anesthesia care is my preferred technique for cataract surgery with implantation of a multifocal IOL. This technique minimizes the risks associated with retrobulbar anesthesia, such as orbital hemorrhage, myotoxicity, and ptosis. Topical anesthesia is also beneficial in enabling intraoperative motility and optic nerve function such that the microscope light is visible to the patient, and may be used in aiding lens centration.

A dispersive viscoelastic may be preferable for protection of the corneal endothelium. Although controversial, the femtosecond laser may reduce ultrasound time and endothelial cell trauma, potentially providing more rapid visual recovery. A well-centered round capsulorrhexis is critical in achieving consistent refractive outcomes. The capsulotomy should be centered on the visual axis, which is slightly nasally decentered in most patients. This is more easily visualized and achieved with femtosecond laser visualization. The size of the capsulorrhexis should be small enough to achieve complete overlap of the lens optic and to reduce the potential for lens tilt. A 5.2-mm capsulotomy provides adequate room for phacoemulsification and enables excellent lens centration and 360-degree overlap of the lens optic.

An endocapsular technique for phacoemulsification may be favorable in reducing endothelial compromise, providing for less corneal edema, and more rapid visual rehabilitation. Options include divide and conquer, phaco chop, or a quick chopping technique. Phaco flip and other supracapsular techniques may be associated with more corneal edema and slower visual recovery.

Meticulous cortical cleanup to provide a pristine capsular bag may reduce early formation of posterior capsule opacification and reduce the need for yttrium-aluminum-garnet (YAG) laser capsulotomy in the early postoperative period. Ideally, YAG capsulotomy should not be performed in the early postoperative period if there is any possibility of an IOL exchange due to visual dissatisfaction. Additionally, meticulous cortical cleanup and anterior capsular polishing may make any potential IOL exchange technically less difficult due to less capsular phimosis and less vigorous cellular proliferation around the haptics within the capsular bag.

Intraoperative aberrometry is helpful in verifying lens power, especially in eyes with unusual anatomy. After insertion of the

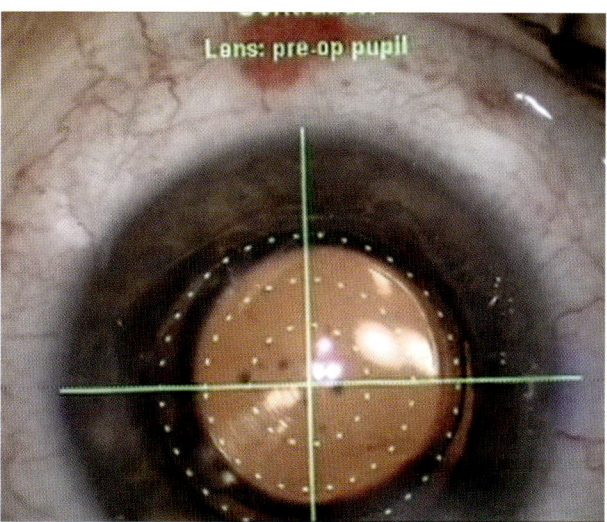

Fig. 46.5   Alcon Verion system, with centration markers based on preoperative imaging. (Courtesy of Elizabeth Yeu, MD.)

multifocal IOL, the patient should be asked to look at the center of the microscope light to help in achieving optimal lens centration. The surgeon then attempts to align the corneal light reflex with the center of the IOL. This may help to minimize the effect of a large angle kappa, which along with IOL decentration, has been shown to contribute to poor vision quality and suboptimal outcomes with implantation of multifocal IOLs.[18] Image guidance systems such as Verion™ (Alcon) may facilitate centration and alignment based on preoperative imaging, taking angle kappa into account, with an intraoperative display in the surgical microscope **(Fig. 46.5)**. At this point, after insertion of the IOL, the eye may be physiologically inflated with BSS to allow intraoperative aberrometry to be repeated. This pseudophakic measurement may allow residual astigmatism to be identified. If consistent measurement of significant (>0.5 D) is noted, previously placed femtosecond LRI's may be opened, or aberrometry-guided LRI's or PLRI/OCCI may be placed. With an adjustable depth LRI blade, careful extension of a femtosecond LRI may be carried out. Performing an LRI enhancement intraoperatively may reduce the need for postoperative refractive enhancement.[19]

Overcorrection is possible with manual LRI's, and care should be taken to be somewhat conservative, with a mild undercorrection being preferred, vs an overcorrection or 180 degree axis flip.

Intraocular miotics do not provide physiological constriction of the pupil, and are not advisable for estimation of ideal centration of a multifocal lens. At the close of the procedure, intracameral antibiotics are instilled to reduce the risk of postoperative endophthalmitis.

Postoperative Care

A topical steroid may be used postoperatively for several weeks on a tapering schedule. Use of a topical nonsteroidal anti-inflammatory drug (NSAID) preoperatively for 2 to 3 days and postoperatively for 4 to 6 weeks may be helpful in reducing intraoperative discomfort, maintaining pupillary dilation, and reducing the risk of postoperative cystoid macular edema (CME).[20] Even subclinical CME may potentially impact contrast sensitivity and quality of vision, reducing effectiveness of a multifocal IOL. Immediately after surgery it is important to tell patients that they will experience blurred vision for up to a week, and to expect blurry vision for near work as well. This helps to reduce the patients' anxiety if they are unable to see clearly in the early postoperative period due to normal healing issues such as cell, flare, and corneal edema.

At the 1-day postoperative visit, both distance and near acuity should be tested, and patients should be reassured that reduced acuity is normal. These patients tend to have high expectations, and during the early postoperative period it is important to provide copious amounts of reassurance. Patients are instructed that they can begin to use their new eye immediately, with the understanding that multifocality is a new and different way of seeing than what they were accustomed to. It is important to make them aware of the typical focal distance of the multifocal lens, depending on the IOL implanted. Patients may be accustomed to holding their reading material farther away, and may have to adjust to finding their new "sweet spot" for vision. The sweet spot should be demonstrated to patients during their postoperative visit so that they understand the importance of placing reading material at the focal distance dictated by the optics of the lens.

For patients receiving a 4.0 diopter add power multifocal lens, intermediate vision may be suboptimal, especially early in the postoperative period. Patients should be instructed that a +1.00 D reading glass may help with computer work, or the computer may need to be moved closer to find the more optimal reading distance of the multifocal lens. The intermediate vision does tend to improve over time and with neuroadaptation. With a hybrid refractive/diffractive lens such as Restor, it is important to advise the patient to find adequate direct light to aid in reading. This will help to facilitate miosis and effective utilization of the central reading zone of the IOL. A smartphone provides patients with easy access to a cell phone flashlight, which may be used in dim lighting to aid near acuity. Patients are discouraged from using reading glasses during the early postoperative period, as this may delay or prevent proper neuroadaptation.

For low-add multifocals, it is important to query the patient regarding satisfaction with distance and intermediate vision, as this is the anticipated optimal functional zone based on the reduction in add power. If the patient is unhappy with the requirement for some reading correction at this stage, consideration may be given to placing a higher-powered add power MFIOL in the contralateral eye. The patient should be counseled, however, that a higher-add MFIOL may be associated with more halo and glare, or some reduction in visual quality, particularly at distance. In my experience, patients who choose a low-add multifocal do so to minimize the risk of nighttime halo, and therefore do not want a higher-add MFIOL in the second eye.

In the early postoperative period, there may be difficulty tolerating the visual imbalance of having a multifocal IOL in one eye, and a cataract or significant refractive error in the other eye. Counseling patients to remove the spectacle lens from the glasses for their new eye may be helpful for monofocal IOL patients, but for multifocal lens patients it is more helpful to have them discontinue glasses completely as soon as the new multifocal lens provides good enough vision to function. This may eliminate confusion between the two eyes utilizing two different vision systems until the second eye surgery may be performed.

If the second eye does not have a visually significant cataract, there are several strategies that may be utilized. The most ideal scenario is to use a multifocal contact lens in the other eye to provide similar vision and binocular near acuity. However, a distance contact lens may be well tolerated in the phakic eye, and the multifocal lens may provide satisfactory near acuity. Patient satisfaction with a unilateral multifocal lens has been reported to be high, and spectacle independence levels are close to the levels achieved with bilateral implantation.[21]

Late Postoperative Issues

Patient dissatisfaction with the vision provided by multifocal lenses is a recognized risk of utilizing this technology. It is difficult to predict which patients may be unable to neuroadapt to a multifocal IOL. Some patients may have moderate to severe difficulty with neuroadaptation in the first 6 months postoperatively. However, even patients who are slow to neuroadapt, or never fully tolerate multifocality, typically will be happy enough with their unaided near acuity to elect not to undergo lens exchange. There is a small contingent of patients who are so unhappy with their vision quality, or photic phenomena, that they may consider lens exchange. This group of patients can be most challenging to care for.

It is important to reassure patients who complain about vision quality that it is completely normal to take weeks to months to adjust to multifocality. However, other potential causes of blurred vision should be addressed during this time as well. Dry eye is an underrecognized contributor to blurred vision in the cataract age group. Any unhappy multifocal patient who is evaluated should be considered a potential dry-eye patient. Frequent artificial tears should be a minimum recommendation to ensure the corneal surface can support high-quality vision. Preservative and medication toxicity from perioperative medications, particularly some generic NSAIDs, can delay vision recovery. For this reason, branded medications may be preferred in multifocal IOL patients.

Other reasons for reduced vision in the postoperative period include corneal edema, posterior capsule opacity, unrecognized macular pathology, unrecognized mild amblyopia, and unrecognized residual refractive error. At the 1-week visit, if the cornea is normal, a macula OCT should be obtained if the best corrected visual acuity (BCVA) is not correctable to 20/25. If macular pathology is identified, such as a previously unrecognized epiretinal membrane, a frank discussion regarding explantation of the lens, or proceeding with surgery in the second eye, is necessary. Proceeding with surgery in the second eye is a viable option, and good vision function may be achieved in this scenario, if the second eye has a normal retinal examination. Alternatively, the first lens may be explanted, although this is a major decision, and should be delayed or deferred if possible.

The issue of performing YAG laser capsulotomy after cataract surgery becomes more complex in the unhappy multifocal IOL patient. The presence of any capsular striae or fibrosis may sufficiently degrade and scatter incident light rays to reduce optical quality in a multifocal IOL patient. If there is no other pathology to explain reduced vision, and corneal surface issues have been addressed, then proceeding with YAG capsulotomy is reasonable 2 to 3 months after cataract surgery. An extensive discussion with the patient regarding IOL exchange is mandatory, however, before proceeding with YAG capsulotomy, as the capsular opening significantly complicates surgical planning for IOL exchange, as a vitrectomy will likely be required. Fortunately, if patients are sufficiently motivated by the desire for unaided near vision, it is extremely unlikely that they will elect to have their multifocal IOL removed. The lack of near vision with monofocal lenses can be simulated with –3.00 lenses prior to any consideration of a lens exchange.

Uncorrected refractive error may significantly reduce vision quality in the multifocal IOL patient. If uncorrected refractive error is identified, the patient may be encouraged to obtain temporary spectacles, or wear a low-power contact lens, to see if vision quality is sufficiently improved. If patients are happy enough to tolerate their multifocal vision while wearing a pair of glasses or contact lenses, laser vision correction may be performed to duplicate the refractive correction. In some cases, however, patients may be willing to wear a low-power pair of glasses for the occasions in which their unaided acuity is not sufficient, in lieu of undergoing another surgical procedure. Specifically, when night driving is the primary complaint, this option should be presented. Some patients are not optimal candidates for refractive surgery, and instead of undergoing further surgery with some risk involved, they may elect to wear a pair of glasses for certain tasks. Performing an LRI is an option for a refractive enhancement as well, and in patients with residual astigmatism and a plano spherical equivalent, this option should be considered. It is prudent to wait a minimum of 2 to 3 months for refractive stabilization to attempt any refractive enhancements after cataract surgery.

Conclusion

Fortunately, with good patient selection, meticulous biometry, careful surgical technique, and patience with neuroadaptation, most patients do very well with diffractive multifocal IOLs. Patient satisfaction and spectacle independence rates are very high with these lenses.[22] Continued advances in surgical instrumentation and lens design may be expected.

References

1. Pieh S, Marvan P, Lackner B, et al. Quantitative performance of bifocal and multifocal intraocular lenses in a model eye: point spread function in multifocal intraocular lenses. Arch Ophthalmol 2002;120:23–28

2. Stangos N, Voutas S, Topouzis F, Karampatakis V. Contrast sensitivity evaluation in eyes predisposed to age-related macular degeneration and presenting normal visual acuity. Ophthalmologica 1995;209:194–198

3. McKendrick AM, Sampson GP, Walland MJ, Badcock DR. Contrast sensitivity changes due to glaucoma and normal aging: low-spatial-frequency losses in both magnocellular and parvocellular pathways. Invest Ophthalmol Vis Sci 2007;48:2115–2122

4. Braga-Mele R, Chang D, Dewey S, et al; ASCRS Cataract Clinical Committee. Multifocal intraocular lenses: relative indications and contraindications for implantation. J Cataract Refract Surg 2014;40:313–322

5. Visser N, Nuijts RMMA, de Vries NE, Bauer NJV. Visual outcomes and patient satisfaction after cataract surgery with toric multifocal intraocular lens implantation. J Cataract Refract Surg 2011;37:2034–2042

6. Liu Z, Pflugfelder SC. Corneal surface regularity and the effect of artificial tears in aqueous tear deficiency. Ophthalmology 1999;106:939–943

7. Choi J, Schwiegerling J. Optical performance measurement and night driving simulation of ReSTOR, ReZoom, and Tecnis multifocal intraocular lenses in a model eye. J Refract Surg 2008;24:218–222

8. Cerviño A, Hosking SL, Montés-Micó R, Alió JL. Retinal straylight in patients with monofocal and multifocal intraocular lenses. J Cataract Refract Surg 2008;34:441–446

9. Prakash G, Agarwal A, Prakash DR, Kumar DA, Agarwal A, Jacob S. Role of angle kappa in patient dissatisfaction with refractive-design multifocal intraocular lenses. [letter] J Cataract Refract Surg 2011;37:1739–1740, author reply 1740

10. Muftuoglu O, Dao L, Mootha VV, et al. Apodized diffractive intraocular lens implantation after laser in situ keratomileusis with or without subsequent excimer laser enhancement. J Cataract Refract Surg 2010;36:1815–1821

11. Ianchulev T, Hoffer KJ, Yoo SH, et al. Intraoperative refractive biometry for predicting intraocular lens power calculation after prior myopic refractive surgery. Ophthalmology 2014;121:56–60

12. Petermeier K, Messias A, Gekeler F, Szurman P. Effect of +3.00 diopter and +4.00 diopter additions in multifocal intraocular lenses on defocus profiles, patient satisfaction, and contrast sensitivity. J Cataract Refract Surg 2011;37:720–726

13. Vogel A, Dick HB, Krummenauer F. Reproducibility of optical biometry using partial coherence interferometry: intraobserver and interobserver reliability. J Cataract Refract Surg 2001;27:1961–1968

14. Jasvinder S, Khang TF, Sarinder KKS, Loo VP, Subrayan V. Agreement analysis of LENSTAR with other techniques of biometry. Eye (Lond) 2011;25:717–724

15. Rabsilber TM, Jepsen C, Auffarth GU, Holzer MP. Intraocular lens power calculation: clinical comparison of 2 optical biometry devices. J Cataract Refract Surg 2010;36:230–234

16. Hoffman R, Allen Q, Vasavada A, Devgan U, Snyder M. Cataract surgery in the small eye. J Cataract Refract Surg 2015;41:2565–2575

17. Ouchi M. High-cylinder toric intraocular lens implantation versus combined surgery of low-cylinder intraocular lens implantation and limbal relaxing incision for high-astigmatism eyes. Clin Ophthalmol 2014;8:661–667

18. Karhanová M, Marešová K, Pluháček F, Mlčák P, Vláčil O, Sín M. [The importance of angle kappa for centration of multifocal intraocular lenses]. Cesk Slov Oftalmol 2013;69:64–68

19. Packer MJ. Effect of Intraoperative Aberrometry on the rate of postoperative enhancement: retrospective study. Cataract Refractive Surgery. 2010; May 747–755

20. Wittpenn JR, Silverstein S, Heier J, et al, for the Acular Cystoid Macular Edema (ACME) Study Group. A masked comparison of topical ketorolac 0.4% plus steroid vs. steroid alone for the prevention of macular thickening following cataract surgery. Poster presented at the American Academy of Ophthalmology, Las Vegas, November 2006

21. Cionni RJ, Osher RH, Snyder ME, Nordlund ML. Visual outcome comparison of unilateral versus bilateral implantation of apodized diffractive multifocal intraocular lenses after cataract extraction: prospective 6-month study. J Cataract Refract Surg 2009;35:1033–1039

22. Allen Q. Comparing Presbyopic Visual Systems: Visual Satisfaction Survey Comparing Toric Distance, Toric Monovision, Accommodating, and Multifocal Lens Technology. San Diego, CA: American Society of Cataract and Refractive Surgery; November 2011

XVII   Combined Phacoemulsification and Glaucoma Surgery

47 Combined Phacoemulsification and Glaucoma Procedures

Jeff S. Maltzman and Brock K. Bakewell

Cataract surgeons face many challenges when performing combined glaucoma procedures, as well as many options, including standard trabeculectomy, EX-PRESS™ (Alcon, Fort Worth, TX) shunt surgery, glaucoma drainage devices, canaloplasty, and the new minimally invasive procedures. Each of these offerings has a unique set of preoperative considerations, as well as intraoperative and postoperative challenges and possible complications. This ever-expanding armamentarium of options provides the cataract surgeon with greater flexibility in matching the proper glaucoma procedure to the individual needs of the patient.

This chapter discusses the preoperative planning and surgical techniques for combined procedures, as well as the ways to avoid common pitfalls. Intraoperative and postoperative complications are separately discussed for each procedure, and procedures are compared and contrasted in terms of common challenges. The reader will acquire a detailed understanding of how each procedure impacts the patient, and how surgeons can develop a surgical plan to meet the needs of any patient suffering both cataract and glaucoma.

More than 12 years have passed since the publication of the first edition of this book, and in those years much has changed in the realm of glaucoma surgery, just as it has with phacoemulsification. Preferred techniques have evolved; new surgical implants and adjunctive devices have been developed. The surgeon wishing to combine a glaucoma procedure with cataract surgery has more and, arguably, better options today. Nonpenetrating canal-based procedures such as deep sclerectomy and viscocanalostomy have mostly given way to canaloplasty. Glaucoma drainage devices, or tube shunts, are gaining popularity. Microinvasive glaucoma surgery (MIGS) is rapidly progressing (see Chapter 47). Even the time-honored trabeculectomy, which remains the gold standard for surgical intraocular pressure (IOP) reduction, has seen significant improvements over the last decade.

Preoperative Consideration and Factors that Predispose to Complications

Surgeons must recognize and manage complications as they arise, but avoidance of complications is always preferable. Awareness of potential issues enables the surgeon to take the necessary steps preoperatively to limit intraoperative complications and achieve a successful outcome.

Bleeding

Although not normally a concern in routine cataract surgery, bleeding can be a significant problem during glaucoma procedures. Bleeding complications range from a substantial nuisance during conjunctival and scleral dissection to severe intraocular or subconjunctival bleeding that can affect other aspects, or even the ultimate success, of the procedure. Numerous systemic medications routinely used by patients contribute significantly to risk of intraoperative bleeding. All forms of blood thinners, including warfarin, aspirin, nonsteroidal anti-inflammatory drugs (NSAIDs), platelet aggregation inhibitors, and even perhaps vitamin E in high doses potentially increase bleeding during surgery.[1] Warfarin exerts its anticoagulant effect via interference with vitamin K–dependent synthesis of clotting factors II, VII, IX, and X.[2] Aspirin irreversibly inhibits platelet aggregation for the 8- to 10-day life span of the affected platelets.[3] Oral NSAIDs, such as ibuprofen and naproxen, reversibly prevent platelet aggregation via inhibition of cyclooxygenase, with platelet function restored as the medication is eliminated from the body.[4] Vitamin E interferes with platelet adhesion by reducing stimulation-induced pseudopodia formation, and may further exacerbate the effects of other blood thinners.[5] Medications such as Ticlid (ticlopidine), Plavix (clopidogrel), and Effient (prasugrel) are thienopyridines, which selectively target the adenosine diphosphate (ADP)-2 receptor on the platelet surface, thereby preventing platelet activation.[6] Newer anticoagulants continue to be developed, with variable mechanisms of action. Pradaxa (dabigatran) directly inhibits thrombin, whereas Xarelto (rivaroxaban) and Eliquis (apixaban) inhibit factor Xa.[7]

Bleeding is undesirable in glaucoma surgery, as it increases postoperative inflammation and scarring, and may also temporarily occlude the flow of aqueous at the surgical site. Some surgeons routinely recommend discontinuing some or all anticoagulant medications for several days to 2 weeks prior to glaucoma surgery, depending on the drug type and anticipated duration of action. This practice, however, must be cautiously considered, as discontinuation of such treatment could lead to thromboembolic events with potentially serious consequences.[8] Hemorrhagic complications may occur more commonly in patients taking warfarin than in patients taking aspirin, with a greater risk of surgical failure in the former.[9] There is little good data on risks associated with other anticoagulant medications. A survey of British glaucoma specialists found that approximately one third of surgeons routinely stopped warfarin or aspirin prior to glaucoma procedures, whereas the majority stopped neither.[10]

There is clearly no consensus on this issue. We generally prefer to discontinue aspirin and NSAIDs, but not warfarin or other agents, with the consent of the patient's primary physician or cardiologist.

Other Considerations

The effects of previous ocular surgery must be taken into account when planning a glaucoma procedure. Prior procedures involving the conjunctiva and sclera may limit options and increase the risk of certain complications. Significant conjunctival and episcleral scarring can impede conjunctival dissection and creation of a flap, with the risk of tears or buttonholes. Scleral dissection may also be affected, with the risk of thin or torn flaps. Evidence also suggests that prior surgery that violates the conjunctiva may limit the success of future trabeculectomy.[11] Conjunctival biopsies taken distant from the site of apparent scarring in patients having undergone prior surgery were noted to contain more fibroblasts, macrophages, and lymphocytes in the conjunctival stroma.[12] Additionally, alterations in the composition of aqueous humor and exposure of the conjunctiva to aqueous may permanently alter the tissue, leading to more vigorous wound healing and scarring.[13] Extensive superior scarring, therefore, might lead the surgeon to choose a drainage device over trabeculectomy. Inferior trabeculectomy should be avoided, as the risk of complications, particularly blebitis/endophthalmitis, is significantly higher with an inferior limbal bleb.[14,15] Nonpenetrating procedures, such as canaloplasty, generally do not lead to the formation of significant blebs and can be positioned more freely, including temporally or even inferiorly, although operating inferiorly can be technically and ergonomically more challenging.

Prior use of topical ophthalmic medications, particularly chronic use, may increase postoperative inflammation and influence surgical success.[16,17] Studies have shown increased numbers of conjunctival fibroblasts, macrophages, and lymphocytes, as well as a decrease in goblet cell density and loss of epithelial cell microvilli, in conjunctival tissue exposed to topical medications.[18–20] The majority of the evidence implicates benzalkonium chloride, the most commonly used preservative in topical ophthalmic preparations, as the primary cause of these changes.[21,22] Decreased success of trabeculectomy in patients previously treated with topical glaucoma medications has indeed been noted.[16,23] One recent study, however, failed to identify any effect of either number of topical medications or duration of use on the outcome of trabeculectomy.[24] Thus, the degree to which topical glaucoma therapy affects surgical outcome remains somewhat unclear. It seems reasonable to treat an inflamed eye that has received numerous injections with topical steroids for 1 to 2 weeks preoperatively to reduce the risk of failure due to possible chronic conjunctival inflammatory changes.

Young age and darkly pigmented skin may also be risk factors for failure of filtering surgery.[25,26] Surgical considerations that may improve success include increased dose or application time of intraoperative antimetabolite, as well as more frequent and aggressive postoperative follow-up, with early lysis or removal of scleral flap sutures and injections of subconjunctival 5-fluorouracil, as indicated.

Spectrum of Glaucoma Procedures

Before entering into a discussion of complications, it is first necessary to review the current spectrum of glaucoma surgery as well as the details of the newer procedures. Following its introduction by Cairns[27] in 1968, trabeculectomy quickly became the procedure of choice for IOP reduction that could not be achieved by nonsurgical therapy, and it remains the gold standard today. Nonetheless, even modern, guarded filtration surgery entails substantial risk of complications, including hyphema, conjunctival leaks, hypotony with possible maculopathy, suprachoroidal hemorrhage, and endophthalmitis.[28] The relatively high rate of complications in filtering surgery has prompted the development of nonpenetrating techniques such as nonpenetrating trabeculectomy/deep sclerectomy,[29] vicsocanalostomy,[30] and canaloplasty.[31,32] The hunt for safer, less technically challenging, and more effective surgery continues with the introduction of the MIGS series of procedures. Ideal for combination with phacoemulsification and generally performed through a clear corneal incision, these procedures are addressed comprehensively in Chapter 47.

Trabeculectomy Procedure

Since its introduction by Cairns, the trabeculectomy has undergone numerous modifications, including use of antimetabolites, adjustable and releasable scleral flap sutures, and the EX-PRESS™ shunt.

Although traditionally performed with a retrobulbar block, topical anesthesia augmented with intraoperative sub-Tenon's anesthetic is gaining popularity. Initially, a conjunctival flap is fashioned in either fornix-based or limbus-based fashion, extending posteriorly toward the superior fornix, with care to avoid tears or buttonholes. Light cautery is applied to avoid excessive bleeding. An approximately one-half scleral thickness flap is created, based at and extending into the limbus, maintaining even thickness throughout. There is no consensus on the size or shape of flap necessary to provide adequate IOP control,[33] and this remains the surgeon's preference. Antimetabolite, if indicated, is applied. Alternatively, antimetabolite may be injected into the subconjunctival space prior to the procedure, a technique that is becoming popular with some surgeons. The ocular surface is irrigated and a paracentesis is created to allow for instillation of balanced salt solution (BSS) or viscoelastic into the anterior chamber (AC). If desired, scleral flap sutures can be pre-placed for quick closure of the flap following sclerectomy.

At this point the surgeon may choose to proceed with traditional trabeculectomy or consider the use of the EX-PRESS glaucoma shunt. If the traditional approach is taken, the AC is entered at the base of the scleral flap and a block sclerectomy is made with a blade, a scissors, or a Descemet's punch. It is generally recommended that an iridectomy be made to avoid incarceration of peripheral iris within the sclerostomy, although this may not be necessary in the pseudophakic patient if the chamber is fairly deep. Alternatively, if the EX-PRESS shunt is to be implanted, the surgeon creates a tract for the device using a needle or blade, starting at the scleral blue line and remaining parallel with the iris plane. The EX-PRESS device can then be easily implanted via the inserter by turning it sideways and using gentle rocking pressure until the flange is captured by the internal scleral wall. An iridectomy is not necessary with the EX-PRESS. Scleral flap sutures are then placed and tied, the tightness adjusted to facilitate appropriate transscleral flow of aqueous. The conjunctiva is then sutured, with care taken to achieve a completely watertight closure. This is best achieved with a running double-layer closure of a limbus-based flap, or a running horizontal mattress closure of a fornix-based flap. The AC is pressurized with BSS and a bleb should form. The wound is checked for leaks, and these are repaired as necessary.

Releasable Suture Techniques

Various releasable suture techniques have been reported, initially by Shaffer et al,[34] and subsequently by Cohen and Osher,[35]

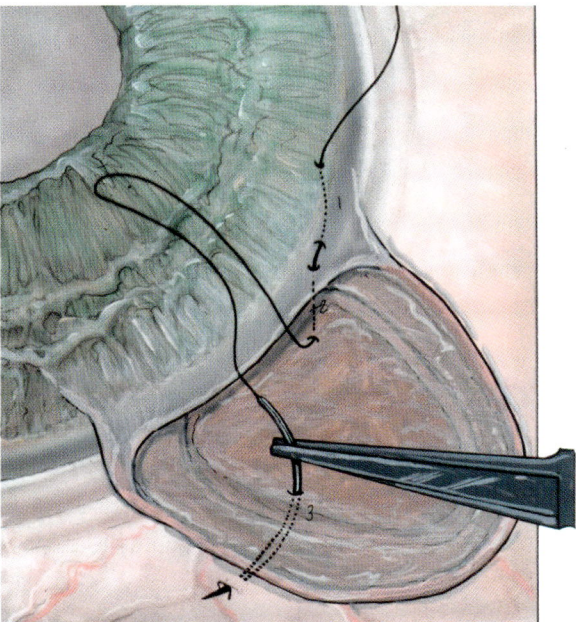

a

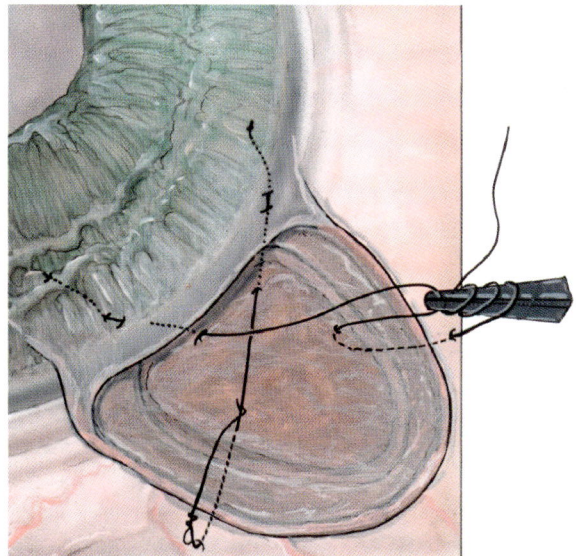

b

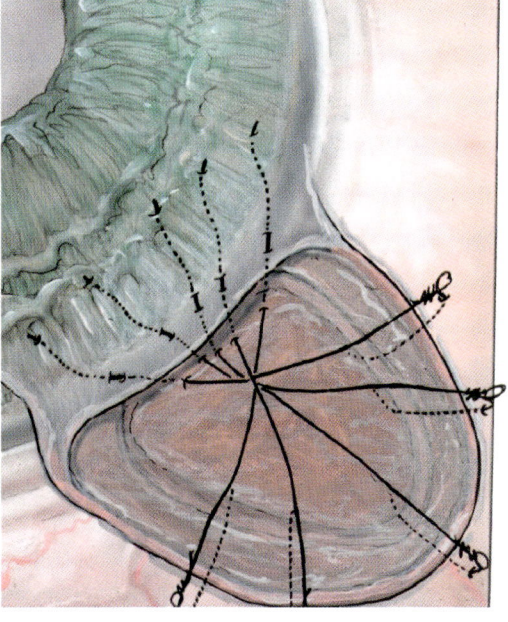

c

Fig. 47.1   (a) Cohen and Osher externalized releasable sutures to close a trabeculectomy flap. The first suture bite is a 2- to 3-mm superficial intracorneal bite that is almost parallel to the limbus. The second suture bite enters the cornea one-half millimeter away from the exit site of the first suture bite. The suture passes into the cornea, into the corneoscleral limbus and out through the trabeculectomy flap (close to the base of the flap). The third suture bite passes through the edge of the trabeculectomy flap into the adjacent sclera. **(b)** The suture is then tied tightly with a four-throw slipknot. The loop is made smaller by pulling on the corneal aspect of the suture. This will facilitate later release. **(c)** All sutures are in position. The excess suture is excised at the entrance of the intracorneal bite to ensure epithelialization of the suture.

Wilson,[36] Shin,[37] Johnstone and coworkers,[38] Hsu and Yarng,[39] and Maberley and coworkers.[40] These suture techniques may be used with either limbus- or fornix-based conjunctival flaps. The Cohen and Osher technique consists of multiple four-throw slipknots of 10-0 or 9-0 nylon, which are used to close the trabeculectomy flap (**Fig. 47.1**). This suturing technique consists of taking three bites and proceeding from the cornea posterior through the scleral flap and emerging from the sclera. The free end of each slipknot is buried within the corneal stroma. In our experience, 9-0 nylon is less likely to break during removal and is preferred.

The Wilson releasable technique also involves taking three suture bites with a square knot (3–1–1–1). This is tied on the epithelial surface of the cornea (**Fig. 47.2**). It is important to cut off the excess suture flush with the knot with a 15-degree blade. This promotes epithelialization of the knot, which is important

for patient comfort postoperatively. This suture often produces some astigmatism until it is either released or the nylon relaxes. However, it may achieve a tighter closure, and is easier to release, than the Cohen and Osher suture. The Wilson suture cannot be easily used at the apex of a triangular trabeculectomy flap, whereas the Cohen and Osher suture can. Therefore, it may be helpful to use both suturing techniques in closing trabeculectomy flaps.

In addition to releasable sutures, an adjustable suturing technique has been introduced by Peng Khaw's group.[41] Rather than the absolute approach of releasable sutures, this technique allows for a titrated increase in transscleral aqueous flow postoperatively. It does, however, require the use of a specially designed forceps (the Khaw Transconjunctival Adjustable Suture Forceps No. 2–502, Duckworth and Kent, Baldock, United Kingdom) to adjust tension on the sutures. The required manipulation can

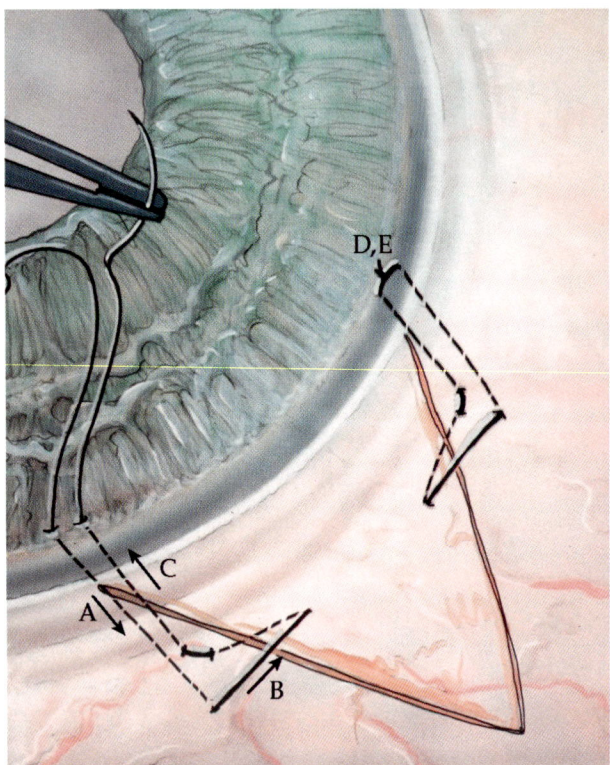

Fig. 47.2 Wilson externalized releasable suture. *A,* bite 1 enters the cornea 1 mm from the conjunctival reflection and passes into the corneoscleral limbus and out the sclera adjacent to the trabeculectomy flap. *B,* bite 2 enters the sclera of the trabeculectomy flap near the edge of the flap and into the sclera adjacent to the trabeculectomy flap. *C,* bite 3 enters the sclera adjacent to the trabeculectomy flap, passes through the corneoscleral limbus, and exits the cornea 1 mm posterior to the conjunctival reflection and 1 to 2 mm nasal to the entrance site for bite 1. *D,* the suture is tied with a 3–1–1–1 throw pattern. *E,* excess suture is cut on the knot with a 15-degree blade to ensure epithelialization.

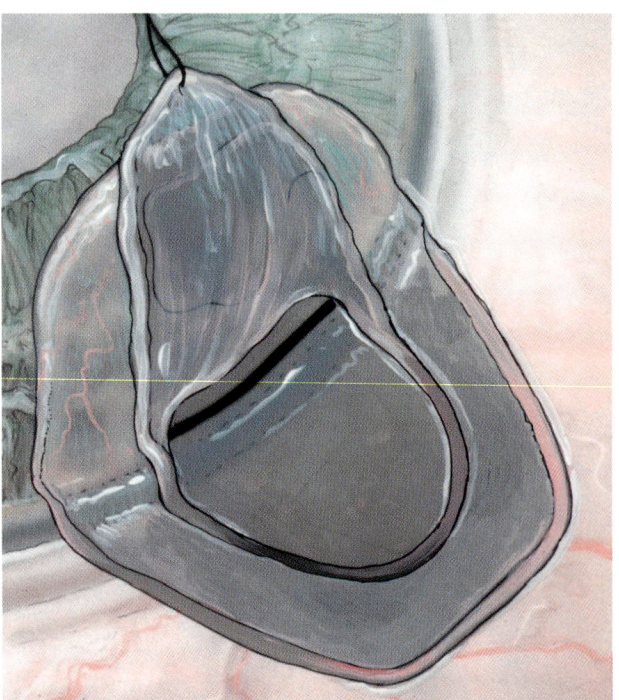

Fig. 47.3 A cataract incision made under a trabeculectomy flap should enter the anterior chamber 1 mm anterior to the anterior edge of the flap to avoid iris prolapse.

lead to conjunctival injury and buttonholes, particular where the conjunctiva is thin and Tenon's is minimal. The technique is best avoided in these cases.

Postoperatively these sutures should be released only if the IOP is higher than desired, and then only after some conjunctival and episcleral healing has occurred. Otherwise, hypotony may result. These releasable suture techniques are a valuable adjunct to trabeculectomy surgery and help to decrease the incidence of postoperative hypotony. They offer the distinct benefit of not having to lyse sutures via laser, an option that may be limited by poor visibility due to blood or thick Tenon's, or by lack of access to an appropriate laser.

One-Site Versus Two-Site Surgery

When combined with trabeculectomy, phacoemulsification can be performed either superiorly, under the trabeculectomy flap, or via a separate incision, most commonly by the clear-corneal temporal approach. The single-site technique offers the advantage of not shifting surgeon and microscope positions during the procedure, saving time. However, this approach requires that phacoemulsification be performed superiorly, a position that may be ergonomically challenging for the surgeon not accustomed to doing so (**Fig. 47.3**).

There has been some debate regarding the outcome of trabeculectomy via the one-site versus two-site approach. Several

studies have found no difference in efficacy in terms of IOP reduction and the postsurgical requirement for glaucoma medication use.[42,43] Others, however, have concluded that two-site surgery offers better long-term IOP reduction and surgical success.[44] In the absence of conclusive data, the surgeon's comfort and familiarity with technique should dictate the surgical approach.

Canaloplasty Procedure

Canaloplasty is essentially an evolution of viscocanalostomy, in which Schlemm's canal is cannulated with a microcatheter that serves to both deliver viscoelastic, dilating the canal over 360 degrees, as well as to position a stenting suture within the canal. The procedure begins with a small limbal peritomy. A superficial scleral flap of approximately one-third to one-half depth is then fashioned, taking care to maintain fairly uniform thickness throughout. This flap need not be of a specific shape or size; however, its width will determine the potential size of the intrascleral lake, and should therefore be at least 4 or 5 mm. Additionally, surgeons unfamiliar with dissection of the deep flap will benefit by starting more posteriorly, then decreasing the radial dimension of the superficial flap as they become more comfortable with the procedure. The deep dissection is then outlined approximately one-half millimeter inside the superficial flap, leaving a small shelf. A deep scleral flap is carefully dissected forward, working in a plane 50 to 100 μm above the choroid. It is important to maintain this plane at the proper depth, or Schlemm's canal will be missed. Once the scleral fibers appear to become more organized, a paracentesis incision is made and the eye is depressurized to 5 to 10 mm Hg. Inadvertent perforation of Descemet's membrane is less likely with a soft eye. Deep dissection is carefully continued anteriorly, unroofing the canal and exposing Descemet's.

At this point it is helpful to use blunt dissection to disinsert Schwalbe's line and carry the flap into the cornea, forming the

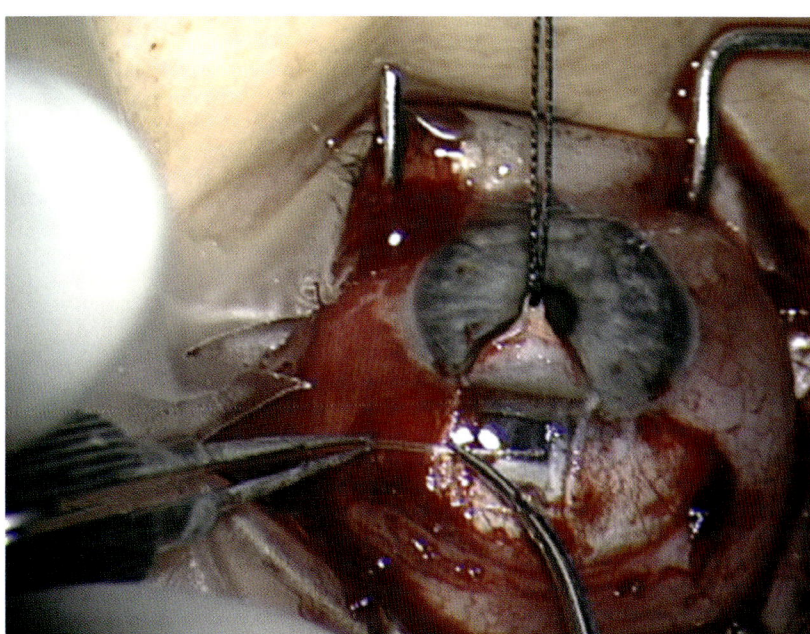

Fig. 47.4 The microcatheter is introduced into Schlemm's canal.

trabeculo-Descemet's window. The window should extend at least 500 µm anterior to Schwalbe's line, as this is the primary means by which aqueous will drain into the scleral lake and canal. The deep flap is then excised, with care taken to not perforate the window. Next, a microcatheter (iTrack-250, Ellex iScience, Menlo Park, CA) is introduced into a cut end of Schlemm's canal, passed 360 degrees, and retrieved from the opposite side (**Figs. 47.4** and **47.5**).

A 9-0 or 10-0 Prolene suture is tied to the end of the catheter, which is then withdrawn as viscoelastic (Healon GV, Abbott Medical Optics, Santa Ana, CA) is slowly but steadily injected to dilate the canal. The suture is cut from the catheter and the ends tightly tied, creating a cerclage-like stent within Schlemm's canal. The tension on this suture is critical, with studies showing that

the ultimate IOP reduction correlates with this tension.[32] The superficial scleral flap is sutured back into place, creating a watertight closure. Finally, the conjunctiva is closed.

Glaucoma Drainage Device Procedure

Drainage devices, or tube shunts, come in two basic forms: valved and nonvalved. Valved shunts offer the advantages of immediate IOP control and, theoretically, prevention of early hypotony. However, the valve mechanism does not always function as intended, sometimes causing hypotony due to excessive flow or late failure due to valve malfunction. Furthermore, early flow

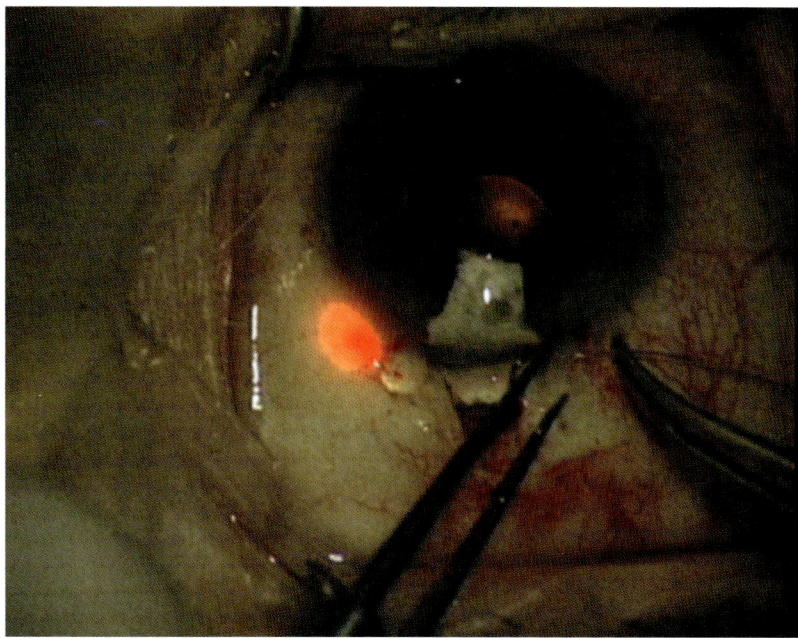

Fig. 47.5 As the catheter passes though Schlemm's canal, the beacon tip can be visualized through the sclera to assist catheter advancement.

of aqueous into the subconjunctival space may cause a more robust encapsulation to develop around the plate, leading to poorer IOP control.[45–47] Nonvalved shunts must be occluded to prevent early flow of aqueous, achieved via placement of ligature sutures that either dissolve or can be removed by the surgeon after plate encapsulation has occurred. These shunts may suffer higher early postoperative IOPs and require more early medication use, but long-term IOP control may be better, with the need for fewer glaucoma medications.[45,46] It has further been suggested that larger plates may lead to lower IOP, but the data on this are unclear. Surgeons must ultimately choose the type of implant with which they are most comfortable and that will achieve the specific treatment goals for the patient.

The procedure is begun with a generous limbal peritomy in the quadrant of shunt placement, with dissection carried posteriorly with tenotomy scissors, creating an adequate pocket for the plate. Lateral relaxing incisions can be helpful for exposure. Light cautery is applied for hemostasis. The shunt is removed from its packaging and inspected. The tube should be irrigated to ensure patency and, in the case of valved shunts, to prime the valve. If the shunt is nonvalved, ligature sutures can be placed at this time. The plate is then slid into the sub-Tenon's pocket and, in the case of a Baerveldt® shunt (Abbott Medical Optics), the wings are captured beneath the surrounding rectus muscles that have been previously hooked. Once in position, the plate is sutured to the sclera with its base at least 10 mm from the limbus. The tube is then placed in its desired position and trimmed to an appropriate size. An anterior bevel will both assist with insertion and help prevent iris incarceration once in the AC. A paracentesis is made, and a 23-gauge needle is then used to create an entry tract, parallel with and close to the iris, starting approximately 2 mm posterior to the limbus. The tube is then inserted into the chamber and its position verified. It is recommended that nonabsorbable sutures secure the tube to the sclera to prevent migration. The tube is then covered with a patch graft of banked sclera, cornea, or several commercially available preparations. Finally, the conjunctiva is closed. The AC is re-formed with BSS and the wounds are checked for any significant leaks.

Intraoperative Complications

Conjunctival Tears and Buttonholes

The creation of a watertight closure in filtering surgery is vital to success and to avoidance of numerous postoperative complications, including hypotony, choroidal effusions, and endophthalmitis. Therefore, great care must be taken when creating the conjunctival flap. Small tears or buttonholes are most likely to occur in the presence of thin, friable tissue, or in areas scarred by prior surgery. Dissection should be performed particularly slowly and methodically in these cases. Proper instrumentation and technique are important, and only non-toothed forceps should be used to manipulate conjunctiva. After the initial incision, blunt dissection should be performed, taking care to handle conjunctiva only along the cut margins. In thin or scarred areas, attention to both sides of the tissue is vital to avoid inadvertent perforation. If a tear or hole is noted, it is best repaired immediately to avoid enlargement as the tissue is further manipulated during the procedure. If a large hole develops in thin conjunctiva prior to scleral dissection, consideration should be given to abandoning that location and identifying healthier tissue before proceeding. Although strict watertight closure is not as important in nonpenetrating surgery, blebs may still form. Furthermore, conversion to a penetrating filtering procedure is occasionally necessary in these procedures. Therefore, similar attention to surgical technique and repair of conjunctival defects is mandatory.

Direct repair of a conjunctival buttonhole can usually be achieved using a 10-0 or 9-0 polyglactin or nylon suture on a tapered needle, either via a purse-string or interrupted technique. If possible, Tenon's capsule should be incorporated into the repair for added strength. For holes or small tears near the limbus in a fornix-based flap, the area may simply be excised and the flap pulled forward for standard closure. Care must be taken, however, with holes in very thin conjunctiva, where Tenon's may also be thin or absent. These holes may form over the scleral flap, particularly when mitomycin has been applied, and must be meticulously repaired to prevent early leaks and hypotony. Thin tissue may be difficult to suture, with "cheese-wiring" and enlargement of the defect. Several novel techniques have been described for dealing with conjunctival holes in such cases. Tissue adhesives, either cyanoacrylate or fibrin-based, have been successfully employed to seal small defects.[48–50] Additionally, intra-bleb injection of sodium hyaluronate 2.3% (Healon 5, Abbott Medical Optics) has been efficacious at closing small buttonholes in thin conjunctiva in a small series.[51] For defects that are not amenable to direct repair by suturing or the use of adhesives, amniotic membrane grafting may enable effective closure.[52]

Scleral Flap Complications

Trabeculectomy

As the primary determinant of aqueous flow and IOP in the early postoperative period, the scleral flap must be fashioned with care. As noted earlier, flap shape is relatively unimportant, but its thickness should be at least one-third to one-half the scleral depth to avoid tearing or avulsing the tissue and to prevent cheese-wiring of sutures. The flap should be dissected anteriorly into clear cornea to create a reasonably anterior sclerostomy, avoiding the ciliary body. However, care should be taken to avoid cutting the lateral flap margins too far beyond the limbus, as this may result in overfiltration and early hypotony.[53] If implanting an EX-PRESS shunt, the flap does not need to be dissected as far anteriorly, as the insertion point is at the scleral spur, posterior to the limbus. Nonetheless, the dissection must be continued slightly beyond the point of insertion to avoid excessive compression of the device and poor resultant flow.

Many complications involving the scleral flap can be avoided by paying attention to risk factors preoperatively and by careful surgical technique. Prior surgery at the intended flap site has already been discussed. In such cases, Tenon's capsule is often scarred and adherent to sclera, and identifying the correct tissue plane can be challenging, leading to irregular flap thickness and margins. High myopia, known to be associated with scleral thinning,[54] may require dissection of a thinner flap, which is more prone to tears or buttonholes, and requires very delicate handling. Other conditions affecting scleral thickness or strength, including scleritis and other autoimmune inflammatory disease, as well as genetic abnormalities such as Ehlers-Danlos and Marfan's syndromes, may predispose to flap complications, and extra care, therefore, must be taken.

The surgeon should attempt to maintain a consistent depth throughout the dissection of the scleral flap. Superficial dissection results in a thin and more easily damaged flap. Overly deep dissection, particularly anteriorly, may lead to premature, posterior entry into the globe with possible bleeding from the ciliary body or iris prolapse. Proper repair of a damaged scleral flap allows the procedure to proceed without significant difficulty in most cases. A thin flap, although not truly a complication, must be handled carefully, as previously noted, to avoid inadvertent tearing or buttonholing. Suture tracts should be a bit longer than usual to prevent cheese-wiring through the edges of the flap.

Should the flap prove too thin to adequately tamponade the flow of aqueous, a patch graft may be necessary to more effectively restrict flow. Small tears, and even complete dehiscence of the scleral flap, can be repaired primarily by suturing using a horizontal mattress technique.[55] The use of donor sclera to create a functional scleral flap has also been described.[56] Again, if primary repair does not adequately strengthen the flap and lead to flow restriction, patch grafting should be performed. Donor scleral or corneal tissue, or a commercially available preparation of sclera, cornea, or pericardium, may be used for this purpose. The use of tissue adhesive, as described in the prior section on conjunctival repair, may also serve as an adjunct to achieving a functional scleral flap.[57]

Canaloplasty/Viscocanalostomy

Superficial Flap

As in trabeculectomy, proper dissection of the scleral flaps, both superficial and deep, is vital in nonpenetrating procedures. The superficial flap is intended to create a watertight closure, eliminating the filtering bleb and its attendant complications. It is therefore important that this flap be of adequate and relatively uniform depth, preferably about one-half scleral thickness. Although the precise size and shape of the flap are not critical, the tangential length should be large enough to allow a reasonably sized scleral lake. At least 4 mm is recommended. Too thin a flap may lead to poor closure, buttonholes, cheese-wiring of sutures, and leaks. An overly thick flap, particularly at the anterior aspect, may cause perforation into the AC. Given the typically large size of this flap, extra care should be taken to maintain the proper tissue plane. A crescent blade may be useful for this dissection, and the surgeon should pay attention to the thickness of the flap margins as well as the central flap. If the flap appears translucent with the blade visible beneath, dissection should be directed more deeply. Tight closure of this flap is necessary at the end of the procedure to prevent formation of a bleb. However, in our experience, a low bleb does occasionally form. These blebs cause no problems, having not been exposed to antimetabolites, and may slightly augment the effect of the procedure.

Deep Flap

Creation of the deep scleral flap necessitates an understanding of and comfort with the surgical anatomy of the AC angle. Dissection of the flap should commence as posteriorly as possible, so that proper depth can be achieved well before Schlemm's canal is approached. Proper depth is determined by either noting the underlying dark choroid though a thin bed of scleral fibers, or by exposing choroid slightly and then backing up 50 to 100 μm. Maintaining this depth as the dissection is carried forward essentially guarantees entry into the canal.

The most common mistake made as the procedure is being learned is dissecting the deep flap too shallowly and passing over the canal. If this occurs, a deeper plane must be established posteriorly. Therefore, dissection should be performed slowly, maintaining a depth just over the choroid. As the limbal blue zone is approached, the deep scleral fibers appear to change direction and become more organized. At this point, the surgeon should create a paracentesis and decompress the eye, thus preventing the soon-to-be-exposed Descemet's membrane from bulging and reducing the risk of inadvertent perforation. Dissection can then be very carefully continued anteriorly, unroofing the canal and exposing trabecular meshwork and Descemet's membrane. The walls of the deep flap should be maintained as vertical as possible at this point, to produce clean Schlemm's canal ostia.

Creation of the trabeculo-Descemet's window is the most delicate aspect of the procedure and involves cautious, sharp dissection of the lateral deep flap margin into clear cornea, while bluntly separating the corneal stroma from Schwalbe's line with a rounded spatula or moistened surgical sponge. Dissection of the lateral margins can be aided by use of a vertically cutting diamond with a specially designed footplate, known as a ZIP blade (model SPDM ZP, Mastel Precision Surgical Instruments, Rapid City, SD), that protects Descemet's membrane as the incision is advanced into the cornea. Blunt dissection is continued until the window is of adequate size, generally at least 400 to 500 μm anterior to Schwalbe's, and the deep flap is excised with a blade or Vannas scissors. A very small perforation of Descemet's at this stage may not be a problem, and the case may proceed normally. Postoperative use of topical pilocarpine may be useful to prevent iris incarceration into the trabeculo-Descemet's window caused by increased flow.[58] A macro-perforation, however, usually necessitates conversion to a trabeculectomy.

Anterior Chamber Entry in Trabeculectomy: Sclerectomy Versus EX-PRESS Shunt

When performing trabeculectomy, the surgeon has the option of standard block/punch sclerectomy or implantation of the EX-PRESS shunt. Block excision, performed with a blade and scissors, offers the least reproducibility and control of sclerectomy size. More commonly, a scleral punch is employed to create an opening of uniform size. Care should be taken to ensure that the full thickness of the scleral lip is engaged, with the punch then turned perpendicular to the eye so that a clean, non-shelved sclerectomy is created. Positioning the punch centrally will help avoid excessive filtration and early hypotony. It has been suggested, however, that the sclerectomy be decentered toward one edge of the scleral flap to improve the likelihood that releasing a flap suture during the postoperative period will result in improved flow and reduced IOP.[59] In this case, care must be taken to ensure adequate flap suture tension to avoid excessive leakage. More recently, Peng Khaw et al[60] have advocated the use of a smaller, 0.5-mm punch to better control aqueous egress, prioritizing the avoidance of early postoperative hypotony.

The development of the EX-PRESS shunt has provided the surgeon with even greater regulation of aqueous flow. Available in two models, with either a 50- or 200-μm lumen, the shunt offers more standardized control of aqueous egress than a sclerectomy. The smaller, 50-μm lumen appears to be adequate in the majority of cases. A prospective randomized study comparing EX-PRESS with standard trabeculectomy reported significantly better control of IOP during the first 3 years of follow-up, with 66.7% of EX-PRESS eyes versus 38.5% of standard trabeculectomy eyes demonstrating an IOP less than 15 mm Hg at 3 years.[61] The trend continued at 5 years, but was not statistically significant. Furthermore, fewer glaucoma medications and postoperative interventions for complications were required following EX-PRESS surgery throughout the 5-year follow-up. Additional studies have confirmed IOP reduction with EX-PRESS that is equal to or better than that with trabeculectomy alone, with significantly reduced rates of complications, particularly early hypotony, as well as fewer required glaucoma medications.[62–64] Our personal experience reflects these findings, with less hypotony, fewer hyphemas, and an overall smoother postoperative course.

Implantation of the EX-PRESS device is relatively straightforward but requires careful attention to anatomic landmarks. The scleral spur and limbal blue zone must be identified, and a 26-gauge needle used to create an entry tract at the junction of these structures, parallel with the iris. Angling the entry anteriorly or posteriorly results in the implant potentially contacting the cornea or iris, respectively. The needle should be inserted and withdrawn smoothly, as excessive lateral movement may allow fluid to escape around the shunt. Additionally, the scleral bed should be of adequate thickness to support the device, as a thin bed may either tear during insertion or may allow for too much movement of the shunt, risking injury to adjacent structures or even a rare dislocation of the device.[65] If a thin bed and unstable shunt are noted after insertion, the shunt should be removed and a standard sclerectomy performed.

Bleeding and Hyphema

Intraoperative bleeding is a common complication in glaucoma surgery, and can range from a mere nuisance to a vision-threatening hemorrhage, though the latter is uncommon. Conjunctival and episcleral bleeding is usually mild and self-limited, but may be greater in patients on anticoagulants, as noted previously. A combination of judicious cautery and localized pressure with a cotton-tipped applicator usually suppresses the bleeding. The development of extensive subconjunctival hemorrhage should be avoided in filtering surgery, as this may plug the scleral flap and hinder bleb formation, increase inflammation, and potentially lead to surgical failure. In the case of canaloplasty, cautery of the scleral surface should be minimized, as this may damage the episcleral vessels that drain the aqueous collector channels, decreasing the efficacy of the procedure.[66] Surface bleeding is primarily a nuisance in drainage device surgery, although significant thickening of Tenon's fascia due to hematoma, although uncommon, can cause difficulty with conjunctival closure.

Intraoperative hyphema is a relatively common complication in filtering surgery, occurring in 8% of trabeculectomies in one large multicenter clinical trial.[67] Bleeding develops most commonly during iridectomy, but may also occur during creation of the sclerectomy or implantation of an EX-PRESS shunt or drainage device tube. When possible, bleeding from the iris base or sclerectomy margins should be cauterized, which is best performed with a fine needle-tipped probe. Direct pressure with a cotton-tipped applicator may also be useful. In most cases, hemorrhaging stops spontaneously, but closing the eye and elevating the IOP, either with BSS or viscoelastic, may be required to tamponade the offending vessels.

Limited hyphema during canaloplasty is also quite common.[32,68] The main source of bleeding appears to be reflux from Schlemm's canal into the depressurized eye.[66] One recent study found that surgical success and degree of IOP reduction correlated positively with presence and height of microhyphema on postoperative day 1, with 88% with hyphema versus 38% without hyphema achieving a 30% or greater reduction in pressure at 24 months.[69] The authors suggest that hyphema in this context should not be considered a complication, but rather an indicator that the collector system is functioning. Small hyphemas in canaloplasty are nearly always self-limited with no adverse consequences, and blood seldom remains in the AC beyond 1 week.

Vitreous Prolapse

The risk factors, etiologies, and management of vitreous loss due to capsular tears or zonular defects are addressed in more detailed discussions in many other chapters in this book. When combined with a glaucoma procedure, care must be taken to remove all lens fragments, cortex, and vitreous according to the principles discussed. This is necessary to minimize postoperative inflammation, which may cause increased scarring and failure of the glaucoma procedure. If vitreous is present in the AC

postoperatively, it may block or form anterior synechiae to Descemet's window in a canaloplasty or to the sclerectomy in a trabeculectomy. In this case, an additional surgical intervention with anterior vitrectomy and lysis of vitreous bands may be required. Sometimes vitreous bands can be lysed with the yttrium-aluminum-garnet (YAG) laser. However, this frequently requires high energy and a large number of pulses. This can increase the inflammation in the AC with a resultant increased risk of failure of the glaucoma procedure. Subconjunctival Depo-Medrol or Kenalog (triamcinolone 20 to 40 mg) should be routinely given after combined phaco–glaucoma procedures, but especially after cases in which more inflammation is anticipated.

If the anterior capsular rim is intact, and a posterior capsular rent cannot be converted into a continuous tear by capsulorrhexis, then a posterior chamber intraocular lens (IOL) should be placed in the ciliary sulcus. If the diameter of the anterior capsulotomy is smaller than that of the IOL optic, the optic of the IOL should be captured within the anterior capsule. This ensures a snug fit between the edge of the capsulorrhexis and the posterior edge of the optic and makes herniation of vitreous into the AC unlikely. Additionally, it also stabilizes the lens implant, making anterior displacement of the lens less likely if postoperative hypotony occurs. The haptics of a posterior chamber lens placed in the ciliary sulcus should be oriented in a meridian perpendicular to the meridian of the glaucoma operation. This prevents iris from being pushed anteriorly at the site of Descemet's window (in a canaloplasty) or the sclerectomy (in a trabeculectomy), thereby reducing the risk of synechiae. If there is an anterior capsular rent in conjunction with an intact posterior capsule, a posterior chamber (PC) IOL can usually be gently placed in the capsular bag. If both the anterior and posterior capsules have been damaged to a significant degree, then a suture fixated PC IOL in the ciliary sulcus or an AC IOL may be necessary. If either a ciliary sulcus suture-fixated PC IOL or an AC IOL is used, it is best to place the haptics away from Descemet's window or the sclerectomy. This helps to minimize inflammation in the immediate area and makes the occurrence of peripheral anterior synechiae, with subsequent failure of the glaucoma procedure, less likely.

Less commonly, vitreous may present during trabeculectomy if the sclerectomy is made too far posteriorly. This typically occurs following iridectomy when the scleral flap has not been dissected far enough into clear cornea, or occasionally if a canaloplasty must be converted to trabeculectomy due to macroperforation of Descemet's window. Vitreous may also present at this location through a zonular defect during an otherwise normal case. Regardless, the principles of meticulous vitreous cleanup must be maintained to prevent vitreous from plugging the sclerectomy and possibly causing surgical failure. Although anterior vitrectomy via the sclerostomy is most straightforward in this situation, it seems reasonable to suggest that a pars plana approach might be more successful, maintaining vitreous posteriorly rather than pulling it anteriorly. Ultimately, this issue is best avoiding by ensuring adequate scleral flap dissection and anterior placement of the sclerectomy.

Intraoperative Complications Unique to Canaloplasty

Although canaloplasty shares many potential complications with other glaucoma surgeries, some problems are unique to the procedure, related to the microcatheter, viscodissection, and stent suture placement.

Although Schlemm's canal has been properly unroofed, the ostia may be difficult to identify and catheterize. This may be due to irregular dissection of the deep flap walls, or simply due to collapse of the canal, causing the ostia to appear as tiny slits. Careful dissection along the lateral flap margin may improve visualization of an ostium. Additionally, there is often slight reflux of blood from the canal ostia, as the IOP has been reduced below episcleral venous pressure. Using the scleral spur and pigmented trabecular meshwork as a landmark and moving laterally, a 30-gauge viscocanalostomy cannula can be used to enter an ostium. Gentle injection of BSS causes blanching of episcleral vessels if the canal has been entered properly. Injecting a small amount of viscoelastic to maintain patency aids in placement of the microcatheter.

Once the microcatheter has been introduced into the canal, it is passed 360 degrees around the chamber using a steady hand-over-hand approach. Occasionally, an obstruction is encountered, preventing further advancement. In this case, the surgeon should back up and attempt passage again, as the catheter may be caught on a septum or the edge of a collector channel. Gentle pressure over the point of resistance while pushing the catheter forward often enables passing the obstruction. A final option is to create a slight bend in the catheter tip, which may enable it to slip around a blockage. If all attempts fail, passage should be restarted from the opposite ostium, which nearly always facilitates successful passage. If, despite all efforts, the canal cannot be fully circumnavigated by the catheter, the surgeon must decide whether to simply perform a viscocanalostomy or to convert to a trabeculectomy.

Observation of the beacon light at the catheter tip is important, as this helps to identify malposition of the device. Occasionally, the catheter appears to be moving through the canal, but the beacon is seen either moving posteriorly or, occasionally, entering the AC. This signifies a false passage into the suprachoroidal space and is seldom a significant problem, though a limited hyphema may occur if the chamber has been breached. Simply retract the catheter slowly, properly identify the canal ostium, and begin passage again.

Viscodilation of Schlemm's canal is performed as the catheter is retracted, with care taken to ensure slow, steady release of viscoelastic. Excessive viscodissection may lead to Descemet's detachment, in which the sub-Descemet's space is filled with viscoelastic or blood, a finding noted in numerous studies.[32,58,70] The occurrence rate of this complication is generally low, with one recent report of 7.4% (12 of 162 eyes).[70] The majority of these were small, measuring less than 3 mm, and resolved spontaneously over 4 to 6 weeks, with no significant sequelae. Three required drainage at the slit lamp, and two of these resolved completely. The final patient ultimately developed corneal decompensation requiring penetrating keratoplasty. Thus, although a relatively uncommon and usually benign complication, Descemet's detachment is best avoided by slow and gentle viscodilation of the canal. Small detachments can be observed and they usually resolve, whereas larger occurrences may require drainage.

Postoperative Complications Common to All Surgeries

Hyphema

Postoperative hyphema is common in glaucoma surgery. Although rates in the literature vary, studies suggest the occurrence of significant bleeding in up to 25% of trabeculectomies.[28,67,71] The incidence of hyphema in drainage device surgery appears to be less, with the majority of hyphemas occurring in patient with neovascular glaucoma.[72,73] Small hyphemas after canaloplasty, a normal and self-limited occurrence, have been discussed previ-

ously. Preoperative considerations regarding anticoagulant use have already been addressed, as has the importance of hemostasis intraoperatively. Nonetheless, significant hyphema continues to plague the surgeon following filtering surgery, although there may have been no evidence of bleeding at the end of the procedure. These delayed hemorrhages may be caused by postoperative hypotony, or may be due to Valsalva maneuver or eye rubbing. Additionally, manipulations performed by the surgeon during the postoperative period, such as digital massage of the bleb, suture lysis/removal, or needle revision of a failing bleb at the slit lamp may cause undesired bleeding.[74,75]

In the event of significant hyphema, the patient should be instructed to limit physical activity and to sleep with the head of the bed elevated to maintain better vision. An eye shield should be worn at all times to prevent accidental trauma. Blood thinning medications must be avoided. The IOP may need to be controlled with topical medications, or possibly with oral carbonic anhydrase inhibitors. Increased topical steroids may be useful to limit the inflammatory reaction and fibrin production stimulated by the blood. With such conservative measures, the majority of smaller hyphemas resolve, usually within 1 to 2 weeks, as the clot hemolyzes. A larger hyphema that is not clearing, however, may require surgical intervention with AC washout. Prolonged presence of blood in the AC may cause elevated IOP due to clogging of the sclerostomy, EX-PRESS shunt, or tube, ultimately leading to surgical failure. Anterior synechiae or corneal blood staining may also result. The amount of blood and the IOP dictate the urgency of intervention.

Hypotony

Although the goal of glaucoma surgery is reduction of the IOP to a low enough level to preserve vision, an overly low tension is not well tolerated by most eyes, leading to changes within ocular structures that can adversely affect visual acuity, including maculopathy and corneal edema.[76] Achieving the appropriate balance surgically can be difficult, and early postoperative hypotony is quite common following filtration surgery, occurring in as many as one third of procedures.[28,77,78] Hypotony may be statistically defined as an IOP below 6 mm Hg, or 3 standard deviations below the mean.[79] As the adverse clinical manifestations of low IOP often occur below this level, 6 mm Hg shall be considered the definition of hypotony for this discussion. The use of antimetabolites, primarily in trabeculectomy, has certainly improved surgical success, but it has also resulted in a significant increase in early hypotony.[78,80] Uncommonly, low IOP is due to decreased aqueous production, which may occur in cases of intraocular inflammation, in the presence of a large choroidal or retinal detachment, or with the concomitant use of aqueous suppressants, such as oral carbonic anhydrase inhibitors or β-blockers.[81] Such conditions are usually easily ruled out. In most cases, hypotony is caused by excessive aqueous outflow. Thus, many cases of postoperative low IOP can be avoided by careful attention to detail during surgery.

Trabeculectomy Hypotony

Overfiltration

The primary determinant of early postoperative IOP following trabeculectomy is the resistance created by the scleral flap.[82] Therefore, strict attention should be paid to the tension on flap sutures prior to closure of the conjunctiva. Inflating the AC with BSS to physiological pressure enables the surgeon to check the rate of transscleral flow as well as the maintenance of chamber depth and globe firmness. It is often best to leave the flap somewhat tight with minimal flow and to make adjustments to sutures postoperatively, particularly in patients at increased risk for hypotony and its complications, such as high myopes or older patients with vascular disease.[83] The use of an AC infusion line has been advocated as a means of maintaining rigidity of the globe intraoperatively, minimizing the risk of choroidal effusions, and facilitating estimation of scleral flow after suturing of the flap.[60] If the chamber fails to remain well formed as flow is monitored, additional sutures should be placed until adequate pressurization of the globe is maintained. Of course, watertight conjunctival closure is also vital to surgical success and the avoidance of hypotony, and any conjunctival defects, whether buttonholes or wound leaks, must be meticulously closed before the procedure is completed.

Beyond the early postoperative period, episcleral and conjunctival healing begin to have a greater impact on aqueous outflow and IOP, and the effects of mitomycin C become more pronounced. A scleral flap that fails to adequately restrict flow initially typically heals via episcleral fibrosis, but this process may be inhibited by mitomycin, leading to more prolonged hypotony.[83] Additionally, postoperative manipulations of the scleral flap, such as suture lysis or removal, or needling of an encapsulated bleb or fibrotic flap, can cause a precipitous drop in IOP that is slow to return to acceptable levels.[75,84–87] Hypotony in these circumstances typically presents with a diffuse, intact, functional bleb. In most cases, resolution comes about with nothing more than routine postoperative care, though more frequent follow-up is recommended to monitor for complications. Some patients tolerate prolonged hypotony with no discernible adverse effects or complaints, and may be monitored indefinitely as long as visual acuity does not suffer. If, however, visual symptoms or significant AC shallowing are present, then treatment is indicated.

Early hypotony may respond to more rapid reduction in topical steroid dosing, allowing episcleral and conjunctival fibrosis to develop. Pressure patching or the use of a scleral shell or large-diameter contact lens flattens the conjunctiva and scleral flap and may promote fibrosis, leading to elevated IOP.[88,89] Autologous blood injection into the bleb, possibly combined with conjunctival compression sutures, may also cause fibrosis and raise IOP.[90–92] As long as the AC remains deep, these relatively conservative measures may suffice. However, if the chamber shallows significantly, additional action may be required. In general, it has been our experience that AC shallowing in pseudophakic eyes is less severe and better tolerated than in phakic eyes, and may be monitored for a more extended period as long as the central chamber is not flat. Pharmacological measures, such as use of topical atropine or other cycloplegics, may help deepen the chamber by restoring the normal anatomy of the iris and ciliary body, lessening iridocorneal contact. If necessary, AC reformation with a viscoelastic, injected via a paracentesis at the slit lamp, is easily performed and may lead to resolution of hypotony, though multiple injections may be required.[93,94]

Ultimately, if persistent hypotony causes continued poor vision, shallow chamber, or evidence of hypotony maculopathy such as choroidal folds or macular edema, then surgical revision is indicated. This may be achieved by opening the conjunctiva and placing additional sutures to tighten the scleral flap.[95,96] Transconjunctival suturing of the scleral flap, as has been recently described,[97,98] has been found to be safe and effective, is less invasive, and can be performed at the slit lamp. Eyes suffering late hypotony, which is often due to progressive thinning of the scleral flap and conjunctiva following exposure to mitomycin, may not be amenable to these techniques. In such cases, more complex revisions involving patch grafts to reinforce the sclera, and either conjunctival advancement or free conjunctival grafts will be required.[99–101] Drainage of choroidal effusion is also often necessary.

Conjunctival Leaks

Wound leaks may occur early following surgery due to inadequate conjunctival closure, or may develop subsequently due to poor healing, particularly following exposure to mitomycin C. Furthermore, mitomycin-exposed conjunctiva may become progressively avascular and thin over time, leading to late bleb leaks and hypotony.[83] All patients with hypotony, particularly when IOP has dropped substantially from the prior visit, must be checked for the presence of conjunctival leaks via the Seidel test, using either moistened fluorescein strips or 2% fluorescein solution. If using a strip, care should be taken to "paint" the entire bleb. Leaks in the hypotonous eye may be intermittent and not immediately apparent, possibly requiring prolonged observation to be identified. Gentle pressure on the globe will raise IOP and may reveal an occult leak. Management of leaks is dependent on the location and the condition of the surrounding tissue.

An early leak, whether a buttonhole or wound-related, can be observed as long as the AC remains formed. Small leaks may respond to conservative therapy, including a decrease in the frequency of topical steroids to allow more rapid fibrosis and wound healing. Aqueous suppressants, including oral carbonic anhydrase inhibitors and topical β-blockers, can decrease the flow of fluid through the leak and may improve the chances of closure.[77–79] Additionally, a large-diameter bandage contact lens or Simmons Shell will cover the defect, protecting it from trauma, and can lead to complete resolution of the leak.[89,102,103] Topical antibiotics should be continued until the leak is fully resolved, and topical steroids increased in frequency to normal levels as soon as possible to diminish inflammation and avoid surgical failure.

Another conservative approach is the use of cyanoacrylate tissue glue, as noted previously for management of intraoperative conjunctival defects.[48–50,103] Care must be taken to apply only a small amount of glue with the wooden end of a cotton-tipped applicator, a small plastic micropipette, or a thin glass rod. The conjunctival surface must be fairly dry to enable the glue to stick, which can be difficult to achieve in the presence of a leak. Finally, a bandage contact lens should be placed to avoid both traumatic dislocation of the adhesive and patient discomfort, and multiple reapplications of glue may be required to achieve resolution.[104]

Fibrin tissue adhesive may also be used to seal an early or late conjunctival leak.[50,105,106] Two products, Tisseel (Baxter International, Deerfield, IL) and Evicel (Johnson & Johnson, Somerville, NJ), are Food and Drug Administration (FDA)-approved and readily available for use in the United States. Both are produced from pooled plasma and share the threat of transmission of blood-borne pathogens, but such risk has been largely mitigated by improved plasma fractionation practices.[107] Alternatively, autologous fibrin can be employed, but production requires equipment and reagents not typically found in the ophthalmologist's office or surgery center, making this approach inconvenient.[50] Compared with cyanoacrylate-based adhesives, fibrin sealants have the advantages of greater ease of application, in layers if necessary, improved biocompatibility with creation of a scaffold for cellular adhesion for improved wound healing, and a nonirritant nature, obviating the need for a bandage contact lens.

Failure of more conservative measures to heal a leak will necessitate surgical repair. An early leak, particularly of the wound margin, can usually be repaired by directly suturing the defect, as the tissue has not become ischemic and thin. As noted previously, conjunctiva is best sutured using 8-0 or 9-0 Vicryl on a tapered needle, which minimizes the size of the holes created.

We have found that a running horizontal mattress technique improves the odds of successful closure. When suturing conjunctiva to either sclera or cornea, such as when repairing the dehiscence of a fornix-based flap, a needle with a small cutting tip (Ethicon VAS 100–4) is helpful, as a tapered needle is quite difficult to pass through firmer tissue. Buttonholes are repaired using a purse-string or interrupted technique, as noted previously.

Late conjunctival leaks often develop in the presence of thin, avascular conjunctiva due to the long-term effects of mitomycin C, and are usually not amenable to direct repair given the friable nature of the tissue. These cases require revision with conjunctival advancement flaps or free autografts, and may necessitate scleral reinforcement with a patch graft if aqueous flow is found to be excessive.[99-101] The conjunctiva should be cut posterior to the area of thinning, within healthy, vascular tissue, followed by blunt dissection posteriorly and laterally to mobilize as much conjunctiva as possible. The atrophic bleb can be retained, but all epithelium should be removed from the ischemic conjunctiva and limbus to promote adhesion and avoid formation of epithelial cysts. The advancement flap is then sutured anteriorly to the limbus. If excessive tension is noted, a relaxing incision can be made posteriorly in the conjunctiva, which can then be sutured to underlying Tenon's fascia. If it is determined that enough healthy conjunctiva does not exist for adequate closure, then a free autograft, typically taken from inferiorly in the same eye, will be necessary. As a whole, these techniques are quite successful at eliminating leaks, resolving hypotony, and maintaining IOP control, but additional glaucoma medications are often necessary.[108,109]

Glaucoma Drainage Devices Hypotony

Hypotony following drainage device surgery may be due to overfiltration, aqueous hyposecretion, or, less commonly, wound leak. The causes of aqueous hyposecretion are the same as those following trabeculectomy, including choroidal or retinal detachment, excessive inflammation, or use of aqueous suppressants. In such cases, treatment of the underlying condition promotes resolution of hypotony.

The primary etiology of hypotony in the early postoperative period following tube shunt surgery is overfiltration, the causes of which vary slightly by type of shunt. Independent of shunt design, leakage around the tube may lead to very low IOP in the days immediately following the procedure, and careful surgical technique will mitigate the risk.[110] Scleral entry with a 23-gauge needle usually results in a tightly fitting tube, with low risk of significant leakage. Creation of a fairly long intrascleral track, preferably at least 2 to 3 mm, also reduces the risk of peritubular leakage.[111] Use of a larger diameter needle, or lateral movements of the needle tip to widen the tract for easier tube insertion, may lead to excessive flow. Occasionally, creation of a second entry tract may be necessary due to poor tube positioning in the AC. In such cases, care must be taken to properly close the initial sclerostomy tightly. Absorbable sutures, such as Vicryl, work well in this role, as any induced astigmatism will resolve as the sutures dissolve. Areas of thin sclera, such as adjacent to a prior trabeculectomy flap, should be avoided when possible, as there is greater risk for aqueous leakage.

The type of drainage device implanted also impacts the risk of postoperative hypotony. Two basic drainage device styles are available: restricted and unrestricted. Restricted devices, also known as valved shunts, have a mechanism within the plate body meant to limit the early postoperative flow of aqueous humor, theoretically reducing the risk of hypotony.[112] Although these shunts offer the advantage of immediate IOP reduction, the flow restrictors do not always function as intended or may be damaged during tube priming, leading to extremely low early postoperative IOP. Unrestricted implants, in contrast, offer no early resistance to aqueous flow and must be completely ligated, typically with an absorbable suture, to avoid early hypotony.[113] The ligature dissolves in 4 to 6 weeks following surgery, allowing the tube to open and drain aqueous. To allow some immediate postoperative flow and avoid significantly elevated IOP, most surgeons create venting incisions within the tube proximal to the ligature using a suture needle or small blade, thus allowing early egress of aqueous. Although generally successful at producing a reasonable postoperative IOP, this practice can lead to excessive flow and hypotony. Furthermore, failure of adequate fibrous encapsulation to develop around the plate by the time the tube opens can cause a sudden drop in IOP.[114]

Hypotony following drainage device implantation can usually be managed relatively conservatively, as most cases resolve as fibrous encapsulation of the plate develops and resistance to aqueous outflow increases.[114] If significant choroidal effusions and AC shallowing develop, injection of a viscoelastic agent into the chamber provides transient deepening, elevation of IOP, and reduced flow through the tube. Repeated injections may be required to stabilize the globe until encapsulation results in maintenance of an adequate pressure. Prolonged instability of the chamber and IOP, particularly in cases at greater risk for more severe hypotony-related complications, should be addressed surgically. Ligature of the tube, although not commonly necessary, is relatively straightforward and effective at resolving hypotony, with greater success found using nonabsorbable versus absorbable sutures.[115]

Elevated Intraocular Pressure and Surgical Failure

Trabeculectomy

Deep Anterior Chamber

Early elevated IOP following trabeculectomy, in the presence of a deep AC, is nearly always due to underfiltration, caused either by overly tight scleral flap sutures or mechanical obstruction of the sclerostomy or EX-PRESS shunt. Careful examination usually reveals the etiology. Extensive subconjunctival hemorrhage may obstruct the scleral flap. The presence of excessive blood or fibrin within the AC may lead to blockage of aqueous outflow. The configuration of the pupil may suggest iris incarceration at the sclerostomy. Gonioscopy should be performed to confirm these findings.

Relatively mild digital massage in the region of the scleral flap typically produces egress of aqueous in the presence of tight sutures, proving this to be the primary issue. In such cases, improved flow may develop spontaneously as tissues stretch over the first couple of weeks postoperatively. Failure to achieve an adequate IOP will prompt either laser suture lysis or removal of releasable sutures. The direction in which the bleb expands during massage often indicates which suture's removal is most likely to effect the greatest improvement in flow. Suture lysis or removal is best avoided during the first 2 weeks postoperatively, as this may cause prolonged hypotony, although long-term reduction in IOP may benefit from earlier intervention.[85,116]

If digital massage is initially unsuccessful, more direct manipulation of the flap margin can be achieved with a cotton-tipped applicator using the Carlo Traverso Maneuver (CTM), named for the physician who initially described it.[117] Under topical anesthesia, a moistened applicator is placed adjacent or posterior to the scleral flap with pressure applied to deform the globe. This maneuver often promotes flow, possibly by dislodging either an internal obstruction or a blood clot at the scleral flap margin. This means of reestablishing aqueous flow may be all that is required to produce effective filtration. In some cases, however, no amount of massage or focal pressure reestablishes outflow. If no clear obstruction is visible on examination, suture lysis or removal should be considered. However, other interventions may be considered if obstructing material is identified. Iris incarceration may be alleviated by use of miotics such as pilocarpine. Blood, fibrin, vitreous, iris tissue, or fragments of Descemet's membrane may be dislodged via gonioscopically directed YAG or argon laser.[118,119] Additionally, tissue plasminogen activator (tPA; Activase®, Genentech, San Francisco, CA), in doses of 6 to 25 µg, may be useful to dissolve blood or fibrin that is obstructing the outflow pathway. Such treatment has been reported to reestablish flow and lower IOP when injected either subconjunctivally for an adherent scleral flap,[120] or intracamerally. Doses less than 12.5 µg appear less likely to cause hyphema.[121] Ultimately, if IOP can be temporarily managed with topical medication, and if the eye can tolerate the level of increased IOP, obstructions due to blood and fibrin tend to resolve spontaneously as reabsorption occurs.

Elevation in IOP may also occur several weeks to months following trabeculectomy due either to fibrous encapsulation of the filtering bleb or to episcleral fibrosis of the flap. Bleb encapsulation tends to present at between 2 and 8 weeks postoperatively as a tense, elevated, often quite vascular elevation of Tenon's capsule and conjunctiva, associated with a significant increase in IOP that is unresponsive to bleb massage. Rates of encapsulation are reported between 2.5% and 18.5%, although the higher incidence is associated with procedures performed prior to the routine use of antimetabolites, specifically mitomycin C.[122,123] Bleb encapsulation may be managed medically, with topical or oral ocular antihypertensive agents and steroids, often with a gradual decline in IOP and improved bleb morphology occurring over several months.[124] If more rapid decompression of the encapsulated bleb is necessary, needle revision can be performed with adjunctive 5-fluorouracil.[125,126] Commonly described as "bleb needling," this procedure can usually be comfortably performed at the slit lamp under topical anesthesia. After placement of a lid speculum and instillation of topical antibiotic and/or povidone-iodine, a 27- or 30-gauge needle is inserted subconjunctivally near the margin of the bleb, outside the encapsulated area. The needle is then advanced into and withdrawn from the encapsulated Tenon's cyst repeatedly, creating numerous perforations, using the needle tip to incise as much of the capsule wall as possible (**Fig. 47.6**). It is common to see the area of encapsulation flatten and a much more diffuse bleb form quite rapidly upon decompression. Then 5-fluorouracil, 0.1 to 0.2 mL of 50 mg/mL solution, is injected into the bleb or, alternatively, in the inferior fornix. If necessary, this procedure can be repeated if encapsulation redevelops. One prospective randomized study comparing needling with medical management found that, although both methods were effective at reducing IOP, bleb needling produced a significantly lower mean IOP at 12 months.[126]

Fibrosis of the scleral flap, often occurring months to years following trabeculectomy, is the most common cause of late IOP elevation and surgical failure, and is heralded by flattening of a previously elevated bleb. Bleb needling is an effective means of managing such late failures.[75,127] The procedure is similar to needling an encapsulated bleb, and has been described using either 5-fluorouracil or mitomycin C. In this case, the antimetabolite is often injected subconjunctivally in the region of the bleb and allowed to diffuse prior to needling. The use of mitomycin C, 0.2 mL of a 0.2 mg/mL solution, has been described as safe and effective.[75] The needle tip is used to perforate the adhesions between the scleral flap and bed, elevating at least one corner of the flap. Some surgeons prefer to introduce the needle into the

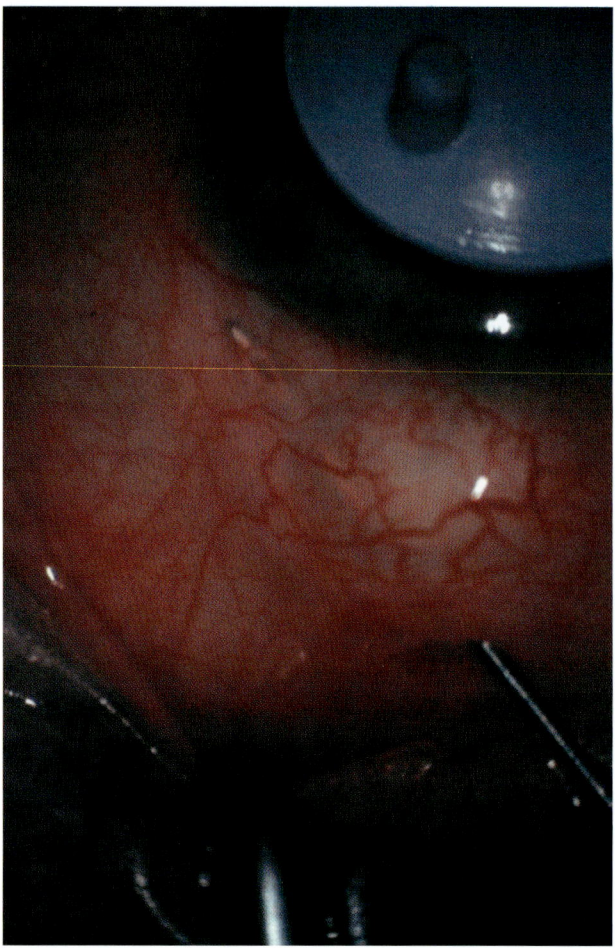

Fig. 47.6 Photograph of the needling of an encysted bleb with a 27-gauge needle. It is important to puncture the fibrous wall of the bleb multiple times with a forward and backward motion of the needle rather than a side-to-side motion.

AC to prove that the sclerostomy is patent, a maneuver that is not possible with an EX-PRESS shunt. Success rates of 64% achieving IOP less than 21 mm Hg[75] and 71% achieving IOP less than 16 mm Hg[128] have been reported for revision with mitomycin, which has been found more effective than 5-fluorouracil.[128]

In late-failing blebs where obstruction to the sclerostomy is thought to be the etiology for failure, internal revision of the ostomy may be possible via neodymium:yttrium-aluminum-garnet (Nd:YAG) laser application.[118,119,129] The success of this procedure may be augmented by injection of subconjunctival 5-fluorouracil.[130]

Ultimately, if the early- or late-failing bleb fails to respond to the above methods, surgical revision in the operating room may be indicated. If, however, successful salvage is deemed unlikely, then consideration should be given to proceeding with another glaucoma procedure at a separate site.

Shallow Anterior Chamber

As noted previously, a shallow AC following trabeculectomy is most commonly due to wound leaks or overfiltration with the development of choroidal effusions, and typically presents with significant hypotony. However, a shallow chamber can also be associated with elevated IOP, the causes of which must be identified and managed expeditiously to avoid loss of vision.

Although less common than in a phakic eye, pupillary block can occur in the pseudophakic eye, developing more often with an AC IOL. However, pupillary block has been reported following implantation of PC IOLs as well.[131,132] In such cases there are often predisposing factors, such as excessive inflammation, short axial length, or sulcus positioning of the lens. If suspected, and posterior segment pathology is ruled out by examination, this condition is managed by iridotomy, which is both diagnostic and therapeutic in this situation.

Suprachoroidal hemorrhage (SCH) can also present with a shallow AC, often associated with elevated IOP, significant pain, nausea, and vomiting. The incidence of postoperative SCH following glaucoma surgery has been reported to be 1.6 to 6.2%, using various diagnostic criteria.[133] Risk factors include high myopia, hypertension, anticoagulation, high preoperative IOP, older age, diabetes, and vitrectomized status. However, the primary risk factor, and often the inciting event, is profound hypotony.[133-135] When operating on patients at significant risk of SCH, it is advisable to take steps to avoid severe acute hypotony. The scleral flap should be sutured with enough tension to maintain adequate postoperative IOP. Additional flap sutures may be placed so that lysis or removal can be performed in a more controlled manner, avoiding sudden, large drops in pressure. Consideration should be given to discontinuing anticoagulants prior to surgery, if possible.[135] Avoidance of postoperative SCH is key, as vision outcomes following such events are typically poor.

If pupillary block and SCH have been ruled out, the finding of significant axial shallowing in the presence of elevated or normal IOP is likely due to malignant glaucoma. This condition, the mechanisms of which are not fully understood, has also been called aqueous misdirection, although posteriorly diverted aqueous may not play a major role in the pathogenesis of the condition. Rather, it has been suggested that choroidal expansion, in the setting of poor vitreous conductivity, leads to anterior movement of the lens–iris diaphragm and closure of the angle.[136,137] The majority of affected eyes have hyperopic refractions preoperatively, with shorter than average axial length. Therefore, this condition should be suspected in such eyes presenting with axial shallowing and elevated IOP. Treatment involves controlling IOP and restoring normal anatomic relationships, often by disrupting the anterior hyaloid face and creating a unicameral eye. A stepwise approach to treatment has been advocated.[137] Medical therapy, with aqueous suppressants and topical cycloplegics, which pull the lens–iris diaphragm posteriorly, may be successful at breaking the cycle. More often, however, surgical intervention is necessary. The Nd:YAG laser can be used to penetrate the iris, the zonules or capsule, and the anterior hyaloid face, allowing normal posterior to anterior movement of aqueous.[138] In one recent series, laser iridozonulohyaloidotomy was successful in 35% of affected eyes.[137] If laser treatment fails to resolve the condition, then additional interventions are required, progressing from reformation of the chamber with viscoelastic and pushback of the IOL to surgical vitrectomy, including disruption of the anterior hyaloid, zonules, and iris.

Glaucoma Drainage Devices

Elevated IOP following drainage device implantation is not uncommon and has numerous possible etiologies. In the early postoperative period, high pressure is usually caused by limited flow through the tube. In a nonvalved implant, inadequate venting of the tube may lead to high pressures until the ligature sutures dissolve, typically at between 4 to 6 weeks postoperatively. Topical or oral glaucoma medications may be required to control IOP until tube opening occurs. Valved shunts, if not properly primed at the time of implantation, may fail to drain effectively, or may become obstructed by blood, fibrin, or debris, requiring

surgical intervention to flush and re-prime the tube. Damage to the valve mechanism during intraoperative handling has also been considered a possible cause of valve obstruction.[139] Nonvalved shunts are also susceptible to tube clogs, with similar intervention needed to promote resolution if the obstruction fails to clear spontaneously.

Elevated IOP is more common several weeks to months following tube shunt surgery, due to development of excessive fibrous encapsulation around the plate. Many eyes experience a "hypertensive phase" following implantation of a drainage device, typically occurring between 4 and 8 weeks postoperatively. This phase of elevated IOP, which is more common in valved than in nonvalved implants,[46,47] often lasts for several months, requiring the prolonged use of ocular antihypertensive medications for adequate control.[140] It has been theorized that exposure to pro-inflammatory cytokines in the glaucomatous aqueous, as well as increased tension on the forming bleb wall, stimulate excessive collagen production leading to a abnormally thickened plate capsule.[141,142] Thus, the hypertensive phase tends to develop later in nonvalved implants, after the tube has opened and aqueous fills the capsule. If IOP cannot be well controlled during the hypertensive phase with medications alone, the removal of aqueous from the bleb with a 30-gauge needle on a syringe may be necessary. This procedure, which usually can be performed at the slit lamp with the patient comfortable under topical anesthesia, may be repeated weekly until the pressure normalizes. Such serial taps of aqueous may also help limit the ultimate thickness of the capsule wall, preventing a pathologically encysted capsule.

A thickened, encysted bleb may persist despite the above efforts, with poor control of IOP. In such cases, needling of the bleb at the slit lamp may be performed with or without 5-fluorouracil, similar to the procedure used for an encapsulated trabeculectomy bleb. Ultimately, should such maneuvers fail to adequately lower IOP, additional surgery, possibly with another drainage device in a separate quadrant, may be needed.

Canaloplasty

Mild elevation of IOP in the first 1 to 2 weeks following canaloplasty is common, probably due to retained viscoelastic or hyphema, and is generally transient and controllable with topical medications.[143] Possible steroid response should also be considered. If IOP remains elevated beyond the first few weeks, Nd:YAG laser goniopuncture may be performed, disrupting the Descemet's window and potentially producing improved outflow. It is not unusual for these eyes to require continued use of glaucoma medication to maintain adequate IOP control.[144,145] Failure of goniopuncture to control IOP may indicate fibrosis of the scleral lake, canal, or collector system. If pressure cannot be controlled medically, additional glaucoma surgery is indicated.

Blebitis and Endophthalmitis

Bleb-associated endophthalmitis is one of the most feared and potentially devastating complications of glaucoma filtering surgery. Endophthalmitis can develop early in the postoperative period or, more commonly, may present years after surgery. Early diagnosis and aggressive management of this condition are vital for a successful visual outcome.

Risk factors for bleb-related infections include use of antimetabolites,[14] bleb leaks,[146] bleb manipulations such as needling,[147] inferior bleb location,[147,148] nasolacrimal duct obstruction,[147] contact lens wear,[149] intermittent or prolonged use of antibiotics,[150] and blepharitis.[149] A distinction can be made between "blebitis," in which only the bleb and AC are affected, and endophthalmitis, where the infection involves the vitreous. The incidence of bleb-related infection is difficult to determine, but one study estimated the 5-year probability of developing a bleb leak, blebitis, or endophthalmitis to be 17.9%, 6.3%, and 7.5%, respectively.[151]

Symptoms of bleb-associated infections include foreign-body sensation or pain, photophobia, tearing, and decreased visual acuity. Signs include prominent hyperemia surrounding the bleb, which may have a milky-white appearance, as well as a very thin-walled bleb or overt bleb leak. Chemosis, corneal edema, AC cell and flare, keratic precipitates, and hypopion may be present. The chamber may be shallow due to leak with hypotony. Alternatively, the IOP may be elevated due to plugging of the outflow pathway with inflammatory debris or to scarring of the bleb. White blood cells in the vitreous define endophthalmitis, and the vitreous may become progressively hazier as the infection advances posteriorly. For this reason, a dilated examination is essential when the postsurgical glaucoma patient presents with significant inflammation.

Most cases of early bleb-related endophthalmitis, occurring within the first 6 weeks postoperatively, are caused by *Staphylococcus epidermidis* or *Staphylococcus aureus*, the same organisms responsible for the majority of post-cataract infections.[152] The most common causative organisms in late infection include *Streptococcus* species, *Haemophilus influenzae,* and other gram-negative bacteria, a spectrum of distinctly different, and often more pathogenic, organisms than found in early infection.[152] Sensitivity of the gram-positive organisms to vancomycin remains nearly 100%, but sensitivity to penicillins, cephalosporins, aminoglycosides, and fluoroquinolones is quite variable, with significant changes in sensitivity rates over the past two decades.[153] Although the bacteria that cause bleb-related infections most likely arise from the ocular surface, conjunctival cultures generally correlate poorly with isolates from intraocular aspirates, suggesting limited utility of such samples.[152]

All patients undergoing glaucoma filtration surgery should be warned about the risks of endophthalmitis and encouraged to seek attention as soon as symptoms develop, particularly patients with thin, ischemic blebs who may be at greater risk for leaks. Identified leaks must be managed expeditiously by one of the methods discussed earlier in this chapter, although it has been found that direct surgical repair by conjunctival advancement decreases the risks of recurrent leaks and infection compared with nonsurgical approaches.[154]

Management of bleb-related infections generally depends on the extent and severity of the condition. Although no study has evaluated treatment patterns of blebitis, an older survey of members of the American Glaucoma Society (AGS) conducted in 1999 found that 51% prescribe a topical fluoroquinolone alone as initial treatment, whereas 23% use a fluoroquinolone in combination with additional topical antibiotics, typically an aminoglycoside, vancomycin, or cephalosporin[155]; 31% preferred a combination of fortified agents as primary therapy. Only 6% of responding AGS members indicated that they would use oral or intravenous antibiotics routinely in these cases. The majority (80%) would treat blebitis as endophthalmitis with increasing inflammatory reaction within the AC. Interestingly, a recent survey of surgeons in the United Kingdom[156] revealed quite different results, with 55% of physicians admitting patients to the hospital for treatment, 69% routinely prescribe oral antibiotics, and 23% treating all cases of blebitis, regardless of AC reaction, as endophthalmitis. Clearly, there is significant variability in treatment regimens and lack of consensus regarding management of blebitis. Our approach is to treat mild blebitis, without significant AC reaction, with frequent topical administration of a current-generation fluoroquinolone (q30m to q1h). If a mild to moderate AC reaction is present, we prefer a combination of topical fortified antibiotics, typically vancomycin (25 mg/mL) and gentamicin (14 mg/mL), alternating every 30 minutes for the first few days until clinical improvement is noted, at which point topical corticosteroids can be added to decrease inflammation and decrease risk of bleb failure.

Once cells are noted in the vitreous, treatment for endophthalmitis should be initiated promptly. Topical fortified antibiotics can be continued, and aqueous and vitreous aspirates should be obtained for culture. Empiric treatment with vancomycin (1 mg/0.1 mL), combined with ceftazidime (2.25 mg/0.1 mL), amikacin (0.4 mg/0.1 mL), or gentamycin (0.1 mg/0.1 mL) has been suggested.[157] A recent study indicates that oral fluoroquinolones, particularly the fourth-generation agents gatifloxacin and moxifloxacin, offer good coverage[153] (and an older study indicates that they offer excellent penetration into the vitreous[158]), and may serve as powerful adjuncts to intravitreal antibiotics, avoiding the possible need for inpatient treatment with intravenous agents. Little data exists regarding the role of vitrectomy versus vitreous tap with injection of intravitreal antibiotics in bleb-related endophthalmitis. The results of the Endophthalmitis Vitrectomy Study (EVS) should not be directly extrapolated to late-onset bleb-related endophthalmitis, as the causative organisms and severity of infection are rather different in this clinical situation than following cataract surgery alone.[152,159]

Two reasonably large studies have evaluated outcomes for bleb-associated infections with respect to treatment modality. Song et al[147] published a series of 49 patients treated with either pars plana vitrectomy (PPV) and intravitreal antibiotics or vitreous tap with antibiotic injection, finding that those undergoing PPV had poorer outcomes. They noted that this was possibly due to selection bias, as the eyes undergoing PPV had more severe infections and poorer visual acuity at the time of diagnosis. Busbee et al[160] also published a separate series of 68 patients with bleb-associated endophthalmitis, finding that patients undergoing PPV were more likely to retain 20/100 vision or better at 1 year when compared with the tap/inject group (33% vs 13%, $p = 0.09$). Regardless of treatment modality, however, and consistent with findings from several other studies, these studies reported very poor visual outcomes overall. Song et al noted recovery of vision better than 20/400 in 53%, whereas Busbee et al found the same in only 34%, and 35% of eyes developed no light perception vision by 1 year.

Endophthalmitis following glaucoma drainage device surgery appears to be far less common than after trabeculectomy, possibly due to the more posterior location of the filtering bleb as well as the lack of antimetabolites used during these procedures. Isolated organisms are similar to those found in post-trabeculectomy infections.[161] In the majority of cases, tube or plate exposure has been identified as the primary risk factor for infection.[161,162] Exposed tubes should be revised using a patch graft. Unfortunately, reexposures are common in these eyes, often necessitating additional procedures.[163] Repositioning the tube into the pars plana, if possible, or rerouting it to another location in the AC may be effective. Plate exposures often prove more difficult to repair, and repeated exposures are not uncommon.[163] In the case of multiple reexposures, or if infection is noted, it is probably best to remove the shunt and consider another procedure for IOP control.

Symptomatic Filtering Blebs

Filtering blebs are generally well tolerated, with most patients aware of a slight conjunctival elevation or "blister." Some, however, experience discomfort related to the bleb, more frequently when it is located nasally, is particularly large or elevated, or extends onto the cornea.[164] Symptomatic patients often show signs of superficial punctate keratopathy or dellen formation, and overhanging blebs are occasionally responsible for blurred vision, field defects, or monocular diplopia.

In many cases, conservative treatment with only topical lubricants provides adequate relief. Persistent symptoms can be managed via several techniques, including chemical irritant therapy with silver nitrate or trichloroacetic acid,[165] use of the argon[166] or Nd:YAG laser,[167] cryotherapy,[168] or cauterization.[169] Successful reduction of symptoms has also been achieved via segmental bleb incision and suturing of the cut margins to underlying sclera.[170] Alternatively, compression sutures, with or without autologous blood injection into the areas to be flattened, may also lead to resolution of symptoms.[171,172] Overhanging blebs lie on the corneal surface rather than within deeper tissue planes and may simply be bluntly or sharply dissected free and cut flush with the limbus, with little concern about leaks.[173,174] The patient should always be warned that revision, regardless of the method, may compromise bleb function and IOP control.

Complications Specific to EX-PRESS Shunts

As noted previously, the EX-PRESS shunt has been found to be a safe and effective alternative to standard trabeculectomy, with a very similar spectrum of complications. The rates of certain issues, such as early hypotony and hyphema, appear to be somewhat lower with the EX-PRESS. There are, however, a few potential problems, directly related to the shunt, that are unique to EX-PRESS procedures.

When initially introduced to the United States market in 2002, the standard technique involved implanting the EX-PRESS in an unguarded fashion directly below the conjunctiva. This resulted in numerous complications including severe hypotony, extrusion, or erosion of the implant.[175–178] The incidence of such complications has been dramatically reduced by the current technique of implantation under a scleral flap,[61,179] but malpositioned or dislocated shunts occasionally occur.[65,179–181] This can best be avoided by paying careful attention to detail at the time of implantation, as discussed previously. Both the scleral flap and scleral bed must be of adequate thickness; otherwise, there is a risk of external exposure or internal erosion. Additionally, proper needle size and entry technique are important, as an overly large track may predispose to dislocation.[65] Entry too far anteriorly or posteriorly may cause insertion of the device in the peripheral cornea or the iris, respectively. Due to openings at both the end as well as the sides of the device, contact of the tip of the EX-PRESS with iris seldom leads to obstruction and appears to be well tolerated, with no significant inflammation or effect on vision.[179] Blockage of the shunt, which can occur early postoperatively or significantly later, can be successfully treated with the Nd:YAG laser. Kanner et al[179] identified obstruction in six of 345 eyes (1.7%), manifested as elevated IOP and flattened bleb that did not respond to laser suture lysis. All six cases responded to Nd:YAG laser treatment to the tip of the tube (1 to 2 mJ), including four eyes where mild chronic inflammation was found but no visible obstruction of the shunt could be seen gonioscopically.

Failure of EX-PRESS shunt surgery occurs via the same mechanisms as standard trabeculectomy, primarily due to episcleral and subconjunctival fibrosis. When another filtration procedure is performed in an adjacent quadrant, the shunt need not be removed unless it is malpositioned or at risk of exposure. If necessary, the shunt can be removed by making a ~ 2-mm incision adjacent to the device, grasping it firmly with a needle holder, and turning it to align the retention spur with the incision.[180,181] The incision is then closed with 10-0 nylon sutures, as needed.

Finally, the economics of the EX-PRESS shunt warrant mention. A recent study by Patel et al[182] evaluated the 1-year cost differential between EX-PRESS and standard trabeculectomy, finding a net greater surgical expense of at least $877 for the EX-PRESS, principally due to the cost of the device. There was no significant difference in overall postoperative cost or the cost of follow-up visits, additional procedures, or glaucoma medications required, despite evidence previously discussed in this chapter suggesting that EX-PRESS surgery benefits from a less complicated postoperative course. No study has yet found any long-term benefit in terms of IOP control or number of medications required. Given the economic pressures we face in medicine today, the individual surgeon must personally weigh the specific benefits of the EX-PRESS against the added "cost to the system" when deciding whether or not to use this technology.

Complications Specific to Glaucoma Drainage Devices

Drainage devices, due to the presence of a large external plate and intraocular silicone tube, are subject to numerous complications not found with other forms of glaucoma surgery. Many of these issues occur months to years following surgery, are challenging to manage, and are often best handled by an experienced glaucoma specialist. Such complications include exposure of the tube or plate (briefly discussed in this chapter), late obstructions of the tube or valve, diplopia and disturbances of ocular motility, and corneal decompensation. There are, however, potential issues that arise intraoperatively that may challenge the cataract surgeon when implanting a drainage device, including malpositioned tubes, inadequate tube length, scleral perforation, and inadequate conjunctival tissue for closure.

Achieving proper tube position at the time of surgery helps to avoid secondary complications postoperatively. A tube that is too far anterior risks injury to the cornea, ultimately leading to edema and decompensation. Placement too far posteriorly, against the iris, may cause chronic low-grade inflammation or lead to tube obstruction by the iris. Optimally, the tube should sit as posteriorly as possible without directly contacting the iris. Achieving this position, however, can be difficult, particularly following cataract surgery when AC depth may not be normal due to prior surgical manipulations. It is advisable to attempt to return the chamber to a normal depth prior to making the entry track with a 23-gauge needle, which should be parallel to the iris plane. Care must be taken during both needle and tube entry to avoid injury to the iris. Inadvertent capture of iris tissue during entry may cause iridodialysis, and tube positioning within iris stroma can lead to obstruction. In such cases the tube should be removed and repositioned through a new entry site. The incorrect track can be closed with a single suture if necessary, or may be sealed by the tamponade effect of the tube placed via a new, immediately adjacent entry. Once the tube is properly positioned in the chamber, its extraocular segment should be fixated to the sclera with nonabsorbable sutures to prevent both lateral and radial movements that could lead to subsequent malposition.

In addition to proper positioning, adequate tube length is important for surgical success. Prior to implantation, the tube should be laid along its intended path without stretching and cut over the cornea with an anterior bevel. It is best to err on the long side, as it is far easier to trim an overly long tube than to add length to one that is too short. Nonetheless, a few options exist to manage a tube that is found to be too short once placed in the AC. Depending on the type of implant, the plate may be amenable to repositioning closer to the limbus, though it should remain at least 7 to 8 mm posterior to the cornea to decrease the risk of plate erosions caused by lid movement.[183] As anterior movement of a Baerveldt shunt is limited by the rectus muscles, suturing the plate to the sclera 1 to 2 mm behind the muscle insertion enables anterior resuturing if extra tube length is needed.

Another option for adding length to a short tube is the use of a commercially available tube extender (New World Medical Tube Extender, New World Medical, Rancho Cucamonga, CA).[184,185] This device, which serves as a "spacer" between the cuts ends of two silicone tube segments, can also be used to reconnect an inadvertently transected tube, as may occur when creating venting slits in a nonvalved implant. The extender has two fixation eyelets at its base to enable suturing to the sclera, which prevents movement or retraction. Another, perhaps less expensive, option that has been reported for lengthening a short tube is the use of a segment of angiocatheter as an extender.[186,187] In this technique, a short segment of 22-gauge catheter is cut from the central, nontapered region and used to join the cut ends of the tube, which fits tightly within the catheter. Each end of the angiocatheter is then fixated to the sclera with nonabsorbable sutures. Although tube dislocation and migration from the catheter extender is uncommon, a 10-0 Prolene suture can be passed through the joined edges of tube and catheter in patients at risk, such as those who squeeze excessively or rub their eyes.[188]

Scleral perforation during drainage device surgery occurs rarely, most commonly as the plate is sutured to the globe. In a report of the Tube Versus Trabeculectomy Study,[189] perforation occurred in three of 107 patients in the tube group, whereas only one of 276 patients in the Ahmed Baerveldt Comparison Study[190] experienced this complication. Most at risk are patients with thin sclera, such as high myopes or those with scarring from prior surgery. The sclera, although reasonably thick near the limbus, becomes progressively thinner posteriorly where the plate is fixated to the globe.[191] Great care must be taken to ensure that scleral suture bites are superficial, ideally visualizing the needle through the entire course of its passage. In high-risk patients, consideration can be given to firmly suturing only the tube anteriorly, where sclera is thicker, allowing fibrosis to fixate the plate during the first few postoperative weeks. If a perforation is identified, intraoperative cryotherapy or indirect laser retinopexy can be performed to limit the risk of retinal detachment.[189,192] The patient should be advised to be aware of symptoms of detachment. Evaluation by a vitreoretinal specialist is recommended.

Successful completion of tube shunt surgery entails full coverage of the device, including the tube and patch graft, by conjunctiva, which must be reapproximated to the limbus. Conjunctival scarring or thinning, often due to prior ophthalmic surgery or inflammation, can cause difficulty with closure. The conjunctiva should be thoroughly assessed preoperatively to identify areas of scarring, which may be avoided by planning surgery in an alternate quadrant. If scarring is extensive, consideration should be given to a different procedure, when possible. Once surgery is underway and the conjunctival flap has been dissected, a mobility check should be performed to ensure adequate tissue for full coverage. Such a check is also advisable after the plate has been sutured to the sclera to ensure that tissue has not been trapped by the device. If the conjunctiva cannot be brought back to the limbus without tension and associated risk of exposure, relaxing incisions may be made posteriorly and laterally allowing for conjunctival advancement. If a larger area of tissue is needed, either a conjunctival pedicle flap or a free autograft may be used, similar to the technique used to repair a dysfunctional bleb.[100,101,108,109]

Conclusion

The cataract surgeon today has numerous options available for the simultaneous surgical treatment of glaucoma. This chapter has evaluated the prevention and management of complications associated with trabeculectomy, canaloplasty, and drainage devices, whereas MIGS is addressed in Chapter 47.

Performed for over 45 years, trabeculectomy remains very popular, in large part due to surgeon familiarity with the procedure and its complications, as refinements along the way have improved safety and success. Broad application of mitomycin C, as promoted by Peng Khaw, has been widely adopted, producing low, diffuse blebs that are less likely to become avascular and develop leaks, thus decreasing the risk of late hypotony and endophthalmitis.[60] The EX-PRESS shunt offers standardization of an important step in the procedure, and has been shown to reduce the rate of some early complications such as hypotony and hyphema while providing better control of IOP within the first several years postoperatively.[61–64] The added cost of the device must be considered,[182] however, and time and experience will tell if the EX-PRESS is truly safer and more cost-effective than standard trabeculectomy.

Although trabeculectomy remains the gold standard for surgical reduction of IOP, the Tube Versus Trabeculectomy (TVT) study has shown that glaucoma drainage devices may offer very similar success and safety.[71] This multicenter randomized trial enrolled 212 eyes of 212 patients who had undergone either previous cataract or glaucoma surgery, comparing trabeculectomy with mitomycin C (0.4 mg/mL for 4 minutes) to tube shunt (350 mm² Baerveldt® glaucoma implant). At 5 years, the mean IOP was in the low to mid-teens in both groups (14.4 ± 6.9 mm Hg in the tube group and 12.6 ± 5.9 mm Hg in the trabeculectomy group), with very similar supplemental use of glaucoma medication. The success rate was higher for tube shunts, with a cumulative probability of failure of 29.8% in the tube group and 46.9% in the trabeculectomy group, and eyes undergoing trabeculectomy were more likely to require an additional glaucoma procedure. Although early postoperative complications were greater in the trabeculectomy group, the incidence of late complications was similar. Another recent report identified the clinical failure rate of tube shunts at ~ 10% per year, very similar to the failure rate of trabeculectomy.[193] A survey of the American Glaucoma Society performed in 2008 comparing practice patterns to those from 1996 identified a very significant increase in drainage device surgery and corresponding decrease in trabeculectomy.[194] Glaucoma drainage devices represent a safe, effective, and increasingly popular means of surgical IOP reduction, and offer the cataract surgeon an excellent alternative to trabeculectomy in patients who would benefit from a filtering procedure.

Although external filtration procedures are generally quite effective at reducing IOP and have been the mainstay of glaucoma surgery for decades, their benefits are tempered by a high rate of associated complications. Searching for safer means of improving aqueous outflow, innovative clinicians such as Robert Stegmann began to reexplore Schlemm's canal, hoping to bypass the obstruction in the trabecular meshwork and to reestablish a functioning, natural outflow system.[30] His viscocanalostomy procedure built upon previous work with nonpenetrating deep sclerectomy,[29] and has now been further refined into modern-day canaloplasty.[31] Numerous studies have found canaloplasty both effective and safe, with IOP reduction rivaling filtration procedures and significantly fewer postoperative complications.[32,66,195]

A retrospective, nonrandomized series comparing trabeculectomy (n = 46) and canaloplasty (n = 33) found mean IOP reductions at 12 months of 43% and 32%, respectively, a difference that did not reach statistical significance.[58] The mean reduction in glaucoma medications as well as rates of failure were also not significantly different. Another series published by the same authors compared phacotrabeculectomy (n = 41) and phacocanaloplasty (n = 36), with similar results, but the phacotrabeculectomy group showed a significantly greater median absolute (8 vs 5 mm Hg) and percent (40% vs 28%) reduction in IOP at 12 months (p = 0.02).[196] Failure rates at 1 year were comparable (22% for phacocanaloplasty vs 20% for phacotrabeculectomy), although phacotrabeculectomy experienced more failures based on complication-related visual loss, whereas phacocanaloplasty failures were primarily due to loss of IOP control.

Brüggemann et al[197] recently reported on a small series of 15 patients who underwent canaloplasty in one eye following trabeculectomy in the fellow eye. Again, IOP reduction from baseline was statistically significant in both groups at 12 months, whereas postoperative IOP did not differ significantly between groups. Of particular note, postoperative interventions were performed in two patients undergoing canaloplasty, whereas eight eyes in the trabeculectomy group required a total of 112 interventions for management of the bleb, including 5-fluorouracil injections, bleb needlings, AC reformations, and revisions of leaking or scarred blebs. The evidence suggests that canaloplasty, particularly when combined with phacoemulsification, is capable of producing IOP levels similar to those of trabeculectomy, with far fewer postoperative complications or necessary interventions. Canaloplasty, therefore, may be an excellent option for patients at higher risk of serious complications of filtering surgery, such as high myopes, or for those who cannot tolerate frequent follow-up or postoperative interventions.

Numerous options exist for the cataract surgeon contemplating surgical comanagement of glaucoma. Both filtering and nonpenetrating options may be combined safely and effectively with cataract surgery, and each offers a specific set of benefits as well as challenges. No single procedure has been found superior to another in terms of efficacy or safety, giving the surgeon significant discretion to tailor the chosen procedure to the specific needs of the individual patient. Ongoing advances in microsurgical technology will, no doubt, continue to improve outcomes and safety.

References

1. Pastori D, Carnevale R, Cangemi R, et al. Vitamin E serum levels and bleeding risk in patients receiving oral anticoagulant therapy: a retrospective cohort study. J Am Heart Assoc 2013;2:e000364

2. Whitlon DS, Sadowski JA, Suttie JW. Mechanism of coumarin action: significance of vitamin K epoxide reductase inhibition. Biochemistry 1978; 17:1371–1377

3. Burch JW, Stanford N, Majerus PW. Inhibition of platelet prostaglandin synthetase by oral aspirin. J Clin Invest 1978;61:314–319

4. Vane JR, Botting RM. Mechanism of action of anti-inflammatory drugs. Scand J Rheumatol Suppl 1996;102:9–21

5. Steiner M. Vitamin E, a modifier of platelet function: rationale and use in cardiovascular and cerebrovascular disease. Nutr Rev 1999;57:306–309

6. Hashemzadeh M, Goldsberry S, Furukawa M, Khoynezhad A, Movahed MR. ADP receptor-blocker thienopyridines: chemical structures, mode of action and clinical use. A review. J Invasive Cardiol 2009;21:406–412

7. Mueck W, Schwers S, Stampfuss J. Rivaroxaban and other novel oral anticoagulants: pharmacokinetics in healthy subjects, specific patient populations and relevance of coagulation monitoring. Thromb J 2013; 11:10

8. Bonhomme F, Hafezi F, Boehlen F, Habre W. Management of antithrombotic therapies in patients scheduled for eye surgery. Eur J Anaesthesiol 2013;30:449–454

9. Cobb CJ, Chakrabarti S, Chadha V, Sanders R. The effect of aspirin and warfarin therapy in trabeculectomy. Eye (Lond) 2007;21:598–603

10. Alwitry A, King AJ, Vernon SA. Anticoagulation therapy in glaucoma surgery. Graefes Arch Clin Exp Ophthalmol 2008;246:891–896

11. Broadway DC, Chang LP. Trabeculectomy, risk factors for failure and the preoperative state of the conjunctiva. J Glaucoma 2001;10:237–249

12. Broadway DC, Grierson I, Hitchings RA. Local effects of previous conjunctival incisional surgery and the subsequent outcome of filtration surgery. Am J Ophthalmol 1998;125:805–818

13. Joseph JP, Grierson I, Hitchings RA. Chemotactic activity of aqueous humor. A cause of failure of trabeculectomies? Arch Ophthalmol 1989; 107:69–74

14. Greenfield DS, Suñer IJ, Miller MP, Kangas TA, Palmberg PF, Flynn HW Jr. Endophthalmitis after filtering surgery with mitomycin. Arch Ophthalmol 1996;114:943–949

15. Caronia RM, Liebmann JM, Friedman R, Cohen H, Ritch R. Trabeculectomy at the inferior limbus. Arch Ophthalmol 1996;114:387–391

16. Broadway DC, Grierson I, O'Brien C, Hitchings RA. Adverse effects of topical antiglaucoma medication. II. The outcome of filtration surgery. Arch Ophthalmol 1994;112:1446–1454

17. Landers J, Martin K, Sarkies N, Bourne R, Watson P. A twenty-year follow-up study of trabeculectomy: risk factors and outcomes. Ophthalmology 2012;119:694–702

18. Sherwood MB, Grierson I, Millar L, Hitchings RA. Long-term morphologic effects of antiglaucoma drugs on the conjunctiva and Tenon's capsule in glaucomatous patients. Ophthalmology 1989;96:327–335

19. Broadway DC, Grierson I, O'Brien C, Hitchings RA. Adverse effects of topical antiglaucoma medication. I. The conjunctival cell profile. Arch Ophthalmol 1994;112:1437–1445

20. Cennamo G, Forte R, Del Prete S, Cardone D. Scanning electron microscopy applied to impression cytology for conjunctival damage from glaucoma therapy. Cornea 2013;32:1227–1231

21. De Saint Jean M, Brignole F, Bringuier A-F, Bauchet A, Feldmann G, Baudouin C. Effects of benzalkonium chloride on growth and survival of Chang conjunctival cells. Invest Ophthalmol Vis Sci 1999;40:619–630

22. Baudouin C, Pisella PJ, Fillacier K, et al. Ocular surface inflammatory changes induced by topical antiglaucoma drugs: human and animal studies. Ophthalmology 1999;106:556–563

23. Lavin MJ, Wormald RPL, Migdal CS, Hitchings RA. The influence of prior therapy on the success of trabeculectomy. Arch Ophthalmol 1990;108: 1543–1548

24. Öztürker ZK, Öztürker C, Bayraktar S, Altan C, Yilmaz OF. Does the use of preoperative antiglaucoma medications influence trabeculectomy success? J Ocul Pharmacol Ther 2014;30:554–558

25. Stürmer J, Broadway DC, Hitchings RA. Young patient trabeculectomy. Assessment of risk factors for failure. Ophthalmology 1993;100:928–939

26. Broadway D, Grierson I, Hitchings R. Racial differences in the results of glaucoma filtration surgery: are racial differences in the conjunctival cell profile important? Br J Ophthalmol 1994;78:466–475

27. Cairns JE. Trabeculectomy. Preliminary report of a new method. Am J Ophthalmol 1968;66:673–679

28. Edmunds B, Thompson JR, Salmon JF, Wormald RP. The National Survey of Trabeculectomy. III. Early and late complications. Eye (Lond) 2002;16: 297–303

29. Fyodorov SN, Kozlov VI, Timoshkina NT, et al. Non-penetrating deep sclerectomy in open-angle glaucoma. Eye Microsurg. 1989;2:52–55

30. Stegmann R, Pienaar A, Miller D. Viscocanalostomy for open-angle glaucoma in black African patients. J Cataract Refract Surg 1999;25:316–322

31. Cameron B, Field M, Field M, Ball S, Kearney J. Circumferential viscodilation of Schlemm's canal with a flexible microcannula during nonpenetrating glaucoma surgery. Digit J Ophthalmol 2006;12

32. Lewis RA, von Wolff K, Tetz M, et al. Canaloplasty: circumferential viscodilation and tensioning of Schlemm canal using a flexible microcatheter for the treatment of open-angle glaucoma in adults: two-year interim clinical study results. J Cataract Refract Surg 2009;35:814–824

33. Kimbrough RL, Stewart RH, Decker WL, Praeger TC. Trabeculectomy: square or triangular scleral flap? Ophthalmic Surg 1982;13:753

34. Shaffer RN, Hetherington J Jr, Hoskins HD Jr. Guarded thermal sclerostomy. Am J Ophthalmol 1971;72:769–772

35. Cohen JS, Osher RH. Releasable scleral flap suture. Ophthalmol Clin North Am 1988;1:187–197

36. Wilson RP. Adjuncts to filtering surgery: releasable sutures. In: McAllister JA, Wilson RP, eds. Glaucoma. Stoneham, MA: Butterworths; 1986:243–250

37. Shin DH. Removable-suture closure of the lamellar scleral flap in trabeculectomy. Ann Ophthalmol 1987;19:51–53, 55

38. Johnstone MA, Wellington DP, Ziel CJ. A releasable scleral-flap tamponade suture for guarded filtration surgery. Arch Ophthalmol 1993;111:398–403

39. Hsu CT, Yarng SS. A modified removable suture in trabeculectomy. Ophthalmic Surg 1993;24:579–584, discussion 584–585

40. Maberley D, Apel A, Rootman DS. Releasable "U" suture for trabeculectomy surgery. Ophthalmic Surg 1994;25:251–255

41. Wells AP, Bunce C, Khaw PT. Flap and suture manipulation after trabeculectomy with adjustable sutures: titration of flow and intraocular pressure in guarded filtration surgery. J Glaucoma 2004;13:400–406

42. Buys YM, Chipman ML, Zack B, Rootman DS, Slomovic AR, Trope GE. Prospective randomized comparison of one- versus two-site Phacotrabeculectomy two-year results. Ophthalmology 2008;115:1130–1133.e1

43. Shingleton BJ, Price RS, O'Donoghue MW, Goyal S. Comparison of 1-site versus 2-site phacotrabeculectomy. J Cataract Refract Surg 2006;32:799–802

44. Liu HN, Li X, Nie QZ, Chen XL. Efficacy and tolerability of one-site versus two-site phacotrabeculectomy: a meta-analysis. Int J Ophthalmol 2010;3:264–268

45. Tsai JC, Johnson CC, Dietrich MS. The Ahmed shunt versus the Baerveldt shunt for refractory glaucoma: a single-surgeon comparison of outcome. Ophthalmology 2003;110:1814–1821

46. Budenz DL, Barton K, Feuer WJ, et al; Ahmed Baerveldt Comparison Study Group. Treatment outcomes in the Ahmed Baerveldt Comparison Study after 1 year of follow-up. Ophthalmology 2011;118:443–452

47. Christakis PG, Tsai JC, Kalenak JW, et al. The Ahmed versus Baerveldt study: three-year treatment outcomes. Ophthalmology 2013;120:2232–2240

48. Zalta AH, Wieder RH. Closure of leaking filtering blebs with cyanoacrylate tissue adhesive. Br J Ophthalmol 1991;75:170–173

49. Grady FJ, Forbes M. Tissue adhesive for repair of conjunctival buttonhole in glaucoma surgery. Am J Ophthalmol 1969;68:656–658

50. Asrani SG, Wilensky JT. Management of bleb leaks after glaucoma filtering surgery. Use of autologous fibrin tissue glue as an alternative. Ophthalmology 1996;103:294–298

51. Higashide T, Tagawa S, Sugiyama K. Intraoperative Healon5 injection into blebs for small conjunctival breaks created during trabeculectomy. J Cataract Refract Surg 2005;31:1279–1282

52. Li G, O'Hearn T, Yiu S, Francis BA. Amniotic membrane transplantation for intraoperative conjunctival repair during trabeculectomy with mitomycin C. J Glaucoma 2007;16:521–526

53. Birchall W, Wakely L, Wells AP. The influence of scleral flap position and dimensions on intraocular pressure control in experimental trabeculectomy. J Glaucoma 2006;15:286–290

54. Curtin BJ, Teng CC. Scleral changes in pathological myopia. Trans Am Acad Ophthalmol Otolaryngol 1958;62:777–788, discussion 788–790

55. Riley SF, Smith TJ, Simmons RJ. Repair of a disinserted scleral flap in trabeculectomy. Ophthalmic Surg 1993;24:349–350

56. Riley SF, Lima FL, Smith TJ, Simmons RJ. Using donor sclera to create a flap in glaucoma filtering procedures. Ophthalmic Surg 1994;25:117–118

57. Bahar I, Lusky M, Gaton D, Robinson A, Avisar R, Weinberger D. The use of fibrin adhesive in trabeculectomy: a pilot study. Br J Ophthalmol 2006;90:1430

58. Ayyala RS, Chaudhry AL, Okogbaa CB, Zurakowski D. Comparison of surgical outcomes between canaloplasty and trabeculectomy at 12 months' follow-up. Ophthalmology 2011;118:2427–2433

59. Wilson R. Advanced phaco and combined glaucoma-phaco surgery. Course on videotape at the American Academy of Ophthalmology meeting, New Orleans, 1998

60. Khaw PT, Chiang M, Shah P, Sii F, Lockwood A, Khalili A. Enhanced trabeculectomy: the Moorfield's Safer Surgery System. Dev Ophthalmol 2012;50:1–28

61. de Jong L, Lafuma A, Aguadé AS, Berdeaux G. Five-year extension of a clinical trial comparing the EX-PRESS glaucoma filtration device and trabeculectomy in primary open-angle glaucoma. Clin Ophthalmol 2011;5:527–533

62. Dahan E, Ben Simon GJ, Lafuma A. Comparison of trabeculectomy and Ex-PRESS implantation in fellow eyes of the same patient: a prospective, randomised study. Eye (Lond) 2012;26:703–710

63. Marzette L, Herndon LW. A comparison of the Ex-PRESS™ mini glaucoma shunt with standard trabeculectomy in the surgical treatment of glaucoma. Ophthalmic Surg Lasers Imaging 2011;42:453–459

64. Maris PJG Jr, Ishida K, Netland PA. Comparison of trabeculectomy with Ex-PRESS miniature glaucoma device implanted under scleral flap. J Glaucoma 2007;16:14–19

65. Teng CC, Radcliffe N, Huang JE, Farris E. Ex-PRESS glaucoma shunt dislocation into the anterior chamber. J Glaucoma 2008;17:687–689

66. Grieshaber MC, Pienaar A, Olivier J, Stegmann R. Clinical evaluation of the aqueous outflow system in primary open-angle glaucoma for canaloplasty. Invest Ophthalmol Vis Sci 2010;51:1498–1504

67. Jampel HD, Musch DC, Gillespie BW, Lichter PR, Wright MM, Guire KE; Collaborative Initial Glaucoma Treatment Study Group. Perioperative complications of trabeculectomy in the collaborative initial glaucoma treatment study (CIGTS). Am J Ophthalmol 2005;140:16–22

68. Matlach J, Freiberg FJ, Leippi S, Grehn F, Klink T. Comparison of phacotrabeculectomy versus phacocanaloplasty in the treatment of patients with concomitant cataract and glaucoma. BMC Ophthalmol 2013;13:1

69. Grieshaber MC, Schoetzau A, Flammer J, Orgül S. Postoperative microhyphema as a positive prognostic indicator in canaloplasty. Acta Ophthalmol (Copenh) 2013;91:151–156

70. Jaramillo A, Foreman J, Ayyala RS. Descemet membrane detachment after canaloplasty: incidence and management. J Glaucoma 2014;23:351–354

71. Gedde SJ, Schiffman JC, Feuer WJ, Herndon LW, Brandt JD, Budenz DL; Tube versus Trabeculectomy Study Group. Treatment outcomes in the Tube Versus Trabeculectomy (TVT) study after five years of follow-up. Am J Ophthalmol 2012;153:789–803.e2

72. Ayyala RS, Zurakowski D, Smith JA, et al. A clinical study of the Ahmed glaucoma valve implant in advanced glaucoma. Ophthalmology 1998;105:1968–1976

73. Netland PA. The Ahmed glaucoma valve in neovascular glaucoma (An AOS thesis). Trans Am Ophthalmol Soc 2009;107:325–342

74. Bhargava S, Choudhari NS, Vijaya L. Intra-bleb hematoma and hyphema following digital ocular compression. Oman J Ophthalmol 2014;7:22–24

75. Shetty RK, Wartluft L, Moster MR. Slit-lamp needle revision of failed filtering blebs using high-dose mitomycin C. J Glaucoma 2005;14:52–56

76. Costa VP, Arcieri ES. Hypotony maculopathy. Acta Ophthalmol Scand 2007;85:586–597

77. Hyung SM, Jung MS. Management of hypotony after trabeculectomy with mitomycin C. Korean J Ophthalmol 2003;17:114–121

78. Zacharia PT, Deppermann SR, Schuman JS. Ocular hypotony after trabeculectomy with mitomycin C. Am J Ophthalmol 1993;116:314–326

79. Pederson JE. Ocular hypotony. In: Ritch R, Shields MB, Krupin T, eds. The Glaucomas, 2nd ed. St. Louis: Mosby; 1996:385–395

80. Tsai JC, Chang HW, Kao CN, Lai IC, Teng MC. Trabeculectomy with mitomycin C versus trabeculectomy alone for juvenile primary open-angle glaucoma. Ophthalmologica 2003;217:24–30

81. Schubert HD. Postsurgical hypotony: relationship to fistulization, inflammation, chorioretinal lesions, and the vitreous. Surv Ophthalmol 1996;41:97–125

82. Lee SJ, Paranhos A, Shields MB. Does titration of mitomycin C as an adjunct to trabeculectomy significantly influence the intraocular pressure outcome? Clin Ophthalmol 2009;3:81–87

83. Elner VM, Newman-Casey PA, Patil AJ, et al. Aberrant wound-healing response in mitomycin C-treated leaking blebs: a histopathologic study. Arch Ophthalmol 2009;127:1036–1042

84. Savage JA, Condon GP, Lytle RA, Simmons RJ. Laser suture lysis after trabeculectomy. Ophthalmology 1988;95:1631–1638

85. Bardak Y, Cuypers MH, Tilanus MA, Eggink CA. Ocular hypotony after laser suture lysis following trabeculectomy with mitomycin C. Int Ophthalmol 1997–1998;21:325–330

86. Simsek T, Citirik M, Batman A, Mutevelli S, Zilelioglu O. Efficacy and complications of releasable suture trabeculectomy and standard trabeculectomy. Int Ophthalmol 2005;26:9–14

87. Zhou M, Wang W, Huang W, Zhang X. Trabeculectomy with versus without releasable sutures for glaucoma: a meta-analysis of randomized controlled trials. BMC Ophthalmol 2014;14:41

88. Villarrubia HJ, Bell NP. Hypotony. In: Feldman RM, Bell NP, eds. Complications of Glaucoma Surgery. New York: Oxford University Press; 2013:85–91

89. Simmons RJ, Kimbrough RL. Shell tamponade in filtering surgery for glaucoma. Ophthalmic Surg 1979;10:17–34

90. Leen MM, Moster MR, Katz LJ, Terebuh AK, Schmidt CM, Spaeth GL. Management of overfiltering and leaking blebs with autologous blood injection. Arch Ophthalmol 1995;113:1050–1055

91. Wise JB. Treatment of chronic postfiltration hypotony by intrableb injection of autologous blood. Arch Ophthalmol 1993;111:827–830

92. Haynes WL, Alward WLM. Combination of autologous blood injection and bleb compression sutures to treat hypotony maculopathy. J Glaucoma 1999;8:384–387

93. Hosoda S, Yuki K, Ono T, Tsubota K. Ophthalmic viscoelastic device injection for the treatment of flat anterior chamber after trabeculectomy: a case series study. Clin Ophthalmol 2013;7:1781–1785

94. de Barros DS, Navarro JB, Mantravadi AV, et al. The early flat anterior chamber after trabeculectomy: a randomized, prospective study of 3 methods of management. J Glaucoma 2009;18:13–20

95. Nuyts RM, Greve EL, Geijssen HC, Langerhorst CT. Treatment of hypotonous maculopathy after trabeculectomy with mitomycin C. Am J Ophthalmol 1994;118:322–331

96. Suñer IJ, Greenfield DS, Miller MP, Nicolela MT, Palmberg PF. Hypotony maculopathy after filtering surgery with mitomycin C. Incidence and treatment. Ophthalmology 1997;104:207–214, discussion 214–215

97. Letartre L, Basheikh A, Anctil JL, et al. Transconjunctival suturing of the scleral flap for overfiltration with hypotony maculopathy after trabeculectomy. Can J Ophthalmol 2009;44:567–570

98. Eha J, Hoffmann EM, Pfeiffer N. Long-term results after transconjunctival resuturing of the scleral flap in hypotony following trabeculectomy. Am J Ophthalmol 2013;155:864–869

99. Bashford KP, Shafranov G, Shields MB. Bleb revision for hypotony maculopathy after trabeculectomy. J Glaucoma 2004;13:256–260

100. Schnyder CC, Shaarawy T, Ravinet E, Achache F, Uffer S, Mermoud A. Free conjunctival autologous graft for bleb repair and bleb reduction after trabeculectomy and nonpenetrating filtering surgery. J Glaucoma 2002;11:10–16

101. Bochmann F, Kaufmann C, Kipfer A, Thiel MA. Corneal patch graft for the repair of late-onset hypotony or filtering bleb leak after trabeculectomy: a new surgical technique. J Glaucoma 2014;23:e76–e80

102. Blok MD, Kok JH, van Mil C, Greve EL, Kijlstra A. Use of the Megasoft Bandage Lens for treatment of complications after trabeculectomy. Am J Ophthalmol 1990;110:264–268

103. Ruderman JM, Allen RC. Simmons' tamponade shell for leaking filtration blebs. Arch Ophthalmol 1985;103:1708–1710

104. Okabe M, Kitagawa K, Yoshida T, et al. Application of 2-octyl-cyanoacrylate for corneal perforation and glaucoma filtering bleb leak. Clin Ophthalmol 2013;7:649–653

105. Panda A, Kumar S, Kumar A, Bansal R, Bhartiya S. Fibrin glue in ophthalmology. Indian J Ophthalmol 2009;57:371–379

106. Chan SM, Boisjoly H. Advances in the use of adhesives in ophthalmology. Curr Opin Ophthalmol 2004;15:305–310

107. Horowitz B, Busch M. Estimating the pathogen safety of manufactured human plasma products: application to fibrin sealants and to thrombin. Transfusion 2008;48:1739–1753

108. Budenz DL, Chen PP, Weaver YK. Conjunctival advancement for late-onset filtering bleb leaks: indications and outcomes. Arch Ophthalmol 1999;117:1014–1019

109. Lin AP, Chung JE, Zhang KS, et al. Outcomes of surgical bleb revision for late-onset bleb leaks after trabeculectomy. J Glaucoma 2013;22:21–25

110. García-Feijoó J, Cuiña-Sardiña R, Méndez-Fernández C, Castillo-Gómez A, García-Sánchez J. Peritubular filtration as cause of severe hypotony after Ahmed valve implantation for glaucoma. Am J Ophthalmol 2001;132:571–572

111. Ozdamar A, Aras C, Ustundag C, Tamcelik N, Ozkan S. Scleral tunnel for the implantation of glaucoma seton devices. Ophthalmic Surg Lasers 2001;32:432–435

112. Eisenberg DL, Koo EY, Hafner G, Schuman JS. In vitro flow properties of glaucoma implant devices. Ophthalmic Surg Lasers 1999;30:662–667

113. Molteno AC, Polkinghorne PJ, Bowbyes JA. The Vicryl tie technique for inserting a draining implant in the treatment of secondary glaucoma. Aust N Z J Ophthalmol 1986;14:343–354

114. Hong CH, Arosemena A, Zurakowski D, Ayyala RS. Glaucoma drainage devices: a systematic literature review and current controversies. Surv Ophthalmol 2005;50:48–60

115. Stein JD, McCoy AN, Asrani S, et al. Surgical management of hypotony owing to overfiltration in eyes receiving glaucoma drainage devices. J Glaucoma 2009;18:638–641

116. Kapetansky FM. Laser suture lysis after trabeculectomy. J Glaucoma 2003;12:316–320

117. Traverso CE, Greenidge KC, Spaeth GL, Wilson RP. Focal pressure: a new method to encourage filtration after trabeculectomy. Ophthalmic Surg 1984;15:62–65

118. Cohn HC, Aron-Rosa D. Reopening blocked trabeculectomy sites with the YAG laser. Am J Ophthalmol 1983;95:293–294

119. Baik AK, Brandt JD. Elevated IOP with a deep anterior chamber. In: Feldman RM, Bell NP, eds. Complications of Glaucoma Surgery. New York: Oxford University Press; 2013:100–106

120. Piltz JR, Starita RJ. The use of subconjunctivally administered tissue plasminogen activator after trabeculectomy. Ophthalmic Surg 1994;25:51–53

121. Lundy DC, Sidoti P, Winarko T, Minckler D, Heuer DK. Intracameral tissue plasminogen activator after glaucoma surgery. Indications, effectiveness, and complications. Ophthalmology 1996;103:274–282

122. Schwartz AL, Van Veldhuisen PC, Gaasterland DE, Ederer F, Sullivan EK, Cyrlin MN, the AGIS investigators. The Advanced Glaucoma Intervention Study (AGIS): 5. Encapsulated bleb after initial trabeculectomy. Am J Ophthalmol 1999;127:8–19

123. Azuara-Blanco A, Bond JB, Wilson RP, Moster MR, Schmidt CM. Encapsulated filtering blebs after trabeculectomy with mitomycin-C. Ophthalmic Surg Lasers 1997;28:805–809

124. Scott DR, Quigley HA. Medical management of a high bleb phase after trabeculectomies. Ophthalmology 1988;95:1169–1173

125. Allen LE, Manuchehri K, Corridan PG. The treatment of encapsulated trabeculectomy blebs in an out-patient setting using a needling technique and subconjunctival 5-fluorouracil injection. Eye (Lond) 1998;12(Pt 1):119–123

126. Suzuki R, Susanna-Jr R. Early transconjunctival needling revision with 5-fluorouracil versus medical treatment in encapsulated blebs: a 12-month prospective study. Clinics (Sao Paulo) 2013;68:1376–1379

127. Broadway DC, Bloom PA, Bunce C, Thiagarajan M, Khaw PT. Needle revision of failing and failed trabeculectomy blebs with adjunctive 5-fluorouracil: survival analysis. Ophthalmology 2004;111:665–673

128. Anand N, Khan A. Long-term outcomes of needle revision of trabeculectomy blebs with mitomycin C and 5-fluorouracil: a comparative safety and efficacy report. J Glaucoma 2009;18:513–520

129. Oh Y, Katz LJ. Indications and technique for reopening closed filtering blebs using the Nd:YAG laser—a review and case series. Ophthalmic Surg 1993;24:617–622

130. Patel SB. Laser goniopuncture for bleb revision. JAMA Ophthalmol 2014;132:286–290

131. Cohen JS, Osher RH, Weber P, Faulkner JD. Complications of extracapsular cataract surgery. The indications and risks of peripheral iridectomy. Ophthalmology 1984;91:826–830

132. Gaton DD, Mimouni K, Lusky M, Ehrlich R, Weinberger D. Pupillary block following posterior chamber intraocular lens implantation in adults. Br J Ophthalmol 2003;87:1109–1111

133. Tuli SS, WuDunn D, Ciulla TA, Cantor LB. Delayed suprachoroidal hemorrhage after glaucoma filtration procedures. Ophthalmology 2001;108:1808–1811

134. Jeganathan VS, Ghosh S, Ruddle JB, Gupta V, Coote MA, Crowston JG. Risk factors for delayed suprachoroidal haemorrhage following glaucoma surgery. Br J Ophthalmol 2008;92:1393–1396

135. Law SK, Song BJ, Yu F, Kurbanyan K, Yang TA, Caprioli J. Hemorrhagic complications from glaucoma surgery in patients on anticoagulation therapy or antiplatelet therapy. Am J Ophthalmol 2008;145:736–746

136. Quigley HA, Friedman DS, Congdon NG. Possible mechanisms of primary angle-closure and malignant glaucoma. J Glaucoma 2003;12:167–180

137. Varma DK, Belovay GW, Tam DY, Ahmed II. Malignant glaucoma after cataract surgery. J Cataract Refract Surg 2014;40:1843–1849

138. Brown RH, Lynch MG, Tearse JE, Nunn RD. Neodymium-YAG vitreous surgery for phakic and pseudophakic malignant glaucoma. Arch Ophthalmol 1986;104:1464–1466

139. Hill RA, Pirouzian A, Liaw L. Pathophysiology of and prophylaxis against late Ahmed glaucoma valve occlusion. Am J Ophthalmol 2000;129:608–612

140. Nouri-Mahdavi K, Caprioli J. Evaluation of the hypertensive phase after insertion of the Ahmed glaucoma valve. Am J Ophthalmol 2003;136:1001–1008

141. Freedman J, Goddard D. Elevated levels of transforming growth factor beta and prostaglandin E2 in aqueous humor from patients undergoing filtration surgery for glaucoma. Can J Ophthalmol 2008;43:370

142. Friedman J. Encysted Bleb. In: Feldman RM, Bell NP, eds. Complications of Glaucoma Surgery. New York: Oxford University Press; 2013:283–288

143. Lewis RA, von Wolff K, Tetz M, et al. Canaloplasty: circumferential viscodilation and tensioning of Schlemm's canal using a flexible microcatheter for the treatment of open-angle glaucoma in adults: interim clinical study analysis. J Cataract Refract Surg 2007;33:1217–1226

144. Grieshaber MC, Fraenkl S, Schoetzau A, Flammer J, Orgül S. Circumferential viscocanalostomy and suture canal distension (canaloplasty) for whites with open-angle glaucoma. J Glaucoma 2011;20:298–302

145. Tam DY, Barnebey HS, Ahmed IIK. Nd: YAG laser goniopuncture: indications and procedure. J Glaucoma 2013;22:620–625

146. Soltau JB, Rothman RF, Budenz DL, et al. Risk factors for glaucoma filtering bleb infections. Arch Ophthalmol 2000;118:338–342

147. Song A, Scott IU, Flynn HW Jr, Budenz DL. Delayed-onset bleb-associated endophthalmitis: clinical features and visual acuity outcomes. Ophthalmology 2002;109:985–991

148. Higginbotham EJ, Stevens RK, Musch DC, et al. Bleb-related endophthalmitis after trabeculectomy with mitomycin C. Ophthalmology 1996;103:650–656

149. Bellows AR, McCulley JP. Endophthalmitis in aphakic patients with unplanned filtering blebs wearing contact lenses. Ophthalmology 1981;88:839–843

150. Jampel HD, Quigley HA, Kerrigan-Baumrind LA, Melia BM, Friedman D, Barron Y; Glaucoma Surgical Outcomes Study Group. Risk factors for late-onset infection following glaucoma filtration surgery. Arch Ophthalmol 2001;119:1001–1008

151. DeBry PW, Perkins TW, Heatley G, Kaufman P, Brumback LC. Incidence of late-onset bleb-related complications following trabeculectomy with mitomycin. Arch Ophthalmol 2002;120:297–300

152. Ciulla TA, Beck AD, Topping TM, Baker AS. Blebitis, early endophthalmitis, and late endophthalmitis after glaucoma-filtering surgery. Ophthalmology 1997;104:986–995

153. Gentile RC, Shukla S, Shah M, et al. Microbiological spectrum and antibiotic sensitivity in endophthalmitis: a 25-year review. Ophthalmology 2014;121:1634–1642

154. Burnstein AL, WuDunn D, Knotts SL, Catoira Y, Cantor LB. Conjunctival advancement versus nonincisional treatment for late-onset glaucoma filtering bleb leaks. Ophthalmology 2002;109:71–75

155. Reynolds AC, Skuta GL, Monlux R, Johnson J. Management of blebitis by members of the American Glaucoma Society: a survey. J Glaucoma 2001;10:340–347

156. Chiam PJT, Arashvand K, Shaikh A, James B. Management of blebitis in the United Kingdom: a survey. Br J Ophthalmol 2012;96:38–41

157. Ceballos EM, Gedde SJ. Bleb infections after glaucoma filtering surgery. Comprehensive Ophthalmology Update 2000;1:287–292

158. Hariprasad SM, Mieler WF, Holz ER. Vitreous and aqueous penetration of orally administered gatifloxacin in humans. Arch Ophthalmol 2003;121:345–350

159. Endophthalmitis Vitrectomy Study Group. Results of the Endophthalmitis Vitrectomy Study. A randomized trial of immediate vitrectomy and of intravenous antibiotics for the treatment of postoperative bacterial endophthalmitis. Arch Ophthalmol 1995;113:1479–1496

160. Busbee BG, Recchia FM, Kaiser R, Nagra P, Rosenblatt B, Pearlman RB. Bleb-associated endophthalmitis: clinical characteristics and visual outcomes. Ophthalmology 2004;111:1495–1503, discussion 1503

161. Al-Torbak AA, Al-Shahwan S, Al-Jadaan I, Al-Hommadi A, Edward DP. Endophthalmitis associated with the Ahmed glaucoma valve implant. Br J Ophthalmol 2005;89:454–458

162. Gedde SJ, Scott IU, Tabandeh H, et al. Late endophthalmitis associated with glaucoma drainage implants. Ophthalmology 2001;108:1323–1327

163. Huddleston SM, Feldman RM, Budenz DL, et al. Aqueous shunt exposure: a retrospective review of repair outcome. J Glaucoma 2013;22:433–438

164. Azuara-Blanco A, Katz LJ. Dysfunctional filtering blebs. Surv Ophthalmol 1998;43:93–126

165. Gehring JR, Ciccarelli EC. Trichloracetic acid treatment of filtering blebs following cataract extraction. Am J Ophthalmol 1972;74:622–624

166. Fink AJ, Boys-Smith JW, Brear R. Management of large filtering blebs with the argon laser. Am J Ophthalmol 1986;101:695–699

167. Lynch MG, Roesch M, Brown RH. Remodeling filtering blebs with the neodymium:YAG laser. Ophthalmology 1996;103:1700–1705

168. Cleasby GW, Fung WE, Webster RG Jr. Cryosurgical closure of filtering blebs. Arch Ophthalmol 1972;87:319–323

169. Kirk HQ. Cauterization of filtering blebs following cataract extraction. Trans Am Acad Ophthalmol Otolaryngol 1973;77:OP573–OP580

170. Anis S, Ritch R, Shihadeh W, Liebmann J. Surgical reduction of symptomatic, circumferential, filtering blebs. Arch Ophthalmol 2006;124:890–894

171. Palmberg P, Zacchei A. Compression sutures—a new treatment for leaking or painful filtering blebs. Invest Ophthalmol Vis Sci 1996;37:S444

172. Morgan JE, Diamond JP, Cook SD. Remodelling the filtration bleb. Br J Ophthalmol 2002;86:872–875

173. Lanzl IM, Katz LJ, Shindler RL, Spaeth GL. Surgical management of the symptomatic overhanging filtering bleb. J Glaucoma 1999;8:247–249

174. Anis S, Ritch R, Shihadeh W, Liebmann J. Sutureless revision of overhanging filtering blebs. Arch Ophthalmol 2006;124:1317–1320

175. Stewart RM, Diamond JG, Ashmore ED, Ayyala RS. Complications following ex-press glaucoma shunt implantation. Am J Ophthalmol 2005;140:340–341

176. Rivier D, Roy S, Mermoud A. Ex-PRESS R-50 miniature glaucoma implant insertion under the conjunctiva combined with cataract extraction. J Cataract Refract Surg 2007;33:1946–1952

177. Tavolato M, Babighian S, Galan A. Spontaneous extrusion of a stainless steel glaucoma drainage implant (Ex-PRESS). Eur J Ophthalmol 2006;16:753–755

178. Garg SJ, Kanitkar K, Weichel E, Fischer D. Trauma-induced extrusion of an Ex-PRESS glaucoma shunt presenting as an intraocular foreign body. Arch Ophthalmol 2005;123:1270–1272

179. Kanner EM, Netland PA, Sarkisian SR Jr, Du H. Ex-PRESS miniature glaucoma device implanted under a scleral flap alone or combined with phacoemulsification cataract surgery. J Glaucoma 2009;18:488–491

180. Stein JD, Herndon LW, Brent Bond J, Challa P. Exposure of Ex-PRESS Miniature Glaucoma Devices: case series and technique for tube shunt removal. J Glaucoma 2007;16:704–706

181. Khouri AS, Khan MN, Fechtner RD, Vold SD. Technique for removal of malpositioned Ex-PRESS glaucoma device. J Glaucoma 2014;23:435–436

182. Patel HY, Wagschal LD, Trope GE, Buys YM. Economic analysis of the Ex-PRESS miniature glaucoma device versus trabeculectomy. J Glaucoma 2014;23:385–390

183. Piovanetti O. Tube misdirection and inadequate tube length. In: Feldman RM, Bell NP, eds. Complications of Glaucoma Surgery. New York: Oxford University Press; 2013:243–249

184. Sarkisian SR, Netland PA. Tube extender for revision of glaucoma drainage implants. J Glaucoma 2007;16:637–639

185. Merrill KD, Suhr AW, Lim MC. Long-term success in the correction of exposed glaucoma drainage tubes with a tube extender. Am J Ophthalmol 2007;144:136–137

186. Smith MF, Doyle JW. Results of another modality for extending glaucoma drainage tubes. J Glaucoma 1999;8:310–314

187. Bansal A, Fenerty CH. Extension of retracted glaucoma drainage tube using a 22-gauge intravenous catheter in complex pediatric glaucoma. J Glaucoma 2010;19:248–251

188. Sheets CW, Ramjattan TK, Smith MF, Doyle JW. Migration of glaucoma drainage device extender into anterior chamber after trauma. J Glaucoma 2006;15:559–561

189. Gedde SJ, Herndon LW, Brandt JD, Budenz DL, Feuer WJ, Schiffman JC. Surgical complications in the Tube Versus Trabeculectomy Study during the first year of follow-up. Am J Ophthalmol 2007;143:23–31

190. Barton K, Gedde SJ, Budenz DL, Feuer WJ, Schiffman J; Ahmed Baerveldt Comparison Study Group. The Ahmed Baerveldt Comparison Study methodology, baseline patient characteristics, and intraoperative complications. Ophthalmology 2011;118:435–442

191. Norman RE, Flanagan JG, Rausch SM, et al. Dimensions of the human sclera: Thickness measurement and regional changes with axial length. Exp Eye Res 2010;90:277–284

192. Morris RJ, Rosen PH, Fells P. Incidence of inadvertent globe perforation during strabismus surgery. Br J Ophthalmol 1990;74:490–493

193. Minckler DS, Francis BA, Hodapp EA, et al. Aqueous shunts in glaucoma: a report by the American Academy of Ophthalmology. Ophthalmology 2008;115:1089–1098

194. Desai MA, Gedde SJ, Feuer WJ, Shi W, Chen PP, Parrish RK II. Practice preferences for glaucoma surgery: a survey of the American Glaucoma Society in 2008. Ophthalmic Surg Lasers Imaging 2011;42:202–208

195. Bull H, von Wolff K, Körber N, Tetz M. Three-year canaloplasty outcomes for the treatment of open-angle glaucoma: European study results. Graefes Arch Clin Exp Ophthalmol 2011;249:1537–1545

196. Schoenberg ED, Chaudhry AL, Chod R, Zurakowski D, Ayyala RS. Comparison of surgical outcomes between phacocanaloplasty and phacotra-beculectomy at 12 months follow-up: a longitudinal cohort study. J Glaucoma 2015;24:543–549

197. Brüggemann A, Despouy JT, Wegent A, Müller M. Intraindividual comparison of Canaloplasty versus trabeculectomy with mitomycin C in a single-surgeon series. J Glaucoma 2013;22:577–583

48 Microinvasive Glaucoma Surgery

Harmanjit Singh and Iqbal Ike K. Ahmed

The development of microinvasive glaucoma surgery (MIGS) over the last decade has brought this field to an exciting new era. MIGS has a highly favorable risk profile compared with traditional surgeries and can easily be performed in conjunction with cataract surgery. The opportunity to improve vision and to reduce both intraocular pressure (IOP) and the need for topical medications with a single surgery is very appealing. This chapter describes MIGS techniques and management strategies, using the micro-stent as the prime example.

Background

Cataract and glaucoma are the leading causes of blindness worldwide.[1] They are often present simultaneously; hence, it is reasonable to treat these diseases together in one combined surgery. Glaucoma and ocular hypertension affect nearly 20% of patients undergoing cataract surgery in the United States.[2]

In the past, glaucoma treatment primarily included topical or systemic medication and lasers before advancing to filtration surgery. The treatment algorithm remained standard regardless of the severity of glaucomatous disease. In addition to the huge safety gap between the nonsurgical and surgical options, the latter options are associated with vision-threatening complications. The Tube Versus Trabeculectomy (TVT) study demonstrated that early and late postoperative complications occurred in 73% of trabeculectomies and 55% of aqueous drainage devices.[3]

To fill this gap, safer options are now available: microinvasive glaucoma surgery. MIGS is defined by five main characteristics: an ab interno conjunctiva-sparing approach, minimal disruption of normal anatomy and physiology, modest to high IOP-lowering efficacy, a positive safety profile, and rapid recovery by the patient.[4] Trabecular micro-bypass surgery is a physiological option as it restores the natural drainage pathway and avoids blebs and its related complications. Furthermore, it preserves potential future treatment options including incisional glaucoma surgery.

After its first introduction in Europe in 2004, the iStent (Glaukos, Laguna Hills, CA), a trabecular micro-bypass stent targeting the conventional outflow system, was approved by the Food and Drug Administration (FDA) in 2012.[5] It is the smallest known medical device to be implanted in the human body. It is made of nonferromagnetic titanium measuring 1 mm by 0.33 mm, and the diameter of the snorkel part is 120 µm **(Fig. 48.1)**.[6] The other trabecular micro-bypass stent targeting the conventional outflow system is the Hydrus microstent (Ivantis, Irvine, CA), which is still undergoing clinical trials.[5] The latest version of this micro-stent is a crescent-shaped 8-mm device designed to scaffold and dilate three clock hour positions of Schlemm's canal (SC). Another FDA-approved MIGS device for performing an ab interno trabeculectomy is the Trabectome (NeoMedix, Tustin, CA). It uses electrocautery to ablate a segment of the trabecular meshwork (TM) and the inner wall of SC

to achieve direct flow of aqueous into the SC and the collector channels. Studies have shown a significant decrease in IOP and medication load with a favorable safety profile for patients with mild to moderate open-angle glaucoma undergoing MIGS in combination with phacoemulsification.[7–11]

Anatomy

Recognizing angle anatomy variations and understanding the physiology of the ocular outflow system are essential for MIGS success. The normal conventional outflow pathway of the aqueous humor is from the anterior chamber to the TM, entering the SC to be further drained by collector channels or aqueous veins to the episcleral venous system.[12] An average of four to six aqueous veins, most commonly found in the inferonasal quadrant, are responsible for most of the eye's outflow system.[13,14] They are of larger caliber, with an average diameter of 50 µm **(Fig. 48.2)**.[13–15] In primary open-angle glaucoma (POAG), the location of highest resistance to outflow is the juxtacanalicular TM.[12] A trabecular micro-bypass stent can thus enhance the conventional, pressure-dependent outflow pathway by allowing aqueous to directly bypass the TM.[16] This causes an increase in the pressure applied on the downstream collector channels and also increases the aqueous drainage, especially in the area where the bypass is located.[16,17] The inferonasal quadrant appears to be the ideal implantation site, as a higher density of collector channels and aqueous veins are typically present.[13,16,17] Therefore, trabecular bypass should optimize outflow, thus reducing the IOP. However, the IOP reduction is limited by the distal outflow system and the episcleral venous pressure (EVP), which is normally between 8 and 11 mm Hg.[12]

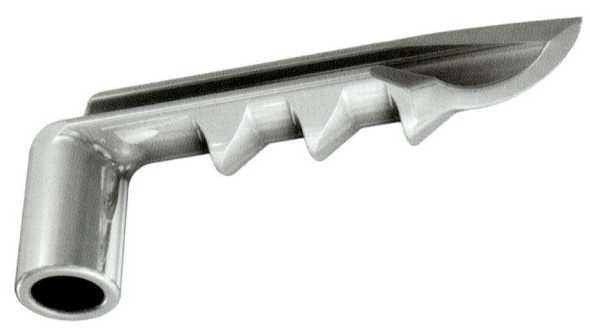

Fig. 48.1 iStent trabecular micro-bypass device (Glaukos). (Courtesy of Glaukos.)

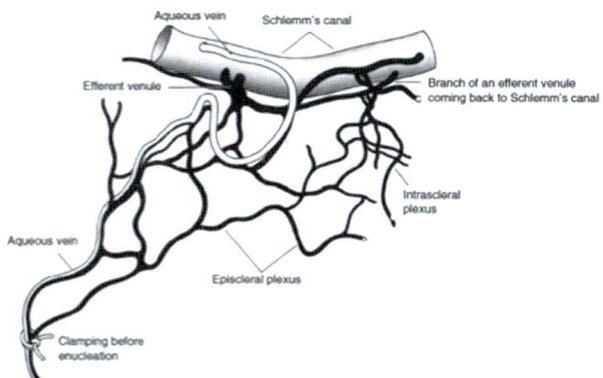

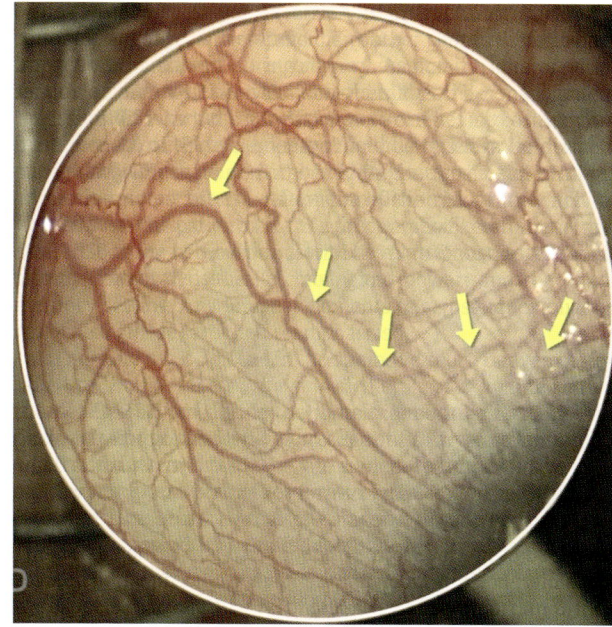

Fig. 48.2 **(a)** Drainage routes of aqueous humor. **(b)** An aqueous vein *(arrows)*. (**a** from Sampaolesi R, Sampaolesi JR, Zárate J. Structure and function of the tissues that are in contact with the aqueous humor. In: Sampaolesi R, Sampaolesi JR, Zárate J. The Glaucomas. Berlin: Springer-Verlag, 2014. Reprinted by permission.)

Preoperative Considerations

Preparation

Performing MIGS is a highly technical procedure with a steep learning curve. Surgical success depends on adequate planning and proper knowledge of anatomic landmarks of the iridocorneal angle. It is imperative to review the gonioscopy findings in the office and essential to learn intraoperative gonioscopy before performing surgery. Practicing in a wet-lab facilitates becoming acquainted with the surgical steps under direct gonioscopic view. The best way to get started with MIGS is to simulate angle surgery with a goniolens in routine cataract surgeries before attempting it on patients. One may manipulate an instrument in the angle to get a feel for the magnification and ergonomics of the maneuvers. One can also practice tilting the microscope and the patient's head. Mastering the steps without the pressure of implanting the device will help make the surgeon more comfortable in preparing for the first surgical procedure. It may also be useful to watch surgical videos of the implantation technique and review the steps in detail.

Instrumentation

Appropriate equipment is key to MIGS success. The micro-bypass stent comes preloaded in a single-use, sterile injector.[6] It has a secure, rotatable grip and reacquisition capability to facilitate manipulation and placement into the SC. The inserter has a button that is pressed to release or disengage the device at the appropriate time. There are two orientations of the micro-stent: the right and the left.[6] The left micro-stent is easier to implant by most right-handed surgeons, as they may feel more comfortable with a forehand insertion technique (**Fig. 48.3**). For right micro-stent, they must use a backhand technique, which may be more challenging (**Fig. 48.4**). If implanting one micro-stent, surgeons should opt for the most comfortable approach, regardless of the design. At our center, two micro-stents per eye are typically implanted, one right and one left.

Use of a cohesive ophthalmic viscoelastic device (OVD) in the anterior chamber (AC) provides the clearest view. If needed, the surgeon should not hesitate to inject more to clear any blood in the angle, making sure to release some from the wound to prevent over pressurization of the AC and collapsing the SC.

Several goniolens prototypes are available, designed to optimize angle visualization including clarity, globe stability, accessibility, and simultaneous surgical manipulation of angle structures.[18] The Swan-Jacob goniolens (Ocular Instruments, Bellevue, WA) is commonly used for manipulation during angle surgery. However, it requires repositioning of the patient's head and the microscope. Thus, access to a surgical microscope with large tilt capabilities is necessary.

Micro-tying forceps (MicroSurgical Technologies, Redmond, WA) are very useful tools in various situations.[19] They may be used for regrasping, repositioning, and ensuring appropriate positioning of the device. It may be easier to manipulate the device with the micro-tying forceps rather than the inserter once it has released the micro-stent.

Patient Selection and Preoperative Management

Indications for MIGS are mild to moderate open-angle glaucoma in the presence of a cataract in patients who are able to tolerate topical medications, if needed postoperatively.[7,11] For initial cases, it is preferable to schedule a combined procedure for patients in whom cataract surgery alone would be sufficient, but who may derive additional benefit from MIGS. If the device cannot be implanted for some reason, the patient can be expected to still do well with or without topical IOP-lowering medication. It is also initially recommended to select patients who have prominent angle landmarks, a well-defined pigmented TM, and wide-open angles. Also, avoid performing the surgery during a busy operative schedule, as the time pressure can lead to added stress.

The sedation must be titrated so that the patient may participate and cooperate as much as possible. A retrobulbar or peribulbar block may be used during the first few cases to minimize patient movement.[5] However, this implies no cooperation from the patient with respect to eye movements during surgery. It is preferable to perform MIGS with the patient under topical anesthesia, as the patient can assist by moving the eye as directed to

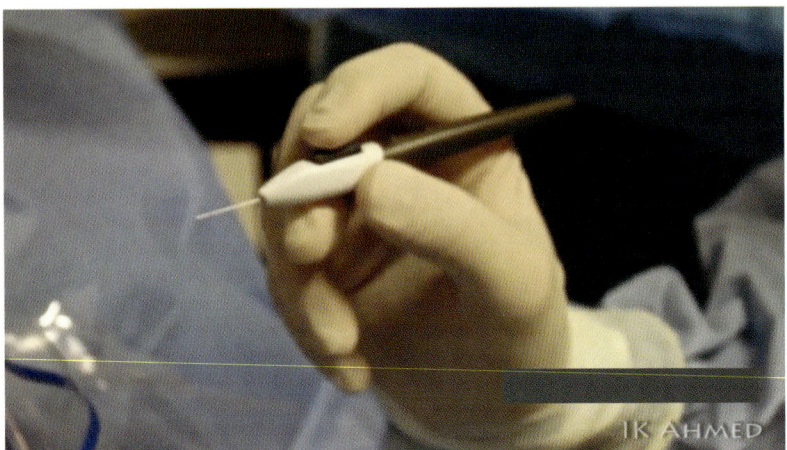

a

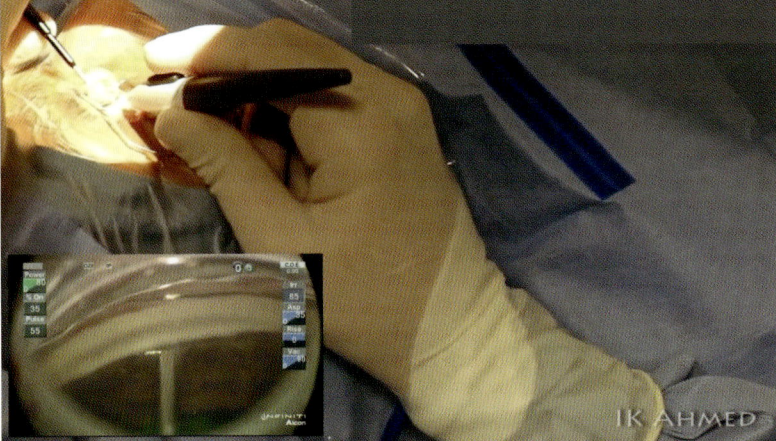

b

Fig. 48.3 **(a)** Forehand insertion technique. **(b)** Left-pointing iStent with forehand grip in counterclockwise rotation.

optimize the surgical view. It therefore is important to select patients who are able to cooperate, who do not have a language barrier, and whose cognitive status is good. The lack of any of these patient factors can compromise the procedure intraoperatively.

Intracameral or preoperative miotics have also been recommended by some surgeons to constrict the pupil and open the angle.[5] In our center, we generally perform MIGS before cataract extraction and have not felt the need to use miotics, as using OVD in the angle usually opens the angle effectively and adequately. If the angle is not sufficiently open, some surgeons prefer implanting the micro-stent after performing phacoemulsification. This order of steps may also prevent the pupil from coming down before phacoemulsification. However, our preference is to implant the micro-stent first as the corneal clarity is maximized, the eye is firmer and the OVD is already in place for phacoemulsification.

Technique Overview

Initial Steps

After performing a standard paracentesis for routine cataract surgery, intracameral anesthesia is achieved by injecting Xylocaine 2% in the anterior chamber. A soft shell technique (see Chapter 17), which entails injecting a dispersive OVD followed by a cohesive, is employed to deepen and maintain the AC. Care must be taken not to overinflate the eye, as this may collapse the SC, making insertion of the micro-stent difficult. Insufficient

OVD may cause Descemet's folds and difficulty with visualization. Then a temporal clear corneal main incision is made, as done in a routine cataract surgery. It is suggested to perform the main incision slightly anterior to the limbus to avoid blood vessels. Even minimal hemorrhage can obstruct the view during gonioscopy, further increasing the difficulty of implantation. However, the incision should not be too anterior as this may obscure visualization of the angle, as the inserter may interfere with the gonioprism.

Patient Positioning

The patient should be reminded to follow instructions and avoid sudden movements of the eyes or head. The patient should be asked to move the eyes very gently and slowly when indicated. The patient's head must be tilted 40 degrees away from the surgeon, and the microscope angled 35 degrees toward the surgeon, to enable the illumination to be directed nasally for a direct gonioscopic view of the angle **(Fig. 48.5)**. The patient is then asked to slightly fixate away from the operated eye. The surgeon then needs to adjust the oculars superiorly and reset the microscope focus and magnification. The cornea should be irrigated with balanced salt solution (BSS) and any blood should be cleared. OVD may be placed on the cornea as a coupling agent to provide the best view. With the dominant hand, insert the micro-stent injector into the AC, entering parallel to the iris plane across the pupillary margin, to avoid capturing the iris. At this point, using your nondominant hand, place the Swan-Jacob gonioprism on

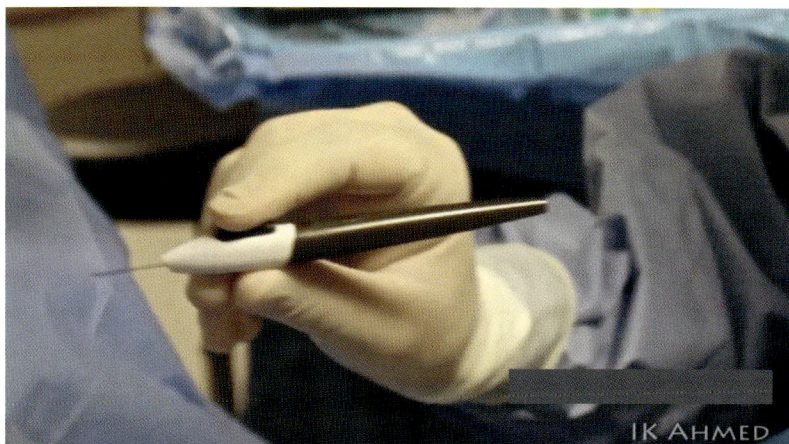

a

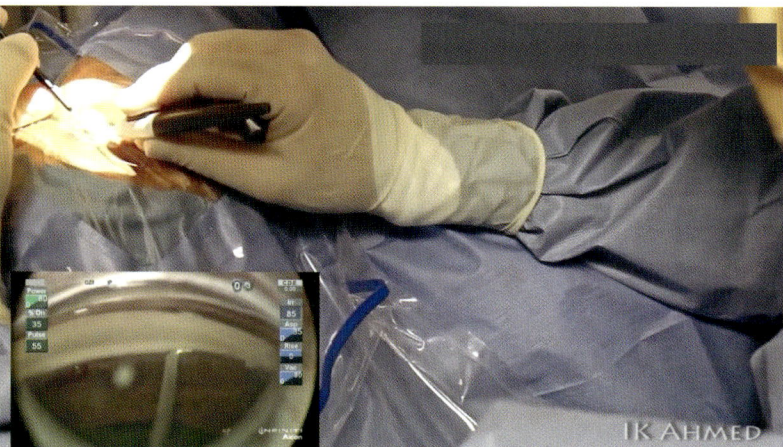

b

the cornea and focus on the angle. Make sure that only gentle pressure is applied on the cornea to avoid any Descemet's folds, which can blur visualization of the angle. Also avoid placing pressure on the wound with the inserter for the same reason. It is recommended to work under high magnification when implanting the micro-stent. Under direct gonioscopic view, advance the micro-stent for visualization in the angle. Furthermore, a direct "en-face" view is favored when performing micro-stent implantation, as opposed to a top-down view.

Micro-Stent Insertion

The TM is identified as a pigmented line between the scleral spur and Schwalbe's line and is the site for device insertion. Advance the micro-stent to position the tip over the superior third of the TM. The micro-stent should engage the TM with a 30-degree approach for easier entry and to be steep enough to thoroughly penetrate the inner wall (**Fig. 48.6**). The TM should be engaged gently to avoid ripping and unnecessary bleeding. Once the tip is

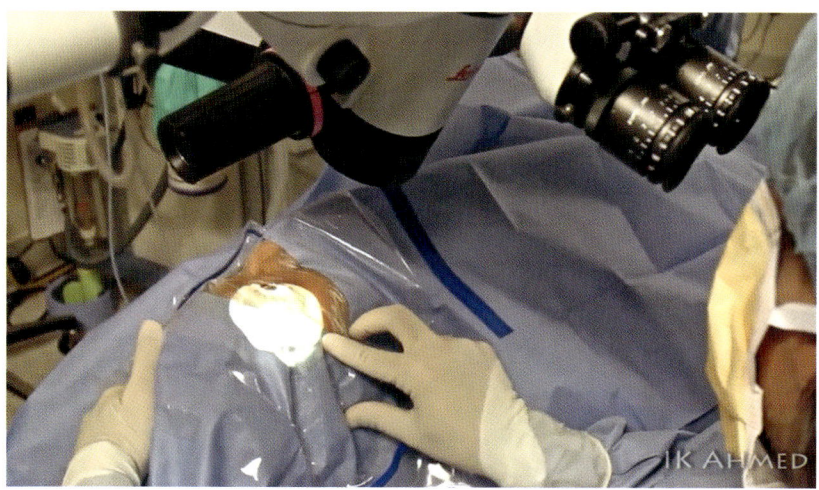

Fig. 48.5 Patient positioning and microscope tilt. The patient's head must be tilted 40 degrees away from the surgeon and the microscope angled 35 degrees toward the surgeon for optimal visualization of angle structures.

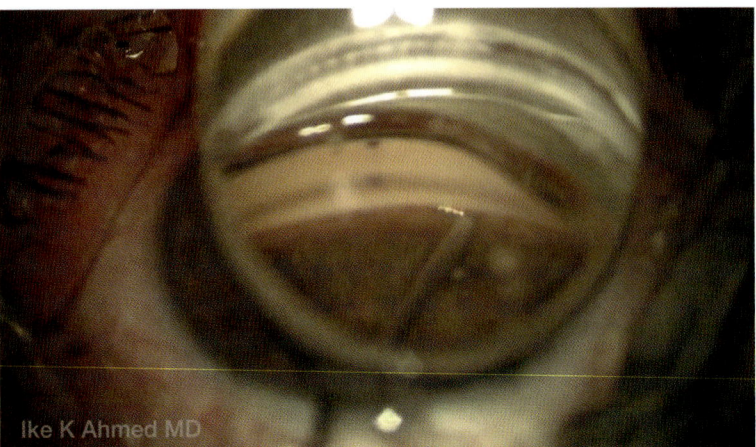

Fig. 48.6 Micro-stent insertion. The micro-stent should engage the trabecular meshwork with a 30-degree approach for easier entry and to be steep enough to thoroughly penetrate the inner wall.

in the SC, one should straighten out the device to follow the curvature of the angle and advance it with a gentle motion, while the base is kept parallel to the TM. It is important at this step to palmar flex one's wrist, instead of advancing one's hand. Using the incision as a fulcrum prevents loss of visualization with corneal striae. It may also be useful to pull the device toward you to avoid the posterior scleral wall. Only minimal resistance should be encountered. The device should be advanced until the snorkel touches the TM. Once it is well placed, make sure that there is no tension on the micro-stent and that the eye is in neutral position before releasing from the inserter. This way, the device should not spring back when released due to torque forces.

After placement, it is recommended to gently tap the side of the snorkel with the inserter to ensure that the device is securely sitting in the SC. The retention arches of the micro-stent appear obscured by the lacy TM when properly inserted, and the TM should completely surround the snorkel (**Fig. 48.7**). If there is heme released from the snorkel, cohesive OVD should be injected in the angle to tamponade and visualize the device and confirm its position. A small intraoperative blood reflux may be a sign of system patency but is an inconsistent finding (**Fig. 48.8**).[5] The second micro-stent is then placed at least two clock hour positions away from the first micro-stent to increase the chance of accessing a different aqueous vein. For the right micro-stent, we recommend using a backhand approach with your dominant hand if right-handed. It is important at this step to flex your elbow, and increasingly pronate your forearm with palmar flex-ion of the wrist (**Fig. 48.4**). Alternatively, you may also use your left hand.

Phacoemulsification

After the stent placement is confirmed gonioscopically, the patient's head and the microscope are repositioned for a standard cataract surgery. OVD may be added if needed to refill the AC and cataract extraction may be performed with the technique of choice. It is essential to remove all the OVD from the AC and the capsular bag at the end of the procedure to prevent IOP spike. Before terminating the procedure, the eye is well pressurized with BSS to prevent any blood reflux from the micro-stent and avoid hyphema postoperatively. Finally, it is important to ensure that the incisions are watertight.

Postoperative Care

Our postoperative regimen and recommendations are similar to those for standard postoperative cataract surgery and include antibiotics, nonsteroidal anti-inflammatory drugs, and steroid drops. A lower potency steroid may be used to prevent steroid response. In addition to the postoperative drops described above, miotics sometimes may be used to keep the iris flat and away from the angle, preventing peripheral anterior synechiae (PAS) formation. One can try tapering topical glaucoma medication anytime postoperatively depending on the target IOP, being mindful

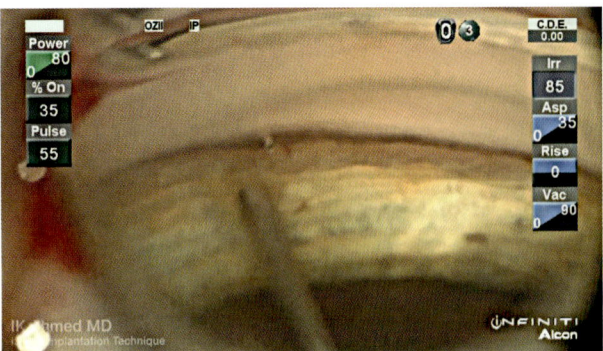

Fig. 48.7 Adequately placed micro-stent with retention arches opaque and covered by the trabecular meshwork.

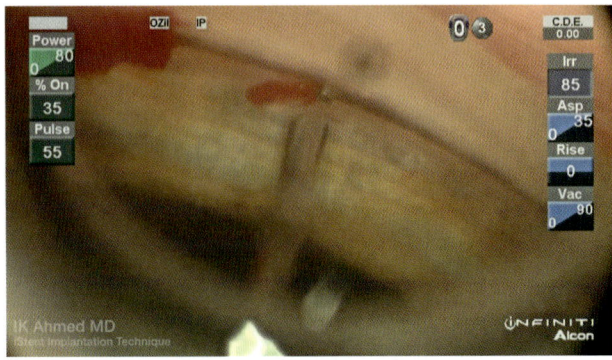

Fig. 48.8 Intraoperative blood reflux.

of a possible steroid response.[5,20] Assessing the new baseline IOP must wait at least 6 to 8 weeks postoperatively. Until then, the patient must be carefully monitored and medications may be added or tapered as needed.

Special Maneuvers

Target Micro-Stents to Aqueous Veins

Although the conventional outflow system is interconnected, it seems to be segmental and a device implanted in a certain region does not necessarily access the entire system.[13] One promising technique is to strategically target micro-stent implantation in areas of preferential flow where aqueous veins may be seen. To do so, meticulous preoperative evaluation of the episcleral venous structure around the limbus is necessary to identify these aqueous veins. At the end of the surgery, one may notice laminar flow in the aqueous vein targeted and blanching in the area where micro-stent has been implanted (**Fig. 48.9**). Using targeted placement of the micro-stents may lead to a greater reduction of IOP. Placement of multiple micro-stents may further increase the number of aqueous veins accessed and potentially further lower the IOP.[20] Multiple micro-stents combined with phacoemulsification were studied. The IOP reduction was similar in the two micro-stent group compared with the three micro-stent group; however, at 1 year, patients in the three micro-stent group were on significantly fewer topical medications.[20]

Identifying Nonpigmented Trabecular Meshwork

At times, the TM may be nonpigmented or very lightly pigmented, making the site of insertion difficult to detect. There are a few ways to circumvent this problem. First, one can look for local, pinpoint red areas in the SC, indicating blood reflux from collector channels. If it is not visible, pressure may be applied on the perilimbal conjunctiva to favor blood reflux in the SC to help identify these sites. Alternatively, hypotony may be induced at the beginning of surgery, allowing blood reflux in the SC. Second, TM placement can be in focal area of hyperpigmentation, which once again indicates areas for higher outflow and greatest density of collector channels.[5] Finally, it is important, as mentioned before, to do a complete gonioscopic examination preoperatively in the office and to make detailed notes to help with intraoperative decision making. Preoperatively, the corneal wedge is a well-described and effective technique to delineate Schwalbe's line, and the TM is located directly posterior to it.

Pearls and Pitfalls

Great care should be taken while manipulating the device in the eye to avoid trauma to adjacent structures, such as the corneal endothelium, the iris, and the lens.

Visualization

Good gonioscopy technique, patient positioning, and microscope tilt are critical for optimal visualization of angle structures. Every step as described previously is integral to the overall success of the procedure. Appropriate inflation of the eye with OVD cannot be undermined. However, it is integral to avoid overinflation, to avoid SC collapse, or underinflation, causing corneal striae that compromise the surgeon's view.[21] It is also important to let the gonioprism float on the corneal surface to avoid corneal striae. One should judiciously use OVD to tamponade any bleeding in the angle to avoid blurring the view.

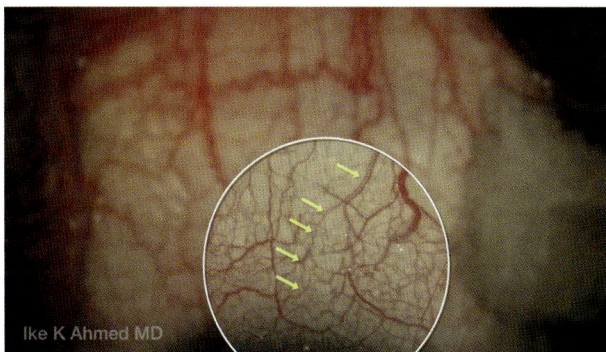

Fig. 48.9 Laminar flow in the aqueous vein targeted by the micro-stent.

Schlemm's Canal Insertion

If significant resistance is felt when entering the SC or if the eye rotates during insertion, inadvertent engagement of the scleral outer wall may occur. One must then relax the pressure on the device, pull toward oneself, and change the direction of the insertion. Alternatively, one can retract the micro-stent and reinsert in the same location or one to two clock hour positions away from the original site.

Superficial Placement

For the micro-stent to be adequately placed, it should be parallel to the TM, and the retention arches should be opaque and covered by the TM, with the snorkel protruding in the AC, perpendicularly to the TM. One can also look at the scleral spur, confirming that the device is seated parallel to it. If the retention arches are easily visible (**Fig. 48.10**), it may be possible that the micro-stent is superficially placed within the inner wall or the TM layers. This problem may occur with overpressurization of the AC with OVD or with a flat approach into the SC. Once recognized intraoperatively, this problem is rectified by regrasping and then reattempting micro-stent implantation. As most of the complications associated with the device are the result of improper placement, the surgeon should be extremely focused and driven about positioning.[7,20]

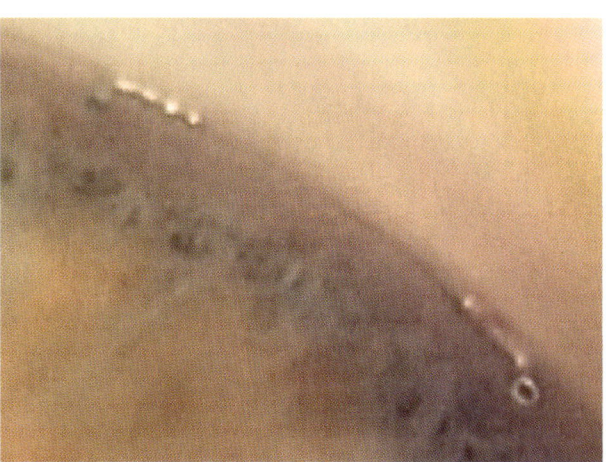

Fig. 48.10 Superficially placed micro-stent with retention arches easily visible.

Micro-Stent Manipulations

If the micro-stent dislodges from the inserter or is inadequately placed, it can easily be regrasped and reloaded. Alternatively, micro-tying forceps may be used to manipulate the stent. OVD may be used to move and present the device for easier grasping with the inserter or the micro-tying forceps.

Postoperative Complications

Complications from MIGS are marginal when compared with traditional filtration surgeries and include obstruction by fibrin or PAS, stent malposition or superficial placement, transient hyphema, IOP spike, and steroid response.[7,9,20]

Some surgeons described relieving stent obstruction by using the yttrium-aluminum-garnet (YAG) laser.[11,20] Stent malposition may be prevented by adequate and compulsive confirmation intraoperatively. Postoperative gonioscopy is also important to recognize any iris tissue or PAS development near the device. If noticed in the early postoperative period, miotics may be useful in maintaining the patency of the micro-stent or the fistula.

Hyphema may occur secondary to blood reflux from the collector channels, indicating free communication with the drainage system.[5] It is usually transitory and no surgical intervention has been reported. If associated with IOP spike, this may be managed medically until the blood resorbs. Other causes of IOP elevation are OVD retention, inflammation, and steroid response. To avoid the latter, steroids must be tapered quickly depending on the inflammation. Alternatively, low-potency steroids may be used to reduce the incidence of steroid response.

To date, there have been no reports of vision-threatening complications, such as choroidal effusion or hemorrhage, persistent hypotony, bleb-related complications, or endophthalmitis.

Conclusion

Microinvasive glaucoma surgery may help fill the safety gap between the medical options, laser treatments, and high-risk filtration procedures. Performing these surgeries has a steep learning curve, and proper technique is crucial for success and low complication rates. MIGS has a highly favorable risk profile compared with traditional surgeries and can be performed in conjunction with phacoemulsification in patients with concurrent cataract and glaucoma.

References

1. Quigley HA, Broman AT. The number of people with glaucoma worldwide in 2010 and 2020. Br J Ophthalmol 2006;90:262–267

2. Centers for Medicare and Medicaid Services. 2002–2007 Medicare Standard Analytical File. Baltimore, MD: Centers for Medicare and Medicaid Services, US Department of Health and Human Services; 2007

3. Gedde SJ, Herndon LW, Brandt JD, Budenz DL, Feuer WJ, Schiffman JC; Tube Versus Trabeculectomy Study Group. Postoperative complications in the Tube Versus Trabeculectomy (TVT) study during five years of follow-up. Am J Ophthalmol 2012;153:804–814

4. Ahmed IIK. Defining MIGS. Cataract Refract Surg Today 2014;October: 57–58

5. Kahook MY. MIGS: Advances in Glaucoma Surgery. Thorofare, NJ: Slack; 2014

6. Glaukos. iStent. http://www.glaukos.com/istent. Accessed December 2014

7. Samuelson TW, Katz LJ, Wells JM, Duh YJ, Giamporcaro JE; US iStent Study Group. Randomized evaluation of the trabecular micro-bypass stent with phacoemulsification in patients with glaucoma and cataract. Ophthalmology 2011;118:459–467

8. Fea AM. Phacoemulsification versus phacoemulsification with micro-bypass stent implantation in primary open-angle glaucoma: randomized double-masked clinical trial. J Cataract Refract Surg 2010;36:407–412

9. Francis BA, Minckler D, Dustin L, et al; Trabectome Study Group. Combined cataract extraction and trabeculotomy by the internal approach for coexisting cataract and open-angle glaucoma: initial results. J Cataract Refract Surg 2008;34:1096–1103

10. Minckler DS, Baerveldt G, Alfaro MR, Francis BA. Clinical results with the Trabectome for treatment of open-angle glaucoma. Ophthalmology 2005;112:962–967

11. Craven ER, Katz LJ, Wells JM, Giamporcaro JE; iStent Study Group. Cataract surgery with trabecular micro-bypass stent implantation in patients with mild-to-moderate open-angle glaucoma and cataract: two-year follow-up. J Cataract Refract Surg 2012;38:1339–1345

12. Ramakrishnan R, Krishnadas S, Khurana M, Robin AL. Diagnosis and Management of Glaucoma. Kerala, India: Jaypee Brothers Medical Publishers; 2013

13. Ascher K. The Aqueous Veins. Springfield, IL: Charles C. Thomas; 1961

14. Schacknow P, Samples J. The Glaucoma Book. New York: Springer; 2010

15. Sampaolesi R, Sampaolesi JR, Zárate J. The Glaucomas. Berlin: Springer Verlag; 2014

16. Zhou J, Smedley GT. Trabecular bypass: effect of Schlemm canal and collector channel dilation. J Glaucoma 2006;15:446–455

17. Bahler CK, Smedley GT, Zhou J, Johnson DH. Trabecular bypass stents decrease intraocular pressure in cultured human anterior segments. Am J Ophthalmol 2004;138:988–994

18. Shareef S, Alward W, Crandall A, Vold S, Ahmed I. Intra-operative gonioscopy: a key to successful angle surgery. Expert Rev Ophthalmol 2014; •••:1–13; early online

19. MicroSurgical Technologies products. http://www.microsurgical.com/products/forceps-and-scissors. Accessed December 2014

20. Belovay GW, Naqi A, Chan BJ, Rateb M, Ahmed II. Using multiple trabecular micro-bypass stents in cataract patients to treat open-angle glaucoma. J Cataract Refract Surg 2012;38:1911–1917

21. Kaplowitz K, Schuman JS, Loewen NA. Techniques and outcomes of minimally invasive trabecular ablation and bypass surgery. Br J Ophthalmol 2014;98:579–585

XVIII Toxic Anterior Segment Syndrome and Endophthalmitis

49 Toxic Anterior Segment Syndrome

Nick Mamalis and Mohammed Aabid Farukhi

Toxic anterior segment syndrome (TASS) is a rare, yet serious complication that typically develops acutely following exposure of a toxic substance to the anterior segment of the eye. It is a sterile, postoperative, inflammatory reaction of the anterior segment. Though cataract surgery is the most common surgery leading to the development of TASS, it can theoretically occur after any anterior segment surgery, including cornea transplant or glaucoma surgeries. Any substance used during or immediately after anterior segment surgery can potentially cause TASS, as the tissues of the anterior segment of the eye are very sensitive structures. The extent and intensity of the inflammatory reaction depends on the type of toxin and the duration the toxin remains in the anterior segment. A common end point of the toxic insult is the widespread breakdown of the blood–aqueous barrier, resulting in significant anterior segment inflammation with increased aqueous cell and flair as well as possible fibrin and hypopyon formation. Prompt recognition and treatment of TASS is critical. It is important to distinguish TASS from other causes of postoperative inflammation, especially infectious endophthalmitis, though this is often difficult. Any uncertainty of diagnosis should result in the collection of vitreous and aqueous fluid for further infectious workup. Although prevention is the most effective method of minimizing the incidence of TASS, topical corticosteroids remain the mainstay of treatment in positive cases. Outcomes vary depending on the type of toxic substance that enters the eye, the duration of exposure to the substance, and the amount of time before initiation of treatment, and can resolve completely or result in significant sequelae including permanent corneal edema, or medically refractive glaucoma.

Toxic anterior segment syndrome typically develops 12 to 48 hours following anterior segment surgery, though a rare, delayed-onset TASS has been reported.[1] The inflammation is sterile and is triggered by a substance that enters the anterior segment of the eye.

The occurrence of TASS is rare, though it is difficult to estimate its exact incidence. A retrospective case series conducted at the Aravind Eye Hospital in India reported an incidence of 0.23% (60 eyes from 26,408 cataract surgeries).[2] Cases of TASS often occur in clusters, though individual cases have been seen. Sporadic cases of TASS are often overlooked, given the lack of awareness of available registries for reporting outbreaks. In response to TASS outbreaks, the American Society of Cataract and Refractive Surgery (ASCRS) created a TASS task force, to educate anterior segment surgeons regarding TASS and to help investigate outbreaks of TASS. Questionnaires are available on the ASCRS Web site to aid in the reporting of TASS cases.[3]

The pathophysiology of TASS involves a toxic insult that damages the corneal endothelial cell layer, iris, or trabecular meshwork, resulting in a marked inflammatory reaction. The extent and intensity of the inflammatory reaction depends on the type of toxin and the duration that the toxin remains in the anterior segment. A common end point of the toxic insult is the wide-spread breakdown of the blood–aqueous barrier, resulting in significant anterior segment inflammation with increased aqueous cell and flair as well as possible fibrin and hypopyon formation.

Etiology

The etiologies of TASS are broad, as any substance used during or immediately after anterior segment surgery can potentially cause TASS. Upon entering the anterior segment, the toxic substance causes injury to the sensitive tissues of the eye, particularly the corneal endothelium, iris, and trabecular meshwork.

A recent retrospective analysis by Bodnar et al[4] of surveys reporting cases of TASS from June 2007 through March 2012 evaluated the most common risk factors for TASS. The study identified inadequate cleaning and sterilization of ophthalmic instruments as the most commonly identified risk factor for TASS. Other causes include the use of medications or solutions containing incorrect formulations or toxic additives, mishandling of intraocular lenses or instrument tips, and poor maintenance of equipment used for cleaning surgical instruments.

The etiologies of TASS can be categorized as (1) intraocular medications and solutions, and (2) cleaning and sterilization of ophthalmic instruments.

Intraocular Medications and Solutions

Balanced Salt Solution

Virtually all cataract procedures use balanced salt solution (BSS) as an irrigating solution intraoperatively. Abnormalities in the composition of BSS, including pH, osmolarity, or ionic composition, can lead to the development of TASS. Specifically, pH values less than 6.5 or greater than 8.5 are toxic to tissues in the anterior chamber. Osmolarity values less than 200 mOsm or greater than 400 mOsm may cause cellular damage to tissues in the anterior chamber. Furthermore, any substance added to BSS during surgery (i.e., epinephrine or antibiotics) may also cause TASS, especially those containing preservatives.

Topical Ophthalmic Eyedrops

Many topical eyedrops contain preservatives or stabilizing agents intended to maintain the efficacy of the medication for an extended period of time. These agents may be toxic to the corneal endothelium if they gain access to the anterior chamber of the eye. The most common preservative in topical ophthalmic drops is benzalkonium chloride. There are reports of patients developing significant corneal edema or endothelial cell damage after being treated with solutions containing this substance.[5] Another preservative to be wary of is methyl paraben, which is used in lidocaine. Though these preservatives are relatively safe when used on the surface of the eye, they are toxic to anterior segment tissue and should be avoided during anterior segment surgery.

Stabilizing Agents

Stabilizing agents, such as bisulfites and metasulfites in a high enough concentration, are also potentially toxic to anterior segment tissues, especially corneal endothelium. Addition of a stabilizing agent, such as bisulfite, to epinephrine prevents the degradation and efficacy of the medication. However, these additives are known to cause corneal endothelial damage, resulting in TASS when not properly diluted. Intracameral epinephrine containing 0.1% bisulfite has been associated with corneal edema, whereas epinephrine containing 0.05% bisulfite does not cause endothelial changes.[6] Given that bisulfite-free epinephrine is not available in the Unites States, and that the need for epinephrine to combat miosis is critical, commercially available epinephrine is appropriate for use, but only when it is diluted at least 1:4 in BSS or in a preservative-free anesthetic.

Intraocular Anesthetics

Intraocular anesthetics are increasingly used to reduce intraoperative and postoperative pain and to supplement topical anesthetics. The most common intracameral anesthetic currently used in surgery is 1% methylparaben-free (MPF) lidocaine. Low concentrations of preservative-free anesthetics do not seem to cause endothelial toxicity. Higher concentrations (i.e., > 2.0% lidocaine) or preservative-containing anesthetics are toxic to endothelial tissue. For example, 2.0% lidocaine has been associated with significant postoperative corneal thickening and opacification. Therefore, it is critical that intracameral anesthetics be preservative-free and of the appropriate concentration.

Intraocular Antibiotics

Although the practice of mixing antibiotics into BSS has largely fallen out of favor due to the unproven efficacy in preventing endophthalmitis, it is still being practiced by numerous surgical centers, as reported by Bodnar et al.[4] The lack of a commercially available injectable solution approved for endophthalmitis prophylaxis increases the risk of developing TASS secondary to improperly mixed, diluted, or prepared antibiotics. In addition, the narrow therapeutic index of antibiotics in general increases the incidence of poor outcomes with intracameral antibiotic use. Antibiotics such as gentamicin and cefuroxime have been associated with anterior and posterior segment inflammation, including TASS, cystoid macular edema, and macular infarction, when inadequately prepared or used in too high a concentration.[7–10]

Because no injectable prophylactic antibiotic solution exists in the United States, any intracameral antibiotic must be mixed, diluted, and prepared appropriately prior to use in surgery. Improper preparation of these antibiotics has been associated with both anterior and posterior segment inflammation.[10] Several studies found intracameral cefuroxime to be associated with a reduction in the occurrence of endophthalmitis when used in the proper concentration (1 mg/0.1 cc).[11–13] However, even with a strict protocol, achieving a consistent dilution for intracameral use is difficult.[14] The Intermountain Ocular Research Center recently became involved in a TASS outbreak in which 12 patients were administered a commercially available 0.5% moxifloxacin product called Moxeza (Alcon, Fort Worth, TX). This topical drug contains ingredients such as xanthan gum, sorbitol, and tyloxapol, which are toxic to sensitive structures within the anterior chamber. Any surgeon considering using intracameral antibiot-

ics must proceed with caution and ensure that any intracameral antibiotic is properly mixed.

Ophthalmic Viscosurgical Devices

Ophthalmic viscosurgical devices (OVDs) are potentially toxic to corneal endothelial cells, especially when residual OVD remains in the anterior segment at the conclusion of surgery. The incidence of retained OVD is higher in cases with posterior capsular rupture and vitreous loss, in which OVD may remain in the remnant capsular bag or posterior to the iris. In addition, poorly flushed and cleaned reusable cannulas and handpieces are a source of contamination. If OVD is retained in phaco equipment and is broken down during sterilization processes and subsequently flushed into the anterior segment during subsequent surgeries, it can cause TASS.

Cleaning and Sterilization of Ophthalmic Instruments

As previously mentioned, problems with the instrument-cleaning process was found to be the most common identified risk factor in a recent retrospective analysis.[4] The instrument cleaning process entails the use of sufficient volume for flushing equipment, flushing of the handpieces and reusable cannulas with deionized/distilled water, and the use of enzymatic detergents and ultrasonic baths.

Small-bore instruments, such as cannulas, ultrasound, and irrigation/aspiration handpieces, are particularly susceptible to retained material, given their small internal diameters and openings. Residual OVD as well as cortex can build up in these instruments and within the equipment's lumen. The OVD that remains within the lumen becomes denatured by autoclaving and could result in TASS when these instruments are used in subsequent surgeries. To avoid OVD and cortical buildup, it is critical to flush reusable cannulas and handpieces with at least 120 mL of deionized/distilled water. Deionized/distilled water ensures that the instruments do not become contaminated with solutes or endotoxins. This flushing should be done either manually with a syringe or an automated unit that is set to deliver the appropriate flush volume. Consideration should be given to using disposable cannulas whenever possible, especially with OVD cannulas.

Enzymatic Detergents and Ultrasound Baths

There are two commonly used methods to remove bioburden from surgical instruments: washing with enzymes and detergents, and placing instruments in an ultrasound bath. However, compared with most other general surgical instruments, ophthalmic instruments accumulate very little bioburden. Therefore, the cleaning process should be different for instruments used in anterior segment surgery. The use of enzymes and detergents remains debatable, but they should be avoided because they have been shown to be toxic to corneal endothelial cells in human and animal studies.[15] Enzymatic detergents are not deactivated during sterilization by autoclave, and can cause inflammation if not thoroughly flushed out of the lumen of handpieces and cannulas.

Similarly, ultrasound baths require strict and regular cleaning. If not maintained adequately, they can become colonized with gram-negative bacteria that produce endotoxin. The heat-stable endotoxin survives despite the autoclave sterilization and can cause TASS when the contaminated instruments are used in subsequent anterior segment surgeries.[4,16]

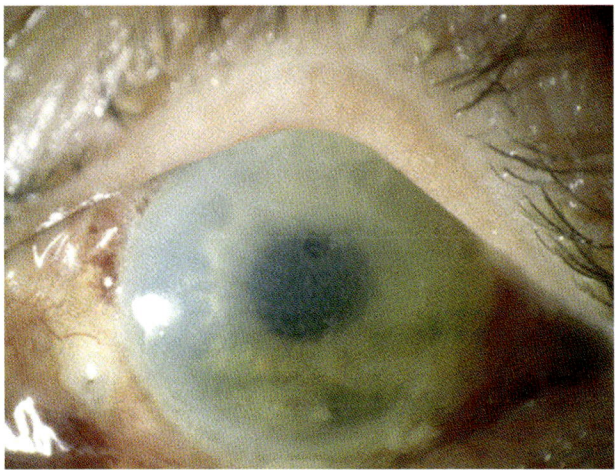

Fig. 49.1   Slit-lamp examination photograph depicting diffuse limbus-to-limbus corneal edema that is characteristic of TASS. (From Mamalis N, Edelhauser HF, Dawson DG, Chew J, LeBoyer RM, Werner L. Toxic anterior segment syndrome. J Cataract Refract Surg 2006;32:324–333. Reprinted by permission of Elsevier.)

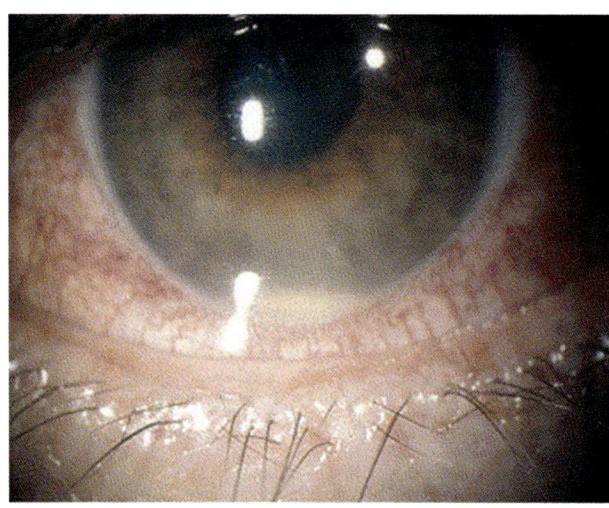

Fig. 49.2   Anterior segment inflammation with inferior hypopyon. (From Mamalis N, Edelhauser HF, Dawson DG, Chew J, LeBoyer RM, Werner L. Toxic anterior segment syndrome. J Cataract Refract Surg 2006;32:324–333. Reprinted by permission of Elsevier.)

Recognition

Prompt recognition and treatment of TASS is critical. It is important to distinguish TASS from other causes of postoperative inflammation, especially infectious endophthalmitis. Though there are numerous similarities in the presentations of both entities, their treatments differ significantly.

The hallmark of TASS is an inflammatory process that begins within 12 to 48 hours following an anterior segment surgery.[1,17] Conversely, infectious endophthalmitis presents 2 to 7 days postoperatively, or even longer, even if infected with the most virulent organism. The most common clinical symptom experienced by TASS patients is blurry vision. Other commonly observed symptoms are irritation and injection of the eye. Pain is notably absent in the presenting symptoms in TASS patients. In contrast, 75% of patients with infectious endophthalmitis present with ocular pain. Furthermore, other signs of infection, such as lid swelling, conjunctival chemosis and discharge, and diffuse ocular injection are often present in cases of infectious endophthalmitis.

The most common clinical finding on slit-lamp examination is a diffuse, limbus-to-limbus corneal edema (**Fig. 49.1**). This finding is due to widespread endothelial cell damage and is distinct from the often-noted focal edema following difficult cataract surgeries. Another common clinical examination finding is marked anterior segment inflammation and hypopyon formation secondary to breakdown of the blood–aqueous barrier (**Fig. 49.2**). This is characterized by increased numbers of inflammatory cells, aqueous flare, and fibrin formation in the anterior chamber. Unfortunately, this finding is common to both severe TASS and infectious endophthalmitis, and does not help distinguish the two disease processes.

The iris and trabecular meshwork are among the other sensitive tissues in the anterior segment that can be damaged during TASS. Slit-lamp findings include a permanently dilated and irregularly shaped iris or pupil that dilates and constricts poorly and a thin iris that can be transilluminated (**Fig. 49.3**). Severe cases of TASS may also be associated with significant damage to the trabecular meshwork, leading to ocular hypertension or secondary glaucoma that is difficult to medically manage.[1,17]

A patient presenting with acute postoperative anterior segment inflammation should have a detailed, focused eye history taken and should be examined for infectious versus noninfectious causes. Any suspicion of an infectious etiology warrants an immediate tap of the vitreous and aqueous fluids with Gram stain and cultures. Given the similarities in presentation of infectious endophthalmitis and TASS (**Fig. 49.4**), it is critical for effective treatment to distinguish between the two as quickly as possible, based on the following general characteristics of the two entities: TASS patients present earlier, typically within 24 hours postoperatively, have diffuse corneal edema, pupil/iris changes, and always have a negative Gram stain and culture. In addition, the inflammatory cells and fibrin are usually limited to the anterior chamber in TASS cases, with rare spillover into the vitreous

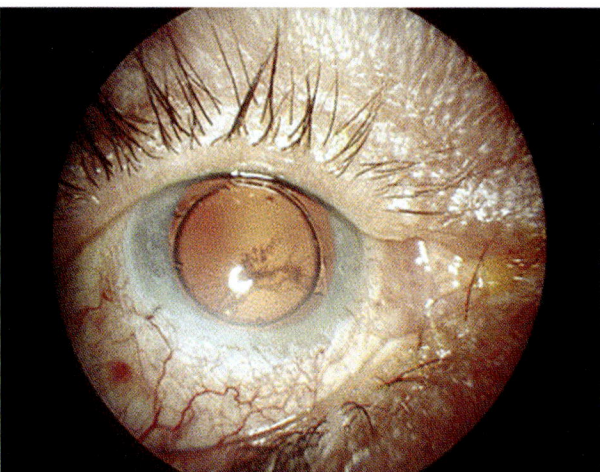

Fig. 49.3   Slit-lamp photograph demonstrating an irregularly shaped pupil and atrophic iris that can be seen in severe cases of TASS. (From Mamalis N, Edelhauser HF, Dawson DG, Chew J, LeBoyer RM, Werner L. Toxic anterior segment syndrome. J Cataract Refract Surg 2006;32:324–333. Reprinted by permission of Elsevier.)

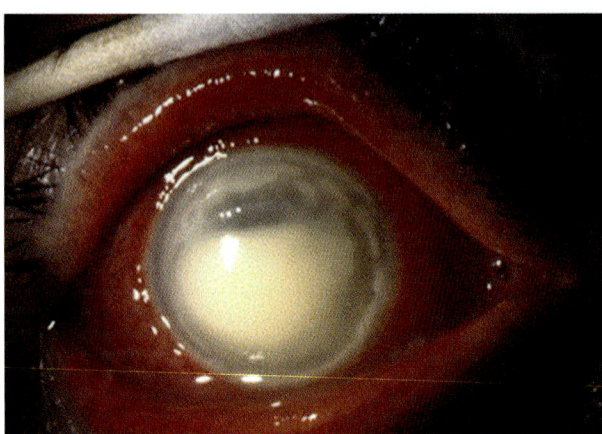

Fig. 49.4 Slit-lamp photograph of bacterial endophthalmitis. There is significant ocular injection, more prominent hypopyon formation, and association with vitreitis. (From Mamalis N, Edelhauser HF, Dawson DG, Chew J, LeBoyer RM, Werner L. Toxic anterior segment syndrome. J Cataract Refract Surg 2006;32:324–333. Reprinted by permission of Elsevier.)

chamber. In contrast, infectious endophthalmitis patients present later, usually 2 to 7 days postoperatively with the exception of highly virulent strains of bacteria, typically do not have diffuse corneal edema or pupil/iris changes, and can have a positive Gram stain or culture. It is important to know that it is possible to obtain vitreous or anterior chamber taps that are negative on Gram stain and culture in a patient with infectious bacterial endophthalmitis.[18,19] Infectious endophthalmitis cases commonly involve the vitreous in addition to the aqueous inflammation.

Treatment

Prevention of TASS is the most effective method of dealing with the syndrome. Once the offending agent is in the eye, damage has likely already occurred and there is little a clinician can do other than to suppress the secondary inflammatory response. Therefore, anterior chamber washout is neither significantly helpful nor recommended, unless there is any retained material within the anterior chamber of the eye.

Once the diagnosis of TASS is made and any infectious etiology is ruled out, the mainstay of treatment is intense topical corticosteroid drops with close observation. A low threshold for vitreous and aqueous taps should be maintained, and antibiotic injection should be considered if there is a lack of clinical improvement.

Topical corticosteroids aimed at decreasing the inflammatory response to the toxic insult are the mainstay of treatment. Prednisone acetate 1% drops every 1 to 2 hours, with careful slit-lamp exams starting hours after treatment initiation, as well as daily for the first several days, is recommended. The extent, and improvement, of anterior segment inflammation and corneal edema should be carefully documented.

Topical nonsteroidal anti-inflammatory drops and systemic steroids have not been evaluated in the treatment of TASS. However, given the theoretical value of nonsteroidal anti-inflammatory drugs in reestablishing the blood–aqueous barrier and minimizing further complications (i.e., cystoid macular edema), nonsteroidal anti-inflammatory drops may be of benefit when used in conjunction with corticosteroids.

Intraocular pressures (IOP) should be monitored frequently, as the trabecular meshwork is susceptible to damage from the toxic insult, resulting in acute trabeculitis. It is important to note

that the IOP may be low following the onset of TASS due to the disruption of aqueous humor production, but it can precipitously spike as the production of aqueous humor by the ciliary body recovers. Therefore, it is critical to monitor the IOP of a patient with TASS for several days after the initial insult. In severe cases, permanent damage to the trabecular meshwork can occur, leading to glaucoma that is refractory to medical treatment. It is recommended to perform a gonioscopic exam to search for peripheral anterior synechiae, which may indicate the presence of chronic trabecular meshwork damage.[20,21]

Outcomes

Clinical outcomes of patients with TASS depend on the severity of the toxic insult to the anterior segment. Three main factors influence the degree of severity: the type of toxic substance that enters the eye, the duration of exposure to the substance, and the time delay before initiation of treatment.

Patients with a mild case of TASS usually experience full recovery. This includes complete clearing of the cornea edema over the course of days to week without any long-term sequelae. Moderate cases of TASS are associated with a more prolonged resolution of the anterior segment inflammation. The cornea edema can take weeks to months to fully clear. In some cases, mild residual corneal edema can persist, and these patients are susceptible to increased IOP after resolution of the inflammation. Patients with severe insult can have permanent damage to the anterior segment of the eye. This includes corneal edema that does not clear, permanent iris damage, and severe glaucoma that is refractory to medical treatment alone. Glaucoma surgery is often necessary to treat elevated IOP including glaucoma valve placement procedures. Typically, severe cases require endothelial keratoplasty such as Descemet's stripping automated endothelial keratoplasty (DSAEK) or penetrating keratoplasty (PKP).[1,14]

References

1. Mamalis N, Edelhauser HF, Dawson DG, Chew J, LeBoyer RM, Werner L. Toxic anterior segment syndrome. J Cataract Refract Surg 2006;32:324–333 Review

2. Sengupta S, Chang DF, Gandhi R, Kenia H, Venkatesh R. Incidence and long-term outcomes of toxic anterior segment syndrome at Aravind Eye Hospital. J Cataract Refract Surg 2011;37:1673–1678

3. TASS Registry. http://www.ascrs.org/tass-registry. Accessed October 12, 2014

4. Bodnar Z, Clouser S, Mamalis N. Toxic anterior segment syndrome: update on the most common causes. J Cataract Refract Surg 2012;38:1902–1910

5. Eleftheriadis H, Cheong M, Sandeman S, et al. Corneal toxicity secondary to inadvertent use of benzalkonium chloride preserved viscoelastic material in cataract surgery. Br J Ophthalmol 2002;86:299–305 ISSN 1468-2079

6. Myers WG, Edelhauser HF. Shortage of bisulfite-free preservative-free epinephrine for intracameral use. J Cataract Refract Surg 2011;37:611

7. Campochiaro PA, Conway BP. Aminoglycoside toxicity—a survey of retinal specialists. Implications for ocular use. Arch Ophthalmol 1991;109:946–950

8. Qureshi F, Clark D. Macular infarction after inadvertent intracameral cefuroxime. J Cataract Refract Surg 2011;37:1168–1169

9. Olavi P. Ocular toxicity in cataract surgery because of inaccurate preparation and erroneous use of 50 mg/ml intracameral cefuroxime. Acta Ophthalmol (Copenh) 2012;90:e153–e154

10. Delyfer MN, Rougier MB, Leoni S, et al. Ocular toxicity after intracameral injection of very high doses of cefuroxime during cataract surgery. J Cataract Refract Surg 2011;37:271–278

11. Barry P, Seal DV, Gettinby G, Lees F, Peterson M, Revie CW; European Society of Cataract and Refractive Surgeons (ESCRS) Endophthalmitis Study Group. ESCRS study of prophylaxis of postoperative endophthalmitis

after cataract surgery: Preliminary report of principal results from a European multicenter study. J Cataract Refract Surg 2006;32:407–410. Erratum in J Cataract Refract Surg 2006;32:709.

12. Gupta MS, McKee HD, Saldaña M, Stewart OG. Macular thickness after cataract surgery with intracameral cefuroxime. J Cataract Refract Surg 2005;31:1163–1166

13. Jensen MK, Fiscella RG, Crandall AS, et al. A retrospective study of endophthalmitis rates comparing quinolone antibiotics. Am J Ophthalmol 2005;139:141–148

14. Lockington D, Flowers H, Young D, Yorston D. Assessing the accuracy of intracameral antibiotic preparation for use in cataract surgery. J Cataract Refract Surg 2010;36:286–289

15. Parikh C, Sippy BD, Martin DF, Edelhauser HF. Effects of enzymatic sterilization detergents on the corneal endothelium. Arch Ophthalmol 2002; 120:165–172

16. Chang DF, Braga-Mele R, Mamalis N, et al; American Society of Cataract and Refractive Surgery (ASCRS) Cataract Clinical Committee. Prophylaxis

of postoperative endophthalmitis after cataract surgery: results of the 2007 ASCRS member survey. J Cataract Refract Surg 2007;33:1801–1805

17. Mamalis N. Toxic anterior segment syndrome. Focal Points (of the American Academy of Ophthalmology) 2009;10:1–13

18. West ES, Behrens A, McDonnell PJ, Tielsch JM, Schein OD. The incidence of endophthalmitis after cataract surgery among the U.S. Medicare population increased between 1994 and 2001. Ophthalmology 2005;112:1388–1394

19. Wallin T, Parker J, Jin Y, Kefalopoulos G, Olson RJ. Cohort study of 27 cases of endophthalmitis at a single institution. J Cataract Refract Surg 2005; 31:735–741

20. Worst JGF. A retrospective view on the sterilization of intraocular lenses and the incidence of sterile hypopyon. J Am Intraocul Implant Soc 1980; 6:10–12

21. Meltzer DW. Sterile hypopyon following intraocular lens surgery. Arch Ophthalmol 1980;98:100–104

50 Endophthalmitis

Francis S. Mah

Despite the tremendous advancements in the technology and techniques of modern cataract surgery, one of the earliest identified complications continues to plague surgeons. Endophthalmitis is arguably the most devastating vision-threatening complication associated with cataract surgery, and its incidence and prevalence have not changed significantly in 50 years. Surgeons are no closer to eliminating this potentially catastrophic complication now than they were in a half-century ago.[1]

Because of the potentially-vision threatening complications of postsurgical endophthalmitis, identifying the risks, refining the methods of infection prophylaxis, and improving treatment have been the subject of ongoing research and debate. Although it is fortunate that postsurgical endophthalmitis is rare, the low incidence makes it difficult to perform prospective clinical trials to definitively determine the causes and the most effective means of preventing postoperative infections. Cataract surgeons must therefore exercise clinical judgment based on the best available published evidence. This chapter discusses the findings in the medical literature, and provides some guidance on current best practices while the research and debate continue.

Incidence and Prevalence

Worldwide, postoperative acute, bacterial endophthalmitis has been reported to occur in 0.04 to 0.2% of cataract surgical cases.[1] Surprisingly, despite reducing complications, making smaller incisions, and reducing surgical times, there appeared to be an increase in the incidence of endophthalmitis reported in the United States at the start of this century.[2] Using Medicare data, two studies from the same group found similar trends. In 2005, West et al[3] reported that the rate of endophthalmitis increased, whereas in the same year Taban et al[2] reported an increased rate of endophthalmitis associated with clear corneal versus scleral tunnel incisions.

Internationally, the Swedish national reporting database identified an endophthalmitis incidence of 0.05% in over 225,000 cases.[4] In India, an analysis of over 42,000 consecutive cases, including manual extracapsular and phacoemulsification techniques, found the incidence of postoperative endophthalmitis was 0.09%.[5] Finally, two studies performed in Canada found similar rates, 0.14% and 0.15%, of endophthalmitis after cataract surgery.[6,7]

Etiology

The normal ocular surface is colonized with a spectrum of pathogens that are considered to be a primary source of infection in endophthalmitis.[8] Conditions altering the normal flora such as contact lens wear, blepharitis, lacrimal system disease, and previous antimicrobial use may increase the risk of postoperative endophthalmitis.[8–10] The normal flora may also be altered in patients who are chronically institutionalized, health care workers, and patients with indwelling catheters or with ileostomies or colostomies.[11]

Certain pathogens may also vary by geographic region. According to the North American Endophthalmitis Vitrectomy Study (EVS), 94.2% of culture-positive acute, postsurgical endophthalmitis cases involved gram-positive bacteria; 70.0% of these isolates were coagulase-negative *Staphylococcus* (CoNS), 9.9% were *Staphylococcus aureus*, 9.0% were *Streptococcus* species, 2.2% were *Enterococcus* species, and 5.9% were gram-positive species.[12] In contrast, a survey from India reported that gram-positive bacteria accounted for only 53% of postoperative endophthalmitis cases, whereas 26% were gram-negative isolates and 17% were fungal.[13] One ominous trend is that evidence suggests that the incidence of methicillin-resistant *S. aureus* (MRSA) ocular infections is rising, both in total numbers and as a percentage of all *S. aureus* infections.[14–16] In the EVS, *S. aureus* was the second most common organism after CoNS. A later longitudinal study by Major et al[16] found that MRSA accounted for 44% of postcataract *S. aureus* endophthalmitis in one institution from 1995 through 2008, whereas not a single case of MRSA had been identified at the same institution from 1984 through 1992. A significant number of *S. aureus* cases were resistant not only to methicillin, but also to the commonly used fourth-generation fluoroquinolones, such as moxifloxacin and gatifloxacin. Fortunately, all *Staphylococcus* species were sensitive to vancomycin, the intravitreal antibiotic of choice to treat gram-positive bacterial infections.[17]

Risk Factors

Identifying patients at risk for acute endophthalmitis after cataract surgery is important from both a public health standpoint and a clinical perspective, as this could possibly prevent the occurrence or at least facilitate earlier intervention before the onset of irreversible vision loss. In one published systematic review and meta-analysis, large-incision extracapsular or intracapsular cataract extraction, a clear corneal incision, silicone intraocular lenses, and intraoperative complications such as posterior capsular rupture were strongly and consistently associated with acute endophthalmitis.[7] All of these factors are easily assessed and do not entail a lengthy medical history or laboratory evaluations. Other significant factors with a lower strength of association in the same meta-analysis were male gender and older age (85 years and older). All of these factors can be measured and monitored in the early postoperative period. The increased risk with age was only true for the older ages (≥ 85 years), and this result might be explained by a reduced natural immunity in this advanced age group.[4,7,18] In addition, a large prospective study identified older patients (≥ 80) as more likely to have normal bacterial flora as well as resistant strains.[19] Several studies have reported increased rates of adverse postsurgical events among men.[7,20] Researchers have noted that men had a 41% increased risk of postoperative endophthalmitis compared with women. Possible explanations for the higher complication rates in men include behavioral differences (e.g., lack of adherence to postoperative instructions and antibiotic use)[21]; differences in bacterial flora between the genders[22]; and use of α-antagonists, which can increase the surgical complexity, as there is a clear relationship between these medications and intraoperative floppy iris syndrome.[23]

Is a clear corneal incision associated with a greater risk of endophthalmitis compared with a scleral tunnel or limbal incision? Controversy exists regarding this question. Theories to account for more frequent infections with sutureless clear corneal incisions are centered on the stability of the surgical wound because its lack of integrity is believed to be a critical factor. A stable, self-sealing incision may be technically more difficult in the cornea than in the sclera. Many reports concluded that postoperative wound defects were a risk factor for the development of endophthalmitis,[24,25] and a corneal incision at least 2.0 mm in length had substantially greater resistance to incision failure.[26] This suggests that the integrity of a self-sealing incision depends to some extent on length. This may be more difficult in a clear corneal incision. If the incision is too short, the cataract wound may be susceptible to a postoperative perturbation (such as rubbing of the eye) and wound abnormality. Two studies showed the rates of adverse events, including endophthalmitis, decreased among patients undergoing small-incision phacoemulsification from 1994 to 2006, due to the innovations in phacoemulsification technology, the types of instruments available to better manage complex cases (pupil stretchers, capsular tension rings, dyes to stain the capsule), increased use of topical anesthesia, improvements in intraocular lenses, changes in preoperative or postoperative medication regimens, and better strategies to deal with intraoperative complications.[7,27] The incision location, structure, and length should be more thoroughly studied in large prospective clinical trials.

Prevention

Operating Room Aseptic Protocols

The combination of povidone-iodine 10% with a detergent remains the compound of choice for effective skin antisepsis. In vitro and in vivo tests show consistent bacterial kill rates of over 99.99%.[28,29] In the event of an iodine allergy, chlorhexidine gluconate is an iodine-free antimicrobial that is as effective as povidone-iodine in bacterial suspension tests, although under practical conditions it may perform slightly less well, and there may also be ocular symptoms and toxicity.[30]

Practice patterns for the prevention of postoperative endophthalmitis almost universally include preoperative sterile preparation of the surgical site. In most cases, this involves the instillation of povidone–iodine 5% solution into the conjunctival cul-de-sac, a practice of proven efficacy in reducing the bacterial load.[31,32] A prospective study demonstrated that topical antibiotics had no significant additive effect on the preoperative reduction of conjunctival bacterial colonization beyond the effect of povidone–iodine 5% solution alone.[33] A 5% concentration of povidone-iodine is more effective than 1% in decreasing the human conjunctival bacterial flora in vivo.[34] There is some evidence that the use of lidocaine gel prior to instillation of povidone–iodine 5% solution diminishes its antimicrobial effect.[35] In cases of documented or suspected iodine allergy, polyhexanide[36] or chlorhexidine gluconate are recommended as effective alternatives, although some ocular symptoms or toxicity may occur with higher concentrations.

Although bacteria may gain intraocular access during surgery,[37,38] it has been demonstrated that povidone–iodine conjunctival irrigation effectively prevents endophthalmitis.[39] An evidence-based assessment of endophthalmitis prophylaxis found that preoperative povidone–iodine antisepsis received the highest rating compared with other preoperative techniques.[40]

Draping and Lashes

Proper draping is critical to ensure that the lashes and lid margins are entirely sequestered by overhanging wraparound flaps from the drape. The potential for microbial contamination from exposed lid margins and lashes is a clear source of pathogens.[41–43]

Antimicrobial Agents and Resistance

Unfortunately, the development of antibiotic resistance is universal. Causative factors include the widespread systemic use of antibiotics and the use of antibiotics in agriculture.[44,45] The emergence of resistant bacteria in ophthalmology has been documented in the evaluation of isolates from keratitis and conjunctivitis.[46,47] Although newer fourth-generation fluoroquinolones theoretically have less susceptibility to the development of resistance and an enhanced spectrum of activity against many gram-positive bacteria,[48] one study found that the majority of MRSA are resistant to ciprofloxacin, levofloxacin, gatifloxacin, and moxifloxacin.[49] The rapid evolution of resistant bacteria has amplified the importance of developing newer and more potent ophthalmic antibiotics. Besifloxacin, a new broad-spectrum fluoroquinolone, is the most recently approved for ophthalmic use. A potential advantage of this medication is that it has no systemic, veterinary, or agricultural uses.[50]

Cefuroxime, a second-generation cephalosporin with bactericidal action, was extensively evaluated in Sweden prior to its widespread use following the European Society of Cataract and Refractive Surgeons (ESCRS) Endophthalmitis Study.[51,52] Two gaps in the coverage of cefuroxime are MRSA and multiresistant Enterococci, such as vancomycin-resistant Enterococci. Vancomycin has also been used as an intracameral antibiotic for the prevention of endophthalmitis. Because vancomycin remains one of the last resorts in the treatment of multidrug-resistant bacteria, there has been controversy and historical concern about whether routine intracameral vancomycin administration could contribute to future resistance to the drug.[53]

Topical Prophylaxis

In addition to preoperative povidone–iodine antisepsis,[53–55] perioperative topical antibiotic prophylaxis is very common in the United States. However, controversy regarding its efficacy remains.[40,56] In the United States, fourth-generation fluoroquinolones have emerged as the most commonly prescribed topical prophylactic therapeutics because of their broad-spectrum activity and superior ocular penetration.[57,58]

The optimal timing and frequency of topical antibiotic prophylaxis has also been the subject of debate. Many surgeons begin dosing antibiotics on the day of surgery. However, based on the pharmacokinetics of fluoroquinolones, starting these 1 to 3 days before surgery may be advantageous.[59] There is evidence that frequent instillation of topical fluoroquinolones immediately before surgery may increase the concentration of drug in the anterior chamber and decrease the bacterial load.[60,61] Preoperative topical antibiotic use reduces the number of bacteria on the ocular surface at the time of surgery; postoperative topical antibiotic use without a taper until the wound is sealed addresses postoperative inoculation.[62] It is common for antibiotic drops to be discontinued 1 week after surgery, although some studies suggest that the average time of presentation of endophthalmitis is 9.3 days after clear corneal incision cataract surgery.[58]

No prospective study has been conducted to provide direct proof that topical antibiotic use decreases the risk of endophthalmitis. In the ESCRS study, perioperative use of topical levofloxacin was associated with a decreased rate of endophthalmitis, but the benefit did not achieve statistical significance. Further studies are needed to evaluate the ideal drug, dosing, and route to prevent postoperative endophthalmitis.

Intracameral Antibiotic Agents

Of the various methods of antibiotic prophylaxis, the strongest evidence supports a direct intracameral bolus at the conclusion of surgery. Two early and large retrospective studies suggested that direct intracameral injections of gentamicin and vancomycin were efficacious.[63,64] A 2002 retrospective study of direct intracameral cefuroxime injection in more than 32 000 cases in Sweden reported an endophthalmitis rate of 0.06%, which was significantly lower than comparable published rates.[51] Twelve of the 13 culture-positive endophthalmitis organisms were cefuroxime resistant, including MRSA, suggesting that this method of administration was protective against organisms sensitive to the drug. Following this review, a 3-year prospective nonrandomized study of more than 225,000 cases in Sweden found a lower rate of endophthalmitis with intracameral cefuroxime than with topical antibiotic use alone.[65]

The landmark multicenter prospective randomized study conducted by the ESCRS enrolled 16,603 patients and provides the strongest support for the efficacy of intracameral antibiotic prophylaxis.[20] The rates of culture-proven endophthalmitis were 0.050% and 0.025% in the two groups receiving intracameral cefuroxime prophylaxis compared with 0.226% and 0.176% in the two groups not receiving intracameral prophylaxis. Overall, direct intracameral cefuroxime injections resulted in a 5.86-fold decrease in the risk for culture-positive endophthalmitis.[20,66] No comparative studies suggest the optimal antibiotic agent for intracameral endophthalmitis prophylaxis.

The peer-reviewed literature generally supports the safety of using intracameral preparations of vancomycin, moxifloxacin, and several cephalosporins.[52,64,67–71] However, both toxic anterior segment syndrome (TASS) and dosing errors are acknowledged risks of compounding medications for intraocular administration.[72] One study concluded that intracameral cefuroxime was more cost-effective than topical fluoroquinolones.[73] Others have suggested that moxifloxacin has theoretical advantages for intracameral prophylaxis because of its potency and bactericidal activity and because the self-preserved commercial formulation avoids the need for compounding.[57] In the only study of its kind,[74] one group used serial aqueous taps following cataract surgery to show that a single intracameral injection of vancomycin 1.0 mg achieved an aqueous drug concentration that was four times the minimum inhibitory concentration for most gram-positive bacteria for longer than 24 hours. This study may represent what might be considered a depot effect, which might be why intracameral bolus of antibiotics is effective.

In 2012, single-use cefuroxime for intracameral use became commercially available in some countries in Europe. This product represents a step forward, as it significantly reduces the safety concerns associated with extemporaneous preparation. However, it does not completely eliminate the potential for dilutional errors and contamination, and there have been reports of anaphylaxis associated with its use. Interestingly, in a survey of ESCRS members published in 2014, only 74% of respondents were always or usually using an intracameral antibiotic in cata-

ract surgery, despite the fact that it is recommended by the ESCRS and various European national ophthalmology societies.

Finally, no prospective clinical trial exists to support mixing antibiotics into the irrigating infusion bottle as a method of intracameral prophylaxis.

Toxic Anterior Segment Syndrome and Intracameral Antibiotic Agents

Toxic anterior segment syndrome is an acute sterile postoperative inflammation that can occur after uncomplicated or complicated cataract surgery and typically presents within 12 to 48 hours of surgery. Although problems with the cleaning and sterilization of instruments remains the most common risk factor associated with TASS, improper preparation of antibiotics for intracameral injection may also entail inaccuracies leading to TASS. Toxic anterior segment syndrome has been associated with the use of intracameral antibiotics in a small number of cases.[75]

To reduce the risk for TASS, intracameral medications must be preservative free and have the proper concentration, pH, osmolarity, and osmolality. With specific regard to cefuroxime, the recommended dose of 1.0 mg in 0.1 mL has been shown to be well tolerated and to cause no ocular toxicity.[52] Because of a misunderstanding in the dilution protocol, an outbreak of TASS was reported following the intracameral injection of cefuroxime mixed to deliver a dose almost 50 times higher than usual. The patients had significant postoperative inflammation of the anterior segment of the eye, with extensive macular edema.[76] Even following a strict dilution protocol under the controlled conditions of a research study, accurate dosage cannot be ensured.[72]

The lack of a commercially available U.S. Food and Drug Administration (FDA)–approved antibiotic preparation for intracameral use means that intracameral antibiotics must be mixed by the surgeon, the operating room nursing staff, or a compounding pharmacy. A 2007 American Society of Cataract and Refractive Surgery (ASCRS) survey,[77] performed 8 months after the preliminary report of the ESCRS study, found that 77% of the more than 1,300 respondents were not using intracameral antibiotics. However, 82% stated that they would likely adopt this practice if a reasonably priced commercial preparation were available. Forty-five percent of the respondents not using intracameral antibiotic prophylaxis expressed concerns about the risk of injecting noncommercially prepared solutions. The survey determined that most respondents were using topical gatifloxacin or moxifloxacin (81%) and were initiating topical prophylaxis at least 1 day preoperatively (78%) and immediately postoperatively (66%). Because its control group did not mirror these practices, the ESCRS study was not able to determine whether intracameral cefuroxime was equal to, superior to, or of adjunctive benefit to the most commonly used topical antibiotic protocols preferred by the ASCRS survey population. The development, clinical investigation, and regulatory approval of a commercially available antibiotic for intracameral use would help eliminate potential toxicity and dilution problems.[78]

Subconjunctival Injection

In the 2007 ASCRS survey,[77] only 13% of respondents were using subconjunctival antibiotic prophylaxis. Although there are no prospective randomized studies to support the use of subconjunctival antibiotic prophylaxis, some clinical evidence suggests a protective benefit. Retrospective studies from Canada,[79] the United Kingdom,[80] and Western Australia[81] found statistically lower rates of endophthalmitis when subconjunctival antibiotics were given. The largest of these studies (Western Australia) was a population-based case-control study from 1980 to 2000.[81] However, because most of the surgeons used topical antibiotics and did not use intracameral antibiotics, there was insufficient statistical power to assess the relative benefits of these methods of antibiotic prophylaxis.

Surgical Technique

Many surgical factors can influence the risk of intracameral bacterial inoculation during routine phacoemulsification. These include incision location, architecture and integrity, aseptic technique, avoidance of ocular surface contact with instruments and the intraocular lens (IOL), and the duration of surgery.

Wound Construction

Regardless of the incision type, any postoperative wound leak increases the risk of endophthalmitis. Wallin et al[82] found that a wound leak on postoperative day 1 was associated with a 44-fold increase in the risk of postoperative endophthalmitis. Meanwhile, most of the debate surrounding wound construction has centered on the relative risk of scleral tunnel incision versus clear corneal incision. In their prospective randomized study of more than 12,000 cataract surgeries, Nagaki et al[83] found an increased risk of postoperative endophthalmitis in patients who had temporal clear corneal incisions than in those who had superior sclerocorneal incisions. This study's findings supported the observations found in other retrospective case-control studies.[22,84] Other studies suggest that there is no increased risk of postoperative endophthalmitis with clear corneal incisions. The largest study looking at the endophthalmitis risk of clear corneal incisions was conducted as part of the National Cataract Registry in Sweden.[4] In that prospective study of 225,471 cataract surgeries, there was a slightly higher rate of postoperative endophthalmitis in eyes with clear corneal incisions (0.053%) than in those with scleral incisions (0.036%) but the difference did not reach statistical significance ($p \leq 0.14$). Of note, 99% of the patients in that study received an intracameral cefuroxime injection, whereas fewer than 5% received postoperative topical antibiotics, so there might have been an overall protective effect that confounded the incisional data.

An important consideration in assessing the risk of clear corneal incisions is the variability in their construction. These wounds can vary in width, radial length, depth, location, angle, anterior and posterior thicknesses, shape, and entry point. Some authors have suggested that the shape of the incision is more important than the size with respect to being self-sealing.[85]

There is also variance in the types of blades used for wound construction. Even if surgeons could create the same incision architecture consistently, wound manipulation during cataract surgery could introduce variability. Most large retrospective studies that have implicated clear corneal incisions as a risk factor for endophthalmitis have not characterized their architecture, which would probably not be uniform or standardized in a large multicenter series. Femtosecond laser technology offers the potential to create even more precise clear corneal incisional architecture. Whether this might impact endophthalmitis risk would be worthy of future study.

In addition to wound construction, wound location has been examined as a possible risk factor. Investigators from the Bascom Palmer Eye Institute[1] observed that 86% of cases of postoperative endophthalmitis at their institution occurred in right eyes with incisions located inferotemporally, in closer proximity to the inferior lid margin and tear meniscus.

One rationale cited for using microcoaxial or microbiaxial phacoemulsification is the possibility that smaller incisions might reduce the risk of postoperative endophthalmitis. As with pro-

phylactic antibiotics, the low incidence of infection makes it difficult to prove the superiority of one incision size over another in a prospective study. Furthermore, improperly constructed incisions or those that are stretched by instrumentation may leak regardless of their width. Despite the controversy over endophthalmitis risk with clear corneal incisions, there is general agreement that a suture or an FDA-approved sealant (ReSure® Sealant, Ocular Therapeutix, Bedford, MA) should be placed if the incision is not watertight at the conclusion of surgery.[86,87]

Treatment
Clinical Picture

Postoperative endophthalmitis presents as two distinct entities: early or acute endophthalmitis, occurring within a few days of the procedure, and chronic or delayed endophthalmitis, which can present several weeks after surgery with more subtle symptoms. The more virulent organisms (e.g., gram-negative bacteria) are associated with the acute type, and the less virulent (e.g., *Propionibacterium acnes*), with the delayed presentation.[88]

Patients with acute postoperative endophthalmitis typically present within 2 weeks of surgery with progressive pain, reduced vision, eyelid edema, conjunctival injection, and chemosis.[88–90] Patients often report a sudden decrease of vision, aching pain, and severe photosensitivity. Because early intervention can save vision, the office staff should be aware of these symptoms in postoperative patients to help speed triage, evaluation, and treatment.

Physical findings of acute endophthalmitis are usually not subtle. Patients present with anterior chamber inflammation ranging from excessive cell and flare to severe inflammation with fibrin and hypopyon. The presence of vitreous cells is characteristic. Patients who present with acute anterior segment inflammation and no vitreitis, especially in the first 24 to 48 hours following surgery, may be more likely to have TASS than endophthalmitis.[78] The decline in vision from acute endophthalmitis is associated with corneal edema, anterior and posterior chamber inflammation, retinal vasculitis, hemorrhage, and inflammation.[88,89,91,92] More severe infections are correlated with loss of the red reflex and less than hand motion vision.[89] Infected eyes may have corneal infiltrates and leaking wounds with fibrin tracking into the anterior chamber.

Chronic delayed-onset endophthalmitis is less common, and the symptoms and findings can be subtle.[88,93] Patients with chronic endophthalmitis may report only mild pain and photosensitivity that may be masked by postoperative corticosteroids. Al-Mezaine et al[93] found an average delay of more than 5 months from surgery to the time of diagnosis.

On examination, these patients may have only rare cellular reaction in the anterior chamber and vitreous, and rarely have keratic precipitates. They sometimes have white plaques on the IOL surface, haptics, or capsule. It is important to rule out retained lens material, which can cause persistent inflammation that mimics chronic endophthalmitis.

Diagnosis and Treatment

The differential diagnosis of acute severe inflammation in the immediate postoperative period includes infection, TASS, surgical trauma, retained lens fragments, and uveitic syndromes. Although the clinical distinction between these conditions can be difficult, infection must be ruled out because severe vision loss can result from even a slight delay in treatment. The differential diagnosis of chronic postoperative endophthalmitis includes endogenous infection and masquerade syndromes.[94]

Acute Endophthalmitis

Ideally, treatment of acute postoperative infectious endophthalmitis is both immediate and tailored to the specific antibiotic sensitivities of the organism involved. However, although symptoms and findings may correlate with the severity of the infection, they do not enable differentiating among infectious organisms.[95] Broad-spectrum antibiotics should be used because of the wide range of potential causative organisms and the requisite delay in obtaining culture results.

As established by the EVS, initial treatment of postcataract-surgery endophthalmitis is twofold: specimen collection and antibiotic administration. A vitreous specimen is preferred, as it roughly doubles the diagnostic yield compared with the aqueous (54.9% vs 22.5%).[96] The EVS concluded that the choice of vitreous tap or biopsy versus three-port vitrectomy should be based on the presenting visual acuity.[12] In patients with visual acuity better than light perception, either method can be used without a clinical difference in the final outcome; however, in patients with light perception vision or worse, a three-port pars plana vitrectomy should be used because this regimen has demonstrated a threefold increase in the likelihood of 20/40 final acuity. The choice of vitreous tap versus vitrectomy does not increase the yield of the culture.[96] Regardless of the presenting visual acuity, diabetic patients present a special situation and have a greater likelihood of achieving a 20/40 acuity with vitrectomy (57%) than with a simple tap or biopsy (40%).[97] The most favorable prognosis for visual acuity is associated with CoNS.[98]

Administration of broad-spectrum antibiotics and dexamethasone into the vitreous cavity should follow specimen collection. Although adjunctive routes of antibiotic administration are used, there is no evidence that supplemental topical and subconjunctival[99] delivery of antibiotics is efficacious in treating endophthalmitis. Intravenous antibiotics have not been shown to change either the final visual acuity or media opacity in this setting.[12] Newer antibiotics, such as systemic fluoroquinolones, however, have not been tested for efficacy in a rigorous manner.[100,101]

Conclusion

Because of the potentially devastating complications of postsurgical endophthalmitis, infection prophylaxis, diagnosis, and treatment have been the subject of ongoing research and debate. Although it is fortunate that postsurgical endophthalmitis is rare, the low incidence also makes it virtually impossible to perform enough prospective randomized clinical trials to determine the most effective means of prophylaxis. Ophthalmologists must therefore exercise clinical judgment based on the best available published evidence.

References

1. Miller JJ, Scott IU, Flynn HW Jr, Smiddy WE, Newton J, Miller D. Acute-onset endophthalmitis after cataract surgery (2000–2004): incidence, clinical settings, and visual acuity outcomes after treatment. Am J Ophthalmol 2005;139:983–987

2. Taban M, Behrens A, Newcomb RL, et al. Acute endophthalmitis following cataract surgery: a systematic review of the literature. Arch Ophthalmol 2005;123:613–620

3. West ES, Behrens A, McDonnell PJ, Tielsch JM, Schein OD. The incidence of endophthalmitis after cataract surgery among the U.S. Medicare population increased between 1994 and 2001. Ophthalmology 2005;112:1388–1394

4. Lundström M, Wejde G, Stenevi U, Thornburn W, Montan P. Endophthalmitis after cataract surgery; a nationwide perspective study evaluating incidence in relation to incision type and location. Ophthalmology 2007; 114:866–870

5. Ravindran RD, Venkatesh R, Chang DF, Sengupta S, Gyatsho J, Talwar B. Incidence of post-cataract endophthalmitis at Aravind Eye Hospital: outcomes of more than 42,000 consecutive cases using standardized sterilization and prophylaxis protocols. J Cataract Refract Surg 2009;35: 629–636

6. Hatch WV, Cernat G, Wong D, Devenyi R, Bell CM. Risk factors for acute endophthalmitis after cataract surgery: a population-based study. Ophthalmology 2009;116:425–430

7. Freeman EE, Roy-Gagnon M-H, Fortin E, Gauthier D, Popescu M, Boisjoly H. Rate of endophthalmitis after cataract surgery in Quebec, Canada, 1996–2005. Arch Ophthalmol 2010;128:230–234

8. Miño de Kaspar H, Shriver EM, Nguyen EV, et al. Risk factors for antibiotic-resistant conjunctival bacterial flora in patients undergoing intraocular surgery. Graefes Arch Clin Exp Ophthalmol 2003;241:730–733

9. Proença-Pina J, Ssi Yan Kai I, Bourcier T, Fabre M, Offret H, Labetoulle M. Fusarium keratitis and endophthalmitis associated with lens contact wear. Int Ophthalmol 2010;30:103–107

10. Lopez PF, Beldavs RA, al-Ghamdi S, et al. Pneumococcal endophthalmitis associated with nasolacrimal obstruction. Am J Ophthalmol 1993;116: 56–62, erratum 780

11. Klevens RM, Morrison MA, Nadle J, et al; Active Bacterial Core surveillance (ABCs) MRSA Investigators. Invasive methicillin-resistant Staphylococcus aureus infections in the United States. JAMA 2007;298:1763–1771

12. Endophthalmitis Vitrectomy Study Group. Results of the Endophthalmitis Vitrectomy Study. A randomized trial of immediate vitrectomy and of intravenous antibiotics for the treatment of postoperative bacterial endophthalmitis. Arch Ophthalmol 1995;113:1479–1496

13. Kunimoto DY, Das T, Sharma S, et al; Endophthalmitis Research Group. Microbiologic spectrum and susceptibility of isolates: part I. Postoperative endophthalmitis. Am J Ophthalmol 1999;128:240–242

14. Blomquist PH. Methicillin-resistant Staphylococcus aureus infections of the eye and orbit (an American Ophthalmological Society thesis). Trans Am Ophthalmol Soc 2006;104:322–345

15. Freidlin J, Acharya N, Lietman TM, Cevallos V, Whitcher JP, Margolis TP. Spectrum of eye disease caused by methicillin-resistant Staphylococcus aureus. Am J Ophthalmol 2007;144:313–315

16. Major JC Jr, Engelbert M, Flynn HW Jr, Miller D, Smiddy WE, Davis JL. Staphylococcus aureus endophthalmitis: antibiotic susceptibilities, methicillin resistance, and clinical outcomes. Am J Ophthalmol 2010;149:278–283.e1

17. Gordon YJ. Vancomycin prophylaxis and emerging resistance: are ophthalmologists the villains? The heroes? Am J Ophthalmol 2001;131:371–376

18. Li J, Morlet N, Ng JQ, Semmens JB, Knuiman MW; Team EPSWA. Significant nonsurgical risk factors for endophthalmitis after cataract surgery: EPSWA fourth report. Invest Ophthalmol Vis Sci 2004;45:1321–1328

19. Olson R, Donnenfeld E, Bucci FA Jr, et al. Methicillin resistance of Staphylococcus species among health care and nonhealth care workers undergoing cataract surgery. Clin Ophthalmol 2010;4:1505–1514

20. Endophthalmitis Study Group, European Society of Cataract & Refractive Surgeons. Prophylaxis of postoperative endophthalmitis following cataract surgery: results of the ESCRS multicenter study and identification of risk factors. J Cataract Refract Surg 2007;33:978–988

21. Tordoff JM, Bagge ML, Gray AR, Campbell AJ, Norris PT. Medicine-taking practices in community-dwelling people aged > or = 75 years in New Zealand. Age Ageing 2010;39:574–580

22. Bekibele CO, Kehinde AO, Ajayi BG. Upper lid skin bacterial count of surgical eye patients in Ibadan, Nigeria. Afr J Med Med Sci 2008;37:273–277

23. Speaker MG, Menikoff JA. Prophylaxis of endophthalmitis with topical povidone-iodine. Ophthalmology 1991;98:1769–1775

24. Aaberg TM Jr, Flynn HW Jr, Schiffman J, Newton J. Nosocomial acute-onset postoperative endophthalmitis survey. A 10-year review of incidence and outcomes. Ophthalmology 1998;105:1004–1010

25. Montan PG, Koranyi G, Setterquist HE, Stridh A, Philipson BT, Wiklund K. Endophthalmitis after cataract surgery: risk factors relating to technique and events of the operation and patient history: a retrospective case-control study. Ophthalmology 1998;105:2171–2177

26. Cooper BA, Holekamp NM, Bohigian G, Thompson PA. Case-control study of endophthalmitis after cataract surgery comparing scleral tunnel and clear corneal wounds. Am J Ophthalmol 2003;136:300–305

27. Stein JD, Grossman DS, Mundy KM, Sugar A, Sloan FA. Severe adverse events after cataract surgery among medicare beneficiaries. Ophthalmology 2011;118:1716–1723

28. Ulrich JA. Clinical study comparing Hibistat (0.5% chlorhexidine gluconate in 70% isopropyl alcohol) and Betadine surgical scrub (7.5% povidone-iodine) for efficacy against experimental contamination of human skin. Curr Ther Res 1982;31:27–30

29. Faoagali J, Fong J, George N, Mahoney P, O'Rourke V. Comparison of the immediate, residual, and cumulative antibacterial effects of Novaderm R, Novascrub R, Betadine Surgical Scrub, Hibiclens, and liquid soap. Am J Infect Control 1995;23:337–343

30. Marchetti MG, Kampf G, Finzi G, Salvatorelli G. Evaluation of the bactericidal effect of five products for surgical hand disinfection according to prEN 12054 and prEN 12791. J Hosp Infect 2003;54:63–67

31. Ou JI, Ta CN. Endophthalmitis prophylaxis. Ophthalmol Clin North Am 2006;19:449–456

32. Carrim ZI, Mackie G, Gallacher G, Wykes WN. The efficacy of 5% povidone-iodine for 3 minutes prior to cataract surgery. Eur J Ophthalmol 2009; 19:560–564

33. Halachmi-Eyal O, Lang Y, Keness Y, Miron D. Preoperative topical moxifloxacin 0.5% and povidone-iodine 5.0% versus povidone-iodine 5.0% alone to reduce bacterial colonization in the conjunctival sac. J Cataract Refract Surg 2009;35:2109–2114; errata 2010; 36:535

34. Ferguson AW, Scott JA, McGavigan J, et al. Comparison of 5% povidone-iodine solution against 1% povidone-iodine solution in preoperative cataract surgery antisepsis: a prospective randomised double blind study. Br J Ophthalmol 2003;87:163–167

35. Boden JH, Myers ML, Lee T, Bushley DM, Torres MF. Effect of lidocaine gel on povidone-iodine antisepsis and microbial survival. J Cataract Refract Surg 2008;34:1773–1775

36. Hansmann F, Kramer A, Ohgke H, Strobel H, Müller M, Geerling G. [Lavasept as an alternative to povidone-iodine for preoperative disinfection in ophthalmic surgery; randomized, controlled, prospective double-blind trial.] Ophthalmologe 2005;102:1043–1050

37. Tervo T, Ljungberg P, Kautiainen T, et al. Prospective evaluation of external ocular microbial growth and aqueous humor contamination during cataract surgery. J Cataract Refract Surg 1999;25:65–71

38. Mistlberger A, Ruckhofer J, Raithel E, et al. Anterior chamber contamination during cataract surgery with intraocular lens implantation. J Cataract Refract Surg 1997;23:1064–1069

39. Leong JK, Shah R, McCluskey PJ, Benn RA, Taylor RF. Bacterial contamination of the anterior chamber during phacoemulsification cataract surgery. J Cataract Refract Surg 2002;28:826–833

40. Ciulla TA, Starr MB, Masket S. Bacterial endophthalmitis prophylaxis for cataract surgery: an evidence-based update. Ophthalmology 2002;109: 13–24

41. Chan DG, Francis IC. Effective draping for cataract surgery by using a relieving incision in the operative drape. [letter] Clin Experiment Ophthalmol 2004;32:656

42. Buzard K, Liapis S. Prevention of endophthalmitis. J Cataract Refract Surg 2004;30:1953–1959

43. Miller KM, Glasgow BJ. Bacterial endophthalmitis following sutureless cataract surgery. Arch Ophthalmol 1993;111:377–379

44. Smith DL, Harris AD, Johnson JA, Silbergeld EK, Morris JG Jr. Animal antibiotic use has an early but important impact on the emergence of antibiotic resistance in human commensal bacteria. Proc Natl Acad Sci U S A 2002;99:6434–6439

45. Teuber M. Veterinary use and antibiotic resistance. Curr Opin Microbiol 2001;4:493–499

46. Moshirfar M, Mirzaian G, Feiz V, Kang PC. Fourth-generation fluoroquinolone-resistant bacterial keratitis after refractive surgery. J Cataract Refract Surg 2006;32:515–518

47. Marangon FB, Miller D, Muallem MS, Romano AC, Alfonso EC. Ciprofloxacin and levofloxacin resistance among methicillin-sensitive Staphylococcus aureus isolates from keratitis and conjunctivitis. Am J Ophthalmol 2004;137:453–458

48. Mamalis N. The increasing problem of antibiotic resistance. [editorial] J Cataract Refract Surg 2007;33:1831–1832

49. Asbell PA, Colby KA, Deng S, et al. Ocular TRUST: nationwide antimicrobial susceptibility patterns in ocular isolates. Am J Ophthalmol 2008; 145:951–958

50. Haas W, Pillar CM, Zurenko GE, Lee JC, Brunner LS, Morris TW. Besifloxacin, a novel fluoroquinolone, has broad-spectrum in vitro activity against aerobic and anaerobic bacteria. Antimicrob Agents Chemother 2009;53: 3552–3560

51. Montan PG, Wejde G, Koranyi G, Rylander M. Prophylactic intracameral cefuroxime. Efficacy in preventing endophthalmitis after cataract surgery. J Cataract Refract Surg 2002;28:977–981

52. Montan PG, Wejde G, Setterquist H, Rylander M, Zetterström C. Prophylactic intracameral cefuroxime. Evaluation of safety and kinetics in cataract surgery. J Cataract Refract Surg 2002;28:982–987

53. Jones DB. Emerging vancomycin resistance: what are we waiting for? [editorial] Arch Ophthalmol 2010;128:789–791

54. Miño de Kaspar H, Chang RT, Singh K, Egbert PR, Blumenkranz MS, Ta CN. Prospective randomized comparison of 2 different methods of 5% povidone-iodine applications for anterior segment intraocular surgery. Arch Ophthalmol 2005;123:161–165

55. Wu P-C, Li M, Chang S-J, et al. Risk of endophthalmitis after cataract surgery using different protocols for povidone- iodine preoperative disinfection. J Ocul Pharmacol Ther 2006;22:54–61

56. Bratzler DW, Houck PM; Surgical Infection Prevention Guidelines Writers Workgroup; American Academy of Orthopaedic Surgeons; American Association of Critical Care Nurses; American Association of Nurse Anesthetists; American College of Surgeons; American College of Osteopathic Surgeons; American Geriatrics Society; American Society of Anesthesiologists; American Society of Colon and Rectal Surgeons; American Society of Health-System Pharmacists; American Society of PeriAnesthesia Nurses; Ascension Health; Association of periOperative Registered Nurses; Association for Professionals in Infection Control and Epidemiology; Infectious Diseases Society of America; Medical Letter; Premier; Society for Healthcare Epidemiology of America; Society of Thoracic Surgeons; Surgical Infection Society. Antimicrobial prophylaxis for surgery: an advisory statement from the National Surgical Infection Prevention Project. Clin Infect Dis 2004;38:1706–1715

57. O'Brien TP, Arshinoff SA, Mah FS. Perspectives on antibiotics for postoperative endophthalmitis prophylaxis: potential role of moxifloxacin. J Cataract Refract Surg 2007;33:1790–1800

58. Moshirfar M, Feiz V, Vitale AT, Wegelin JA, Basavanthappa S, Wolsey DH. Endophthalmitis after uncomplicated cataract surgery with the use of fourth-generation fluoroquinolones: a retrospective observational case series. Ophthalmology 2007;114:686–691

59. McCulley JP, Caudle D, Aronowicz JD, Shine WE. Fourth-generation fluoroquinolone penetration into the aqueous humor in humans. Ophthalmology 2006;113:955–959

60. Kowalski RP, Romanowski EG, Mah FS, Yates KA, Gordon YJ. Topical prophylaxis with moxifloxacin prevents endophthalmitis in a rabbit model. Am J Ophthalmol 2004;138:33–37

61. Kim DH, Stark WJ, O'Brien TP, Dick JD. Aqueous penetration and biological activity of moxifloxacin 0.5% ophthalmic solution and gatifloxacin 0.3% solution in cataract surgery patients. Ophthalmology 2005;112:1992–1996

62. Liesegang TJ. Intracameral antibiotics: questions for the United States based on prospective studies. J Cataract Refract Surg 2008;34:505–509

63. Peyman GA, Sathar ML, May DR. Intraocular gentamicin as intraoperative prophylaxis in South India eye camps. Br J Ophthalmol 1977;61:260–262

64. Gimbel HV, Sun R, DeBrof BM. Prophylactic intracameral antibiotics during cataract surgery: the incidence of endophthalmitis and corneal endothelial cell loss. Eur J Implant Refract Surg 1994;6:280–285

65. Wejde G, Montan P, Lundström M, Stenevi U, Thorburn W. Endophthalmitis following cataract surgery in Sweden: national prospective survey 1999–2001. Acta Ophthalmol Scand 2005;83:7–10

66. Barry P, Seal DV, Gettinby G, Lees F, Peterson M, Revie CW; ESCRS Endophthalmitis Study Group. ESCRS study of prophylaxis of postoperative endophthalmitis after cataract surgery: preliminary report of principal results from a European multicenter study. J Cataract Refract Surg 2006; 32:407–410

67. Espiritu CRG, Caparas VL, Bolinao JG. Safety of prophylactic intracameral moxifloxacin 0.5% ophthalmic solution in cataract surgery patients. J Cataract Refract Surg 2007;33:63–68

68. Lane SS, Osher RH, Masket S, Belani S. Evaluation of the safety of prophylactic intracameral moxifloxacin in cataract surgery. J Cataract Refract Surg 2008;34:1451–1459

69. Arbisser LB. Safety of intracameral moxifloxacin for prophylaxis of endophthalmitis after cataract surgery. J Cataract Refract Surg 2008;34: 1114–1120

70. Yoeruek E, Spitzer MS, Saygili O, et al. Comparison of in vitro safety profiles of vancomycin and cefuroxime on human corneal endothelial cells for intracameral use. J Cataract Refract Surg 2008;34:2139–2145

71. Hui M, Lam PTH, Cheung S-W, Pang C-P, Chan C-Y, Lam DSC. In vitro compatibility study of cephalosporin with intraocular irrigating solutions and intracameral medications. Clin Experiment Ophthalmol 2011;39:164–170

72. Lockington D, Flowers H, Young D, Yorston D. Assessing the accuracy of intracameral antibiotic preparation for use in cataract surgery. J Cataract Refract Surg 2010;36:286–289

73. Sharifi E, Porco TC, Naseri A. Cost-effectiveness analysis of intracameral cefuroxime use for prophylaxis of endophthalmitis after cataract surgery. Ophthalmology 2009;116:1887–96.e1

74. Murphy CC, Nicholson S, Quah SA, Batterbury M, Neal T, Kaye SB. Pharmacokinetics of vancomycin following intracameral bolus injection in patients undergoing phacoemulsification cataract surgery. Br J Ophthalmol 2007;91:1350–1353

75. Cutler Peck CM, Brubaker J, Clouser S, Danford C, Edelhauser HE, Mamalis N. Toxic anterior segment syndrome: common causes. J Cataract Refract Surg 2010;36:1073–1080

76. Delyfer M-N, Rougier M-B, Leoni S, et al. Ocular toxicity after intracameral injection of very high doses of cefuroxime during cataract surgery. J Cataract Refract Surg 2011;37:271–278

77. Chang DF, Braga-Mele R, Mamalis N, et al; ASCRS Cataract Clinical Committee. Prophylaxis of postoperative endophthalmitis after cataract surgery: results of the 2007 ASCRS member survey. J Cataract Refract Surg 2007;33:1801–1805

78. Mamalis N. Intracameral medication: is it worth the risk? [editorial] J Cataract Refract Surg 2008;34:339–340

79. Colleaux KM, Hamilton WK. Effect of prophylactic antibiotics and incision type on the incidence of endophthalmitis after cataract surgery. Can J Ophthalmol 2000;35:373–378; discussion 378

80. Kamalarajah S, Ling R, Silvestri G, et al. Presumed infectious endophthalmitis following cataract surgery in the UK: a case-control study of risk factors. Eye (Lond) 2007;21:580–586

81. Ng JQ, Morlet N, Bulsara MK, Semmens JB. Reducing the risk for endophthalmitis after cataract surgery: population-based nested case-control study: endophthalmitis population study of Western Australia sixth report. J Cataract Refract Surg 2007;33:269–280

82. Wallin T, Parker J, Jin Y, Kefalopoulos G, Olson RJ. Cohort study of 27 cases of endophthalmitis at a single institution. J Cataract Refract Surg 2005;31:735–741

83. Nagaki Y, Hayasaka S, Kadoi C, et al. Bacterial endophthalmitis after small-incision cataract surgery. effect of incision placement and intraocular lens type. J Cataract Refract Surg 2003;29:20–26

84. Lertsumitkul S, Myers PC, O'Rourke MT, Chandra J. Endophthalmitis in the western Sydney region: a case-control study. Clin Experiment Ophthalmol 2001;29:400–405

85. Masket S, Belani S. Proper wound construction to prevent short-term ocular hypotony after clear corneal incision cataract surgery. J Cataract Refract Surg 2007;33:383–386

86. Nichamin LD, Chang DF, Johnson SH, et al; American Society of Cataract and Refractive Surgery Cataract Clinical Committee. ASCRS White Paper: What is the association between clear corneal cataract incisions and postoperative endophthalmitis? J Cataract Refract Surg 2006;32:1556–1559

87. Tam DY, Vagefi MR, Naseri A. The clear corneal tongue: a mechanism for wound incompetence after phacoemulsification. Am J Ophthalmol 2007;143:526–528

88. Kernt M, Kampik A. Endophthalmitis: Pathogenesis, clinical presentation, management, and perspectives. Clin Ophthalmol 2010;4:121–135

89. Mamalis N, Kearsley L, Brinton E. Postoperative endophthalmitis. Curr Opin Ophthalmol 2002;13:14–18

90. Anijeet D. Endophthalmitis after cataract surgery [letter]. Ophthalmology 2010;117:853; reply 853–854

91. Godley BF, Folk JC. Retinal hemorrhages as an early sign of acute bacterial endophthalmitis. Am J Ophthalmol 1993;116:247–249

92. Subbiah S, McAvoy CE, Best JL. Retinal vasculitis as an early sign of bacterial post-operative endophthalmitis. [letter] Eye (Lond) 2010;24:1410–1411

93. Al-Mezaine HS, Al-Assiri A, Al-Rajhi AA. Incidence, clinical features, causative organisms, and visual outcomes of delayed-onset pseudophakic endophthalmitis. Eur J Ophthalmol 2009;19:804–811

94. Fox GM, Joondeph BC, Flynn HW Jr, Pflugfelder SC, Roussel TJ. Delayed-onset pseudophakic endophthalmitis. Am J Ophthalmol 1991;111:163–173

95. Johnson MW, Doft BH, Kelsey SF, et al. The Endophthalmitis Vitrectomy Study. Relationship between clinical presentation and microbiologic spectrum. Ophthalmology 1997;104:261–272

96. Barza M, Pavan PR, Doft BH, et al. Evaluation of microbiological diagnostic techniques in postoperative endophthalmitis in the Endophthalmitis Vitrectomy Study. Arch Ophthalmol 1997;115:1142–1150

97. Doft BH, Wisniewski SR, Kelsey SF, Fitzgerald SG; Endophthalmitis Vitrectomy Study Group. Diabetes and postoperative endophthalmitis in the endophthalmitis vitrectomy study. Arch Ophthalmol 2001;119:650–656

98. Endophthalmitis Vitrectomy Study Group. Microbiologic factors and visual outcome in the endophthalmitis vitrectomy study. Am J Ophthalmol 1996;122:830–846

99. Smiddy WE, Smiddy RJ, Ba'Arath B, et al. Subconjunctival antibiotics in the treatment of endophthalmitis managed without vitrectomy. Retina 2005;25:751–758

100. Flynn HW Jr, Scott IU. Legacy of the endophthalmitis vitrectomy study. Arch Ophthalmol 2008;126:559–561

101. Doft BH. Treatment of postcataract extraction endophthalmitis: a summary of the results from the Endophthalmitis Vitrectomy Study. Arch Ophthalmol 2008;126:554–556

XIX Prevention Pearls and Damage Control

51 Residual Astigmatism with Toric Intraocular Lenses

David R. Hardten, Brent A. Kramer, and John P. Berdahl

A toric intraocular lens (IOL) during cataract surgery results in near emmetropia in the nearly one third of patients with significant corneal astigmatism.[1] Early toric designs proved to be rotationally unstable, rotating more than 10 degrees in 50% of cases and more than 30 degrees in 20% of cases.[2] Since, advancements in design have allowed for more rotational stability (**Table 51.1**).[3-6] Damage control, though, is needed in the occasional patient who experiences residual astigmatism and is dissatisfied with the results. Surgeons then need to analyze the residual astigmatism, the underlying cause, and how to move forward with the next steps to get patients back on the road to spectacle independence. This chapter provides pearls to prevent this problem and pearls for damage control when problems occur.

Residual Astigmatism

Residual astigmatism occurs when an implanted toric IOL is not in the ideal position or does not have the correct power and therefore does not neutralize the corneal astigmatism. There are many questions to consider when determining the cause of residual astigmatism:

- Was the patient not a good candidate for a toric IOL implant? That is, did the patient have irregular astigmatism or anterior basement membrane corneal dystrophy?
- Was there a measurement, calculation, or transcription error?
- Was there an error made during preoperative marking?
- Was surgically induced astigmatism (SIA) considered, or was there a surprising amount of SIA?
- Was there a significant amount of posterior corneal astigmatism that was not considered?
- Was there postoperative toric IOL rotation?

Successful Implementation of Toric IOLs

Choose Patients Who Desire Spectacle Independence

The vision goals of the patient are very important to understand. Toric IOLs are generally intended for patients with regular astigmatism who desire greater spectacle independence for distance vision, yet patients may have the goal of monovision with near vision in one eye and also benefit from reduced astigmatism. In Ahmed et al's[4] 2010 study, 54 of 78 patients (69%) with bilateral toric implants were spectacle independent for distance vision.

Choose Patients with Regular Astigmatism

Toric IOLs available in the United States enable correction of regular anterior corneal astigmatism between 0.75 and 4.1 D after astigmatic changes from the surgical incisions. Although astigmatism greater than 4.1 D can be reduced with a single implanted toric IOL, residual astigmatism should be expected.

Reasons that Problems Occur

Patients Who Do Not Value Spectacle Independence

The patient's postoperative vision goals may not necessarily include reduction of dependence on glasses. The increase in cost, extra tests, and surgical procedures to obtain spectacle independence may not be worth it for these patients, and glasses may be preferred.

Table 51.1 Recent Toric Intraocular Lens (IOL) Alignment Studies

Reference	Year	Study Population	Misalignment (Mean ± Standard Deviation)	> 10 Degrees	IOL Model	Follow-Up (Months)
Holland et al[3]	2010	256	2 ± 2	7	AcrySof T3-T5	12
Ahmed et al[4]	2010	234	3.0	0	AcrySof T3-T5	6
Chang[5]	2008	100	3.4 ± 3.4	1	AcrySof T3-T5	1
Visser et al[6]	2011	67	3.2 ± 2.8	1	AcrySof T6-T9	6

Patients Who Have Irregular Astigmatism

Toric IOLs do not eliminate irregular corneal astigmatism. For example, patients with ectatic diseases such as keratoconus, or other nonectatic irregular astigmatism, such as prior refractive surgery, keratoplasty, corneal scars, significant anterior basement membrane dystrophy, or Salzmann's nodular degeneration, often have poorer results with toric IOL implantation. Although case studies have demonstrated the benefit of toric IOLs in some eyes with keratoconus[7,8] and pellucid marginal degeneration,[9] it is important to note the likelihood of residual irregular astigmatism or unpredictable results. In ectatic irregular astigmatism cases, it is also important to assess the risk of disease progression. Additionally, because there is now intraocular toricity in addition to the irregular corneal astigmatism, specialty contact lens fitting, if necessary, would be more difficult and likely require a front toric contact lens.

Patients Who Have Poor Visual Potential

Patients with advanced macular degeneration, glaucoma, or amblyopia may not have enough improvement in vision to justify the cost of a toric IOL.

Patients Who Have Weak Zonules

Pseudoexfoliation syndrome, phacodonesis, prior vitrectomy, or other causes of lax zonules can be relative contraindications of toric IOL implantation. Abnormal capsular integrity decreases the IOL stability and therefore increases the probability of a misaligned toric IOL.

Preoperative Measurement and Calculation Pearls

Discontinuation of contact lens use and upright head positioning during testing and marking facilitate making accurate measurements. Using two or more confirmatory keratometry sources such as topography, optical biometry, or manual keratometry is important because there can be variability in measurements (**Box 51.1**). The topography is also used to assess the regularity of the astigmatism, as keratometry can often miss irregular astigmatism. It is also important to note the opportunity for

human error when transcribing measurements and using toric IOL calculators.

When using a toric calculator to determine the correct toric IOL, it is important to consider the estimated residual astigmatism given with the calculations. Because this is the amount of astigmatism that can be expected if the IOL is in the optimal position and corneal astigmatism is unchanged after surgery, it should be used as a baseline when predicting the potential amount of residual astigmatism. There are many toric IOL calculators, but the one that we find most useful preoperatively is the Barrett Toric Calculator that is now available on the American Society of Cataract and Refractive Surgery (ASCRS) Web site (http://www.ascrs.org/barrett-toric-calculator).

Determining Axis Alignment

Many methods have been described for determining the axis of alignment. These range from simple marking of the ocular meridians and then aligning a secondary device intraoperatively to intraoperative photographic comparisons, to intraoperatively measuring preinsertion and postinsertion ocular astigmatism[10–12] (**Figs. 51.1** and **51.2**).

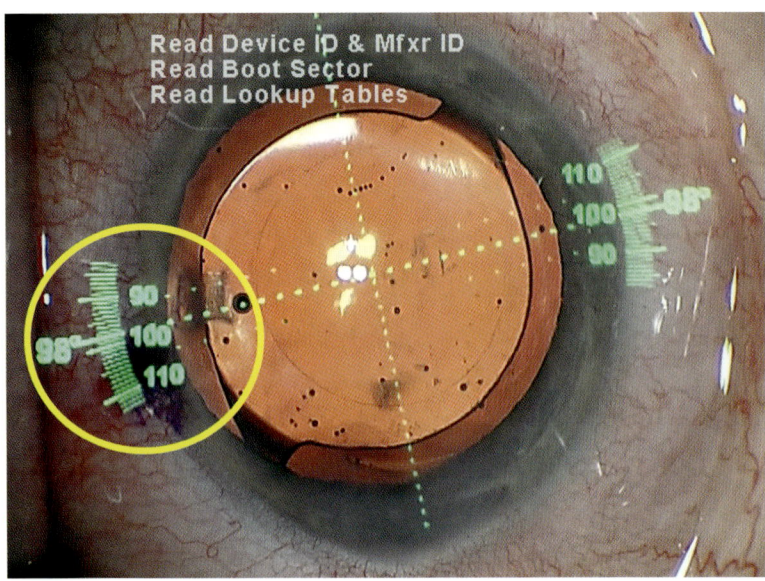

Fig. 51.1　Intraoperative guidance via the Verion device (Alcon, Fort Worth, TX).

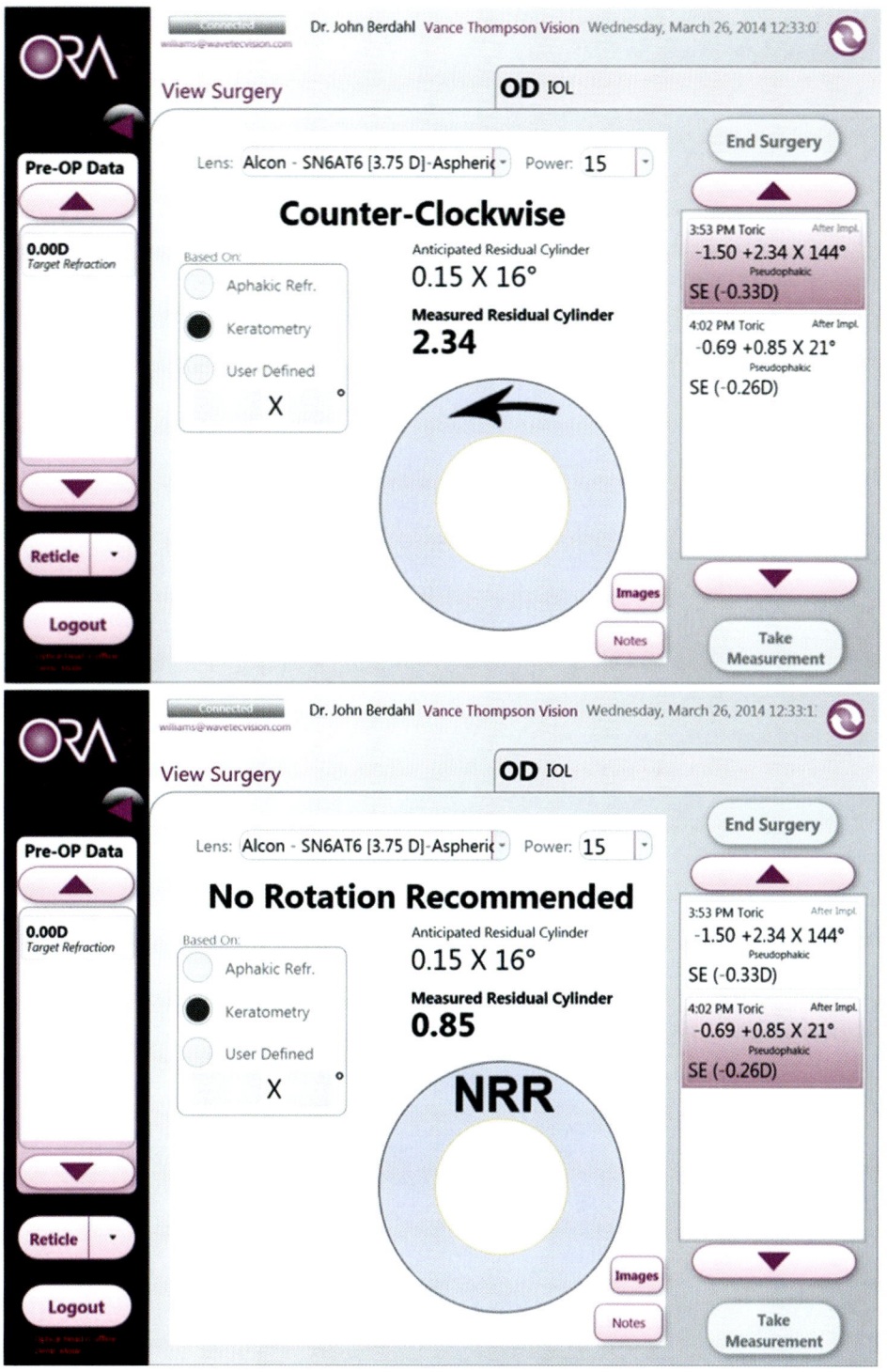

Fig. 51.2 Intraoperative aberrometry performed by Optiwave Refractive Analysis (ORA) (WaveTec Visions, Aliso Viejo, CA), showing the proper alignment and astigmatism reduction.

Determination of Anticipated Surgically Induced Astigmatism

Accurate determination of the surgically induced astigmatism can improve the accuracy of toric IOLs.[13] The amount of SIA induced depends on the size and location of the incision and the biomechanical properties of the cornea. Warren Hill has developed the Surgically Induced Astigmatism Calculator (http://www.sia-calculator.com/) to help surgeons calculate the SIA.

Posterior Corneal Astigmatism

About 9% of eyes have greater than 0.50 D of posterior corneal astigmatism, and if not taken into consideration it can lead to the overcorrection of with-the-rule (vertical steep meridian) anterior corneal astigmatism and undercorrection of against-the-rule (horizontal steep meridian) anterior corneal astigmatism[14,15] (**Fig. 51.3**).

Treatment of Residual Astigmatism After Toric IOL Placement

Treatment methods of residual astigmatism are as follows (also see the treatment algorithm in **Fig. 51.4**):

1. Rotation of the toric IOL
2. Exchange of the toric IOL
3. Astigmatic keratotomy
4. Excimer laser ablation
5. Glasses or contacts

Toric IOL Rotation

If the toric IOL is not aligned with the corneal astigmatism, its ability to correct corneal astigmatism is diminished by about 3.3% for every degree of mismatch between the corneal astigmatism and the IOL toricity. If the IOL is 90 degrees away from the ideal axis, the astigmatism is doubled.[16] **Table 51.2** shows this loss of function and how the absolute loss is greater in IOLs with higher power (**Fig. 51.5**).

A misaligned toric IOL can leave postimplant patients unsatisfied with their uncorrected distance vision acuity because of residual astigmatism. When this happens, surgeons should consider rotating the toric IOL to its optimal position. In doing so, several questions can help determine the course of action.

What Is the Current Location of the Toric IOL?

It is important to check the current axis of the toric IOL. Although the normal angular markings on a slit lamp typically do

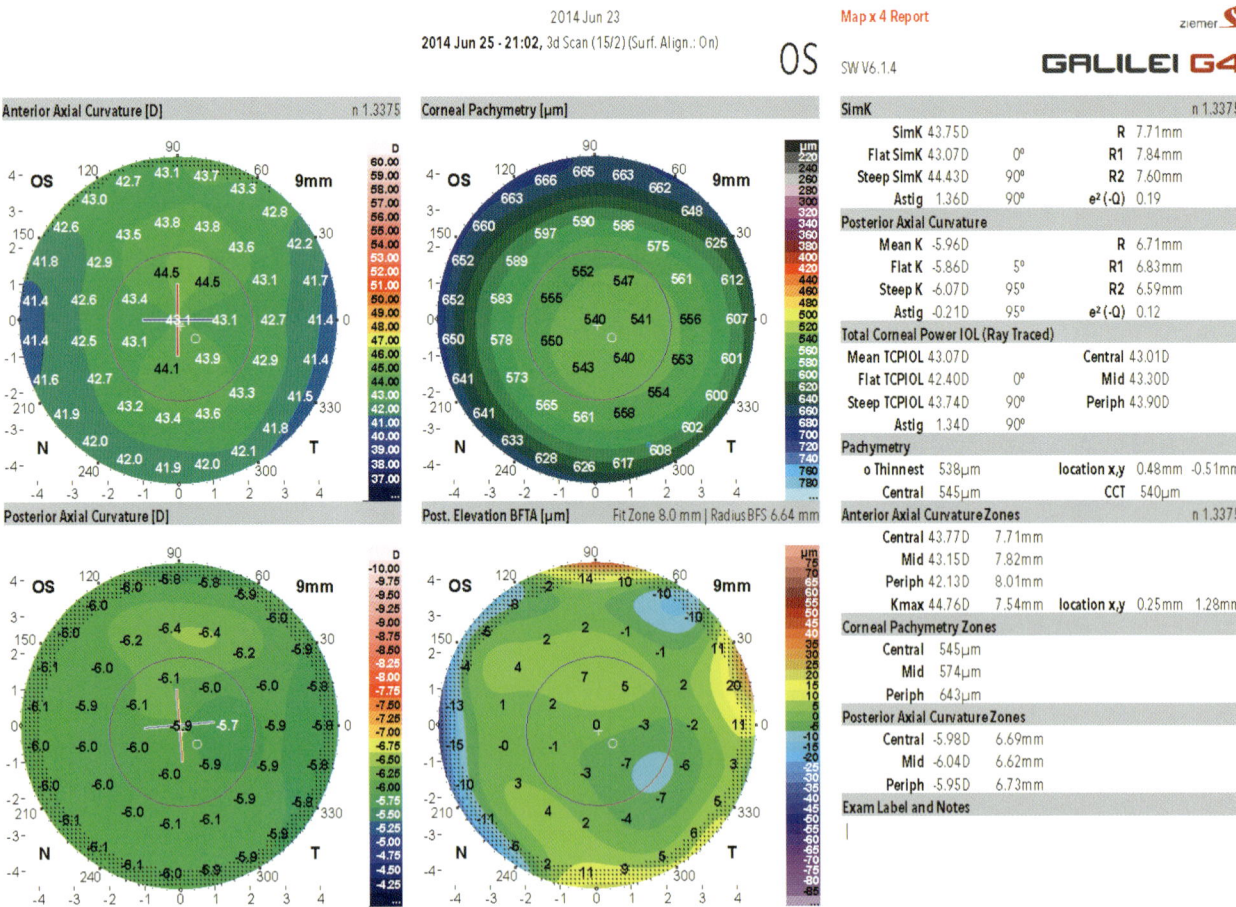

Fig. 51.3 Posterior corneal measurements (*bottom left panel*), among others, via the Galilei system. (Courtesy of Ziemer, Alton, IL.)

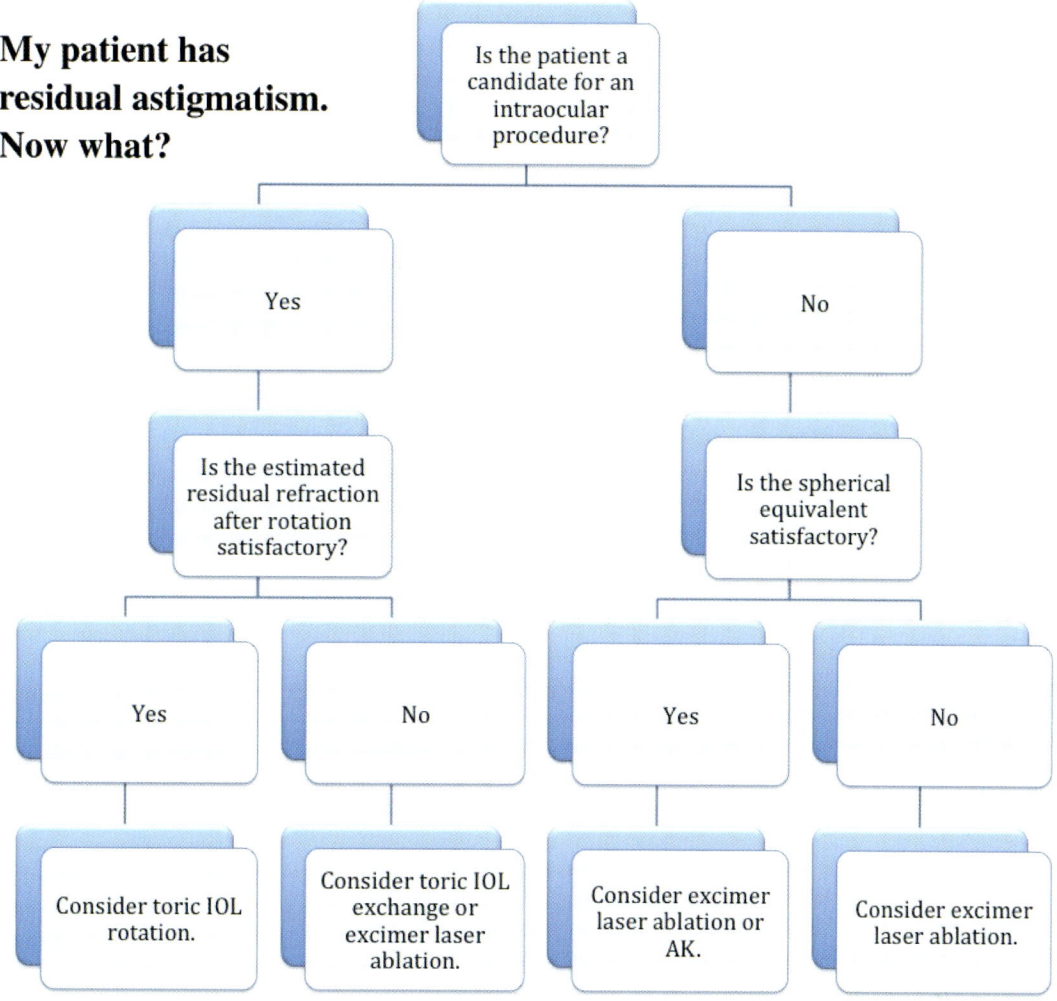

Fig. 51.4   Treatment algorithm for residual astigmatism. AK, astigmatic keratotomy.

not offer the precision necessary to determine the exact IOL location, there are a few methods that can be used.

A simple method identified by Roger Steinert utilizes smartphone technology. Once dilated, align the slit-beam light on the slit lamp with the patient's toric IOL markings (**Fig. 51.6**). Then, using a level app on a smartphone that displays degrees of rotation, align the smartphone with the slit-beam lamp to determine the toric IOL location.

Another high technology method can be performed with wavefront aberrometry and corneal topography in a device such as the OPD Scan III (Nidek). The internal OPD shows the angulation and power of the toric IOL and can be used for calculations. (**Fig. 51.7**).[17]

Does the Toric IOL Need to Be Rotated?

Once the location of the IOL is measured, the next steps are as follows:

1. Determine if the toric IOL is not in its intended location due to inaccurate placement or postprocedure rotation.
2. Determine if the intended location or power is not correct due to inaccurate measurements, inaccurate markings, or surprising surgically induced astigmatism, or unaccounted for posterior corneal astigmatism.

Although the primary treatment for residual astigmatism is to rotate the toric IOL into its optimal location, the task of calculating the optimal toric IOL location can be difficult. This process is

Table 51.2   Loss of Refractive Power Upon Toric IOL Rotation

Misalignment (Degrees)	Loss (%)	Absolute Loss (Diopters)	
		AcrySof Model SN60T3 (1.03 D)	AcrySof Model SN60T9 (4.11 D)
0	0	0	0
5	17.5	0.18	0.71
10	35	0.36	1.43
15	50	0.51	2.05
30	100	1.03	4.11

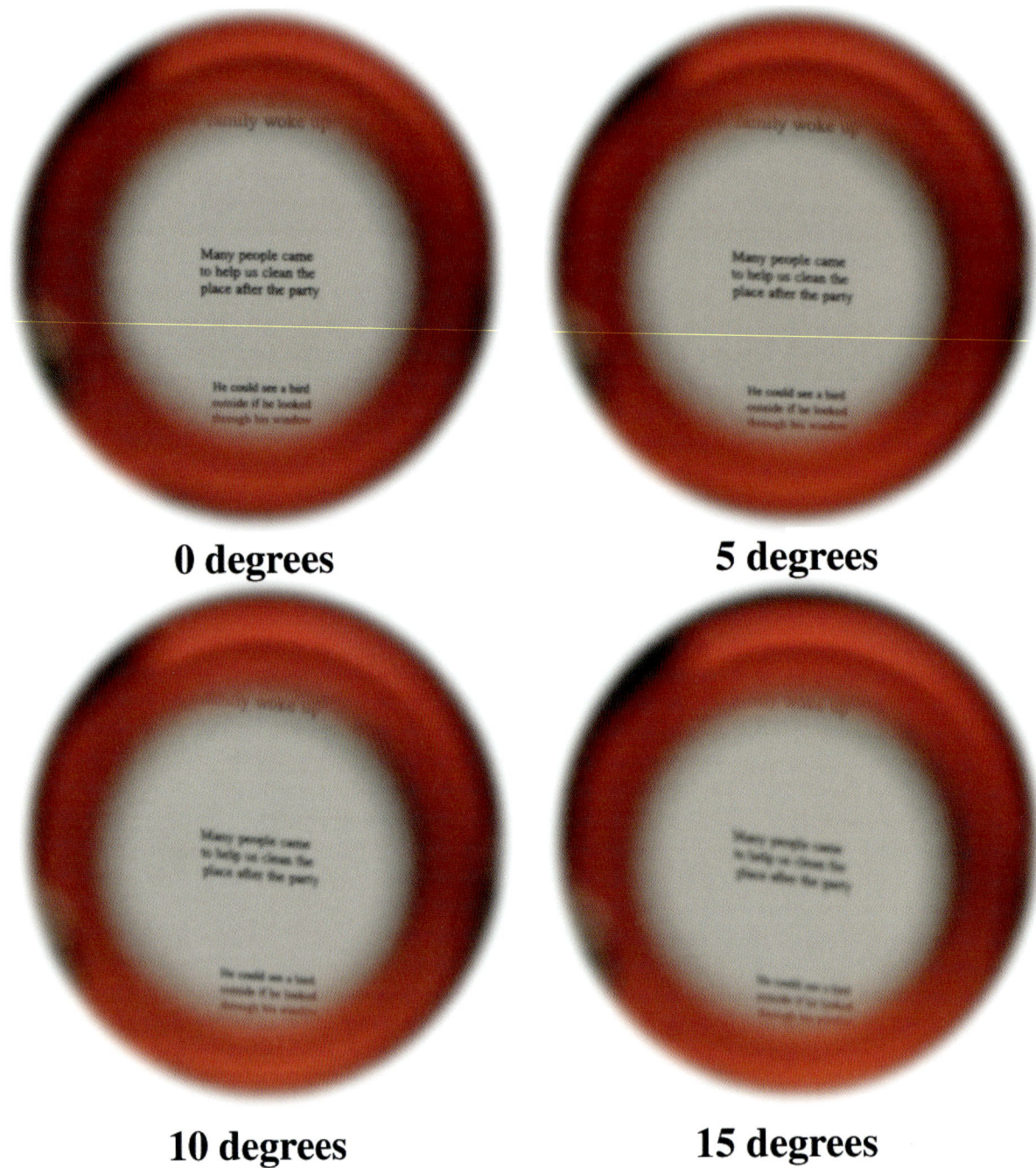

0 degrees

5 degrees

10 degrees

15 degrees

Fig. 51.5   The effects of a misaligned SN60T9 AcrySof toric IOL (Alcon, Fort Worth, TX.)

simplified with the Toric Results Analyzer (http://astigmatism fix.com), designed by Berdahl and Hardten (**Fig. 51.8**). The surgeon enters the patient's current refraction along with the toric IOL location and power, and the Web site calculates the ideal toric IOL position and the expected residual refraction.

Is There a Reasonable Chance of Clinical Success If the IOL Is Rotated?

It is typically not worth rotating the IOL unless it will correct at least 0.5 D of astigmatism. Additionally, unless the residual astigmatism will be below 0.5 D, the patient will still likely have unacceptable uncorrected visual acuity. If there is significant residual myopia or hyperopia, then rotation of the IOL will not solve the vision problem as the spherical equivalent will not change with IOL rotation.

When Should the Toric IOL Rotation Surgical Procedure Occur?

The optimal timeframe in which to rotate the toric IOL is between 2 and 12 weeks postsurgery. This allows enough time for the refraction to normalize but still enables easy rotation because complete fibrotic healing has not yet occurred.

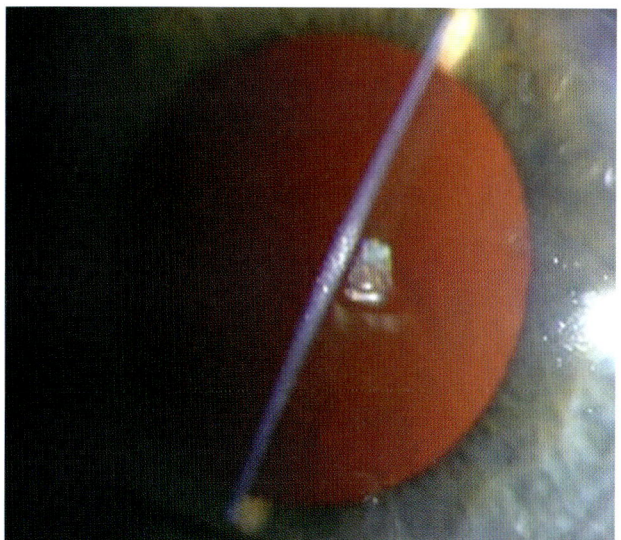

Fig. 51.6 Aligning the slit beam of a slit lamp with a toric IOL to determine its location.

How Is a Toric IOL Rotated?

The cornea can be marked with the current location of the toric IOL and then the ideal location (typically, the amount of rotation required in the clockwise direction). Note that when utilizing this method of marking, there is no need to worry about cyclorotation because the IOL itself is the reference point. Reopen the incisions used during cataract surgery to reduce the introduction of new SIA. Inflate the capsular bag with viscoelastic and place new viscoelastic posterior to the IOL to loosen it from the posterior capsule. Free the capsule–capsule, capsule–IOL, and capsule–haptic adhesions. Rotate the IOL (usually clockwise) into the correct position, aligning the corneal marks with the IOL alignment marks. Consider performing aberrometry to confirm that astigmatism has been minimized (**Fig. 51.2**). If the configuration of the capsular bag originally allowed rotation insertion of a capsular tension ring, then the Henderson ring with undulating contour may be especially useful to reduce the risk of rotation of the IOL. Once the IOL is aligned, remove the viscoelastic from the eye and behind the IOL. Gently push the IOL posteriorly to create contact between the posterior capsule and the IOL. Ensure that the IOL is centered and all edges are covered by the capsulorrhexis (**Box 51.2**).

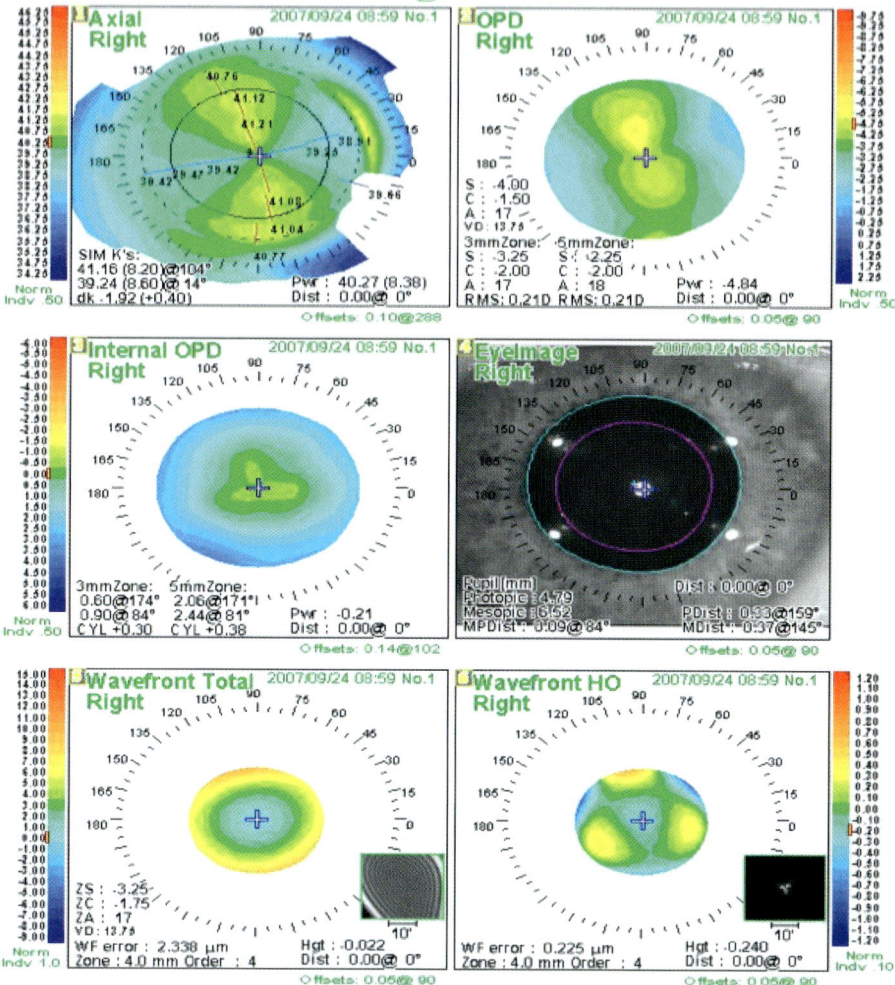

Fig. 51.7 The internal optical path difference (OPD) of this OPD Scan III (Nidek, Fremont, CA) measurement (upper right panel) shows the power and axis of the lenticular astigmatism. The other panels help to confirm the overall astigmatism, any other higher order aberrations, and the overall regularity of the astigmatism.

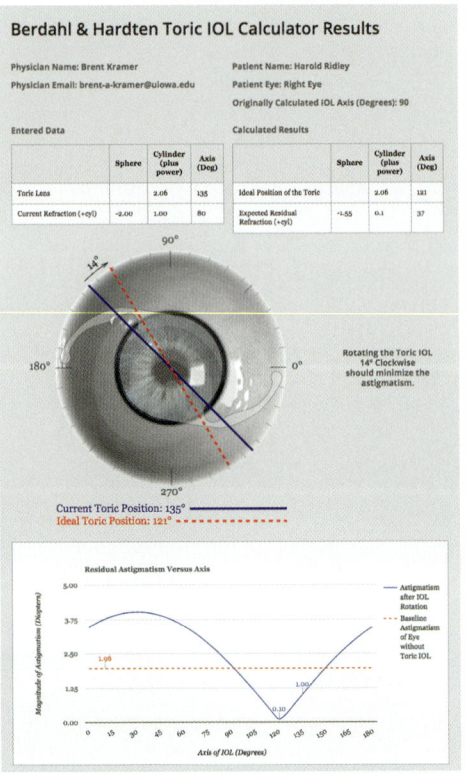

Fig. 51.8 The data entry and results page of the Toric Results Analyzer.

IOL Exchange

If rotation of the IOL is not enough to reduce the astigmatism to an acceptable level, exchanging the toric IOL for one with a different power may be a viable treatment option. The Toric Results Analyzer can help with this decision.

Box 51.2 Rotating a Toric IOL

1. Prep and drape the patient.
2. Mark the current location of the IOL on the cornea.
3. Mark the ideal location of the toric IOL on the cornea.
4. Open the prior incision (reduces the risk of new induction of SIA).
5. Instill intracameral lidocaine.
6. Instill viscoelastic.
7. Free the capsule–IOL and capsule–capsule adhesions.
8. Free the haptics from the capsule.
9. Rotate the IOL to the ideal position (consider aberrometry to confirm astigmatism neutralization).
10. Remove all viscoelastic from the eye, including from behind the IOL.
11. Gently push the IOL posteriorly, creating contact with the posterior capsule.
12. Hydrate and seal the incision.

Corneal Surgical Correction

If a patient is unable to tolerate an intraocular procedure, if the capsular bag is compromised, or if rotation alone will not solve the problem adequately, then corneal refractive surgery may be preferred. This is especially the case if there are surprising changes in corneal astigmatism, especially the induction of irregular astigmatism through the initial incision. Astigmatic keratotomy, laser-assisted in situ keratomileusis (LASIK), or photorefractive keratectomy (PRK) are options depending on the amount and degree of myopia, hyperopia, or astigmatism.

Glasses or Contacts

Patients who have elected to receive toric IOL implants during cataract surgery are usually striving for spectacle independence at distance. However, many patients are happy enough with the improvement in their vision from the cataract surgery and some reduction in the refractive error that glasses or contacts may also be a viable option.

Conclusion

For any procedure, there are potential pitfalls, and yet by learning pearls to improve the chances for success, and by having tools for damage control when surgery does not go as planned, the surgeon can provide a final outcome with which the patient will be satisfied. Future designs of IOLs, range of powers, and even combination of multifocality and astigmatism will increase the use of toric IOLs and the importance of having a plan for success when using these IOLs. When residual astigmatism does occur, managing the problem effectively can help patients achieve better vision and spectacle independence. To review, here are the key points that this chapter discussed:

1. Residual astigmatism occurs when toric IOLs are aligned or powered in a manner that does not neutralize corneal astigmatism.
2. Each degree of misalignment yields about 3.3% of diminished correcting function.
3. Rotating the IOL to its optimal position does not always remove residual astigmatism.
4. The Toric Results Analyzer (http://astigmatismfix.com/) is a key tool in managing residual astigmatism.
5. Other options for treating residual astigmatism include excimer laser ablation with LASIK or PRK, astigmatic keratotomies, IOL exchange, and glasses or contact lenses.

References

1. Hoffmann PC, Hütz WW. Analysis of biometry and prevalence data for corneal astigmatism in 23,239 eyes. J Cataract Refract Surg 2010;36:1479–1485

2. Shimizu K, Misawa A, Suzuki Y. Toric intraocular lenses: correcting astigmatism while controlling axis shift. J Cataract Refract Surg 1994;20:523–526

3. Holland E, Lane S, Horn JD, Ernest P, Arleo R, Miller KM. The AcrySof toric intraocular lens in subjects with cataracts and corneal astigmatism: a randomized, subject-masked, parallel-group, 1-year study. Ophthalmology 2010;117:2104–2111

4. Ahmed IIK, Rocha G, Slomovic AR, et al; Canadian Toric Study Group. Visual function and patient experience after bilateral implantation of toric intraocular lenses. J Cataract Refract Surg 2010;36:609–616

5. Chang DF. Comparative rotational stability of single-piece open-loop acrylic and plate-haptic silicone toric intraocular lenses. J Cataract Refract Surg 2008;34:1842–1847

6. Visser N, Ruíz-Mesa R, Pastor F, Bauer NJC, Nuijts RMMA, Montés-Micó R. Cataract surgery with toric intraocular lens implantation in patients with high corneal astigmatism. J Cataract Refract Surg 2011;37:1403–1410

7. Navas A, Suárez R. One-year follow-up of toric intraocular lens implantation in forme fruste keratoconus. J Cataract Refract Surg 2009;35:2024–2027

8. Jaimes M, Xacur-García F, Alvarez-Melloni D, Graue-Hernández EO, Ramirez-Luquín T, Navas A. Refractive lens exchange with toric intraocular lenses in keratoconus. J Refract Surg 2011;27:658–664

9. Luck J. Customized ultra-high-power toric intraocular lens implantation for pellucid marginal degeneration and cataract. J Cataract Refract Surg 2010;36:1235–1238

10. Ma JJK, Tseng SS. Simple method for accurate alignment in toric phakic and aphakic intraocular lens implantation. J Cataract Refract Surg 2008;34:1631–1636

11. Tjon-Fo-Sang MJ, de Faber J-THN, Kingma C, Beekhuis WH. Cyclotorsion: a possible cause of residual astigmatism in refractive surgery. J Cataract Refract Surg 2002;28:599–602

12. Wiley WF, Bafna S. Intra-operative aberrometry guided cataract surgery. Int Ophthalmol 2011;52:119–129

13. Hill W. Expected effects of surgically induced astigmatism on AcrySof toric intraocular lens results. J Cataract Refract Surg 2008;34:364–367

14. Koch DD, Ali SF, Weikert MP, Shirayama M, Jenkins R, Wang L. Contribution of posterior corneal astigmatism to total corneal astigmatism. J Cataract Refract Surg 2012;38:2080–2087

15. Cheng LS, Tsai CY, Tsai RJF, Liou SW, Ho JD. Estimation accuracy of surgically induced astigmatism on the cornea when neglecting the posterior corneal surface measurement. Acta Ophthalmol (Copenh) 2011;89:417–422

16. Felipe A, Artigas JM, Díez-Ajenjo A, García-Domene C, Alcocer P. Residual astigmatism produced by toric intraocular lens rotation. J Cataract Refract Surg 2011;37:1895–1901

17. Carey PJ, Leccisotti A, McGilligan VE, Goodall EA, Moore CBT. Assessment of toric intraocular lens alignment by a refractive power/corneal analyzer system and slitlamp observation. J Cataract Refract Surg 2010;36:222–229

52 General Treatment Guidelines

Roger F. Steinert

This chapter describes the key steps that I take for complication avoidance. Even so, complications do occur, so I also describe the less common but most helpful maneuvers I favor to minimize damage and regain control of the situation. The discussion is not comprehensive. Rather, I present my personal favorites. These pearls work well with my current technique, but I am always looking for new and better pearls. As in any human endeavor, a surgeon will benefit from skills that add to strengths and compensate for weaknesses. Read this chapter with an open mind, and try to identify elements that resonate with your own current technique and skill set.

Preoperative Evaluation

Some special steps in the preoperative evaluation help ensure a good surgical outcome. In addition to a comprehensive preoperative examination, including a dilated lens and fundus exam, the surgeon must evaluate the patient from the perspective of preparedness for surgery. Is the patient well oriented and able to cooperate? Do medical conditions, such as respiratory distress or spinal deformity, make supine positioning impossible? If topical anesthesia is being considered, does the patient exhibit a high level of anxiety, or squeeze uncontrollably during applanation pressure measurement? Before focusing on the slit-lamp exam, take a moment to look at the orbital configuration. Deep-set eyes, high orbital rims, or a narrow palpebral fissure all argue for a temporal incision.

In the eagerness to examine the lens, do not forget to note the presence of blepharitis and to institute preoperative treatment. A history of epiphora may indicate lacrimal outflow obstruction and risk of infection; press on the lacrimal sac.

Keratitis sicca has been linked to an ever more prominent role in interfering with accurate keratometry and A-Scan measurements for intraocular lens (IOL) power. The preoperative office visit is an excellent time to make note of this potential problem and institute treatment in an attempt to enhance preoperative measurement and postoperative outcomes.

Corneal guttae must be carefully considered; if present, preoperative pachymetry and evaluation of cellular morphology are good indicators of endothelial function. Specular microscopy is helpful for both the diagnostic information it provides and from a medicolegal perspective. In any case, the patient needs to be informed of the increased risk of postoperative corneal decompensation and of the possibility of Descemet's stripping automated endothelial keratoplasty (DSAEK) or *Descemet's membrane endothelial keratoplasty* (DMEK). Additionally, the surgeon should put a prominent reminder in the admission note to be particularly vigilant, and take such steps as extra dispersive ophthalmic viscosurgical device (OVD), and low power in the bag phaco, to protect the depleted endothelium.

The dilation of the pupil must be noted. Synechiae from prior surgery or inflammation need to be lysed at the beginning of the surgery. A poorly dilating pupil may mask the presence of underlying pseudoexfoliation, with the combined operative risks of poor dilation and potentially weak zonular support. If pseudoexfoliation material cannot be seen on the limited amount of visible anterior capsule, look carefully for pseudoexfoliation dandruff at the edge of the pupil and on the endothelium. Even if none is seen, the surgeon should note the potential in the admission note as a reminder to look carefully for pseudoexfoliation once the pupil is mechanically stretched at surgery.

Preoperative accurate assessment of the cataract itself is very helpful in preparation for a smooth operative procedure. Use of the Lens Opacities Classification System (LOCS), devised by Leo T. Chylack, Jr. and coworkers,[1,2] helps obtain consistent grading of the cataract and encourages a disciplined approach to lens evaluation. The published grading system was devised as a cataract research tool, but I keep a copy in each examination lane as a clinical guide.

The key insight of the grading scheme is the separation of nuclear brunescence from nuclear opacification. Each of these aspects is graded on a scale of 1 to 6. Most clinicians pick up the habit in residency of simply glancing at a cataract and jotting down "3+ NS" for a moderately advanced senile cataract that is well along in nuclear sclerosis (hardening). Yet we cannot directly judge nuclear hardness at the slit lamp. A patient may complain of multiplopia and have progressive myopic shifting of the spectacle correction, with a modest amount of green-brown coloration but a high degree of haze in the central nucleus and less haze in the periphery. The rating would then be NC 2 (minimal color) and NO 5 (very significant opalescence). An elderly patient with 20/40 distance and J 1 near vision might have a dark brown but relatively clear lens, similar to the color of Coca-Cola. The rating might be NC 6 or NO 3. In both cases, the rating is much more meaningful than 2+ NS or 4+ NS, respectively. The first patient needs surgery; the second may not.

The remainder of the LOCS classification deals with anterior (A) and posterior (P) opacities on a scale of 1 to 4. I have modified this to AC (anterior cortical), PC (posterior cortical), and PSC (posterior subcapsular) to differentiate these types of changes because PSC cataracts typically cause more glare symptoms.

This rating system is not an empty exercise. In addition to sharpening the observations of the clinician, the ratings prepare the surgeon for the likely behavior of the nucleus during phacoemulsification. I use nuclear color and the patient age together to select which combinations of fluidics to employ. My phacoemulsification unit is programmed with five memory settings, and my admission note tells the operating room staff which memory setting to set up before I enter the room. This is both more efficient and safer than having the nurse ask, in mid-capsulorrhexis, "Is 200 OK?"

Each surgeon needs to develop phaco memory settings appropriate for the technique and for the machine. For my high-vacuum phaco chop technique with the AMO Surgical Signature Unit (Abbott Medical Optics [AMO], Abbott Park, IL), each memory setting represents a 100 mm Hg increment in the high vacuum setting, with corresponding increases in maximum phaco power and intravenous (IV) pole height. In all cases, flow is set at 28 cc/min. For example, Memory 3 is 300 mm Hg vacuum, 80% maximum phaco power. I also add in a setting for WhiteStar™ (AMO) power modulations (micro-pulse phaco) and a setting for elliptical power. Each has its own vacuum and flow setting.

Table 52.1 demonstrates the complexity of exploiting the settings for reliable outcomes. It lists the configurations used by William J. Fishkind, and demonstrates the complexity of the machine settings for one machine. Every machine, by virtue of its pump dynamics, software, tubing, foot pedal, venting, and tuning, will have distinctive settings. The optimum approach to define the settings that would be most advantageous to the surgeon is to work with the manufacturer's surgical representative to fine-tune the settings.

Admission Note and Operative Note

The admission note and the operative note are key elements that can defend you or damage you in the event of legal action. Accordingly, they should be fastidiously prepared to explain your plan and accurately convey the events of the surgery. Most importantly, the surgeon must use the admission note as a tool to maximize the potential for a complication-free surgery. The admission note is the surgeon's opportunity to alert anesthesia and nursing personnel to key issues. These include the usual items such as medical allergies, systemic diseases, and medications, but

also relevant issues such as anxiety, claustrophobia, back pain, tremors, language barriers, and many other factors that can have impact on the patient during surgery. As noted in the previous section on preoperative evaluation, the surgeon has many potential issues for which the admission note can be used as memory freshener. All of these elements should be typed in **bold** and, if particularly unusual or critical, ***bold italics.*** At the end of all my admission notes, after a statement of the risks that were reviewed with the patient, I list the preoperative keratometry and desired location of the wound, with the plan for astigmatic keratotomy if indicated; the IOL model and power; and the phaco memory setting. Any unusual elements (e.g., pseudoexfoliation or corneal guttae) are then reemphasized.

This note can be placed in the operative chart, or even better, taped to the IV stand or the side of the phaco machine so that it can be consulted during the initial time out and at any time during the surgery (**Fig. 52.1**).

Standard Operative Procedure

The details of the standard operative procedure have been well covered in the preceding chapters. Individual surgeons will adopt the aspects that suit their technique. The most important principle is that a surgeon may be pleased with the current techniques and results, but should never be satisfied. The history of cataract surgery has proven that a highly successful procedure may always be improved.

Often neglected are the aspects of surgery prior to the first incision that may well determine the success or failure of the procedure itself. This begins with the preoperative evaluation discussed previously, and continues with the preoperative care of the overall patient, which must result in a maximally relaxed, comfortable, and confident patient who is medically stable.

At surgery, the patient must be positioned to be comfortable and simultaneously accessible to the surgeon. For example, the patient can be placed in the supine position, with one or two pillows under the knees to avoid lower back pain. The surgeon must take the time to examine overall patient positioning at the outset of the procedure. For example, to expose the superior cornea adequately, does the patient just need to be reminded to lift the chin, or should the headrest be adjusted or should the head pillow be removed? Reverse Trendelenburg positioning is helpful, as it facilitates the patient's breathing by removing the pressure from the abdominal contents on the diaphragm.

An important advance in cataract surgical access, in my opinion, has been the shift to temporal incisions. A superior incision requires rotation of the eye downward, with degradation of the optics, loss of red reflex, and often an arcus senilis or superior pannus obscuring the surgeon's view. The temporal incision, in contrast, enables the eye to be positioned with a vertical optical access aligned with the operating microscope. A deep-set eye or prominent orbital rim no longer presents an obstacle. In setting up for surgery, the surgeon must observe the position of the operating microscope itself; the optical axis of the microscope must be precisely vertical if the eye is to be properly positioned (**Fig. 52.2**).

Table 52.1 Example of Phaco Settings

Fishkind Ellipse FX	Aspiration Rate	Vacuum	Power	Notes
Hard chop				
Unoccluded	32 cc/min panel Ramp 35%	340 mm Hg panel	50% linear	WS Kick 6–12 (0 to 80%) 90-cm bottle height
Occluded Threshold 200	28 cc/min 30% ramp speed	340 mm Hg linear	50% linear 6 long pulses/sec	90-cm bottle height
Chop				
Unoccluded	32 cc/min panel Ramp 30%	325 mm Hg linear	40% linear WS On/off = 8/4 PPS = 83 Duty cycle 67%	Kick 5 fixed 0–80% 92-cm bottle height
Occluded Threshold 200	30 cc/min linear Ramp 30%		40% linear 6 long pulse/sec	90-cm bottle height
Soft chop				
Unoccluded	30 cc/min panel Ramp 40%	260 mm Hg linear	35% linear Variable WS On/off = 10/12, 10/10,10/6,10/4 PPS = 45,50,62,71 Duty cycle = 45,50, 63,71	90-cm bottle height Kick 6–12 (0–80%)
Occluded Threshold 200	28 cc/min panel	20% ramp speed 90 cm bottle height Occlusion threshold 175 mm Hg	35% linear 6 LPPS	
Epinucleus				
Unoccluded	30 cc/min panel	300 mm Hg linear	10% linear	90-cm bottle height Kick 6–12 (0–80)
Occluded Threshold 150	22 cc/min panel	300 mm Hg linear	10% linear 4 LPPS	
I/A 1 (max vac)	26 linear Ramp 75% Nonzero start 10 cc/min	600 linear Nonzero start 50 mm Hg		80-cm bottle height
I/A 2 (cap vac)	5 panel Ramp 25%	5 linear		50-cm bottle height
I/A 3 (visco removal)	38 panel Ramp 80%	500 linear Nonzero start 50 mm Hg		90-cm bottle height
Vitrectomy 1			CPM, cuts/minute	
	20 panel	300 linear	1500 panel	Bottle 90 cm CIA (Cut-IA)
Vitrectomy 2	20 panel	300 linear	1500 panel	Bottle 90 cm IAC (IA-Cut)
Diathermy (rarely used)	50% linear			
Foot-pedal settings	0–5% foot position zero	5–19% foot position 1	19–72% foot position 2	72–100% foot position 3

Abbreviations: I/A, irrigation and aspiration; LPPS, long pulse per second; PPS, short pulse per second; WS, WhiteStar.

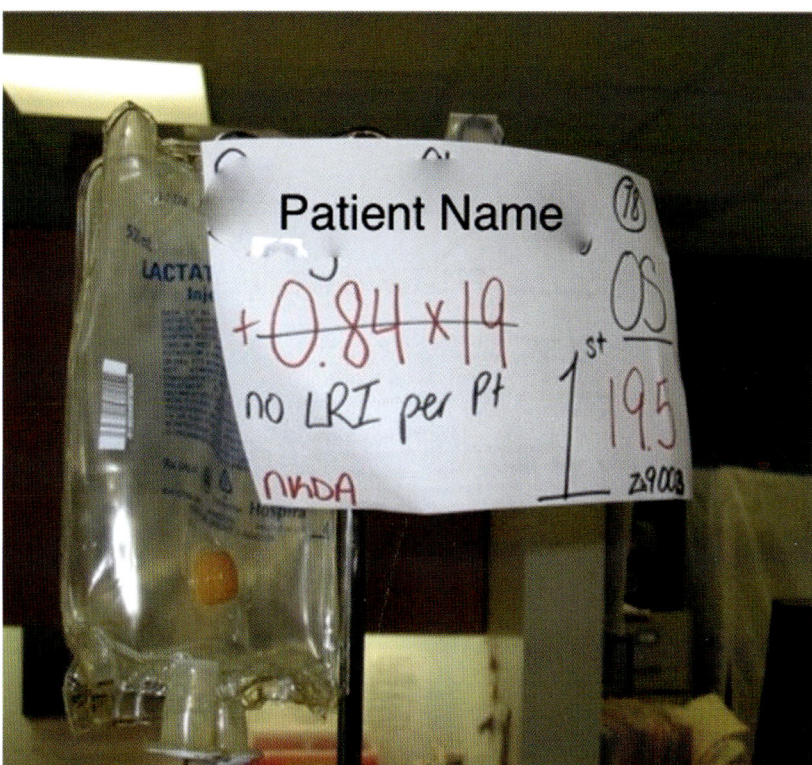

Fig. 52.1 A basic phaco note taped to the IV pole. Much information can be easily visualized and verified.

New microscope models have significantly improved visualization of the procedure. For example, the Zeiss OPMI microscopes (Carl Zeiss, Jena, Germany) have stereo coaxial illumination (SCI) **(Fig. 52.3)** The traditional Zeiss OPMI illumination is a single beam aligned 2 degrees off truly coaxial viewing alignment. This near-coaxial orientation provides a standard red reflex, but enough oblique lighting to provide depth, such as detail in three-dimensions (3D) of a nuclear fragment. The Lumera microscope (Zeiss) has two separate illumination beam angles that can be combined together in differing proportions. One beam is a 6-degree

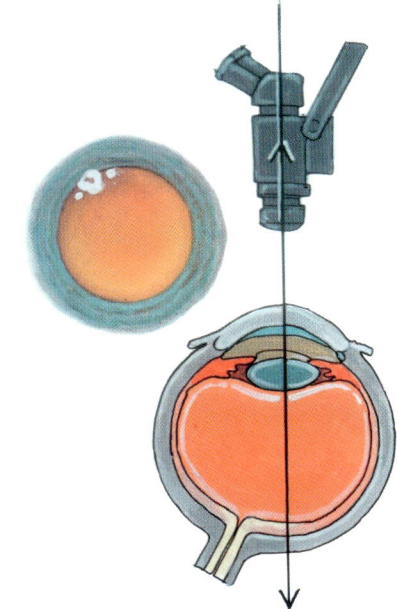

a

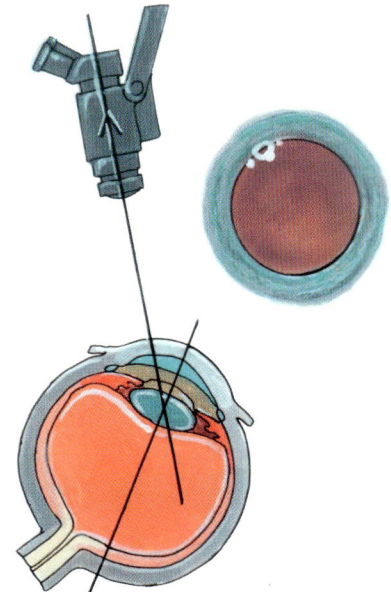

b

Fig. 52.2 **(a)** Coaxial alignment of the microscope and the optical axis of the eye is critical in obtaining a bright red reflex and good surgical visualization. A temporal approach improves the ability to achieve this alignment. **(b)** Tilt of the microscope and/or the eye markedly reduces visibility with surgeon foot pedal control. If I find that my preoperative prediction is inaccurate, then the memory setting is readily adjusted, but the preoperative evaluation system is highly accurate.

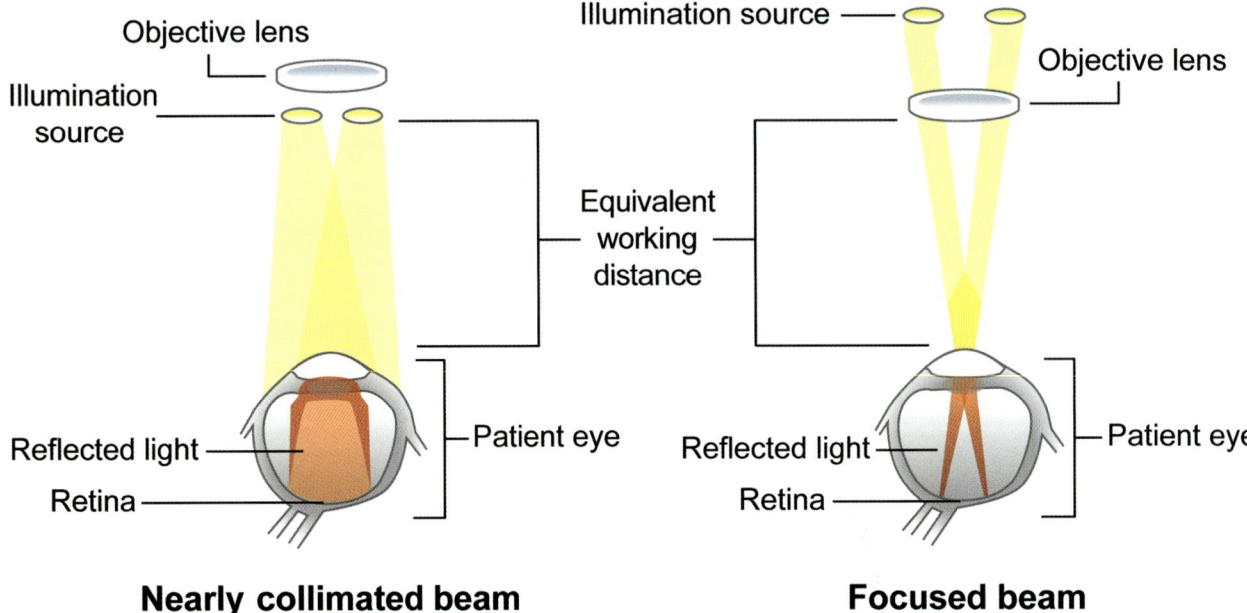

Fig. 52.3 A comparison of the conventional illumination beam aligned 2 degrees off truly coaxial. The Lumera has two separate illumination beams so that each ocular is coaxially aligned. Retroillumination is therefore maximized.

oblique field illumination. The other is split into two separate coaxial beams aligned with the oculars which provides 0-degree illumination. This is called stereo coaxial illumination by Zeiss. The result of this illumination is constant brilliance and brightness; every detail of the patient's eye becomes visible.

Chang[3] provides a thorough discussion of how to maximize the red reflex. Clearly, spending some time with the microscope manufacturer's representative is the best way to refine the features of the microscope to take full advantage of the enriched imaging.

Refractive Cataract Surgery

I believe that the trend to consider every cataract surgery a refractive surgery is a good one. I obtain corneal topography on every patient and determine the best approach to manage both astigmatism and spherical outcomes. Presently I am correcting the cylinder with a limbal relaxing incision (LRI) by hand, with a Nichamin nomogram, or by the femtosecond laser, for ¾ diopter to 1.25 D. I use toric IOLs for more than 1.25 D. I aim for a –0.50 D spherical result with no more than +0.50 D of cylinder. I also incorporate the posterior corneal cylinder into my calculations.

Special Maneuvers

One of the most important things a surgeon can do to minimize a complication is to remain calm and focused; in fact, the surgeon must be calmer during a crisis than when things are going well. Surgeons must personally assume an aura of complete control. To do that, they must have not only technical mastery of the procedure, including complication management, but also the combination of mental strength and confidence to enable their technical competence and creativity to be applied for a positive outcome.

The most critical techniques for salvaging a phacoemulsification cataract extraction that is going badly are the steps that stabilize the nucleus when the capsular bag has a posterior rupture:

1. Maintain integrity of the anterior capsule.
2. Inject OVD through the paracentesis to stabilize the anterior chamber before withdrawing the phaco tip (**Fig. 52.4**).
3. Inject more OVD around and behind the nucleus (**Fig. 52.5**).
4. As soon as access allows, insert a narrow Sheets' glide behind the remaining nuclear fragments that have been elevated by the viscoelastic[4] (**Fig. 52.6**).
5. Alternatively, if the anterior capsule is intact, elevate the remaining cataractous fragments above the capsular bag and insert the IOL with the haptics in the ciliary sulcus. The remaining fragments can then be emulsified with the IOL performing the role of the Sheets' glide preventing loss of nucleus into the vitreous. Once nucleus and cortex is removed, the IOL optic can be captured by the anterior capsule
6. Another alternative is the Viscoat posterior assisted levitation (PAL) technique (Alcon, Fort Worth, TX). A sclerotomy is created 3.5 mm posterior to the limbus. Viscoat, which has the smallest OVD cannula produced, is positioned through the sclerotomy and a small quantity of Viscoat is used to buoy up the nucleus. The nucleus is also manipulated with the cannula itself to reposition it in the anterior chamber. A large volume of OVD

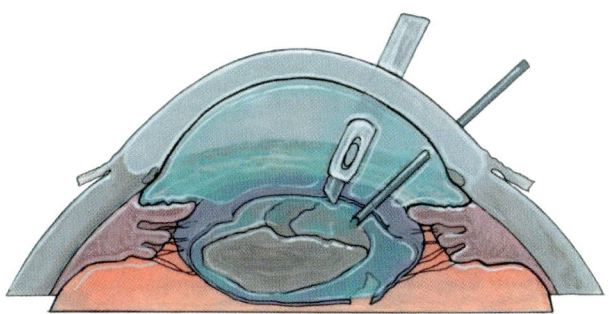

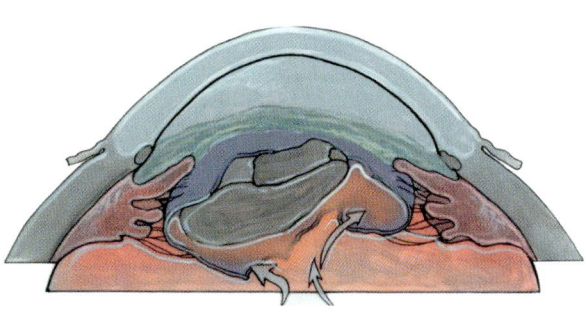

a

b

Fig. 52.4 **(a)** If a posterior capsular break or zonular dehiscence is suspected, viscoelastic should be injected through the paracentesis before withdrawing the phaco tip and infusion to prevent shallowing of the anterior chamber. **(b)** If the anterior chamber shallows, vitreous will herniate through the posterior capsular tear, often extending the tear.

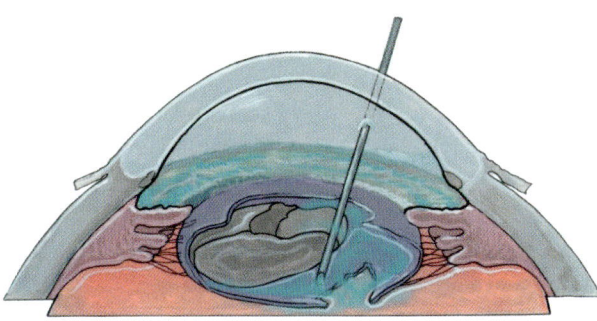

Fig. 52.5 Injecting a retentive, low molecular weight viscoelastic behind the nucleus will help block vitreous from herniating through the posterior capsule defect and slightly elevate the nucleus.

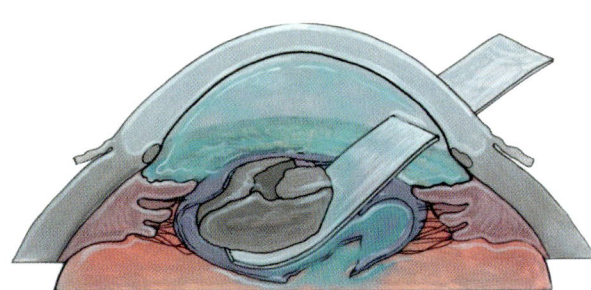

Fig. 52.6 A Sheets'-type glide is then passed between the posterior capsule and remaining nucleus. The phaco tip with very low flow settings can then be reintroduced to remove the remaining nuclear and epinuclear fragments.

should be avoided, as it may result in overinflation of the globe and expulsion of more vitreous.[5]

7. Reduce irrigation flow by lowering the bottle, and reduce vacuum and aspiration rates to very low levels. These settings can always be increased if needed as the surgery progresses, but high settings may cause irreversible extension of a capsular tear or loss of nucleus into the vitreous cavity (**Fig. 52.7**).

Do not hesitate to make a pars plana sclerotomy ~ 3.0 to 3.5 mm posterior to the limbus. This opening enables the introduction of viscoelastic behind the nucleus to lift it anteriorly, enables an instrument to support and elevate lens fragments, and enables a pars plana vitrectomy (with infusion through the limbal paracentesis), which will be more thorough and less likely to extend the capsular damage than a limbal vitrectomy (**Fig. 52.8**).

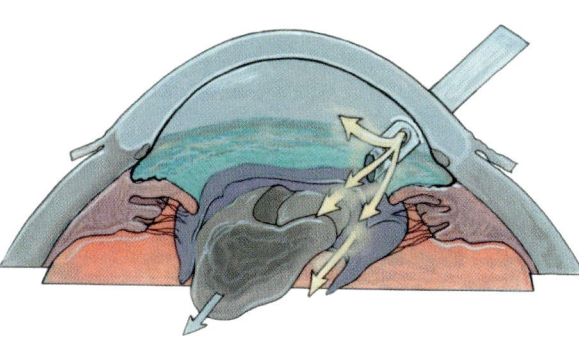

Fig. 52.7 Failure to lower the height of the irrigation bottle before reintroducing the phaco tip causes downward pressure, leading to extension of the capsular defects and/or zonular breaks, and the possible loss of the nucleus into the vitreous.

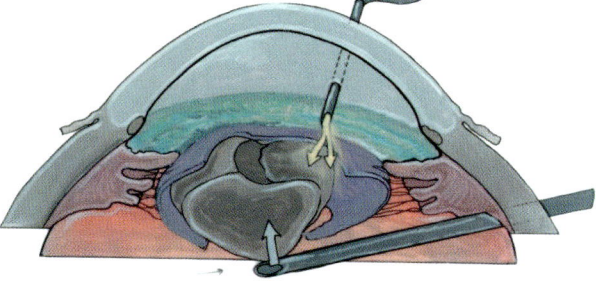

Fig. 52.8 A single sclerotomy through the pars plana 3.0 mm posterior to the limbus has many advantages. Infusion is performed through the limbus. A vitrectomy performed in this manner will pull vitreous out of the anterior chamber and not enlarge the capsular defect. If lens fragments threaten to fall posteriorly, the vitrector or another instrument passed through the pars plana enables the surgeon to apply a posterior force to prolapse the fragments into the anterior chamber.

Conclusion

Advancement of surgical skills is a never-ending search for solutions. This chapter described some of my personal pearls, but there are many more. The most important pearls are the ones that improve outcomes for our patients. No limit exists on creativity.

References

1. Chylack LT Jr, Ransil BJ, White O. Classification of human senile cataractous change by the American Cooperative Cataract Research Group (CCRG) method: III. The association of nuclear color (sclerosis) with extent of cataract formation, age, and visual acuity. Invest Ophthalmol Vis Sci 1984;25:174–180

2. Chylack LT Jr, Wolfe JK, Singer DM, et al; The Longitudinal Study of Cataract Study Group. The Lens Opacities Classification System III. Arch Ophthalmol 1993;111:831–836

3. Chang DF, ed. Phaco Chop and Advanced Phaco Techniques. Thorofare, NJ: Slack; 2013:175–177

4. Michelson MA. Use of a Sheets' glide as a pseudoposterior capsule in phacoemulsification complicated by posterior capsule rupture. Eur J Implant Surg 1993;570–572

5. Chang DF, Packard RB. Posterior assisted levitation for nucleus retrieval using Viscoat after posterior capsule rupture. J Cataract Refract Surg 2003;29:1860–1865

53 The Challenges with Phacoemulsification

David M. Dillman

Cataract surgery has changed for the better in the 12 years since the publication of the first edition of this book. Preoperative testing and imaging, the phaco machines, the microscopes, intraoperative aberrotomy, and femtosecond laser–assisted surgery are just a few of the advances that have been made.

But in other ways, not much has changed in cataract surgery since the first edition. Most of the issues that were discussed in the first edition remain issues for discussion in this edition. The factors that surgeons considered then as they prepared for cataract surgery are the factors they still consider today.

Thus, this chapter addresses some of the issues that were addressed 12 years ago but now in the context of the new technologies that are available today.

Controversies

There are two technologies that remain controversial. They have already been discussed in other chapters, with some authors having positive feelings about them and others negative. These are technologies that I use, and they are part of my current approach to complication prevention and management.

The first controversial technology is femtosecond laser–assisted cataract surgery (FLACS). Like many other surgeons, I was initially skeptical about FLACS. But then I consulted the surgeons who were the early adapters. I observed five surgeons performing FLACS in about one hundred surgeries, and then discussed the procedure with them. I concluded that FLACS was a positive advance, and 3 years ago I learned to perform it.

As my understanding of the technology and my ability to apply it has improved over time, I have become increasingly more reliant on it to help prevent complications. FLACS facilitates performing routine cases, and is especially helpful with difficult cases, such as dense lenses, weak zonules, and poor surgical visualization. If a patient's insurance does not cover FLACS, I deeply discount my fees or, in a few cases a month, I assess no fee at all. I lose money on these cases, but that indicates how highly I value the technology of FLACS in preventing complications.

The second controversial technology is intraoperative aberrotomy. Initially, it was not very good; it was cumbersome to use and not very reliable. But, as with other technologies, it quickly improved, and now I find it to be much easier and faster to perform and quite reliable. I cannot imagine doing cases involving a post-refractive intraocular lens (IOL), a multifocal IOL, a toric IOL, or even a distance vision monovision IOL without the availability of intraoperative aberrotomy. It also helps avoid IOL power and orientation (toric) complications.

Granted, both technologies add time and cost to each cataract surgery. But I am convinced that the benefits easily outweigh those downside factors.

Two Basic Philosophies

Two basic philosophies underpin my approach to cataract surgery and complication prevention. Although technologies have changed over time, these philosophies have not; if anything, they have strengthened, because as technology advances it is more and more tempting to hide behind it.

The first philosophy is to "major in the minors," that is, to pay a lot of attention to seemingly small details. The second philosophy, closely aligned with the first, is to focus on what is important at each step of the procedure. This helps prevent complications.

Surgical Procedures

One-Handed Two-Hand Phaco

The success of the phaco procedure depends on the surgeon's ability to understand and control the phaco fluidics. Many variables are involved, and today's phaco machines are very good at self-regulating them. But they cannot control incisional leakage.

Phaco fluidics have been discussed elsewhere in this book, so I am going to focus on just one aspect—incisional leakage, and especially leakage through the side-port incision. By side-port incision, I am referring to the incision made a few clock hour positions to the side of the primary phaco incision for traditional coaxial phaco.

Incisional leakage has an untoward effect on phaco fluidics, regardless of the location of the leakage. We can create a well-balanced phaco incision and still negatively influence fluidics by creating an unnecessarily large side-port incision. When we create a side-port incision, how large should it to be: 0.5 mm? 1.0 mm? 1.5 mm? One of the advantages of FLACS is that this incision will be the exact size we want. But what is the appropriate size? It depends on what is used as the second instrument. It should be just big enough to allow entry and exit of the second instrument. I have used many of the choppers, manipulators, and rotators available today, and I find that a side-port incision no greater than 0.5 mm is a very close approximation of the appropriate size. And yes, there is a meaningful difference between a 0.5-mm and a 1.0-mm side-port incision in performing a successful surgery.

However, I also recommend not using a side-port incision, even a properly sized one, unless it makes a significant contribution to the surgery. For too many years, I would place the second instrument through the side-port incision at the beginning of the phaco process and leave it in the eye until the end. But I eventually realized that even with a properly sized side-port incision, there is going to be some leakage, and it was the presence of the second instrument (especially through a too large side-port incision) that was causing the side incision leakage and thus causing the

457

posterior capsule to come forward. So I ask myself constantly, "Is my second instrument really advancing this phacoemulsification in a safe and positive fashion, or am I leaving it in the eye simply because it is convenient to do so?" Although at first it may seem to be a hassle to be putting your second instrument in and out of the eye, you will notice improved fluidics with it *out* of the eye. This will result in improved followability and chamber stability, both of which will lead to fewer complications. Thus, I recommend being a one-handed two-handed surgeon as much as possible.

The No-Excuse Hydrodissection

The Colvard Maneuver

Excellent mobility of the cataract within the capsular bag is an essential precursor to all endocapsular phaco techniques, even those that are a part of FLACS. Mobility of the lens within the capsular bag is a function of hydrodissection, thus making hydrodissection a crucial (but often underappreciated) step. It is an excellent way to help prevent complications.

The presence of a posterior fluid wave is not proof that the hydrodissection has been successful. The only way to be assured of successful hydrodissection is to actually test for and prove mobility. There are many ways to do so; I simply use my hydrodissection cannula before removing it from the eye. But what if the nucleus will not spin easily, that is, without putting stress on the zonules or posterior capsule. What if you have tried straight cannulas and curved cannulas, and you have tried it inferiorly and superiorly, and still the nucleus will not spin! This happens more frequently with FLACS, because of the gas bubbles between the cataract and the central posterior capsule, so I tend to be less aggressive in using hydrodissection. The answer is what I have termed the "Colvard maneuver."

In the early days of phaco, Michael Colvard developed an ingenious little device, the phaco shield, that was placed between the cataract and the central posterior capsule. When the shield is properly placed, it becomes impossible to break the posterior capsule by phacoing through the cataract. By placing the phaco shield, we create space between the cataract and anterior capsule. I applied the concept to hydrodissection—hence, the Colvard maneuver.

The Colvard maneuver is simple; all we are doing is creating space. In situations in which we cannot obtain good hydrodissection, and cortical and epinuclear material is fluffing up, making visualization increasingly difficult, we should simply refrain from further efforts. Instead, we should ask for the phaco handpiece, and in foot position 2, aspiration, simply remove as much cortex and epinucleus as we can, not just centrally, but as far out into the periphery as possible. The peripheral material can be approached by gently putting the phaco tip just short of the capsulorrhexis/capsulotomy.

Once this is done, it is often possible to easily rotate the cataract within the bag with the phaco tip in foot position 1, irrigation. If not, simply re-form the anterior chamber with the viscoelastic of your choice, and complete the hydrodissection with the cannula of your choice. I have so much faith in the Colvard maneuver that the first patient I used it on was my mother; I tried and tried to hydrodissect, and her cataract did not respond. So I did the Colvard maneuver, and lo and behold, I obtained excellent hydrodissection with excellent mobility of the lens.

The Clandestine Wraparound Tear

The Little Dutch Boy Maneuver

In my experience, the most underrecognized etiology for a posterior capsular tear is an anterior capsular tear that has become a wraparound tear. One current criticism of the FLACS capsulotomy is that there are more anterior capsule tears than with traditional capsulorrhexis, but that has not been my experience. Nonetheless, regardless of how it occurred, it is very important that we keep anterior capsular tears anterior only and not allow them to wrap around to the equator and posterior capsule. I find that the best way to do this is to prevent the capsular bag from sudden decompression. This often happens when the phaco handpiece or irrigation and aspiration (I/A) handpiece is removed from the eye. I vividly remember a case I did in 1996 in which I knew there was a tear in the anterior capsule early on. I was able to do the phaco. I was able to remove all of the cortex without difficulty. However, as I pulled the I/A handpiece out of the eye, I could see the anterior capsular tear wrap around and create a significant tear in the posterior capsule. I vowed I would never let that happen again.

What I learned to do is simple but effective. In the presence of a known anterior capsule tear, or even if I suspect an anterior capsule tear, I do not allow the capsular bag to suddenly decompress. I make sure it always has support. I call this the "Little Dutch Boy" maneuver with the analogy of trying to keep a small hole from becoming a huge hole with bad consequences.

Each time I feel it is necessary to remove either the phaco handpiece or the I/A handpiece (commonly at the conclusion of the phaco or cortex removal, but occasionally at other times as well), I switch to foot position 1 and pause with the phaco tip or I/A tip resting gently in the center of the anterior chamber. I then ask the scrub nurse for a viscoelastic agent (all these agents work well for this application). With my dominant right hand I hold the phaco tip or I/A tip in the eye, again in foot position 1, and I hold the viscoelastic syringe in my left hand. I insert its cannula through the side-port incision and inject the viscoelastic **(Fig. 53.1)**. Sometimes it is easier for me to hold the syringe and have the scrub nurse depress the plunger and insert the viscoelastic. After a moderate amount of viscoelastic has been injected, I switch to foot position 0; that is, the irrigation inflow has stopped, but the phaco or I/A handpiece stays in the eye, "plugging" the phaco incision. More viscoelastic is injected until I feel the capsular bag has been stabilized. Then I remove the

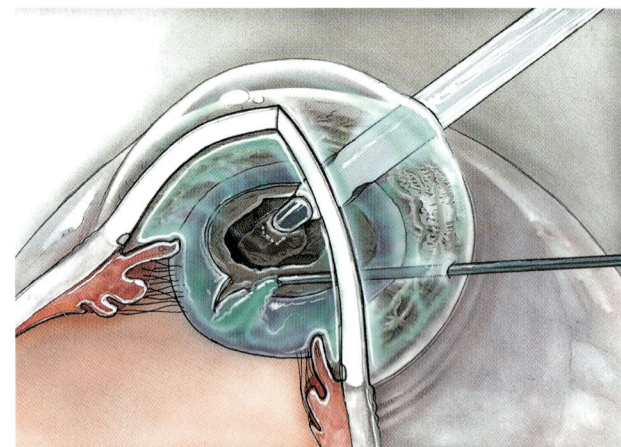

Fig. 53.1   To prevent an anterior capsular tear, I keep the bag from decompressing. Therefore, before removing either the phaco or the irrigation and aspiration (I/A) handpiece, I switch to foot position 1 (inflow) and allow the handpiece to rest gently within the phaco wound. The outer silicone sleeve helps plug the wound. Through the side-port incision, viscoelastic is slowly placed into the bag. Once I can see the bag forming, I switch to foot position 0, but leave the handpiece in the eye, while viscoelastic continues to be gently injected. Once the bag is formed, both instruments can be removed from the eye.

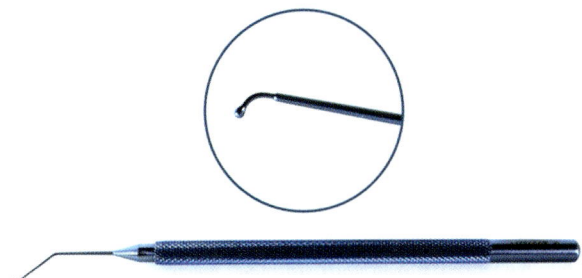

Fig. 53.2 The Connor wand. (Courtesy of Accutome, Malvern, PA.)

phaco or I/A handpiece and return it to the scrub nurse. At that point I may or may not add additional viscoelastic.

I repeat that series of maneuvers, using viscoelastic to prevent forward movement of the capsular bag as often as necessary until the IOL has been implanted into the capsular bag. The IOL provides the added support necessary to keep the anterior capsular tear anterior from that point on.

Other Techniques

Phaco prechop is my fastball technique and has been for years. For lenses that are too dense for prechopping, I use quick chopping (vertical chopping). For lenses that are too dense for quick chopping, I do some form of divide and conquer (I do these cataracts with the assistance of FLACS). One thing these techniques all have in common is that occasionally one or more pieces are stuck and cannot be moved with conventional maneuvers. Years ago I broke a capsule or two trying to get them out.

Christopher Connor designed a device that can serve as the second instrument that became known as the "Connor wand." It is unique in that it has a blunt, rounded end (**Fig. 53.2**). The concept behind it is that it can be placed under parts of the cataract and if it comes into contact with the posterior capsule, the bluntness of the instrument would cause no harm. If this is done safely, it can be beneficial to work behind the cataract. I never felt comfortable having a second instrument of any kind in contact with the posterior capsule, but I still was intrigued by the idea of working behind the cataract when I was not making progress from in front of the cataract. So I learned to do the over/under maneuver.

The Over/Under Maneuver

There are two premises to performing this maneuver: (1) the phaco handpiece must be out of the eye; and (2) there must be a through and through division, a through and through chop or crack of some sort, to work through to gain access to the back side of the cataract. Once done, I simply place my viscoelastic cannula over the chop/crack (**Fig. 53.3a**). I then start to slowly but steadily inject viscoelastic and watch for a subtle but definite widening of the gap in the chop/crack. Then I continually inject viscoelastic as I slowly advance the cannula through the gap. The viscoelastic will push the posterior capsule posteriorly and will create a good space, a safe zone, in which to work behind the cataract but also away from the posterior capsule. We are now under the cataract (**Fig. 53.3b**). I then use that same cannula as a second instrument to back-crack the piece, and lift it up to facilitate gaining access for the phaco (**Fig. 53.3c**). I use the viscoelastic to go over and then under, and in my hands this has proven to be a consistently safe and reliable way to gain access to and then remove pieces that are stuck. I use this maneuver regularly.

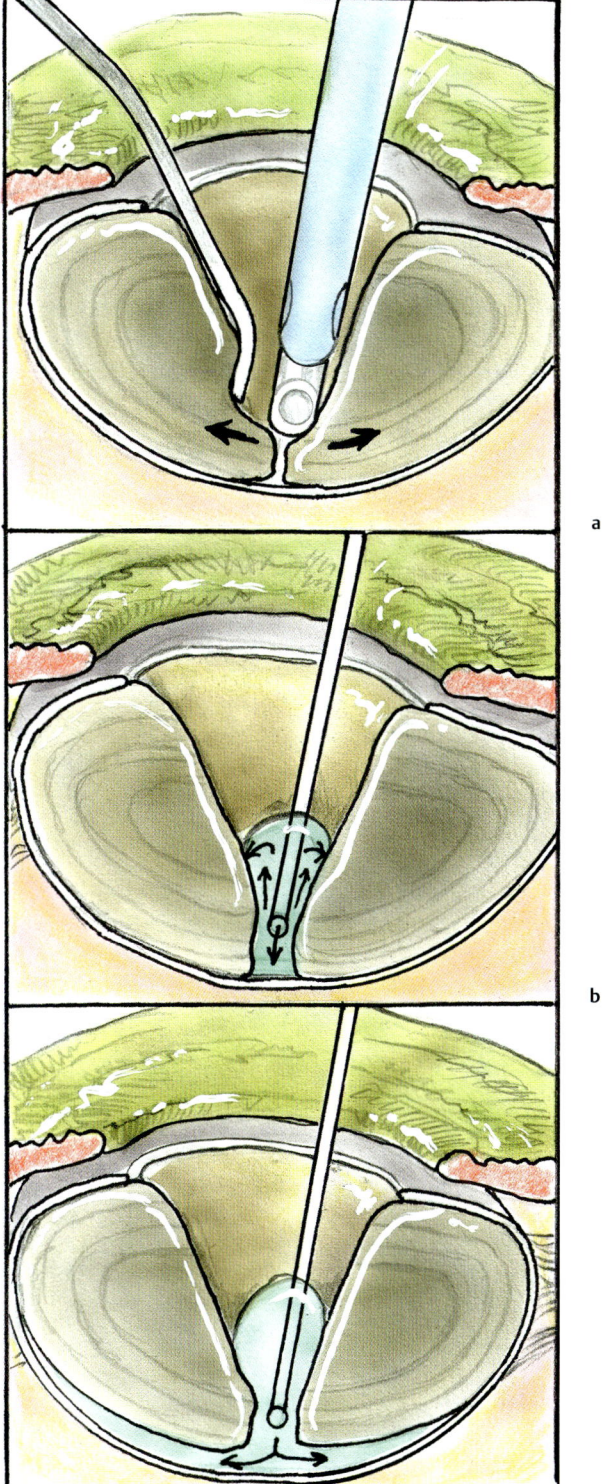

Fig. 53.3 **(a)** When I can identify a through and through chop or crack, I place my viscoelastic cannula into the eye and begin to inject viscoelastic as I approach the chop/crack. Then, when just on top of the chop/crack, I continue to slowly but steadily inject and watch for a widening of the gap in the chop/crack. **(b)** I continually inject viscoelastic as I slowly advance the cannula through the gap. The viscoelastic will gently and safely push the posterior capsule posteriorly, creating a safe zone in which to work behind the cataract. **(c)** Then use the same canula to either back-crack or lift a piece way up off the posterior capsule so that there will now be easy and safe access with the phaco.

Sticky, Recalcitrant Cortex

In the first edition of this book I stated my opinion that more capsules are broken during the I/A of cortex than during the phacoemulsification. Back then it was not uncommon for surgeons to use a metal irrigating sleeve on their I/A handpiece, which combined with the larger incisions of that time (3.0 to 3.2 mm), resulted in poor fluidics and compromised control. Most surgeons used metal aspirating tips, which were rather unforgiving if the posterior capsule was aspirated.

However, since then, most surgeons use silicone irrigating sleeves and the incisions have gotten smaller (2.2 to 2.4 mm). The result is much improved fluidics and thus improved control. Just as important, there are now polymer material aspirating tips that are very forgiving if the posterior capsule is aspirated.

Thus, the removal of cortex is now much easier. But there are still cases in which we are confronted with sticky, recalcitrant cortex, as commonly occurs following a capsulotomy made by the femtosecond laser, because the laser neatly "amputates" the cortex immediately under the capsulotomy for 360 degrees. For the most part this eliminates the "tags" of cortex that we had been so accustomed to; we were able to grab those tags with the I/A tip. With these tags the cortex seemingly "came to us," making removal of the cortex often simple and straightforward. Now, with those tags gone, we have to seek the cortex; we go to it, it no longer comes to us.

So, whether it is post–traditional capsulorrhexis or post–laser capsulotomy, how do we best deal with sticky, recalcitrant cortex? We can use a series of simple maneuvers to assist in the taming of sticky, recalcitrant cortex. The first is the most difficult: simply leave it alone. For some reason, there seems to be an almost macho attitude when it comes to removing cortex. It is almost as if the cortex has thrown done the gauntlet, and we must conquer it at all costs. But leave it alone for the moment. Instead, use the viscoelastic agent to viscodissect the stubborn cortex off the posterior capsule and up into the fornix. Because it is often the subincisional cortex that is recalcitrant, this maneuver is almost always best accomplished through the side-port incision. The objective is to get under the leading edge of the remaining cortex (**Fig. 53.4a**). Then create an advancing wave of viscoelastic that will peel the cortex off and deposit it in the fornix (**Fig. 53.4b**). Next, continue with the viscoelastic injection until the capsular bag is well filled and ready for the next step, which is IOL implantation. The IOL will assist in keeping the bag filled and the posterior capsule posterior.

The next step is optional and is determined by just how "sticky" the cortex was to begin with. If I feel it was really socked in, even though I loosened it with viscodissection, then I loosen it more by employing manual *irrigation*, not manual aspiration. Next, I gently squirt balanced salt solution into its belly. The objective is to both loosen and hydrate the cortex to greatly improve its accessibility. I learned this technique from a demonstration film by Harold Ridley, the inventor of the IOL in the 1950s. Once he removed the nucleus, he removed all of the cortex by gentle irrigation. He used no aspiration whatsoever! Many cannula styles can be used to accomplish this irrigation, approached through both the phaco and side-port incisions. As a general rule of thumb, for subincisional cortex I use a U-shaped cannula through the phaco incision. When this last step is completed, I use the automated I/A handpiece to remove the remaining cortex. Often this is best accomplished with one of the curved or angled aspiration tips.

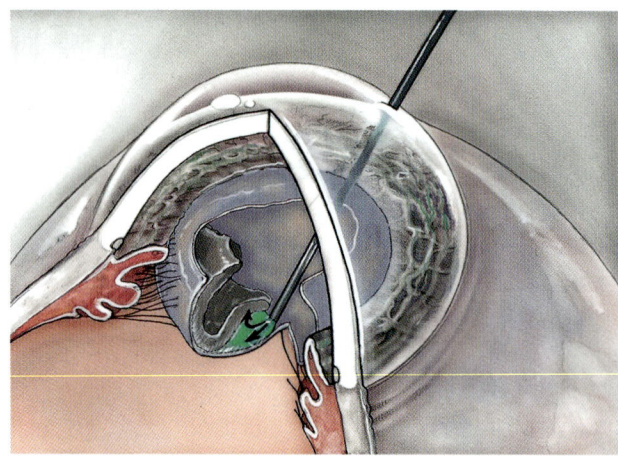

a

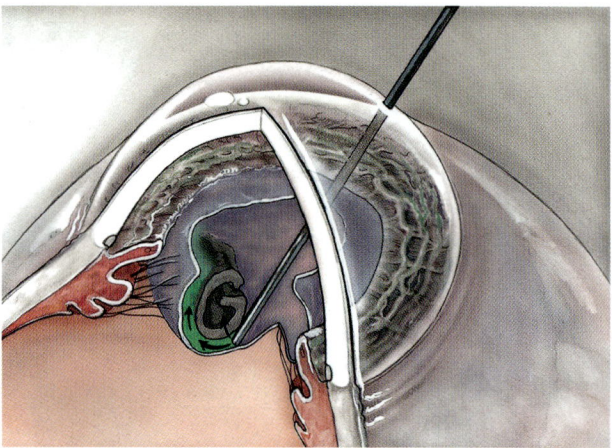

b

Fig. 53.4 **(a)** This side view illustrates viscodissection of stubborn cortex. The viscoelastic cannula tip is placed just in front of the leading edge of the remaining cortex. The viscoelastic is slowly injected, pushing the underlying posterior capsule backward to create space between it and the cortex. **(b)** Once this space has been created, viscoelastic is continually injected and the cannula advanced toward the fornix as the cortex obligingly retreats.

Almost always this series of maneuvers will successfully address recalcitrant cortex. But occasionally I find it necessary to manually re-irrigate, to "fluff it up" some more. In rare situations I leave a little cortex rather than risk a more serious problem, such as breaking the posterior capsule trying to remove a little stubborn cortex.

Conclusion

How can we minimize damage when, regardless of our best preventive measures, we hit a snag? We simply deal with it. Denial might well be the single greatest cause of complications, and yet it is also the most preventable. By using the techniques and maneuvers discussed in this chapter, surgeons can achieve successful outcomes and minimize complications.

54 Microincision Phaco Surgery

Louis D. "Skip" Nichamin

This chapter discusses routine microincision phaco surgery, which is the technique I currently perform. The discussion focuses on subtle points of the procedure that facilitate performing it, help avoid complications, and lead to successful and reproducible outcomes. I also review several common difficult situations faced by today's implant surgeon, and discuss the principles and pearls that can facilitate dealing with these trying situations.

Routine Phaco Surgery

When one observes true masters of phacoemulsification perform surgery, one cannot help but wonder, as I have, how it is that they achieve seemingly flawless results with such aplomb and ease. The answer, of course, is to be found in their attention to detail. The following discussion addresses the basic components of the procedure, providing details that I have learned from my teachers that facilitate performing the procedure and avoiding complications.

Anesthesia

The advantages of noninjection anesthesia to both patient and surgeon are well recognized. A common denominator for success, for both the novice as well as experienced surgeon, is proper patient selection. In fact, after many years of performing topical (and later intracameral) anesthesia, my percentage of noninjection cases began to approach the 98% level; however, I realized that my surgery had become less enjoyable and more trying for both me and my patients. This was due to "pushing the envelope," as I was operating on many patients who were simply not appropriate candidates. By becoming more selective (and returning to more frequent use of injection anesthesia), I was able to be more efficient, and both my patient and I enjoyed a better experience. One's selection criteria will vary based on experience and case variety, but I base my decision on a few simple elements of the preoperative exam and how the patient reacts to them.

Noninjection Anesthesia: Selection Criteria

If the patient exhibits unusual blepharospasm or a marked Bell's phenomenon during biomicroscopy and, in particular, indirect ophthalmoscopy, the patient is almost always deemed an inappropriate candidate for topical anesthesia. I further empower my surgical assistants who perform our biometric measurements to designate on the chart that the patient exhibited poor cooperation, and I adhere to their recommendations. Also, once in the operating room, if the nursing or anesthesia personnel voice doubt about the patient's ability to cooperate, then we convert to some form of injection anesthesia. I have rarely regretted opting for a deeper anesthetic, but I have often regretted not doing so.

When utilizing noninjection anesthesia, draping of the patient's eyelids may become more challenging. I am a firm believer in compulsively sequestering the entire lid margin under the protection of a plastic drape to enhance "barrier" prophylaxis against infection. This requires extra effort when orbicularis function is intact. If the patient shows an unusual reaction to draping and the insertion of the speculum, it is the final chance to "bale out" by converting to injection anesthesia.

Anesthetic Timing and Application

Surprisingly, it actually requires very little topical anesthesia to adequately anesthetize an eye for intraocular surgery. I have found that nearly any common topical anesthetic agent will suffice, but the important point is not to overdo it. Administering a single drop prior to instillation of the dilating regimen, followed by a drop at the time of the prep, and then again immediately prior to commencing surgery, is generally more than adequate. If instilled too early or too often, despite insisting that patients keep their eyes closed, troublesome drying and a punctate surface keratopathy may result; most patient's anxious and inquisitive state prior to surgery may cause them to gaze about the room, curious about the unfamiliar situation and surroundings. This may potentially compromise intraoperative visualization as well as increase postoperative discomfort. Topical gel anesthetics are also useful to prolong the anesthetic effect and aid in lubrication throughout the procedure. Many surgeons further supplement the topical agent through the use of an intracameral agent such as 1% sterile nonpreserved lidocaine.

Another important clinical point is that the sensation that is most profound to the patient while under anesthesia involves stretching of the zonular apparatus. This is most likely to occur in high myopes and in patients who have had previous vitreous surgery. I find that noninjection anesthesia may still be used in these cases, but great care must be taken to gradually deepen the anterior chamber (AC), trying to avoid a sudden and severe stretch placed upon the zonules. Even in routine cases, patients may note some sensation when the irrigation and aspiration (I/A) is first placed into the eye following phacoemulsification. It is at this point during the procedure that the greatest hydrostatic tension is placed on the zonules. Therefore, I find it helpful to instill additional intracameral anesthesia during the exchange of the phaco to I/A instrumentation. The increase in AC volume due to the additional anesthetic and balanced salt solution (BSS) also helps to blunt the sudden pressure and volume rise that occurs upon reentering the eye.

The surgeon should be aware of an interesting phenomenon that occurs in an eye that has previously undergone vitrectomy surgery. Shortly after adopting noninjection anesthesia, I was surprised to learn that in the post-vitrectomized state, intracameral anesthesia can very efficiently diffuse back to the retina and cause amaurosis despite an intact posterior capsule. Similarly, if a capsular rent occurs intraoperatively, and particularly if a vitrectomy is required, diffusion may again occur. Patients should be warned of a temporary diminution or loss of their vision. To my knowledge, no untoward sequelae have ever been documented following this phenomenon. In fact, I have personally employed topical and intracameral anesthesia in planned posterior vitrectomy cases.

Exposure and Instrumentation

It is well recognized that one of the greatest advantages of the temporal approach is better access to the globe and improved exposure and intraoperative visualization. In fact, once surgeons who had previously utilized a superior approach have accomplished this somewhat challenging transposition, they will likely find that they dislike working from any other approach. In transitioning to the temporal position, several challenges arise: positioning one's knees under the operating table, acquiring adequate wrist support, and shifting personnel and equipment into a new workable configuration. Once these hurdles are met, several additional subtle challenges may be recognized; for example, access to the side-port incision, which is now either at the 6 or 12 o'clock position, may be awkward, especially in patients with deeply set eyes.

Several specialized specula have been designed to aid with the temporal approach. I use a modification of the classic Kratz-Barraquer wire lid speculum, which works well in most patients. It is made of a heavier gauge metal, making it more resistant to blepharospasm. In addition, the temporal aspect is angulated posteriorly, over the lateral canthus, such that it is out of the way of incoming instrumentation. I also use a similar design with a locking mechanism for those patients who are truly squeezers; however, if I have adhered to the preoperative selection criteria, this situation rarely arises because the squeezing patient should have been scheduled to receive injection anesthesia.

Another important issue is fixation of the globe, particularly under noninjection anesthesia and when utilizing a clear corneal incision. My preference is to use a modified Fine-Thornton fixation ring. The upper surface has 10-degree markings to aid in placement of limbal relaxing incisions, and the undersurface of the ring has been highly polished to minimize conjunctival trauma. Mild downward pressure of the ring is typically all that is necessary to stabilize the globe. Other surgeons find it helpful to place an instrument through the side port to fixate the globe, or simply using a gloved finger placed over the bulbar surface may gently stabilize the eye.

As noted above, a potentially challenging peculiarity of the temporal approach is access to the side-port incision. When operating superiorly there is typically unencumbered access to the paracentesis (at the 3 or 9 o'clock position). Now, however, access to the 6 or 12 o'clock position may be hampered by either the lid speculum or the orbital rim, particularly in deep-set eyes or in individuals with narrow palpebral fissures. For this reason, additional modifications to conventional instrumentation may be of help. These include nuclear manipulators that have a more vertical angulation to better fit down into a deep-set eye. Also, modified irrigating cannulae with shortened tips facilitate placement through side-port incisions.

Always important is the detail of patient positioning. One must ensure that the patient's neck is neither hyper- nor hypoextended (the elderly tend toward the former, and younger patients toward the latter). I encourage our operating room personnel to labor over this detail, as proper and consistent positioning leads to more efficient and reproducible surgery. This holds true also for the surgeon's chair, pedals, and microscope. I further

employ a subtle but helpful maneuver taught to me by Bruce Wallace, a cataract surgeon in Alexandria, Louisiana. By slightly tilting the patient's head temporally toward the side that the surgeon is sitting on, there is significant improvement of visualization as well as more ergonomic positioning of the microscope. There is a tendency during surgery for the patient to move away from the surgeon, so we routinely place a very light strip of tape over the patient's forehead as a friendly reminder to maintain the desired position.

Lastly, to improve efficiency and logistics in the operating room, an attempt is made to schedule all right eyes together and similarly left eyes are grouped together to avoid having to make unnecessary changes to the positioning of equipment and instrumentation.

Incision

One need not extol the many virtues and efficiency of clear corneal incisions; however, studies and early experience provided evidence that there may be an increased tendency toward wound leakage and a higher risk for infection with this approach, particularly during one's learning curve. Through the work of Paul Ernest and others,[1–3] it has become clear that the key to creating a wound with sufficient integrity to avoid leakage is to strive toward a "square" architecture, such that the incision's depth approximates its width. With today's smaller incision sizes, such wound construction is readily accomplished.

Another point to consider is proper sizing of an incision in relation to the phaco needle and sleeve combination that is used, as this is of paramount importance to achieve optimal fluidics.[4] Too tight an incision risks impeded infusion with loss of AC volume, or worse yet, a corneoscleral burn[5]; however, the more common tendency is to use an incision size that is too large and therefore leads to unnecessary leakage and chamber instability. It should be noted that a grooved incision tends to gape more and will therefore behave as if it were a slightly larger incision, and tends to induce slightly more wound flattening and hence surgically induced astigmatism. Many surgeons ignore the importance of the side-port paracentesis incision. Most manipulators will pass through an incision of 0.5 to 0.7 mm, thus making the standard 1-mm side-port incision too large and, hence, leaky.

Capsulorrhexis

The key to performing a consistent capsulorrhexis is maintenance of a deep AC. Fortunately, today's microincisions help to inhibit loss of viscoelastic and aid in retention of AC depth. In difficult cases, such as intraoperative floppy iris syndrome (IFIS) or an unusually shallow AC, performing the rhexis through a separate smaller incision may be helpful, and proper use of viscoelastics is fundamental in promoting and maintaining chamber depth and iris stability. Though my preference is to use actuating microcapsulorrhexis forceps in most cases, yet another trick in difficult eyes is to create the rhexis through a small paracentesis utilizing a cystotome, placed upon the a viscoelastic syringe, such that the chamber may be immediately deepened should shallowing occur or excursion of the tear be encountered.

My standard incision is placed temporally, is single plane (unless a relaxing incision is needed for preexisting astigmatism), measures 1.8 mm to correspond to my preferred micro-coaxial phaco tip and sleeve combination, and is created at the posteriormost extent of the limbus. As such it typically produces a trace amount of bleeding. I find that this approach seals consistently well. In performing the rhexis through this microincision, I have found that the Seibel micro-actuating forceps (Micro-Surgical Technologies [MST], Redmond, WA) are very useful. The tear is begun by pinching the anterior capsule centrally, and is immediately followed by a circumlinear movement clockwise, such that the flap is folded over upon itself and advanced using a shearing rather than a stretching force. Following completion of the tear, the capsular segment is removed from the AC to ensure that the rhexis has been completed 360 degrees. Additionally, when removing the torn capsule, gentle pressure on the posterior lip of the incision enables decompression of the AC, helping prevent over-pressurization during subsequent hydrodissection. This decompression should be performed slowly and gently in cases of IFIS.

Hydrosteps

Thorough hydrodissection is important to ensure trouble-free phacoemulsification for most forms of intracapsular surgery. I find it helpful to confirm adequate hydrodissection by visualizing free and easy rotation of the lens within the capsular bag before proceeding with lens removal. I personally prefer the technique of cortical cleaving hydrodissection as taught by Howard Fine, a surgeon in Eugene, Oregon: without irrigation, a flattened hydrodissection tip is placed under the anterior capsular leaflet and injection is gently performed in one or two locations. After each injection the lens is lightly balloted in a posterior direction, causing the injected fluid to pass in a wave-like fashion around the equatorial region, lysing cortical capsular adhesions.

Hydrodelineation, on the other hand, may be considered an optional step by some surgeons, but I personally employ this maneuver in all endocapsular techniques. This hydro-maneuver enables one to work within the safe confines of the epinuclear shell, affording better capsular protection. Also, with modern chopping techniques, I find it easier to remove the chopped segments of the hydrodelineated nucleus, as they are smaller and easier to purchase. Some surgeons may initially struggle with removal of the outer epinucleus. This is in actuality easily accomplished, again as taught by Fine, by simply trimming the epinuclear bowl in all four quadrants using aspiration and then allowing it to collapse and flip in upon itself.

Phacoemulsification

There are now many variations on the original Nagahara phaco chop technique, originally described in 1993.[6] My personal preference is for a technique that was originally referred to as "Quick Chop," a term coined by David Dillman (Danville, IL), and is now more widely referred to as vertical chop. This technique, with slight variations, was described contemporaneously by several surgeons, including Thomas Neuhann (Germany),[7] Vladimir Pfeifer (Slovenia),[8] Abhay Vasavada (India),[9] and Hideharu Fukasaku (Japan). Several key points pertain to all phaco chop techniques.

First, one should get in the habit of exposing more of the phaco needle (beyond the leading edge of the silicone sleeve) to enable a deeper purchase of the nucleus. I personally find that a 15- to 30-degree bevel tip is optimal. After chopping, the purchase of cleaved segments may be aided by tipping up the central tip or "apex" of the chopped segment anteriorly, and then sliding the phaco tip beneath the undersurface, rather than allowing the segment to tumble forward. This may be facilitated by using the manipulator to push the chopped segment out toward the equator of the bag, which in turn causes the posterior apical aspect to slide upward. If the phaco needle or chopper is positioned too high, it will skim over the surface of the nucleus. If the chopper is inadvertently placed over the capsular bag, it will tear the bag or the zonule (**Fig. 54.1**).

Another helpful hint involves rotation of the bevel such that optimal apposition occurs with chopped segments. This requires rotation of the phaco instrument along its long axis, and will in essence create a 0-degree tip when the bevel is placed parallel to the presenting surface or facet of the chopped segment. Occlusion is thus maximized.

Perhaps the most important point in all disassembly techniques involves the discipline to ensure that each successive cleavage plane is complete in its separation from one pole of the nucleus to the other and from anterior to posterior. This may require placement of the instruments deeply into the fault line that has been created, and then lateral separation in several different locations to ensure that the division plane propagates entirely through the posterior nuclear plate. Complete separation is confirmed by visualization of the red reflex. This separation should occur on each successive chop and division, or the result will be multiple, partly separated, peripheral segments connected centrally and posteriorly—a conformation that resembles a tulip or garlic clove.

One of the most common complaints voiced during the transition to the traditional Nagahara phaco chop technique involves placement of the chop instrument around the edge of the nucleus in the capsular bag periphery. Upon examination of the bag anatomy and curvature and design of most choppers, it becomes apparent that this potentially dangerous maneuver may be safely performed by carefully angulating the instrument such that the proximal handle of the instrument is brought back toward the surgeon, causing the distal tip of the chop instrument to assume a plane parallel to the iris (**Fig. 54.2a**). At this point, excursion out under the anterior capsule to the periphery may be safely made without snagging the capsule or prematurely engaging the nucleus. Once out and around the endonucleus, the handle of the instrument is brought upright once again, thus causing the distal tip to pass around the equator of the lens (**Fig. 54.2b**). The chop can then be made against the impaled phaco tip.

Alternatively, this maneuver may be obviated by adopting the vertical chop technique described above. Again, in this approach the chop instrument is placed just in front of or to the side of the centrally impaled phaco needle. The chop instrument is pressed downward, toward the optic nerve, and then outward (or laterally). The phaco tip, impaled in the bulk of the nucleus, is slightly elevated, providing counterforce to the downward force of the vertical chopper (**Fig. 54.3**). One subtle key with these maneuvers is to use the side-port incision as a fulcrum such that the heel of the instrument—that portion outside of the incision—elevates as the distal tip passes downward into the lens. Otherwise, depression of the paracentesis site will cause a distorted view of the AC. Additionally, a more pointed or faceted tip, as opposed to the blunted tip designed for safety during traditional phaco chop, is best for this technique.

Preplacement of a groove or central sculpting can be quite helpful to the surgeon making the transition from a standard divide-and-conquer approach to a chopping technique. The veteran phaco chop surgeon generally utilizes only central debulking when dealing with extremely dense nuclear cataracts. This enables the initial chop to be performed on less nuclear bulk, thus creating more space and requiring less physical energy to create the initial cleavage plane.

Irrigation and Aspiration

Many surgeons continue to utilize bare-metal I&A instrumentation without a silicone sleeve and therefore incur unnecessary incisional leakage. This leads to collapse of the capsular fornix, thereby creating greater difficulty accessing and removing cortical material. I find that a 45-degree angled diamond-dusted tip, used with an appropriate incision-sized silicone sleeve, provides excellent access to 360 degrees of the capsular bag. Rarely, recalcitrant, usually subincisional, cortex may remain, and I use a

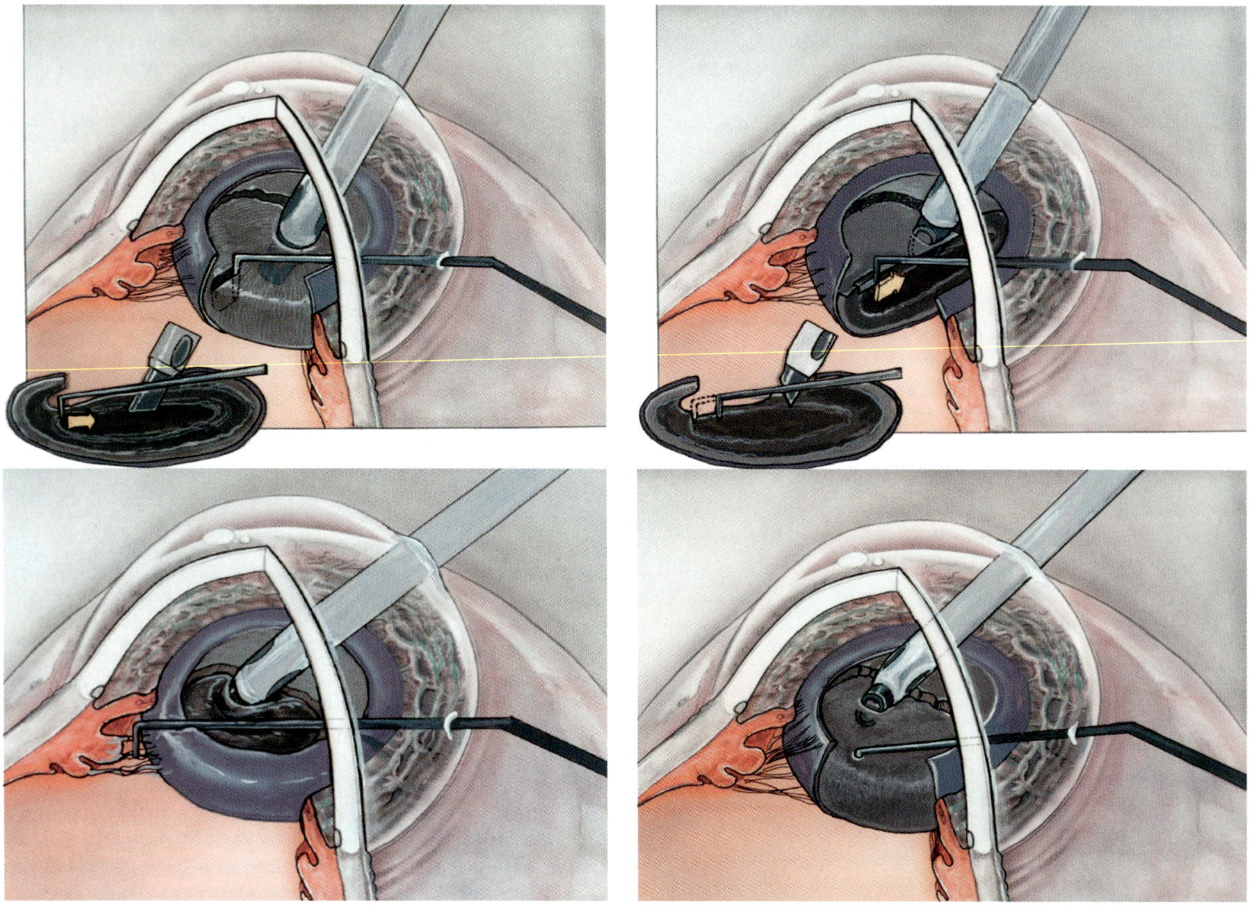

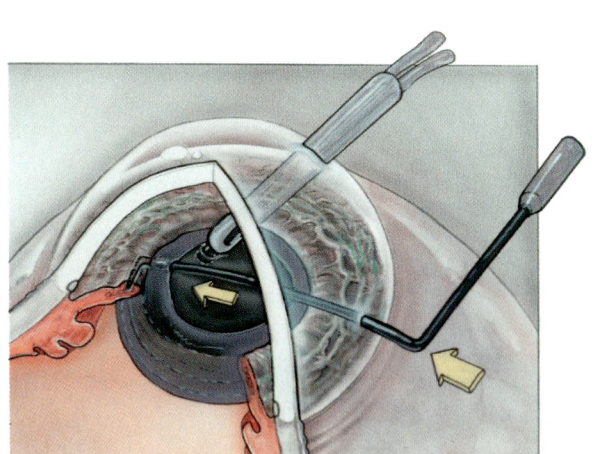

Fig. 54.1 Examples of incorrect positioning. **(a)** The chopper is positioned too high. It will skim over the nucleus. An adequate chop is therefore impossible. **(b)** Both the chopper and phaco tip are too high. **(c)** The chopper is placed outside the capsular bag, which will create a zonular dialysis on attempted chopping. **(d)** The phaco tip is not deep enough into the nuclear material, and in addition is too central to adequately create a chop.

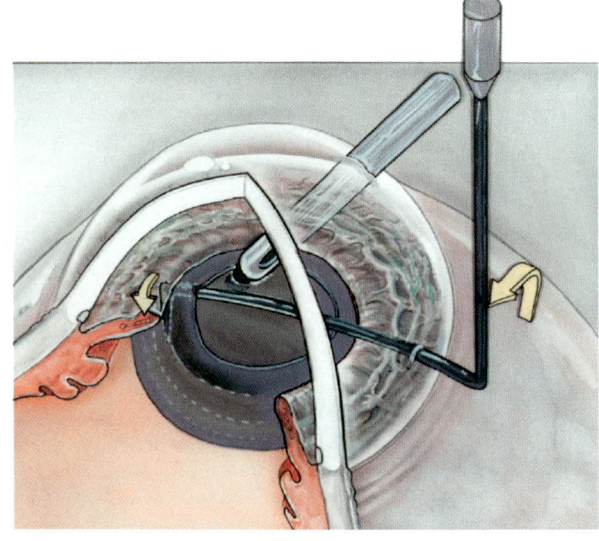

Fig. 54.2 **(a)** The handle of the chopping instrument is rotated toward the surgeon, resulting in rotation of the tip so that it is parallel to the nucleus and can be easily passed under the anterior capsule. **(b)** Once past the equator, bringing the handle vertically enables the tip to pass around the nucleus equator.

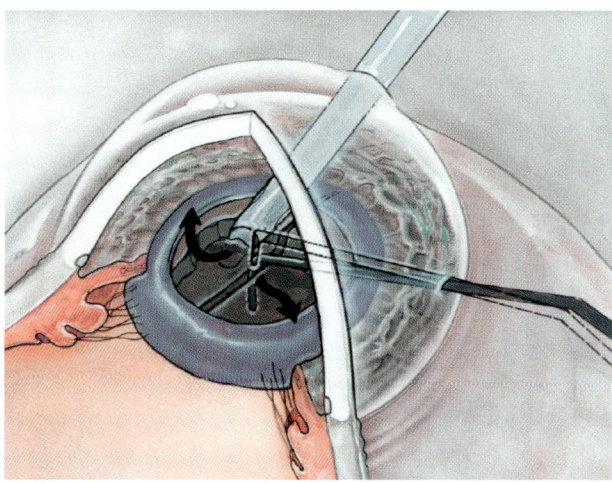

Fig. 54.3 The chopper tip is placed left of but near the embedded phaco tip. The chopper is pushed posteriorly into the nucleus while the nucleus is held in place or elevated with the phaco tip. Simultaneously, the chopper is moved down and left while the phaco tip is moved up and right. This creates a split in the entire nucleus between both instruments.

simple manual maneuver to remove this material. Viscoelastic is first used to push the posterior capsule downward in the area of the cortex. A double-bent 27-gauge cannula attached to a tuberculin (TB) syringe half filled with BSS is then placed through a side-port incision. The double-bent cannula can easily reach the subincisional area. Light pressure on the plunger of the syringe enables delicate loosening of the cortex by irrigation, which is then followed by purchase and stripping from the fornix by lightly pulling back on the plunger and aspirating. The cortex is then brought up and into the AC, where removal may then be completed with the I/A tip. This same technique is used to remove cortex when faced with a breach in the posterior capsule or when dealing with weakened zonules (see below).

Bimanual instrumentation is also very useful in achieving complete 360 degree cortical cleanup, and the separation of the aspirating force from infusion flow may be preferred in complex situations.

Intraocular Lens Insertion

Historically, the most common problems incurred during placement of an intraocular lens (IOL) involved either poor loading of the foldable implant or an attempt to place the lens through too small an incision. Improved injector delivery systems have greatly reduced such problems, though attention to detail is still required in this regard. Given the reduced size of contemporary incisions, one really has no need to force the injector tip into too tight a wound, which may result in stretching of the tissue and potential wound leak. However, some injector tips are designed for "wound-assisted" delivery, wherein the tip is just barely placed into the outermost aspect of the incision, and the corneal tunnel then serves as a conduit for delivery. Again, one should always avoid the temptation to implant through too small an incision, which not only may disrupt the wound architecture, but also may lead to premature IOL release, damage to the implant, or a Descemet's detachment.

If undue resistance is encountered during insertion, it is best to stop, remove the device, and inspect the IOL and injector, and consider reloading the device. Resistance to IOL passage often is

secondary to malposition of the IOL or overriding of the plunger or obturator. Blythe persistence in this situation may end in delivery of a damaged IOL or undue trauma and injury to intraocular structures.

Two of the more frustrating situations that one may encounter during lens implantation is delivery of an inverted IOL or, as noted, a damaged implant. In the case of the latter, depending on the extent of the problem, the lens may be left in situ, but when in doubt it is generally best to remove and exchange the implant.

In the case of an upside-down delivery, following generous deepening of the AC with viscoelastic, the optic can be flipped over, right side up, using two manipulators placed through side-port incisions. The axis of rotation of the lens optic should be at the plane of the iris within a viscoelastic deepened chamber. Given an optic radius typically of 3.0 mm, and a viscoelastic-filled AC depth of 4 to 5 mm, there should be a space of at least 1.0 to 1.5 mm between the endothelium and the edge of the optic as it is repositioned. One can use a dispersive ophthalmic viscosurgical device (OVD) to protect the endothelium and an additional cohesive agent to optimize deepening of the capsular bag.

When faced with the need to remove a foldable IOL, the optic does not always need to be entirely bisected to preserve the small incision. Rather, by just obtaining a cut 2.0 to 3.0 mm in length and then firmly grasping an edge, the optic will elongate and pass through the incision (especially more pliable biomaterials such as silicone). Alternatively, specialized instrumentation is available to aid in bisecting a lens (Rhein Medical, St. Petersburg, FL, or MST), which may be preferable for stiffer, acrylic implants.

Alternatively, after appropriate positioning within the AC, the IOL may be folded intracamerally over a thin spatula placed through a paracentesis port 180 degrees away from the main incision and then removed through the unenlarged wound.

Wound Closure

As noted, clear corneal incision integrity has been a topic of debate. As discussed above, if incision architecture approximates a square configuration, with the width not being much greater than the depth of the tunnel, wound integrity is typically adequate and self-sealing will occur. I do find stromal hydration helpful even if the incision appears to be watertight. By bringing the roof and floor of the tunnel into strict apposition, a more secure closure is obtained. I also take time to hydrate the side-port incision. This incision, if checked, often leaks more than the main phaco incision due to intraoperative manipulation at this less accessible site. Another pearl for obtaining good closure is to slightly hyperinflate the chamber and then slowly release fluid through the side-port incision until a normal intraocular pressure is obtained. This maneuver helps to close the internal lip of the phaco incision to promote a watertight seal.

Difficult Situations

Of all the benefits that contemporary clear corneal small incision surgery offers, none is greater than the markedly reduced rate of complications. Nonetheless, even the most experienced surgeon will on occasion encounter trouble. What then distinguishes master surgeons is their ability to retain a sense of equipoise and methodically work through the challenge. By utilizing proper instrumentation, technique, and most importantly maintaining a closed-chamber environment, the surgeon retains control over the intraocular milieu and can thereby dictate the eventual outcome.

Armed with a thorough understanding of these surgical strategies, this sense of confidence and equanimity may be engendered by both novice as well as experienced phaco surgeons.

Management of the Broken Posterior Capsule and Advanced Vitrectomy Technique

Admittedly, each case and anatomic scenario involving a broken posterior capsule is unique; however, several fundamental surgical principles apply universally. When followed, these principles enable surgeons to achieve the following goals: (1) safe and thorough removal of all lens material; (2) as indicated, removal of presenting vitreous without imparting unnecessary retinal traction forces; and (3) avoidance of further enlargement of the posterior capsular tear.

First, one must have the discipline to stop working as soon as a problem is sensed. This does not necessarily mean removal of instruments from within the eye because abrupt shallowing of the AC may extend the tear. Rather, filling of the AC with viscoelastic through the side-port incision may then permit removal of the phaco or I/A instrument without incurring sudden hypotony. At the same time, viscoelastic is used to tamponade the anterior hyaloid face and stabilize any remaining lens material. Time then exists for careful assessment of the pathology, which will then dictate subsequent surgical strategy (**Fig. 54.4**). It should be noted that a low-viscosity, less cohesive, and highly dispersive viscoelastic helps to form a better "plug" in a capsular break and tamponade the anterior hyaloid face (**Fig. 54.5**). When faced with this challenging situation, well-prepared surgeons are able to quickly avail themselves of the necessary (often multiple) viscoelastic agents and a pre-prepared set of instruments for such rare events (an "emergency" kit).

In an effort to avoid enlarging the capsular tear, one must strive toward the maintenance of a truly closed-chamber environment. Although aided by small, self-sealing incisions, further maneuvers in the face of an open capsule must utilize truly watertight incisions. This intraocular state helps permit the next surgical principle to take place, that is, the minimizing or eliminating infusion. These two concepts are the essence of avoiding extension of the capsular tear (**Fig. 54.6**).

If significant nuclear material is present, a decision must be made regarding further phacoemulsification. This depends on the surgeon's experience and the anatomic particulars of the case; however, if conversion is thought to be necessary, generously enlarge the incision. Astigmatic concerns may be addressed at a later time. Care should also be taken to avoid pressure on the

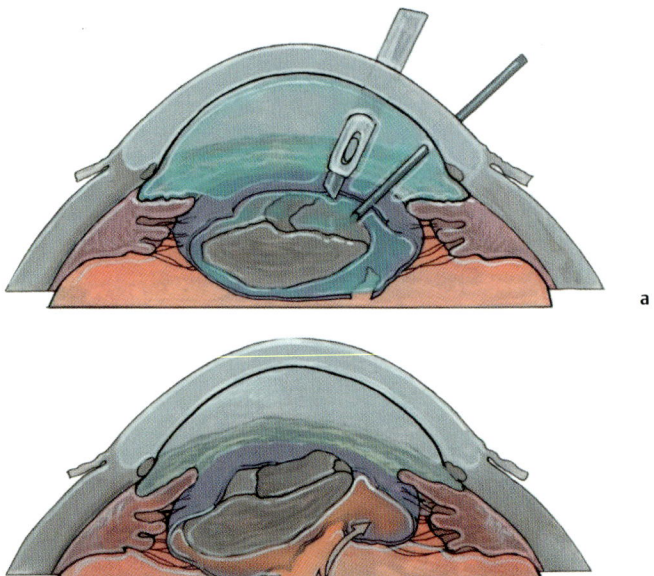

Fig. 54.4 **(a)** If a posterior capsular break or zonular dehiscence is suspected, viscoelastic should be injected through the paracentesis before withdrawing the phaco tip, and infusion should be performed to prevent shallowing of the anterior chamber. **(b)** If the anterior chamber shallows, vitreous will herniate through the posterior capsular tear, often extending the tear.

globe when removing lens material; viscodissection and instrument-aided nucleus removal is preferable. A modified lens glide (Beaver Visitec, Waltham, MA) may be called into use to both support and aid in removal. Alternatively, the lens glide may be used as a "pseudoposterior capsule," allowing further phacoemulsification to be performed. This must be performed in a low-flow state (**Fig. 54.7**).[10]

For residual cortex, I strongly advocate a manual technique of removal, or at least mobilization, followed by automated I/A after the implant has been placed and the pupil constricted. If the I/A handpiece is used in a routine fashion, the associated high flow will undoubtedly cause extension of the tear. Alternatively, if the anterior hyaloid face has been broken, cortex may be removed utilizing the vitrectomy instrument. The manual technique first employs viscodissection between the cortex and the posterior capsule, and then placement of a double-angled

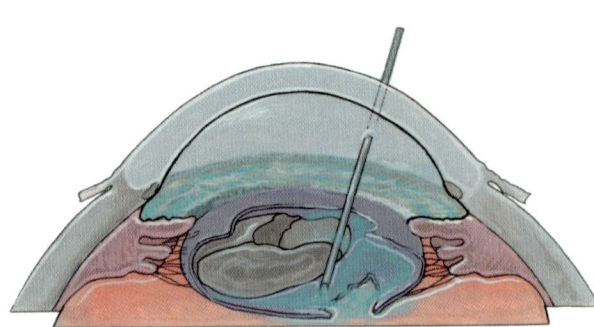

Fig. 54.5 Injecting a retentive, low molecular weight viscoelastic behind the nucleus helps block vitreous from herniating through the posterior capsule defect, and slightly elevates the nucleus.

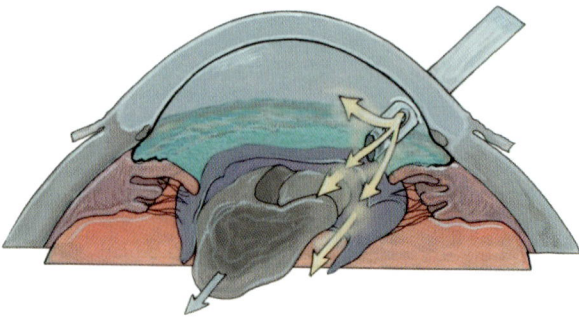

Fig. 54.6 Failure to lower the height of the irrigation bottle before reintroducing the phaco tip causes downward pressure, leading to extension of the capsular defects and/or zonular breaks, and the possible loss of the nucleus into the vitreous.

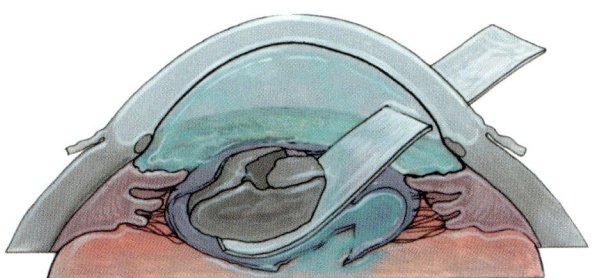

Fig. 54.7   A Sheets'-type glide is then passed between the posterior capsule and remaining nucleus. The phaco tip with very low flow settings can then be reintroduced to remove the remaining nuclear and epinuclear fragments.

27-gauge cannula through side-port incisions. Simcoe or Binkhorst cannulas may be substituted. As noted previously, the cannula is attached to a BSS-filled TB syringe, which can provide for gentle infusion to loosen cortex, followed by exquisitely controlled manual aspiration enabling one to gently strip remaining cortex from the capsular fornix without further extension of the capsular rent. The cortex need only be brought up into the AC, not completely drawn into the syringe; after lens implantation and constriction of the pupil, the liberated cortical material within the AC may then be removed with automated instrumentation (I/A, or preferably a vitrector). Additional viscoelastic is placed as necessary during this process to tamponade the anterior hyaloid face and maintain chamber volume.

If vitreous is present within the AC, a vitrectomy is mandated. Many authors (including Fishkind, Koch, Osher, and Arbisser[11]) have expounded the virtues of a bimanual, two-port vitrectomy, yet many cataract surgeons still rely on what is familiar and superficially easier to use—a unimanual, coaxial vitrectomy instrument. Unfortunately, this approach is inefficient, potentially more dangerous, and much more likely to lead to enlargement of the capsular rent. By simply separating the infusion line from the vitrectomy instrument, a more controlled and effective vitrectomy can be performed. Various AC maintainers are available. Self-maintaining cannulas have the advantage of freeing-up one hand, but I prefer to maintain bimanual control over the eye, and I have found that a blunt-ended specifically designed 21-gauge

infusion cannula is ideal (model E4421-S21, Bausch and Lomb Storz, El Segundo, CA; **Fig. 54.8**). The standard infusion line connects easily to this simple instrument, and is then placed through the side-port incision. The infusion rate is lowered to a level that simply maintains volume as material is removed. A microvitreoretinal (MVR) blade is then used to make a separate stab incision either at the limbus (**Fig. 54.9**) or through the pars plana (**Fig. 54.10**) to permit placement of the vitrectomy cutter. These incisions must be snug and watertight. If not self-sealing, the phaco incision must be sutured. Vitreous removal should be performed at low (50 to 100 mm Hg) vacuum settings with high (500 to 5000 cpm) cutting rates. If lens material is to be removed, the cutting rate is reduced and vacuum carefully and gradually increased as needed.

Though most anterior-segment surgeons opt for a limbal approach for placement of the vitrectomy instrument, which is perfectly acceptable when performed in a bimanual fashion, alternatively one may utilize the pars plana to perform potentially a more efficient anterior vitrectomy (**Fig. 54.10**). This technique has the advantage of better accessing the subincisional area where residual lens material often resides, and permits efficient removal of AC vitreous by drawing it down posteriorly from the AC, rather than continuously pulling it up, thereby potentially limiting the total amount of vitreous that is removed and minimizing dangerous vitreoretinal traction forces.

Although anterior-segment surgeons may be understandably averse to performing it, an incision placed through the pars may be safely and easily accomplished. Following a small conjunctival peritomy, calipers are used to carefully measure 3.0 to 3.5 mm posterior to the limbus. An appropriate MVR blade (matched to the vitrectomy cutter's gauge) is then used to make a stab incision, keeping the blade perpendicular to the eye wall. The metal tip of the blade should be visualized through the pupil to be sure that entry is complete. Once the vitrectomy is completed, the incision is freed of any remaining vitreous and closed with a suture. Following IOL placement, a miotic is gradually instilled. Viscoelastic is removed with the vitrectomy instrument, with meticulous attention directed toward the pupil and wounds to be sure that all vitreous has been removed. Late shallowing of the AC must be avoided to prevent further vitreous prolapse; temporary air injection followed by a gradual manual fluid–air exchange may be useful in this regard. Rapid stromal hydration of limbal incisions is also helpful. Watertight wounds, as always,

ANTERIOR CHAMBER MAINTAINERS

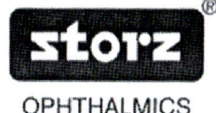

OPHTHALMICS

Nichamin Side Port Cannula

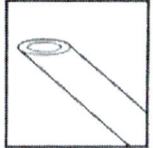

E4421 S
E4421 S21

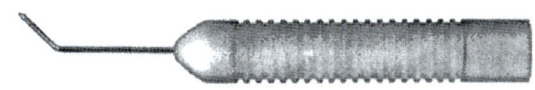

Cannula designed for maintaining the anterior chamber. Angled 45° 7mm from tip. Handle design allows for connection to the irrigation line. Overall length (including handle) 72mm, 2.8

E4421 S21   21 Gauge

Fig. 54.8   This 21-gauge blunt-tip cannula from Bausch and Lomb Storz (model E4421-S21) is perfect to provide infusion for bimanual vitrectomy.

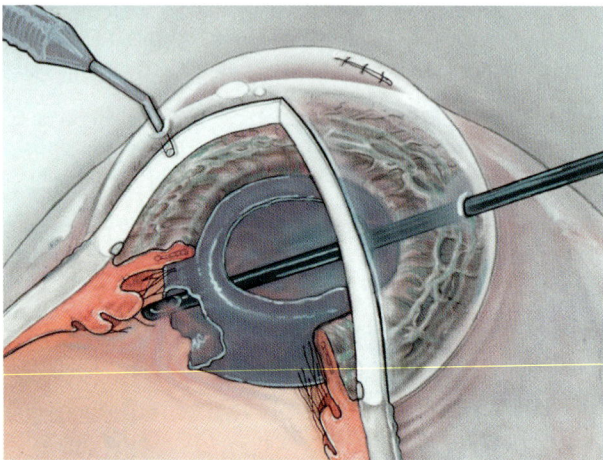

Fig. 54.9 Maximal control during anterior vitrectomy is obtained through the use of a closed-chamber system. The inflow and vitrectomy are performed through separate paracenteses. If the main incision is not watertight, it should be sutured.

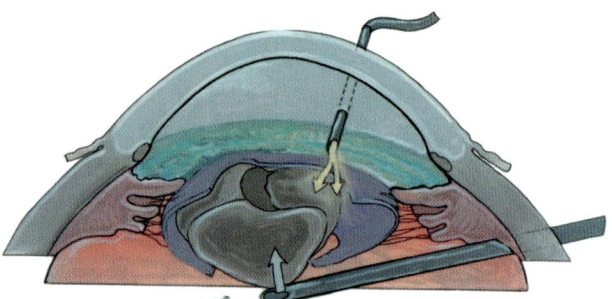

Fig. 54.10 A single incision measuring 3 mm posterior to the limbus has many advantages. A vitrectomy performed in this manner may be useful to draw vitreous back behind the plane of the posterior capsule and not enlarge the capsular rent. If a lens fragment threatens to fall posteriorly, the vitrector, or another instrument, may be utilized to elevate the fragment into the anterior chamber for stabilization. In addition, the pars plana port may be used to remove subincisional cortex.

should be confirmed. Postoperatively, steroid and nonsteroidal anti-inflammatories should be vigorously employed, and cycloplegic and antihypertensive agents considered.

Smaller gauge vitrectomy instrumentation is now available, and may be used by the anterior segment. Initially somewhat "flimsy" in their tensile strength, making their use in complex surgery difficult, recent improvements in both 25- and 27-gauge instruments, along with much higher cutting rates, now afford the lens surgeon greater control and efficiency in this setting, and may help limit the amount of vitreous removal that is required. Use of a suture-less trocar entry system, however, may not be appropriate in an "open" eye setting.

Lastly, intracameral triamcinolone is now recognized as an important adjunct in helping the surgeon to visualize prolapsed vitreous, and commercial preparations are now readily available. In addition, use of this intraocular steroid may help to suppress postoperative inflammation.

The Mature Cataract

Though often challenging, advanced and even mature cataracts can be efficiently managed today through the use of advanced surgical equipment, instrumentation, technique, and viscoelastic use. Preoperative planning, including the setting of appropriate patient expectations, and intraoperative patience is key in these cases.

It is important to differentiate between the white or intumescent cataract, and the rock-hard dark brown or even black nuclear cataract (see Chapters 14 and 15). The white cataract, typically seen in younger patients, is a fairly straightforward condition once the capsulorrhexis is completed. These lenses divide nicely with minimal force or difficulty. On the other hand, the rock hard nuclear cataract, more often occurring in the elderly, can be more difficult and is often accompanied by weak zonules and a thin tenuous posterior capsule.

When facing these cases, it is important to be armed with contingency plans. Depending on the surgeon's experience, one may opt to approach such eyes through a scleral tunnel incision, making conversion easier should it become necessary. The more experienced surgeon, however, may feel comfortable working through their standard clear corneal incision, and if a change in strategy becomes necessary, the corneal incision can be closed

and a second separate scleral incision crafted to enable manual extraction.

Obtaining an adequate capsulorrhexis is perhaps the most important step when dealing with these difficult cases. The use of capsular dye, specifically trypan blue, has had a profound effect upon the ease by which this step can now be performed, as the red reflex is usually severely compromised in such cases. Instillation of the dye is typically performed under an air bubble, and a small amount of viscoelastic placed just inside of the wound may aid in its retention. The dye is "painted" onto the anterior capsule using the cannula provided with the dye's syringe. Other options to aid in enhanced visualization are more of a historical note and include working under very high magnification, slowing the zoom speed of the microscope, turning the operating room lights off for better illumination, and utilizing an oblique lighting source placed outside of the eye.

In the case of an intumescent or swollen white lens, initial puncturing of the capsule may present with the "Argentinian flag sign," wherein the dyed anterior capsule suddenly splits out to the periphery (so named because of the blue-white-blue appearance of the torn anterior capsule), which can then easily wrap around the equator, jeopardizing the posterior capsule and the stability of the lens. Options to avoid this predicament include minimizing external pressure on the eye from the lid speculum and excessive anesthetic volume, use of a highly cohesive viscoelastic to maintain a deep AC, and initially creating a very small and controlled opening in the central anterior capsule and slowly aspirating the milky lens material, thereby decompressing the capsular bag. Others have recommended using the phaco tip in a bevel-down position to open the intact anterior capsule and then immediately aspirate lens material. In some of these cases a second opening and tear in the opposite direction may become necessary, or conversion to a can-open style opening will be needed.

For a capsulorrhexis in the case of a brunescent cataract, again capsular staining may be necessary to optimize visualization, and proper use of viscoelastic(s) is of key importance for maintenance of a deep AC. One should be familiar with the varying physical characteristics of dispersive (coating and barrier formation) versus cohesive (space maintenance) agents. The brunescent lens is typically very large with a convex anterior curvature. If the tear begins to veer peripherally, pulling back centrally utilizing a stretching force as described by Brian Little can be very helpful.[12] Phacoemulsification times in these cases can be lengthy, and attention should be directed toward extra protection of the corneal endothelium. Many surgeons find that

Arshinoff's soft-shell technique is particularly helpful in this setting wherein a highly dispersive viscoelastic is placed to protect the corneal endothelium, and a more cohesive material is placed below to maintain space (see Chapter 33).[13,14] Although some surgeons prefer to make a smaller than average rhexis in such cases to help prevent peripheral extension, it is my preference to err on the larger side to aid in subsequent nucleus removal.

Mature lenses are typically loose within the capsular bag. However, hydrodissection should not be ignored. It is performed gently and slowly as zonular and capsular strength is often compromised.

Because of the extreme mass and density of these lenses, central debulking is commonly needed. Creating a preliminary groove or sculpting a central crater will weaken the core of the nucleus, making subsequent cracking or chopping easier and safer on the capsule and zonule. When sculpting, adequate phaco power should be used such that the lens does not chatter and is not pushed about. This can be aided by utilizing a more highly beveled or Kelman-style angulated phaco needle. Continuous phaco power rather than pulse or burst mode may be preferred for efficient sculpting, along with lower flow and vacuum, though one must have enough infusion and aspiration present to avoid the possibility of thermal damage to the wound during this step.

The lens is debulked as far posteriorly as possible. Breaking through the posterior nuclear plate and visualizing the red reflex under high magnification facilitates creation of additional division planes.

At this point, one can choose to commence cracking or chopping. I find, as with most cases, that a combination of both vertical and horizontal chop is most efficient, with the initial divisional planes created with vertical forces, followed by sequential segmentation performed with horizontal chop maneuvers. For nuclear segment removal, one may need to increase vacuum, decrease phaco power, and switch to a pulse or burst mode. The greater the nuclear density, the greater the number of segments that are created as smaller, more bite-sized pieces that can be more efficiently phaco-aspirated. Even more importantly than with routine cases, with each successive division plane, one must confirm separation through the dense posterior nuclear plate and be able to visualize the red reflex. It is remarkable how resistant the leathery posterior nuclear fibers may be. During these final nuclear removal steps, one may wish to place additional viscoelastic posteriorly to act as a "pseudo-epinucleus" to protect the capsule, and anteriorly to prevent damage to the endothelium from mobile nuclear particles.

Cortical removal is typically straightforward in these cases except that dense, adherent posterior plaques or pearls are often encountered. Because of weak zonules and a generally floppy posterior capsule, it may be necessary to temper aggressive maneuvers, and consideration should be given to placing an endocapsular tension ring. For similar reasons, the implant should be carefully chosen because of the increased tendency for capsular fibrosis and shrinkage due to weakened zonules.

Zonular Dialysis

Zonular weakness or dialysis (see Chapters 25 and 26) remains one of the more challenging situations confronted by today's cataract surgeon. In years past, phacoemulsification was often considered to be contraindicated in this setting, and surgeons opted (and referred) for a pars plana lensectomy approach, or even considered intracapsular techniques. Today, with improvements in instrumentation and equipment, along with refinements in surgical technique, most cases involving compromised zonules may be safely managed by phacoemulsification. However, these challenging cases require several important modifications in technique.

Although seemingly awkward, incision placement may be best located 180 degrees away from the area of dialysis. This reduces intraoperative stress to the area of the weakened zonules. Otherwise, the to-and-fro motion that occurs with the phaco instrument will cause further damage to the already weakened zonular capsular attachments.

Immediately following creation of the paracentesis, a dispersive viscoelastic is placed within the AC and over the area of zonular weakness and exposed hyaloid face. Hypotony is to be avoided. A small amount of presenting vitreous may be buttressed by the viscoelastic, avoiding an immediate vitrectomy. If significant vitreous is present anterior to the plane of the lens capsule, then a closed compartment, two-port vitrectomy should be performed, preferably through the pars plana. Following stabilization of the vitreous face, the AC is filled further with a more viscous cohesive agent, to take advantage of the characteristic space maintenance and optical clarity.

The capsulorrhexis is then begun with an initial tear directed toward the area of weakened zonules, thus avoiding further disinsertion at this early stage of the operation. Gentle, slow tearing of the capsule is then performed, possibly aided by the use of intraocular scissors. In cases of severe laxity, capsular hooks should be placed once the initial capsulotomy is created. The number and location of the stabilizing hooks is determined by the location and severity of the zonular defect. Many surgeons prefer to create a "mini-capsulorrhexis" to prevent extension of the tear and reduce infusion-related turbulence; however, with generous use of viscoelastic, chamber stability can be maximized and it is my preference to opt for a standard or even large capsulorrhexis, thus facilitating lens removal. Gentle but very thorough hydrodissection is then performed.

The use of endocapsular tension rings (ECRs) and segments has revolutionized the efficacy and safety of these cases. Each patient's anatomy is unique and will dictate what type and the number of devices that should be utilized. In general, one should opt to place the supporting element no sooner than is necessary, as it can interfere with subsequent lens removal, but to do so as soon as it is needed to prevent further zonular loss and lens dislocation. The degree of zonular laxity encountered intraoperatively is typically greater than that which is anticipated based on the preoperative exam (which must include careful gonioscopy). One should also be mindful of the type of zonular pathology that is present. For example, is it likely to be of a stable nature (traumatic) or more likely to be progressive (Marfan's syndrome) and thereby require more extensive long-term support? Cionni and Ahmed devices that have eyelets for suturing are much more likely to provide better long-term stability in advanced cases.

Phacoemulsification should be performed slowly, avoiding excess turbulence and maneuvering. Modern phaco instrumentation with enhanced fluidics is essential in these cases. One must be extremely careful carrying out rotational maneuvers, watching closely for imparted stress to the zonules. Nonrotational techniques (Fine's chip-and-flip, Gimbel's phaco sweep, etc.) may be preferable. Softer lenses may be completely hydro- or visco-maneuvered out of the capsule and into the AC, avoiding further capsule manipulation and possible extension of the dialysis; however, collapse of the bag must be avoided through the use of endocapsular support elements, or vitreous prolapse will undoubtedly ensue.

Removal of cortex is best performed in a manual or at least automated bimanual fashion utilizing low vacuum settings. I have found cortical viscodissection to be very helpful, followed by manual stripping of cortical fibers out of the capsular fornix using an angled cannula placed through side-port incisions as described above. Again, endocapsular support devices and capsular hooks are indispensable in this setting.

The choice of IOL in this setting is important. Silicone should likely be avoided within the capsular bag as increased capsular fibrosis and shrinkage is anticipated. Larger and more robust acrylic IOLs are typically preferred, and one must be circumspect when considering the use of a toric lens based on the need for intraoperative (and possibly postoperative) lens dialing and positioning, as well as long-term capsular stability issues. Implantation off multifocal lens technology should probably be avoided or reserved for only the mildest of cases along with the use of an ECR.

Conclusion

Modern microincision phaco and implant surgery is capable of achieving unprecedented results and has changed the lives of countless cataract patients. The safety and efficacy of the procedure, however, remains contingent on the surgeon's level of preparation and attention to detail. Though complications are becoming increasingly rare with contemporary surgery, management techniques are still very important. By employing proper techniques and technology, surgeons will find that the vast majority of these challenging situations result in outcomes that rival or are even indistinguishable from that of routine cases.

References

1. Ernest PH, Lavery KT, Kiessling LA. Relative strength of scleral corneal and clear corneal incisions constructed in cadaver eyes. J Cataract Refract Surg 1994;20:626–629.

2. Ernest PH, FenzlR, Lavery KT, Sensoli A. Relative stability of clear corneal incisions in a cadaver eye model. J Cataract Refract Surg 1995;21:39–42

3. Ernest PH, Tipperman R, Eagle R et al. Is there a difference in incision healing based on location? J Cataract Refract Surg 1998;24:482–486

4. Mamalis N. Incision width after phacoemulsification with foldable intraocular lens implantation J Cataract Refract Surg 2000;26:237–241

5. Fine IH. Special Report to ASCRS Members: Phacoemulsification Incision Burns. Letter to American Society of Cataract and Refractive Surgery Members, 1997

6. Nagahara K, Phaco Chop Video, ASCRS Film Festival, May 1993, Seattle, Washington.

7. Gimbel HV, Neuhann T. Divide and conquer nucleofractis phacoemulsification-developmaent and variations. J Cataract Refract Surg 1991;17: 281–291

8. Vasavada AR, Desai JP: Stop, chop, chop and stuff. J Cataract Refract Surg 1996;22:526–529

9. Vasavada AR, Singh R; Step by Step chip in situ and separation of a very dense cataract. J Cataract Refract Surg 1998;24:156–159

10. Michelson MA. Use of a Sheets' glide as a pseudo posterior capsule in phacoemulsification complicated by posterior capsule rupture. Eur J Implant Surg 1993;570–572.

11. Arbisser LB, Charles S, Howcroft M Werner L. Management of vitreous loss and dropped nucleus during cataract surgery. Ophthalmol Clin North Am 2006;19(4):495–506 Review.

12. Little Brian C., Jennifer H. Smith, MD, Mark Packer, MD Capsulorhexis tear-out rescue J Cataract Refract Surg 2006; 32:1420–1422 Q 2006 ASCRS and ESCRS

13. Arshinoff Steve A. Dispersive-cohesive viscoelastic soft shell technique. J. Cataract Refract Surg 1999;25(2):167–173

14. Arshinoff Steve A. Using BSS with viscoadaptives in the ultimate soft-shell technique. J Cataract Refract Surg 2002;28(9):1509–1514

55 Divide-and-Conquer Technique

James A. Davison

This chapter discusses prevention of clinically significant complications during the divide-and-conquer phacoemulsification technique through excellent preparation, disciplined routine, and early recognition of aberrant situations accompanied by strategies to resolve them.

Review of the Patient's Record

Patients and families are normally somewhat anxious in the preoperative area. Review their personal information before you see them and then extend a warm greeting and a friendly smile. Patients need to feel that you recall their office visit and examination as if it were just yesterday, and that you remember them and know them, and that sufficient medication will be administered in the operating room to make them feel relaxed and comfortable and that everything will be fine.

Review of their clinical examination is important. Specifically we need to remind ourselves about previous eye surgery or trauma and anatomic details including the Lens Opacity Classification System (LOCS III) cataract rating, the presence or absence of pseudoexfoliation (PXF), and the dilated pupil size achieved in clinic. We need to verify which eye we are treating, what the refractive goal is, and which intraocular lens (IOL) we are implanting, along with any special needs, such as anticipated difficult positioning because of previous neck surgery.

Preparation in the Operating Room

Your machine settings should be confirmed (**Fig. 55.1**), and the microscope should be adjusted to your preference. The staff should review the record, confirm the patient's identity, verify the eye to be operated, and review any special anticipated requirements.

The patient should be placed on the surgical bed so that he or she is comfortable and so that the face is oriented toward the ceiling with the brow and cheek bone at the same height to give symmetrical access to the globe without impingement from those boney structures. I like turning the patient's head toward

me slightly. The patient's forehead should be taped to the bed (**Fig. 55.2**).

Relaxing medication is given while the prepping and draping occur. When you enter the room and sit down, make sure that the bed is adjusted so that the face is oriented properly and you have the same amount of sclera showing above and below, that is, a neutral position (**Fig. 55.3**). Make sure that the wrist rest does not impede your movement or positioning. Make sure that the eye is the right height for you and matches the patient eye level (PEL) setting on the machine, and that there is room for your legs and feet on the pedals. This is your final opportunity to create an optimized playing field for the surgical event. You can make adjustments during surgery if absolutely necessary but force yourself to try to make it perfect before you start. Make sure the microscope is in neutral position and angled properly for you. Turn off the overhead fluorescent lights to eliminate their reflection, enabling you to minimize the amount of light you need to use, which reduces the risk of light toxicity and creates maximum patient comfort and cooperation. Start with low light and ask the patient to look at it. Get an idea of the red reflex and adjust the blend of the microscope light so that the mix is what will be desired for the continuous curvilinear capsulorrhexis (CCC) portion of the procedure, usually about two thirds to three fourths of the total from the zero-degree source and one third to one fourth from the 6-degree source, depending on the microscope being used. More dense cataracts or highly pigmented *retinal pigment epithelium* (RPE) will yield less red reflex from zero-degree light and may require more 6-degree light during CCC and phacoemulsification as well. Different phases of surgery yield different red reflex illumination, and the ratio can be adjusted during the procedure to optimize the detailed view. Give the patient time to become adjusted to the light and to become comfortable. Ask the patient if he or she feels sufficiently relaxed and ready to proceed, or if more medication is needed for the patient to feel adequately relaxed. Do this as you drizzle more preservative-free lidocaine 1% to test sensation and relaxation and to further anesthetize. With the patient's confirmation that he or she is adequately relaxed and comfortable, verify that you have adequate light and that the patient's eye has steady fixation. If so, you are now ready to start surgery.

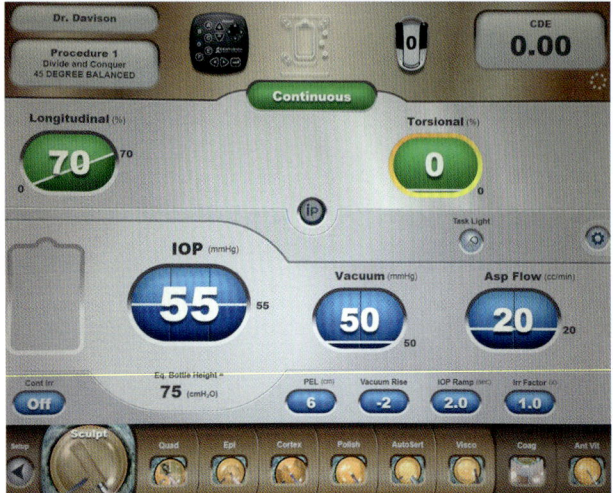

a

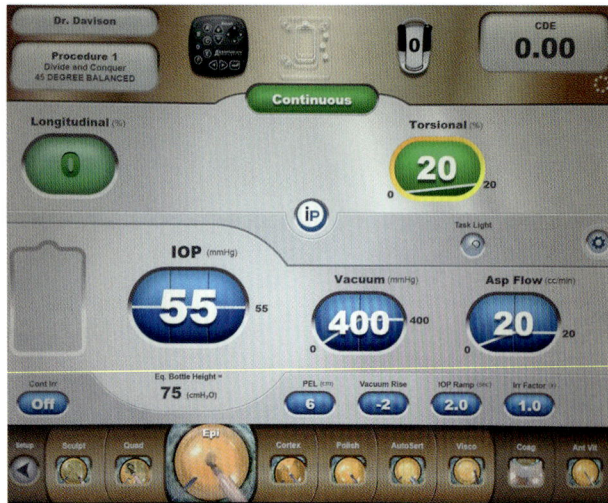

b

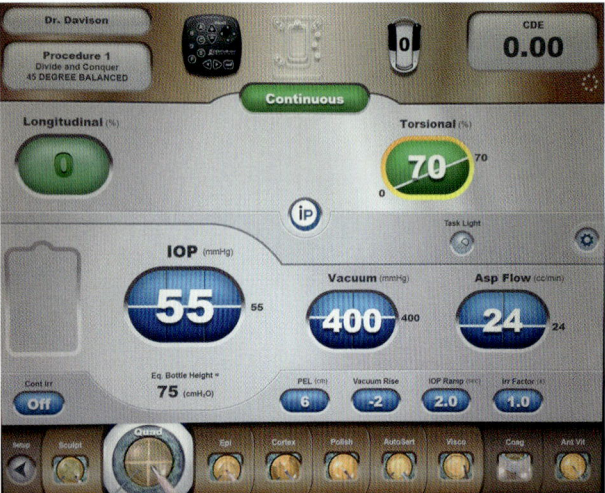

c

Fig. 55.1 Centurion (Alcon, Fort Worth, TX) phacoemulsification settings for **(a)** Sculpt, **(b)** Epinucleus, and **(c)** Quadrant Removal. Longitudinal and torsional tip movement maximums are set at 70%.

Surgical Procedure

It is best to engage in a circular one-way traffic pattern with your technician. I receive new instruments from the right and pass off the used ones to the left. Blades are always passed and released handle first. Your arms and hands should be in comfortable natural positions while holding the 2.4-mm keratome and 22.5-degree paracentesis blade. For me, the target for each is the slightly vascularized corneal limbus. My primary incision usually ends up being ~ 10 degrees above midline in right eyes and 17 degrees above midline in left eyes. Penetrate with the paracentesis blade first. Aim toward the lens's central anterior surface. The 22.5-degree blade creates a larger external opening that accommodates full movement without oar locking while creating a smaller internal opening that accommodates the lens manipulator and that seals easily. After reaching proper depth, use the top back of that blade to slightly pull toward and upward to stabilize the eye as you enter with the keratome. It is important not to waver on the way in or out with the keratome so the incision does not become enlarged (**Figs. 55.4, 55.5, 55.6**). Subtle angulation adjustments of the blade handle can help create limbal symmetric, parallel external and internal incisions as the blade is slowly driven forward. The shelf length is usually ~ 1.75 mm, perhaps slightly longer in high myopes so overinflation is not necessary during stromal hydration and pressurization at the end of surgery. The external incision seems to be less irritating that one made in clear cornea. Also, the incision is cosmetically desirable in that the external entry eventually is invisible and the internal entry is very peripheral and not immediately noticeable.

The blades should not be removed from their packaging until you are ready to use them. The keratome blade may become dull if it rolls over even once on the Mayo stand. Get a new blade if either one seems dull at the initiation of the incision. Incision perfection is very important. A dull blade can create irregularities in the superficial stromal entry and deep exit into the anterior chamber. And there is nothing worse than a dull blade bursting through the cornea (usually too central), hitting the lens, and then being withdrawn in an uncontrolled fashion. The inadvertently extended incision with longer shelf length will make all subsequent maneuvers and infusion balance difficult. There would likely be corneal distortion during phaco from the depressed midperipheral cornea, making visibility poor, and the additional trauma will result in early pupillary miosis as well. The lens penetration will need to be included central to the CCC border. This is not a good way to start a case.

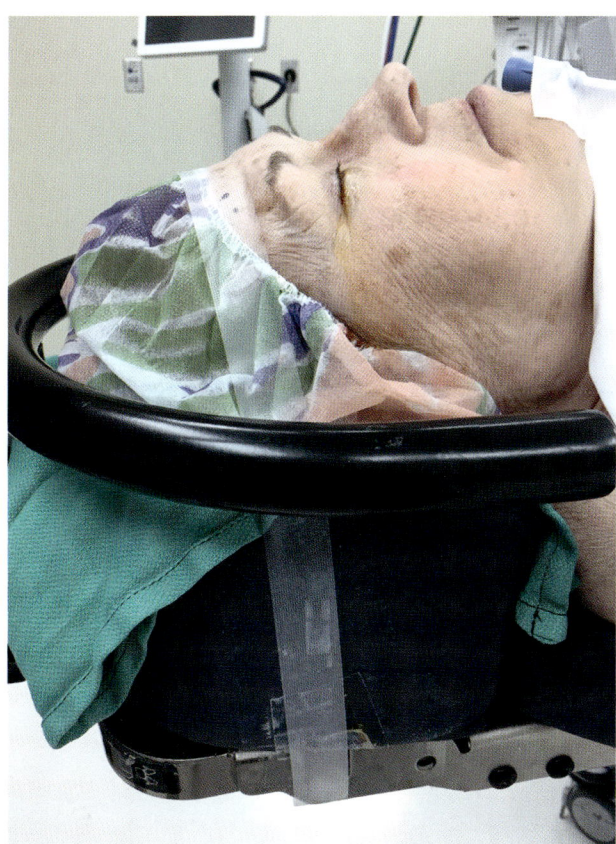

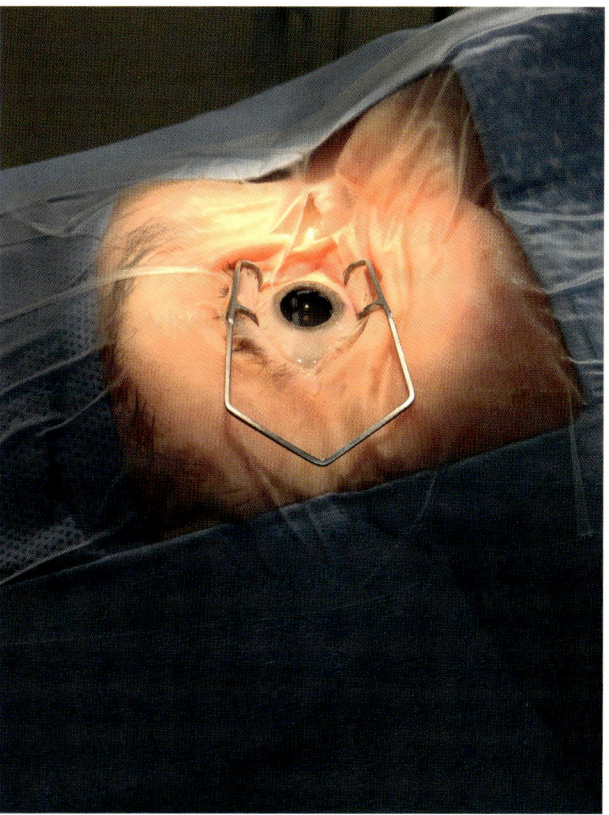

Fig. 55.2 The bed, the articulated headrest, and the foam headrest have all been adjusted so that the patient is comfortable and so that the cheek-bone and forehead are at the same height. The patients' head is turned slightly toward the surgeon. Tape goes all the way around the head and headrest and its adhesive applied to the forehead and cap. The wrist rest is at about the height of the front of the patient's ear.

Fig. 55.3 A similar amount of sclera is visible superior and inferior. This neutral position is easy for the patient to maintain and it facilitates access for instruments. The opaque drape aligns with the bridge of the nose and leaves a generous portion of skin for the plastic drape to stick to without tissue bunching or globe compression. Painting the eyebrow using a Weck Cell Sponge saturated with BSS helps prevent hair loss when the drape is removed.

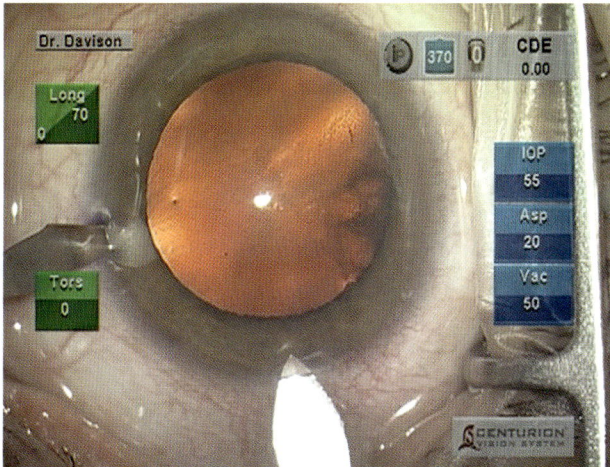

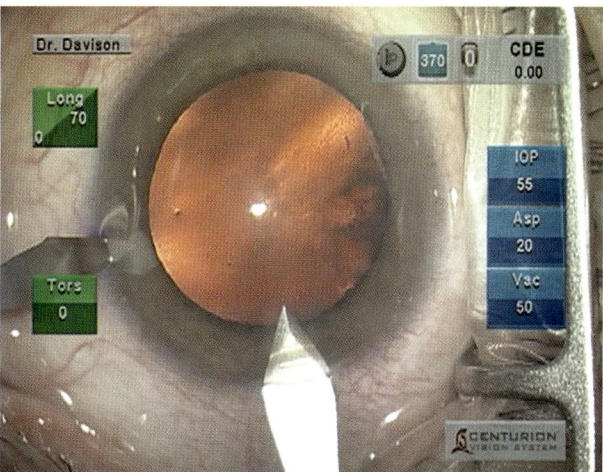

Fig. 55.4 The 22.5-degree paracentesis blade has penetrated the limbal cornea and is being drawn upward and toward the surgeon slightly to stabilize the globe as the 2.4-mm keratome is being driven into the slightly vascularized limbal cornea.

Fig. 55.5 The Descemet's level entry is slightly imperfect as it is not quite parallel to the external entry. The etched mark on the keratome is 2.0 mm from the tip, so the incision shelf length extends for ~ 1.75 mm.

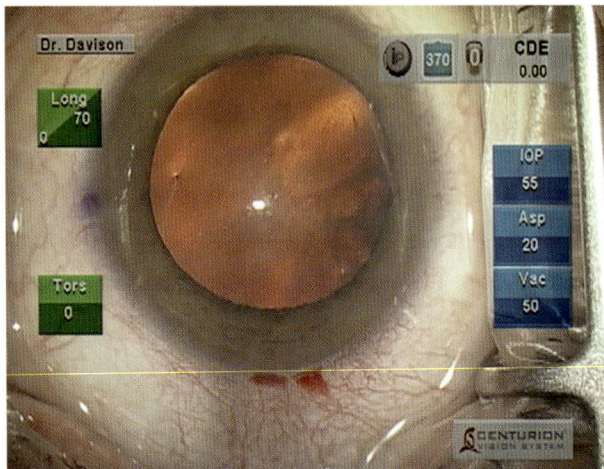

Fig. 55.6 The desired light bleeding from the limbal vessels is seen as well as the almost parallel internal entry.

If four-cut or eight-cut radial keratotomy incisions are present, carefully go between them. If 16-cut or more incisions are present, perform a small fornix-based flap and use a more scleral incision. Also, if you prefer to use manual blade–created incisions when using the femtosecond laser as I do, be careful to identify and avoid the transverse arcuate incisions made by the laser for astigmatism reduction.

In my technique, preservative-free lidocaine 1% is injected slowly through a 30-gauge cannula, a little inside and then over the globe's surface with several repeats so it does not cause pain as it affects the iris. Then fill one third to one half of the anterior chamber with Viscoat (Alcon, Fort Worth, TX), and then finish filling with Provisc (Alcon) underneath until some of it just starts to egress from the incision. This egress is not usually necessary especially in high myopes where the lens will just be pushed far posterior. You just get a feeling when the chamber ii full and egress is about to happen. This pressure creates a flat anterior capsular surface, which is the best configuration for capsulorrhexis.

For a 6.0-mm-diameter optic, a 5.0-mm-diameter capsulorrhexis is accomplished with a cystotome starting in the center and spiraling left and peripherally. The final radius will be set as

the CCC is nearing the surgeon on the left side, thereby ensuring an accurate radius and a start/finish junction that will be in the proximal half, that is, not located in the distal half, where most of the surgical maneuvering will be (**Figs. 55.7** and **55.8**). A 4.6-mm diameter is better at preventing postoperative rotation or toric IOLs in high myopes, especially when receiving vertically oriented toric IOLs that can rotate off axis after surgery. This diameter can be better ensured by using an electronic overlay or femtosecond laser.

Hydrodissection is accomplished using a Chang cannula, usually with one injection of balanced salt solution (BSS) near the surgeon to the right. Lift the anterior capsular edge slightly during injection. If the usual fluid wave is not apparent, try the same maneuver on the left side. After hydrodissection, I embed the Chang cannula tip into the left side of the midperipheral lens and dislodge the nucleus attachments with a gentle downward and rotational motion. I then do the same on the right side (**Figs. 55.9** and **55.10**). I can see the nucleus slowly separating from the cortex. I want the dissection plane to be between the epinucleus and cortex (hydrodissection), not between the nucleus and epinucleus (hydrodelineation). When done, the nucleus and epinucleus, as an uninterrupted unit, should be easily turned by the embedded Chang cannula within the cortex and capsule. If hydrodelineation has occurred, rotation becomes more difficult, especially in soft lenses. If good symmetrical dissection planes cannot be created, then one quadrant can be isolated through two grooves and fractures and then removed; movement of the remaining quadrants should be easier even with disjunctive planes.

The sleeve position on the phaco tip is confirmed. There should be enough tip extended so that nuclear material will not be pushed away by the sleeve edge as the material is aspirated. The infusion openings should be 90 degrees from the tip's bevel.

Phacoemulsification

To perform my usual micro-coaxial phacoemulsification, I use a 45-degree balanced tip with the ultra-sleeve and a specially modified cyclodialysis spatula. I use the shorter end of a 0.5-mm spatula that has been custom thinned to 0.35 mm, because the standard 0.25 mm is too thin and penetrates the nucleus too easily, making it difficult to push the surface, whereas the 0.5 mm is too thick and awkward and requires too large an incision. Its

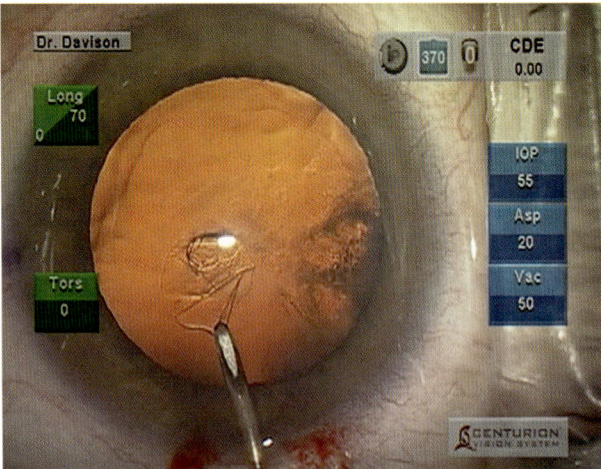

Fig. 55.7 The cystotome initially penetrates the center of the lens. It is then swept to the left and toward the surgeon, achieving the final desired radius in the proximal left quadrant.

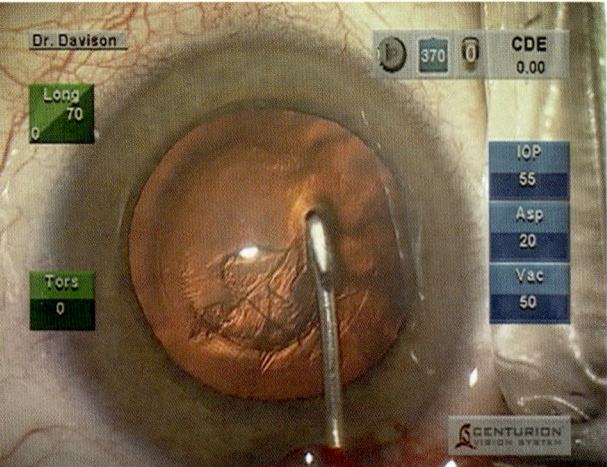

Fig. 55.8 The continuous curvilinear capsulorrhexis (CCC) is completed by guiding the capsule tear through the origination of the initial radius. Continue to draw it through to make sure that the tear is complete. Usually the junction of the origination and finishing point is not visible.

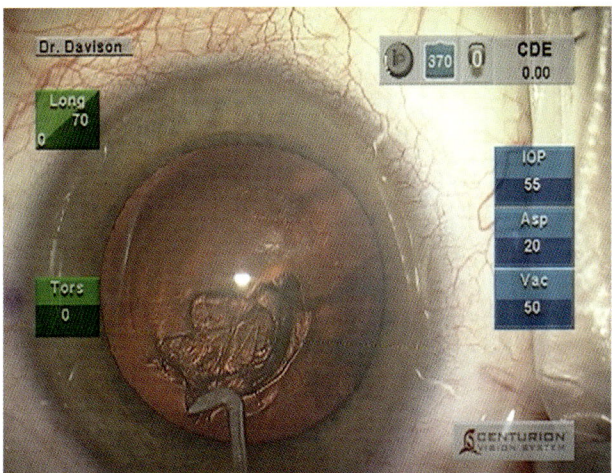

Fig. 55.9 The Chang cannula is pulling up slightly against the anterior capsular rim.

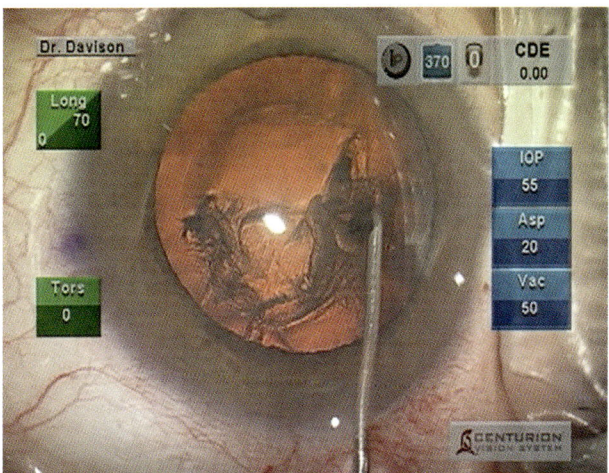

Fig. 55.10 The Chang cannula is penetrating into the lens on the right side after already penetrating on the left. In both positions it is being used to push down slightly and rotate the lens so that nucleus–cortex adhesion will be slowly and gradually disrupted. The nucleus will then rotate easily within the cortical pillow.

single-piece construction can withstand inadvertent contact with an active phacoemulsification tip, and its shape is ideal for manipulation and quick insertion and withdrawal through the incision.

The infusion is turned off as the cyclodialysis spatula protects the internal aspect of the incision as the tip enters the eye. The phaco tip traumatizes least when it enters slightly sideways (**Fig. 55.11**). The infusion is usually turned on as the tip enters the anterior chamber but it can be turned on before or after entry, depending on the situation and anatomy.

The machine is placed on the Sculpt setting. Continuous longitudinal tip movement is used to aspirate the anterior capsule and shave away a superficial layer of the nucleus. Before shaving, this layer is difficult to see through because of the irregularity created by the two penetrations of the Chang cannula. With better clarity, deeper nuclear detail can then be appreciated as lens dissection progresses (**Fig. 55.12**). With each quarter turn while creating nuclear quadrants, we create a kind of "spiral" deepening pattern as sculpting shaves through progressively deeper surface levels. An adequate final depth can be reached sometimes in three, but usually five, quarter rotations, but maybe more in very

hard cataracts. We try to sculpt symmetrical grooves and thus create symmetrical remaining quadrants. It is important to continually adjust the microscope's focus as sculpting continues. It is important to maintain a sharp view of the cutting edge of the phaco tip as it encounters the surfaces of the posterior nuclear plate. It takes a total of about 50 microscope pedal adjustments to accomplish an average cataract-IOL surgery.

Grooving starts at the surface and descends to about one-half depth becoming about two tips wide depending on lens hardness (thinner grooves with softer lenses). The initial groove length extends through about half of the distal hemisphere and one third of the proximal. The nucleus is rotated, and a similar process occurs in the newly presented proximal and distal hemispheres, only this time we can go deeper and more peripheral. The groove in the distal half is deep enough when it reaches about a three-fourths depth. The proximal needs to be deepened concurrently to accommodate the needle's shaft to slide through, but care must be taken not to insult the proximal CCC border in

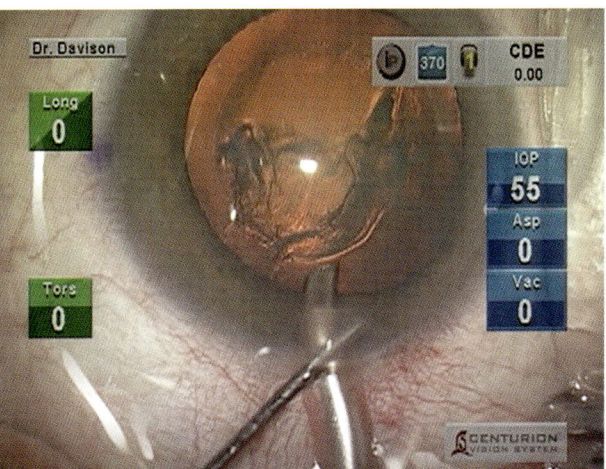

Fig. 55.11 To protect the Descemet's membrane attachment at the incision edge, the cyclodialysis spatula is lifting the anterior cornea away from the entering phacoemulsification tip.

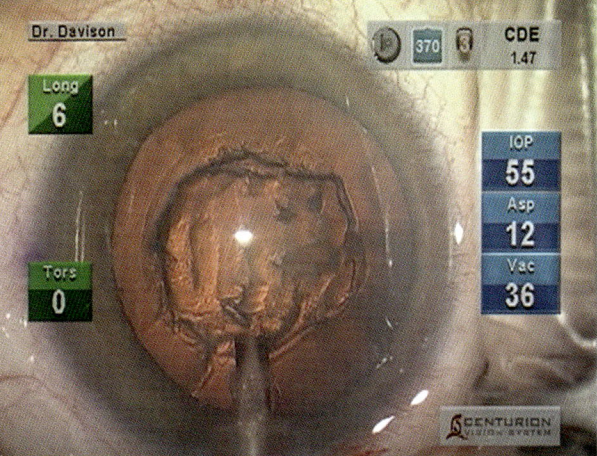

Fig. 55.12 Removal of the penetration irregularities created by the Chang cannula has been accomplished by anterior surface sculpting and removal of anterior cortex. An even surface provides a clear view of the deeper lens.

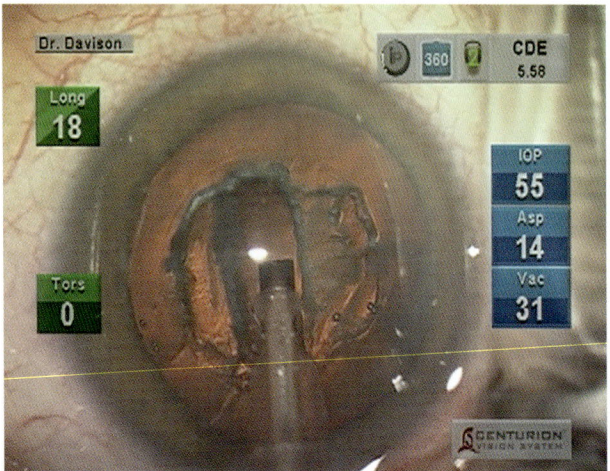

Fig. 55.13 An initial groove has been sculpted to about one-half depth.

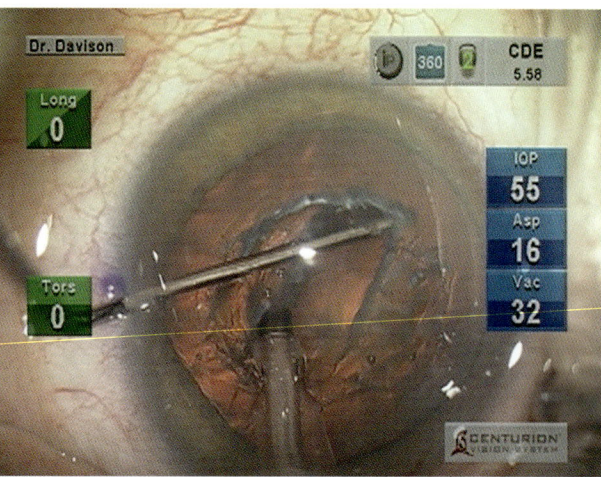

Fig. 55.14 Bimanual rotation is quick and minimizes zonular stress.

the process. The nucleus is quarter turned and the sequence repeated to three-fourths depth once again. One more quarter turn and that usually completes the deep grooving. For the deeper grooving phase, I find that I always orient the tip obliquely with the tip aperture away from my left shoulder so that I get the best three-dimensional view of the edge of the tip and its aperture and the posterior nuclear plate, which is being approached as well as the portion of the plate that has just been thinned. The spiral down process of creating progressively deeper more peripheral grooves has now been completed (**Figs. 55.13, 55.14, 55.15, 55.16**).

Fracture of the posterior plate and separation of the quadrants can now be accomplished from the outside toward the center with a cross-hand motion (**Figs. 55.17** and **55.18**). If the center does not tear through and separate, good visualization with an obliquely oriented 45-degree tip enables even deeper central nucleus thinning. (We think that we sculpt almost to the posterior capsule sometimes but we really never get thinner than 500 μm, as can be demonstrated when sculpting a lens that has been dissected to that level with the femtosecond laser chop cyl-

inder pattern. We hardly ever penetrate that preset laser dissection level.)

In virtually all lenses, I then turn the tip 90 degrees for a different oblique position, with the tip aperture toward my left shoulder, and I shave away the interior corners of the nuclear quadrants, creating a generous bowl composed of four relatively thin two-dimensional plates (**Figs. 55.19** and **55.20**). The large resulting space enables quadrant removal to occur mostly behind the iris plane in the confines of the capsular bag, well away from the corneal endothelium. When using the femtosecond laser, I like to create a pattern that is similar to that created by hand, that is, a four-quadrant chop. This yields the same quadrant dimensions that are easily manipulated and emulsified just like the manual cases.

The machine is now placed on the Quadrant Removal setting. Higher vacuum and aspiration flow rates will withdraw nuclear material into the tip while it is in a central position within the nuclear bowl. The continuous torsional movement with intermittent injected longitudinal (Intelligent Phaco [IP]: 10-ms longitudinal pulse duration, 95% vacuum threshold, 1.0 longitu-

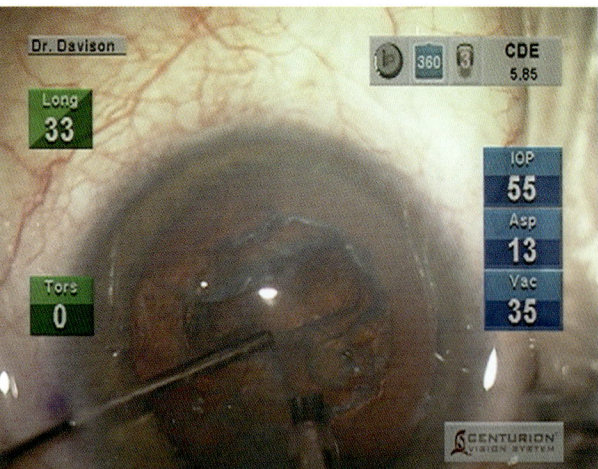

Fig. 55.15 The proximal groove is being sculpted. The cyclodialysis spatula holds the lens in place to create four equal quadrants and helps reduce zonular stress.

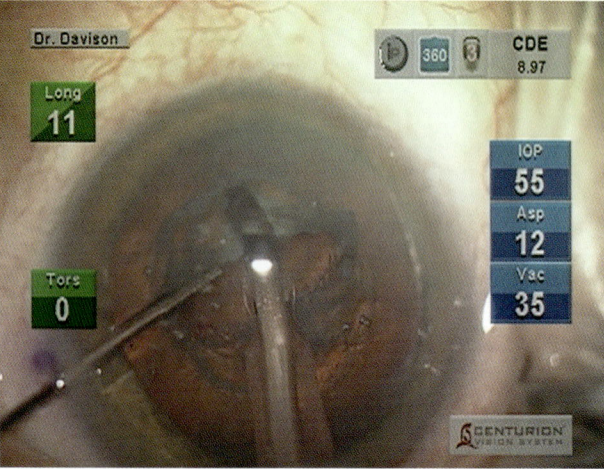

Fig. 55.16 The shaft of the tip slides within the proximal groove, enabling it to cut deeper into the distal half. The balanced tip is turned obliquely with the aperture away from the surgeon's left shoulder to maximize visibility of its leading edge against the deeper nuclear surface.

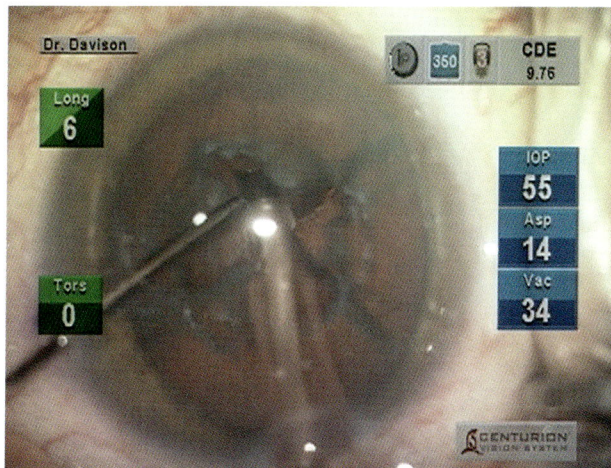

Fig. 55.17 Deep sculpting has been completed. The instruments are poised to initiate the first posterior and peripheral nuclear crack. The tip is turned slightly obliquely with the aperture away from the surgeon.

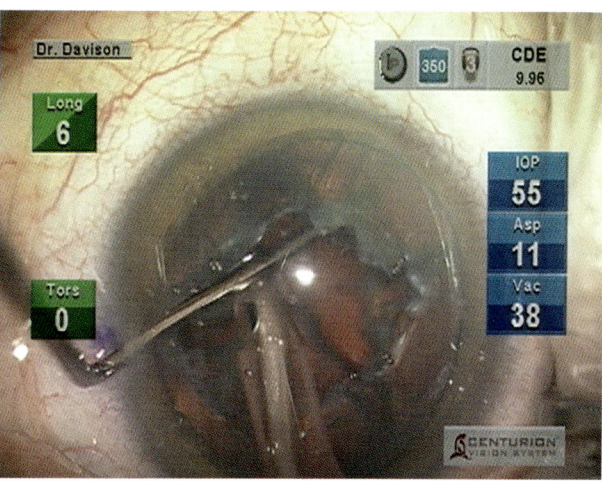

Fig. 55.18 The crack is propagated from peripheral to central by a cross-hand action of the tip and cyclodialysis spatula against the deep quadrant walls.

dinal/torsional ratio) keeps material on the tip for efficient removal. But for extremely hard lenses, the longitudinal tip motion may still be more efficient. I always try IP first, but if it seems that it is taking too long, I switch over to longitudinal. For extremely hard lenses, I even may have to bimanually "smash" material into the tip's aperture with the cyclodialysis spatula as emulsification continues.

I like to orient the tip obliquely, with the tip aperture toward my left shoulder, to engage the left corner of the distal first quadrant (quadrant 1) to be removed. With that tip aperture-corner orientation, an inadvertent pop through of the tip occurs to an open space rather than to the peripheral cortex and posterior capsule, which could happen if the quadrant were to be grasped at the center or right edge. I push the adjacent left quadrant (quadrant 2) edge away with the cyclodialysis spatula to create an open space (kind of like holding the door open for quadrant 1), which facilitates the centralizing motion of the tip as it acts on the adherent left nuclear edge of quadrant 1. The creation of adherence with vacuum is virtually simultaneous and continuous

throughout the centralizing motion. It happens very quickly, within a fraction of a second. We switch the machine to the Epinucleus setting if it happens too quickly. (See later discussion of soft cataract.) This "unlocks the puzzle," and the right edge of quadrant 1 follows centrally, and the whole thing is removed within the confines of the capsular bag. Clockwise rotations expose the second and third quadrants, which are drawn centrally as well. They come central very easily, so the tip can bond to the right edge of the quadrant. For removal of the first three quadrants, the remaining underlying nuclear plates form a protective but progressively narrower bench on which to support the quadrant that is being removed and to protect the posterior capsule. The last quadrant is always held higher within the iris plane to protect the posterior capsule from inadvertent aspiration (**Figs. 55.21, 55.22, 55.23, 55.24, 55.25, 55.26**). In very firm lenses, additional Viscoat can be injected (leave the phaco tip in but turn off the infusion during Viscoat injection) at any point in the procedure to push the posterior capsule back and protect the cornea, especially before aspiration of the last quadrant.

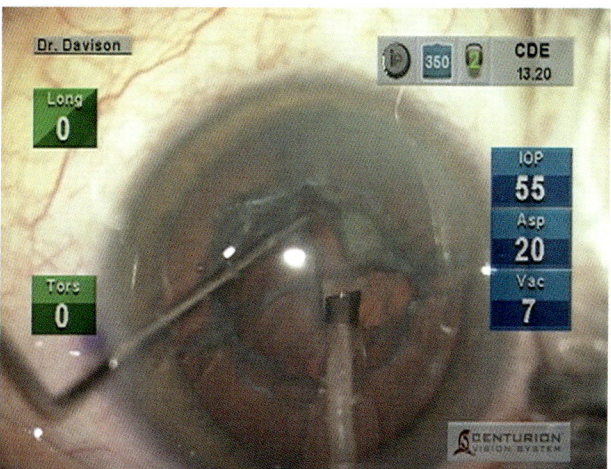

Fig. 55.19 Three of the internal corners have been shaved away as the tip approaches the fourth.

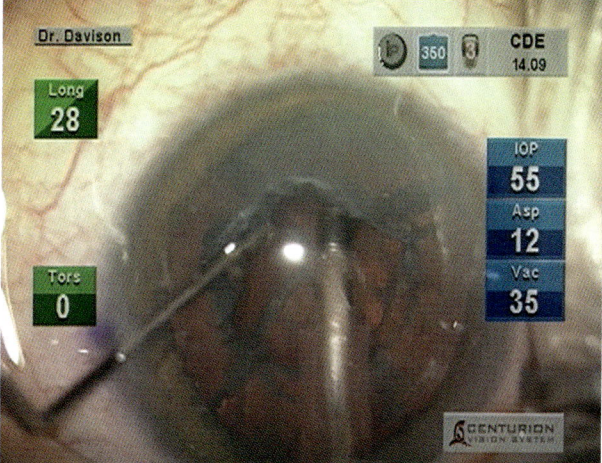

Fig. 55.20 The obliquely oriented tip with the aperture toward the surgeon is shaving away the last corner projection.

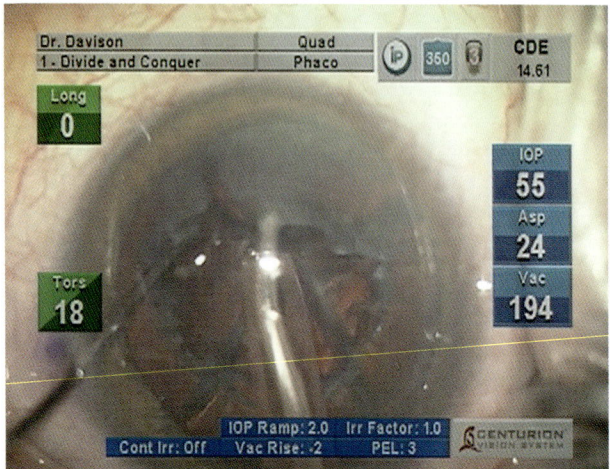

Fig. 55.21 In the first phase of the Quadrant Removal setting, the cyclodialysis spatula is pushing back the right edge of quadrant 2 (Q2) so the phacoemulsification tip burrow into, adhere to, and draw central the left edge of quadrant 1 (Q1).

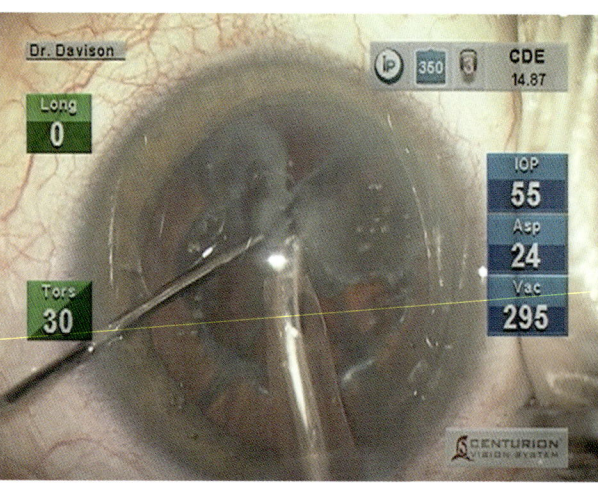

Fig. 55.22 Q1 has been partially centralized and is being emulsified within the nuclear bowl well away from the cornea. Torsional tip movement and high vacuum can be safely applied for efficient removal of nuclear substance in this central location.

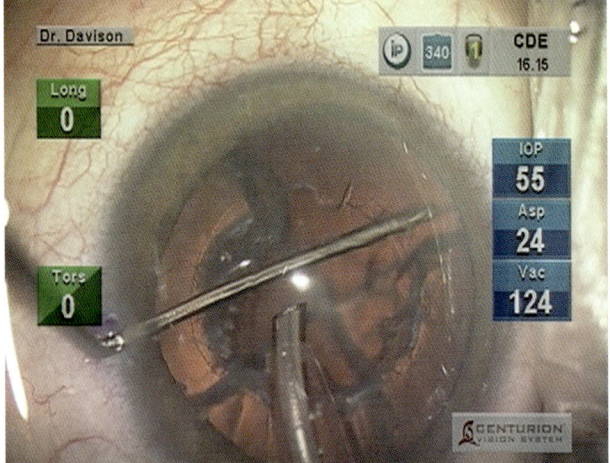

Fig. 55.23 Q1 has been removed. The cyclodialysis spatula will push against the left edge of quadrant 4 (Q4) to rotate Q2 into position for removal.

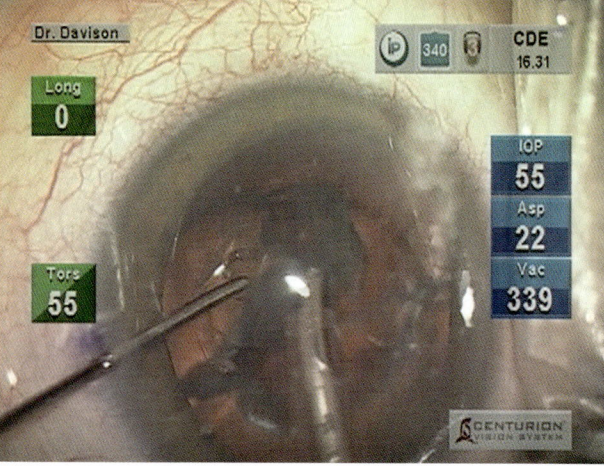

Fig. 55.24 Q2 has been mostly removed in its centralized position within the nuclear bowl.

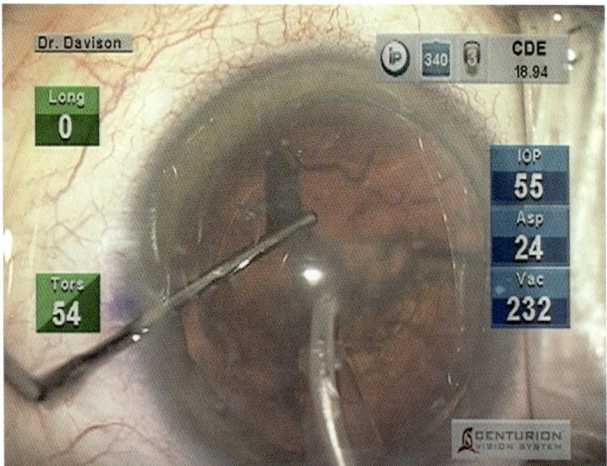

Fig. 55.25 Quadrant 3 (Q3) is being removed centrally. Q4 is providing the last "work bench" buffer to help stabilize Q3 and protect the posterior capsule.

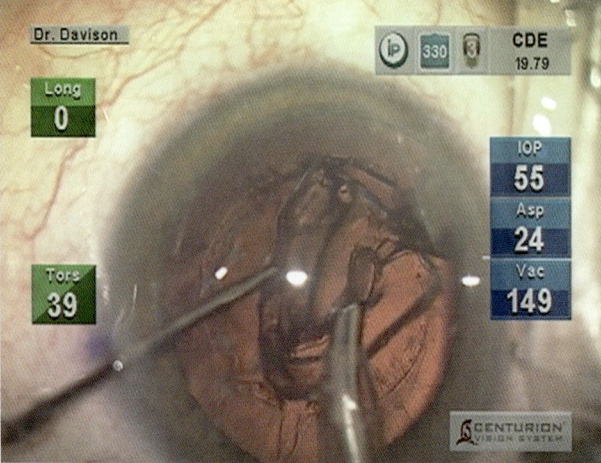

Fig. 55.26 Q4 is stabilized by the spatula as it is guided into the tip aperture. The latter part of this process usually occurs at a more anterior level within the iris plane or anterior chamber.

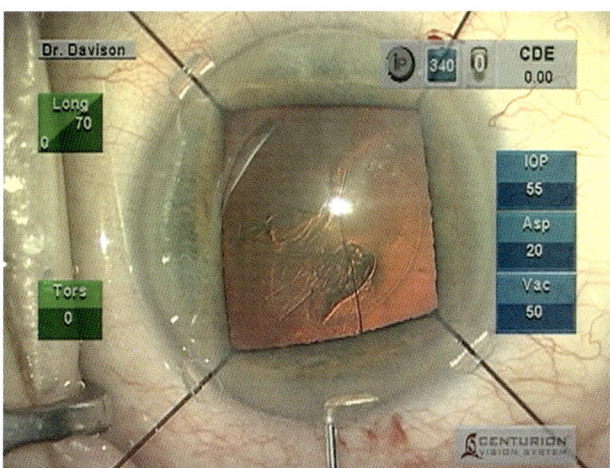

Fig. 55.27 As the Chang cannula enters the incision, the tension on the iris is the same for all four retractors.

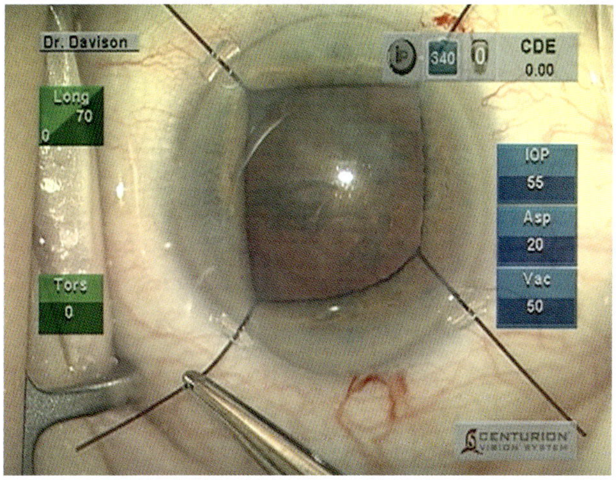

Fig. 55.28 A tying forceps is going to push the iris retractor central ~ 1.5 mm so that the iris will fall to a more posterior position. This has already been done for the retractor on the right side.

Special Considerations

Small Pupil

The pupil needs to be mechanically dilated if it does not permit the creation of a 5.0-mm-diameter CCC. The need is more critical if the lens is hard (make sure to check the preoperative LOCS III nuclear opalescence [NO] and nuclear color [NC] estimates while making decisions about mechanical dilation. Values of 3.8 or greater in either category suggest mechanical dilation if the pupil is borderline.) or if PXF exists. Mechanical dilation might be advisable in 5.5-mm or even 6.5-mm pupils if those features are combined. Remember, pupils hardly ever get bigger as procedures progress.

I prefer to use Grieshaber iris retractors (Alcon) for mechanical dilation. These single-use devices are minimally traumatic to the iris, and also to the zonule, as they require no downward motion on the lens to engage, are easy to install, and are relatively inexpensive. I usually make the four required incisions first aiming at the pupillary border with the 22.5-degree blade,

and then the paracentesis and main incision together afterward as usual. Then I inject 1% preservative free lidocaine, viscoelastics and install the retractors. But, they need to be installed prior to the injection of dye for capsular staining, which, remember, occurs prior to viscoelastic injection. For toric IOLs, they can be left in after viscoelastic removal to facilitate final IOL orientation under BSS only. Prior to phacoemulsification, I always relax the proximal retractors so that the iris can fall posterior and be less likely to be chafed by the phacoemulsification tip (**Figs. 55.27, 55.28, 55.29, 55.30**). Most of the phacoemulsification is done in the distal half, but the shaft (through the sleeve) will be vibrating against the proximal half's iris. We just need to minimize contact as much as possible. Also, with the balanced tip, it is important not to withdraw it so far that the curved portions encounter the iris or cornea any more than necessary. When activated, these portions move much more than the simple rotational motion of the shaft. Use only low power necessary localizing maneuvers when in semi-withdrawn positions. Relaxing the proximal retractors also makes IOL insertion easier and safer for the iris.

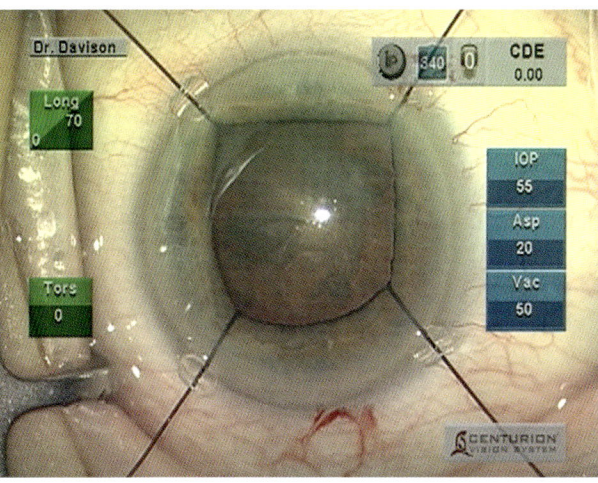

Fig. 55.29 Tension has been released from both proximal iris retractors, enabling the iris to fall away posterior from the cornea. Make sure that the retractors do not engage the anterior capsule border.

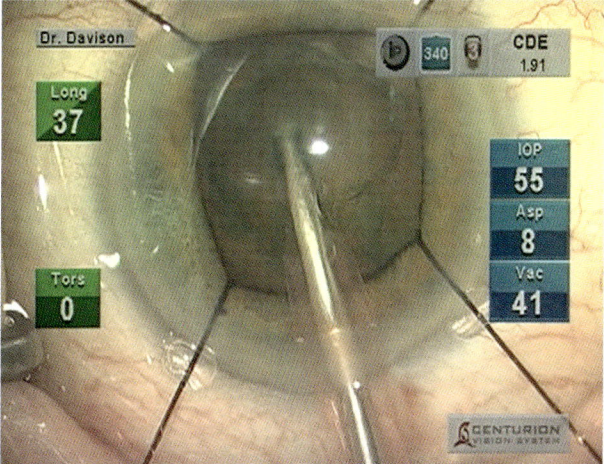

Fig. 55.30 The initial groove is being sculpted. By falling posterior, the iris is being contacted less by the sleeve and shaft of the phacoemulsification tip. Note the tip's central location within the incision. Visualization of the distal nucleus has not been affected by relaxation of the proximal retractors.

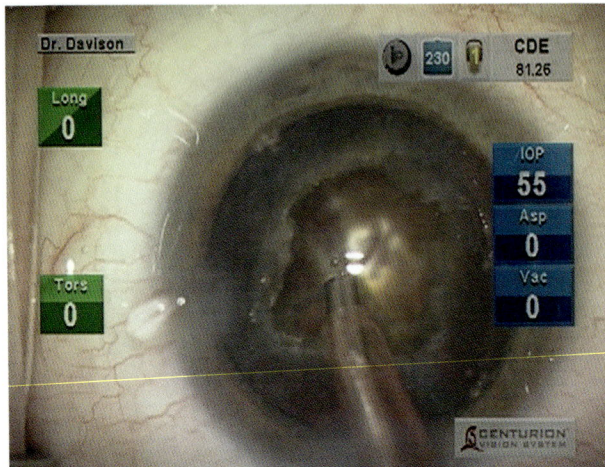

Fig. 55.31 A relatively thin-walled nuclear bowl is being created in this mature cataract by sculpting away a substantial amount of central nuclear volume. The cumulative dissipated energy measurement (CDE) is high but all of the tip movement has occurred deep within the nucleus away from the corneal endothelium.

If the pupil gets smaller during the procedure or if iris is aspirated, I sometimes install iris retractors even late in the procedure, for example, even prior to IOL implantation. We just have to be careful not to engage the anterior capsule rim and damage it in the process. This is also especially true with miosis after femtosecond laser treatment.

Hard Cataract

Give sufficient consideration to the retractors and the dye, make a good CCC, and be sure that the CCC is not too small; take your time, and reinject Viscoat especially before the last quadrant removal. Do not use longitudinal power greater than 70% with a balanced tip. Even though the cumulative dissipated energy (CDE) on the machine may measure lower with this tip (because it measures movement of the shaft), the distal end has dramatically more movement than other tips; that is, considerably more acoustic energy is actually being experienced at the tip than is measured at the shaft. The longitudinal movement at very high percentages of maximum seems violent and disorganized, creates cavitation bubbles, vibrates the iris, thus shrinking the pupil, and does not actually facilitate organized nuclear dissection. Take more lower power swipes. Let the incision cool between swipes. The goal of sculpting is to create a very thin bowl by sculpting away as much central volume as possible so that the nuclear plates can be as thin as possible during quadrant removal (**Fig. 55.31**). For quadrant removal, consider longitudinal tip motion in quadrant removal if torsional motion with IP is too inefficient. Avoid the seemingly natural tendency to pull up on the tip. Be aware of the tip's three-dimensional presence in the incision

throughout. Keep it central. Don't panic; take your time. Keep the patient comfortable with extra doses of sedation and preservative-free lidocaine if needed. Have a three-piece backup IOL calculated for ciliary sulcus placement with or without optic capture. Use generous stromal hydration if needed in both incisions, and use a 10-0 nylon closure or sealant glue if there is any doubt about the competence of an incision which may have been heated and the tissue and deformed.

Mature Cataract

Mature dark brown cataracts are really no different from normal hard ones except that no red reflex exists, so dye is necessary to create the capsulorrhexis. The texture of the capsule may be brittle and tear slightly irregularly. Going slow helps. Make sure that the anterior chamber is filled with viscoelastic so that there is downward pressure on the anterior capsule. If the lens is just hard, go slow; do not penetrate so deeply as to move the lens. Push lightly with the cystotome because the lens material will not deform and sink in as easily as normal. This can cause a triangular tear in the anterior capsule underneath the flap of anterior capsule as the CCC is being made. If that happens, the tear needs to be incorporated into the CCC. If the lens is white and intumescent, make the initial anterior capsule penetration slightly to the right of center, and tear across the lens quickly as you approach the radius adjustment to the final diameter location on the central left side. This larger opening helps relieve internal intracapsular pressure over a larger area so as to avoid inadvertent tear extensions seen with positive intracapsular pressure, which could produce the "Argentinian flag sign." A white cloud of liquid cortex may puff through the opening and obscure any view of the capsule. The I/A tip should be used to clear the cloud and with it the Provisc. This usually reveals a shrunken hard brown freely mobile nucleus which and an otherwise empty capsule. Dye can then be re-instilled and then more viscoelastic so that the anterior capsulotomy can be completed. Be careful not to penetrate the anterior capsule which could allow the cystitome to penetrate the posterior capsule as well. In both brown and white cataracts, try to make a generous 5.0-mm capsulotomy. Too small will encourage anterior radial tear (ART) formation. Reinject Provisc to maintain pressure dynamics so as to avoid a peripheral extension tendency with the CCC. Mechanical pupil dilation is necessary if a generous pupil is not present at the start. In order for dye to be absorbed by the anterior capsule, iris retractors need to be placed prior to dye application, which needs to be accomplished prior to viscoelastic instillation. Anterior chamber pressure can be maintained by injecting BSS into it and performing some early incisional stromal hydration.

Soft Cataract

Evaluation of the LOCS III NO and NC ratings helps plan ahead for the Epinucleus setting on the machine. NO and NC values of 3.6 or less usually lend themselves to the slower Epinucleus setting. An Akahoshi prechopper (Katena Products, Denville, NJ) is most easily used to create four quadrants. The cracks in the nucleus are then sculpted into grooves, the four fractures of the posterior nuclear plate are confirmed and completed if necessary using the cyclodialysis spatula and phaco tip as usual. The bulk of the deeper nucleus is sculpted away as always and then the quadrants can be aspirated starting with the Epinucleus mode and advancing to Quadrant Removal mode as usual. Alternatively a deep circular midperipheral deep grooving with very low phaco power can be employed. The need for the Epinucleus setting is indicated by the inability to create quadrants by making the usual cracks in the posterior nuclear plate. The Epinucleus setting lets me control the quadrant removal process in very similar fashion to cortex irrigation and aspiration (I/A). I refer to it as "phaco assisted I/A" because the feedback process is mentally almost identical. As I push down on the pedal through foot position 2, I increase vacuum and flow, and then as I push down through foot position 3, I add torsional tip motion but only to a 20% limit. I simply groove deep in the Sculpt setting, try to rotate the nucleus, and perform the crack, but if cracking is not possible, then I just thin the deep midperipheral rim 360 degrees. I can then rotate and aspirate the nuclear periphery until there is only posterior material, which usually flips anterior as it is drawn forward (**Figs. 55.32, 55.33, 55.34, 55.35, 55.36**).

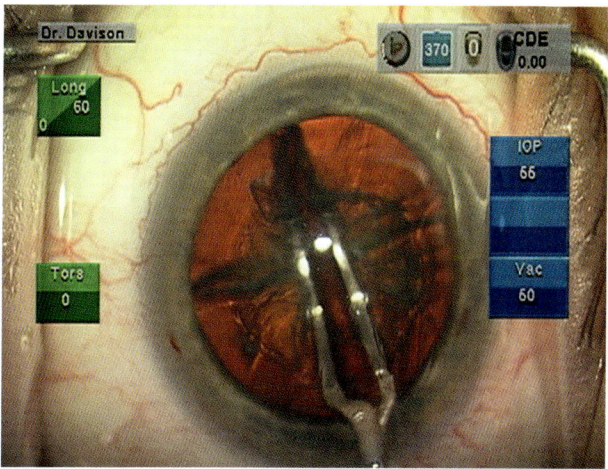

Fig. 55.32 The Akahoshi Pre-chopper has been driven into the nucleus and is making the chop between the two right and left nuclear halves. The nucleus has been rotated 90 degrees with the Chang Cannula to this position after the first pre-chopper bisection.

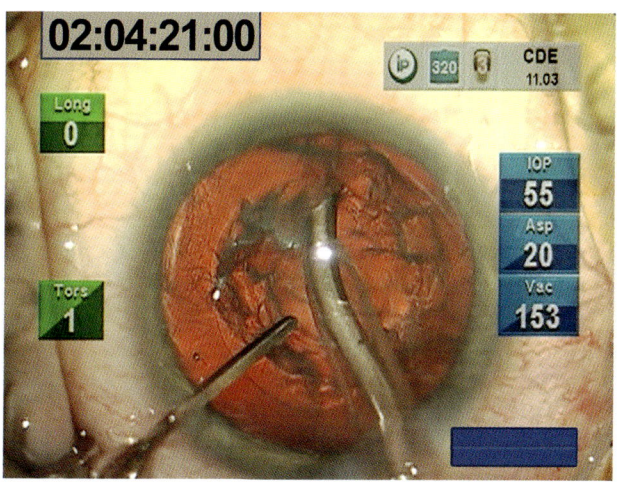

Fig. 55.33 A standard 30 frame per second video timer, which started with a case-independent arbitrary number on the hard drive, reads 2 hours, 4 minutes, 21 seconds, and 0 thirtieths of a second. Nuclear cracking was not possible, so the midposterior nuclear wall has been thinned all the way around by the obliquely oriented tip that is now poised to begin higher vacuum nucleus aspiration using a torsional motion.

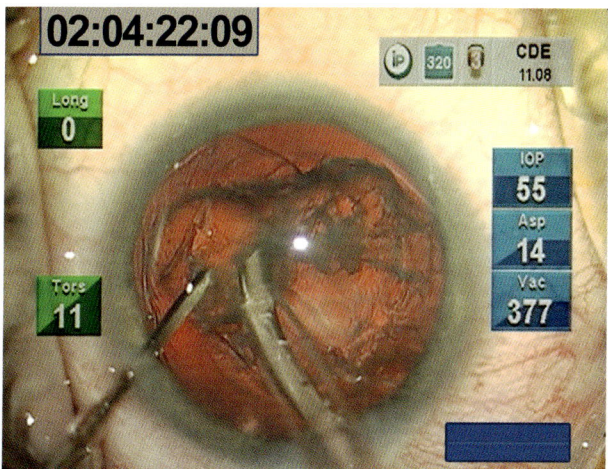

Fig. 55.34 In approximately one second, the first grasp of the nuclear rim has occurred and the lens has rotated slightly. The second grasp will draw more new peripheral material central. Surgeon control of torsional amplitude, vacuum, and aspiration flow enables the material to be accessed and slowly withdrawn in a very controlled fashion with the same feeling as experienced in cortex removal with the irrigation and aspiration (I/A) handpiece and silicone tip.

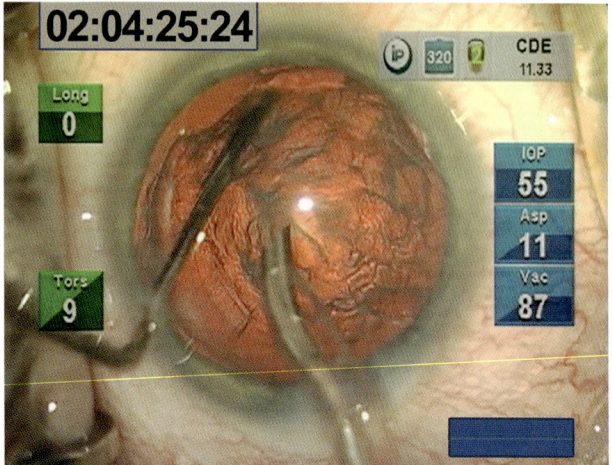

Fig. 55.35 The lens is rotated with the spatula so that a new section of peripheral material will be available. As the diameter of the nuclear disk is reduced, the peripheral material can be more centrally drawn for more aggressive aspiration.

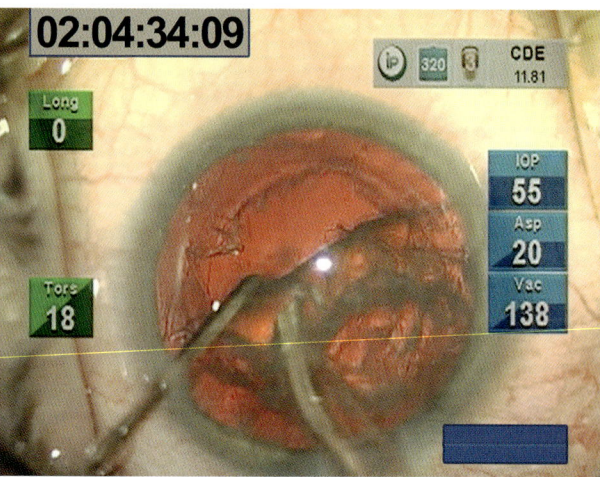

Fig. 55.36 The posterior nuclear plate is about to flip over into the iris plane as it is simultaneously being aspirated and drawn anterior by the tip's attachment to the midperipheral nucleus. The cyclodialysis spatula helps keep the posterior plate from falling back.

Average Cataract

During the unlocking process of first quadrant removal, sometimes chunks of the quadrant just get sucked off and are aspirated during attempted quadrant acquisition rather than the whole quadrant being mobilized centrally. This is especially true while trying to unlock the first quadrant, and if that fails rotating, trying the second, and if that fails, trying the third, and so on. Things just seem to happen too fast in the Quadrant Removal Setting because of the immediate physical changes being accomplished on the nuclear surface and deeper to it by high-performance tip movement and high vacuum and flow rate parameters, even with a –2 vacuum rise. Sometimes we just keep aspirating pieces away from the quadrant or subsequent quadrants as we try to acquire and centralize. If that happens to Q1, I switch to the Epinucleus setting to acquire and unlock the second quadrant and remove it. Its lower flow rate and finer foot switch control of vacuum, flow rate, and small amplitude torsional tip movement enable me to acquire the quadrant's accessible surfaces and, with controlled adherence, centralize and then slowly remove nuclear material. Once one quadrant has been unlocked and removed, I can usually switch back to the Quadrant Removal setting to draw out and emulsify the remaining quadrants more quickly. But if things seem to still be happening too quickly, I can switch back to the Epinucleus setting (**Figs. 55.37, 55.38, 55.39, 55.40, 55.41, 55.42**). It's just like driving a car. Start with the slow-speed first gear to pull away from the curb, then shift to second gear to increase speed. The acquisition and centralization process can be stretched from the usual 0.5 seconds in the Quadrant Removal

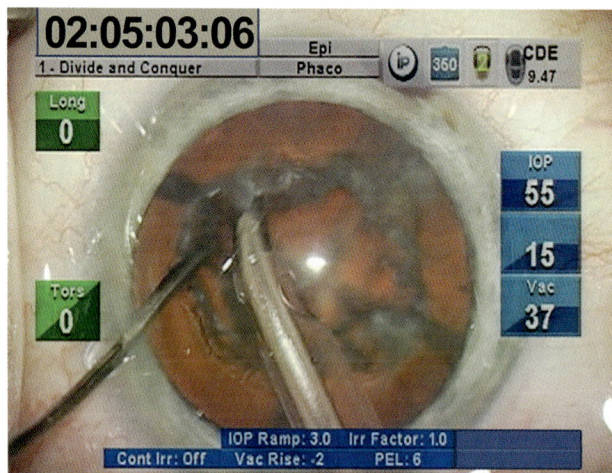

Fig. 55.37 A 30 frame per second standard case–independent timer has been running and registers 5 minutes, 3 seconds, and 6/30ths of a second. Initial contact of the tip to Q1 is occurring. The Epinucleus setting has been engaged. Simultaneous control of torsional tip motion, vacuum, and aspiration flow rate (AFR) will result in a much slower acquisition of the edge of Q1, thus enabling the tip to burrow in enough to maintain vacuum, as it becomes adherent to the nuclear material, and the quadrant to be drawn centrally. The cyclodialysis spatula is pushing the right edge of Q4 away from the left edge of Q1. Torsional tip motion has not yet been activated, and the flow rate and vacuum are just starting to increase; that is, the pedal is in foot position 2.

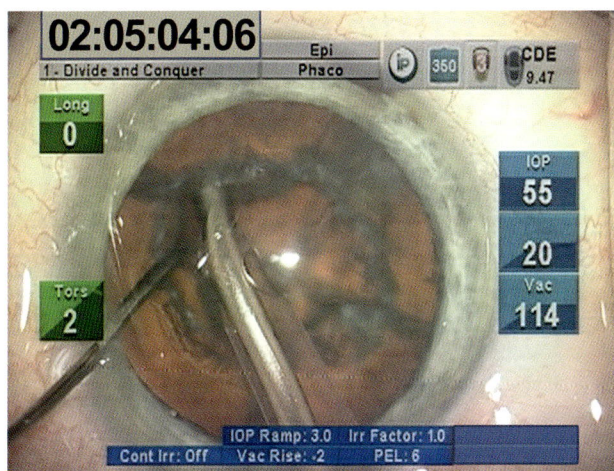

Fig. 55.38 One second from initial contact, vacuum is building as the minimally moving tip starts to burrow into Q1 using foot position 3.

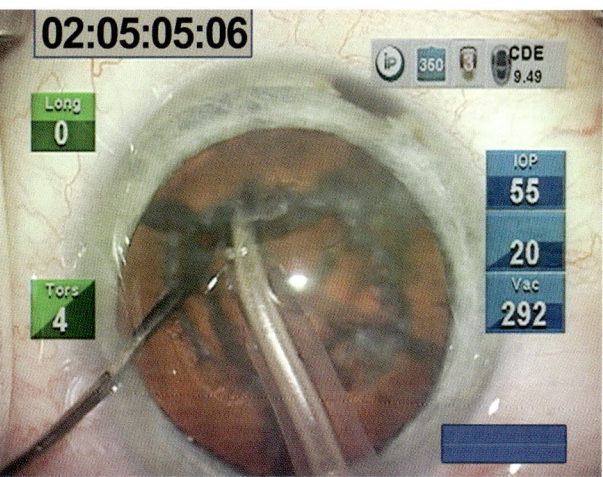

Fig. 55.39 Two seconds from initial contact, with the tip vibrating minimally, vacuum has built to a higher degree, enabling the left edge of Q1 to begin to be drawn centrally.

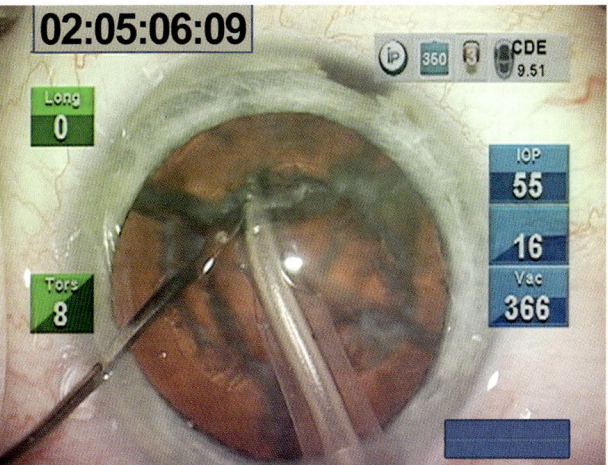

Fig. 55.40 Three seconds from initial contact, the high vacuum level and minimally vibrating tip are providing enough suction contact to draw Q1 more centrally.

setting to typically 1.5 seconds or longer using the Epinucleus setting. That strategy keeps things from happening too fast and prevents iris or posterior capsule aspiration.

Corneal Endothelial Dystrophy

Be gentle throughout and go slowly. Use a little more Viscoat in the initial DuoVisc mix. Add more Viscoat during the procedure if it is prolonged. Use low power. Be diligent to keep the entire process low in the capsular bag.

Aberrant Situations

Moving Patients

A taped head and appropriate consciousness will help, but sometimes patients move suddenly or sometimes they have a tremor or restless body syndrome. A lead apron from radiology can dampen movement from restless legs. Your assistant can steady the head while you keep your fingers and hands in good contact with the patient's face. Do not let a space develop between your

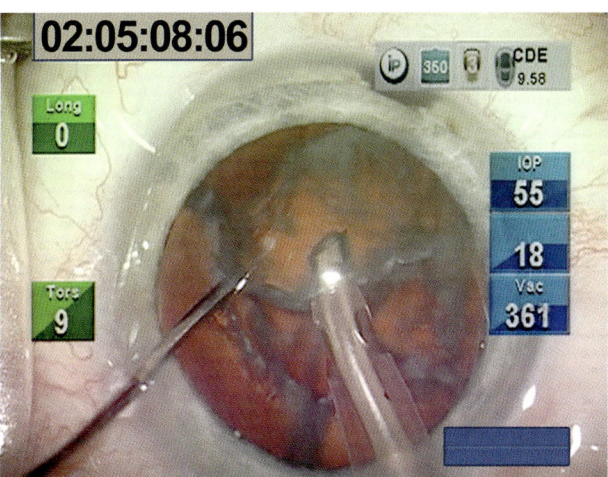

Fig. 55.41 Five seconds from initial contact, the left portion of Q1 has been centralized.

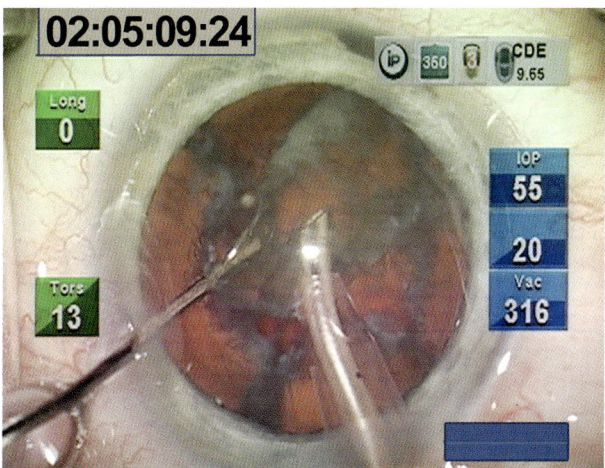

Fig. 55.42 Six seconds from initial contact, the more central portion of Q1 has been drawn centrally and is held in place with high vacuum and being emulsified with a higher level of torsional vibration amplitude.

hands and the patient's face. Think of a rodeo rider who tries to stay in contact with his horse by letting no space develop between him and the saddle.

Moving Eyes

Nystagmus patients usually have a point of gaze that displays less motion. If motion is minimal, surgery can be accomplished with the usual topical/intracameral anesthesia. The globe may be steadied by a second instrument, a Weck-Cel sponge (Beaver Visitec, Waltham, MA), or gloved finger. The incision and CCC are the hard parts. Phacoemulsification is usually uneventful.

Deaf Patients

Deaf patients are cooperative, gentle, and usually very good patients. Good preoperative preparations make these cases uneventful. Sometimes a gentle tap with your finger on their forehead will remind them to look at the microscope light.

Conjunctival Balloon

Incisions placed in the vascularized corneal limbus may bleed a little, which is no problem. But conjunctival tissue may become elevated because of the pressure from exiting BSS. This almost always happens only at the primary incision and if it does, and fluid seems to be collecting quickly, the 22.5-degree paracentesis blade can be used to create one or two conjunctival vents so that the fluid will drain through them, thus preventing subconjunctival accumulation. It is more effective to do this early rather than late when lots of fluid has collected and good visualization is threatened from the "swimming pool effect" of the contained BSS within a raised pillow of conjunctiva (**Fig. 55.43**).

Torn Anterior Capsular

Tears in the anterior capsule are commonly called anterior radial tears (ARTs) because they are always radial in nature. Subincisional ARTs used to be the norm when we had to prolapse the proximal edge of the lens into the iris plane for emulsification. They are now quite unusual but can be more consequential because of their location and contemporary nuclear dissection techniques. The main cause of ARTs is too small a capsulorrhexis, so it is important to be vigilant for such tears especially if a small rhexis is created. Once one is identified, it is important not to propagate the tear through the equator and into the posterior capsule. This can occur in proximal (toward the surgeon) ARTs but is more of a danger with distal ARTs (away from the surgeon) because most of the action, including cracking and quadrant removal, happens in the distal half of the lens. Be mindful of the ART and try to locate nuclear manipulation to another location.

Posterior Capsule Tear

Posterior capsular tears in normal cases are infrequent. They occur usually because of an extension of an ART or because of aspiration of the posterior capsule. It is not the cutting edge of the phaco tip that creates the defect but rather the sudden unexpected aspiration of the capsule. This is caused by vacuum and flow, which creates an attractive hydraulic force that is projected

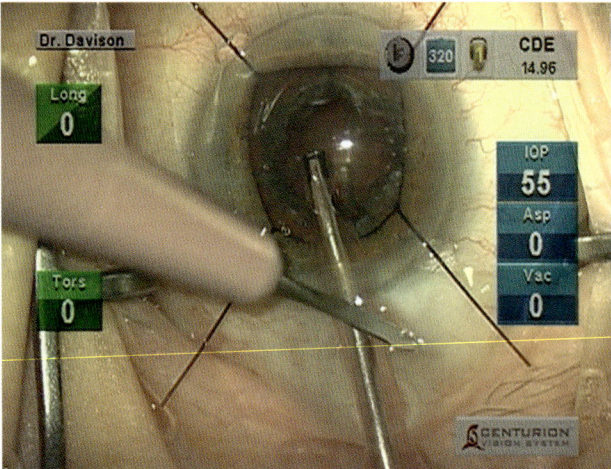

Fig. 55.43 To prevent a large conjunctival balloon, a "conjunctival vent" is being created by the 22.5-degree paracentesis blade.

from the phaco tip. This vortex projects an attractive force that reaches out to draw in material distant from the tip itself. If the capsule is near, it may be drawn and deformed enough that a hole is created even if the capsule itself has not actually entered the phaco tip's aperture. This can happen very quickly, literally in the blink of an eye (**Figs. 55.44, 55.45, 55.46, 55.47, 55.48, 55.49**). Modern machines have much less postocclusion surge, but a relative partial surge after release of partial occlusion can still be generated nonetheless. The key to prevent such a problem is to avoid higher vacuum or flow when near the capsule. The problem is actually more likely in softer lenses because of the homogeneity of the nucleus, cortex, and capsule; that is, they consist of one continuous gelatinous mass.

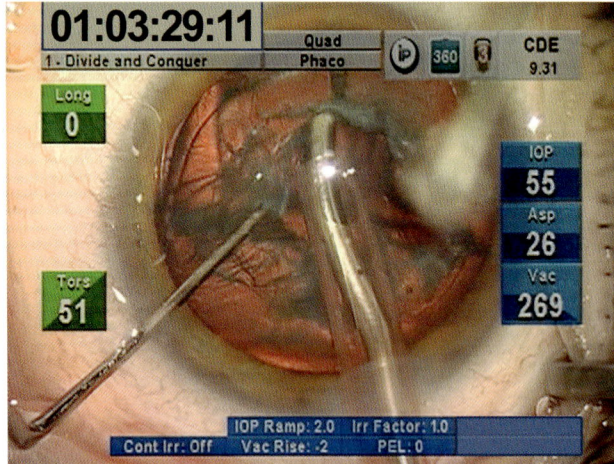

Fig. 55.44 A standard 6 frame per second video case-independent timer reads 1 hour, 3 minutes, 29 seconds, and 11/30ths of a second. Tip contact with Q1 of this soft lens (LOCS III: NO, 3.6; NC, 3.6) has just been made, the quadrant partially centralized and material is just starting to be aspirated using the Quadrant Removal setting. Torsional amplitude is high, and a high level of vacuum has been achieved.

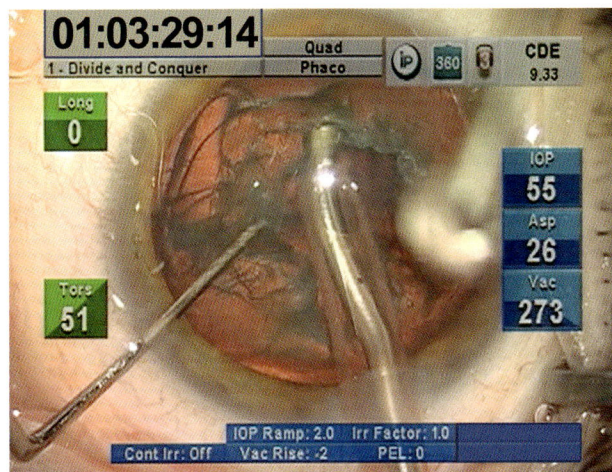

Fig. 55.45 Three frames (1/30th of a second later, a dimpling of nuclear material is seen as it is flowing into the tip aperture, which is in a position between peripheral and central, ~ 1.5 mm from the peripheral posterior capsule. High levels of torsional movement and vacuum are indicated.

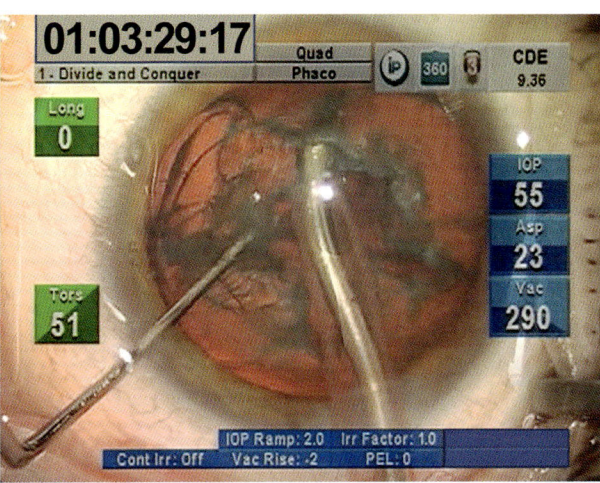

Fig. 55.46 Six frames (6/30ths or 0.2 of a second) after initial contact and partial centralization, a cylinder of nucleus, cortex, and posterior capsule have been aspirated. The small punched out hole in the posterior capsule is partially visible under the word "Phaco."

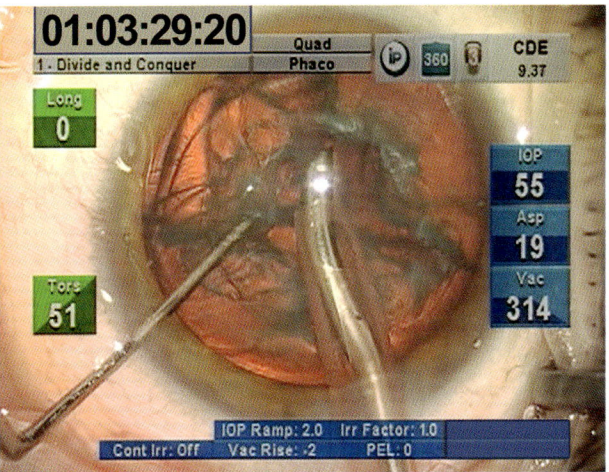

Fig. 55.47 Nine frames (9/30ths or one third of a second) after initial contact and partial centralization, even though vacuum is still registering, zonular traction has pulled the capsule and adjacent cortex and nucleus back into their normal positions.

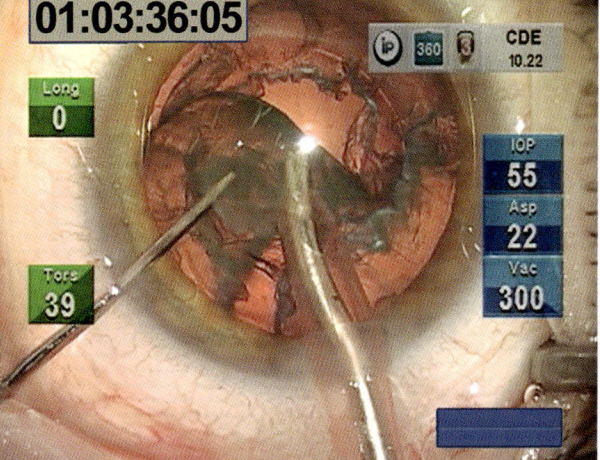

Fig. 55.48 Q4 is being aspirated. The hole had been recognized and phacoemulsification carefully continued away from it. Enough fluid was present between the posterior capsule and anterior hyaloids membrane so that no vitreous was aspirated in this case.

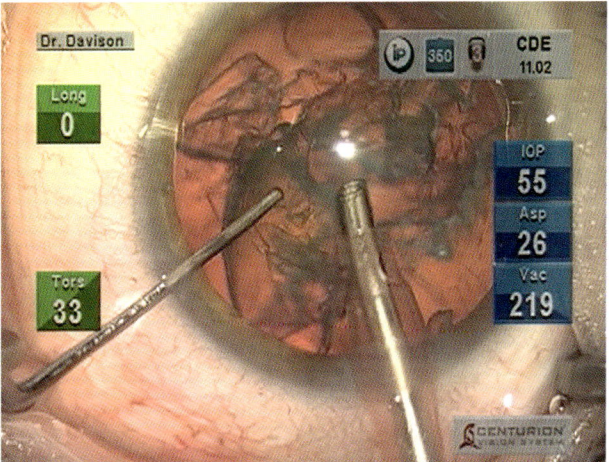

Fig. 55.49 The hole has enlarged (but is still circular), as fluid is finally driven through it and deepens the anterior chamber.

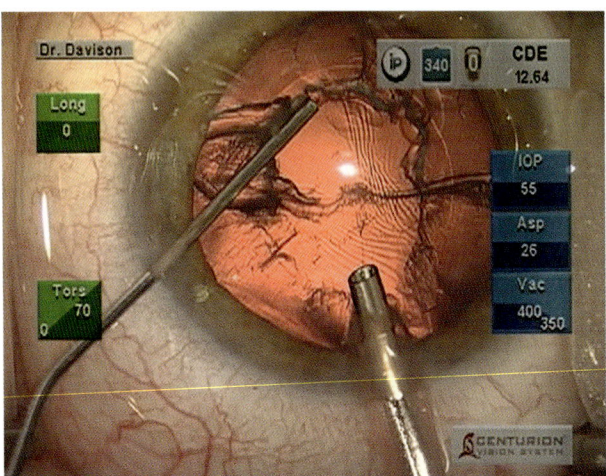

Fig. 55.50 The tip has remained in the anterior chamber with the infusion running, while the Viscoat syringe and cannula have been put into position. Simultaneously when turning the infusion off, Viscoat is injected over the hole. Cortex removal can progress starting away from the defect working toward it. Reinjection of Viscoat over the defect will keep the anterior hyaloid membrane insulated from the cortex removal process.

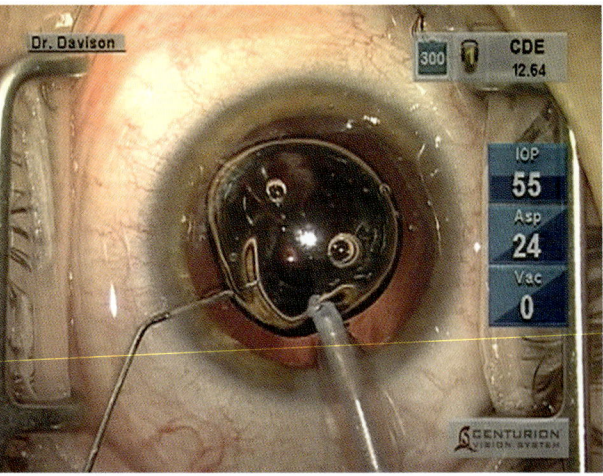

Fig. 55.51 A 3.0-cc air-filled syringe with a 30-gauge cannula is injecting air into the anterior chamber while the balanced salt solution (BSS) infusion is still on. The infusion will be turned off and the I/A tip withdrawn as air continues to be injected, allowing it to fill the anterior chamber. Continuous positive pressure and surface tension between the anterior hyaloid membrane and air will keep vitreous from coming forward through the capsular defect.

If a posterior capsular opening can be identified early, Viscoat can be used to plug the hole, allowing surgery to proceed relatively normally, and then using air to create surface tension and pressure to keep the anterior hyaloid membrane intact and vitreous back (**Figs. 55.50, 55.51, 55.52, 55.53, 55.54, 55.55**). If vitreous is drawn in, an anterior vitrectomy is needed to cut vitreous strands and to enable the remaining vitreous to fall back. Usually the earlier the vitrectomy and the briefer it is, the less of a vitrectomy will be required. Most machines do not provide a low enough infusion pressure. Too much fluid just mixes with the vitreous and brings it forward, thus requiring a greater vitrectomy than should be needed. Clamping the inflow line with a hemostat about three fourths of the way across reduces the flow effectively. You want to see the smallest stream possible to balance the low aspiration rate. Not just drops, but a stream.

Compartmentalization with Viscoat, using air in transitions and minimal vitrectomy featuring high cutting rates and very low infusion flow (sometimes none) and very low flow, usually enables surgery to proceed fairly normally. It is imperative to try to save the anterior capsule rim and keep it intact, as a posterior chamber lens with optic capture can be implanted. If the rim is not intact, a McCannel suture or double McCannel is usually required because the haptics of a posterior chamber lens can dial through the communicating openings.

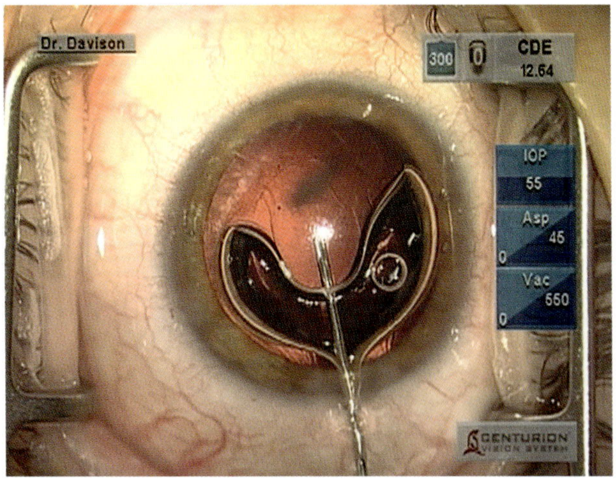

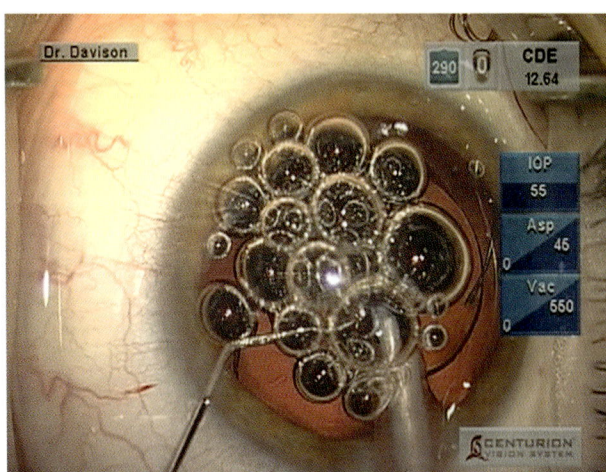

Fig. 55.53 A three-piece intraocular lens (IOL) has been injected and placed with the haptics in the ciliary sulcus and the optic captured by the CCC border within the capsule. The I/A tip has withdrawn Provisc and replaced it with BSS. With it in place and with the infusion on, a syringe injects air through a 30-gauge cannula into the anterior chamber, thus maintaining a positive anterior chamber pressure. As the I/A tip is removed with the infusion still running the air continues to fill and maintain the anterior chamber.

Fig. 55.52 Provisc injection keeps vitreous back while expelling air from the incision. Positive pressure is continuously maintained.

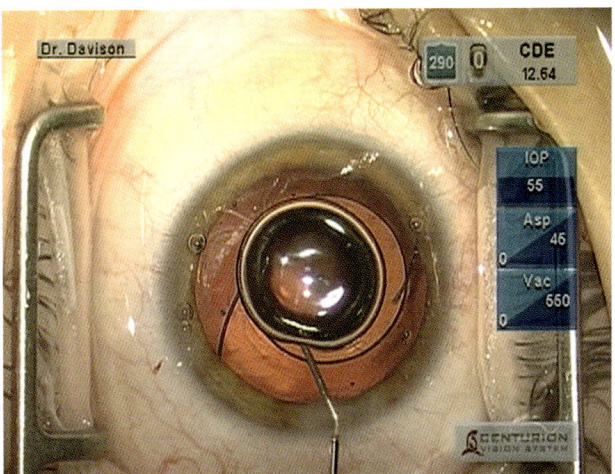

Fig. 55.54 Air is serially exchanged for BSS by aspirating small amounts of air with the air syringe and using another 3.0-cc syringe filled with BSS tipped with another 30-gauge cannula to then inject compensatory amounts of BSS. This continues to keep positive pressure in the anterior chamber keeping the vitreous *anterior hyaloid membrane* (AHM) back and preserving normal anatomic relationships. Air is just about to be aspirated in this photo.

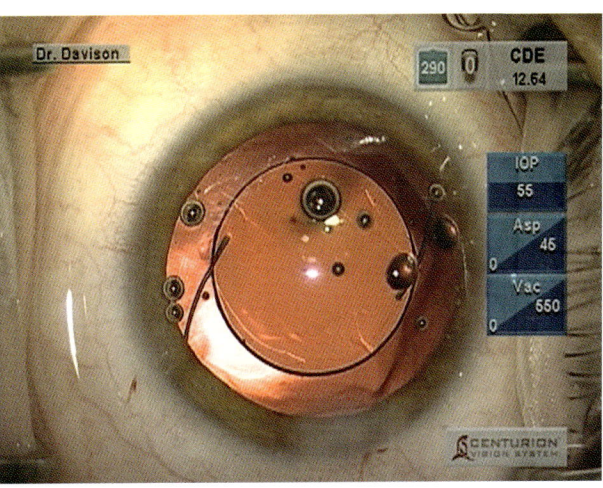

Fig. 55.55 With the haptics in the ciliary sulcus, the optic has been captured by the CCC border and is in good position. A few small bubbles remain and will be absorbed quickly.

Loose Zonule (Generalized)

Pseudoexfoliation is the usual problem. One can predict difficulty by observing minimal phacodonesis at the preoperative examination. But the zonule may be very weak even if no phacodonesis exists. Cases with minimal to moderate phacodonesis need Mackool retractors (Storz, El Segundo, CA) during cataract removal and IOL implantation, followed by two Ahmed segments and perhaps a capsular tension ring (CTR) before IOL implantation. One usually realizes the problem during creation of the CCC. The whole lens moves and does not spring back well. Mackool hooks can be placed after CCC. They can support the capsular bag during phacoemulsification and cortex aspiration. An in-the-bag posterior chamber IOL can usually be placed that ideally will be functional for a long time. Regular inspections should be exercised to detect progressive postoperative dislocation. If zonular tension looks hopeless during surgery, then two Ahmed segments and maybe a capsular tension ring can be placed before IOL implantation to stabilize the capsular bag/IOL complex.

Loose Zonule (Localized)

Trauma is usually the etiology of this situation. If three clock hour positions or less are involved, usually surgery can proceed normally. Viscoat can act as a temporary capsule retractor. If more than three but less than five clock hour positions are involved, a CTR may be all that is required. If greater than that, an Ahmed segment and maybe a CTR should yield the best support during phacoemulsification and IOL implantation.

Iris Aspiration

It is wise to place iris retractors if the iris is even briefly aspirated into the phacoemulsification tip. Many times it is the second aspiration that creates significant damage to the sphincter muscle, a poor cosmetic appearance, and perhaps significant other problems.

Final Inspection for Nuclear Fragments

Look very carefully for these fragments, especially if iris retractors have been used and the cataract is hard, and especially if multiple injections of Viscoat were needed. Irrigate into the paracentesis incision, inspect the others as well, remove all viscoelastic, and irrigate under the iris and over it to dislodge fragments. If you see a fragment, get it early before it hides under the iris.

Index

Note: Page numbers followed by *f* or *t* indicate figures or tables, respectively.